Red Book:

2018–2021 REPORT OF THE COMMITTEE ON INFECTIOUS DISEASES

31ST EDITION

Author: Committee on Infectious Diseases,
American Academy of Pediatrics

David W. Kimberlin, MD, FAAP, Editor

Michael T. Brady, MD, FAAP, Associate Editor
Mary Anne Jackson, MD, FAAP, Associate Editor
Sarah S. Long, MD, FAAP, Associate Editor

American Academy of Pediatrics
345 Park Blvd
Itasca, IL 60143

Suggested citation: American Academy of Pediatrics. [Chapter title.] In: Kimberlin DW, Brady MT, Jackson MA, Long SS, eds. *Red Book: 2018 Report of the Committee on Infectious Diseases.* 31st ed. Itasca, IL: American Academy of Pediatrics; 2018:[chapter page numbers]

31st Edition
1st Edition – 1938
2nd Edition – 1939
3rd Edition – 1940
4th Edition – 1942
5th Edition – 1943
6th Edition – 1944
7th Edition – 1945
8th Edition – 1947
9th Edition – 1951
10th Edition – 1952
11th Edition – 1955
12th Edition – 1957
13th Edition – 1961
14th Edition – 1964
15th Edition – 1966
16th Edition – 1970
16th Edition Revised – 1971
17th Edition – 1974
18th Edition – 1977
19th Edition – 1982
20th Edition – 1986
21st Edition – 1988
22nd Edition – 1991
23rd Edition – 1994
24th Edition – 1997
25th Edition – 2000
26th Edition – 2003
27th Edition – 2006
28th Edition – 2009
29th Edition – 2012
30th Edition – 2015

ISSN No. 1080-0131
ISBN No. 978-1-61002-146-3
MA0858

Quantity prices on request. Address all inquiries to:
American Academy of Pediatrics
345 Park Blvd
Itasca, IL 60143

or Phone:
1-888-227-1770 Publications

The recommendations in this publication do not indicate an exclusive course of treatment or serve as a standard of medical care. Variations, taking into account individual circumstances, may be appropriate.

Publications from the American Academy of Pediatrics benefit from expertise and resources of liaisons and internal (AAP) and external reviewers. However, publications from the American Academy of Pediatrics may not reflect the views of the liaisons of the organizations or government agencies that they represent.

The American Academy of Pediatrics has neither solicited nor accepted any commercial involvement in the development of the content of this publication.

3-341/0418
1 2 3 4 5 6 7 8 9 10

Committee on Infectious Diseases, 2015–2018

Collaborators

Francisca Abanyie, MD, MPH, Centers for Disease Control and Prevention, Atlanta, GA

Mark J. Abzug, MD, University of Colorado School of Medicine and Children's Hospital Colorado, Aurora, CO

Anna M. Acosta, MD, Centers for Disease Control and Prevention, Atlanta, GA

Edward P. Acosta, PharmD, University of Alabama at Birmingham, Birmingham, AL

Paula Ehrlich Agger, MD, MPH, Food and Drug Administration, Silver Spring, MD

Andrés Esteban Alarcón, MD, MPH, Food and Drug Administration, Silver Spring, MD

Grace Aldrovandi, MD, David Geffen School of Medicine at UCLA, Mattel Children's Hospital UCLA, Los Angeles, CA

John J. Alexander, MD, MPH, Food and Drug Administration, Silver Spring, MD

Maria C. Allende, MD, Food and Drug Administration, Silver Spring, MD

Mandy A. Allison, MD, MSPH, University of Colorado, Anschutz Medical Campus, Children's Hospital Colorado, Aurora, CO

Jon Kim Andrus, MD, Sabin Vaccine Institute, Washington, DC

Jorge Arana, MD, MPH, Centers for Disease Control and Prevention, Atlanta, GA

Paul M. Arguin, MD, Centers for Disease Control and Prevention, Atlanta, GA

Paige Armstrong, MD MHS, Centers for Disease Control and Prevention, Atlanta, GA

Stephen S. Arnon, MD, MPH, California Department of Public Health, Richmond, CA

David M. Asher, MD, Food and Drug Administration, Silver Spring, MD

Negar Ashouri, MD, Children's Hospital of Orange County, Orange, CA

John William Baddley, MD, MSPH, University of Alabama at Birmingham, Birmingham, AL

Bethany Baer, MD, Food and Drug Administration, Silver Spring, MD

Carol J. Baker, MD, Baylor College of Medicine, Texas Children's Hospital, Houston, TX

M. Douglas Baker, MD, Johns Hopkins University School of Medicine, Baltimore, MD

Robert S. Baltimore, MD, Yale University School of Medicine, New Haven, CT

Margaret C. Bash, MD, MPH, Food and Drug Administration, Silver Spring, MD

Judy A. Beeler, MD, Food and Drug Administration, Silver Spring, MD

Karlyn D. Beer, MS, PhD, Centers for Disease Control and Prevention, Atlanta, GA

Ermias Belay, MD, Centers for Disease Control and Prevention, Atlanta, GA

Ozlem Belen, MD, MPH, Food and Drug Administration, Silver Spring, MD

Yodit Belew, MD, Food and Drug Administration, Silver Spring, MD

Melissa Bell, MS, Centers for Disease Control and Prevention, Atlanta, GA

Roy Benaroch, MD, Emory University, Dunwoody, GA

Kaitlin Benedict, MPH, Centers for Disease Control and Prevention, Atlanta, GA

William E. Benitz, MD, Stanford University, Palo Alto, CA

Daniel K. Benjamin, Jr, MD, PhD, Duke University, Durham, NC

Casidhe-Nicole Bethancourt, BA, Cohen Children's Medical Center of New York, New Hyde Park, NY

Stephanie R. Bialek, MD, MPH, Centers for Disease Control and Prevention, Atlanta, GA

Holly Biggs, MD, MPH, Centers for Disease Control and Prevention, Atlanta, GA

Jessica M. Biggs, PharmD, BCPPS, University of Maryland Medical Center, Severna Park, MD

David Blaney, MD, MPH, Centers for Disease Control and Prevention, Atlanta, GA

Karen C. Bloch, MD, MPH, Vanderbilt University Medical Center, Nashville, TN

Joseph A. Bocchini, Jr, MD, Louisiana State University Health Sciences Center-Shreveport, Shreveport, LA

Suresh B. Boppana, MD, University of Alabama at Birmingham, Birmingham, AL

Anna Bowen, MD, MPH, Centers for Disease Control and Prevention, Atlanta, GA

Michael D. Bowen, PhD, Centers for Disease Control and Prevention, Atlanta, GA

William Bower, MD, Centers for Disease Control and Prevention, Atlanta, GA

Mary Adetinuke Boyd, MD, Food and Drug Administration, Gaithersburg, MD

John S. Bradley, MD, University of California San Diego, Rady Children's Hospital San Diego, San Diego, CA

Joseph Bresee, MD, Centers for Disease Control and Prevention, Atlanta, GA

Elizabeth Briere, MD, MPH, Centers for Disease Control and Prevention, Atlanta, GA

William J. Britt, MD, University of Alabama at Birmingham Medical Center, Birmingham, AL

Karen R. Broder, MD, Centers for Disease Control and Prevention, Atlanta, GA

Patricia C. Brown, MD, Food and Drug Administration, Silver Spring, MD

Kevin Edward Brown, MD, MRCP, FRCPath, Public Health England, London, United Kingdom

Sarah K. Browne, MD, Food and Drug Administration, Silver Spring, MD

Beau B. Bruce, MD, PhD, Centers for Disease Control and Prevention, Atlanta, GA

Gary Brunette, MD, MS, Centers for Disease Control and Prevention, Alpharetta, GA

Heather Burke, MA, MPH, Centers for Disease Control and Prevention, Atlanta, GA

Gale R. Burstein, MD, MPH, Erie County Department of Health, Buffalo, NY

Diego H. Caceres, BSc, MSc, Centers for Disease Control and Prevention, Atlanta, GA

Carlos C. Campbell, MD, MPH, Program for Appropriate Technology in Health (PATH), Tucson, AZ

Maria V. Cano, MD, MPH, Centers for Disease Control and Prevention, Atlanta, GA

Paul Cantey, MD, MPH, Centers for Disease Control and Prevention, Atlanta, GA

Michael Cappello, MD, Yale School of Medicine, New Haven, CT

Cristina V. Cardemil, MD, MPH, Centers for Disease Control and Prevention, Atlanta, GA

Mary T. Caserta, MD, University of Rochester School of Medicine and Dentistry, Rochester, NY

Corey Casper, MD, MPH, University of Washington, Seattle, WA

Jessica R. Cataldi, MD, MSCS, University of Colorado School of Medicine, Aurora, CO

Robert Maccabee Centor, MD, University of Alabama at Birmingham, Birmingham, AL

Larisa Cervenakova, MD, PhD, American National Red Cross, Rockville, MD

Ellen G. Chadwick, MD, Northwestern University Feinberg School of Medicine, Chicago, IL

Rana Chakraborty, MD, MSc, FRCPCH, DPhil, Emory University, Atlanta, GA

Kirk M. Chan-Tack, MD, Food and Drug Administration, Silver Spring, MD

Kevin Chatham-Stephens, MD, MPH, Centers for Disease Control and Prevention, Atlanta, GA

Archana Chatterjee, MD, PhD, University of South Dakota, Sanford School of Medicine, Sioux Falls, SD

Rana Chattopadhyay, PhD, Food and Drug Administration, Silver Spring, MD

Preeti Chhabra, PhD, Centers for Disease Control and Prevention, Atlanta, GA

Brian Chow, MD, Tufts Medical Center, Boston, MA

John C. Christenson, MD, Indiana University School of Medicine, Indianapolis, IN

Paul R. Cieslak, MD, Oregon Health Authority, Portland, OR

Kevin L. Clark, MD, Food and Drug Administration, Silver Spring, MD

Shannon S. Cleary, BA, Cohen Children's Medical Center of New York, New Hyde Park, NY

Susan E. Coffin, MD, MPH, Children's Hospital of Philadelphia, Philadelphia, PA

Melissa Gerhart Collier, MD, MPH, Centers for Disease Control and Prevention, Atlanta, GA

Wayne Conlan, PhD, National Research Council Canada, Ottawa, Ontario, Canada

Laura Cooley, MD, MPHTM, Centers for Disease Control and Prevention, Atlanta, GA

Jennifer R. Cope, MD, MPH, Centers for Disease Control and Prevention, Atlanta, GA

Margaret M. Cortese, MD, Centers for Disease Control and Prevention, Atlanta, GA

Christina M. Coyle, MD, MS, Albert Einstein College of Medicine, Bronx, NY

Tamera Coyne-Beasley, MD, MPH, University of North Carolina, Chapel Hill, NC

Sam J. Crowe, PhD, MPH, Centers for Disease Control and Prevention, Atlanta, GA

James E. Crowe, Jr, MD, Vanderbilt University Medical Center, Nashville, TN

F. Scott Dahlgren, MSPH, Centers for Disease Control and Prevention, Atlanta, GA

Lara Danziger-Isakov, MD, MPH, Cincinnati Children's Hospital Medical Center, Cincinnati, OH

Lee (Toni) A. Darville, MD, University of North Carolina School of Medicine, Chapel Hill, NC

Alma C. Davidson, MD, Food and Drug Administration, Silver Spring, MD

Roberta L. DeBiasi, MD, MS, Children's National Health System, The George Washington University School of Medicine, Washington, DC

Melissa Del Castillo, MD, Food and Drug Administration, Mackinaw, IL

Penelope Hill Dennehy, MD, Alpert Medical School of Brown University and Hasbro Children's Hospital, Providence, RI

Carmen C. Deseda, MD, Sociedad Latinoamericana de Infectología Pediátrica (SLIPE), San Juan, Puerto Rico

Simon Dobson, MBBS, MD, FRCPC, BC Children's Hospital, University of British Columbia, Canada, Vancouver, British Columbia, Canada

Sheila Dollard, PhD, Centers for Disease Control and Prevention, Atlanta, GA

Kenneth Dominguez, MD, MPH, Centers for Disease Control and Prevention, Atlanta, GA

Naomi A. Drexler, MPH, Centers for Disease Control and Prevention, Atlanta, GA

Christine Dubray, MD, MSc, Centers for Disease Control and Prevention, Atlanta, GA

Gueorgui (George) Dubrocq, MD, Food and Drug Administration, Silver Spring, MD

Jonathan Duffy, MD, MPH, Centers for Disease Control and Prevention, Atlanta, GA

Daniel E. Dulek, MD, Monroe Carell Jr. Children's Hospital at Vanderbilt, Nashville, TN

Judith K. Eckerle, MD, University of Minnesota, Minneapolis, MN

Morven S. Edwards, MD, Baylor College of Medicine, Houston, TX

Sean P. Elliott, MD, University of Arizona College of Medicine, Tucson, AZ

Delia Alcira Enría, MD, MPH, Instituto Nacional de Enfermedades Virales Humanas, Pergamino, Argentina

Roselyn E. Epps, MD, Food and Drug Administration, Silver Spring, MD

Rachel Epstein, MD, MA, Boston Medical Center, Boston, MA

Dean Erdman, DrPH, Centers for Disease Control and Prevention, Atlanta, GA

Susan Even, MD, University of Missouri Student Health Center, Columbia, MO

Darcie Everett, MD, MPH, Food and Drug Administration, Silver Spring, MD

Anat R. Feingold, MD, MPH, Cooper Medical School of Rowan University, Camden, NJ

Meghan Ferris, MD, MPH, Food and Drug Administration, Silver Spring, MD

Patricia I. Fields, PhD, Centers for Disease Control and Prevention, Atlanta, GA

Doran L. Fink, MD, PhD, Food and Drug Administration, Silver Spring, MD

Theresa M. Finn, PhD, Food and Drug Administration, Silver Spring, MD

Margaret C. Fisher, MD, Unterberg Children's Hospital at Monmouth Medical Center, Long Branch, NJ

Collette Fitzgerald, PhD, Centers for Disease Control and Prevention, Atlanta, GA

Elaine W. Flagg, PhD, MS, Centers for Disease Control and Prevention, Atlanta, GA

Katherine E. Fleming-Dutra, MD, Centers for Disease Control and Prevention, Atlanta, GA

Patricia M. Flynn, MD, MS, St. Jude Children's Research Hospital, Memphis, TN

Monique A. Foster, MD, MPH, Centers for Disease Control and Prevention, Atlanta, GA

LeAnne Fox, MD, MPH, DTM&H, Centers for Disease Control and Prevention, Atlanta, GA

Louise K. Francois Watkins, MD, MPH, Centers for Disease Control and Prevention, Atlanta, GA

Sheila F. Friedlander, MD, University of California San Diego School of Medicine, San Diego, CA

Sara Gagneten, PhD, Food and Drug Administration, Silver Spring, MD

Renee L. Galloway, MLS(ASCP)^{CM}, MPH, Centers for Disease Control and Prevention, Atlanta, GA

Hayley A. Gans, MD, Stanford University Medical Center, Stanford, CA

Paul A. Gastañaduy, MD, MPH, Centers for Disease Control and Prevention, Atlanta, GA

Julianne Gee, MPH, Centers for Disease Control and Prevention, Atlanta, GA

Bob Geng, MD, University of California San Diego, San Diego, CA

Noel J. Gerald, PhD, Food and Drug Administration, Silver Spring, MD

Susan Gerber, MD, Centers for Disease Control and Prevention, Atlanta, GA

Anne A. Gershon, MD, Columbia University College of Physicians and Surgeons, New York, NY

Francis Gigliotti, MD, University of Rochester School of Medicine and Dentistry, Rochester, NY

Jessica Gillon, PharmD, Monroe Carell Jr. Children's Hospital at Vanderbilt, Nashville, TN

Janet R. Gilsdorf, MD, University of Michigan Medical Center, Ann Arbor, MI

Brittany Goldberg, MD, MS, Food and Drug Administration, Silver Spring, MD

Gerardo A. Gomez, BS, BA, Centers for Disease Control and Prevention, Atlanta, GA

Ramya Gopinath, MBBS, FRCP(C), Food and Drug Administration, Silver Spring, MD

Rachel J. Gorwitz, MD, MPH, Centers for Disease Control and Prevention, Atlanta, GA

Elizabeth B. Gray, MPH, Centers for Disease Control and Prevention, Atlanta, GA

Greg Greene, MSPH, Centers for Disease Control and Prevention, Marietta, GA

Patricia M. Griffin, MD, Centers for Disease Control and Prevention, Atlanta, GA

Charles F. Grose, MD, University of Iowa, Iowa City, IA

Alice Y. Guh, MD, MPH, Centers for Disease Control and Prevention, Atlanta, GA

Julie R. Gutman, MD, MSc, Centers for Disease Control and Prevention, Atlanta, GA

Penina Haber, MPH, Centers for Disease Control and Prevention, Atlanta, GA

Aron Hall, DVM, MSPH, Centers for Disease Control and Prevention, Atlanta, GA

Scott A. Halperin, MD, Dalhousie University, Canadian Center for Vaccinology, Halifax, Nova Scotia, Canada

Theresa Harrington, MD, MPH&TM, Centers for Disease Control and Prevention, Atlanta, GA

Jason B. Harris, MD, Massachusetts General Hospital, Boston, MA

Joshua D. Hartzell, MD, Walter Reed National Military Medical Center, Bethesda, MD

C. Mary Healy, MD, Baylor College of Medicine, Houston, TX

Katherine Hendricks, MD, MPH&TM, Centers for Disease Control and Prevention, Atlanta, GA

Thomas Hennessy, MD, MPH, Centers for Disease Control and Prevention, Anchorage, AK

Adam L. Hersh, MD, PhD, University of Utah, Salt Lake City, UT

Barbara L. Herwaldt, MD, MPH, Centers for Disease Control and Prevention, Atlanta, GA

Beth Hibbs, RN, MPH, Centers for Disease Control and Prevention, Atlanta, GA

Sheila M. Hickey, MD, University of New Mexico, Albuquerque, NM

Hiwot Hiruy, MD, PhD, Food and Drug Administration, Silver Spring, MD

Michele Hlavsa, RN, MPH, Centers for Disease Control and Prevention, Atlanta, GA

Scott Holmberg, MD, MPH, Centers for Disease Control and Prevention, Atlanta, GA

Katherine Hsu, MD, MPH, Massachusetts Department of Public Health, Boston University Medical Center, Jamaica Plain, MA

Christine M. Hughes, MPH, Centers for Disease Control and Prevention, Atlanta, GA

Dmitri Iarikov, MD, PhD, Food and Drug Administration, Silver Spring, MD

Joseph P. Icenogle, PhD, Centers for Disease Control and Prevention, Atlanta, GA

Martha Iwamoto, MD, MPH, Centers for Disease Control and Prevention, Atlanta, GA

Brendan R. Jackson, MD, MPH, Centers for Disease Control and Prevention, Atlanta, GA

Preeti Jaggi, MD, Nationwide Children's Hospital, Columbus, OH

Ruth A. Jajosky, DMD, MPH, Centers for Disease Control and Prevention, Atlanta, GA

Renée R. Jenkins, MD, Howard University College of Medicine, Washington, DC

Ling Jing, BA, Cohen Children's Medical Center of New York, New Hyde Park, NY

Caroline J. Jjingo, MD, MPH, Food and Drug Administration, Silver Spring, MD

Chandy C. John, MD, Indiana University School of Medicine, Riley Hospital for Children at IU Health, Indianapolis, IN

Jeffrey L. Jones, MD, MPH, Centers for Disease Control and Prevention, Atlanta, GA

Sheldon L. Kaplan, MD, Baylor College of Medicine, Houston, TX

Rama Kapoor, MD, Food and Drug Administration, Silver Spring, MD

Ben Z. Katz, MD, Northwestern University Feinberg School of Medicine, Ann & Robert H. Lurie Children's Hospital of Chicago, Chicago, IL

Carol A. Kauffman, MD, VA Ann Arbor Healthcare System, University of Michigan Medical School, Ann Arbor, MI

Gilbert Kersh, PhD, Centers for Disease Control and Prevention, Atlanta, GA

David L. Kettl, MD, Food and Drug Administration, Silver Spring, MD

Grishma Kharod, MPH, Centers for Disease Control and Prevention, Atlanta, GA

Bharat Khurana, DVM, PhD, Food and Drug Administration, Silver Spring, MD

Sarah Kidd, MD, MPH, Centers for Disease Control and Prevention, Atlanta, GA

Lindsay Kim, MD, MPH, Centers for Disease Control and Prevention, Atlanta, GA

Peter W. Kim, MD, MS, Food and Drug Administration, Silver Spring, MD

Charles H. King, MD, Case Western Reserve University, Cleveland, OH

Miwako Kobayashi, MD, MPH, Centers for Disease Control and Prevention, Atlanta, GA

Larry K. Kociolek, MD, MSCI, Ann & Robert H. Lurie Children's Hospital of Chicago and Northwestern University Feinberg School of Medicine, Chicago, IL

Andreas G. Konstantopoulos, MD, PhD, Athens University, Greece, Athens, Greece

Athena P. Kourtis, MD, PhD, MPH, Centers for Disease Control and Prevention, Atlanta, GA

Phyllis E. Kozarsky, MD, Centers for Disease Control and Prevention, Atlanta, GA

Philip R. Krause, MD, Food and Drug Administration, Silver Spring, MD

Kristen Kreisel, PhD, Centers for Disease Control and Prevention, Atlanta, GA

Andrew Thaddeus Kroger, MD, MPH, Centers for Disease Control and Prevention, Atlanta, GA

Madan Kumar, DO, Food and Drug Administration, Silver Spring, MD

Preeta Krishnan Kutty, MD, MPH, Centers for Disease Control and Prevention, Atlanta, GA

Adam J. Langer, DVM, MPH, Centers for Disease Control and Prevention, Atlanta, GA

Gayle Langley, MD, MPH, Centers for Disease Control and Prevention, Atlanta, GA

Paul M. Lantos, MD, MS, GIS, Duke University School of Medicine, Greensboro, NC

Tatiana Lanzieri, MD, MPH, Centers for Disease Control and Prevention, Atlanta, GA

Rotem Lapidot, MD, Boston Medical Center, Boston, MA

Ralph E. LeBlanc, MD, MPH, DTMH, PhD, Food and Drug Administration, Silver Spring, MD

Joohee Lee, MD, Food and Drug Administration, Silver Spring, MD

Lucia Lee, MD, Food and Drug Administration, Silver Spring, MD

Myron M. Levine, MD, DTPH, Center for Vaccine Development, University of Maryland School of Medicine, Baltimore, MD

Felicia M. T. Lewis, MD, Centers for Disease Control and Prevention, Philadelphia, PA

Linda L. Lewis, MD, Food and Drug Administration, Bethesda, MD

Jennifer L. Liang, DVM, MPVM, Centers for Disease Control and Prevention, Atlanta, GA

Jill A. Lindstrom, MD, Food and Drug Administration, Silver Spring, MD

John J. LiPuma, MD, University of Michigan, Ann Arbor, MI

Anastasia P. Litvintseva, PhD, Centers for Disease Control and Prevention, Atlanta, GA

Lindy Liu, MPH, Centers for Disease Control and Prevention, Atlanta, GA

Eloisa Llata, MD MPH, Centers for Disease Control and Prevention, Atlanta, GA

Mark Lobato, MD, Centers for Disease Control and Prevention, Atlanta, GA

Cortland Lohff, MD, MPH, Chicago Department of Public Health, Chicago, IL

Bennett Lorber, MD, MACP, Temple University School of Medicine, Philadelphia, PA

Benjamin D. Lorenz, MD, Food and Drug Administration, Silver Spring, MD

Carolina Lúquez, PhD, Centers for Disease Control and Prevention, Atlanta, GA

Jessica R. MacNeil, MPH, Centers for Disease Control and Prevention, Atlanta, GA

Ryan A. Maddox, PhD, Centers for Disease Control and Prevention, Atlanta, GA

Mario J. Marcon, PhD, Ohio State University College of Medicine, Westerville, OH

Mona Marin, MD, Centers for Disease Control and Prevention, Atlanta, GA

Lauri Markowitz, MD Centers for Disease Control and Prevention, Atlanta, GA

Gary S. Marshall, MD, University of Louisville School of Medicine, Louisville, KY

Diana Martin, PhD, Centers for Disease Control and Prevention, Atlanta, GA

Jessica R. Marus, MPH, Centers for Disease Control and Prevention, Atlanta, GA

Susan Maslanka, PhD, Centers for Disease Control and Prevention, Atlanta, GA

Janet C. McAllister, PhD, Centers for Disease Control and Prevention, Ft. Collins, CO

Orion McCotter, BS MPH, Centers for Disease Control and Prevention, Atlanta, GA

Anita K. McElroy, MD, PhD, Emory University, Atlanta, GA

Michael M. McNeil, MD MPH, Centers for Disease Control and Prevention, Atlanta, GA

John McQuiston, PhD, Centers for Disease Control and Prevention, Atlanta, GA

H. Cody Meissner, MD, Tufts University School of Medicine, Weston, MA

Elissa Meites, MD, MPH, Centers for Disease Control and Prevention, Atlanta, GA

Sarah Meyer, MD, MPH, Centers for Disease Control and Prevention, Atlanta, GA

Joette M. Meyer, PharmD, Food and Drug Administration, Silver Spring, MD

Ian C. Michelow MD, DTM&H, Warren Alpert Medical School of Brown University, Providence, RI

Amy Middleman, MD, MSEd, MPH, University of Oklahoma Health Sciences Center, Oklahoma City, OK

Peter Miele, MD, Food and Drug Administration, Silver Spring, MD

Elaine R. Miller, RN, MPH, Centers for Disease Control and Prevention, Atlanta, GA

Alexander J. Millman, MD, Centers for Disease Control and Prevention, Atlanta, GA

Eric D. Mintz, MD, MPH, Centers for Disease Control and Prevention, Atlanta, GA

John F. Modlin, MD, Bill and Melinda Gates Foundation, Seattle, WA

Tina Khoie Mongeau, MD, MPH, Food and Drug Administration, Silver Spring, MD

Susan P. Montgomery, DVM, MPH, Centers for Disease Control and Prevention, Atlanta, GA

José G. Montoya, MD, Stanford University School of Medicine, Stanford, CA

Pedro Moro, MD, MPH, Centers for Disease Control & Prevention, Atlanta, GA

Charu Mullick, MD, Food and Drug Administration, Silver Spring, MD

Julia M. Murphy, DVM, MS, DACVPM, Virginia Department of Health, Richmond, VA

Henry W. Murray, MD, Weill Cornell Medical College, New York, NY

Oidda Ikumboka Museru, MSN, MPH, Centers for Disease Control and Prevention, Atlanta, GA

Angela L. Myers, MD, MPH, Children's Mercy, Kansas City, Kansas City, MO

Sumathi Nambiar, MD, MPH, Food and Drug Administration, Silver Spring, MD

Srinivas Acharya Nanduri, MBBS, MD, MPH, Centers for Disease Control and Prevention, Atlanta, GA

James P. Nataro, MD, PhD, MBA, University of Virginia Children's Hospital, Charlottesville, VA

Mark S. Needles, MD, Food and Drug Administration, Silver Spring, MD

Maria E. Negron Sureda, DVM, PhD, MS, Centers for Disease Control and Prevention, Atlanta, GA

Noele Nelson, MD, PhD, MPH, Centers for Disease Control and Prevention, Atlanta, GA

Danielle Nesbit, BS, Duke University, Durham, NC

Steven R. Nesheim, MD, Centers for Disease Control and Prevention, Atlanta, GA

Jason G. Newland, MD, MEd, Washington University School of Medicine, St Louis, MO

Megin Nichols, DVM, MPH, Centers for Disease Control and Prevention, Atlanta, GA

Kristen Nichols Heitman, MPH, Centers for Disease Control and Prevention, Brookhaven, GA

William Nicholson, MS, PhD, Centers for Disease Control and Prevention, Atlanta, GA

Obianuju N. Nsofor, PhD, Food and Drug Administration, College Park, MD

Thomas B. Nutman, MD, National Institutes of Health, Bethesda, MD

Steve Oberste, PhD, Centers for Disease Control and Prevention, Atlanta, GA

Theresa J. Ochoa, MD, Instituto de Medicina Tropical "Alexander von Humboldt," Lima, Peru

Miguel Luis O'Ryan Gallardo, MD, Universidad de Chile, Santiago, Chile

Elizabeth O'Shaughnessy, MB, BCh, Food and Drug Administration, Silver Spring, MD

Gary D. Overturf, MD, University of New Mexico School of Medicine, Los Ranchos, NM

Sherry Michele Owen, PhD, Centers for Disease Control and Prevention, Atlanta, GA

Chris D. Paddock, MD, MPHTM, Centers for Disease Control and Prevention, Atlanta, GA

Mark A. Pallansch, PhD, Centers for Disease Control and Prevention, Atlanta, GA

Zoi Dorothea Pana, MD, MSc, PhD, Johns Hopkins Hospital, Baltimore, MD

Manisha Patel, MD, Centers for Disease Control and Prevention, Atlanta, GA

Sheral S. Patel, MD, Food and Drug Administration, Silver Spring, MD

Thomas F. Patterson, MD, University of Texas Health Science Center at San Antonio, South Texas Veterans Health Care System, San Antonio, TX

Andrew T. Pavia, MD, University of Utah, Salt Lake City, UT

Jessica R. Payne, MPH, California Department of Public Health, Richmond, CA

Stephen Ira Pelton, MD, Boston University Schools of Medicine and Public Health and Boston Medical Center, Boston, MA

Teresa C. T. Peret, PhD, Centers for Disease Control and Prevention, Atlanta, GA

Joe F. Perz, DrPH, MA, Centers for Disease Control and Prevention, Atlanta, GA

Thomas A. Peterman, MD, MSc, Centers for Disease Control and Prevention, Atlanta, GA

Larry K. Pickering, MD, Emory University School of Medicine, Atlanta, GA

Andreas Pikis, MD, Food and Drug Administration, Silver Spring, MD

Tamara Pilishvili, MPH, Centers for Disease Control and Prevention, Atlanta, GA

Ana Yecê das Neves Pinto, MD, Evandro Chagas Institute, Ananindeua City, Para, Brazil

Alice Pong, MD, University of California San Diego, Rady Children's Hospital San Diego, San Diego, CA

Claudette Lapage Poole, MBChB, University of Alabama at Birmingham, Birmingham, AL

Drew L. Posey, MD, MPH, Centers for Disease Control and Prevention, Atlanta, GA

Susan M. Poutanen, MD, MPH, FRCPC, Mount Sinai Hospital, Toronto, Ontario, Canada

R. Douglas Pratt, MD, MPH, Food and Drug Administration, Silver Spring, MD

Nathan Price, MD, University of Iowa Children's Hospital, Iowa City, IA

Gary W. Procop, MD, MS, Cleveland Clinic, Twinsburg, OH

Amol Purandare, MD, Food and Drug Administration, Silver Spring, MD
Ronald E. Pust, MD, University of Arizona College of Medicine, Tucson, AZ
Roshan Ramanathan, MD, MPH, Food and Drug Administration, Silver Spring, MD
Octavio Ramilo, MD, Nationwide Children's Hospital and The Ohio State University, Columbus, OH
Anuja Rastogi, MD, MHS, Food and Drug Administration, Silver Spring, MD
Jennifer S. Read, MD, MS, MPH, DTM&H, Centers for Disease Control and Prevention, San Juan, Puerto Rico
Susan Reef, MD, Centers for Disease Control and Prevention, Atlanta, GA
Mary G. Reynolds, PhD, Centers for Disease Control and Prevention, Atlanta, GA
Brian Rha, MD, MSPH, Centers for Disease Control and Prevention, Atlanta, GA
Frank O. Richards, Jr, MD, The Carter Center, Atlanta, GA
Nicholas S. Rister, MD, Food and Drug Administration, Silver Spring, MD
Jeffrey N. Roberts, MD, Food and Drug Administration, Silver Spring, MD
Candice L. Robinson, MD, MPH, Centers for Disease Control and Prevention, Atlanta, GA
Dawn M. Roellig, MS, PhD, Centers for Disease Control and Prevention, Atlanta, GA
Pierre E. Rollin, MD, Centers for Disease Control and Prevention, Atlanta, GA
José Rafael Romero, MD, University of Arkansas for Medical Sciences and Arkansas Children's Hospital, Little Rock, AR
Paul A. Rota, PhD, Centers for Disease Control and Prevention, Atlanta, GA
Anne H. Rowley, MD, Northwestern University Feinberg School of Medicine, Chicago, IL
Steven A. Rubin, PhD, Food and Drug Administration, Silver Spring, MD
Lorry G. Rubin, MD, Cohen Children's Medical Center of New York of Northwell Health, New Hyde Park, NY, and Hofstra Northwell School of Medicine, New Hyde Park, NY
Hari Cheryl Sachs, MD, Food and Drug Administration, Silver Spring, MD
Marco Aurelio P. Safadi, MD, PhD, Santa Casa de São Paulo School of Medical Sciences, São Paulo, Brazil
Hugh A. Sampson, MD, Icahn School of Medicine at Mount Sinai, New York, NY
Kim Sapsford-Medintz, PhD, Food and Drug Administration, Silver Spring, MD
Jason B. Sauberan, PharmD, Rady Children's Hospital San Diego, San Diego, CA
Ilana J. Schafer, DVM, MSPH, Centers for Disease Control and Prevention, Atlanta, GA
Sarah Schillie, MD, MPH, MBA, Centers for Disease Control and Prevention, Atlanta, GA
Julia A. Schillinger, MD, MSc, Centers for Disease Control and Prevention, New York, NY
Scott Schmid, BA, MS, PhD, Centers for Disease Control and Prevention, Atlanta, GA
Eileen Schneider, MD, MPH, Centers for Disease Control and Prevention, Atlanta, GA
Gordon E. Schutze, MD, Baylor College of Medicine, Houston, TX
Ann Talbot Schwartz, MD, Food and Drug Administration, Silver Spring, MD
Robert A. Schwartz, MD, MPH, DSc (Hon), Rutgers New Jersey Medical School, Newark, NJ
Kathleen B. Schwarz, MD, Johns Hopkins University School of Medicine, Baltimore, MD
Dorothy E. Scott, MD, Food and Drug Administration, Silver Spring, MD
Justin B. Searns, MD, Children's Hospital Colorado, University of Colorado, Aurora, CO

William Evan Secor, PhD, Centers for Disease Control and Prevention, Atlanta, GA

Isaac See, MD, Centers for Disease Control and Prevention, Atlanta, GA

Rangaraj Selvarangan, BVSc, PhD, D(ABMM), Children's Mercy Hospital, Kansas City, MO

Samir S. Shah, MD, MSCE, Cincinnati Children's Hospital Medical Center, Cincinnati, OH

Hala Shamsuddin, MD, Food and Drug Administration, Silver Spring, MD

Andi L. Shane, MD, MPH, MSc, Emory University School of Medicine and Children's Healthcare of Atlanta, Atlanta, GA

Alan M. Shapiro, MD PhD, Food and Drug Administration, Silver Spring, MD

Devindra Sharma, MSN, MPH, Centers for Disease Control and Prevention, Atlanta, GA

Tyler M. Sharp, PhD, Centers for Disease Control and Prevention, San Juan, PR

Tom T. Shimabukuro, MD, MPH, MBA, Centers for Disease Control and Prevention, Atlanta, GA

Timothy R. Shope, MD, MPH, Children's Hospital of Pittsburgh of UPMC, Pittsburgh, PA

Stanford T. Shulman, MD, Ann & Robert H. Lurie Children's Hospital of Chicago, Northwestern University Feinberg School of Medicine, Evanston, IL

Upinder Singh, MD, Stanford University, Stanford, CA

Anders Sjöstedt, MD, PhD, Umeå University, Sweden

Tami Skoff, MS, Centers for Disease Control and Prevention, Atlanta, GA

Thomas D. Smith, MD, Food and Drug Administration, Silver Spring, MD

P. Brian Smith, MD, MPH, MHS, Duke University Medical Center, Durham, NC

Kirk Smith, DVM, MS, PhD, Minnesota Department of Health, St Paul, MN

Donna L. Snyder, MD, Food and Drug Administration, Silver Spring, MD

Sunil Kumar Sood, MD, Cohen Children's Medical Center, Northwell Health, Hofstra North Shore-LIJ School of Medicine, Bay Shore, NY

Paul W. Spearman, MD, Cincinnati Children's Hospital Medical Center, Cincinnati, OH

Stanley M. Spinola, MD, Indiana University School of Medicine, Indianapolis, IN

Arjun Srinivasan, MD, Centers for Disease Control and Prevention, Atlanta, GA

Joseph W. St. Geme III, MD, The Children's Hospital of Philadelphia, Philadelphia, PA

William M. Stauffer, MD, MSPH, FASTMH, University of Minnesota, Minneapolis, MN

Irving Steinberg, PharmD, University of Southern California, Keck School of Medicine and School of Pharmacy, Los Angeles, CA

Shannon Stokley, DrPH, Centers for Disease Control and Prevention, Atlanta, GA

Anne M. Straily, DVM, MPH, Centers for Disease Control and Prevention, Atlanta, GA

Raymond Strikas, MD, MPH, Centers for Disease Control and Prevention, Atlanta, GA

Tara W. Strine, PhD, Centers for Disease Control and Prevention, Atlanta, GA

Nancy A. Strockbine, PhD, Centers for Disease Control and Prevention, Atlanta, GA

John R. Su, MD, PhD, MPH, Centers for Disease Control and Prevention, Atlanta, GA

Lakshmi Sukumaran, MD, MPH, Centers for Disease Control and Prevention, Atlanta, GA

Wellington Sun, MD, Food and Drug Administration, Silver Spring, MD

Jacqueline E. Tate, PhD, Centers for Disease Control and Prevention, Atlanta, GA

Eyasu Habtu Teshale, MD, Centers for Disease Control and Prevention, Atlanta, GA

Beth Kristine Thielen, MD, PhD, University of Minnesota, Minneapolis, MN

Tejpratap S. P. Tiwari, MD, Centers for Disease Control and Prevention, Atlanta, GA

Melissa Tobin-D'Angelo, MD, MPH, Georgia Department of Public Health, Atlanta, GA

Sean Trimble, MPH, Centers for Disease Control and Prevention, Atlanta, GA

Richard W. Truman, PhD, Louisiana State University School of Veterinary Medicine, Baton Rouge, LA

Ronald B. Turner, MD, University of Virginia School of Medicine, Charlottesville, VA

Elizabeth R. Unger, PhD, MD, Centers for Disease Control and Prevention, Atlanta, GA

Snigdha Vallabhaneni, MD, MPH, Centers for Disease Control and Prevention, Atlanta, GA

Chris A. Van Beneden, MD, MPH, Centers for Disease Control and Prevention, Atlanta, GA

John A. Vanchiere, MD, PhD, Louisiana State University, Health Sciences Center, Shreveport, LA

Marietta Vázquez, MD, Yale University School of Medicine, New Haven, CT

Claudia Vellozzi, MD, MPH, Centers for Disease Control and Prevention, Atlanta, GA

Joseph M. Vinetz, MD, University of California San Diego School of Medicine, LaJolla, CA

Jan Vinje, PhD, Centers for Disease Control and Prevention, Atlanta, GA

Prabha Viswanathan, MD, Food and Drug Administration, Silver Spring, MD

Duc J. Vugia, MD, MPH, California Department of Public Health, Richmond, CA

Ken B. Waites, MD, University of Alabama at Birmingham, Birmingham, AL

Tiffany Walker, MD, Centers for Disease Control and Prevention, Atlanta, GA

Tiffany Wang, BA, Cohen Children's Medical Center of New York New, Hyde Park, NY

Richard L. Wasserman, MD, PhD, Medical City Children's Hospital, Dallas, TX

John T. Watson, MD, MSc, Centers for Disease Control and Prevention, Atlanta, GA

Donna L. Weaver, RN, MN, Centers for Disease Control and Prevention, Atlanta, GA

Michelle Weinberg, MD, MPH, Centers for Disease Control and Prevention, Atlanta, GA

Edward A. Weinstein, MD, PhD, Food and Drug Administration, Silver Spring, MD

Eric Weintraub, MPH, Centers for Disease Control and Prevention, Atlanta, GA

Emily J. Weston, MPH Centers for Disease Control and Prevention, Atlanta, GA

A. Clinton White, Jr, MD, University of Texas Medical Branch, Galveston, TX

Mary Beth White-Comstock, DNP, RN, CIC, Centers for Disease Control and Prevention, Atlanta, GA

Richard J. Whitley, MD, University of Alabama at Birmingham, Birmingham, AL

Rodney E. Willoughby, Jr, MD, Medical College of Wisconsin, Milwaukee, WI

Jessie S. Wing, MD, MPH, Centers for Disease Control and Prevention, Atlanta, GA

Amber Haynes Winn, MPH, Centers for Disease Control and Prevention, Atlanta, GA

Carla A. Winston, PhD, MA, Centers for Disease Control and Prevention, Atlanta, GA

A. Patricia Wodi, MD, Centers for Disease Control and Prevention, Atlanta, GA

JoEllen Wolicki, BSN, RN, Centers for Disease Control and Prevention, Atlanta, GA

Karen K. Wong, MD, MPH, Centers for Disease Control and Prevention, Atlanta, GA

Emily Jane Woo, MD, MPH, Food and Drug Administration, Silver Spring, MD

Kimberly Ann Workowski, MD, Centers for Disease Control and Prevention, Atlanta, GA

Gary P. Wormser, MD, New York Medical College, Valhalla, NY

Alexandra S. Worobec, MD, Food and Drug Administration, Silver Spring, MD

Mary A. Worthington, PharmD, BCPS, McWhorter School of Pharmacy, Samford University, Birmingham, AL

Albert C. Yan, MD, The Children's Hospital of Philadelphia - University of Pennsylvania School of Medicine, Philadelphia, PA

Yuliya, Yasinskaya, MD, Food and Drug Administration, Silver Spring, MD

AAP Committee on Adolescence
AAP Committee on Child Abuse and Neglect
AAP Committee on Coding and Nomenclature
AAP Committee on Fetus and Newborn
AAP Committee on Medical Liability and Risk Management
AAP Committee on Native American Child Health
AAP Committee on Nutrition
AAP Committee on Pediatric AIDS
AAP Committee on Pediatric Emergency Medicine
AAP Committee on Practice and Ambulatory Medicine
AAP Council on Children With Disabilities
AAP Council on Early Childhood
AAP Council on Environmental Health
AAP Council on Foster Care, Adoption, and Kinship Care
AAP Council on School Health
AAP Disaster Preparedness Advisory Council
AAP Section on Administration and Practice Management
AAP Section on Adolescent Health
AAP Section on Breastfeeding
AAP Section on Cardiology and Cardiac Surgery
AAP Section on Child Abuse and Neglect
AAP Section on Critical Care
AAP Section on Early Career Physicians
AAP Section on Emergency Medicine
AAP Section on Epidemiology, Public Health, and Evidence
AAP Section on Hematology/Oncology
AAP Section on Home Care
AAP Section on Hospital Medicine
AAP Section on Infectious Diseases
AAP Section on Neonatal-Perinatal Medicine
AAP Section on Nephrology
AAP Section on Neurology
AAP Section on Oral Health
AAP Section on Orthopaedics
AAP Section on Otolaryngology – Head and Neck Surgery
AAP Section on Pediatric Pulmonology and Sleep Medicine
AAP Section on Rheumatology

Committee on Infectious Diseases, 2015–2018

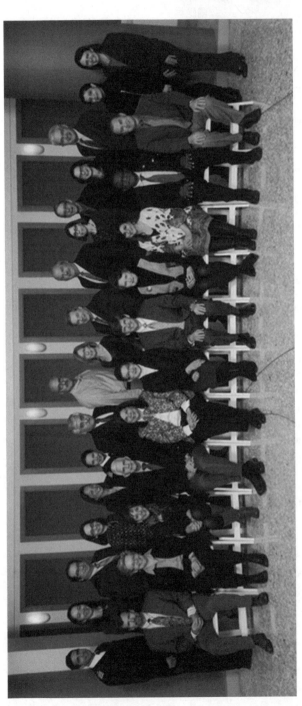

SEATED, LEFT TO RIGHT: Sean T. O'Leary, Ann-Christine Nyquist, Mary Anne Jackson, Michael T. Brady, Yvonne A. Maldonado, Carrie L. Byington, David W. Kimberlin, Sarah S. Long, Natasha B. Halasa, H. Dele Davies, William J. Steinbach

STANDING, LEFT TO RIGHT: Marc Fischer, Dawn Nolt, Geoffrey R. Simon, Karen M. Farizo, Tina Q. Tan, Amanda C. Cohn, Mobeen H. Rathore, Theoklis E. Zaoutis, Joan L. Robinson, Henry H. Bernstein, R. Phillips Heine, Elizabeth D. Barnett, Mark H. Sawyer, Ruth Lynfield, James D. Campbell, Flor M. Munoz, Jennifer M. Frantz

NOT PICTURED: Ritu Banerjee, Douglas Campos-Outcalt, Jamie Deseda-Tous, Kathryn M. Edwards, Bruce G. Gellin, Jeffrey S. Gerber, Richard L. Gorman, Nicole Le Saux, H. Cody Meissner, Scot Moore, Neil S. Silverman, Jeffrey R. Starke, James J. Stevermer, Kay M. Tomashek

2018 Red Book Dedication for Larry K. Pickering, MD, FAAP, and Carol J. Baker, MD, FAAP

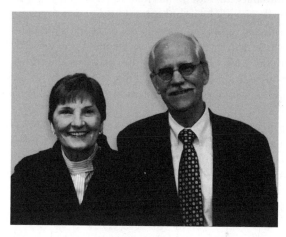

Partnerships have been foundational to the American Academy of Pediatrics (AAP) since its establishment in 1930. At the individual level, pediatricians have partnered with one another to improve the lives of the children for whom they care. At the organizational level, the AAP has partnered with groups that impact children's health, such as the Centers for Disease Control and Prevention (CDC), the American College of Obstetricians and Gynecologists (ACOG), the American Academy of Family Physicians (AAFP), and the US Food and Drug Administration (FDA). And at the governance level, the Academy has partnered with local and national leaders across party lines to advance policies that benefit children. At their core, partnerships have been the fundamental reason for the Academy's success in advancing the health and well-being of children for almost 90 years.

The 2018 *Red Book: Report of the Committee on Infectious Diseases* is dedicated to two of the Academy's most influential partners, Larry K. Pickering, MD, and Carol J. Baker, MD. Drs. Pickering and Baker personify the highest ideals of effective collaboration and partnership. Both are passionate advocates for children who have harnessed their energies and friendship to achieve more together than would have been accomplished separately. As Editor and Associate Editor, respectively, for 5 editions of the *Red Book* spanning 15 years, Drs. Pickering and Baker worked side by side to create a product that is used the world over by pediatricians caring for children. To be sure, the editions of the *Red Book* that they led in 2000, 2003, 2006, 2009, and 2012 were very much a group effort, with several skilled associate editors and scores of Committee on Infectious Diseases (COID) members and liaisons also guiding the development of great *Red Books*. But it was Larry and Carol who inspired and led this group to achieve truly remarkable things.

Carol Baker entered medicine in an era when women physicians were rare. She was the only woman in her medical school class at Baylor College of Medicine from 1964 to 1968. Following graduation, she completed an internship in pediatrics at the University of Southern California before returning to Baylor for residency and pediatric infectious disease fellowship training. She then spent two years at Harvard Medical School as a research fellow and instructor before accepting a faculty position at Baylor College of Medicine in 1975, where she has remained for her entire career. Carol is responsible for generating an extraordinary amount of information regarding *Streptococcus agalactiae*. She performed the seminal epidemiologic and natural history investigations of the role this pathogen plays in neonatal sepsis and meningitis, correlated maternal colonization of group B streptococcus at delivery with risk to the neonate, and devised the screening plan, in collaboration with the AAP, CDC, and ACOG, that is used worldwide for the prevention of early-onset group B streptococcal disease, whereby women are universally screened for colonization with the bacteria near the end of pregnancy and treated perinatally if positive.

Larry Pickering completed medical school at West Virginia University School of Medicine in 1970 and then completed his residency and pediatric infectious diseases fellowship training at Washington University in St. Louis. He was recruited to the University of Texas School of Medicine at Houston in 1974, where he began a long career focusing on viral, bacterial, and protozoal enteric diseases. His research explored the protective factors against enteric pathogens that are present in human milk, contributing to the resurgence of breastfeeding across the country in the 1980s and 1990s. Larry's work on the pathophysiology of enteric diseases was truly bench to bedside to bench and laid the groundwork for outbreak investigations, diagnostic advances, therapeutic interventions, and prevention of enteric diseases through hygienic improvements and vaccine development.

Although at separate institutions, the environment in Houston was inclusive and collaborative as well as a bit competitive. Drs. Baker and Pickering would see each other at least weekly at the citywide infectious disease conference, where representatives of the participating institutions would prepare and present cases for the meeting. At many, if not most, of these weekly meetings, Larry would present a patient for the stated purpose of stumping Carol, or vice versa. They forged a deep friendship based on profound respect for the clinical acumen, scientific rigor, and ethical underpinnings of the other. Their first publication together was in 1981, the case of a child with group A streptococcal meningitis. It was the first of many collaborative efforts.

After leaving UT Houston in 1992, Larry moved to Eastern Virginia Medical School, where he was vice chair for pediatric research. In 2001, he moved to the CDC to serve as the Senior Advisor to the Director and the Executive Secretary of the Advisory Committee on Immunization Practices (ACIP). Larry served on the AAP COID from 1990–1996 and was an Associate Editor of the 1994 and 1997 editions of the *Red Book*. Following publication of the 1997 *Red Book*, Larry was named Editor of the 2000 edition, and he immediately recruited Carol to serve as an Associate Editor. Carol served as a COID member from 1999–2005, and together she and Larry produced five editions of the *Red Book*. Their partnership extended to the CDC as well when Dr. Baker joined the ACIP in 2006 as a member and ascended to Chair of the ACIP from 2009–2012. Whether sitting side by side at ACIP meetings or around the conference room table at COID meetings, Drs. Pickering and Baker modeled respect for one another as they worked tirelessly toward the better health of all children. Their thoughtful and informed leadership at the AAP and CDC helped establish the current era of historically low rates of most vaccine-preventable diseases.

There is an old African proverb that if you want to go fast, go alone; but if you want to go far, go together. Larry and Carol have always gone together, and children across the world have benefited from how far they traveled. This edition of the *Red Book* is dedicated to Larry and Carol as a small token of thanks and appreciation on behalf of all of the children and pediatricians whose lives are better because of their partnership.

PREVIOUS RED BOOK DEDICATION RECIPIENTS:

2015 Stanley Plotkin, MD, FAAP
2012 Samuel L. Katz, MD, FAAP
2009 Ralph Feigin, MD, FAAP
2006 Caroline Breese Hall, MD, FAAP
2003 Georges Peter, MD, FAAP
2000 Edgar O. Ledbetter, MD, FAAP
1997 Georges Peter, MD, FAAP

Preface

The *Red Book*, now in its 31ˢᵗ edition, has been a unique and valuable source of information on infectious diseases and immunizations for pediatric practitioners since 1938. In the 21ˢᵗ century, with the practice of pediatric infectious diseases changing rapidly and the limited time available to the practitioner, the *Red Book* remains an essential resource to quickly obtain current, accurate, and easily accessible information about vaccines and vaccine recommendations, emerging infectious diseases, diagnostic modalities, and treatment recommendations. The Committee on Infectious Diseases of the American Academy of Pediatrics (AAP), the editors of the *Red Book*, and the 500 *Red Book* contributors are dedicated to providing the most current and accurate information available in the concise, practical format for which the *Red Book* is known.

For the first time since the 2006 edition, the print version of the *Red Book* will be provided to every AAP member as part of their member benefit. This change reflects the Academy's strong interest in its members' needs. In a series of AAP Periodic Surveys conducted of its members, pediatricians expressed that the ease of retrieval of information from the book format is highly valued in the midst of busy practices.

As with each of the last 4 editions, AAP members also will continue to have access to *Red Book* content on *Red Book* Online (**www.aapredbook.org**). AAP policy statements, clinical reports, and technical reports and recommendations endorsed by the AAP are posted on *Red Book* Online as they become available during the 3 years between *Red Book* editions, and online chapters are modified as needed to reflect these changes. *Red Book* users also are encouraged to sign up for e-mail alerts on **www.aapredbook.org** to receive new information and policy updates between editions.

Another important resource is the visual library of *Red Book* Online, which is continually updated and expanded to include more images of infectious diseases, examples of classic radiologic and other findings, and recent information on epidemiology of infectious diseases.

The Committee on Infectious Diseases relies on information and advice from many experts, as evidenced by the lengthy list of contributors to *Red Book*. We especially are indebted to the many contributors from other AAP committees, sections, and councils; the American Academy of Family Physicians; the American College of Obstetricians and Gynecologists; the American Thoracic Society; the Canadian Paediatric Society; the Centers for Disease Control and Prevention; the US Food and Drug Administration; the National Institutes of Health; the National Vaccine Program Office; the Pediatric Infectious Diseases Society; la Sociedad Latinoamericana de Infectología Pediátrica; the World Health Organization; and many other organizations and individuals who have made this edition possible. In addition, suggestions made by individual AAP members to improve the presentation of information on specific issues and on topic selection have been incorporated whenever possible.

Most important to the success of this edition is the dedication and work of the editors, whose commitment to excellence is unparalleled. This new edition was made possible under the able leadership of David W. Kimberlin, MD, editor, along with associate editors Michael T. Brady, MD, Mary Anne Jackson, MD, and Sarah S. Long, MD. We also are indebted to H. Cody Meissner, MD, for his untiring efforts to gather and organize the slide materials that make up the visual library of *Red Book* Online and are part of the electronic versions of the *Red Book*, and to Henry H. Bernstein, DO, MHCM, for his continuous efforts to maintain up-to-date content as editor of *Red Book* Online.

As noted in previous editions of the *Red Book*, some omissions and errors are inevitable in a book of this type. We ask that AAP members continue to assist the committee actively by suggesting specific ways to improve the quality of future editions. The committee membership and editorial staff hope that the 2018 *Red Book* will enhance your practice and benefit the children you serve.

Carrie L. Byington, MD, FAAP
Chair, Committee on Infectious Diseases

Introduction

The Committee on Infectious Diseases (COID) of the American Academy of Pediatrics (AAP) is responsible for developing and revising guidance from the AAP for management and control of infectious diseases in infants, children, and adolescents. Every 3 years, the COID issues the *Red Book: Report of the Committee on Infectious Diseases,* which contains a composite summary of current recommendations representing the policy of the AAP on various aspects of infectious diseases, including updated vaccine recommendations for the most recent US Food and Drug Administration (FDA)-licensed vaccines for infants, children, and adolescents. These recommendations represent a consensus of opinions based on consideration of the best available evidence by members of the COID, in conjunction with liaison representatives from the Centers for Disease Control and Prevention (CDC), the FDA, the National Institutes of Health, the National Vaccine Program Office, the Canadian Paediatric Society, the American Thoracic Society, the Pediatric Infectious Diseases Society, the American Academy of Family Physicians, the American College of Obstetricians and Gynecologists, *Red Book* consultants, and scores of collaborators. This edition of the *Red Book* is based on information available as of February 2018. The *Red Book* is your own personal infectious disease consultant, on your bookshelf and ready for you 24 hours a day, 7 days a week. Arguably, it is most valuable in those circumstances in which definitive data from randomized controlled trials are lacking. It is in those situations that guidance from experts in the field is most critical, and the COID has literally hundreds of years of cumulative expertise to bring to bear on such recommendations. The *Red Book* is formatted as hard copy, mobile app, and online Web version, with the electronic versions containing links to supplemental information, including visual images, graphs, maps, and tables.

Preparation of the *Red Book* is a team effort in the truest sense of the term. Within weeks following the publication of each *Red Book* edition, all *Red Book* chapters are sent for updates to primary reviewers who are leading national and international experts in their specific areas. For the 2018 *Red Book,* one quarter of primary reviewers were new to this process, ensuring that the most up-to-date information has been included in this new edition. Following review by the primary reviewer, each chapter is returned to the assigned Associate Editor for incorporation of the reviewer's edits. The chapter then is disseminated to content experts at the CDC and FDA and to members of all AAP Sections, Committees, and Councils that agree to review specific chapters for their additional edits as needed, after which it again is returned to the assigned Associate Editor for harmonization and incorporation of edits as appropriate. Two designated COID reviewers then complete a final review of the chapter, and it is returned to the assigned Associate Editor for inclusion of any needed additional modifications. Finally, each chapter is discussed and debated by the full COID at its "Marathon Meeting," held at the AAP during the spring of the year prior to publication, where it is finalized. Copyediting by the Editor and senior medical copy editor follows, and the book then is reviewed by the *Red Book* reviewers appointed by the AAP Board of Directors. In all, 1000 hands have touched the 2018 *Red Book* prior to its publication! That so many contributors dedicate so much time and expertise to this product is a testament to the role the *Red Book* plays in the care of children.

Through this deliberative and inclusive process, the COID endeavors to provide current, relevant, evidence-based recommendations for the prevention and management of infectious diseases in infants, children, and adolescents. Seemingly unanswerable scientific questions, the complexity of medical practice, ongoing innovative technology, continuous new information, and inevitable differences of opinion among experts all are addressed during production of the *Red Book*. In some cases, other committees and experts may differ in their interpretation of data and resulting recommendations, and occasionally no single recommendation can be made because several options for management are equally acceptable. In such circumstances, the language incorporated in the chapter acknowledges these differing acceptable management options by use of the phrases "most experts recommend..." and "some experts recommend..." Both phrases indicate valid recommendations, but the first phrase signifies more agreement and support among the experts. Inevitably in clinical practice, questions arise that cannot be answered easily on the basis of currently available data. When this happens, the COID still provides guidance and information that, coupled with clinical judgment, will facilitate well-reasoned, clinically relevant decisions. Through this process of lifelong learning, the committee seeks to provide a practical guide for physicians and other health care professionals in their care of infants, children, and adolescents.

To aid physicians and other health care professionals in assimilating current changes in recommendations in the *Red Book*, a list of major changes between the 2015 and 2018 editions has been compiled (see Summary of Major Changes, p XXXV). However, this list only begins to cover the many in-depth changes that have occurred in each chapter and section. Throughout the *Red Book*, Internet addresses enable rapid access to new information. In addition, new information between editions from the COID, in the form of Policy Statements, Clinical Reports, and Technical Reports, are posted on *Red Book* Online (**www.aapredbook.org**)**,** and online chapters are modified as needed with clear indications of where changes have been made. These completed work products are a result of the continuous reassessment by the COID of its current positions across the spectrum of pediatric infectious diseases, and demonstrate the dynamic process by which the Committee's deliberations always are inclusive of new data and perspectives.

Information on use of antimicrobial agents is included in the package inserts (product labels) prepared by manufacturers, including contraindications and adverse events. The *Red Book* does not attempt to provide this information comprehensively, because it is available readily in the Physicians' Desk Reference (**www.pdr.net**) and in package inserts. As in previous editions of the *Red Book*, recommended dosage schedules for antimicrobial agents are provided (see Section 4, Antimicrobial Agents and Related Therapy) and may differ from those of the manufacturer as provided in the package insert. Antimicrobial agents recommended for specific infections in the *Red Book* may or may not have an FDA indication for treatment of that infection. Physicians also can reference additional information in the package inserts of vaccines licensed by the FDA (which also may differ from COID and ACIP/CDC recommendations for use) and of immune globulins, as well as recommendations of other committees (see Sources of Vaccine Information, p 0), many of which are included in the *Red Book*.

Likewise, we strive to utilize the accurate terminology for licensure, approval, or clearance of drugs and devices by the FDA. The correct term used depends on the classification of the product (eg, drug, biological product, or device) and, for devices, whether a "premarket notification" or a "premarket application" has been submitted.

Drugs are approved by the FDA. Biologic products (eg, vaccines, immunoglobulin preparations) are licensed by the FDA, and vaccines are approved for use in certain populations and age groups. The FDA "clears" devices after reviewing premarket notifications, but "approves" devices after reviewing a premarket application. Whether a premarket notification or premarket application needs to be filed depends on the classification of the medical device. "Cleared" devices (also called "510 (k)" or "premarket notification" devices) can be searched at **www.fda.gov/MedicalDevices/ ProductsandMedicalProcedures/DeviceApprovalsandClearances/ 510kClearances/ucm089319.htm.** Devices@FDA (**www.accessdata.fda.gov/ scripts/cdrh/devicesatfda/index.cfm**) is more comprehensive and includes both "cleared" and "approved" tests and other devices. Where we fail in the *Red Book* to select the appropriate term for a given product, we apologize for any (additional) confusion this adds to this regulatory structure.

This book could not have been prepared without the dedicated professional competence of many people. The AAP staff has been outstanding in its committed work and contributions, particularly Jennifer Frantz, senior manager, who served as the administrative director for the COID and coordinated preparation of the *Red Book;* Jennifer Shaw, senior medical copy editor; Linda Rutt, division coordinator; Theresa Wiener, manager of publishing and production services; and all of the directors and staff of the AAP publishing and marketing groups who make the full *Red Book* product line possible.

Marc Fischer, MD, of the CDC, and Karen M. Farizo, MD, of the FDA, devoted time and effort in providing significant input from their organizations. Meg Fisher, MD, and Renée Jenkins, MD, served as *Red Book* reviewers appointed by the AAP Board of Directors, spending scores of hours reviewing the final chapters for consistency and accuracy. I am especially indebted to the Associate Editors Michael T. Brady, MD, Mary Anne Jackson, MD, and Sarah S. Long, MD, for their expertise, tireless work, good humor, and immense contributions in their editorial and committee work. Members of the COID contributed countless hours and deserve appropriate recognition for their patience, dedication, revisions, and reviews. The COID appreciates the guidance and dedication of Carrie L. Byington, MD, COID Chairperson, whose knowledge, dedication, insight, and leadership are reflected in the quality and productivity of the committee's work. I thank my wife, Kim, for always being there and for her patience, understanding, and never-ending support as this edition of the *Red Book* came to fruition.

I also would like to personally thank Karen Remley, MD, for her leadership of the AAP and for her support of the COID and the *Red Book*. In her travels across the country, Dr. Remley has heard first-hand the value that the *Red Book* brings to the treatment of children. These experiences mirror her own as a pediatric emergency medicine physician earlier in her luminous career. Dr. Remley has provided keen insights into the design of the new *Red Book* cover to be inclusive of the years that it will be current, between now and 2021. She also has tirelessly supported efforts across the AAP to be responsive to members' stated desire to have access to the printed version of the *Red Book*, culminating in the AAP Board of Directors' approval of providing a hard copy of the book to all AAP members as part of their member benefit. Her tireless fight for the welfare of all children is inspiring to all who look to the AAP for leadership.

There are many other contributors whose professional work and commitment have been essential in the committee's preparation of the *Red Book*. Of special note are the individuals to whom this edition of the *Red Book* is dedicated, Larry K. Pickering, MD, and

Carol J. Baker, MD. I have learned so much from each of them, and the legacies that they leave in pediatrics and the *Red Book* will endure for generations to come.

David W. Kimberlin, MD, FAAP
Editor

Table of Contents

SECTION 2
RECOMMENDATIONS FOR CARE OF CHILDREN IN SPECIAL CIRCUMSTANCES

SECTION 3
SUMMARIES OF INFECTIOUS DISEASES

SECTION 4
ANTIMICROBIAL AGENTS AND RELATED THERAPY

SECTION 5
ANTIMICROBIAL PROPHYLAXIS

APPENDICES

Summary of Major Changes in the 2018 *Red Book*

MAJOR CHANGES: GENERAL

1. All chapters in the last edition of the *Red Book* were assessed for relevance in the dynamic environment that is the practice of pediatric medicine today. This assessment led to the elimination of 27 chapters from the 2018 *Red Book*. At the same time, 3 chapters were added (Chikungunya, Coagulase-Negative Staphylococcal Infections, and Zika). This results in a 9% overall decrease in the number of chapters in the 2018 *Red Book* compared with the last edition.

2. Every chapter in the 2018 *Red Book* has been modified since the last edition. The listing below outlines the more major changes throughout the 2018 edition.

3. To ensure that the information presented in the *Red Book* is based on the most accurate and up-to-date scientific data, the primary reviewers of each *Red Book* chapter were selected for their specific academic expertise in each particular area. In this edition of the *Red Book*, 24% of the primary reviewers were new for their assigned chapters. This ensures that the *Red Book* content is viewed with fresh eyes with each publication cycle.

4. All Diagnostic Tests portions of the pathogen-specific chapters in Section 3 were reviewed by 2 microbiology laboratory experts to ensure that they include state-of-the-art diagnostic modalities.

5. Throughout the *Red Book*, the number of Web sites where additional current and future information can be obtained has been updated. All Web sites are in bold type for ease of reference, and all have been verified for accuracy and accessibility.

6. Reference to evidence-based policy recommendations from the American Academy of Pediatrics (AAP), the Advisory Committee on Immunization Practices (ACIP) of the Centers for Disease Control and Prevention (CDC), and other select professional organizations have been updated throughout the *Red Book*.

7. Standardized approaches to disease prevention through immunizations, antimicrobial prophylaxis, and infection-control practices have been updated throughout the *Red Book*.

8. Recommendations for the use of doxycycline have been liberalized. Recent comparative data in younger children suggest that doxycycline is not likely to cause visible teeth staining or enamel hypoplasia in children younger than 8 years. These reassuring data support the revised recommendation of the AAP that doxycycline can be administered for short durations (ie, 21 days or less) without regard to the patient's age. When used, patients should be careful to avoid excess sun exposure because of the photosensitivity associated with doxycycline (see Tetracyclines, p 905).

9. Mebendazole is available again in the United States beginning in 2016, after being unavailable for a number of years. It has been added back into the relevant chapters as a therapeutic option.

10. Policy updates released after publication of this edition of the *Red Book* will be posted on *Red Book* Online.

11. Appropriate chapters throughout the *Red Book* have been updated to be consistent with 2018 AAP and CDC vaccine recommendations, CDC recommendations for immunization of health care personnel, and drug recommendations from *2018 Nelson's Pediatric Antimicrobial Therapy*.[1]

12. Several tables and figures have been added for ease of information retrieval.

SECTION 1. ACTIVE AND PASSIVE IMMUNIZATION

1. **Information sources about immunization** have been updated and added. A resource for the names of international vaccines also has been added, as has a quick reference table for Web site addresses for reliable information on immunization.

2. Information from the 2016 AAP clinical report "Countering Vaccine Hesitancy" has been incorporated in the **Discussing Vaccines With Patients and Parents** chapter.

3. New vaccines approved since 2015 have been added to the **Active Immunization** chapter, and those removed from the market have been deleted.

4. New information on pharmacologic options, including over-the-counter topical medications, for **Managing Injection Site Pain** has been added.

5. Guidance on timing of administration of Menactra (MCV4-D, Sanofi Pasteur) and Daptacel (DTaP, Sanofi Pasteur) in children 4 through 6 years of age has been added to the **Timing of Vaccines and the Immunization Schedule** chapter, based on recent data indicating that administration of Menactra 1 month after Daptacel reduces meningococcal antibody response to Menactra.

6. The epidemiology of increased risk of seizure among recipients of concurrent influenza vaccine and conjugate pneumococcal vaccine has been updated in the chapter on **Simultaneous Administration of Multiple Vaccines.**

7. HibMenCY has been removed from the **Combination Vaccines** chapter following its removal from the US market.

8. The **Unknown or Uncertain Immunization Status** chapter now includes recent guidance on reconciling documentation of adequate poliovirus vaccination in refugee or immigrant children immunized internationally.

9. Oral typhoid vaccine has been added to the chapter on **Active Immunization of People Who Recently Received Immune Globulin and Other Blood Products.** The table detailing the suggested intervals between IG administration and active immunization with MMR, MMRV, or monovalent varicella vaccines has been updated to account for a new BabyBIG formulation, recent changes to the measles IG prophylaxis recommendations, and inclusion of the time interval following CMV hyperimmune globulin.

10. The **Vaccine Adverse Event Reporting System** chapter has updated information on monitoring of VAERS reports and reporting of adverse events.

11. Information on 21st Century Cures and on pregnant women has been added to the **Vaccine Injury Compensation** chapter.

---

[1]Bradley JS, Nelson JD, Barnett ED, et al, eds. *2018 Nelson's Pediatric Antimicrobial Therapy*. 24th ed. Elk Grove Village, IL: American Academy of Pediatrics; 2018

12. Clarification on when referral to immunology is warranted following an allergic reaction to a vaccine has been added in the **Hypersensitivity Reactions After Immunization** chapter, as has information on gelatin.

13. Preference of MMR vaccine over IGIM in vaccine-eligible measles nonimmune people, if it can be administered within 72 hours of initial exposure to measles, has been added to the **Immune Globulin Intramuscular** chapter.

14. The upper amount of IGIV dosing as replacement therapy in antibody-deficiency disorders has been increased in the **Immune Globulin Intravenous** chapter. Management options for patients who have had reactions to IGIV have been expanded.

15. The 4 IGSC products licensed for use in the United States have been added to the **Immune Globulin Subcutaneous** chapter. A table has been added to aid in determination of which route of IG administration is most appropriate for a given patient.

16. The **Immunization in Pregnancy** chapter has been harmonized with American College of Obstetricians and Gynecologists (ACOG) recommendations. Recommendations for timing ot Tdap administration have been added, and recommendations on breastfeeding following yellow fever vaccine have been incorporated.

17. The chapter on **Immunization and Other Considerations in Immunocompromised Children** has been extensively rewritten. Information on inactivated vaccines, primary and secondary immunodeficiencies, household members of immunocompromised patients, and biologic response modifiers (including rotavirus vaccination in infants exposed to biologic response modifiers in utero) has been updated. The table detailing immunization of children and adolescents with primary and secondary immune deficiencies has been expanded. The chapter and table are fully harmonized with the recommendations of the Infectious Diseases Society of America and the CDC.

18. Information on febrile seizures associated with inactivated influenza vaccine has been added to the **Immunization in Children With a Personal or Family History of Seizures** chapter.

19. Immunization of HIV-infected children with quadrivalent meningococcal conjugate vaccine (MCV4) beginning at 2 months of age has been added to the **Immunization in Children With Chronic Diseases** chapter. This harmonizes AAP recommendations with those of the ACIP.

20. In the **Immunization in American Indian/Alaska Native Children and Adolescents** chapter, permissive language for chemoprophylaxis of close contacts of an index case with *Haemophilus influenzae* type a (Hia) has been added. The epidemiology of rotavirus and HPV in this population also was added.

21. Emphasis on the acceptability of starting the HPV vaccine series as early as 9 years of age has been added to the chapter on **Immunization in Adolescent and College Populations.**

22. The option to give a single dose of HepB vaccine to health care personnel who fail to serologically respond to a first vaccination series and then test again for anti-HBs (rather than immediately commit to an additional full 3 doses of vaccine) has been added to the **Immunization in Health Care Personnel** chapter. Information on meningococcal vaccine also has been added.

23. In the chapter **Children Who Received Immunizations Outside the United**

States or Whose Immunization Status is Unknown or Uncertain, interpretation of polio vaccines received outside the United States has been updated. Criteria for acceptance of records of immunizations received outside of the United States have been modified.

24.   Information on booster dose recommendations for yellow fever vaccine and for Japanese encephalitis vaccine has been added to the **International Travel** chapter. Information on the new oral cholera vaccine (Vaxchora) also has been incorporated.

SECTION 2. RECOMMENDATIONS FOR CARE OF CHILDREN IN SPECIAL CLINICAL CIRCUMSTANCES

1.   Information on yellow fever vaccine and on Zika virus in human milk has been added to the **Human Milk** chapter. Discussion of inadvertent human milk exposure has been enhanced and harmonized with CDC recommendations. Presentation of donor human milk has been expanded to include recommendations in the 2017 AAP policy statement on this topic. Discussion of breastfeeding when the mother is receiving biologic response modifiers has been added, and resources regarding drugs and lactation have been provided.

2.   The **Children in Out-of-Home Child Care** chapter has been extensively rewritten and reorganized. Recommendations on return to school after diarrheal diseases have been harmonized with the AAP's Purple Book,[1] and across the relevant pathogen-specific chapters in Section 3 of the 2018 Red Book. The recommendation for return to school with group A streptococcal pharyngitis has been shortened from 24 hours to 12 hours after initiation of antimicrobial therapy. Specific animals that should be excluded from child care facilities have been identified in the chapter.

3.   The time to return to school following initiation of antimicrobial therapy for group A streptococcal pharyngitis has been shortened from 24 hours to 12 hours in the **School Health** chapter. Topics related to organized sports have been updated to reflect the content of the new AAP policy statement on that topic.

4.   The **Infection Control and Prevention in Ambulatory Settings** chapter has been expanded and updated with data and recommendations from the revised AAP policy statement of the same name published in 2017.

5.   The **Sexually Transmitted Infections in Adolescents and Children** chapter has been streamlined substantially, with approximately a 20% decrease in length, to aid in rapid retrieval of needed information.

6.   The **Medical Evaluation for Infectious Diseases for Internationally Adopted, Refugee, and Immigrant Children** chapter has been reorganized to better delineate recommendations among these 3 population groups.

7.   Recommendations in the **Bite Wounds** chapter have been modified to take into account the recent guidelines relating to this area published by the Infectious Diseases Society of America and endorsed by the Pediatric Infectious Diseases Society.

---

[1]*Managing Infectious Diseases in Child Care and Schools, 4th Ed. A Quick Reference Guide.* Aronson SS, Shope TR, eds. Elk Grove Village, IL: American Academy of Pediatrics; 2017

8. The **Prevention of Mosquitoborne and Tickborne Infections** chapter is a combination of 2 separate chapters, one on mosquitoborne and one on tickborne infections, in prior editions of the Red Book. Recommendations on use of DEET (maximal concentration, minimal age, etc) have been updated, and new products (eg, undecanone) have been added. Recommendations also have been harmonized with those in the AAP publication Pediatric Environmental Health, 4th Edition (the Green Book).

SECTION 3. SUMMARIES OF INFECTIOUS DISEASES

1. Mention of brincidofovir as a therapeutic option has been removed from the **Adenovirus** chapter after disappointing results of the AdVise study were presented at the IDWeek 2016 meeting.
2. Treatment recommendations for **Amebiasis** have been harmonized with the Drugs for Parasitic Infections table in Section 4, and more specificity with respect to dosages has been added.
3. *Sappinia* species have been added to the **Amebic Meningoencephalitis and Keratitis** chapter. Contact information for guidance from the CDC on the diagnosis and management of primary amebic meningoencephalitis caused by *Naegleria fowleri* has been added.
4. Obiltoxaximab, approved in March 2016 for the treatment of inhalational anthrax and the prevention of inhalational anthrax, has been added to the **Anthrax** chapter.
5. Both chikungunya and Zika have been separated from the **Arbovirus** chapter into their own chapters of the 2018 *Red Book*. Yellow fever vaccine has been updated both in terms of booster dose (which generally is not needed) and current vaccine shortage (resources provided). The durability of protection following Japanese encephalitis vaccine has been updated as well.
6. The epidemiology and treatment of ***Arcanobacterium haemolyticum* Infections** has been updated and expanded.
7. The **Aspergillosis** chapter has been harmonized with the 2016 guidelines from the Infectious Diseases Society of America. The diagnosis portion of the chapter has been updated.
8. The clinical manifestations of **Astrovirus Infections** have been broadened to include central nervous system disease, primarily in immunocompromised hosts. Molecular diagnostics have also been updated.
9. Discussion of molecular diagnostics for **Babesiosis** has been expanded, and discussion of coinfection with *Borrelia burgdorferi* or *Anaplasma phagocytophilum* has been added. Treatment of babesiosis in severely immunocompromised individuals has been added.
10. Information on ***Bacillus cereus*** enterotoxins causing emetic and diarrheal disease have been added to that chapter.
11. The chapter on *Bacteroides* and *Prevotella* has been expanded to include other anaerobic bacteria as the ***Bacteroides, Prevotella,* and Other Anaerobic Gram-Negative Bacilli Infections** chapter. Information on antibiotic resistance has been added, and therapeutic options have been updated.
12. Greater specificity about the serologic diagnosis and the treatment of cat scratch

disease has been added to the ***Bartonella henselae*** chapter.

13. Tinidazole has been added as an alternative treatment for **Infections With *Blastocystis hominis* and Other Subtypes.**

14. The epidemiology of **Blastomycosis** has been expanded. Use of an enzyme immunoassay that detects *Blastomyces* antigen in urine for diagnosis and monitoring response to therapy has been updated. Treatment durations have been arranged to improve ease of access.

15. The clinical manifestations of **Bocavirus** have been updated to reflect new data that more strongly suggest primary infection causes respiratory disease. Information on duration of shedding has been added.

16. Discussion of *Borrelia miyamotoi* has been added to the ***Borrelia* Infections Other Than Lyme Disease (Relapsing Fever)** chapter. The epidemiology of soft- and hard-bodied ticks has been expanded.

17. Guidance for mothers with active brucellosis not to breastfeed their infants has been added to the **Brucellosis** chapter.

18. Sources of health care-associated ***Burkholderia* Infections** have been updated. Clinical manifestations of melioidosis in children have been added based on recent data. Information on *Burkholderia gladioli* disease in cystic fibrosis and lung transplant patients has been added.

19. Molecular assays available for the diagnosis of ***Campylobacter* Infections** have been updated. Current resistance rates of *Campylobacter* species to macrolides and quinolones have been added. Recommendations on return to school have been harmonized with the AAP's Purple Book.[1]

20. The **Candidiasis** chapter has been harmonized with the 2016 candidiasis guideline published by the Infectious Diseases Society of America and endorsed by the AAP. *Candida auris* also has been added to the chapter. Molecular diagnostic advancements have been incorporated as well.

21. Recent data implicating *Haemophilus ducreyi* as a major cause of cutaneous ulcers in children in equatorial regions have been added to the **Chancroid and Cutaneous Ulcers** chapter.

22. **Chikungunya** has been separated out into its own chapter. It previously was included in the Arbovirus chapter.

23. The duration of therapy for ***Chlamydia pneumoniae*** infections has been harmonized with the community-acquired pneumonia guidelines published by the Pediatric Infectious Diseases Society.

24. Diagnosis of ***Chlamydia psittaci*** infections has been harmonized with the 2017 compendium published by the National Association of State Public Health Veterinarians.

25. The epidemiology of ***Chlamydia trachomatis***, especially among adolescents, has been updated. The diagnostic section of the chapter also has been updated.

26. The number of cases of **Botulism and Infant Botulism (*Clostridium botulinum)*** has been updated. Additional guidance on avoidance of honey in prepared cereals during the first year of life has been added.

[1]*Managing Infectious Diseases in Child Care and Schools, 4th Ed. A Quick Reference Guide.* Aronson SS, Shope TR, eds. Elk Grove Village, IL: American Academy of Pediatrics; 2017

27. In the ***Clostridium difficile*** chapter, clinical manifestations and therapeutic options have been updated. Treatment recommendations have been assembled into a table for easier reference and have been harmonized with the 2017 guidelines from the Infectious Diseases Society of America. Updated information on community-associated *C difficile* disease has been added.

28. The **Coccidioidomycosis** chapter has been harmonized with the 2016 guidelines from the Infectious Diseases Society of America.

29. The epidemiology and clinical manifestations of **Coronaviruses, Including SARS and MERS** have been updated.

30. The epidemiology, diagnosis, and treatment of **Cryptosporidiosis** has been modified, with harmonization with the Infectious Diseases Society of America guidelines for the diagnosis and management of infectious diarrhea in the final stages of development.

31. *Isospora belli* is now named *Cystoisospora belli*, and the **Cystoisosporiasis** chapter is now among the chapters beginning with C in Section 3.

32. Saliva polymerase chain reaction assay as the preferred diagnostic tool for screening for **Cytomegalovirus** has been emphasized. Treatment recommendations for symptomatic congenital cytomegalovirus disease have been harmonized with international guidelines published in 2017.

33. New information on development of a vaccine to prevent **Dengue Fever** and on diagnostic testing has been added.

34. Laboratory abnormalities seen with **Ehrlichia, Anaplasma, and Related Infections** and duration of antimicrobial therapy have been updated.

35. The newly renamed **Serious Bacterial Infections Caused By *Enterobacteriaceae* (With Emphasis on Septicemia and Meningitis in Neonates)** chapter includes new information on the epidemiology and treatment of extended-spectrum beta-lactamases (ESBLs).

36. New data on the epidemiology and clinical manifestations of EV-D68 have been incorporated in the **Enterovirus (Nonpoliovirus) Infections** chapter.

37. The clinical manifestations, epidemiology, and diagnostic modalities for ***Escherichia coli* Diarrhea** have been updated.

38. Table 3.7 for **Other Fungal Diseases** has been modified and enhanced.

39. Abdominal manifestations of ***Fusobacterium* Infections** have been added to the chapter.

40. Discussion of molecular diagnostic tests for *Giardia intestinalis* (formerly *Giardia lamblia* and *Giardia duodenalis*) Infections (Giardiasis) have been added to the chapter.

41. The epidemiology of and molecular diagnostic testing for **Gonococcal Infections** have been updated. Treatment of adolescents and young adults with gonorrhea has been consolidated into a new table, separate from treatment of infants and children.

42. The incidence of typeable and nontypeable ***Haemophilus influenzae* Infections** has been updated. Nucleic acid amplification tests have been incorporated into the diagnostic approach to *Haemophilus* infections. The chapter has been modified to account for 2 Hib vaccines that have been removed from the market. Permissive language has been added for chemoprophylaxis of contacts of invasive *Haemophilus influenzae* type a infections.

43. Laboratory and clinical findings that suggest **Hantavirus Pulmonary Syndrome** have been more clearly stated.

44. Clinical manifestations and antibiotic resistance in ***Helicobacter pylori Infections*** have been added to the chapter. Diagnostic groups and treatment recommendations have been harmonized with the 2016 update of the joint ESPGHAN/NASPGHAN guidelines for children and adolescents.

45. Vectors and hosts for Hemorrhagic Fevers Caused by Arenaviruses have been added.

46. The epidemiology and diagnostic approach to **Hemorrhagic Fevers Caused by Bunyaviruses** have been updated and expanded. Ribavirin has been identified as increasing the likelihood of central nervous system disease in Rift Valley fever and, therefore, should be avoided.

47. The **Hemorrhagic Fevers Caused by Filoviruses: Ebola and Marburg** chapter was first included in the 2015 edition of the *Red Book*. The chapter in the 2018 edition provides updated epidemiologic data from the 2014-2015 Ebola pandemic as well as new information on virus transmission (eg, human milk). Guidance from the AAP clinical report "Parental Presence During Treatment of Ebola or Other Highly Consequential Infection" has been included, and contact information for therapeutic options at the CDC has been added.

48. Diagnostic and epidemiologic updates have been provided to the **Hepatitis A** chapter.

49. The interval for postvaccination testing of infants born to HBsAg-positive mothers has been modified in the **Hepatitis B** chapter. A figure and table have been added, providing guidance for evaluating health care personnel for hepatitis B virus protection and for administering postexposure management. The recent emphasis of the AAP and CDC on giving the first HepB vaccination within 24 hours of birth has been added. Molecular diagnostic testing options have been updated.

50. The diagnostic testing and treatment options for **Hepatitis C** have been modified to match this rapidly changing field.

51. Clinical trial data suggesting a possible therapeutic advance in the management of **Hepatitis D** has been incorporated in the chapter.

52. The clinical manifestations, etiology, and diagnosis of **Hepatitis E** have been updated.

53. **Herpes simplex virus.** Treatment of genital herpes has been harmonized with sexually transmitted infections guidelines from the CDC. The chapter has been shortened.

54. Target itraconazole trough concentrations and interpretation of laboratory results thereof have been updated in the **Histoplasmosis** chapter.

55. Methods for distinguishing chromosomally integrated HHV-6 have been added to the **Human Herpesvirus 6 (Including Roseola) and 7** chapter.

56. The **Human Immunodeficiency Virus Infection** chapter has been reduced in length by approximately 25%. Testing information has been updated. Management and prevention of opportunistic infection have been harmonized with the AIDSInfo recommendations, including for meningococcal vaccination. Breastfeeding information has been added.

57. The **Kawasaki Disease** chapter has been updated and harmonized with the 2017 guidelines from the American Heart Association.

58. The diagnosis section has been updated with information on mass spectrometry of bacterial cellular components that may be used for rapid identification, and the

treatment section has been updated with information on TEM-1 β-lactamase production, for the ***Kingella kingae* Infections** chapter.

59. The clinical manifestations ***Legionella pneumophila* Infections** have been updated. The availability of a polymerase chain reaction diagnostic assay that has been cleared by the US Food and Drug Administration (FDA) has been added. Levofloxacin (or another fluoroquinolone) has been added to intravenous azithromycin as the drug of choice for treatment of disease in immunocompetent patients.

60. The **Leishmaniasis** chapter has been harmonized with the 2016 practice guidelines published by the Infectious Diseases Society of America and the American Society of Tropical Medicine and Hygiene.

61. The serovar and serogroup criteria for **Leptospirosis** has been modified, and this newer nomenclature supersedes the former division of these organisms into 2 species. The global impact of disease has been updated.

62. Sources of acquisition of ***Listeria monocytogenes* Infections** have been added to the chapter. Diagnostic assays for central nervous system infections have been expanded.

63. The epidemiology and treatment of **Lyme Disease** has been updated, including the recently discovered *Borrelia mayonii*. Management recommendations have been harmonized with advanced drafts of the updated guidelines under development by the Infectious Diseases Society of America.

64. The clinical manifestations of **Lymphatic Filariasis** have been expanded.

65. A table listing drugs available for prophylaxis, including dosing, timing, and adverse effects, has been added to the **Malaria** chapter.

66. Recent outbreaks of **Measles** have been added to the epidemiology portion of the chapter. The diagnostic evaluation of suspected measles cases has been updated and streamlined.

67. Changes have been added for vaccine recommendations in **Meningococcal Infections.** These include a 2-dose schedule for Trumenba in some patient populations, and removal of MenHibRix and the polysaccharide MenACWY vaccines, which have been removed from the US market. Increased risk of meningococcal disease in patients receiving eculizumab has been added, and antibiotic prophylaxis in addition to vaccination in these patients is suggested. Recommendations for vaccinating HIV-infected children down to 2 months of age have been harmonized with those of the ACIP.

68. The **Microsporidia Infections** chapter has been harmonized with the updated the "Guidelines for Prevention and Treatment of Opportunistic Infections in HIV-Exposed and HIV-Infected Children" on the AIDSInfo Web site and the 2016 infectious diarrhea guidelines from the Infectious Diseases Society of America. A table of clinical manifestations by microsporidia species has been added.

69. Correlation between DOCK8 deficiency and more extensive **Molluscum Contagiosum** has been added. Risk factors for transmission have been expanded.

70. Information on the new and ongoing outbreaks in Marshallese populations and on college campuses has been added to the **Mumps** chapter.

71. Diagnostic assays and specific treatment recommendations have been added to the ***Mycoplasma pneumoniae* and Other *Mycoplasma* Species Infections** chapter.

72. Discussion of antimicrobial resistance in the management of **Nocardiosis** has been added.

73. The epidemiology and diagnostic sections of the **Norovirus and Sapovirus Infections** chapter have been updated.

74. A 2-dose schedule for HPV vaccination for children younger than 15 years has been added to the **Human Papillomaviruses** chapter. The 9-valent HPV vaccine is now the only vaccine on the US market. The AAP is emphasizing that children as young as 9 years of age can start their HPV vaccination series, so it is acceptable not to wait until the adolescent platform at 11 through 12 years of age to administer the vaccine.

75. A new species causing **Paracoccidioidomycosis** has been added to the chapter. Target itraconazole trough concentrations and interpretation of laboratory results thereof have been updated.

76. The clinical and laboratory manifestations of **Paragonimiasis** are presented in greater detail.

77. Fascioliasis has been added to the table in the **Parasitic Diseases** chapter.

78. Clinical manifestations and diagnostic assays for **Human Parechovirus Infections** have been updated.

79. Detailed information on the molecular detection of **Parvovirus B19** has been added.

80. The clinical presentations and epidemiology of ***Pasteurella* Infections** has been updated.

81. The **Pediculosis Capitis** chapter has been updated with information from the AAP's 2015 Clinical Report. The table of pediculicides available for use has been expanded for quick reference by health care providers. Control measures have been updated.

82. Discussion of diagnosis of **Pelvic Inflammatory Disease** has been expanded in greater detail.

83. Azithromycin has been reinforced as the drug of choice for treatment or prophylaxis of **Pertussis (Whooping Cough).** Some information on treatment of *Bordetella parapertussis* also has been added. Vaccination with Tdap during pregnancy is now recommended to occur earlier in the window of 27 to 36 weeks' gestational age. Recommendations are now provided on how to respond to inadvertent administration of Tdap instead of DTaP, or vice versa.

84. Treatment options for **Pinworm Infections** have been updated, including the reintroduction of mebendazole to the US market and use of ivermectin.

85. The epidemiology of **Pneumococcal Infections** in the 7 years following introduction of the 13-valent conjugate pneumococcal vaccine in 2010 has been updated. Diagnostic assays for the detection of *Streptococcus pneumoniae* also have been expanded. Specific therapeutic recommendations for pneumonia have been added.

86. Recommendations for the treatment of ***Pneumocystis jirovecii* Infections** have been harmonized with recommendations on AIDSInfo, including treatment durations (now 21 days instead of 14-21 days). A new table has been added to guide utilization of steroids in the management of *Pneumocystis* pneumonia.

87. Worldwide eradication efforts for **Poliovirus Infections** have been updated. Polio vaccination requirements for immigrants and refugees to the United States has been clarified, given the eradication efforts' movement toward bivalent oral polio vaccine.

88. The epidemiology, diagnosis, and treatment of **Polyomaviruses** has been updated. This includes more detailed discussion of polyomaviruses other than BK virus and JC virus.

89. Newer diagnostics for Prion Diseases: Transmissible Spongiform Encephalopathies have been added.

90. The numbers of cases of **Rabies** has been updated. Information on expertise at the level of the states has been added. The discussion of rabies diagnostic testing has been expanded.

91. The description of diagnostic tests for **Rat-Bite Fever** has been expanded. The limited availability of streptomycin has been added.

92. Considerations for when to test patients for **Respiratory Syncytial Virus** in the outpatient and inpatient settings have been added. Recommendations for populations in which palivizumab should be used have not changed from the 2015 *Red Book*. An increased risk for RSV disease in pediatric liver transplant recipients has been reported in a review of the national transplantation database.

93. The clinical manifestations and epidemiology of, and diagnostic tests for, **Rhinovirus Infections** have been updated.

94. The list of causes of other rickettsial spotted fever infections has been expanded in the **Rickettsial Infections** chapter. The importance of prompt initiation of treatment with doxycycline for all patients in all age groups with suspected Rocky Mountain spotted fever or ehrlichiosis, without waiting for confirmative diagnostic testing, is emphasized.

95. The diagnosis and treatment of **Rocky Mountain Spotted Fever** has been harmonized with those of the CDC on tickborne rickettsial diseases.

96. The epidemiology of **Rotavirus Infections** in the postvaccine era has been updated. Clinical manifestations have been expanded. Avoidance of rotavirus vaccine for infants born to mothers who received biologic response modifiers during pregnancy has been added to the chapter.

97. ***Salmonella* Infections** have been substantially reorganized and separated into nontyphoid and typhoid/paratyphoid portions throughout the chapter. Treatment recommendations for both typhoid fever and nontyphoid bacteremia have been modified. Recommendations on return to school have been harmonized with those in the AAP Purple Book.[1]

98. Emerging data on antibiotic resistance in ***Shigella* Infections** have been added to the chapter. Molecular diagnostic tests have been updated. Recommendations on return to school have been harmonized with those in the AAP Purple Book.[1]

99. The ***Staphylococcus aureus*** chapter has been separated from the coagulase-negative *Staphylococcus* chapter, and has been shortened. Disease incidence and diagnostic approaches have been updated. Data on drainage plus antimicrobial therapy for skin and soft tissue abscesses have been added. Treatment recommendations have been streamlined.

100. The **Coagulase-Negative Staphylococcal Infections** chapter is a new chapter in the 2018 *Red Book*.

101. Several changes have been made to the **Group A Streptococcal Infections**

[1]*Managing Infectious Diseases in Child Care and Schools, 4th Ed. A Quick Reference Guide.* Aronson SS, Shope TR, eds. Elk Grove Village, IL: American Academy of Pediatrics; 2017

chapter. The diagnosis of rheumatic fever, including the modified Jones criteria, has been harmonized with the 2015 scientific statement from the American Heart Association. Time to return to school following initiation of treatment for streptococcal pharyngitis has been modified, from 24 hours to 12 hours. In addition, language has been strengthened discouraging antimicrobial treatment or prophylaxis, IGIV, or plasmapheresis for children with symptoms suggestive of pediatric autoimmune neuropsychiatric disorders associated with streptococcal infections (PANDAS) or pediatric acute-onset neuropsychiatric syndrome (PANS).

102. The **Non-Group A or B Streptococcal and Enterococcal Infections** chapter has been harmonized with the updated endocarditis guidelines published by the American Heart Association and endorsed by the Infectious Diseases Society of America. Clinical manifestations of infection have been expanded.

103. The **Syphilis** chapter has been shortened substantially. "Reverse-sequence screening" has been added to the algorithm for the diagnostic approach of infants born to mothers with reactive serologic tests. A table detailing the approach to the evaluation and treatment of infants with possible, probable, or confirmed congenital syphilis has been added. The epidemiology of syphilis, including recent increases in disease incidence, has been updated.

104. The option for use of combination therapy for neurocysticercosis has been added to the **Tapeworm Disease** chapter. The recommendation has been added to screen household members of patients with cysticercosis for taeniasis.

105. The etiology and number of cases of **Tetanus** worldwide have been updated. Global efforts to eliminate maternal and neonatal tetanus have been added. The Control Measures portion of the chapter has been reorganized for easier retrieval of recommendations following exposure to *Clostridium tetani*.

106. The epidemiology of **Tinea Capitis** is presented in greater detail, including racial differences by pathogen and genetic predisposition to infection.

107. A new table listing products for topical treatment of tinea infections has been added to the **Tinea Corporis** chapter. This table applies to tinea cruris and pedis as well. A differential diagnosis for tinea corporis has been added.

108. The differential diagnosis for **Tinea Cruris** has been incorporated in the Clinical Manifestations portion of the chapter.

109. The epidemiology of **Tinea Pedis and Tinea Unguium** is presented in greater detail, including racial differences by pathogen, genetic predisposition to infection, and incidence rates. Options for topical management of tinea unguium have been expanded.

110. The chapter on ***Toxoplasma gondii* Infections** has been harmonized with the 2017 AAP technical report addressing the diagnosis, treatment, and prevention of congenital toxoplasmosis. It has been shortened to increase ease of use in retrieving diagnostic and treatment recommendations.

111. The epidemiology, including increasing rates of antimicrobial resistance, and diagnostic testing modalities for ***Trichomonas vaginalis* Infections** have been updated.

112. Data on the endemic occurrence of **American Trypanosomiasis (Chagas Disease)** in the United States has been added to the chapter. The approval of benznidazole by the US FDA in August 2017 for the treatment of Chagas disease in children 2 through 12 years of age has been incorporated as well.

113. The recommended age for use of interferon gamma release assays (IGRAs) for the diagnosis of **Tuberculosis** has been decreased from 5 years to 2 years. For treatment of latent *Mycobacterium tuberculosis* infection (LTBI), 3 treatment options are offered and considered adequate, depending on the circumstances for individual patients: (1) 12 weeks of isoniazid plus rifapentine, once a week; (2) 4 months of rifampin, once a day; or (3) 9 months of isoniazid, once a day. In addition, the chapter has been shortened to more easily locate and utilize information for the management of a patient in the office, clinic, or hospital.

114. Discussion of *Mycobacterium chimaera* contamination of heater-cooler units used in open heart surgery has been added to the **Nontuberculous Mycobacteria** (NTM) chapter. Medical and surgical management options for NTM lymphadenitis have been expanded, and the overall length of the chapter has been shortened.

115. The epidemiology of **Tularemia** infections has been updated to include recent increases in cases in Colorado, Nebraska, South Dakota, and Wyoming. Wording discouraging the use of doxycycline has been added because of the increased likelihood of relapse when this antibiotic is used.

116. Lack of transmission of wild-type and vaccine-strain **Varicella Zoster Virus** in human milk has been added, and discussion of both administration of expressed human milk and isolation of infants born to mothers with varicella in the perinatal period has been provided in greater detail. Use of the vaccine in immunocompromised patients has been harmonized with the guidelines of the Infectious Diseases Society of America. The option of using oral acyclovir as postexposure prophylaxis when VariZIG is not available has been liberalized. The chapter has been shortened to increase ease of use in retrieving diagnostic and treatment recommendations.

117. The new single-dose, live-attenuated monovalent oral **Cholera *(Vibrio cholerae)*** vaccine, Vaxchora, has been added to the chapter. This vaccine is approved by the US FDA and is available in the United States for use for travelers 18 through 64 years of age who are traveling to areas where cholera is a risk.

118. Disease manifestations and risk factors for **Other *Vibrio* Infections** have been added to the chapter. Monotherapy for severe diarrhea using doxycycline or ciprofloxacin has been added as well.

119. Description of **West Nile Virus** transmission via human milk has been expanded. The number of cases has been updated, along with infection incidence rates in more heavily affected states. A Web link to a review summarizing potential treatments (including Immune Globulin Intravenous with or without a high titer of WNV antibody, WNV recombinant humanized monoclonal antibody, interferon, corticosteroid, ribavirin) has been added.

120. The number of species constituting the genus Yersinia has been updated (increased) in the ***Yersinia enterocolitica* and *Yersinia pseudotuberculosis* Infections** chapter. The etiology of infection has been expanded to discuss differences in virulence gene distribution among *Yersinia* species, and correlating with clinical manifestations.

121. **Zika** is a new chapter in the 2018 *Red Book*. Its development has been carefully coordinated to include input from Zika experts and to harmonize with diagnostic recommendations from the CDC, including partnership between the AAP and CDC on the evaluation and management of infants with possible congenital Zika

virus infection as the case incidence decreased in 2017. This chapter was early released online by the AAP in 2017 to aid in management.

SECTION 4. ANTIMICROBIAL AGENTS AND RELATED THERAPY

1. The **Introduction to Antimicrobial Agents and Related Therapy** has incorporated the information from the 2016 AAP clinical report "Use of Systemic and
   Topical Fluoroquinolones." It also explains the rationale for the liberalization of
   recommendations on use of doxycycline in children younger than 8 years.

2. The chapter on **Antimicrobial Resistance and Antimicrobial Stewardship:
   Appropriate and Judicious Use of Antimicrobial Agents** has been updated
   to reflect the current recommendations from the CDC addressing antimicrobial
   stewardship core elements as well as guidelines from the Infectious Diseases Society
   of America and the Society for Healthcare Epidemiology of America published in
   2016.

3. The **Tables of Antimicrobial Drug Dosages** have been updated throughout.
   Dosing in neonates has been modified to take into account variables such as gestational age, postnatal age, and postmenstrual age, that best guide neonatal dosing for
   a given group of agents. Maximum dosages for infants and children have been
   added to emphasize that higher dosages generally are used in more severe infections.

4. The **Sexually Transmitted Infections** tables have been separated to include
   older children, adolescents, and young adults in one table and younger (smaller)
   children in a separate table for ease of use.

5. *Candida auris* has been added to the **Antifungal Drugs for Systemic Fungal
   Infections** chapter. Route of administration, cerebrospinal fluid penetration,
   therapeutic drug monitoring requirements, and adverse reactions have been added
   to the table in this chapter as well.

6. Micafungin dosing in neonates and posaconazole dosing in children have been
   added to the **Recommended Doses of Parenteral and Oral Antifungal
   Drugs** table. The new antifungal drug isavuconazole has been added.

7. The **Drugs for Parasitic Infections** table has been revised to reflect drugs that
   currently are accessible in the United States, with specific drugs added or removed
   since the 2015 edition. Recommendations in the table also have been harmonized
   with published guidelines from professional societies (eg, the *Leishmania* guideline
   from the Infectious Diseases Society of America) or technical reports from the AAP
   (eg, toxoplasmosis).

SECTION 5. ANTIMICROBIAL PROPHYLAXIS

1. The **Antimicrobial Prophylaxis in Pediatric Surgical Patients** chapter
   has been harmonized with the surgical site infections portion of the National
   Healthcare Safety Network, which is the CDC's health care-associated infection
   tracking system.

2. In the chapter on **Prevention of Neonatal Ophthalmia,** the AAP begins
   the process of advocating for repeal of state mandates for topical prophylaxis for
   neonatal ophthalmia. Specific alternative approaches to successfully prevent

gonococcal ophthalmia are provided. Nongonococcal and nonchlamydial causes of neonatal ophthalmia have been expanded.

APPENDICES

1. Telephone and Web site addresses for organizations listed in the **Directory of Resources** have been updated.
2. ICD9 codes have been removed from the **Codes for Commonly Administered Pediatric Vaccines/Toxoids and Immune Globulins** appendix. The table of codes for commonly administered vaccines has been replaced with a Web link to an AAP Web site with the same that is regularly updated.
3. The **Vaccine Injury Table** has been modified to include combine VAERS reporting and the vaccine injury listings.
4. The diseases listed in the **Nationally Notifiable Infectious Diseases in the United States** table are those required for 2017, and include the addition of Zika virus since the last *Red Book*.
5. Terminology used throughout the table of Guide to Contraindications and Precautions to Immunizations, 2018 has been standardized.

Active and Passive Immunization

PROLOGUE

The ultimate goal of immunization is control of infection transmission, elimination of disease, and eventually, eradication of the pathogen that causes the infection and disease; the immediate goal is prevention of disease in people or groups. To accomplish these goals, physicians must make timely immunization a high priority in the care of infants, children, adolescents, and adults. The global eradication of smallpox in 1977, elimination of poliomyelitis disease from the Americas in 1991, elimination of endemic measles transmission in the United States in 2000 and in the Americas in 2002, elimination of rubella and congenital rubella syndrome from the United States in 2004 and from the Americas in 2015, and global eradication of type 2 wild poliovirus in 2015 serve as models for fulfilling the promise of disease control through immunization. These accomplishments were achieved by combining a comprehensive immunization program providing consistent, high levels of vaccine coverage with intensive surveillance and effective public health disease-control measures. The resurgence of measles and mumps in the United States, however, illustrates how precarious the substantial gains to date can be without vigilant commitment by physicians, public health officials, and members of the public. Worldwide eradication of polio, measles, and rubella remains possible through implementation of proven prevention strategies, and in the case of polio is tantalizingly close, but diligence must prevail until eradication is achieved, or success itself is imperiled.

High immunization rates, in general, have reduced dramatically the incidence of all vaccine-preventable diseases (see Tables 1.1 and 1.2, p 2) in the United States. Yet, because pathogens that cause vaccine-preventable diseases persist in the United States and elsewhere around the world, ongoing immunization efforts must be not only maintained but also strengthened. All vaccine-preventable diseases are, at most, 18 hours away by air travel from any part of the world.

Discoveries in immunology, molecular biology, and medical genetics have resulted in groundbreaking advances in vaccine research. Licensing of new, improved, and safer vaccines; establishment of an adolescent immunization platform; development of vaccines against cancer (eg, human papillomavirus and hepatitis B vaccines); and application of novel vaccine-delivery systems promise to continue the advances in preventive medicine achieved during the latter half of the 20th century. The advent of population-based postlicensure studies of vaccines facilitates detection of rare adverse events temporally associated with immunization that were undetected during large prelicensure clinical trials, as well as detection of changes over time in vaccine effectiveness (eg, live attenuated influenza vaccine [LAIV]) that directly inform recommendations on use of specific vaccines.

Table 1.1. Comparison of Prevaccine Era Estimated Average Annual Morbidity with Current Estimates: Vaccines Approved Before 1980

Disease	20th Century Average Annual Morbidity[a]	2016 Reported Cases[b]	Percent Decrease
Smallpox	29 005	0	100
Diphtheria	21 053	0	100
Measles	530 217	85	>99
Mumps	162 344	2 539	99
Pertussis	200 752	15 737[c]	92
Polio (paralytic)	16 316	0	100
Rubella	47 745	1	>99
Congenital rubella syndrome	152	0	100
Tetanus	580	28	98
Haemophilus influenzae	20 000	30[d]	>99

[a]Roush SW, Murphy TV, Vaccine-Preventable Disease Table Working Group. Historical comparisons of morbidity and mortality for vaccine-preventable diseases in the United States. *JAMA.* 2007;298(18):2155–2163
[b]Centers for Disease Control and Prevention. Notifiable diseases and mortality tables. *MMWR Morb Mortal Wkly Rep.* 2017;66(20). Available at: **www.cdc.gov/mmwr/volumes/66/wr/mm6639md.htm**
[c]Centers for Disease Control and Prevention. Notifiable diseases and mortality tables. *MMWR Morb Mortal Wkly Rep.* 2017;65(52). Available at: **www.cdc.gov/mmwr/volumes/65/wr/mm6552md.htm?s_cid=mm6552md_w**
[d]*Haemophilus influenzae* type b (Hib) in children younger than 5 years.

Table 1.2. Comparison of Prevaccine Era Estimated Average Annual Morbidity With Current Estimates: Vaccines Approved Since 1980

Disease	Prevaccine Era Annual Estimate	2015 Estimate	Percent Decrease
Hepatitis A	117 333[a]	2 800[b]	98
Hepatitis B (acute)	66 232[a]	21 900[b]	67
Pneumococcus (invasive)			
All ages	63 067[a]	29 500[c]	53
<5 y	16 069[a]	1 793[d]	89
Rotavirus (hospitalizations, <3 y)	62 500[e]	11 250[f]	82
Varicella	4 085 120[a]	126 639[g]	97

[a]Roush SW, Murphy TV, Vaccine-Preventable Disease Table Working Group. Historical comparisons of morbidity and mortality for vaccine-preventable diseases in the United States. *JAMA.* 2007;298(18):2155–2163
[b]Centers for Disease Control and Prevention. Viral Hepatitis Surveillance – United States, 2015. Available at: **www.cdc.gov/hepatitis/statistics/2015surveillance/commentary.htm**
[c]Centers for Disease Control and Prevention. Active Bacterial Core Surveillance Provisional Report; *Streptococcus pneumoniae,* 2015. Available at: **www.cdc.gov/abcs/reports-findings/survreports/spneu15.html**
[d]Calculated from data from **www.cdc.gov/abcs/reports-findings/survreports/spneu15.html** and **www.census.gov/quickfacts/table/PST045216/00**
[e]Centers for Disease Control and Prevention. Prevention of rotavirus gastroenteritis among infants and children: recommendations of the Advisory Committee on Immunization Practices (ACIP). *MMWR Recomm Rep.* 2009;58(RR-02):1–25
[f]Payne DC. A decade of documenting the impact of rotavirus vaccination in the United States: understanding the post-rotavirus vaccine introduction era. 5th European Expert Meeting on Rotavirus Vaccination (EEROVAC); Utrecht, Netherlands, March 21, 2017
[g]Centers for Disease Control and Prevention. Varicella Program 2015 data (unpublished).

Each edition of the *Red Book* provides recommendations for immunization of infants, children, adolescents, and young adults. These recommendations, which are harmonized among the American Academy of Pediatrics (AAP), the Advisory Committee on Immunization Practices (ACIP) of the Centers for Disease Control and Prevention (CDC), and the American Academy of Family Physicians (AAFP), are based on careful analysis of disease epidemiology, benefits, and risks of immunization; feasibility of implementation; and cost-benefit analysis. ACIP recommendations utilize Grading of Recommendations Assessment, Development and Evaluation (GRADE), when feasible, in evaluating the evidence of benefits and risks for a given vaccine, further ensuring that the recommendations are evidence-based and objectively assessed.

Use of trade names and commercial sources in the *Red Book* is for identification purposes only and does not imply endorsement by the AAP. Internet sites referenced in the *Red Book* are provided as a service to readers and may change without notice; citation of Web sites does not constitute AAP endorsement.

SOURCES OF INFORMATION ABOUT IMMUNIZATION

In addition to the latest print edition of the *Red Book*, the following sources can assist providers in remaining up-to-date with immunization recommendations and finding answers to questions that arise in practice. For many of these resources, providers can sign up for e-mail alerts to receive new information as soon as it is available.

- **American Academy of Pediatrics (AAP)—Red Book Online** includes the print edition content plus updates and is available on the Internet (**http://redbook.solutions.aap.org/Redbook.aspx**) and as a mobile app for iOS and Google Play to AAP members and subscribers. The Web site has links to the latest policy updates, current immunization schedules, and the Vaccine Status Table, which provides the status of recently submitted, approved, and recommended vaccines and licensed biologics. New recommendations are summarized in **AAP News** (**www.aappublications.org/news**), the official newsmagazine of the AAP, and are published in **Pediatrics** (**http://pediatrics.aappublications. org**), the official journal of the Academy (both periodicals are issued monthly). The AAP also maintains a Web site (**www.aap.org/en-us/advocacy-and-policy/aap-health-initiatives/immunization/Pages/default.aspx**) that contains useful links to immunization resources for providers as well as a Web site with information geared toward parents (**https://healthychildren.org**).
- **Centers for Disease Control and Prevention (CDC)**—The CDC immunization Web site (**www.cdc.gov/vaccines/**) contains a wealth of information, including annually updated, routine immunization schedules; vaccine safety information; recommendations from the Advisory Committee on Immunization Practices (ACIP); vaccine supply updates; vaccine coverage and disease surveillance data; recommendations for specific patient populations; information about storage, handling, and administration of vaccines; legal requirements; and education and training. ACIP recommendations become "official" when they are published in the

Morbidity and Mortality Weekly Report (MMWR). Noteworthy CDC Internet resources are listed in Table 1.3. CDC experts also are available to answer immunization-related questions by email at **nipinfo@cdc.gov.**

- **Immunization Action Coalition (IAC)**—The IAC is the most visible nongovernmental source of immunization resources for health care professionals in the United States. Working in partnership with the CDC, the IAC maintains a Web site (**www.immunize.org**) replete with copyright-free information about virtually every aspect of vaccine practice. Unique content includes Vaccine Information Statement (VIS) translations in over 40 languages; *Ask the Experts*, a repository of answers to challenging immunization questions; handouts for patients and staff; *Unprotected People Reports*, containing personal accounts of encounters with vaccine-preventable diseases; updated information about state mandates and exemptions; expansive image and video libraries; and screening tools for contraindications and precautions. The IAC also maintains Web sites for the public (**www.vaccineinformation.org**) and for immunization coalitions (**www.immunizationcoalitions.org**). The IAC's weekly e-mail newsletter, *IAC Express*, and its periodicals, *Needle Tips* and *Vaccinate Adults*, are available free of charge.

- **Vaccine Manufacturers**—Major vaccine manufacturers (Table 1.4) maintain Web sites with current information concerning new products, changes in labeling, contact information for medical questions, and updated package inserts. The package insert (also referred to as the "label," "prescribing information," or "product information") is a document approved by the US Food and Drug Administration (FDA) that specifies product indications and usage, dosage and administration, formulations, contraindications, warnings and precautions, adverse reactions, results from clinical trials, and other information about the vaccine. The FDA maintains a repository of current package inserts on its Web site (**www.fda.gov/BiologicsBloodVaccines/Vaccines/ApprovedProducts/ucm093833.htm**). The indications listed in the package insert are based on data submitted to the FDA as part of the approval process. It is important to understand that the FDA does not issue guidelines or recommendations for vaccine use. In some instances, recommendations of the AAP and ACIP may differ from a vaccine's labeled indications.

- **Other Resources**—Table 1.5 lists major national and international organizations that are involved in immunization policy, education, implementation, and advocacy, along with their respective Web sites. The Directory of Resources in Appendix I (p 1051) also is a source of contact information for these and other organizations.

Table 1.3. CDC Immunization Web Page Quick Reference

Content	URL
National Center for Immunization and Respiratory Diseases (NCIRD)	**www.cdc.gov/ncird**
Information for health care professionals	**www.cdc.gov/vaccines/hcp.htm**
Information for parents	**www.cdc.gov/vaccines/parents/index.html**
Provider resources for vaccine conversations with parents	**www.cdc.gov/vaccines/hcp/conversations/index.html**
ACIP recommendations	**www.cdc.gov/vaccines/hcp/acip-recs/index.html**

Table 1.3. CDC Immunization Web Page Quick Reference, continued

Content	URL
Schedules	www.cdc.gov/vaccines/schedules/index.html
Instant Childhood Immunization Schedule	www2a.cdc.gov/nip/kidstuff/newscheduler_le/
Vaccine Information Statements	www.cdc.gov/vaccines/hcp/vis/index.html
Vaccines for Children Program	www.cdc.gov/vaccines/programs/vfc/index.html
Travel	wwwnc.cdc.gov/travel/destinations/list
Vaccine names in other language	www.cdc.gov/vaccines/pubs/pinkbook/downloads/appendices/B/foreign-products-tables.pdf
CDC Health Information for International Travel (also known as the Yellow Book)	wwwnc.cdc.gov/travel/yellowbook/2016/table-of-contents
Epidemiology and Prevention of Vaccine-Preventable Diseases (also known as the Pink Book)	www.cdc.gov/vaccines/pubs/pinkbook/index.html
Manual for the Surveillance of Vaccine-Preventable Diseases	www.cdc.gov/vaccines/pubs/surv-manual/index.html
Morbidity and Mortality Weekly Report (MMWR)	www.cdc.gov/mmwr/index.html

Table 1.4. Major Vaccine Manufacturers in the United States

Company	URL
GlaxoSmithKline	www.gsk.com
MedImmune (Member of AstraZeneca Group)	www.medimmune.com or www.astrazeneca.com/our-science/MedImmune.html
Merck	www.merck.com
Pfizer	www.pfizer.com
Sanofi Pasteur	www.sanofipasteur.com
Seqirus	www.seqirus.com

Table 1.5. Internet Resources for Vaccine Information for Health Care Professionals and Parents

Resource	URL
Government	
Centers for Disease Control and Prevention: Vaccines & Immunization	www.cdc.gov/vaccines/
Clinical Immunization Safety Assessment (CISA) Project	www.cdc.gov/vaccinesafety/ensuringsafety/monitoring/cisa
National Institute of Allergy and Infectious Diseases	www.niaid.nih.gov
US Food and Drug Administration: Vaccines, Blood & Biologics	www.fda.gov/BiologicsBloodVaccines/default.htm

Table 1.5. Internet Resources for Vaccine Information for Health Care Professionals and Parents, continued

Resource	URL
National Vaccine Injury Compensation Program	www.hrsa.gov/vaccinecompensation/index.html
Vaccine Adverse Event Reporting System	vaers.hhs.gov/index
National Vaccine Program Office	www.hhs.gov/nvpo
National Vaccine Advisory Committee	www.hhs.gov/nvpo/nvac
International	
Pan American Health Organization	www.paho.org/hq
World Health Organization	www.who.int/en
Professional Associations	
American Academy of Pediatrics	www.aap.org/en-us
American Academy of Family Physicians	www.aafp.org
American Medical Association	www.ama-assn.org/ama
American College of Physicians	www.acponline.org
American College of Obstetricians and Gynecologists	www.acog.org
American Pharmacists Association	www.pharmacist.com
American Public Health Association	www.apha.org
Association for Prevention Teaching and Research	www.aptrweb.org
Society of Teachers of Family Medicine	www.immunizationed.org
Association of Immunization Managers	www.immunizationmanagers.org
Infectious Diseases Society of America	www.idsociety.org
Pediatric Infectious Diseases Society	www.pids.org
Advocacy and Implementation	
Children's Hospital of Philadelphia Vaccine Education Center	www.chop.edu/centers-programs/vaccine-education-center
Every Child by Two	www.ecbt.org
	www.vaccinateyourfamily.org
Families Fighting Flu	www.familiesfightingflu.org
Global Alliance for Vaccines and Immunization	www.gavi.org
Immunization Action Coalition	www.immunize.org
Immunization for Women (American College of Obstetricians and Gynecologists)	www.immunizationforwomen.org
National Foundation for Infectious Diseases	www.nfid.org
National Meningitis Association	www.nmaus.org
Parents of Kids With Infectious Diseases	www.pkids.org
Texas Children's Hospital Center for Vaccine Awareness and Research	www.texaschildrens.org/departments/center-vaccine-awareness-and-research-cvar
Value of Vaccination	www.valueofvaccination.org
Vaccinate Your Family	www.vaccinateyourfamily.org
Voices for Vaccines	www.voicesforvaccines.org

DISCUSSING VACCINES WITH PATIENTS AND PARENTS

Patients and their families should be informed about both the benefits and risks of vaccines.[1] The importance of confident and strong support by the health care professional for all recommended vaccines cannot be overemphasized. The single most important factor in parents' acceptance of vaccines is the recommendation of a well-informed, caring, and concerned pediatrician. Questions should be encouraged, and adequate time should be allowed so that the information provided is understood (**www.cdc.gov/vaccines/hcp/conversations/index.html**). Parents should receive a clear message that vaccines are safe and effective and that serious disease can occur when children are not immunized.

Addressing Parents' Questions About Vaccine Safety and Effectiveness

Although parents receive information about vaccines from multiple sources, they consider health care professionals—their primary care physician as well as all members of the health care team in clinical practice settings—to be the their most trusted source of health information. The child's need for a routinely scheduled vaccine should be announced in a confident, assertive manner. Acknowledging parents' concerns, listening respectfully, and providing accurate information about both benefits and risks of vaccines helps forge a trusting relationship. Identifying the specific issue(s) that parents may have about particular vaccines may help to focus the discussion. Several factors contribute to parental concerns about vaccines, including: (1) lack of information about the vaccine being administered and about immunizations in general; (2) lack of understanding of the severity and communicability of vaccine-preventable diseases; (3) opposing information and misinformation from other sources (eg, alternative medicine practitioners, antivaccination organizations, and Web sites); (4) perceived risk of serious vaccine adverse effects; and (5) mistrust of the source of information regarding vaccines (eg, vaccine manufacturer, the government). Some people view the risk involved with immunization as disproportionately greater than the risk of disease, in part because of the relative infrequency of vaccine-preventable diseases in the United States because of the success of the immunization program. Others may dwell on sociopolitical issues, such as mandatory immunization, informed consent, and the primacy of individual rights over that of societal benefit.

Common Misconceptions About Immunizations and the Institute of Medicine Findings

Misconceptions and misinformation regarding vaccines should be addressed clearly and

---

[1]Edwards KM, Hackell JM; American Academy of Pediatrics, Committee on Infectious Diseases, Committee on Practice and Ambulatory Medicine. Countering vaccine hesitancy. *Pediatrics*. 2016;138(3):e20162146

specifically. Table 1.6 includes facts that refute common misconceptions and myths about immunizations. In 2011, the Institute of Medicine (IOM), now called the National Academy of Medicine, reviewed evidence on the safety of 8 individual vaccines (**www.nap.edu/catalog/13164/adverse-effects-of-vaccines-evidence-and-causality**) and, in 2013, the safety of the immunization schedule (**www.nap.edu/catalog/13563/the-childhood-immunization-schedule-and-safety-stakeholder-concerns-scientific-evidence**). Its conclusions were: (1) few health problems are caused by or clearly associated with individual vaccines; and (2) there is no evidence that the immunization schedule is unsafe. The IOM specifically found no links between the immunization schedule and autoimmune diseases, asthma, hypersensitivity, seizures, child developmental disorders, learning or developmental disorders, or attention deficit or disruptive disorders. Additionally, use of nonstandard schedules is harmful, because it increases the period of risk of acquiring vaccine-preventable diseases and increases the risk of incomplete immunization. (Also see Institute of Medicine Reviews of Adverse Events after Immunization, p 43.)

Parents may be aware through the media, social media, or information from alternative Web sites about issues that may be portrayed as controversial regarding scheduled vaccines. Many issues about childhood vaccines communicated by these means are presented incompletely, inaccurately, and in an inflammatory way. When a parent initiates discussion about an alleged vaccine controversy, the health care professional should listen carefully and then nonjudgmentally but confidently and definitively discuss specific concerns using factual information and language appropriate for parents and other care providers.

It is important for the health care professional to articulate clearly the message that vaccines are safe and effective, and serious disease can occur if the child and family are not immunized. Safety information must be presented in a nonconfrontational dialogue with the parents while listening to and acknowledging their concerns. Providing specific examples and anecdotes about the effects of diseases prevented by immunization and sharing personal choices and experiences can provide parents with a compelling message on the confidence and support of the provider on the safety of vaccines. Misconceptions should be corrected, because both parents and pediatricians are in agreement in wanting the best for children's health and well-being.

Resources for Optimizing Communications With Parents About Vaccines

Vaccine information is available that can help health care professionals respond to questions and misconceptions about immunizations and vaccine-preventable diseases (see Table 1.3 and Table 1.5). Helpful credible information sources that can be provided to parents or to which parents can be directed include the "Parent's Guide to Childhood Immunization" (**www.cdc.gov/vaccines**), the Centers for Disease Control and Prevention (CDC) Internet hotline service (**www.cdc.gov/info**), the American Academy of Pediatrics (AAP) Immunization Initiative Web site (**www2.aap.org/immunization/**), and the Vaccine Education Center at Children's Hospital of Philadelphia (**www.chop.edu/centers-programs/vaccine-education-center**).

Table 1.6. Common Misconceptions/Myths About Immunizations[a,b]

Claims	Facts
Natural methods of enhancing immunity are better than vaccinations.	The only "natural way" to be immune is to have the disease. Immunity from a preventive vaccine provides protection against disease when a person is exposed to it in the future. That immunity is usually similar to what is acquired from natural infection, although several doses of a vaccine may have to be administered for a child to develop an adequate immune response.
Giving multiple vaccines at the same time causes an "overload" of the immune system.	Vaccination does not overburden a child's immune system; the recommended vaccines use only a small portion of the immune system's "memory." Although the number of unique vaccines administered has risen over recent decades, the number of antigens administered has decreased because of changes in manufacturing. The Institute of Medicine (IOM) has concluded that there is no evidence that the immunization schedule is unsafe (see text).
Vaccines are ineffective.	Vaccines have spared millions of people the effects of devastating diseases.
Prior to the use of vaccinations, these diseases had begun to decline because of improved nutrition and hygiene.	In the 19th and 20th centuries, some infectious diseases began to be better controlled because of improvements in sanitation, clean water, pasteurized milk, and pest control. However, vaccine-preventable diseases decreased dramatically after the vaccines for those diseases were approved and were administered to large numbers of children.
Vaccines cause poorly understood illnesses or disorders, such as autism, sudden infant death syndrome (SIDS), immune dysfunction, diabetes, neurologic disorders, allergic rhinitis, eczema, and asthma.	These claims are false. Multiple, high-quality studies have failed to substantiate any link between vaccines and these health conditions. See IOM reports.
Vaccines weaken the immune system.	Vaccines actually strengthen the immune system. Vaccinated children have decreased risk of infections. Importantly, natural infections like influenza, measles, and chickenpox can weaken the immune system, increasing the risk of other infections.

Table 1.6. Common Misconceptions/Myths About Immunizations,[a,b] continued

Claims	Facts
Giving many vaccines at the same time is untested.	Concomitant use studies require all new vaccines to be tested with existing vaccines. These studies are performed to ensure that new vaccines do not affect the safety or effectiveness of existing vaccines administered at the same time and that existing vaccines administered at the same time do not affect the safety or effectiveness of new vaccines.
Vaccines can be delayed, separated, and spaced out without consequences.	Many vaccine-preventable diseases occur in early infancy. Optimal vaccine-induced immunity may require a series of vaccines over time. Any delay in receiving age-appropriate immunization increases the risk of diseases that vaccines are administered to prevent.

Adapted from: Myers MG, Pineda D. *Do Vaccines Cause That? A Guide for Evaluating Vaccine Safety Concerns.* Galveston, TX: Immunizations for Public Health; 2008:79.
[a]See Institute of Medicine Reviews of Adverse Events After Immunization (p 43).
[b]Other common misconceptions are detailed online (**www.cdc.gov/vaccines/pubs/parents-guide/parents-guide-part4.html**).

The CDC, the AAP, and the American Academy of Family Physicians developed "Provider Resources for Vaccine Conversations with Parents" (**www.cdc.gov/vaccines/hcp/conversations/index.html**). These educational materials build on the latest research in vaccine and communication science and are designed to help health care professionals remain current on vaccine topics, strengthen communication and trust between health care professionals and parents, and share with parents up-to-date, easy-to-use information about vaccines and vaccine-preventable diseases. People can download these materials and enroll to receive e-mail updates when new resources are posted. The materials include the following:

- Strategies on Talking with Parents about Vaccines for Infants.
- Current vaccine safety topics, such as Understanding MMR and Vaccine Safety; Understanding Thimerosal, Mercury, and Vaccine Safety; Ensuring the Safety of US Vaccines; The Childhood Immunization Schedule; and more.
- Basic and in-depth fact sheets on 14 vaccine-preventable diseases for parents. Fact sheets are available in English and Spanish for a variety of reading levels, and many include stories of families whose children have experienced a vaccine-preventable disease.
- If You Choose Not to Vaccinate Your Child, Understand the Risks and Responsibilities shares the risks for parents who choose to delay or decline a vaccine and offers steps for parents to take to protect their child, family, and others.
- Interactive, online childhood immunization scheduler and waiting room videos, such as Get the Picture: Childhood Immunization Video.

Parental Refusal of Immunizations

Many parents have concerns related to 1 or 2 specific vaccines. Pediatricians and other health care providers should discuss benefits and risks of each vaccine, because a parent who is reluctant to accept administration of one vaccine may be willing to accept others. Parents who have concerns about administering multiple vaccines to a child in a single visit may have their concerns addressed by using methods to reduce the pain of injection (see Managing Injection Pain, p 30) or by using combination vaccines. Any schedule should adhere to age ranges of vaccine administration provided in the "Recommended Immunization Schedule for Children and Adolescents Aged 18 Years or Younger" **(http://redbook.solutions.aap.org/SS/Immunization_Schedules.aspx)**. Physicians also should explore the possibility that cost is a reason for refusing immunizations.

Parents who refuse vaccines for their child should be advised that all states have laws prohibiting unimmunized children from attending school during outbreaks of vaccine-preventable diseases. Parents should be encouraged to read the applicable law(s) in their state. Information on state-specific religious, philosophical, and nonmedical exemptions for immunization is available online **(http://vaccinesafety.edu/cc-exem.htm)**. Discussions about vaccine delay and refusal should be documented in the patient's health record. If one or more scheduled vaccines is refused, a signed *informed refusal* document should note that the parent was informed about why the immunization was recommended, the benefits and risks of immunization, and the possible consequences of not being immunized. Parents also should be encouraged to inform health care professionals when children who are not immunized are seeking care for an acute illness, because they are at risk of acquiring the vaccine-preventable disease themselves and because they, therefore, could be a risk to other vulnerable children who might also be in the health care facility. A sample Refusal to Vaccinate form can be found on the AAP Web site **(www2.aap.org/immunization/pediatricians/pdf/RefusaltoVaccinate.pdf)**.

For cases in which parents refuse vaccine administration for their child, pediatricians should revisit the immunization discussion on subsequent visits. Continued refusal after adequate discussion should be documented in the heath record and no further action taken unless the child is put at additional risk of serious harm (eg, during an epidemic). Only then should state agencies be involved to override parental discretion on the basis of medical neglect. When significant differences in philosophy of care and concerns about practice of care emerge or poor quality of communication persists, a substantial level of distrust may develop. The individual pediatrician may consider dismissal of families who refuse vaccination as an acceptable option. The physician must provide medical care for a reasonable period until a new physician can be secured, in accordance with local and state regulations.

The National Childhood Vaccine Injury Act (NCVIA) of 1986 included requirements for notifying *all* patients and parents about vaccine benefits and risks. Whether vaccines are purchased with private or public funds, this legislation mandates that a current vaccine information statement (VIS) be provided *each* time a vaccine covered under the National Vaccine Injury Compensation Program (VICP), established by the NCVIA, is administered (see Table 1.7, p 12). The VIS must be provided at the time of the immunization and for take-away, if desired. Copies of current VISs in English, Spanish, and other languages are available online from the CDC (**www.cdc.gov/vaccines/ hcp/vis/index.html**). In addition, the Immunization Action Coalition (**www.immunize.org**) includes the VIS documents as well as translations of many of the VIS into more than 40 languages. Every attempt should be made to provide a VIS in the patient or caregivers' native language. If the translated VIS version is older than the current VIS, it is acceptable to give the translated VIS even though it is not the most current. Online availability of the VIS provides the opportunity for the parent/legal guardian to review the information provided before the routine immunization visit, which might be preferred by parents.

The NCVIA requires that personnel administering VICP-covered vaccines, whether purchased with private or public funds, record in the patient's health record the information shown in Table 1.8, as well as confirmation that the relevant VIS was provided to the patient or parent/legal guardian at the time of each immunization. The AAP also recommends recording the site and route of administration and vaccine expiration date when administering any vaccine. Parents' or patients' signatures are not required by the federal NCVIA statute but may be required by state law to indicate that they have read and understood material in the VIS.

If vaccination is not administered according to the recommended immunization schedule because of refusal from the parent/legal guardian, a vaccine refusal waiver should be signed by the parent.

Table 1.7. Guidance in Using Vaccine Information Statements (VISs)[a]

Distribution:

Must be provided each time a VICP-covered vaccine is administered.[b]

Must be provided to and discussed with the patient (nonminor), parent, and/or legal representative.[b,c]

Must be the current version.[d]

Providers can add (not substitute) other written materials or audiovisual aids in addition to VISs.[e]

VICP indicates Vaccine Injury Compensation Program.

[a]VISs are available on the Centers for Disease Control and Prevention (CDC) Web site (**www.cdc.gov/vaccines/hcp/vis/index.html**).

[b]Required under the National Childhood Vaccine Injury Act.

[c]Definition of a consenting adolescent may vary by state.

[d]Required by CDC regulations for vaccines purchased through CDC contract. See the VIS Web site for current versions.

[e]An electronic version of the VIS can be transmitted to the patient's electronic device.

Table 1.8. Documentation Requirements Under the National Childhood Vaccine Injury Act

Document in the Patient's Health Record

Vaccine manufacturer, lot number, and date of administration[a]

Name, title, and business address of the health care professional administering the vaccine and date that the VIS is provided (and VIS publication date)[a]

Site (eg, deltoid area) and route (eg, intramuscular) of administration and expiration date of the vaccine[b]

[a]Required under the National Childhood Vaccine Injury Act.

[b]Recommended by the American Academy of Pediatrics and the Centers for Disease Control and Prevention (CDC).

ACTIVE IMMUNIZATION

Active immunization involves administration of all or part of a microorganism or a modified product of a microorganism (eg, a toxoid, a purified antigen, or an antigen produced by genetic engineering) to evoke an immunologic response and clinical protection that mimics that of natural infection but usually presents little or no risk to the recipient. Immunization can result in antitoxin, antiadherence, anti-invasive, or neutralizing activity or other types of protective humoral or cellular responses in the recipient. Some vaccines provide nearly complete and lifelong protection against disease, some provide protection against the more severe manifestations and/or consequences of the infection if exposed, and some must be readministered periodically to maintain protection. The immunologic response to vaccination is dependent on the type and dose of antigen, the effect of adjuvants, and host factors related to age, preexisting antibody, nutrition, concurrent disease, or genetics of the host. The effectiveness of a vaccine is assessed by evidence of protection against the natural disease. Induction of antibodies is an indirect measure of protection (eg, antitoxin against *Clostridium tetani* or neutralizing antibody against measles virus), but for some infectious diseases, an immunologic response that correlates with protection is understood poorly, and serum antibody concentration does not always predict protection.

Vaccines are categorized as live (viral or bacterial, which almost always are attenuated) or inactivated. The term "inactivated vaccines," for simplicity, includes antigens that are toxoids or other purified proteins, purified polysaccharides, protein-polysaccharide or oligosaccharide conjugates, inactivated whole or partially purified viruses, recombinant proteins, and proteins assembled into virus-like particles. Recommendations for vaccines routinely advised for immunocompetent and immunocompromised individuals are updated annually in the harmonized schedule developed by the AAP, Centers for Disease Control and Prevention (CDC), the American Academy of Family Physicians (AAFP), and the American College of Obstetricians and Gynecologists (ACOG) **(http://redbook.solutions.aap.org/SS/Immunization_Schedules.aspx),** and for simplicity are referred to as being "on the annual immunization schedule." Vaccines approved for use in the United States are listed in Table 1.9 (p 14). The US Food and Drug Administration (FDA) maintains and updates a Web site listing vaccines and all components approved for immunization and distribution in the United States with supporting documents **(www.fda.gov/BiologicsBloodVaccines/Vaccines/ApprovedProducts/ucm093833.htm).** Appendix II provides the codes for commonly administered pediatric vaccines and toxoids used for vaccine administration.

Among currently approved vaccines in the United States, there are 3 live attenuated bacterial vaccines (oral typhoid, oral cholera, and bacille Calmette-Guérin vaccines) and several live attenuated viral vaccines. Although active bacterial or viral replication ensues after administration of these vaccines, because the pathogen has been attenuated, few or no symptoms of illness occur. Sufficient antigenic characteristics of the virus or bacteria are retained during attenuation so that a protective immune response develops in the vaccine recipient.

Table 1.9. Vaccines Approved for Immunization and Distributed in the United States and Their Routes of Administration[a]

Vaccine	Type	Route of Administration
Adenovirus	Live viruses	Oral
Anthrax	Inactivated[b]	IM or SC
BCG	Live bacteria	ID (preferred) or SC
Cholera	Live attenuated bacteria	Oral
Diphtheria-tetanus (DT, Td)	Toxoids	IM
DTaP	Toxoids and inactivated bacterial components	IM
DTaP, hepatitis B, and IPV	Toxoids and inactivated bacterial components, recombinant viral antigen, inactivated virus	IM
DTaP-IPV	Toxoids and inactivated bacterial components, inactivated virus	IM
DTaP-IPV/Hib (PRP-T reconstituted with DTaP-IPV)	Toxoids and inactivated bacterial components, polysaccharide-protein conjugate, inactivated virus	IM
Hepatitis A (HepA)	Inactivated virus	IM
Hepatitis B (HepB)	Recombinant viral antigen	IM
Hepatitis A-hepatitis B	Inactivated virus and recombinant viral antigens	IM
Hib (*Haemophilus influenzae* type b) conjugate (tetanus toxoid)[c]	Bacterial polysaccharide-protein conjugate	IM
Hib conjugate (meningococcal protein conjugate)	Bacterial polysaccharide-protein conjugate	IM

Table 1.9. Vaccines Approved for Immunization and Distributed in the United States and Their Routes of Administration,[a] continued

Vaccine	Type	Route of Administration
Human papillomavirus (9vHPV)	Recombinant viral antigens	IM
Influenza (IIV)	Inactivated viral components	IM
Influenza (IIV)	Inactivated viral components	ID[d]
Influenza (LAIV)	Live attenuated viruses	Intranasal
Japanese encephalitis	Inactivated virus	IM
Meningococcal ACWY conjugate (MCV4 or MenACWY)	Bacterial polysaccharide-protein conjugate	IM
Meningococcal serogroup B (MenB)	Bacterial recombinant protein	IM
MMR	Live attenuated viruses	SC
MMRV	Live attenuated viruses	SC
Pneumococcal polysaccharide (PPSV23)	Bacterial polysaccharide	IM or SC
Pneumococcal conjugate (PCV13)	Bacterial polysaccharide-protein conjugate	IM
Poliovirus (IPV)	Inactivated viruses	SC or IM
Rabies	Inactivated virus	IM
Rotavirus (RV1 and RV5)	Live attenuated virus	Oral
Tdap	Toxoids and inactivated bacterial components	IM

Table 1.9. Vaccines Approved for Immunization and Distributed in the United States and Their Routes of Administration,[a] continued

Vaccine	Type	Route of Administration
Tetanus	Toxoid	IM
Typhoid	Bacterial capsular polysaccharide	IM
Typhoid	Live attenuated bacteria	Oral
Varicella (VAR)	Live attenuated virus	SC
Yellow Fever	Live attenuated virus	SC
Zoster (ZOS)	Live attenuated virus	SC
Zoster (HZ/su)	Recombinant viral antigens	IM

BCG indicates bacille Calmette-Guérin; ID, intradermal; SC, subcutaneous; DT, diphtheria and tetanus toxoids (for children younger than 7 years of age); Td, diphtheria and tetanus toxoids (for children 7 years of age or older and adults); IM, intramuscular; DTaP, diphtheria and tetanus toxoids and acellular pertussis, adsorbed; IPV, inactivated poliovirus; Hib, *Haemophilus influenzae* type b; PRP-T, polyribosylribitol phosphate-tetanus toxoid; HPV, human papillomavirus; MMR, live measles-mumps-rubella; MMRV, live measles-mumps-rubella-varicella (monovalent measles, mumps, and rubella components are not being produced in the United States); Tdap, tetanus toxoid, reduced diphtheria toxoid, and acellular pertussis.

[a] Other vaccines approved in the United States but not distributed include anthrax, smallpox, H5N1 influenza vaccines, influenza A (H1N1) monovalent 2009 vaccine, JE-virus vaccine (JE-VAX), pneumococcal conjugate vaccine (PCV7), and HepB-Hib (Comvax). The FDA maintains a Web site listing currently approved vaccines in the United States (**www.fda.gov/BiologicsBloodVaccines/Vaccines/ApprovedProducts/ucm093833.htm**). The AAP maintains a Web site (**http://aapredbook.aappublications.org/news/vaccstatus.dtl**) showing status of licensure and recommendations for newer vaccines.

[b] **http://pediatrics.aappublications.org/content/pediatrics/early/2014/04/22/peds.2014-0564.full.pdf**. Anthrax vaccine is not approved for use in children. Federal/state authorities would oversee emergency use under an investigational new drug application for children, should the need arise.

[c] See Table 3.13, p 372.

[d] Intradermal influenza vaccine is recommended only for persons 18 through 64 years of age.

Vaccines for some viruses (eg, hepatitis A, hepatitis B, human papillomavirus) and most bacteria are inactivated, component, subunit (purified components) preparations or inactivated toxins. Some vaccines contain purified bacterial polysaccharides conjugated chemically to immunobiologically active proteins (eg, tetanus toxoid, nontoxic variant of mutant diphtheria toxin, meningococcal outer membrane protein complex). Viruses and bacteria in inactivated, subunit, and conjugate vaccine preparations are not capable of replicating in the host; therefore, these vaccines must contain sufficient antigen content and possibly include an adjuvant to stimulate a desired response. In the case of conjugate polysaccharide vaccines, the linkage between the polysaccharide and the carrier protein enhances vaccine immunogenicity by converting the vaccine from a T-lymphocyte–independent antigen to a T-lymphocyte–dependent antigen. Maintenance of long-lasting immunity with inactivated viral or bacterial vaccines and toxoid vaccines may require periodic administration of booster doses. Although inactivated vaccines may not elicit the range of immunologic response provided by live attenuated agents, efficacy of approved inactivated vaccines in children is high. For example, an injected inactivated viral vaccine may evoke sufficient serum antibody or cell-mediated immunity but evoke only minimal mucosal antibody in the form of secretory immunoglobulin (Ig) A. Mucosal protection after administration of inactivated vaccines generally is inferior to mucosal immunity induced by live attenuated vaccines. Nonetheless, the demonstrated efficacy for such vaccines against invasive infection is high. Bacterial polysaccharide conjugate vaccines (eg, *Haemophilus influenzae* type b and pneumococcal conjugate vaccines) reduce nasopharyngeal colonization through exudated IgG. Viruses and bacteria in inactivated vaccines cannot replicate in or be excreted by the vaccine recipient as infectious agents and, thus, do not present the same safety concerns for immunosuppressed vaccine recipients or contacts of vaccine recipients as might live attenuated vaccines. However, only the oral poliovirus vaccine (OPV), which no longer is approved or recommended for use in the United States, is contraindicated for administration to someone living in the home of an immunosuppressed person.

Recommendations for dose, vaccine storage and handling (see Vaccine Handling and Storage, p 20), route and technique of administration (see Vaccine Administration, p 26), and immunization schedules should be followed for predictable, effective immunization (also see disease-specific chapters in Section 3). Adherence to recommended guidance is critical to the success of immunization practices at both the individual and the societal levels.

Vaccine Ingredients

A vaccine's principal constituents are listed in its package insert. As part of the licensure process, the FDA considers all of a vaccine's ingredients—the antigen/immunogen as well as vaccine additives that have specific purposes (eg, stabilizers that protect the vaccine's integrity, preservatives that prevent the growth of bacteria or fungi, and residual components from the manufacturing process) (**www.cdc.gov/vaccines/pubs/pinkbook/downloads/appendices/B/excipient-table-2.pdf**).

ACTIVE IMMUNIZING ANTIGENS/IMMUNOGENS

Some vaccines consist of a single antigen that is a highly defined constituent (eg, tetanus or diphtheria toxoid). Other vaccines consist of multiple antigens, which vary substantially in chemical composition, structure, and number (eg, acellular pertussis components, pneumococcal and meningococcal polysaccharide protein conjugate vaccines [PCV, MCV], serogroup B meningococcal recombinant vaccine [MenB], and pneumococcal polysaccharide vaccine [PPSV]). Other vaccines contain live attenuated viruses (eg, measles-mumps-rubella [MMR], measles-mumps-rubella-varicella [MMRV], varicella [VAR], oral poliovirus vaccine [OPV], live attenuated influenza vaccine [LAIV], oral rotavirus vaccine [RV]), killed viruses or portions of virus (eg, enhanced inactivated poliovirus [IPV], hepatitis A, and inactivated influenza vaccines), or recombinant viral proteins (eg, hepatitis B vaccine, human papillomavirus [HPV] vaccine, and recombinant influenza vaccine.

CONJUGATING AGENTS

Vaccines based solely on bacterial polysaccharides have limited immunogenicity in children younger than 18 months and fail to induce immunologic memory. To overcome these limitations and to facilitate polysaccharide processing by antigen-presenting cells, vaccine antigens for some vaccines (*Haemophilus influenzae* type b [Hib], pneumococcal, and meningococcal vaccines) are chemically conjugated to a protein carrier with proven immunologic potential (eg, tetanus toxoid, nontoxic variant of diphtheria toxin, meningococcal outer membrane protein complex) to improve the immune response.

NONANTIGENIC VACCINE COMPONENTS

Some substances may be included in a vaccine for a specific purpose, including preservatives and stabilizers. Allergic reactions may occur if the recipient is sensitive to one or more of these additives. Whenever feasible, these reactions should be anticipated by a careful screening for a known allergy to specific vaccine components. Porcine gelatin, a stabilizing agent used in several vaccines, is the additive most likely to induce an allergic reaction. Standardized screening checklists are available to assist clinicians in screening for allergies and other potential contraindications to immunization (**www.immunize.org/catg.d/p4060.pdf**).

ADJUVANTS. From the Latin word for "to help," adjuvants are materials that are included in a vaccine to improve the immune response to the antigen. Aluminum salts, the most commonly used adjuvants, have been used in vaccines for more than 80 years and often are used in vaccines containing inactivated microorganisms, subunits, or toxoids (eg, hepatitis B vaccine [HepB] and diphtheria and tetanus toxoids). Despite the well-known clinical effect of adjuvants, their mechanism of action of stimulating an immune response via cytokine release was demonstrated only recently. New adjuvants include molecules that stimulate innate immune responses to enhance the immunogenicity of vaccine antigens—for example, deacylated monophosphoryl lipid A plus aluminum hydroxide (ASO4), as used in the bivalent HPV vaccine; oil-in-water emulsions (MF59, as used in Fluad influenza vaccine [Seqirus Inc, Holly Springs, NC]; and ASO3, which is used in Q-Pan, an approved pandemic influenza vaccine [GlaxoSmithKline, Research Triangle Park, NC]). In addition to improving both the magnitude and the breadth of the immune response to antigens, adjuvants also can have the benefit of "antigen sparing," in which a reduced dose of antigen can stimulate an equivalent immune response and thereby permit availability of more vaccine doses when vast numbers of people require immunization and there might otherwise be a vaccine shortage (eg, pandemic influenza).

PRESERVATIVES. Preservatives are included in multidose vials as a safety feature to prevent the growth of bacteria or fungi that may be introduced into the vaccine following repeated penetrations of a vial to withdraw a dose. In some cases, these compounds are used during the vaccine manufacturing process to inhibit microbial growth, which can leave trace amounts in the final product.

Thimerosal, an ethyl mercury-containing organic compound, is an organomercurial that has been widely used as a preservative in a number of biological and drug products, including many vaccines, since the 1930s to help prevent potentially life-threatening contamination. All routinely recommended vaccines for infants and children in the United States are available as single-dose, preservative-free (eg, thimerosal-free) formulations or contain only trace amounts of thimerosal. Inactivated influenza vaccines for pediatric use are available as thimerosal-free formulation, trace thimerosal-containing formulation, and thimerosal preservative-containing formulation. Information about the thimerosal content of vaccines is available from the FDA (**www.fda.gov/cber/vaccine/thimerosal.htm**). Thimerosal has been studied extensively and is associated with only rare, mild allergic reactions or other adverse events.

Independent safety reviews by the Institute of Medicine (now called the National Academy of Medicine, or NAM) regarding thimerosal-containing vaccines as well as vaccines and autism (**www.nap.edu/catalog/10997/immunization-safety-review-vaccines-and-autism?onpi_newsdoc05182004=**) support the safety of thimerosal in vaccines. It is clear that the use of thimerosal in vaccines does not put vaccine recipients at increased risk of neurodevelopmental problems. The AAP also extended its strongest support for the recommendations of the World Health Organization's Strategic Advisory Group of Experts on immunization to retain the use of thimerosal in the global vaccine supply (**www.who.int/wer/2012/wer8721.pdf**). More information on thimerosal in vaccines is available (**www.fda.gov/BiologicsBloodVaccines/Vaccines/QuestionsaboutVaccines/ucm070430.htm** and **www.cdc.gov/vaccinesafety/Concerns/thimerosal/index.html**).

STABILIZERS. Stabilizers are added to vaccines to ensure that their potency is not affected by adverse conditions during the manufacturing process (eg, freeze drying) or during transport and storage. Stabilizers commonly included in vaccines for this purpose include sugars (sucrose or lactose), amino acids (eg, glycine), or proteins (eg, gelatin).

OTHER INGREDIENTS

Although steps in the manufacturing process are designed to remove nonessential constituents (formaldehyde, glutaraldehyde, antibiotics, and bacterial or cell culture components), small residual amounts may remain in the final product. Such ingredients are noted in the package label.

SUSPENDING FLUID

Sterile water for injection or saline solution are used commonly as a vaccine vehicle or suspending fluid. Some vaccine products use more complex suspending fluids, such as tissue-culture fluid, which may contain proteins or other constituents derived from the growth medium or from the biological system in which the vaccine was produced (eg, egg antigens, gelatin, or cell culture-derived antigens). These are also considered in the licensing process; therefore, for suspension of vaccines supplied in lyophilized form, it is important to use only the diluents supplied by the manufacturer of each vaccine.

ANTIMICROBIAL AGENTS

Certain vaccines contain trace amounts of neomycin, polymyxin B, or streptomycin. Penicillins, cephalosporins, and fluoroquinolones are not present in vaccines.

Vaccine Handling and Storage

For vaccines to be optimally effective, they must be stored properly from the time of manufacturing until they are administered. Immunization providers are responsible for proper storage and handling from the time the vaccine arrives at their facility until the vaccine is administered. All staff should be knowledgeable about the importance of proper storage and handling of vaccines and the implications of improper storage and handling. The administration of improperly stored and handled vaccines is a frequent error reported to the Vaccine Adverse Event Reporting System (VAERS) (see Vaccine Safety, p 41) and can cause disruption in practices and anxiety for parents whose children may receive such vaccines and are uncertain of their effectiveness and/or safety.

A written vaccine-specific storage and handling plan should be available for reference by all staff members and kept on or near the unit used for storing vaccines. This plan should be updated annually. It should detail both routine management of vaccines and emergency measures for vaccine retrieval and storage and for standard operating procedures for documenting these activities.

Most vaccines are designated for optimal storage between 2°C and 8°C (36°F and 46°F), and such vaccines are referred to as "refrigerated vaccines." Of vaccines routinely used in pediatric offices, only those containing varicella virus are required to be stored frozen between −50°C and −15C° (−58°F and +5°F). These are referred to as "freezer vaccines." There is only 1 vaccine, MMR, that can be stored in either location with a safe temperature range between −50°C and 8°C (−58°F and +46°F).

It is imperative that great care be taken to avoid exposing "refrigerated vaccines" to freezing temperatures, even for brief periods. Such exposure can compromise the integrity of refrigerated vaccines even without generating ice crystals or other changes in physical appearance of the vaccine. Visual inspection cannot reliably detect a vaccine that has been compromised by freeze exposure; thus, only careful monitoring of the temperatures used to store these vaccines will allow identification of potentially altered vaccines. It is recommended that refrigerators be set to maintain approximately 5°C (40°F) for storage of these vaccines.

"Refrigerated vaccines" may tolerate limited exposure to elevated temperatures, but care should be taken to maintain storage temperatures within the approved safe storage temperature ranges.

Vaccines exposed to temperatures outside their approved storage ranges should be segregated in a bag or container that is kept in an environment safe for storing these vaccines. They should not be used until specifics of the temperature excursion are reviewed. Protocols after the event vary depending on individual state or agency policies. Providers should contact their state immunization program, vaccine manufacturer, or both for guidance. Advice regarding disposition of improperly handled or stored vaccines should be documented. Vaccines stored outside the recommended temperature range should not be administered unless guidance from the state immunization program and/or the vaccine manufacturer indicates the vaccine can be used.

Some vaccines, including HPV and MMR, must be protected from light exposure of more than 30 minutes. Protection from light exposure can be accomplished by keeping each vial or syringe in its original carton while in recommended storage and until immediate use. Contact phone numbers of the manufacturers are available online (**www.cdc.gov/vaccines/hcp/admin/storage/downloads/manufact-dist-contact.pdf**) as well as in the package inserts and the annual *Physicians' Desk Reference*.

Recommendations for handling and storage of vaccines are summarized in the package insert for each product (**www.immunize.org/fda**). The most accurate information about recommended vaccine storage conditions, handling instructions, and usability for specific temperature excursions must be obtained directly from manufacturers. The following guidance is suggested as part of a quality-control system for safe handling and storage of vaccines in an office or clinic setting. The CDC Vaccine Storage and Handling toolkit is a useful resource for providers (**www.cdc.gov/vaccines/hcp/admin/storage/toolkit/storage-handling-toolkit.pdf**).

PERSONNEL

A primary staff vaccine coordinator and an alternate vaccine coordinator should be trained and responsible for vaccine storage and handling. In addition, a physician or manager with understanding of the importance of appropriate vaccine storage should be engaged with the responsible vaccine coordinating staff. The CDC offers online training on vaccine storage and handling, and information can be found at **www2a.cdc.gov/nip/isd/ycts/mod1/courses/sh/ce.asp.** The vaccine coordinator should be responsible for:

- Ordering vaccines.
- Overseeing proper receipt and storage of shipments.
- Creating and maintaining a vaccine log book.
- Organizing vaccines in storage units.
- Temperature monitoring of storage units at least twice daily and, if using a data logger, monitoring of minimum and maximum temperatures daily, preferably in the morning.
- Recording temperature readings on a log.
- Daily physical inspection of the storage unit.
- Rotating stock so that vaccines closest to expiration date are used first.
- Contacting the state Vaccines for Children (VFC) program vaccine coordinator if it appears that VFC vaccines will expire before they will be used in the practice.
- Monitoring expiration dates and ensuring expired vaccines are removed from the refrigerator/freezer.
- Responding to potential storage temperature excursions and calling the manufacturer, VFC program, or both to obtain guidance for temperature excursion events.
- Overseeing proper vaccine transport, either routine or in an emergency.
- Maintaining all appropriate vaccine storage and handling documentation, including temperature excursion responses.
- Maintaining storage equipment and records, including VFC program documentation.

- Informing all people who will be handling vaccines about specific storage requirements and stability limitations of the products they will encounter. The details of proper storage conditions should be posted on or near each refrigerator or freezer used for vaccine storage or should be readily available to staff. Receptionists, mail clerks, and other staff members who also may receive shipments should be educated in these matters as well.

EQUIPMENT

- Ensure that refrigerators and freezers in which vaccines are to be stored are working properly and are capable of meeting storage requirements.
- Do not connect refrigerators or freezers to a computer uninterrupted power supply or an outlet controlled by a ground fault circuit interrupter or one activated by a wall switch. Use plug guards and warning signs to prevent accidental dislodging of the wall plug. Post "**Do Not Unplug**" warning signs on circuit breakers.
- Store vaccines in refrigerator and freezer units that can maintain the appropriate temperature range and are large enough to maintain the largest anticipated inventory without crowding, along with temperature-buffering water bottles. Stand-alone units are recommended; these are self-contained units that only refrigerate or only freeze and are suitable for vaccine storage. For refrigerated vaccine storage, medical-grade units with an electronic thermostat and digital display are preferred. Household combination refrigerator/freezer units with separate exterior doors and separate thermostats are considered acceptable by the CDC at this time to store refrigerated vaccines only, with careful monitoring and certain cautionary notes. The risk of freeze damage to refrigerated vaccines is increased greatly in combination refrigerator/freezer units. By design, super cold air from the freezer is circulated in the refrigerator to cool that space. This subfreezing air can freeze temperature-sensitive vaccines. In addition, the freezer portion of many combination units is insufficiently cold to store freezer vaccines and, thus, is not permitted for storage of vaccines covered by the VFC program. A separate stand-alone freezer should be used to store freezer vaccines. Use of dormitory or bar-style refrigerator/freezer units with 1 exterior door is not recommended for any vaccine storage and is not allowed for vaccine storage of VFC program products.
- Use refrigerators with wire—not glass—shelving to improve air circulation in the unit. Do not use the top shelf of domestic combination refrigerator-freezer units for vaccine storage. Do not use the refrigerator door for vaccine storage. To improve air circulation, place vaccine storage trays used to separate different vaccines away from the walls and rear of the refrigerator. The CDC recommends that each vaccine storage unit should be monitored by a digital data logger with accuracy of +/− 0.5°C (1°F). The temperature monitoring device should be capable of continuous frequent measurements (with a detachable probe in a temperature buffer [eg, biosafe glycol, glass beads, sand, Teflon]), should display daily maximum and minimum temperatures, and should be readable without opening the unit door. The buffered probes should be located near the vaccines, away from the walls, vents, and floor of the vaccine storage unit. Temperature data should be displayed graphically and should be able to be stored for 3 years. The graphic data should be reviewed and corrective efforts documented if daily maximum and minimum values are found to be

outside of acceptable ranges.

- Use a temperature-monitoring device with a Certificate of Calibration Testing (also known as Report of Calibration). Such temperature-monitoring devices have been individually tested for accuracy against a recognized reference standard by a laboratory with accreditation from an International Laboratory Accreditation Cooperation (ILAC) Mutual Recognition Arrangement (MRA) signatory body or by a laboratory or manufacturer with documentation that calibration testing performed meets ISO/IEC 17025 international standards for calibration testing and traceability. These devices are sold with an individually numbered certificate documenting this testing. Old certified glass thermometers should be replaced by calibrated data-logging devices with a detachable probe that is kept in a bottle filled with a buffering material. This type of probe can provide a more accurate reading of actual vaccine temperature than one that measures air temperature. Providers who receive VFC vaccines or other vaccines purchased with public funds should consult their immunization program regarding the required methods and timeframe for temperature monitoring device calibration testing. The National Institute of Standards and Technology maintains a Web site devoted to vaccine storage education (**www.nist.gov/pml/div685/ grp01/vaccines.cfm**). Calibration testing and traceability must be performed every 1 to 2 years from the last calibration testing date (date certificate issued) or using suggested calibration timelines from the manufacturer of the device. Temperature accuracy of temperature monitoring devices can be checked using an ice melting point test (**www.nist.gov/pml/div685/grp01/upload/Ice-Melting-Point- Validation-Method-for-Data-Loggers.pdf**). Providers should check with their state VFC program for specific requirements related to calibration testing of temperature-monitoring devices.

PROCEDURES

- Maintain a vaccine log, which should include vaccine name, number of doses, arrival condition of the vaccine, manufacturer and lot numbers, and expiration date.
- Formally accept vaccine on receipt of shipment:
  - ◆ Ensure that the expiration date of the delivered product has not passed.
  - ◆ Examine the merchandise and its shipping container for any evidence of damage during transport.
  - ◆ Consider whether the interval between shipment from the supplier and arrival of the product at its destination is excessive (more than 48 hours) and whether the product has been exposed to excessive heat or cold that might alter its integrity. Review vaccine time and temperature indicators, both chemical and electronic, if included in the vaccine shipment.
  - ◆ Find and inspect any temperature excursion devices (electronic or temperature-tape) found in the shipment for evidence of temperature excursions. Do not accept the shipment if reasonable suspicion exists that the delivered product may have been damaged by environmental insult or improper handling during transport.
    - – For VFC providers, do not refuse any vaccine shipments. If the provider believes that a vaccine shipment is compromised or there is a problem with the temperature monitors, the provider must contact the McKesson Specialty Contact Center immediately using the telephone number dedicated to receiving

provider calls about vaccine usability: 1-877-TEMP123).

- ◆ Contact the vaccine supplier or manufacturer when unusual circumstances raise questions about the stability of a delivered vaccine. Store suspect vaccine under proper conditions and label it "**Do Not Use**" until the usability has been determined.
- Inspect the refrigerator and freezer:
  - ◆ If using a combination refrigerator-freezer, determine the placement of the cold air vents and do not put vaccines on the top shelf or near the vents. Measure the temperature of the central part of the storage compartment twice a day, and record this temperature on a temperature log. A minimum-maximum temperature-monitoring device in a thermal buffer is preferred to record extremes in temperature fluctuation and reset to baseline daily. Consider use of an alarm system capable of phone/text message/e-mail notification if there is equipment failure, power outage, or temperature excursion. The refrigerator temperature should be maintained between 2°C and 8°C (36°F and 46°F), with a target temperature of approximately 5°C (40°F), and the freezer temperature should be −15°C (5°F) or colder. A "**Do Not Unplug**" sign should be affixed directly next to the refrigerator electrical outlet and to the circuit breaker controlling that circuit.
- Train and designate staff to respond immediately to temperature recordings outside the recommended range and to document response and outcome.
  - ◆ Inspect the unit weekly for outdated vaccine and either dispose of or return expired products appropriately.
- Establish routine procedures:
  - ◆ Store vaccine where temperature remains constant.
  - ◆ Store vaccines according to temperatures specified in the package insert.
  - ◆ Rotate vaccine supplies so that the shortest-dated vaccines are in front to reduce wastage because of expiration.
  - ◆ Promptly remove expired (outdated) vaccines from the refrigerator or freezer and dispose of them appropriately or return to manufacturer to avoid accidental use.
  - ◆ Store both opened and unopened vials in the original packaging, which facilitates temperature stability, inventory management, and rotation of vaccine by expiration date and avoids light exposure. Mark the outside of boxes of opened vaccines with a large "X" to indicate that it has been opened.
  - ◆ Keep opened vials of vaccine in a tray so that they are readily identifiable.
  - ◆ Indicate on the label of each vaccine vial the date and time the vaccine was reconstituted or first opened.
  - ◆ Unless immediate use is planned, avoid reconstituting multiple doses of vaccine or drawing up multiple doses of vaccine in multiple syringes. Predrawing vaccine increases the possibility of medication errors and causes uncertainty of vaccine stability.
  - ◆ Because different vaccines can share similar components/names (eg, diphtheria and tetanus and acellular pertussis vaccines [DTaP and Tdap] or meningococcal conjugate vaccine [MCV4] and serogroup B meningococcal recombinant vaccine [MenB]), care should be taken during storage to ensure that the different products are stored separately in a manner to avoid confusion and possible medication errors.

◆ Each vaccine and diluent vial should be inspected carefully for damage or contamination prior to use. The expiration date printed on the vial or box should be checked. Vaccine can be used through the last day of the month indicated by the expiration date unless otherwise stated on the package labeling. The expiration date or time for some vaccines changes once the vaccine vial is opened or the vaccine is reconstituted. This information is available in the product package insert. Regardless of expiration date, vaccine and diluent should only be used as long as they are normal in appearance and have been stored and handled properly. Expired vaccine or diluent should never be used.

◆ Discard reconstituted live-virus and other vaccines if not used within the time interval specified in the package insert. Examples of discard times following reconstitution include a varicella-containing vaccine after 30 minutes and MMR vaccine after 8 hours. All reconstituted vaccines should be refrigerated during the interval in which they may be used.

◆ Always store vaccines in the refrigerator or freezer as indicated until immediately prior to delivery. Do not open more than 1 vial of a specific vaccine at a time.

◆ Do not keep food or drink in refrigerators in which vaccine is stored; this will limit frequent opening of the unit that leads to thermal instability.

◆ Do not store radioactive materials in the same refrigerator in which vaccines are stored.

◆ Discuss with all clinic or office personnel any violation of protocol for handling vaccines or any accidental temperature excursion. Segregate the affected vaccine to avoid use until the vaccine manufacturers can be contacted to determine the disposition of the affected vaccine.

SUMMARY

To summarize, best equipment and practices for storage of refrigerated vaccines are as follows:

1. Medical refrigerator with electronic thermostat and an external digital display, set to approximately 5°C (40°F).
2. Wire shelving and an interior circulating fan.
3. One or more data-logging certified continuous temperature monitoring devices with a detachable or wireless probe in a thermal buffer located near the vaccine.
4. Displays with current temperature and resettable maximum and minimum temperatures visible on the outside of the unit.
5. Audible temperature alarm with capability for rapid user notification via phone/text message/e-mail should temperature excursion be detected.
6. Extra space in the unit should be filled with water bottles to serve as a cold mass and to prolong safe storage in the event of refrigerator failure. (Providers should check with manufacturer's guidance, because this may not be necessary for some medical-grade units.)

EMERGENCY VACCINE RETRIEVAL AND STORAGE

Practices should develop a written plan for emergency storage of vaccine in the event of a catastrophic event, train personnel, and make the plan easily accessible. Refrigerators can maintain their 2°C to 8°C temperature for only 2 to 3 hours without power. Refrigerated vaccines should be transported in thick insulated coolers using conditioned frozen water bottles for coolant. A certified digital data logging thermometer should accompany each container of vaccine until appropriate storage facilities are reached. Special care must be taken to avoid freezing refrigerated vaccine either by transport coolant or by environment (as in the winter). Portable powered refrigerators greatly increase the risk of exposing vaccine to freezing temperatures and should be avoided. Frozen vaccine is difficult to transport at under −15°C. Appropriate passive cooling can be achieved by use of specialized phase change material packs rated at −23°C that are on site and maintained frozen for emergency transportation. These packs in a thick-walled cooler will maintain <15°C for transport of less than a few hours. A portable freezer prechilled and known to maintain temperatures of under −15°C is a good option. Vaccine always should be transported with a certified digital data logging thermometer that is reviewed once safe storage has been reached. Frozen water bottles and gel packs are unable to chill a transport container to −15°C and should not be used. If no other choice is available, vaccine should be transported with a data logger and quarantined until the data can be reviewed with appropriate authorities.

After a power outage or mechanical failure, it should not be assumed that vaccine exposed to temperature outside the recommended range is unusable without first contacting the vaccine manufacturer (or, for VFC vaccines, the McKesson Specialty Contact Center at 1-877-TEMP123) for guidance before discarding vaccine. Guidance on vaccine transport is available from the AAP (**www.aap.org/en-us/advocacy-and-policy/aap-health-initiatives/immunization/Pages/vaccine-storage-and-handling-guidance.aspx**) and the CDC (**www.cdc.gov/vaccines/hcp/admin/storage/toolkit/index.html**).

Vaccine Administration

GENERAL CONSIDERATIONS FOR VACCINE ADMINISTRATION

Proper vaccine administration is a critical component of a successful immunization program to ensure that vaccination is as safe and effective as possible. Health care personnel who administer vaccines should be knowledgeable regarding proper vaccine administration, including vaccine preparation and administration techniques.

STAFF TRAINING AND EDUCATION. Competency-based training should be integrated into existing staff education programs such as new staff orientation and annual education requirements.

INFECTION CONTROL. Personnel administering vaccines should take appropriate precautions to minimize risk of spread of disease to or from patients. Hand hygiene should be used before preparing and administering vaccines as well as before and after each new patient contact. Gloves are not required when administering vaccines unless the health care professional has open hand lesions or will come into contact with potentially infectious body fluids. If gloves are worn, they should be changed between patients.

Syringes and needles must be sterile and disposable. To prevent inadvertent needlesticks or reuse, a needle should **not** be recapped after use, and disposable needles and syringes should be discarded promptly in puncture-proof, labeled containers located in the room where the vaccine is administered.

VACCINE PREPARATION. Only vaccines that have been stored and handled correctly should be administered. Vaccines should be prepared just prior to administration using aseptic technique. A separate needle and syringe should be used for each injection. If the vaccine requires reconstitution, the diluent supplied by the manufacturer should be used. Each vaccine and diluent vial should be inspected carefully for damage or contamination prior to use. The expiration date printed on the vial or box should be checked. Expired vaccine or diluent should not be administered. Some vaccines in multidose vials should be used within a certain time frame after the vial is first entered, referred to as the beyond use date. If present, vaccines should not be used after the beyond use date. Information regarding a beyond use date (if applicable) can be found in the approved product information. Different vaccines should not be mixed in the same syringe unless specifically approved and labeled for such use. Changing needles between drawing a vaccine into a syringe and injecting the child is not necessary.

PATIENT CARE BEFORE, DURING, AND AFTER VACCINE ADMINISTRATION. A patient should be restrained adequately, if indicated, before any injection (see Managing Injection Pain, p 30). Information about positioning, comfort restraint, and comfort care is available (**www.cdc.gov/vaccines/parents/tools/holds-factsheet.pdf** and **http://eziz.org/assets/docs/IMM-686ES.pdf**).

Because of the rare possibility of a severe allergic reaction to a vaccine component, people administering vaccines or other biologic products should be prepared to recognize and treat allergic reactions, including anaphylaxis (see Hypersensitivity Reactions After Immunization, p 52). Personnel and equipment should be available for treating immediate allergic reactions. This recommendation does not preclude administration of vaccines in school-based or other nonclinic settings.

Syncope can occur following any immunization, particularly in adolescents and young adults. Personnel should be aware of presyncopal manifestations and take appropriate measures to prevent injuries if weakness, dizziness, or loss of consciousness occurs. However, syncope can occur without any presyncopal symptoms. The relatively rapid onset of syncope in most cases suggests that health care personnel should consider observing adolescents for 15 minutes after they are immunized. Adolescents should be seated or lying down during vaccination, and having vaccine recipients *sit or lie down for at least 15 minutes* after immunization could avert many syncopal episodes and secondary injuries. If syncope develops, the patient should be observed until symptoms resolve.[1] Syncope following receipt of a vaccine is not a contraindication to subsequent doses of that or other vaccines.

SITE AND ROUTE OF IMMUNIZATION (ACTIVE AND PASSIVE)

ORAL VACCINES. Rotavirus vaccines (RV1 [Rotarix], RV5 [RotaTeq], both liquid formulations) and oral typhoid vaccine (TY21a [Vivotif], a capsule formulation) are the only FDA-approved vaccines for children that are administered by the oral route. Oral vaccines generally should be administered prior to administering injections or performing other procedures that might cause discomfort. The liquid RV1 and RV5 vaccines should

---

[1]Centers for Disease Control and Prevention. Syncope after vaccination—United States, January 2005–July 2007. *MMWR Morb Mortal Wkly Rep.* 2008;57(17):457–460

be administered slowly down one side of the inside of the cheek (between the cheek and gum) toward the back of the infant's mouth, but not so far as to initiate the gag reflex. Never administer or spray (squirt) the vaccine directly into the throat. Detailed information on oral delivery of these vaccines is included in FDA-approved prescribing information. Breastfeeding does not appear to diminish response to rotavirus vaccines. If a dose of rotavirus vaccine is regurgitated, spit out, or vomited during or after administration of vaccine, the dose should not be readministered. No data exist on the benefits or risks of repeating the dose. The infant should receive the remaining recommended doses of rotavirus vaccine following the routine schedule (with a 4-week minimum interval between doses).

INTRANASAL VACCINE. Live attenuated influenza vaccine is the only vaccine currently approved for intranasal administration. This vaccine is approved for healthy, nonpregnant people 2 through 49 years of age. The vaccine dose (0.2 mL) is inside a special sprayer device. A plastic clip on the plunger divides the dose into 2 equal parts. With the recipient in the upright position, approximately 0.1 mL (ie, half of the total sprayer contents) is sprayed into 1 nostril. An attached dose-divider clip is removed from the sprayer to administer the second half of the dose into the other nostril. If the recipient sneezes after administration, the dose should not be repeated. The vaccine can be administered during minor illnesses. However, if clinical judgment indicates that nasal congestion might impede delivery of the vaccine to the nasopharyngeal mucosa, consider administering injectable influenza vaccine if the patient is eligible, or deferral can be considered until resolution of the illness. For the 2016–2017 and 2017–2018 influenza seasons, LAIV was not recommended for use in any population because of issues with vaccine effectiveness. For current recommendations on use of LAIV, please refer to the current AAP influenza policy statement, which is updated annually and published in August or September each year.[1]

PARENTERAL VACCINES.[2] Injectable vaccines should be administered using aseptic technique at a site as free as possible from risk of local neural, vascular, or tissue injury. Approved routes of administration are included in package inserts of vaccines and are listed in Table 1.9 (p 14). The approved route for a particular vaccine is based on clinical studies of safety and effectiveness. To minimize untoward local or systemic effects and to ensure optimal efficacy of the immunizing procedure, vaccines should be administered by the approved route. For intramuscular (IM) injections, the choice of site (thigh or arm) depends on the age of the vaccine recipient, the degree of muscle development, and the thickness of adipose tissue at the injection site. In children younger than 2 years, the anterolateral aspect of the upper thigh provides the largest muscle and is the preferred site. In older children, the deltoid muscle usually is large enough for IM injection. A 22- to 25-gauge needle is recommended for IM injections. Decisions on needle length must be made for each person on the basis of the size of the muscle and the thickness of adipose tissue at the injection site. Suggested needle lengths are shown in Table 1.10

---

[1] American Academy of Pediatrics, Committee on Infectious Diseases. Recommendations for prevention and control of influenza in children, 2017–2018. *Pediatrics*. 2017; 140(4):e20172550

[2] For a review on intramuscular injections, see Centers for Disease Control and Prevention. *Epidemiology and Prevention of Vaccine-Preventable Diseases (Pink Book)*. Atlanta, GA: Centers for Disease Control and Prevention; 2015 (**www.cdc.gov/vaccines/pubs/pinkbook/index.html**). For hard copies, contact the Public Health Foundation at 877-252-1200.

Table 1.10. Site and Needle Length by Age for Intramuscular Immunization

Age Group	Needle Length, inches (mm)[a]	Suggested Injection Site
Newborns (preterm and term) and infants <1 mo of age	⅝–1 (16–25 mm)[b]	Anterolateral thigh muscle
Term infants, 1–12 mo of age	⅝–1 (16–25 mm)	Anterolateral thigh muscle
Toddlers and children	⅝–1 (16–25 mm)[b]	Deltoid muscle of the arm
	1–1¼ (25–32 mm)[c]	Anterolateral thigh muscle
Adults		
Female and male, weight <130 lb	⅝–1 (25 mm)[d]	Deltoid muscle of the arm
Female and male, weight 130–152 lb	1 (25 mm)	Deltoid muscle of the arm
Female, weight 153–200 lb	1–1½ (25–38 mm)	Deltoid muscle of the arm
Male, weight 153–260 lb	1–1½ (25–38 mm)	Deltoid muscle of the arm
Female, weight >200 lb	1½ (38 mm)	Deltoid muscle of the arm
Male, weight >260 lb	1½ (38 mm)	Deltoid muscle of the arm

[a]Assumes that needle is inserted fully.
[b]If the skin is stretched tightly and subcutaneous tissues are not bunched.
[c]1½ in (38 mm) needle is an option when administering vaccine in the anterolateral thigh to children 11–18 years of age.
[d]Some experts recommend a ⅝-inch needle for men and women who weigh less than 130 lb.

(p 29). Needles should be long enough to reach the muscle mass and prevent vaccine from seeping into subcutaneous tissue and causing local reactions, yet not so long as to reach underlying nerves, blood vessels, or bone.

Ordinarily, the upper, outer aspect of the buttocks should not be used for active immunization, because the gluteal region is covered by a significant layer of subcutaneous fat. Because of diminished immunogenicity, hepatitis B and rabies vaccines should not be administered in the buttocks at any age.

In general, vaccines containing adjuvants (eg, aluminum present in certain vaccines recommended for IM injection) must be injected deep into the muscle mass. These vaccines should not be administered subcutaneously or intracutaneously, because they can cause local irritation, inflammation, granuloma formation, and tissue necrosis. Adjuvanted vaccines licensed for subcutaneous injection, such as anthrax vaccine adsorbed (AVA), may be given as recommended (see Anthrax, p 214).

Serious complications resulting from IM injections are rare. Reported adverse events include broken needles, muscle contracture, nerve injury, bacterial (eg, staphylococcal, streptococcal, or clostridial) abscesses, sterile abscesses, skin pigmentation changes, hemorrhage, cellulitis, tissue necrosis, gangrene, local atrophy, periostitis, cyst or scar formation, inadvertent injection into a joint space, and shoulder injury related to vaccine administration (SIRVA).

For patients with a known bleeding disorder or people receiving anticoagulant therapy, bleeding complications following IM immunization can occur. The patient or family should be instructed about the risk of hematoma formation from the injection. A finer needle (23-gauge or smaller bore needle and of appropriate length for IM administration) should be used for those patients. Apply firm pressure at the injection site for at least 2 minutes. The site should not be rubbed or massaged. If the patient receives antihemophilia or similar therapy periodically, IM vaccines should be scheduled shortly after such therapy is administered.

Subcutaneous injections should be administered at a 45° angle into the subcutaneous tissue above the muscle of the anterolateral aspect of the thigh or the upper outer triceps area by inserting the needle in a pinched-up fold of skin and subcutaneous tissue. A 23- to 25-gauge needle of ⅝ inch length is recommended. Immune responses after subcutaneous administration of hepatitis B or recombinant rabies vaccine are decreased compared with those after IM administration of either of these vaccines; therefore, these vaccines should not be administered subcutaneously.

No intradermal vaccine is approved for use in people younger than 18 years of age because they may not have sufficient skin thickness for intradermal administration. One manufacturer's intradermal inactivated influenza vaccine is approved for adults 18 through 64 years of age.

When multiple vaccines are administered, separate sites should be used. When necessary, 2 or more vaccines can be administered in the same limb at a single visit. For infants and young children, the anterolateral aspect of the thigh is the preferred site for multiple IM injections because of its greater muscle mass. For older children and adolescents, the deltoid muscle may be used for more than one intramuscular injection. The injections should be separated by at least 1 inch, if possible, so that local reactions can be differentiated if they should develop. Multiple vaccines should not be mixed in a single syringe. A new, sterile needle and syringe should be used for each injection.

Aspiration (ie, pulling back on the syringe plunger after needle insertion, before injection) is not recommended, because no large blood vessels are located at the preferred injection sites and because the process of aspiration has been demonstrated to increase pain (see Managing Injection Pain, p 30).

A brief period of bleeding at the injection site is common and usually can be controlled by applying gentle pressure.

Additional information on vaccine administration and safe injection practices is available on the CDC Web site (**cdc.gov/vaccines/recs/vac-admin/default.htm** and **www.cdc.gov/injectionsafety/providers.html**).

Managing Injection Pain

A planned approach to decreasing the child's anxiety before, during, and after immunization and to decreasing pain from the injection is helpful for children of any age.[1] The Canadian Medical Association has updated its clinical practice guideline for Canadian physicians and families,[2] and guidance from the World Health Organization

---

[1]Schechter NL, Zempsky WT, Cohen LL, McGrath PJ, McMurtry CM, Bright NS. Pain reduction during pediatric immunizations: evidence-based review and recommendations. *Pediatrics.* 2007;119(5):e1184-e1198

[2]Taddio A, McMurtry M, Shah V, et al. Reducing pain during vaccine injections: clinical practice guideline. *CMAJ.* 2015;187(13):975–982

also is available.[1] Parents, children 3 years and older, and health care providers administering vaccine injections should be educated about techniques for reducing injection pain or distress. Combination vaccines should be used when feasible to reduce the number of injections and their attendant pain.

PHYSICAL AND PSYCHOLOGICAL TECHNIQUES FOR MINIMIZING INJECTION PAIN AND ANXIETY

Strategies to reduce pain include holding the child upright, administering the most painful vaccine last, and providing tactile stimulation. The needle should be plunged rapidly through the skin without aspiration. Aspiration before injection is not necessary, because large blood vessels are not present at the recommended injection sites and pain may be increased because of longer needle dwelling time in the tissue and wiggling of the needle. Breastfeeding, feeding sweet-tasting solutions, and applying topical anesthetics are other tools that can be used before vaccine administration to decrease pain. Distraction strategies, including pinwheels, deep breathing exercises, and toys, can be used in older children to decrease anxiety and pain. Although rigorously controlled studies of these techniques have not been performed, studies of use during other painful procedures lend support to their use in vaccination. Adolescents should be seated or lying down during vaccination to reduce the risk of injury should syncope develop. Warming a vaccine by rubbing it between the hands is not recommended because of concern for altering vaccine effectiveness.

PHARMACOLOGIC TECHNIQUES FOR MINIMIZING INJECTION PAIN

If topically applied anesthetic is used, planning ahead is necessary so that the anesthetic is applied to allow the minimum 30 to 60 minutes required to provide optimal anesthesia. Strategies can include applying the anesthetic en route to the office visit or immediately on arrival. Lidocaine 4% (LMX4) is approved by the US Food and Drug Administration (FDA) for children older than 2 years, is available over the counter, and takes effect 30 minutes after application. Lidocaine 2.5%/prilocaine 2.5% (EMLA), available by prescription, is approved by the FDA for neonates >37 weeks' estimated gestational age, infants, and children, and takes effect 60 minutes after application. Topical application of ethyl chloride, sprayed onto a cotton ball that is then placed over the injection site for 15 seconds prior to administering the injection, also has been shown to decrease injection pain in school-aged children. Routine preemptive administration of acetaminophen is not recommended because of concern of overuse of antipyretics, the potential detrimental effect on the immune response to the vaccine(s) being administered, and the false sense of security that acetaminophen can prevent febrile seizures. Acetaminophen can be used after immunizations to treat pain and to reduce discomfort of fever, should either occur.

Timing of Vaccines and the Immunization Schedule

A vaccine is intended to be administered to a person capable of an appropriate immunologic response and likely to benefit from the protection provided. However, the

---

[1]World Health Organization. Reducing pain at the time of vaccination: WHO position paper – September 2015. *Wkly Epidemiol Rec.* 2015;90(39):505–510

optimal immunologic response for a person must be balanced against the need to achieve timely protection against disease. This balance is the basis of the childhood immunization schedule. For this reason, the timing of immunizations in different countries may vary.

With parenterally administered live-virus vaccines, the inhibitory effect of residual specific maternal antibody determines the optimal age of administration. For example, live-virus measles-containing vaccine in use in the United States provides suboptimal rates of seroconversion during the first year of life because of a combination of interference by transplacentally acquired maternal antibody and an immature immune system. If a measles-containing vaccine is administered before 12 months of age (eg, because of travel or increased risk of exposure), the child should receive 2 additional doses of measles-containing vaccine at the recommended ages and interval (see Measles, p 537).

An additional factor in determining the timing of immunizations is the need to optimize the immune response. With some products, an immune response is achieved after 1 dose. For example, live-virus rubella vaccine evokes a predictable response at high rates after a single dose. With many inactivated or component vaccines, a primary series of several doses is necessary to achieve an optimal initial response in recipients. Some people require multiple doses to respond to all included antigens. For some vaccines, periodic booster doses (eg, with tetanus and diphtheria toxoids and acellular pertussis antigen) are required to maintain protection.

ADMINISTRATION OF MULTIPLE VACCINES. In general, simultaneously administered vaccines (ie, >1 inactivated or >1 live-virus or inactivated plus live-virus vaccines) are safe and effective and are recommended routinely in the childhood and adolescent immunization schedule to ensure optimal age-important protection and reduced medical visits. In addition, simultaneous administration of vaccines is particularly important for scheduling immunizations for children with lapsed or missed immunizations, for children requiring early or rapid protection, and for people preparing for international travel (see Simultaneous Administration of Multiple Vaccines, p 35). Data indicate possible impaired immune responses when 2 or more parenterally administered live-virus vaccines are not given simultaneously but within 28 days of each other; therefore, live-virus vaccines not administered on the same day should be given at least 28 days (4 weeks) apart whenever possible (Table 1.11, p 33. No minimum interval is required between administration of different inactivated vaccines, with a few exceptions. In people with functional or anatomic asplenia, the MCV4-D quadrivalent meningococcal conjugate vaccine (Menactra [Sanofi Pasteur, Swiftwater, PA]) should not be given until at least 4 weeks after all doses of 13-valent pneumococcal conjugate vaccine (PCV13) have been administered because of interference with the immune response to the PCV13 series, since both vaccines are conjugated to diphtheria toxin carrier protein. When Menactra and Daptacel (DTaP, Sanofi Pasteur) are being administered to children 4 through 6 years of age, preference should be given to simultaneous administration of the 2 vaccines or administration of Menactra prior to administration of Daptacel, because administration of Menactra 1 month after Daptacel has been shown to reduce meningococcal antibody response to Menactra.

THE RECOMMENDED IMMUNIZATION SCHEDULE. The Recommended Immunization Schedule for Children and Adolescents Aged 18 Years or Younger for the United States represents a consensus of the American Academy of Pediatrics (AAP), the Advisory Committee on Immunization Practices (ACIP) of the Centers for Disease Control and

Prevention (CDC), and the American Academy of Family Physicians (AAFP). The schedule is reviewed regularly, and the updated schedule is issued annually in February. Schedules are available at **www.cdc.gov/vaccines/schedules/index.html** and are posted at *Red Book Online* (**http://redbook.solutions.aap.org/SS/ Immunization_Schedules.aspx**). Interim recommendations occasionally may be made when issues such as a shortage of a product or a safety concern occur, or a new recommendation may be added to incorporate a new vaccine or vaccine indication. Special attention should be given to footnotes on the schedule, which summarize major recommendations for routine childhood immunizations.

Combination vaccine products may be administered whenever any component of the combination is indicated and its other components are not contraindicated, provided they are approved by the FDA for that dose in the schedule for each component and for the child's age. The use of a combination vaccine generally is preferred over separate injections of its equivalent component vaccines.

Web-based childhood immunization schedulers using the current vaccine recommendations are available for parents, caregivers, and health care professionals to facilitate making schedules for children 0 through 6 years of age (**www.cdc.gov/ vaccines**). Most state and regional immunization information systems (also known as immunization registries) also will forecast immunizations that are due according to the immunization schedule.

The immunization schedule issued by the AAP, ACIP, and AAFP primarily is intended for children and adolescents in the United States. In many instances, the guidance may be applicable to children in other countries, but individual pediatricians and recommending committees in each country are responsible for determining the appropriateness of the recommendations for their settings. The schedule recommended by the Expanded Programme on Immunization of the World Health Organization (**www.who.int**) also can serve as a resource, with modifications made by the ministries of health in individual countries on the basis of local considerations. Recommendations for vaccine schedules in Europe are available from the European Center for Disease Prevention and Control (**www.ecdc.europa.eu**).

Table 1.11. Guidelines for Spacing of Live and Inactivated Antigens

Antigen Combination	Recommended Minimum Interval Between Doses
2 or more inactivated[a]	None; can be administered simultaneously or at any interval between doses
Inactivated plus live	None; can be administered simultaneously or at any interval between doses
2 or more live[b]	28-day minimum interval if not administered simultaneously

[a]See text for exceptions.
[b]An exception is made for live oral vaccines (ie, Ty21a typhoid vaccine, oral poliovirus vaccine, oral rotavirus vaccine) that can be administered simultaneously or at any interval before or after inactivated or live parenteral vaccines.

Minimum Ages and Minimum Intervals Between Vaccine Doses

Immunizations generally are recommended for members of the youngest age group at risk of experiencing the disease for whom efficacy, effectiveness, immunogenicity, and safety of the vaccine have been demonstrated. Most vaccines in the childhood and adolescent immunization schedule require 2 or more doses for stimulation of an adequate and persisting immune response. Studies have demonstrated that the recommended age and interval between doses of the same antigen(s) (**www.cdc.gov/vaccines/ schedules/index.html**) provide optimal protection.

Vaccines generally should not be administered at intervals less than the recommended minimum or at an earlier age than the recommended minimum (ie, accelerated schedules). Administering doses of a multidose vaccine at intervals shorter than those recommended in the childhood and adolescent immunization schedule might be necessary in circumstances in which an infant or child is behind schedule and needs to be brought up to date quickly or when international travel is anticipated. For example, during a measles outbreak or for international travel, measles vaccine may be administered as early as 6 months of age. However, if a measles-containing vaccine is administered before 12 months of age, the dose is not counted toward the 2-dose measles vaccine series, and the child should be reimmunized at 12 through 15 months of age with a measles-containing vaccine; a third dose of a measles-containing vaccine then is indicated at 4 through 6 years of age but can be administered as early as 4 weeks after the second dose (see Measles, p 537).

Certain circumstances, such as the need for an additional office visit or a patient or parent poorly adherent to scheduled visits, could lead to consideration of administering a vaccine up to 4 days before the minimum interval or age. In general, vaccine doses administered (intentionally or inadvertently) 4 days or fewer before the minimum interval or age can be counted as valid. Health care professionals should be aware that state and school guidelines may consider such doses invalid and require additional vaccinations. Doses administered 5 days or more before the minimum interval or age should not be counted as valid doses and should be repeated as age appropriate. The repeat dose should be spaced by the recommended minimum interval after the invalid dose. Because of the unique schedule for rabies vaccine, consideration of days of a shortened interval between doses must be individualized.

The latest recommendations can be found in the annual immunization schedule (**http://redbook.solutions.aap.org/SS/Immunization_Schedules.aspx**).

Interchangeability of Vaccine Products

Similar vaccines made by different manufacturers can differ in the number and amount of their specific antigenic components and formulation of adjuvants and conjugating agents, thereby eliciting different immune responses. When possible, effort should be made to complete a series with vaccine made by the same manufacturer. Although data documenting the effects of interchangeability are limited, most experts have considered vaccines interchangeable when administered according to their recommended schedule and dosing regimen. Approved vaccines that may be used interchangeably during a vaccine series from different manufacturers, according to recommendations from the AAP or ACIP, include diphtheria and tetanus toxoids vaccines, hepatitis A vaccines, hepatitis B vaccines, and rabies vaccines.

An example of similar vaccines that are not recommended as interchangeable is the adult formulation of Recombivax HB (Merck and Co Inc, Whitehouse Station, NJ; see Hepatitis B, p 401), which is approved for adolescents 11 through 15 years of age; adolescent patients who start their hepatitis B schedule with this vaccine are not candidates to complete their series with the adult formulation of Engerix-B (GlaxoSmithKline, Research Triangle Park, NC). Likewise, because there are no data on the interchangeability of the 2 meningococcal B vaccines and each vaccine uses very different protein antigens, the same vaccine must be used for all doses to complete the full meningococcal B series.

Approved rotavirus (RV) vaccines (RV5, RotaTeq [Merck and Co Inc]; RV1, Rotarix [GlaxoSmithKline]) are considered interchangeable as long as recommendations concerning conversion from a 2-dose regimen (RV-1) to a 3-dose regimen (RV-5) are followed (see Rotavirus, p 700). Similarly, approved *Haemophilus influenzae* type b (Hib) conjugate vaccines are considered interchangeable as long as recommendations for a total of 3 doses in the first year of life are followed (ie, if 2 doses of Hib-OMP are not administered, 3 doses of a Hib-containing vaccine are required). When a vaccine with increased serotype content replaces a previously recommended product (eg, PCV13 for PCV7 or 9vHPV for 4vHPV), the vaccines are considered interchangeable, so the series can be completed with the broader serotype product.

Minimal data on safety and immunogenicity and no data on efficacy are available for interchangeability of DTaP vaccines from different manufacturers. When feasible, DTaP from the same manufacturer should be used for the primary series (see Pertussis, p 620). However, in circumstances in which the DTaP product received previously is not known or the previously administered product is not readily available, any of the DTaP vaccines may be used according to licensure for dose and age. Matching of booster doses of DTaP and adolescent Tdap by manufacturer is not necessary. Single-component vaccines from the same manufacturer of combination vaccines, including DTaP-HepB-IPV and DTaP-IPV/Hib are interchangeable (see Combination Vaccines, p 36).[1]

Simultaneous Administration of Multiple Vaccines

Simultaneous administration of most vaccines is safe, effective, and recommended. Infants and children have sufficient immunologic capacity to respond to multiple vaccines administered at the same time. There is no contraindication to simultaneous administration of multiple vaccines routinely recommended for infants and children, with 2 exceptions: (1) MCV4-D (Menactra [Sanofi Pasteur, Swiftwater, PA]) should not be given for at least 4 weeks after all doses of PCV13 have been administered because of interference with the immune response to certain serotypes in the PCV13 vaccine, because both vaccines are conjugated to diphtheria toxin carrier protein; and (2) for high-risk children for whom both PCV13 and PPSV23 are recommended, the dose of PPSV23 at 2 years or older should be administered at least 8 weeks after PVC13. When PCV13 is indicated, despite receipt of PPSV23, there should be a minimum interval of 8 weeks

---

[1]Kroger AT, Duchin J, Vázquez M. General best practice guidelines for immunization. Best practices guidance of the Advisory Committee on Immunization Practices (ACIP). Available at: **www.cdc.gov/vaccines/hcp/acip-recs/general-recs/downloads/general-recs.pdf**

between vaccines.

The immune-response to 1 vaccine generally does not interfere with responses to other vaccines. Simultaneous administration of IPV, MMR, varicella, or DTaP vaccines results in rates of seroconversion and of adverse events similar to those observed when vaccines are administered at separate visits. A slightly increased risk of febrile seizures is associated with the first dose of MMRV compared with MMR and monovalent varicella administered simultaneously at separate sites among children 12 through 23 months of age; after dose 1 of MMRV vaccine, 1 additional febrile seizure is expected to occur per approximately 2300 to 2600 young children immunized, compared with MMR and monovalent varicella. During the 2 influenza seasons between 2010–2012, there were reports of febrile seizures in the United States in young children who received inactivated influenza vaccine (IIV) and PCV13 concurrently. One additional febrile seizure is expected to occur per approximately 2200 doses. Vaccine Safety Datalink (VSD) data from the 2013–14 and 2014–15 influenza seasons describe an increased risk of seizure among children 6 through 24 months of age 0 to 1 day after concurrent receipt of IIV3 and PCV13. Simultaneous administration of IIV and PCV13 continues to be recommended when both vaccines are indicated because of the preponderance of benefit relative to the risk.

Because simultaneous administration of routinely recommended vaccines is not known to alter the effectiveness or safety of any of the recommended childhood vaccines, simultaneous administration of all vaccines that are appropriate for the age and immunization status of the recipient is recommended.[1] When vaccines are administered simultaneously, separate syringes and separate sites should be used, and injections into the same extremity should be separated by at least 1 inch so that any local reactions can be differentiated. Simultaneous administration of multiple vaccines can increase immunization rates significantly. Individual vaccines should never be mixed in the same syringe unless they are specifically approved and labeled for administration in 1 syringe. If an inactivated vaccine and an Immune Globulin product are indicated concurrently (eg, hepatitis B vaccine and Hepatitis B Immune Globulin, rabies vaccine and Rabies Immune Globulin, tetanus-containing vaccine and Tetanus Immune Globulin), they should be administered at separate anatomic sites.

Combination Vaccines

Combination vaccines represent one solution to the issue of increased numbers of injections during single clinic visits and generally are preferred over separate injections of equivalent component vaccines. Table 1.12 lists combination vaccines approved for use in the United States. Factors that could be considered by the provider, in consultation with the parent, include the potential for improved vaccine coverage, the number of injections needed, vaccine safety, vaccine availability, interchangeability, storage and cost issues, and whether the patient is likely to return for follow-up.

---

[1] Kroger AT, Duchin J, Vázquez M. General best practice guidelines for immunization. Best practices guidance of the Advisory Committee on Immunization Practices (ACIP). Available at: **www.cdc.gov/vaccines/hcp/ acip-recs/general-recs/downloads/general-recs.pdf**

Table 1.12. Combination Vaccines Approved by the US Food and Drug Administration (FDA)[a]

Vaccine[b]	Trade Name (Year Approved)	FDA Licensure Age Group	Use in Immunization Schedule
HepA-HepB	Twinrix (2001)	≥18 y	Three doses on a 0-, 1-, and 6-mo schedule
DTaP-HepB-IPV	Pediarix (2002)	6 wk through 6 y	Three-dose series at 2, 4, and 6 mo of age
MMRV	ProQuad (2005)	12 mo through 12 y	Two doses (see Varicella-Zoster Infections, p 869)
DTaP-IPV	Kinrix (2008)	4 y through 6 y	Booster for fifth dose of DTaP and fourth dose of IPV in children who have received 3 doses of Pediarix or Infanrix and a fourth dose of Infanrix
DTaP-IPV/Hib	Pentacel (2008)	6 wk through 4 y	Four-dose series administered at 2, 4, 6, and 15 through 18 mo of age
DTaP-IPV	Quadracel (2015)	4 through 6 y	Single dose approved for use in children 4 through 6 years of age as a fifth dose in DTaP series and as a fourth or fifth dose in IPV series, in children who have received 4 doses of Pentacel and/or Daptacel vaccine

HepA indicates hepatitis A vaccine; HepB, hepatitis B vaccine; DTaP, diphtheria and tetanus toxoids and acellular pertussis vaccine; IPV, inactivated poliovirus vaccine; MMRV, measles-mumps-rubella-varicella vaccine; Hib, *Haemophilus influenzae* type b vaccine.

[a]Excludes measles-mumps-rubella (MMR), DTaP, Tdap, Td, and IPV vaccines, for which individual components are not available. DTaP/Hib (TriHIBit) no longer is manufactured.

[b]Dash (-) indicates products in which the active components are supplied in their final (combined) form by the manufacturer; slash (/) indicates products in which active components must be mixed by the user.

Combination vaccines should not be used outside the age groups for which they are approved. Some of these vaccine components also are available for separate administration (eg, MMRV also is available as MMR and varicella vaccine, although single-component measles, mumps, or rubella vaccines are not available in the United States). All available types or brand-name products do not need to be stocked by each health care professional, and it is recognized that the decision of health care professionals to implement use of new combination vaccines involves complex economic and logistical considerations.

When patients have received the recommended immunizations for some of the components in a combination vaccine, administering the extra antigen(s) in the combination vaccine is permissible, if they are not contraindicated (**www.cdc.gov/mmwr/preview/mmwrhtml/rr6002a1.htm?s_cid=rr6002a1_e**) and doing so will reduce the number of injections required. Excessive doses of toxoid vaccines (diphtheria and tetanus) may result in extensive local reactions. To overcome the potential for recording errors and ambiguities in the names of vaccine combinations, electronic systems including bar codes that minimize the potential for recording errors have been developed and are being implemented to enhance the convenience and accuracy of transferring vaccine-identifying information into health records and immunization information systems.

Lapsed Immunizations

A lapse in the immunization schedule does not require reinitiating the entire series or addition of doses to the series for any vaccine in the recommended schedule. If a dose of vaccine is missed, subsequent immunizations should be administered at the next visit as if the usual interval has elapsed. For RV vaccine, the doses to be administered are age limited, so catch-up may not be possible (see Rotavirus Infections, p 700). See specific influenza vaccine recommendations in the Influenza chapter (p 476) and annual influenza policy statement (**https://redbook.solutions.aap.org/ss/influenza-resources.aspx**) for children younger than 9 years whose first 2 doses were not administered in the same season, because recommendations can vary depending on the formulation of each season's vaccine. The health records of children for whom immunizations have been missed or postponed should be flagged to remind health care professionals to resume the child's immunization regimen at the next available opportunity. Minimum age and interval recommendations should be followed for administration of all doses. An interactive app developed by the CDC is available for downloading and has up-to-date information on the childhood immunization schedule, including timing of missed or skipped vaccines (**www.cdc.gov/vaccines/schedules/hcp/schedule-app.html**).

Unknown or Uncertain Immunization Status

Many children, adolescents, and young adults do not have adequate documentation of their immunizations, which reinforces the need to include all vaccinations in state-based immunization information systems. Parent or guardian recollection of a child's immunization history may not be accurate. Only written/electronic, dated, authentic records should be accepted as evidence of immunization. In general, when in doubt, a person with unknown or uncertain immunization status should be considered disease susceptible, and recommended immunizations should be initiated without delay on a schedule commensurate with the person's current age. If the primary series has been started but not completed, the series should be completed, but there is no need to repeat doses or restart the full course.

Serologic testing is an alternative to vaccination for certain antigens (eg, measles, rubella, hepatitis A, and tetanus). However, commercial serologic testing takes time, can lead to a failed immunization opportunity, and may not always be sufficiently sensitive to indicate protection. Importantly, no evidence suggests that administration of vaccines to already immune recipients is harmful.

Vaccine Dose

Recommended vaccine doses are those that have been determined to be both safe and effective for their specified indication in prelicensure clinical trials; no other alternative doses have been determined to be both safe and effective. Reducing or exceeding a recommended dose volume or collecting residual volumes to make up a dose is never recommended. Reducing or dividing doses of any vaccine, including vaccines administered to preterm or low birth weight infants, can result in inadequate immune responses. A previous immunization with a dose that was less than the standard dose or one administered by a nonstandard route should not be counted as valid, and the person should be reimmunized as recommended for age.

Active Immunization of People Who Recently Received Immune Globulin and Other Blood Products

Certain live-virus vaccines may have diminished immunogenicity when administered within 2 weeks before or up to 11 months following receipt of immune globulin (IG) (either standard or hyperimmune globulins following intramuscular, intravenous, or subcutaneous administration). In particular, IG administration inhibits the response to measles vaccine for up to 11 months. Inhibition of immune response to rubella vaccine also has been demonstrated, but the effect on response to mumps or varicella vaccines is not known. The appropriate interval between IG administration and measles immunization varies with the dose of IG and the specific product used. Suggested intervals are provided in Table 1.13 but may be shortened if exposure to measles is likely (see Measles, p 537). Because of potential interference with the immune response, varicella, mumps, or rubella vaccine administration should be delayed as recommended for measles vaccine (see Table 1.13). If IG must be given within 14 days after administration of measles- or varicella-containing vaccines, these vaccines should be administered again after the interval specified in Table 1.13. One exception to this rule is when serologic testing at an appropriate interval after IG administration documents seroconversion.

Administration of IG preparations (either standard or hyperimmune globulins following intramuscular, intravenous, or subcutaneous administration) does not interfere with antibody responses to yellow fever, oral poliovirus (OPV), live attenuated influenza vaccine (LAIV), oral Ty21a typhoid, or oral rotavirus vaccines. Hence, these live vaccines can be administered simultaneously with or at any time before or after administration of IG.

In contrast to the effect on some live-virus vaccines, administration of an IG preparation does not significantly inhibit the immune responses to inactivated vaccines or toxoids. Concurrent administration of recommended doses of Hepatitis B Immune Globulin (HBIG), Tetanus Immune Globulin, or Rabies Immune Globulin (RIG) and standard doses of the corresponding inactivated vaccine or toxoid for postexposure prophylaxis provides immediate protection and long-term immunity and does not impair the efficacy of the vaccine. Vaccines should be administered at a separate anatomic site from that of intramuscularly administered IG. For additional information, see chapters on specific diseases in Section 3.

Respiratory syncytial virus monoclonal antibody (palivizumab) does not interfere with the response to any vaccines.

Table 1.13. Suggested Intervals Between Immune Globulin Administration and Active Immunization with MMR, MMRV, or Monovalent Varicella Vaccines

Indications or Product	Route	Dose U or mL	Dose mg IgG/kg	Interval, mo[a]
Blood transfusion				
Washed RBCs	IV	10 mL/kg	Negligible	0
RBCs, adenine-saline added	IV	10 mL/kg	10	3
Packed RBCs	IV	10 mL/kg	20–60	6
Whole blood	IV	10 mL/kg	80–100	6
Plasma or platelet products	IV	10 mL/kg	160	7
Botulinum Immune Globulin Intravenous (Human [as BabyBIG])	IV	1 mL/kg	50	6
Cytomegalovirus IGIV (hyperimmune globulin)	IV	...	150 (maximum)	6
Hepatitis A prophylaxis (as IG)				
Contact prophylaxis	IM	0.1 mL/kg	...	3
International travel	IM	0.1 or 0.2 mL/kg	...	3
Hepatitis B prophylaxis (as HBIG)	IM	0.06 mL/kg	10	3
Measles prophylaxis (as IG) for people not pregnant or severely immunocompromised[b]	IM	0.5 mL/kg	80	6
Measles prophylaxis for pregnant women and severely immunocompromised host[b] (as IGIV)	IV	...	400	8
Rabies prophylaxis (as RIG)	IM	20 IU/kg	22	4
Replacement (or therapy) of immune deficiencies (as IGIV)	IV	...	300–400	8
RSV prophylaxis (palivizumab monoclonal antibody)[c]	IM	...	15 (monoclonal)	None
Tetanus prophylaxis (as TIG)	IM	250 U	10	3

Table 1.13. Suggested Intervals Between Immune Globulin Administration and Active Immunization with MMR, MMRV, or Monovalent Varicella Vaccines, continued

Indications or Product	Route	Dose U or mL	Dose mg IgG/kg	Interval, mo[a]
Therapy for ITP (as IGIV)	IV	...	400	8
Therapy for ITP (as IGIV)	IV	...	800–1000	10
Therapy for ITP or Kawasaki disease (as IGIV)	IV	...	1600–2000	11
Varicella prophylaxis (as IGIV)	IV	...	400	8
Varicella prophylaxis (as VariZIG)	IM	125 U/10 kg (maximum 625 U)	20–40	5

MMR indicates measles-mumps-rubella; MMRV, measles-mumps-rubella-varicella; RSV, respiratory syncytial virus; IM, intramuscular; TIG, Tetanus Immune Globulin; IG, Immune Globulin; HBIG, Hepatitis B Immune Globulin; RIG, Rabies Immune Globulin; VariZIG, Varicella-Zoster Immune Globulin; IV, intravenous; RBCs, Red Blood Cells; IGIV, Immune Globulin Intravenous; ITP, immune (formerly termed "idiopathic") thrombocytopenic purpura.

[a] These intervals should provide sufficient time for decreases in passive antibodies in all children to allow for an adequate response to measles vaccine. Physicians should not assume that children are protected fully against measles during these intervals. Additional doses of IG or measles vaccine may be indicated if exposure to measles is likely or has occurred (see text).

[b] IGIV is the recommended IG preparation for pregnant women without evidence of measles immunity and for severely immunocompromised hosts regardless of immunologic or vaccination status, including patients with severe primary immunodeficiency; patients who have received a bone marrow transplant until at least 12 months after finishing all immunosuppressive treatment, or longer in patients who have developed graft-versus-host disease; patients on treatment for ALL within and until at least 6 months after completion of immunosuppressive chemotherapy; individuals who have received a solid organ transplant; and people with human immunodeficiency virus (HIV) infection or acquired immunodeficiency syndrome (AIDS) who have severe immunosuppression defined as CD4+ T-lymphocyte percentage <15% (all ages) or CD4+ T-lymphocyte count <200 lymphocytes/mm³ (older than 5 years) and those who have not received MMR vaccine since receiving effective ART.

[c] RSV monoclonal antibody (palivizumab) does not interfere with the immune response to vaccines.

Vaccine Safety

RISKS AND ADVERSE EVENTS

Prior to licensure, all vaccines in the United States undergo rigorous immunogenicity and safety testing. Occasionally, individuals still may acquire a vaccine-preventable disease despite receiving the corresponding vaccine, and adverse events can occur following the administration of a vaccine. Mild and self-limited adverse events (eg, local pain and tenderness at the injection site) are true, causally associated reactions. Serious causally related adverse events also can occur but are rare. Many adverse events may be coincidental events that occur in temporal association after vaccination but are unrelated to vaccination. The mere occurrence of an adverse event following vaccination does not mean the vaccine caused the symptoms or signs. Highly effective vaccines have dramatically reduced the threat of many infectious diseases, and because of this success, some people now are more concerned about potential vaccine adverse effects than about the illnesses vaccines prevent. As vaccinations successfully control their target diseases, health care providers need to communicate benefits and risks of vaccination to a population whose first-hand experience with vaccine-preventable diseases increasingly is rare.

As with all aspects of medicine, the benefits and risks from vaccines must be weighed against each other, and vaccine recommendations are based on this assessment. Recommendations are made to maximize protection and minimize risk by providing specific advice on dose, route, and timing and by identifying precautions or contraindications to vaccination.

Common vaccine adverse reactions usually are mild to moderate in severity (eg, fever or injection site reactions, such as swelling, redness, and pain) and have no permanent sequelae. Examples include local inflammation after administration of DTaP, Td, or Tdap vaccines, and fever and rash 1 to 2 weeks after administration of MMR or MMRV vaccines. Because many suspected adverse events are merely coincidental with administration of a vaccine, definitive assessment of causality often requires careful epidemiologic studies comparing the incidence of the event in vaccinated versus unvaccinated individuals or other comparison group(s) of similar age and residence, or comparing the incidence of the adverse event in a specific time frame following immunization (the postulated risk interval) with the incidence in other timeframes. Although rare, a causal link with a live-virus vaccine may be established if the vaccine-strain virus can be identified in biologic specimens from an ill child with compatible symptoms (eg, rotavirus vaccine-associated diarrhea in a patient with severe combined immunodeficiency).

The Brighton Collaboration is a nonprofit international voluntary consortium formed to develop globally accepted and standardized case definitions for adverse events following immunization that can be used in vaccine safety surveillance and research. The project began in 2000 with formation of a steering committee and creation of work groups composed of international experts in vaccine safety, patient care, pharmacology, regulatory affairs, public health, and vaccine delivery. It is the world's largest network of vaccine safety science experts. The Brighton Collaboration provides guidelines for collecting, analyzing, and presenting vaccine safety data in a way that facilitates sharing and comparison of vaccine data among professionals working in the area of vaccine safety worldwide. Additional information, including current definitions and updates of progress, can be found online (**https://brightoncollaboration.org/public/resources. html**). As of January 2017, a total of 47 case definitions have been developed and completed, and all definitions can be accessed online.

Health care professionals are mandated by law to report specific adverse events found on the Vaccine Adverse Event Reporting System (VAERS) Vaccine Injury Table (Appendix III, p 1058) and adverse events listed by the vaccine manufacturer as a contraindication to further doses of the vaccine (**http://vaers.hhs.gov/resources/ VAERS_Table_of_Reportable_Events_Following_Vaccination.pdf**). Health care professionals are encouraged to report any clinically significant adverse event following vaccination to VAERS (see p 45). When analyzed in conjunction with other VAERS reports, this information can provide evidence of safety signals for unanticipated, potentially causally related vaccine adverse events (Appendix III, p 1058). It is important to understand that VAERS is not designed to assess whether a vaccine caused an adverse event, but rather as a system to generate hypotheses (to detect signals) to be tested subsequently through well-designed epidemiologic studies. Other vaccine safety monitoring systems, such as the Vaccine Safety Datalink (VSD), which uses large linked databases (**www.cdc.gov/vaccinesafety/ensuringsafety/monitoring/vsd/index.html**), or the Clinical Immunization Safety Assessment (CISA) Project (**www.cdc.gov/vaccinesafety/ensuringsafety/monitoring/cisa/index.html**) provide mechanisms to implement such studies. A nationally notifiable vaccine-preventable disease that occurs in a child or adolescent at any time, including after vaccination (vaccine failure), should be reported to the local or state health department (see Appendix IV, p 1069). An Institute of Medicine report published in January 2013[1] reviewed and affirmed existing data sources and systems involved in vaccine safety surveillance and research (also see Addressing Parents' Questions About Vaccine Safety and Effectiveness [p 7] and Institute of Medicine Reviews of Adverse Events After Immunization [below]).

INSTITUTE OF MEDICINE REVIEWS OF ADVERSE EVENTS AFTER IMMUNIZATION

Through a series of comprehensive reviews, the Institute of Medicine (IOM) (now called the National Academy of Medicine, or NAM) independently concluded that current childhood immunizations and the immunization schedule are safe and that following the complete childhood immunization schedule is associated strongly with a reduction in vaccine-preventable diseases. The committee members for these reviews included individuals with expertise in medicine, medical subspecialties, immunology, immunotoxicology, epidemiology, biostatistics, ethics, law, and other scientific disciplines.

During the years 2001–2004, the Immunization Safety Review Committee of the IOM evaluated 8 existing and emerging vaccine safety concerns. One of these reports examined hypotheses about associations between vaccines and autism. The committee concluded that the evidence favors rejection of a causal relationship between the MMR vaccine and autism and between thimerosal-containing vaccines and autism.[2]

In a subsequent review, the IOM convened a committee of experts to review the epidemiologic, clinical, and biological evidence regarding adverse health events associated with specific vaccines covered by the National Vaccine Injury Compensation Program (VICP). The 2012 IOM report, titled "Adverse Effects of Vaccines: Evidence and Causality,"[3] reviewed 8 different types of vaccines covered by the VICP: combination measles-mumps-rubella (MMR) vaccine; varicella vaccine; influenza vaccine; hepatitis A vaccine; hepatitis B vaccine; human papillomavirus (HPV) vaccine; diphtheria toxoid-, tetanus toxoid-, and acellular pertussis-containing (DTaP-containing) vaccines other than those containing whole-cell pertussis component; and meningococcal vaccines. The review also covered the injection related adverse events of complex regional pain

---

[1]Institute of Medicine. *The Childhood Immunization Schedule and Safety: Stakeholder Concerns, Scientific Evidence, and Future Studies.* Washington, DC: National Academies Press; 2013

[2]**www.nationalacademies.org/hmd/Reports.aspx?filters=inmeta:activity=Immunization Safety Review**

[3]**www.nationalacademies.org/hmd/Reports/2011/Adverse-Effects-of-Vaccines-Evidence-and-Causality.aspx**

syndrome, deltoid bursitis, and syncope. Two lines of evidence supported the committee's causality conclusions: epidemiologic evidence and mechanistic evidence. The benefit and effectiveness of vaccines were not assessed during this review. The IOM committee developed 158 specific vaccine-adverse event pairings and assigned each to 1 of 4 categories of causation. Several category 1 and category 2 causal relationships were found for anaphylaxis and injection-related events. A summary of the IOM committee's causality conclusions regarding evidence for a causal relationship between the specific vaccines and other adverse event is as follows:

Category 1: Evidence convincingly supports a causal relationship between vaccines and some adverse events:

- Varicella vaccines and 4 specific adverse events:
  - disseminated vaccine-strain varicella-zoster virus (VZV) infection without other organ involvement
  - disseminated vaccine-strain VZV infection with other organ involvement, including pneumonia, meningitis, or hepatitis, in immunodeficient individuals
  - vaccine-strain viral reactivation without other organ involvement
  - vaccine-strain viral reactivation with subsequent infection resulting in meningitis or encephalitis
- MMR vaccine and 2 specific adverse events:
  - measles inclusion body encephalitis in immunodeficient individuals
  - febrile seizures

Category 2: Evidence favors acceptance of a causal relationship (evidence is strong and generally suggestive but not firm enough to be described as convincing):

- Certain inactivated influenza vaccines previously used in Canada and oculorespiratory syndrome
- MMR vaccine and transient arthralgia in women and in children

Category 3: Evidence favors rejection of a causal relationship:

- MMR vaccine and autism
- MMR vaccine and type 1 diabetes mellitus
- DT, TT, or acellular pertussis-containing vaccines and type 1 diabetes mellitus
- Inactivated influenza vaccines and Bell's palsy
- Inactivated influenza vaccines and exacerbation of asthma or reactive airways disease in children and adults

Category 4: Evidence is inadequate to accept or reject a causal relationship for the vast majority (135 vaccine-adverse event pairs).

In response to a recommendation by the National Vaccine Advisory Committee, in 2013 the IOM issued a report, "The Childhood Immunization Schedule and Safety: Stakeholder Concerns, Scientific Evidence, and Future Studies."[1] The committee reviewed scientific findings and stakeholder concerns related to the safety of the recommended childhood immunization schedule and identified potential research approaches, methodologies, and study designs that could inform this question, considering strengths, weaknesses, as well as the ethical and financial feasibility of each

---

[1]www.nationalacademies.org/hmd/~/media/Files/Report%20Files/2013/Childhood-Immunization-Schedule/ChildhoodImmunizationScheduleandSafety_RB.pdf

approach. The IOM committee concluded that the recommended childhood immunization schedule is safe. The committee based its conclusion on a "lack of conclusive evidence linking adverse events to multiple immunizations" and recommended continued research on the safety of the childhood immunization schedule. In this report, the committee also concluded that following the complete childhood immunization schedule is associated strongly with reducing vaccine-preventable diseases.

VACCINE ADVERSE EVENT REPORTING SYSTEM

The Vaccine Adverse Event Reporting System (VAERS) is a national passive surveillance system that monitors the safety of US vaccines. Jointly administered by the CDC and the FDA, VAERS accepts reports of adverse events occurring in temporal association following administration of vaccines. The strengths of VAERS are that it is national in scope, can detect signals of possible safety problems, and can detect rare and unexpected adverse events. VAERS is intended to:

- Detect new, unusual, or rare vaccine adverse events;
- Monitor increases in known adverse events;
- Identify potential patient risk factors for particular types of adverse events;
- Assess the safety of newly licensed vaccines;
- Determine and address possible reporting clusters (eg, suspected localized [temporally or geographically] or product-/batch-/lot-specific adverse event reporting); and
- Recognize persistent safe-use problems and administration errors.

Like all passive surveillance systems, VAERS is subject to limitations, including reporting biases such as underreporting, stimulated reporting, inconsistent data quality and completeness, lack of denominator data, and absence of an unvaccinated comparison group. Because of these limitations, it is generally not possible to determine whether a vaccine caused an adverse event through VAERS reports alone. VAERS encourages the reporting of any medically important health event, even if the reporter is not certain the vaccine caused the event. A reported adverse event may be coincidental or causal (related to the vaccine).

The National Childhood Vaccine Injury Act of 1986 requires physicians and other health care professionals who administer vaccines covered under the National Vaccine Injury Compensation Program to maintain permanent vaccination records. Additionally, the Act requires reporting to VAERS any condition listed in the VAERS Vaccine Injury Table (see Appendix III, p 1058) or listed in the product package insert as a contraindication to further doses. Vaccines covered under this act include all those that are recommended by the CDC for routine administration to children. Health care professionals are encouraged to report any medically important health event occurring after vaccination, regardless of whether or not it is listed on the VAERS Vaccine Injury Table. People other than health care professionals, including patients and parents, also may submit a report of a suspected adverse event to VAERS. Vaccine manufacturers also are required to report any adverse event that comes to their attention. In 2016, approximately 45 000 reports were submitted to VAERS from health care providers (27%), vaccine manufacturers (51%), other sources (12%), and vaccinated patients or parents of vaccinated children (10%). In addition to adverse events, vaccine failure, vaccine product problems, and vaccine administration errors can be reported to VAERS. The Health Insurance Portability and Accountability Act (HIPAA) Privacy Rule permits reporting of protected health information to public health authorities. A patient's consent is not required to release medical records to VAERS. All patient-identifying information and reporter-identifying information is kept confidential. Submission of a VAERS report does not necessarily indicate that the vaccine or vaccination procedure caused or contributed to the event. Notification that the report has been received is provided to the person submitting the report.

On June 30, 2017, the CDC and FDA implemented VAERS 2.0, which includes a new VAERS reporting form (Fig 1.1) and new submission processes. Instructions for reporting to VAERS are available at **https://vaers.hhs.gov/reportevent.html.** Additional assistance is available via e-mail at **info@vaers.org** or by phone at 1-800-822-7967.

Information in VAERS reports is evaluated and analyzed by the CDC and FDA to determine whether there are unusual or unexpected patterns of adverse event reporting (ie, safety signals). Reports are classified as serious according to a regulatory definition when at least 1 of the following outcomes is documented: death, life-threatening illness, hospitalization, prolongation of an existing hospitalization, permanent disability, or congenital anomaly/birth defect. Medical records are requested for serious reports and other reports of special interest and are reviewed by FDA and CDC physicians.

After licensure of a vaccine for use in children, the FDA presents a summary of the first 18 months of safety data to an independent pediatric advisory committee. Vaccine safety data are presented routinely to the Advisory Committee on Immunization Practices (ACIP) of the CDC to inform deliberations around vaccine recommendations. Periodically, reviews of vaccine and adverse event-specific surveillance summaries from VAERS data are published by CDC and FDA staff. These summary reports often provide reassurance of the safety of a vaccine. However, they also may describe findings of possible safety concerns that require further evaluation. Vaccine safety concerns identified in VAERS as sentinel events usually require further studies for confirmation using established systems, such as the Vaccine Safety Datalink or other controlled epidemiologic methods. At a minimum, determination of causality requires the demonstration that the incidence of an adverse event following immunization is significantly higher than would be expected in an unvaccinated population, or that the incidence in a specific time frame following vaccination is higher than would be expected in an unexposed time frame (in the case of self-controlled designs) and not attributed to other factors.

VACCINE SAFETY DATALINK PROJECT

To supplement the VAERS program, which is a passive surveillance system, the CDC formed partnerships with several large managed-care organizations in 1990 to establish the Vaccine Safety Datalink (VSD) project, an active surveillance system designed to monitor and evaluate vaccine safety, especially when new vaccines are approved or when there are new vaccine recommendations. The VSD project has been one of the most important sources of scientifically based information about the safety of vaccines.

FIG 1.1 VAERS FORM (FOR DIRECTIONS FOR COMPLETING FORM AND FOR A NEW ELECTRONIC REPORTING FORM, SEE HTTPS://VAERS.HHS.GOV/REPORTEVENT.HTML)

VAERS Vaccine Adverse Event Reporting System
www.vaers.hhs.gov

Adverse events are possible reactions or problems that occur during or after vaccination. Items 2, 3, 4, 5, 6, 17, 18 and 21 are **ESSENTIAL** and should be completed. Patient identity is kept confidential. Instructions are provided on the last two pages.

INFORMATION ABOUT THE PATIENT WHO RECEIVED THE VACCINE (Use **Continuation Page** if needed).

1. Patient name: (first) (last)
Street address:
City: State: County:
ZIP code: Phone: ( ) Email:

2. Date of birth: (mm/dd/yyyy)   3. Sex: ☐ Male ☐ Female ☐ Unknown

4. Date and time of vaccination: (mm/dd/yyyy)   Time: hh:mm ☐ AM ☐ PM

5. Date and time adverse event started: (mm/dd/yyyy)   Time: hh:mm ☐ AM ☐ PM

6. Age at vaccination: Years Months   7. Today's date: (mm/dd/yyyy)

8. Is the report about vaccine(s) given to a pregnant woman?: ☐ No ☐ Unknown ☐ Yes
(If yes, describe the event, any pregnancy complications, and estimated due date if known in item 18).

9. Prescriptions, over-the-counter medications, dietary supplements, or herbal remedies being taken at the time of vaccination:

10. Allergies to medications, food, or other products:

11. Other illnesses at the time of vaccination and up to one month prior:

12. Chronic or long-standing health conditions:

INFORMATION ABOUT THE PERSON COMPLETING THIS FORM

13. Form completed by: (name)

Relation to patient: ☐ Healthcare professional/staff ☐ Patient (yourself) ☐ Parent/guardian/caregiver ☐ Other:

Street address: ☐ Check if same as item 1.
City: State: ZIP code:
Phone: ( ) Email:

14. Best doctor/healthcare professional to contact about the adverse event: Name:
Phone: ( ) Ext:

INFORMATION ABOUT THE FACILITY WHERE VACCINE WAS GIVEN

15. Facility/clinic name:
Fax: ( )
Street address: ☐ Check if same as item 13.
City:
State: ZIP code:
Phone: ( )

16. Type of facility: (Check one).
☐ Doctor's office or hospital
☐ Pharmacy or drug store
☐ Workplace clinic
☐ Public health clinic
☐ Nursing home or senior living facility
☐ School/student health clinic
☐ Other:
☐ Unknown

WHICH VACCINES WERE GIVEN? WHAT HAPPENED TO THE PATIENT?

17. Enter all vaccines given on the date listed in item 4: (Route is HOW vaccine was given, Body site is WHERE vaccine was given). Use **Continuation Page** if needed.

Vaccine (type and brand name)	Manufacturer	Lot number	Route	Body site	Dose no. in series
select			select	select	select
select			select	select	select
select			select	select	select
select			select	select	select

18. Describe the adverse event(s), treatment, and outcome(s), if any: (symptoms, signs, time course, etc.)

Use **Continuation Page** if needed.

19. Medical tests and laboratory results related to the adverse event(s): (include dates)

Use **Continuation Page** if needed.

20. Has the patient recovered from the adverse event(s)?: ☐ Yes ☐ No ☐ Unknown

21. Result or outcome of adverse event(s): (Check all that apply).
☐ Doctor or other healthcare professional office/clinic visit
☐ Emergency room or emergency department visit
☐ Hospitalization: Number of days (if known)
  Hospital name:
  City: State:
☐ Prolongation of existing hospitalization (vaccine received during existing hospitalization)
☐ Life threatening illness (immediate risk of death from the event)
☐ Disability or permanent damage
☐ Patient died: Date of death (mm/dd/yyyy)
☐ Congenital anomaly or birth defect
☐ None of the above

ADDITIONAL INFORMATION (Use **Continuation Page** if needed).

22. Any other vaccines received within one month prior to the date listed in item 4:

Vaccine (type and brand name)	Manufacturer	Lot number	Route	Body site	Dose no. in series
select			select	select	select
select			select	select	select

23. Has the patient ever had an adverse event following any previous vaccine?: (If yes, describe adverse event, patient age at vaccination, vaccination dates, vaccine type, and brand name).
☐ No ☐ Unknown ☐ Yes

24. Patient's race: (Check all that apply).
☐ American Indian or Alaska Native ☐ Asian ☐ Black or African American ☐ Native Hawaiian or Other Pacific Islander
☐ White ☐ Unknown ☐ Other:

25. Patient's ethnicity: ☐ Hispanic or Latino ☐ Not Hispanic or Latino ☐ Unknown   26. Immuniz. proj. report no.: (Health Dept use only).

COMPLETE ONLY FOR U.S. MILITARY/DEPARTMENT OF DEFENSE (DoD) RELATED REPORTS

27. Status at vaccination: ☐ Active duty ☐ Reserve ☐ National Guard ☐ Beneficiary ☐ Other:

28. Vaccinated at Military/DoD site: ☐ Yes ☐ No

FORM FDA VAERS-2.0 (6/17)   SAVE

VAERS

CONTINUATION PAGE (Use only if you need more space from the front page).

17. Enter all vaccines given on the date listed in item 4 (continued):					Dose no. in series
Vaccine (type and brand name)	Manufacturer	Lot number	Route	Body site	
select			select	select	select
select			select	select	select
select			select	select	select
select			select	select	select

22. Any other vaccines received within one month prior to the date listed in item 4 (continued):					Dose no. in series
Vaccine (type and brand name)	Manufacturer	Lot number	Route	Body site	
select			select	select	select
select			select	select	select
select			select	select	select
select			select	select	select
select			select	select	select
select			select	select	select

Use the space below to provide any additional information (indicate Item number):

RETURN TO PAGE 1

SAVE

The VSD project provides access to comprehensive medical and immunization histories on more than 9 million people. The VSD project allows for both retrospective and prospective observational vaccine safety studies as well as for timely investigations of newly approved vaccines or emerging vaccine safety concerns and has the ability to assess rates of potential adverse events following immunization compared with background rates of these same events or with rates in a historical cohort, or in other unexposed populations in the VSD cohort, as feasible.

The VSD uses electronic health data from each participating site. These data include information on vaccines, including the kind of vaccine that is administered to each patient, date of vaccination, and other vaccinations administered on the same day. The VSD also uses information on medical illnesses that have been diagnosed during doctors' office visits, urgent care visits, emergency department visits, and hospitalizations. The VSD project conducts vaccine safety studies based on questions or concerns raised in the medical literature and from reports to the VAERS. When a new vaccine has been recommended for use in the United States or when there is a change in how a vaccine is recommended, the VSD will monitor the safety of these vaccines.

The VSD project has a long history of monitoring and evaluating the safety of vaccines. Since 1990, investigators from the VSD have published many studies to address vaccine safety concerns. Examples of the work of the VSD project include the following:

- White Paper on Studying the Safety of the Childhood Immunization Schedule
- Are vaccines that contain additives safe for children? How about vaccines with preservatives?
- Are rotavirus vaccines safe for infants?
- Do vaccines cause febrile seizures?
- Are there safety concerns following HPV vaccine?

The VSD has been a critical part of the public health immunization system in the United States, and VSD studies should be used by pediatricians to address vaccine safety concerns in their practices. Information about the VSD can be found on the CDC Web site (**www.cdc.gov/vaccinesafety/Activities/vsd.html**).

POST-LICENSURE RAPID IMMUNIZATION SAFETY MONITORING (PRISM)

The VSD is complemented by the vaccine safety portion of the FDA's Sentinel Initiative (**www.fda.gov/safety/FDAsSentinelInitiative/ucm2007250.htm**), called the Post-licensure Rapid Immunization Safety Monitoring (PRISM) system. As of August 2015, through participation of a number of large, national data partners in the United States, PRISM has data on >170 million people, of whom 31 million currently are enrolled and for whom new data are being accumulated (**www.sentinelinitiative. org/**). In addition, linkages have been established between health plans, academic centers, and state immunization information systems to enhance data on vaccine exposure. PRISM currently is conducting retrospective vaccine safety evaluations and is preparing for prospective, active surveillance of FDA-approved vaccines in the United States.

CLINICAL IMMUNIZATION SAFETY ASSESSMENT (CISA) PROJECT

Serious and other uncommon clinically important adverse events (AEs) following immunization rarely occur in prelicensure clinical trials, and health care professionals may see them too infrequently to be able to provide standardized evaluation. In addition, high-quality studies are needed to identify risk factors for AEs following immunization, especially in special populations, and to develop strategies to prevent or reduce the severity of AEs following immunization. The CDC established the CISA Project to improve the understanding of AEs following immunization at the individual-patient level. The CISA Project's goals are: (1) to serve as a vaccine safety resource for consultation on clinical vaccine safety issues, including individual case reviews, and to assist with immunization decision making; (2) to assist the CDC in developing strategies to assess individuals who may be at increased risk of AEs following immunization; and (3) to conduct studies to identify risk factors and preventive strategies for AEs following immunization, particularly in special populations. The CISA Project is a collaboration among the CDC, 7 medical research centers, and other federal partners. The medical research centers have expertise in vaccines and vaccine safety, epidemiology, biostatistics, clinical trials, and a wide range of specialty areas, such as allergy, immunology, neurology, infectious diseases, and obstetrics and gynecology.

The CISA Project advises health care providers who have vaccine safety questions about specific patients residing in the United States involving US-approved vaccines that are not readily answered by Advisory Committee on Immunization Practices (ACIP) or professional medical society guidelines. For example, CISA may provide an opinion on whether a patient who had an AE following immunization after 1 dose of a vaccine should receive a future dose of the same vaccine. In a CISA evaluation, vaccine safety experts from the CDC's Immunization Safety Office and the CISA medical centers meet via scheduled teleconferences to review complex vaccine safety cases from US health care providers. The experts discuss the findings from the case, review the literature on the topic, and form a general assessment and plan. These conclusions are then shared with the health care provider. Advice from the CDC and CISA is meant to assist in decision making rather than provide direct patient management, because patient-management decisions are the responsibility of the treating health care provider. The CISA Project also conducts clinical research to advance knowledge of vaccine safety after licensure. National strategic plans and public health needs guide the research priorities of the CISA Project. Current priority areas for CISA research studies (registered at **www.ClinicalTrials.gov**) include influenza vaccine safety, vaccine safety in people with autoimmune diseases and other special populations, and vaccine safety in pregnant women. The CISA studies complement vaccine safety surveillance systems and usually address clinical vaccine safety questions by prospectively enrolling up to hundreds of subjects. Whereas large linked database systems like the VSD are best used to assess risk for rare, medically attended events in vaccinated populations, CISA is designed to study more common, nonmedically attended events (eg, fever or injection-site reactions) and to collect biological specimens after vaccination. CISA investigators also have access to special populations (eg, people with autoimmune diseases) and links to specialists who care for these patients.

US health care providers who have a vaccine safety question about a specific patient residing in the United States can contact the CDC (**CISAeval@cdc.gov**) to request a

CISA evaluation. All requests are reviewed by CDC medical officers with expertise in vaccine safety, who will determine whether each inquiry should be forwarded to CISA for an in-depth evaluation. Only selected inquiries will be forwarded for a CISA evaluation, and providers will be notified, usually within 1 to 2 weeks, after submission of a request. Clinical vaccine safety questions that are not accepted for a CISA consultation will be addressed through other channels. If the case will be reviewed by CISA, there is no cost to the provider for a CISA evaluation. Current information about the CISA Project is available online (**www.cdc.gov/vaccinesafety/Activities/CISA.html**).

VACCINE INJURY COMPENSATION

The Vaccine Injury Compensation Program (VICP) was established in 1988 as a means to stabilize the nation's vaccine supply by reducing excess liability that could lead vaccine manufacturers to exit the US market. It was developed as an alternative to civil litigation to simplify the process of settling vaccine injury claims. The VICP is a no-fault system in which compensation may be sought if people are thought to have suffered death or other injury as a result of administration of a covered vaccine. It was developed as an alternative to civil litigation to simplify the process of settling vaccine injury claims.

The VICP evaluates injuries that have occurred following administration of a vaccine routinely recommended for children from birth through 18 years of age, although the vaccine recipient and beneficiary can be of any age. Vaccines not routinely recommended for children, including zoster vaccines, pneumococcal polysaccharide vaccine (PPSV23), and the meningococcal B vaccines, are not covered by the VICP. Claims must be filed within 36 months after the first symptom appeared following immunization, and death claims must be filed within 3 years after the first symptom of the vaccine injury or within 2 years of a death and 4 years after the start of the first symptom of the vaccine injury that resulted in the death (**www.hrsa.gov/vaccinecompensation/fileclaim.html**). People seeking compensation for alleged injuries from covered vaccines must first file claims with the VICP before pursuing civil litigation against manufacturers or vaccine providers. For a death or other injury, reasonable fees for legal representation and related costs may be paid if the claim was filed on a reasonable basis and in good faith. To ensure that legal expenses are not a barrier to entry into the program, and assuming that certain minimal requirements are met, the VICP may pay lawyer's fees and other legal costs related to a claim, regardless of whether the claimant is paid for a vaccine injury or death. If the claimant accepts the judgment of the VICP, neither vaccine providers nor manufacturers can be sued in civil litigation. If the claimant rejects the VICP judgment, he or she has the option of filing a claim against the health care professional on such grounds as failure to adequately warn, negligent vaccine administration, or negligent postvaccination care.

The VICP is based on the Vaccine Injury Table (VIT [see Appendix III, p 1058] or **www.hrsa.gov/vaccinecompensation/vaccinetable.html**), which lists the vaccines covered by the program as well as injuries, disabilities, illnesses, and conditions (including death) for which compensation may be awarded. The VIT defines the time during which the first symptoms or significant aggravation of an injury must appear after immunization. If an injury listed in the VIT is proven, claimants receive a "legal presumption of causation," thus avoiding the need to prove causation in an individual case. If the claim pertains to conditions not listed in the VIT, claimants may prevail if they prove causation.

In 2009 a separate program, the Countermeasure Injury Compensation Program, was created to cover medical countermeasures developed and/or used in response to public health emergencies, such as in an influenza pandemic or a bioterrorism attack (eg, smallpox, anthrax, or botulism). The 21st Century Cures Act, signed into law in December 2016, amended the legislation that created the VICP to include coverage for vaccines recommended for routine use in pregnant women, ensuring that both a woman who received a covered vaccine while pregnant and her child (in utero at the time) are covered by the program.

Information about the VICP and the VIT can be obtained from the following: Parklawn Building, 5600 Fishers Lane, Room 11C-26, Rockville, MD 20857; telephone: 800-338-2382; Web site: **www.hrsa.gov/vaccinecompensation.**

People wishing to file a claim for a vaccine injury should telephone or write to the following:

United States Court of Federal Claims
717 Madison Place, NW
Washington, DC 20005-1011
Telephone: 202-357-6400.

Information on the VICP is available to parents or guardians through Vaccine Information Statements (**www.cdc.gov/vaccines/hcp/vis/index.html**), which are required to be provided before administering each dose of vaccines covered through the program.

HYPERSENSITIVITY REACTIONS AFTER IMMUNIZATION

Anaphylaxis to a vaccine or vaccine constituent generally is a contraindication to future vaccination (see Treatment of Anaphylactic Reactions, p 64). However, these and other hypersensitivity reactions to constituents of vaccines are rare. Medications, equipment, and competent staff necessary to respond to these medical emergencies to maintain patency of the airway and to manage cardiovascular collapse should be available to treat anaphylaxis in all settings in which vaccines are administered. This recommendation includes administration of vaccines in schools, pharmacies, or other complementary settings.

Children who have experienced an immediate-type hypersensitivity reaction to a vaccine or vaccine constituent should be evaluated by an allergist before receiving subsequent doses of the suspect vaccine or other vaccines containing one or more of the same ingredients. This evaluation and appropriate allergy testing may determine whether the child currently is allergic to a vaccine component, which vaccines pose a risk, and whether alternative vaccines (without the allergen) are available. Even when the child truly is allergic and no alternative vaccines are available, in almost all cases the risk of remaining unimmunized exceeds the risk of careful vaccine administration under observation where personnel, medications and equipment are available to treat anaphylaxis, should it occur.

Hypersensitivity reactions related to vaccine constituents can be immediate or delayed and often are attributable to an excipient rather than the immunizing agent itself.

IMMEDIATE-TYPE ALLERGIC REACTIONS

Immediate allergic reactions may be caused by the vaccine antigen, residual animal protein, antimicrobial agents, preservatives, stabilizers, or other vaccine components. Almost all anaphylactic reactions to vaccines occur within minutes to 1 to 2 hours after vaccination.

ALLERGIC REACTIONS TO EGG PROTEIN (OVALBUMIN). Current measles and mumps vaccines (and some rabies vaccines) are derived from chicken embryo fibroblast tissue cultures and do not contain significant amounts of egg proteins. Studies indicate that children with egg allergy, even children with severe hypersensitivity, are at low risk of anaphylactic reactions to these vaccines, singly or in combination (eg, measles-mumps-rubella [MMR] or measles-mumps-rubella-varicella [MMRV]), and skin testing with the vaccine may not be predictive of an allergic reaction to immunization. Most immediate hypersensitivity reactions after measles or mumps immunization appear to be reactions to other vaccine components, such as gelatin. Therefore, children with egg allergy may receive MMR or MMRV vaccines without special precautions.

Although both inactivated influenza vaccine (IIV) and live attenuated influenza vaccine (LAIV) are produced in eggs, data have shown that these vaccines are well tolerated by essentially all recipients who have an egg allergy, including severely egg-allergic patients, likely because the volume of ovalbumin in these vaccines is well below the threshold required to induce an allergic reaction. More conservative approaches, such as skin testing or a 2-step graded challenge, no longer are recommended.[1]

Yellow fever vaccine may contain a larger amount of egg protein than influenza vaccines, and there are fewer reports on administering the vaccine to egg-allergic patients. The vaccine package insert describes a protocol involving skin testing the patient with the vaccine and if positive, giving the vaccine in graded doses. Such a procedure would best be performed by an allergist.

ALLERGIC REACTIONS TO GELATIN. Some vaccines, such as MMR, MMRV, varicella, yellow fever, zoster, and some influenza and rabies vaccines, contain gelatin as a stabilizer. The Vero cell culture-derived Japanese encephalitis (JE-VC) vaccine available in the United States does not contain gelatin stabilizers. People with a history of food allergy to gelatin may develop anaphylaxis after receipt of gelatin-containing vaccines. Additionally, people without any apparent clinical allergy to oral ingestion of gelatin may experience an immediate hypersensitivity reaction following injection of a vaccine containing gelatin. In either case, such a patient should be evaluated by an allergist before receiving gelatin-containing vaccines to confirm the gelatin allergy with immediate-type allergy skin testing. If gelatin is found to be the triggering allergen, the vaccine should be administered in graded doses under observation, with competent personnel, medications, and equipment available to manage anaphylaxis.

ALLERGIC REACTIONS TO YEAST. Hepatitis B and human papillomavirus (9vHPV) vaccines are manufactured using recombinant technology in *Saccharomyces cerevisiae* (baker's or brewer's yeast). In theory, vaccine recipients with hypersensitivity to yeast could experience an allergic reaction to these vaccines. Allergy to yeast is rare; however, patients claiming such an allergy should be evaluated by an allergist before receiving

---

[1]American Academy of Pediatrics, Committee on Infectious Diseases. Recommendations for prevention and control of influenza in children, 2017–2018. *Pediatrics.* 2017; 140(4):e20172550

yeast-containing vaccines to confirm the yeast allergy. If the history and testing suggest immediate hypersensitivity, the vaccine should be administered, possibly in graded doses, under observation, with competent personnel, medications, and equipment available to manage anaphylaxis.

ALLERGIC REACTIONS TO LATEX. Dry natural rubber latex contains native proteins that may be responsible for allergic reactions. Some vaccine vial stoppers and syringe plungers contain latex. Other vaccine vials and syringes contain synthetic rubber, which does not pose risk to the latex-allergic child. Information about latex used in vaccine packaging is available in the manufacturer's package inserts or on the CDC Web site (**www.cdc.gov/vaccines/pubs/pinkbook/downloads/appendices/B/latex-table.pdf**). Latex-allergic patients should be evaluated by an allergist before receiving vaccines with natural rubber latex in the packaging to confirm the latex allergy and to administer the vaccine, possibly in graded doses, under observation, with competent personnel, medications, and equipment available to manage anaphylaxis.

DELAYED-TYPE ALLERGIC REACTIONS

As with most cell-mediated, delayed-type allergic reactions, the allergens usually are small molecules. The small molecules present in vaccines include thimerosal, aluminum, and antimicrobial agents.

ALLERGIC REACTIONS TO THIMEROSAL. Most patients with localized or delayed-type hypersensitivity reactions to thimerosal tolerate injection of vaccines containing thimerosal uneventfully or with only temporary swelling at the injection site. This is not a contraindication to receive a vaccine that contains thimerosal.

ALLERGIC REACTIONS TO ALUMINUM. Sterile abscesses or persistent nodules have occurred at the site of injection of certain inactivated vaccines. These abscesses may result from a delayed-type hypersensitivity response to the vaccine adjuvant, aluminum (alum). In some instances, these reactions may be caused by inadvertent subcutaneous inoculation of a vaccine intended for intramuscular use (Table 1.9, p 14). Alum-related abscesses recur frequently with subsequent dose(s) of vaccines containing alum. Only if such reactions were severe would they constitute a contraindication to further vaccination with aluminum-containing vaccines.

ALLERGIC REACTIONS TO ANTIMICROBIAL AGENTS. Many vaccines contain trace amounts of streptomycin, neomycin, and/or polymyxin B. Some people have delayed-type allergic reactions to these agents and may develop an injection site papule 48 to 96 hours after vaccine administration. This minor reaction is not a contraindication to future doses of vaccines containing these agents. People with a history of an anaphylactic reaction to one of these antimicrobial agents should be evaluated by an allergist before receiving vaccines containing them. No vaccine currently approved for use in the United States contains penicillin or its derivatives, cephalosporins, or fluoroquinolones.

OTHER VACCINE REACTIONS

People who have high serum concentrations of tetanus immunoglobulin (Ig) G antibody, usually as the result of frequent booster immunizations, may have an increased incidence of large injection site swelling after vaccine administration, presumed to be immune complex mediated (Arthus reaction). These reactions are self-limited and do not contraindicate future doses of vaccines at appropriate intervals. Such reactions had been thought to be common with tetanus-containing vaccines, but studies suggest that the reactions are uncommon, even with short intervals between immunizations. Therefore, when indicated, Tdap should be administered regardless of interval since the last tetanus-containing vaccine.

Reactions resembling serum sickness have been reported in approximately 6% of patients after a booster dose of human diploid rabies vaccine, probably resulting from sensitization to human albumin that had been altered chemically by the virus-inactivating agent. Such patients should be evaluated by an allergist but likely will be able to receive additional vaccine doses.

Passive Immunization

Passive immunization entails administration of preformed antibody to a recipient and, unlike active immunization, confers immediate protection but for only a short period of time. Passive immunization is indicated in the following general circumstances for prevention or amelioration of infectious diseases:

- As replacement, when people are deficient in synthesis of antibody as a result of congenital or acquired antibody production defects, alone or in combination with other immunodeficiencies (eg, immunosuppressive therapy, severe combined immunodeficiency, or human immunodeficiency virus [HIV] infection).
- Prophylactically, when a person susceptible to a disease is exposed to or has a high likelihood of exposure to a specific infectious agent, especially when that person has a high risk of complications from the disease or when time does not permit adequate protection by active immunization alone (eg, Rabies Immune Globulin, Varicella Zoster Immune Globulin, Hepatitis B Immune Globulin).
- Therapeutically, when a disease already is present, whereby administration of preformed antibodies (ie, passive immunization) may ameliorate or aid in suppressing the effects of a toxin (eg, foodborne, wound, or infant botulism; diphtheria; or tetanus), ameliorate or suppress clinical disease (eg, anthrax, vaccinia, post-transplantation hepatitis B, post-transplantation cytomegalovirus [CMV]), or suppress the inflammatory response (eg, Kawasaki disease).

Passive immunization can be accomplished with several types of products. The choice is dictated by the types of products available, the type of antibody desired, the route of administration, timing, and other considerations. These products include standard Immune Globulin (IG) for intramuscular (IM) use; standard Immune Globulin Intravenous (IGIV); hyperimmune globulins, some of which are for intramuscular use (eg, hepatitis B, rabies, tetanus, varicella) and some of which are for intravenous use (eg, botulism, CMV, vaccinia); antibodies of animal origin (eg, foodborne botulism, black widow spider, coral snake, rattlesnake, and scorpion antitoxins); and monoclonal antibodies (eg, respiratory syncytial virus [RSV]). Although the use of Immune Globulin Subcutaneous (Human [IGSC]) for replacement has become increasingly common, IGSC usually is not preferred for prophylactic or therapeutic use because of the slower absorption and diminished bioavailability compared with IGIV.

Indications for administration of IG preparations other than those relevant to infectious diseases or Kawasaki disease are not reviewed in the *Red Book*.

Immune Globulin Intramuscular (IGIM)

IGIM is derived from pooled plasma of adults by a cold ethanol fractionation procedure (Cohn fraction II). IGIM consists of at least 90% immunoglobulin (Ig) G with trace amounts of IgA and IgM, is treated with solvent/detergent to inactivate lipid-enveloped viruses, is sterile, and is not known to transmit any virus or other infectious agent. IGIM is a concentrated protein solution (approximately 16.5% or 165 mg/mL) containing specific antibodies that reflect the infectious and immunization experience of the population from whose plasma the IGIM was prepared. Many donors (1000 to 60 000 donors per lot of final product) are used to include a broad spectrum of antibodies. Products sold in the United States are derived from plasma collected exclusively in US-licensed facilities.

IGIM is licensed and recommended for IM administration. Therefore, IGIM should be administered deep into a large muscle mass (see Site and Route of Immunization, p 27). Ordinarily, no more than 5 mL should be administered at one site in an adult, adolescent, or large child; a lesser volume per site (1–3 mL) should be given to small children and infants. Health care professionals should refer to the package insert for total maximal dose at one time. Peak serum concentrations usually are achieved 2 to 3 days after IM administration.

Standard human IGIM should not be administered intravenously. Intradermal use of IGIM is not recommended. Specific preparations of subcutaneous IG have been shown to be safe and effective in children and adults with primary immune deficiencies (see Immune Globulin Subcutaneous, p 62).

INDICATIONS FOR THE USE OF IGIM

REPLACEMENT THERAPY IN ANTIBODY DEFICIENCY DISORDERS. Most experts no longer consider IGIM appropriate for replacement therapy in immunodeficiency because of the pain of administration and the inability to achieve therapeutic blood concentrations of IgG. If IGIM is used for this indication, the usual dose (limited by muscle mass and the volume that should be administered) is 100 mg/kg (equivalent to 0.66 mL/kg) every 3 weeks. Customary practice is to administer twice this dose initially and to adjust the interval between administration of the doses (2–4 weeks) on the basis of trough IgG concentrations and clinical response (absence of or decrease in infections).

HEPATITIS A PROPHYLAXIS. In people 12 months through 40 years of age, hepatitis A immunization is preferred over IGIM for postexposure prophylaxis against hepatitis A virus infection, for people not previously vaccinated against hepatitis A. Hepatitis A vaccination anytime before departure is recommended for protection of travelers going to areas with high or intermediate hepatitis A endemicity. For people younger than 12 months or older than 40 years, immunocompromised people of all ages, and people with chronic liver disease, IGIM is preferred, because adequate responses to vaccination cannot be guaranteed (see Hepatitis A, p 392). IGIM is not indicated for people with clinical manifestations of hepatitis A infection or for people exposed to hepatitis A more than 14 days earlier.

MEASLES PROPHYLAXIS. IGIM administered to exposed, measles-susceptible (not previously vaccinated or immunocompromised) people will prevent or attenuate infection if administered within 6 days of exposure (see Measles, p 537). The effectiveness of IGIM is titer-dependent. Vaccine eligible people 12 months or older exposed to measles should preferably receive MMR vaccine, if it can be administered within 72 hours of initial exposure. Vaccination with MMR is recommended in nonimmune people exposed to measles who received IG. Measles vaccine and IGIM should not be administered at the same time. The appropriate interval between IGIM administration and measles immunization varies with the dose of IGIM and the specific product (see Table 1.13, p 40).

RUBELLA PROPHYLAXIS. IGIM administered to rubella-susceptible pregnant women after rubella exposure may decrease the risk of fetal infection but should only be offered to women who decline a therapeutic abortion (see Rubella, p 705). Infants with congenital rubella syndrome have been born to women who received IG shortly after exposure. IG has not been shown to prevent rubella or mumps infection after exposure and is not recommended for these purposes.

ADVERSE REACTIONS TO IGIM

- Almost all recipients experience local discomfort, and many experience pain at the site of IGIM administration that is related to the volume administered per injection site. Discomfort is lessened if the preparation is at room temperature at the time of injection. Less common reactions include flushing, headache, chills, and nausea.
- Serious reactions are uncommon; these reactions can be anaphylactic or anaphylactoid in nature and manifest as chest pain or constriction, dyspnea, or hypotension and shock. An increased risk of systemic reaction results from inadvertent intravenous administration. Standard IGIM should not be administered intravenously. People requiring repeated doses of IGIM have been reported to experience systemic reactions, such as fever, chills, sweating, and shock.
- IGIM should not be administered to people with known selective IgA deficiency (serum IgA concentration <7 mg/dL; IgG and IgM concentrations normal). Because IGIM contains trace amounts of IgA, people who have selective IgA deficiency may develop anti-IgA antibodies on rare occasions and on a subsequent dose of IGIM may experience an anaphylactic reaction with systemic symptoms such as chills, fever, and shock. In rare cases in which reactions related to anti-IgA antibodies have occurred, subsequent use of a licensed IGIV preparation with the lowest IgA concentration may decrease the likelihood of further reactions. Because these reactions are rare, routine screening for IgA deficiency is not recommended.

PRECAUTIONS FOR THE USE OF IGIM

- Caution should be used when administering IGIM to a patient with a history of adverse reactions to IGIM. In this circumstance, some experts recommend administering a test dose (1%–10% of the intended dose) before the full dose.
- Although systemic reactions to IGIM are rare (see Adverse Reactions to IGIM, above), epinephrine and other means of treating serious, acute reactions (eg, saline for intravenous administration) should be immediately available. Health care professionals administering IGIM should have training in the management of emergencies (particularly anaphylactic shock).
- Unless the benefit will outweigh the risk, IGIM should not be used in patients with severe thrombocytopenia or any coagulation disorder that would preclude IM injection. In such cases, use of IGIV is recommended.

Table 1.14. Uses of Immune Globulin Intravenous (IGIV) for Which There is Approval by the US Food and Drug Administration[a]

Primary immunodeficiency disorders such as common variable immunodeficiency, X-linked agammaglobulinemia, Wiskott-Aldrich syndrome

Kawasaki disease, for prevention of coronary aneurysms

Immune-mediated thrombocytopenia, to increase platelet count

Secondary immunodeficiency attributable to therapy for B-cell chronic lymphocytic leukemia or autoimmunity

Chronic inflammatory demyelinating polyneuropathy, to improve neuromuscular disability

Multifocal motor neuron neuropathy, to improve muscle strength

Reduction of serious bacterial infection in children with HIV infection

[a]Not all IGIV products are approved by the FDA for all indications.

Immune Globulin Intravenous (IGIV)

IGIV is a highly purified preparation of IgG antibodies extracted from the pooled plasma of 1000 to 60 000 qualified adult donors using methods that vary by manufacturer. IGIV comprises more than 95% IgG, with trace amounts of IgA and IgM. IGIV is available as a lyophilized powder or as a formulated liquid solution, with final concentrations of IgG ranging from 3% to 12%, depending on the product. IGIV does not contain thimerosal or any other preservative. IGIV products vary in their sodium content, type of stabilizing excipients (eg, sugars, amino acids), osmolarity/osmolality, pH, IgA content, and recommended infusion rate. Each of these factors may contribute to tolerability and the risk of serious adverse events. All IGIV preparations must have a minimum concentration of antibodies to measles virus, *Corynebacterium diphtheriae* toxoid, poliovirus, and hepatitis B virus. Antibody concentrations against other pathogens, such as *Streptococcus pneumoniae*, cytomegalovirus, and respiratory syncytial virus, vary widely among products and even between lots from the same manufacturer.

INDICATIONS FOR THE USE OF IGIV

IGIV preparations available in the United States currently are licensed by the US Food and Drug Administration (FDA) for use in 7 conditions (Table 1.14). IGIV products may be useful for other conditions, although demonstrated efficacy from controlled trials is not available for many of them. Blood sample(s) needed for diagnostic serologic tests for infectious diseases or to evaluate for immunologic disorders must be obtained before IGIV administration, because antibodies present in IGIV will confound test interpretation.

All IGIV products are licensed to prevent serious infections in primary immunodeficiency, but not all licensed products are approved for the other indications listed in Table 1.14. In some cases, only a single product has certain indications. Therapeutic differences among IGIV products from different manufacturers may exist, but there are no comparative clinical trials of currently available products. Most experts believe that licensed IGIV and IGSC products are therapeutically equivalent. Among the licensed IGIV products, but not necessarily for each product individually, indications for prevention or treatment of infectious diseases in children and adolescents include the following:

- **Replacement therapy in antibody-deficiency disorders.** The typical dose of IGIV in primary immune deficiency is 400 to 600 mg/kg but may be as much as 800 mg/kg or more, administered by IV infusion approximately every 21 to 28 days. Dose and frequency of infusions should be based on clinical effectiveness in an individual patient and in conjunction with an expert on primary immune deficiency disorders. When possible, the same brand of IGIV should be administered longitudinally, because changing products is associated with an increased risk of adverse reactions.

- **Kawasaki disease.** Administration of IGIV at a dose of 2 g/kg as a single dose within the first 10 days of onset of fever, when combined with salicylate therapy, decreases the frequency of coronary artery abnormalities and shortens the duration of symptoms. IGIV treatment for children with symptoms of Kawasaki disease for more than 10 days is recommended, although data on efficacy are not available (see Kawasaki Disease, p 490). Repeat doses of IGIV may be indicated for refractory Kawasaki disease.

- **Pediatric HIV infection.** In children with HIV infection and hypogammaglobulinemia, IGIV may be used to prevent serious bacterial infection.[1] IGIV also might be considered for HIV-infected children who have recurrent serious bacterial infection but is recommended only in unusual circumstances (see Human Immunodeficiency Virus Infection, p 459).

- **Varicella postexposure prophylaxis.** If Varicella-Zoster Immune Globulin (VariZIG) is not available, IGIV can be considered for use in certain seronegative people up to 10 days after exposure to a person with varicella or zoster (see Varicella-Zoster Infections, p 869). For maximum benefit, it should be administered as soon as possible after exposure. It is preferable to use licensed VariZIG, because varicella titers in IGIV are not tested or controlled and may be significantly lower than those in VariZIG.

IGIV has been used for many other conditions, some of which are listed below.

- **Low birth weight infants.** Results of most clinical trials have indicated that IGIV does not decrease the incidence or mortality rate of late-onset infections in infants who weigh less than 1500 g at birth. IGIV is not recommended for routine use in preterm infants to prevent early-onset or late-onset infection.

- **Guillain-Barré syndrome, chronic inflammatory demyelinating polyneuropathy, and multifocal motor neuropathy.** In Guillain-Barré syndrome, chronic inflammatory demyelinating polyneuropathy, and multifocal motor neuropathy, IGIV treatment has been demonstrated to have efficacy equivalent to that of plasmapheresis and is easier to manage.

- **Toxic shock syndrome.** IGIV has been administered to patients with severe staphylococcal or streptococcal toxic shock syndrome and necrotizing fasciitis. Therapy appears most likely to be beneficial when used early in the course of illness.

- **Other potential uses.** IGIV may be useful for sustained hypogammaglobulinemia

---

[1]Panel on Opportunistic Infections in HIV-Exposed and HIV-Infected Children. *Guidelines for the Prevention and Treatment of Opportunistic Infections in HIV-Exposed and HIV-Infected Children.* Washington, DC: Department of Health and Human Services; 2013. Available at: **https://aidsinfo.nih.gov/guidelines/html/5/pediatric-oi-prevention-and-treatment-guidelines/0**

secondary to anti-B cell therapy for autoimmunity or malignancy, severe anemia caused by parvovirus B19 infection, neonatal autoimmune thrombocytopenia that is unresponsive to other treatments, immune-mediated neutropenia, decompensation in myasthenia gravis, dermatomyositis, polymyositis, and severe thrombocytopenia that is unresponsive to other treatments.

SAFETY OF IGIV

Following an outbreak of hepatitis C virus infection associated with IGIV in the United States in 1993, changes in the preparation of IGIV, including additional viral inactivation steps (such as solvent/detergent exposure, pH 4 incubation, trace enzyme exposure, nanofiltration, and heat treatment), have been instituted to prevent transmission of hepatitis C virus and other enveloped viruses, nonenveloped viruses, and prions via IG preparations. Most manufacturers use 3 or 4 different pathogen removal/inactivation procedures. All products currently available in the United States are believed to be free of known pathogens. HIV infection never has been transmitted by any IGIV product licensed in the United States.

ADVERSE REACTIONS TO IGIV

INFUSION REACTIONS. Reactions such as fever, headache, myalgia, chills, nausea, and vomiting often are related to the rate of IGIV infusion and may occur in as many as 25% of patients. These systemic adverse events usually are mild to moderate and self-limited (Table 1.15, p 61). The cause of most acute reactions, however, is uncertain. Product-to-product variations in adverse effects occur among individual patients, but it is not possible, at this time, to predict the reactogenicity of one product relative to others.

SERIOUS ADVERSE REACTIONS. Acute, severe reactions including hypersensitivity and anaphylactoid reactions occur infrequently and are marked by flushing, changes in blood pressure, tachycardia, and shock. Anaphylactic reactions induced by anti-IgA are very rare and only occur in some patients with selective IgA deficiency (ie, total absence of circulating IgA, IgA <7 mg/dL, with normal anti-protein antibody forming ability) who have been previously sensitized to IgA or rarely in patients with common variable immunodeficiency who develop IgE antibodies to IgA and a small number of patients with primary humoral immunodeficiency. Infusion of licensed IGIV products with a low concentration of IgA may reduce the likelihood of further reactions but rarely is needed. Because of the extreme rarity of these reactions, screening for IgA deficiency is not recommended. An assay for anti-IgA antibodies is not available.

Potentially life-threatening adverse reactions include thrombosis, isoimmune hemolysis, renal insufficiency and failure, aseptic meningitis, noncardiogenic pulmonary edema, and transfusion-related acute lung injury. Products are screened for antibody to A and B blood group antigens (hemolysis risk) and coagulation factor 11 (FXIa) contamination (thrombosis risk). Although products now are tested for presence of thrombotic substances, occasional events still may occur, particularly in patients with underlying thrombosis risk factors. Renal failure occurs mainly in patients with preexisting renal dysfunction and diabetes mellitus. Renal failure also may occur secondary to acute hemolysis mediated by isoagglutinins.

Table 1.15. Managing IGIV Reactions[a]

Timing	Symptoms	Management
During infusion	Anaphylactic/ anaphylactoid	Stop the infusion. Administer epinephrine and fluid support, diphenhydramine, and glucocorticoid.
	Headache, fever, chills, sinus tenderness, cough, mild hypotension	Slow the infusion until symptoms resolve. Administer diphenhydramine, NSAID; consider glucocorticoid. When symptoms resolve, the infusion rate may be increased. Pretreatment with NSAID, diphenhydramine, or glucocorticoid or a combination may lessen or prevent a reaction.
After infusion	Headache	Administer NSAID, tryptan, glucocorticoid. Consider an alternative product if there are repeated reactions.
	Myalgia/malaise	Administer NSAID, glucocorticoid. Consider an alternative product if there are repeated reactions.

NSAID indicates nonsteroidal anti-inflammatory drug.
[a]There are no studies of the management of IGIV adverse effects, only expert opinion.

Hemolytic events are observed mainly in patients with A, B, or AB blood types receiving high doses of IGIV (approximately 80% of patients received ≥1.5 g/kg). Patients receiving high doses of IGIV should be monitored for hemolysis, which can be acute or can evolve over 5 to 10 days. Complications of severe hemolysis include need for transfusion, renal failure, and rarely, disseminated intravascular coagulation. If transfusion is needed, type O blood cells are recommended. Aseptic meningitis syndrome beginning several hours to 2 days following IGIV treatment may be associated with severe headache, nuchal rigidity, fever, nausea, and vomiting. Pleocytosis frequently is present in the cerebrospinal fluid.

Clinicians should be mindful of risk factors for these adverse reactions including hypertension, diabetes mellitus, history of thrombosis, other thrombotic risk factors, prior renal compromise, and underlying hyperviscosity. The risk of some reactions can be mitigated by limiting the dose and infusion rate or by subcutaneous administration (see Immune Globulin Subcutaneous, p 62).

The rate and type of adverse events is one factor that should be considered when deciding on a mode of IG administration.

PRECAUTIONS FOR THE USE OF IGIV

- Caution should be used when administering IGIV to a patient with a history of adverse reactions to IG.
- Because acute anaphylactic or anaphylactoid reactions to IGIV can occur (see Adverse Reactions to IGIV, p 60), experienced personnel, medications, and equipment to manage anaphylaxis should be immediately available. If an anaphylactic or anaphylactoid reaction occurs, the risk versus benefit of further infusions should be evaluated. If IG therapy is continued, IGSC or enzyme-facilitated subcutaneous

infusion (see Immune Globulin Subcutaneous, p 62) is recommended because of the decreased incidence of systemic adverse events compared with IGIV. Whichever modality of administration is used, the product that elicited the reaction should not be used again.

- As practitioners have gained experience with IGSC (see Immune Globulin Subcutaneous, p 62), many experts recommend a change to subcutaneous administration instead of manipulating methods of IV infusion or administering premedications to patients who have had reactions.

- Reducing either the rate of infusion or the IGIV dose often can alleviate mild to moderate infusion-related nonallergic adverse reactions (excluding life-threatening subacute adverse events). Patients sensitive to one product often tolerate alternative products. Although there are no studies to support the practice, most experts pretreat patients who have experienced significant reactions with a nonsteroidal anti-inflammatory agent such as ibuprofen or aspirin, acetaminophen, diphenhydramine, or a glucocorticoid (prednisone, 1 mg/kg; solucortef, 5–6 mg/kg in children or 100–150 mg in adults; or solumedrol, 1–2 mg/kg in children or 40–60 mg in adults) to modify or relieve symptoms. Significant adverse effects of IGIV administration should prompt consultation with an immunologist or other specialist experienced in managing this problem.

- Seriously ill patients with compromised cardiac function who are receiving large volumes of IGIV may be at increased risk of vasomotor or cardiac complications manifested as elevated blood pressure, cardiac failure, or both. In this setting, a low-sodium, high-IgG concentration product should be used if available.

- Screening for selective IgA deficiency is not recommended routinely for potential recipients of IGIV (see Adverse Reactions to IGIV, p 60).

Immune Globulin Subcutaneous (IGSC)

Subcutaneous (SC) administration of IG using manual syringe push, mechanical, or battery-driven pumps has been shown to be safe and effective in adults and children with primary immunodeficiencies. Many experts prefer IGSC, particularly in small children, because SC administration obviates the need for intravenous access and avoids implanted venous access devices. Smaller doses, administered more frequently (ie, daily to biweekly), result in markedly less fluctuation of serum IgG concentrations between infusions. For IGIV, there are troughs and peaks in serum IgG concentration, but IGSC achieves a more consistent concentration following achievement of steady-state. The efficacy of IGSC in preventing infection is at least comparable with that of IGIV.

Both mild and severe systemic reactions are substantially less frequent than with IGIV therapy, and most parents or patients can be taught to infuse at home. The most common adverse effects of IGSC are infusion-site reactions, including local swelling, redness, itching, soreness, induration, and local heat, which most often occur soon after completion of infusion and generally resolve over the next 1 to 2 days. Such reactions occur more frequently during the first months of treatment. The most common systemic reaction is headache. Systemic infusion reactions should be treated as discussed for IGIV (p 60). Infusing daily to several times a week decreases or eliminates systemic adverse effects in most patients.

Table 1.16. Choosing a Route of IG Administration

Attribute	IGIV	Conventional IGSC	IGHY
Infusion frequency	Typically every 3–4 weeks	Most often daily to every 2 weeks	Every 2–4 weeks
Administration requirements	IV access, usually by a health care provider	No IV access, self-administered	No IV access, self-administered or by a health care provider
Dose (relative to IV)	100%	137%	100%
Sites/month	1	4–30	1–2
Systemic adverse events	Higher than with IGSC	Lower than with IGIV	Lower than IGIV
Local adverse events	Infrequent	Common	Similar to conventional IGSC

Factors involved in selection of IGSC versus IGIV are listed in Table 1.16. Four products are licensed in the United States for conventional SC use (Hizentra 20% IG [CSL Behring, King of Prussia, PA], Gammagard 10% IG [Baxalta/Shire, Bannockburn, IL], Cuvitru 20% IG [Baxalta/Shire], and Gamunex-C 10% IG [Grifols USA, LLC, Los Angeles, CA]). There are limited data on the efficacy of IGSC for conditions requiring high-dose IG. Only IGIV should be used for the treatment of Kawasaki disease. There is limited evidence on the use of high-dose IGSC for immunomodulation for autoimmune neurologic conditions, and clinical trials are currently underway for these indications. There are reports that IGSC is well tolerated in thrombocytopenic and patients receiving anticoagulant therapy.

Because the subcutaneous space limits infusion volume (typically to a maximum of 30 mL/site), multiple infusion sites and frequent infusions are needed to achieve an adequate IG dose using conventional IGSC. Pretreatment with recombinant human hyaluronidase (IGHY) permits the subcutaneous infusion of large volumes (up to 600 mL) of IG at a single site. The efficacy of IGHY products is comparable with that of standard IGSC and of IGIV. The infusion frequency and number of needle sticks for IGHY approach those for IGIV; the rate of systemic adverse events is less than half that following IGIV. One IGHY product is licensed in the US (HyQvia [Baxalta, Bannockburn, IL]). The serum IgG peak achieved following IGHY administration occurs several days following infusion and the level is far lower than that of IGIV. Unlike the consistent steady-state serum concentration achieved following IGSC, trough concentrations associated with IGHY are comparable with those following administration of IGIV.

PRECAUTIONS FOR THE USE OF IGSC AND IGHY

- Caution should be used when administering IGSC to a patient with a history of adverse reactions to IGSC. In this circumstance, most experts recommend use of an alternate product. Some suggest administering a fraction (1/30) of the monthly dose daily.

- Although immediate, systemic reactions to IGSC are substantially less common and usually less severe than with IGIV (see Adverse Reactions to IGIV, p 60), epinephrine should be immediately available (ie, epinephrine autoinjector). Health care professionals administering IGSC should have training in the management of emergencies (particularly anaphylactic shock). Parents and patients should be trained on the use of epinephrine autoinjector in case of anaphylaxis.
- Life-threatening, subacute systemic adverse reactions (thrombosis, hemolysis, renal injury) appear to be less common following IGSC than with IGIV but do occur (see Adverse Reactions to IGIV, p 60). Clinicians should be mindful of risk factors for adverse reactions (hypertension, diabetes mellitus, history of thrombosis, renal compromise, and hyperviscosity), because high-dose, IV route, and rapid rate of administration are additive risk factors as well.

Treatment of Anaphylactic Reactions

Health care professionals administering biologic products or serum must be able to recognize and be prepared to treat systemic anaphylaxis. Medications, equipment, and competent staff necessary to maintain the patency of the airway and to manage cardiovascular collapse must be available.[1] In the event of a severe reaction requiring interventions beyond the capacity of the initial treatment team, emergency medical services should be requested to initiate additional emergency care prior to and during transport to a site for higher level of care.

The emergency treatment of systemic anaphylactic reactions is based on the type of reaction. In all instances, epinephrine is the primary drug. Delayed administration of epinephrine is thought to be the major contributor to fatalities. Mild manifestations, such as skin reactions alone (eg, pruritus, erythema, urticaria, or angioedema), may be the first signs of an anaphylactic reaction, but intrinsically and in isolation are not dangerous and can be treated with antihistamines. However, using clinical judgment, an injection of epinephrine may be given, depending on the clinical situation (Table 1.17, p 65). Epinephrine should be injected promptly (eg, goal of <4 minutes) for anaphylaxis, which is likely (although not exclusively) occurring if the patient has 2 or more organ systems involved: (1) skin and mucosal involvement (generalized hives, flush, swollen lips/tongue/uvula); (2) respiratory compromise (dyspnea, wheeze, bronchospasm, stridor, or hypoxemia); (3) low blood pressure; or (4) gastrointestinal tract involvement (eg, persistent crampy abdominal pain or vomiting). If a patient is known to have had a previous severe allergic reaction to the biologic product/serum, onset of skin, cardiovascular, or respiratory symptoms alone may warrant treatment with epinephrine.[2] Epinephrine should be administered IM, because higher in vivo concentrations are achieved more rapidly after IM administration. Use of readily available commercial epinephrine autoinjectors (available in 2 dosages by weight; 0.15 and 0.3 mg/dose) are preferred and have been shown to reduce time to drug administration. Aqueous epinephrine (1:1000 dilution, 0.01 mg/kg; maximum dose, 0.5 mg) or autoinjector can be

[1]Hegenbarth MA; American Academy of Pediatrics, Committee on Drugs. Preparing for pediatric emergencies: drugs to consider. *Pediatrics*. 2008;121(2):433–443 (Reaffirmed September 2011, February 2016)

[2]Lieberman P, Nicklas RA, Randolph C, et al. Anaphylaxis–a practice parameter update 2015. *Ann Allergy Asthma Immunol*. 2015;115(5):341–384

administered intramuscularly every 5 to 15 minutes, as necessary, to control symptoms and maintain blood pressure. Repeat doses of epinephrine are required in up to 35% of cases of anaphylaxis. Injections can be given at shorter than 5-minute intervals if deemed necessary. Most patients being treated for anaphylaxis should be placed in a supine position. If a patient is having difficulty breathing, he or she may be asked to sit up. When the patient's condition improves and remains stable, oral antihistamines and possibly oral corticosteroids (1.5–2.0 mg/kg per day of prednisone; maximum, 60 mg/day) can be given for an additional 24 to 48 hours.

Maintenance of the airway and administration of oxygen should be instituted promptly. Administration of oxygen is the second most important therapeutic intervention in the treatment of anaphylaxis, after administration of epinephrine. Severe or potentially life-threatening systemic anaphylaxis involving severe bronchospasm, laryngeal edema, other airway compromise, shock, and cardiovascular collapse necessitates additional therapy. Rapid IV infusion of physiologic saline solution, lactated Ringer solution, or other isotonic solution adequate to maintain blood pressure must be instituted to compensate for the loss of circulating intravascular volume.

Epinephrine is administered intramuscularly immediately while IV access is being established. IV epinephrine (note further dilution: 1:10 000 dilution) may be indicated for bolus infusion and is provided in most emergency carts (see Table 1.17). Administration of epinephrine intravenously can lead to lethal arrhythmia; cardiac monitoring is recommended. A slow, continuous, low-dose infusion is preferable to repeated bolus administration, because the dose can be titrated to the desired effect, and accidental administration of large boluses of epinephrine can be avoided. Nebulized albuterol is indicated for bronchospasm (see Table 1.18, p 66). In some cases, the use of other inotropic agents, such as dopamine (see Table 1.18), may be necessary for blood pressure support. The combination of histamine H_1 and H_2 receptor-blocking agents (see Table 1.18) may be synergistic in effect and could be used as adjunctive therapy. Corticosteroids have no role in the acute treatment of anaphylaxis but generally are recommended for most cases of anaphylaxis to decrease the likelihood of a biphasic or prolonged reaction, although the evidence for this practice is weak (see Table 1.18).

Table 1.17. Epinephrine in the Treatment of Anaphylaxis[a]

Intramuscular (IM) administration
Epinephrine 1:1000 (1 mg/mL)(aqueous): IM (anterolateral thigh), 0.01 mL/kg per dose, up to 0.5 mL, repeated every 5–15 min, up to 3 doses[b]

Intravenous (IV) administration
An initial bolus of IV epinephrine is given to patients not responding to IM epinephrine using a dilution of 1:10 000 (0.1 mg/mL) rather than a dilution of 1:1000. This dilution can be made using 1 mL of the 1:1000 dilution in 9 mL of physiologic saline solution. The dose is 0.01 mg/kg or 0.1 mL/kg of the 1:10 000 dilution. A continuous infusion should be started if repeated doses are required. One milligram (1 mL) of 1:1000 dilution of epinephrine added to 250 mL of 5% dextrose in water, resulting in a concentration of 4 μg/mL, is infused initially at a rate of 0.1 μg/kg per minute and increased gradually to 1 μg/kg per minute to maintain blood pressure.

[a] In addition to epinephrine, maintenance of the airway and administration of oxygen are critical.
[b] If agent causing anaphylactic reaction was given by injection, epinephrine can be injected into the same site to slow absorption.

Table 1.18. Dosages of Commonly Used Secondary Drugs in the Treatment of Anaphylaxis

Drug	Dose
H₁ receptor-blocking agents (antihistamines)	
Diphenhydramine	Oral, IM, IV: 1–2 mg/kg, every 4–6 h (40 mg, maximum single dose <12 y; 100 mg, maximum single dose for 12 y and older)
Hydroxyzine	Oral, IM: 0.5–1 mg/kg, every 4–6 h (100 mg, maximum single dose)
Cetirizine	Oral: 2.5 mg, 6–23 mo; 2.5–5 mg, 2–5 y; 5–10 mg, >5 y (single dose daily)
H₂ receptor-blocking agents (also antihistamines)	
Cimetidine	IV: 5 mg/kg, slowly over a 15-min period, every 6–8 h (300 mg, maximum single dose)
Ranitidine	IV: 1 mg/kg, slowly over a 15-min period, every 6–8 h (50 mg, maximum single dose)
Corticosteroids	
Methylprednisolone	IV: 1 mg/kg, every 4–6 h (125 mg, maximum single dose)
Prednisone	Oral: 1.5–2 mg/kg, single morning dose (60 mg, maximum single dose); use corticosteroids as long as needed
B₂-agonist	
Albuterol	Nebulizer solution: 0.5% (5 mg/mL), 0.05–0.15 mg/kg per dose in 2–3 mL isotonic sodium chloride solution, maximum 5 mg/dose every 20 min over a 1-h to 2-h period, or 0.5 mg/kg/h by continuous nebulization (15 mg/h, maximum dose)
Vasopressor	
Dopamine	5–20 µg/kg/min IV drip

IM indicates intramuscular; IV, intravenous.

All patients showing signs and symptoms of systemic anaphylaxis, regardless of severity, should be observed for several hours in an appropriate facility, even after remission of immediate symptoms. Anaphylactic reactions can be uniphasic, biphasic, or protracted over 24 to 36 hours despite early and aggressive management. Although a specific period of observation has not been established, a reasonable period of observation would be 4 hours for a mild episode and as long as 24 hours for a severe episode.

Anaphylaxis occurring in people who are taking beta-adrenergic–blocking agents can be more profound and significantly less responsive to epinephrine and other beta-adrenergic agonist drugs. More aggressive therapy with epinephrine may override receptor blockade in some patients. For epinephrine-refractory anaphylaxis, some experts recommend use of IV glucagon (20–30 mg/kg in children; maximum 1 g, administered intravenously over 5 minutes, followed by an infusion at 5 to 15 mg/min titrated to clinical response). Inhaled atropine sometimes is used for management of bradycardia or bronchospasm in these patients. At the time of discharge, all patients should be provided with an epinephrine autoinjector, a written emergency plan to treat future reactions, and a referral to a physician with expertise in managing anaphylaxis and in identifying the etiology, if unknown.

IMMUNIZATION IN SPECIAL CLINICAL CIRCUMSTANCES

Immunization in Preterm and Low Birth Weight Infants

Infants born preterm (at less than 37 weeks of gestation) or of low birth weight (less than 2500 g) who are clinically stable should, with few exceptions, receive all routinely recommended childhood vaccines at the same chronologic age as term and normal birth weight infants. Although studies have shown decreased immune responses to several vaccines administered to neonates with very low birth weight (less than 1500 g) and neonates of very early gestational age (less than 29 weeks of gestation), most preterm infants, including infants who receive dexamethasone for chronic lung disease, produce sufficient vaccine-induced immunity to prevent disease. Vaccine dosages administered to term infants should not be reduced or divided when given to preterm or low birth weight infants.

Preterm and low birth weight infants tolerate most childhood vaccines as well as do term infants. Some studies show that cardiorespiratory events may increase in extremely (less than 1000 g) and very (less than 1500 g) low birth weight infants who receive selected vaccines. Apnea within 24 hours prior to immunization, younger age, or weight less than 2000 g at the time of immunization and 12-hour Score for Neonatal Acute Physiology II[1] greater than 10 have been associated with development of postimmunization apnea, and it may be prudent to monitor infants with these characteristics for 48 hours after immunization if they are still in the hospital. However, these postimmunization cardiorespiratory events do not appear to have a detrimental effect on the clinical course of immunized infants.

Medically stable preterm infants who remain in the hospital at 2 months of chronologic age should receive all inactivated vaccines recommended at that age (see Recommended Immunization Schedule for Children and Adolescents Aged 18 Years or Younger [**http://redbook.solutions.aap.org/SS/Immunization_Schedules. aspx**]). A medically stable infant is defined as one who does not require ongoing management for serious infection; metabolic disease; or acute renal, cardiovascular, neurologic, or respiratory tract illness and who demonstrates a clinical course of sustained recovery and a pattern of steady growth. All immunizations required at 2 months of age can be administered simultaneously to preterm or low birth weight infants, except for oral rotavirus vaccine, which should be deferred until the infant is being discharged from the hospital (see Rotavirus, p 700) to prevent the potential health care-associated spread of this live vaccine virus. The same volume of vaccine used for term infants is appropriate

---

[1]Zupancic JAF, Richardson DK, Horbar JD, Carpenter JH, Lee SK, Escobar GJ. Vermont Oxford Network SNAP Pilot Project Participants. Revalidation of the Score for Neonatal Acute Physiology in the Vermont Oxford Network. *Pediatrics*. 2007;119(1):e156-e163

for medically stable preterm infants. The number of injections of other vaccines at 2 months of age can be minimized by using combination vaccines. When it is difficult to administer 3 or 4 injections simultaneously to hospitalized preterm infants because of limited injection sites, the vaccines recommended at 2 months of age can be administered at different times. Any interval between doses of individual inactivated parenteral vaccines is acceptable. However, to avoid superimposing local reactions, 2-week intervals may be reasonable. The choice of needle lengths used for IM vaccine administration is determined by available muscle mass of the preterm or low birth weight infant (see Table 1.10, p 29).

Hepatitis B vaccine administered to preterm or low birth weight infants weighing 2000 g or more at birth produces an immune response comparable to that in term infants. Medically stable and thriving infants weighing less than 2000 g demonstrate a lower hepatitis B antibody response. Hepatitis B vaccine schedules for infants weighing <2000 g and infants weighing ≥2000 g born to mothers with positive, negative, and unknown hepatitis B surface antigen (HBsAg) status are provided in Hepatitis B, Special Considerations, including Tables 3.24 (p 420) and 3.25 (p 422). Only monovalent hepatitis B vaccine should be used for preterm or term infants younger than 6 weeks. Administration of a total of 4 doses of hepatitis B vaccine is permitted when a combination vaccine containing hepatitis B vaccine is administered after the birth dose.

Because all preterm infants are considered at increased risk of complications of influenza, 2 doses of inactivated influenza vaccine, administered 1 month apart, should be offered for all preterm infants beginning at 6 months of chronologic age as soon as influenza vaccine is available (see Influenza, p 476). Because preterm infants younger than 6 months and infants of any age with chronic complications of preterm birth are extremely vulnerable to influenza virus infection, it is very important that household contacts, child care providers, and hospital nursery personnel caring for preterm infants receive influenza vaccine annually (see Influenza, p 476).

Preterm infants younger than 6 months, who are too young to have completed the primary immunization series, are at increased risk of pertussis infection and pertussis-related complications. Tetanus toxoid, reduced diphtheria toxoid, and acellular pertussis (Tdap) vaccine should be administered to all pregnant women (optimally, early in the interval between weeks 27 and 36 of gestation, to yield high antibody levels in the infant) during every pregnancy. Tdap should be administered immediately postpartum for women who never have received a previous dose of Tdap. Health care personnel caring for pregnant women and infants, and household contacts and child care providers of all infants who have not previously received Tdap, also should be vaccinated (see Pertussis, p 620).

Preterm infants born before 29 weeks, 0 days of gestation; infants born with certain congenital heart defects; and certain infants with chronic lung disease of prematurity or hemodynamically significant heart disease may benefit from monthly immunoprophylaxis with palivizumab (respiratory syncytial virus monoclonal antibody) during respiratory syncytial virus season (see Respiratory Syncytial Virus, p 682). Routine childhood immunizations should be administered on schedule in infants receiving palivizumab.

Preterm infants can receive the first dose of rotavirus vaccine under the following circumstances: the infant is between 6 and 14 weeks, 6 days of chronologic age; the infant is medically stable; and the first dose is administered at the time of or after hospital discharge (see Rotavirus, p 700).

Immunization in Pregnancy[1]

No evidence indicates that routinely recommended vaccines have detrimental effects on the fetus. Increased recognition of the severity of some vaccine-preventable diseases during pregnancy and of the potential benefit of some vaccines to the pregnant woman and to her newborn infant through reducing exposure to the vaccine-preventable disease and/or providing protection through maternally acquired antibodies has led to recommendations for administration of selected vaccines during pregnancy.[2]

Two vaccines now are recommended for routine administration during pregnancy in the United States: tetanus and diphtheria toxoids and acellular pertussis (Tdap) vaccine and inactivated influenza vaccine (IIV).

- **Tdap Vaccine With Each Pregnancy.** The Centers for Disease Control and Prevention (CDC), the American Academy of Pediatrics (AAP), the American College of Obstetricians and Gynecologists (ACOG), and the American Academy of Family Physicians (AAFP) recommend administration of Tdap during every pregnancy to ensure that all newborn infants have the opportunity to receive high concentrations of pertussis-specific antibodies at the time of birth. Administration of Tdap earlier in the interval between 27 and 36 weeks' gestation is preferred to maximize antibodies transferred to the baby, although it may be administered at any time during pregnancy.[3] For women never previously vaccinated with Tdap, if Tdap was not administered during the current pregnancy, Tdap should be administered immediately postpartum. Pregnant women who are unimmunized or only partially immunized against tetanus should complete the primary series, using Tdap for only 1 of the doses. If a Td booster is indicated for wound management during pregnancy, Tdap should be administered if the woman has not already received Tdap during the current pregnancy (see Pertussis, p 620). Studies have not demonstrated safety concerns with administration of Tdap in pregnancy, administration of Tdap concurrently with influenza vaccine during pregnancy, or administration of Tdap after recent receipt of a tetanus-containing vaccine. Observational studies of vaccine effectiveness have demonstrated that Tdap administered during the third trimester of pregnancy reduces pertussis infection in young infants.

- **Inactivated Influenza Vaccine Each Influenza Season.** Studies indicate that women who are pregnant, including those with or without underlying medical conditions, are at increased risk of complications and hospitalization from influenza and that inactivated influenza vaccine (IIV) in pregnancy is beneficial. Studies also have shown that administering IIV in pregnancy can protect infants younger than 6 months who cannot be immunized themselves. Therefore, IIV, using any of the approved vaccines, should be administered to all women who are or will be pregnant during each influenza season, regardless of trimester (see Influenza, p 476). The immunogenicity of IIV has been demonstrated in human immunodeficiency virus (HIV)-infected pregnant women. Live attenuated influenza vaccine (LAIV) should not

---

[1]See adult immunization schedule available at **www.cdc.gov/vaccines/schedules/hcp/adult.html**

[2]**www.cdc.gov/vaccines/pubs/preg-guide.htm**

[3]Centers for Disease Control and Prevention. Updated recommendations for use of tetanus toxoid, reduced diphtheria toxoid, and acellular pertussis vaccine (Tdap) in pregnant women—Advisory Committee on Immunization Practices (ACIP), 2012. *MMWR Morb Mortal Wkly Rep.* 2013;62(7):131–135

be administered to pregnant women at any time.

LIVE-VIRUS VACCINES

Pregnancy is a contraindication to administration of all live-virus vaccines, except when susceptibility and exposure are highly probable and the disease to be prevented poses a greater threat to the pregnant woman or fetus than does the theoretical risk of the vaccine. The background rate of fetal anomalies in otherwise uncomplicated pregnancies may result in a defect that could be attributed inappropriately to a vaccine. Women should be counseled to avoid pregnancy for 4 weeks after receiving live-virus vaccines, although inadvertent administration is not a reason to terminate the pregnancy.

- **Measles, Mumps, Rubella Vaccine.** Measles, mumps, rubella, and varicella vaccines are contraindicated for pregnant women. Efforts should be made to immunize women without evidence of immunity against these illnesses before they become pregnant or in the immediate postpartum period. No case of embryopathy caused by live rubella vaccine has been reported; however, a rare theoretical risk of embryopathy from inadvertent administration cannot be excluded. Because pregnant women might be at higher risk for severe measles and complications, Immune Globulin Intravenous (IGIV) should be administered to pregnant women without evidence of measles immunity who have been exposed to measles. The IGIV dose should be high enough to achieve estimated protective levels of measles antibody titers (see Measles, p 537).

- **Varicella Vaccine.** The effect of the live attenuated varicella vaccine (Oka strain) on the fetus, if any, is unknown. However, because exposure of a nonimmune pregnant woman to wild-type varicella-zoster virus (VZV) might result in congenital varicella syndrome in her fetus, vaccines that contain live, attenuated VZV are contraindicated during pregnancy. Data collected by a Pregnancy Registry to monitor the fetal outcomes of women who inadvertently were given VZV-containing vaccines (VARIVAX, ProQuad, and ZOSTAVAX) during the 3 months before or at any time during pregnancy for more than 18 years (VARIVAX) and 7 years (ProQuad, ZOSTAVAX) found no cases of congenital varicella syndrome and no increased prevalence of other birth defects among women vaccinated. A small, theoretical risk for congenital varicella syndrome (confidence interval, 0%–3.7%) could not be ruled out, because the number of exposures of seronegative women registered each year was low. The registry was discontinued for new enrollments in October 2013 (**www.merckpregnancyregistries.com/varivax.html**).

  A pregnant woman living in the same household is not a contraindication for varicella immunization of a child or other household member. Transmission of vaccine virus from an immunocompetent vaccine recipient to a susceptible person has been reported only rarely and only when a vaccine-associated rash develops in the vaccine recipient (see Varicella-Zoster Infections, p 869). Breastfeeding is not a contraindication for immunization of varicella-susceptible women after pregnancy. Varicella-Zoster Immune Globulin (VariZIG) is recommended for pregnant women without evidence of immunity who have been exposed to natural varicella infection (see Varicella-Zoster Virus Infections, p 869). If VariZIG is not available, some experts suggest use of IGIV; use of acyclovir in this circumstance has not been evaluated.

- **Yellow Fever Vaccine.** Yellow fever vaccine (YF-VAX) is a live attenuated virus vaccine. Whenever possible, pregnant women and nursing mothers should avoid travel to an area where there is high risk of yellow fever. If travel of a pregnant woman cannot be postponed, yellow fever immunization, followed by serologic testing to document the immune response, should be considered. Three cases of YF-VAX–associated neurologic disease (meningoencephalitis and seizures) in exclusively breastfed infants of vaccinated mothers have been reported. Therefore, administration of YF-VAX is a precaution in breastfeeding mothers of infants younger than 9 months because of potential of transmission of vaccine virus in human milk.

- **Smallpox Vaccine.** Vaccinia virus vaccine is a live-virus vaccine and should be administered only when there is a definite exposure to smallpox virus. Because smallpox causes more severe disease in pregnant than nonpregnant women, the risks to the mother and fetus from experiencing the disease may substantially outweigh the risks of immunization. Breastfeeding is contraindicated because of the theoretical risk of contact transmission to the infant. If a woman receives smallpox vaccine during pregnancy or while breastfeeding, she should avoid breastfeeding or handling her infant until the vaccination scab has separated from the vaccination site (approximately 3 weeks). Women who are pregnant should avoid close contact with anyone who has received a smallpox vaccine in the last 28 days, including anyone living in the household.

- **Typhoid Vaccine.** No information is available on the safety of any live or inactivated typhoid vaccines in pregnancy; therefore, generally, it is prudent to avoid vaccinating pregnant women.[1] With consideration of the benefit-to-risk ratio, polysaccharide typhoid vaccine could be considered if the pregnant woman is at high risk for exposure.

INACTIVATED VACCINES

- **Pneumococcal Vaccines.** Pregnant women with underlying conditions that warrant immunization, such as asplenia, diabetes, or others listed in the Recommended Immunization Schedule for Children and Adolescents, may be vaccinated when the benefit of the vaccination is considered to outweigh any potential risks.

- **Meningococcal Vaccines.** Quadrivalent meningococcal conjugate vaccine (MenACWY) may be administered to a pregnant woman when there is increased risk of disease, such as during outbreaks or before travel to an area with hyperendemic infection. Because of lack of information about serogroup B meningococcal vaccine (MenB) in pregnant women, MenB vaccine should be administered during pregnancy only if the woman is at increased risk and if, after consultation with her health care provider, the benefit of vaccination is considered to outweigh the potential risks (**www.cdc.gov/mmwr/preview/mmwrhtml/mm6441a3.htm**).

- **Hepatitis A and Hepatitis B Vaccines.** Infection with hepatitis A virus or hepatitis B virus can result in severe disease in a pregnant woman and, in the case of hepatitis B, chronic infection in the newborn infant. Hepatitis A or hepatitis B immunizations, if indicated, can be administered to pregnant women.

---

[1] wwwnc.cdc.gov/travel/yellowbook/2016/infectious-diseases-related-to-travel/typhoid-paratyphoid-fever

- **Inactivated Poliovirus Vaccine.** Although data on safety of inactivated poliovirus (IPV) vaccine for a pregnant woman or developing fetus are limited, no adverse effect has been found, and no risk would be expected. IPV vaccine can be administered to pregnant women who never have received poliovirus vaccine, are immunized partially, or are immunized completely but require a booster dose (see Poliovirus Infections, p 657). Oral poliovirus (OPV) vaccine should not be administered to pregnant women.

- **Human Papillomavirus Vaccine.** Human papillomavirus (HPV) vaccines are not recommended during pregnancy. Pregnancy testing is not needed before vaccination. If a woman is determined to be pregnant after initiating the immunization series, the remainder of the 2 or 3-dose regimen, as appropriate for age, should be delayed until after completion of the pregnancy. If a vaccine dose has been administered during pregnancy, no intervention is needed.

- **Rabies Virus Vaccine.** Rabies vaccine should be administered to pregnant women after exposure to rabies under the same circumstances as nonpregnant women. No association between rabies immunization and adverse fetal outcomes has been reported. If the risk of exposure to rabies is substantial, preexposure prophylaxis also may be indicated.

- **Anthrax Vaccine.** Anthrax vaccine has not been evaluated for safety in pregnant women, so it should be avoided unless in a postevent situation with a high risk of exposure (see Anthrax, p 214).

- **Japanese Encephalitis Virus Vaccine.** No specific information is available on the safety of Japanese encephalitis virus vaccine for pregnant women. Women should be immunized before conception, if possible. Immunization during pregnancy or while breastfeeding may be considered if travel to an endemic area is unavoidable and the risk of disease outweighs the risk of adverse events in the pregnant woman and fetus (see Arboviruses, p 220).[1]

Immunization and Other Considerations in Immunocompromised Children

The safety and effectiveness of vaccines in people with an immune deficiency depends on the nature and degree of immunosuppression. Because immunocompromised individuals vary in their extent of immunosuppression and susceptibility to infection, they represent a heterogeneous population with regard to immunization. Immunodeficiency conditions can be classified into 2 main disorders: primary and secondary. Primary disorders of the immune system generally are inherited, usually as single-gene disorders; can involve any part of the immune defenses, including B-lymphocyte (humoral) immunity, T-lymphocyte (cell)-mediated immunity, complement and phagocytic function, natural killer cell function, and other innate immunity; and share the common feature of increased susceptibility to infections.[2] Secondary disorders of the immune system are acquired, including in people with HIV infection/acquired immunodeficiency syndrome (AIDS);

---

[1]Centers for Diseases Control and Prevention. Japanese encephalitis virus vaccines—recommendations of the Advisory Committee on Immunization Practices (ACIP). *MMWR Recomm Rep.* 2010;59(RR-01):1–27

[2]Centers for Disease Control and Prevention. Applying public health strategies to primary immunodeficiency diseases: a potential approach to genetic disorders. *MMWR Recomm Rep.* 2004;53(RR-1):1–29

malignant neoplasm; stem cell or solid organ transplantation; functional asplenia (such as in sickle cell disease) or anatomic absence (ie, surgical splenectomy or congenital absence of spleen); people receiving certain biologic response-modifying agents, immunosuppressive, antimetabolic, or radiation therapy; and people with severe malnutrition, protein loss, chronic inflammatory conditions, or uremia (see Table 1.19, p 75). The Infectious Diseases Society of America (IDSA), in conjunction with the American Academy of Pediatrics (AAP), Centers for Disease Control and Prevention (CDC), and other professional societies and organizations, has developed immunization guidelines for children and adults with primary and secondary immune deficiencies[1] (**www.idsociety.org/Templates/Content.aspx?id=32212256011**), which should be consulted for specific conditions, unusual circumstances (eg, international travel), vaccinations for adults, and recommendations for vaccination of hematopoietic stem cell or solid organ transplant recipients. This chapter includes general principles and specific recommendations when the primary care physician is more likely to deliver care without the patient's continuous management by a subspecialist. Subspecialists who care for immunocompromised patients share responsibility with the primary care physician for ensuring appropriate vaccinations for immunocompromised patients, and they share responsibility for recommending appropriate vaccinations for members of patients' households.

GENERAL PRINCIPLES

Certain generalizations regarding degree of immune impairment in patients with a primary or secondary immunodeficiency are useful for the practitioner and were adopted in the IDSA guideline.[1]

High-level immunosuppression includes patients:

- With combined B- and T-lymphocyte primary immunodeficiency (eg, severe combined immunodeficiency [SCID]);
- Receiving cancer chemotherapy;
- Receiving chemotherapeutic agents (eg, cyclophosphamide, methotrexate, mycophenolate) and combination immunosuppressive drugs for rheumatologic conditions
- With HIV infection and a CD4+ T-lymphocyte percentage <15% for children 1 through 13 years, or a CD4+ T-lymphocyte count <200 lymphocytes/mm^3 in adolescents ≥14 years;
- Receiving daily corticosteroid therapy at a dose ≥20 mg (or >2 mg/kg/day for patients weighing <10 kg) of prednisone or equivalent for ≥14 days;
- Receiving certain biologic immune modulators, for example, tumor necrosis factor-alpha (TNF-α) antagonists (eg, adalimumab, certolizumab, infliximab, etanercept, and golimumab), anti–B-lymphocyte monoclonal antibodies (eg, rituximab), or anti-T-lymphocyte monoclonal antibodies (eg, alemtuzumab);
- Within 2 months after receipt of solid organ transplant (SOT); and
- Within 2 months after receipt of hematopoietic stem cell transplant (HSCT) and frequently for a much longer period; HSCT recipients can have prolonged high

[1]Rubin LG, Levin MJ, Ljungman P, et al. 2013 IDSA clinical practice guideline for vaccination of the immunocompromised host. *Clin Infect Dis.* 2014;58(3):309–318. Available at: **www.idsociety.org/Templates/Content.aspx?id=32212256011**

degrees of immunosuppression, depending on type of transplant (longer for allogeneic than for autologous), type of donor and stem cell source, and post-transplant complications, such as graft versus host disease (GVHD) and their treatments. Low-level immunosuppression includes patients:

- With HIV infection without symptoms and with a CD4+ T-lymphocyte percentage ≥15% for children 1 through 13 years, or a CD4+ T-lymphocyte count ≥200 lymphocytes/mm^3 in adolescents ≥14 years;
- Receiving a lower daily dose of systemic corticosteroid than for high-level immunosuppression for ≥14 days, or receiving alternate-day corticosteroid therapy; and
- Receiving methotrexate at a dosage of ≤0.4 mg/kg/week, azathioprine at a dosage of ≤3 mg/kg/day, or 6-mercaptopurine at a dosage of ≤1.5 mg/kg/day.

TIMING OF VACCINES. For patients in whom initiation of immunosuppressive medication is planned, vaccinations should be administered before immunosuppression, when feasible. Live vaccines should be administered as indicated well in advance, and no closer than 4 weeks before initiation of immunosuppression or transplantation. Inactivated vaccines should be administered well in advance and at least 2 weeks before immunosuppression or transplantation. If administration is not possible within these time restrictions, immunization should be deferred.

Certain vaccines may be administered to children while they are modestly immunosuppressed, especially when the immunosuppressed state is likely to be lengthy or lifelong. Examples include inactivated and live vaccines in some HIV-infected children and inactivated vaccines during maintenance chemotherapy for acute leukemia or 2 to 6 months after solid organ transplantation. However, as described further later in this chapter, significant caution is warranted when considering live attenuated vaccine in immunocompromised people. Expert consultation is warranted.

The interval until immune reconstitution following cessation of immunosuppressive therapy varies with the intensity and type of immunosuppressive therapy, radiation therapy, underlying disease, and other factors. Therefore, often it is not possible to make a definitive recommendation for an interval after cessation of immunosuppressive therapy when inactivated vaccines can be administered effectively or when or whether live-virus vaccines can be administered safely and effectively. Immunodeficiency that follows use of certain recombinant human proteins with anti-inflammatory properties, such as the anti–B-lymphocyte monoclonal antibody rituximab, is prolonged such that treated patients are unlikely to respond to vaccines for at least 6 months and often much longer after the last dose (see Biologic Response Modifying Drugs Used to Decrease Inflammation, p 85).

Resumption of vaccinations after reduction or cessation of immunosuppression following transplantation varies depending on the vaccine, underlying disorder, specific immunosuppressive therapy, and presence or absence of GVHD.[1] Timing for inactivated and live-virus vaccines could vary from as early as 3 months after cessation of chemotherapy for acute leukemia to as long as 24 months for measles-mumps-rubella

[1]Rubin LG, Levin MJ, Ljungman P, et al. 2013 IDSA clinical practice guideline for vaccination of the immunocompromised host. *Clin Infect Dis.* 2014;58(3):309–318. Available at: **www.idsociety.org/Templates/Content.aspx?id=32212256011**

Table 1.19. Immunization of Children and Adolescents With Primary and Secondary Immune Deficiencies

Category	Example of Specific Immunodeficiency	Vaccine Contraindications[a]	Comments
Primary			
B lymphocyte (humoral)	Severe antibody deficiencies (eg, X-linked agammaglobulinemia and common variable immunodeficiency)	OPV,[b] BCG, smallpox, YF, and live-bacteria vaccines[c]; no data for rotavirus vaccines	Effectiveness of any vaccine is uncertain if dependent only on humoral response (eg, PPSV23). Replacement IG therapy interferes with response to live vaccines MMR and VAR. Annual IIV is the only vaccine administered routinely to patients receiving IG replacement therapy. All inactivated vaccines are safe to administer as part of immune response assessment prior to instituting IG therapy.
	Less severe antibody deficiencies (eg, selective IgA deficiency and IgG subclass deficiencies)	OPV,[a] BCG, YF; other live-virus vaccines[d] (except YF) appear to be safe	All inactivated and live-virus vaccines on the standard annual schedule are safe, likely are effective (although responses may be attenuated), and should be administered.[e] PPSV23 should be administered beginning at 2 years of age.[f]
T lymphocyte (cell-mediated and humoral)	Complete defects (eg, severe combined immunodeficiency, complete DiGeorge syndrome)	All live-bacteria and live-virus vaccines (including rotavirus vaccine)[c,d,g]	All inactivated vaccines probably are ineffective. Annual IIV is the only vaccine administered routinely to patients receiving IG replacement therapy, if there is some residual antibody-producing capacity.

Table 1.19. Immunization of Children and Adolescents With Primary and Secondary Immune Deficiencies, continued

Category	Example of Specific Immunodeficiency	Vaccine Contraindications[a]	Comments
T lymphocyte (cell-mediated and humoral)	Partial defects (eg, most patients with DiGeorge syndrome, hyperIgM syndrome, Wiskott-Aldrich syndrome, ataxia telangiectasia)	All live-bacteria and live-virus vaccines[c,d,g]	All inactivated vaccines on the standard annual schedule are safe, may be effective depending on the degree of the immune defect, and should be administered.[c] Those with ≥500 CD3+ T lymphocytes/mm³, ≥200 CD8+ T lymphocytes/mm³, and normal mitogen response could be considered to receive MMR and VAR vaccine (but not MMRV). PPSV23 should be administered beginning at 2 years of age.[f] Consider MenACWY-CRM series beginning in infancy[h]; and the MenB series beginning at 10 years of age depending on splenic dysfunction.
	Interferon-alpha; interferon-gamma; interleukin 12 axis deficiencies; STAT1 deficiencies	All live-bacteria vaccines[c] and YF vaccine; other live-virus vaccines[d] if severely lymphopenic	All inactivated vaccines on the standard annual schedule are safe, likely are effective, and should be administered.[c] Based on experience in HIV-infected children with the measles vaccine, MMR and VAR (but not MMRV) probably are safe and may be preferable to the risk of disease. Inactivated typhoid vaccine (Typhoid Vi) is considered for people living in areas with endemic typhoid.
Complement	Persistent complement component, properdin, mannan-binding lectin, or factor B deficiency; secondary deficiency because receiving eculizumab (Soliris)	None	All inactivated and live-virus vaccines on the standard annual schedule are safe, likely are effective, and should be administered.[c] PPSV23 should be administered beginning at 2 years of age[f]; MenACWY-CRM series beginning in infancy[h]; and the MenB series beginning at 10 years of age.

Table 1.19. Immunization of Children and Adolescents With Primary and Secondary Immune Deficiencies, continued

Category	Example of Specific Immunodeficiency	Vaccine Contraindications[a]	Comments
Phagocytic function	Chronic granulomatous disease	Live-bacteria vaccines[c]	All inactivated and live-virus vaccines[d] on the standard annual schedule are safe, likely are effective and should be administered.[e,i]
	Phagocytic deficiencies that are ill-defined or accompanied by defects in T-lymphocyte and natural killer cell dysfunction (such as Chediak-Higashi syndrome, leukocyte adhesion defects, and myeloperoxidase deficiency)	All live-bacteria[c] and live-virus vaccines[d]	All inactivated vaccines on the standard annual schedule are safe, likely are effective, and should be administered. PPSV23 should be administered beginning at 2 years of age.[f] Consider MenACWY-CRM series beginning in infancy[h]; and the MenB series beginning at 10 years of age depending on splenic dysfunction.
Secondary			
	HIV/AIDS	OPV,[a] smallpox, BCG, MMRV, MMR, VAR in highly immunocompromised children; YF vaccine may have a contraindication or precaution depending on indicators of immune function[j]	All inactivated vaccines on the standard annual schedule are safe, may be effective, and should be administered.[e] Rotavirus vaccine should be administered on the standard schedule. MMR and VAR are recommended for HIV-infected children who are asymptomatic or have only low-level immunocompromise.[k] PPSV23 should be administered beginning at 2 years of age.[f] MenACWY series should be administered beginning in infancy.[h] Hib is indicated for under-/unimmunized children ≥5 years of age.[l]

Table 1.19. Immunization of Children and Adolescents With Primary and Secondary Immune Deficiencies, continued

Category	Example of Specific Immunodeficiency	Vaccine Contraindications[a]	Comments
	Malignancy, transplantation, autoimmune disease, immunosuppressive or radiation therapy	All live-virus and live-bacteria vaccines, depending on immune status[c,d]	Refer to text for guidance. All inactivated vaccines on the standard annual schedule are safe, and may be effective depending on degree of immunocompromise.[e] Annual IIV is recommended unless receiving intensive chemotherapy or anti-B cell antibodies. PPSV23 should be administered beginning at 2 years of age.[f] Hib vaccine is indicated in under-/unimmunized children <5 years of age only.[e]
	Asplenia (functional, congenital anatomic, surgical)	None	All inactivated and live-virus vaccines on the standard annual schedule are safe, likely are effective, and should be administered.[e] PPSV23 should be administered beginning at 2 years of age[f]; MenACWY-CRM series beginning in infancy[h]; and the MenB series beginning at 10 years of age. Hib vaccine is indicated for under-/unimmunized children ≥5 years of age.[l]
	Chronic renal failure	None	All inactivated and live-virus vaccines on the standard annual immunization schedule are safe, likely are effective, and should be administered.[e] PPSV23 should be administered beginning at 2 years of age.[f] HepB is indicated if not previously immunized.

Table 1.19. Immunization of Children and Adolescents With Primary and Secondary Immune Deficiencies, continued

Category	Example of Specific Immunodeficiency	Vaccine Contraindications[a]	Comments
	CNS anatomic barrier defect (cochlear implant, congenital dysplasia of the inner ear, persistent CSF communication with naso-/oropharynx)	None	All inactivated and live-virus vaccines on the standard annual immunization schedule are safe and effective, and should be administered.[e] PPSV23 should be administered beginning at 2 years of age.[f]

OPV indicates oral poliovirus; BCG, bacille Calmette-Guérin; YF, yellow fever; PPSV23, 23-valent pneumococcal polysaccharide vaccine; IG, Immune Globulin; MMR, measles-mumps-rubella vaccine; VAR, varicella vaccine; IIV, inactivated influenza vaccine; IgA, immunoglobulin A; IgG, immunoglobulin G; MMRV, measles-mumps-rubella-varicella vaccine; MenACWY, meningococcal conjugate vaccine containing serogroups ACWY; MenB, serogroup B meningococcal vaccine; STAT1, signal transducer and activator of transcription 1; HIV, human immunodeficiency virus; AIDS, acquired immune deficiency syndrome; Hib, *Haemophilus influenzae* type b vaccine; HepB, hepatitis B vaccine; CNS, central nervous system; CSF, cerebrospinal fluid.

[a] This table refers to contraindications for nonemergency vaccination (ie, recommendations of the Advisory Committee on Immunization Practices of the Centers for Disease Control and Prevention).

[b] OPV vaccine no longer is available in the United States.

[c] Live-bacteria vaccines: BCG and Ty21a *Salmonella Typhi* vaccine.

[d] Live-virus vaccines: MMR, VAR, MMRV, OPV, YF, vaccinia (smallpox), and rotavirus. Except for severe T-lymphocyte deficiency, data to contraindicate rotavirus vaccine are lacking; the immunocompromised state generally is considered a precaution for rotavirus vaccine. LAIV is not indicated for any person with a potentially immunocompromising condition.

[e] Children who are underimmunized or unimmunized for age should receive routinely recommended vaccines, according to age and the catch-up schedule, with urgency to administer needed Hib and PCV13.

[f] PPSV23 is begun at ≥2 years of age. If PCV13 is required (ie, for children <6 years who have not received all required doses, and for those ≥6 years of age who never received PCV13), PCV13 dose(s) should be administered first, followed by PPSV23 at least 8 weeks later; a second dose of PPSV23 is administered 5 years after the first (see Pneumococcal Infections, p 639).

[g] Regarding T-lymphocyte immunodeficiency as a contraindication to rotavirus vaccine, data only exist for severe combined immunodeficiency syndrome.

[h] Age and schedule of doses depends on the product; repeated doses are required (see Meningococcal Infections, p 550).

[i] Additional pneumococcal vaccine is not indicated for children with chronic granulomatous disease beyond age-based standard recommendations for PCV13, because these children are not at increased risk of pneumococcal disease.

[f]YF vaccine is contraindicated in HIV-infected children younger than 6 years who are highly immunosuppressed (see text). There is a precaution for use of YF vaccine in asymptomatic HIV-infected children younger than 6 years with total lymphocyte percentage of 15% to 24%, and older than 6 years with CD4+ T-lymphocyte counts of 200–499 cells/mm³ (Centers for Disease Control and Prevention. Yellow fever vaccine: recommendations of the Advisory Committee on Immunization Practices [ACIP]. *MMWR Recomm Rep*. 2010;59[RR-07];1–27).

[a]Live-virus vaccines (measles-mumps-rubella [MMR] and varicella) can be administered to asymptomatic HIV-infected children and adolescents without severe immunosuppression (that is, can be administered to children 1 through 13 years of age with a CD4+ T-lymphocyte percentage ≥15% and to adolescents ≥14 years of age with a CD4+ T-lymphocyte count ≥200 lymphocytes/mm³). Severely immunocompromised HIV-infected infants, children, adolescents, and young adults (eg, children 1 through 13 years of age with a CD4+ T-lymphocyte percentage <15% and adolescents ≥14 years of age with a CD4+ T-lymphocyte count <200 lymphocytes/mm³) should not receive measles virus-containing vaccine, because vaccine-related pneumonia has been reported. The quadrivalent measles-mumps-rubella-varicella (MMRV) vaccine should not be administered to any HIV-infected infant, regardless of degree of immunosuppression, because of lack of safety data in this population.

[f]A single dose of Hib vaccine is indicated for unimmunized children and adolescents ≥5 years of age (children and adolescents who have not received a primary series and booster dose or at least 1 dose of Hib vaccine after 14 months of age are considered unimmunized) who have anatomic or functional asplenia (including sickle cell disease), who will undergo splenectomy, or who have HIV infection.

(MMR) or varicella vaccine after HSCT and only in a patient without ongoing immunosuppression or GVHD. Timing also may be delayed for solid organ transplant recipients with graft rejection.

SAFETY OF VACCINES IN PEOPLE WITH CHRONIC INFLAMMATORY DISORDERS. The Institute of Medicine (IOM [now called the National Academy of Medicine, or NAM]) assessed relationships between vaccines (MMR, acellular pertussis-containing diphtheria and tetanus, tetanus toxoid, influenza, hepatitis A, hepatitis B, and HPV vaccines) as potential triggers for a flare or the onset of chronic inflammatory diseases. Evidence was inadequate to establish or refute a causal relationship between each vaccine and onset or exacerbation of multiple sclerosis, systemic lupus erythematosus, vasculitis, rheumatoid arthritis, or juvenile idiopathic arthritis.[1] The IOM review concluded that overall, the preponderance of clinical evidence indicates that vaccines are not important triggers of disease or flares and should not be withheld because of this concern.

LIVE VACCINES. In general, people who are severely immunocompromised or in whom immune function is uncertain should not receive live vaccines, either viral or bacterial, because of the risk of disease caused by the vaccine strains. However, there are particular immune deficiency disorders in which some live vaccines are safe, and for certain immunocompromised children and adolescents, the benefits may outweigh risks for use of particular live vaccines (see Table 1.19, p 75). Children with primary or secondary immune deficiencies and other chronic conditions are not candidates for live attenuated influenza vaccine (LAIV).

INACTIVATED VACCINES. The decision to administer inactivated vaccines to children with immunodeficiencies depends on likelihood of benefit rather than concern of harm. Annual vaccination with inactivated influenza vaccine (IIV) is recommended for immunocompromised patients 6 months and older with primary and secondary immunodeficiencies. Immune responses of immunocompromised children to inactivated vaccines, including IIV, may be limited or even inadequate compared with an immunocompetent host. Inactivated vaccines administered during immunosuppressive therapies generally are not counted as valid in the recommended immunization schedule. Inactivated vaccines on the standard schedule, other than IIV, generally are not administered to patients receiving immunoglobulin therapy for major antibody deficiency disorders or severe combined immunodeficiencies because of lack of added benefit.

Inactivated vaccines not administered universally or at specific ages sometimes may be indicated for children with inherited and acquired conditions because of their high risk for infection. These might include pneumococcal conjugate vaccine (PCV13) doses at the earliest appropriate time on the annual immunization schedule and then 23-valent pneumococcal polysaccharide vaccine (PPSV23) at 2 years or older and at least 8 weeks after PCV, followed by a second PPSV23 dose 5 years later; PCV13 after the age of 6 years if not previously received; meningococcal conjugate vaccine (MenACWY) beginning in infancy; meningococcal serogroup B vaccine (MenB) beginning at 10 years of age; and *Haemophilus influenzae* type b vaccine (Hib) after the age of 5 years.

Table 1.19 (p 75) provides guidance for some conditions (also see "Vaccines That Might Be Indicated for Persons Aged 0 Through 18 Years Based on Medical Conditions" [Figure 3 and footnotes in the Recommended Immunization Schedule for Children and

---

[1]Stratton K, Andrew F, Rusch E, Clayton E. *Adverse Effects of Vaccines: Evidence and Causality*. Washington, DC: National Academies Press; 2012

Adolescents Aged 18 Years or Younger, United States, 2017; **https://redbook.
solutions.aap.org/SS/Immunization_Schedules.aspx]).**

PRIMARY IMMUNODEFICIENCIES

Vaccine recommendations for primary immunodeficiency disorders depend on the
specific immunologic abnormality and degree of impairment (Table 1.19, p 75). The
immunologist caring for the patient is best able to determine the degree of
immunodeficiency, especially for unique and less established disorders. All live-virus
and inactivated vaccines can be administered to children with isolated immunoglobulin A
deficiency. Inactivated vaccines other than IIV are not routinely administered to patients
with major antibody deficiencies or SCID during IG therapy. For these 2 groups,
inactivated vaccines can be administered as part of immunologic assessment prior to
Immune Globulin Intravenous (IGIV) therapy without safety concerns. For patients with
common variable immunodeficiency, in addition to annual IIV, MenACWY is
considered beginning at 2 months of age because of their splenic dysfunction and lack of
substantial meningococcal antibodies in IGIV.

Table 1.19 (p 75) provides a list of exclusions for use of certain live vaccines because
of safety concerns. Live-virus vaccines should not be administered to patients with major
antibody deficiencies, SCID, and T-lymphocyte immunodeficiencies, including any of
the following conditions: DiGeorge syndrome with CD3+ T-lymphocyte count <500
cells/mm^3, other combined immunodeficiencies with similar CD3+ T-lymphocyte
counts, Wiskott-Aldrich syndrome, or X-linked lymphoproliferative disease or familial
disorders that predispose to hemophagocytic lymphohistiocytosis.

Patients with primary complement deficiencies (ie, of early classic pathway, alternate
pathway, or severe mannose-binding lectin deficiency) should receive all routine inactivated
and live vaccines on the annual immunization schedule; none is contraindicated.

Patients with phagocytic cell deficiencies (ie, chronic granulomatous disease [CGD],
leukocyte adhesion deficiency [LAD], Chediak-Higashi syndrome, cyclic neutropenia)
and patients with innate immune defects that result in defects of cytokine
generation/response or cellular activation (eg, defects of interferon-gamma/interleukin
[IL]-12 axis) should receive all inactivated vaccines on the annual immunization schedule.
Live-virus vaccines should be administered to patients with CGD and cyclic neutropenia,
but live-bacterial vaccines should not be administered to these patients. Live-bacterial and
live-virus vaccines should not be administered to patients with LAD, Chediak-Higashi
syndrome, or defects within the interferon-gamma/IL-12 pathway.

SECONDARY (ACQUIRED) IMMUNODEFICIENCIES

Several factors should be considered in immunization of children with secondary
immunodeficiencies (Table 1.19, p 75), including the underlying disease, the specific
immunosuppressive regimen (dose and schedule), and the patient's infectious disease and
immunization history. Live-virus vaccines generally are contraindicated because of a
proven or theoretical increased risk of vaccine virus disease. Exceptions include
administration of MMR and varicella vaccine (but not combined measles-mumps-rubella-
varicella [MMRV]) in children with HIV infection who are not severely
immunosuppressed. Rotavirus vaccine may be administered to infants exposed to or
infected with HIV, irrespective of CD4+ T-lymphocyte percentage or count, according to

the schedule for uninfected infants (see Human Immunodeficiency Virus Infection, p 459). Although varicella vaccine has been studied in children with acute lymphoblastic leukemia in remission during the maintenance phase of chemotherapy, varicella vaccine should not be administered to children with acute lymphocytic leukemia or another malignancy while undergoing therapy, because (1) many children will have received varicella vaccine prior to immune suppression and may retain protective immunity; (2) the risk of acquiring varicella has diminished in countries with universal immunization programs; (3) most deaths from varicella, although rare, occur within the first year of diagnosis and, thus, would not be preventable by immunization; (4) hyperimmune globulin is available for postexposure prophylaxis; (5) antiviral agents are available for treatment; and (6) chemotherapy regimens change frequently and often are more immunosuppressive than regimens under which the safety and efficacy of varicella vaccine was studied (see Varicella-Zoster Infections, p 869).

Because patients with congenital or acquired immunodeficiencies may not have an adequate response to vaccines, they may remain susceptible despite having been immunized. Positive serologic test results are not always reliable markers of protection. Susceptibility generally is assumed when considering potential postexposure strategies.

HOUSEHOLD MEMBERS OF IMMUNOCOMPROMISED PATIENTS

Immunocompetent individuals who live in a household with immunocompromised patients should be current with all routinely recommended immunizations to minimize the exposure of the immunocompromised patient to vaccine-preventable infections. They should receive inactivated vaccines on the annual immunization schedule or for travel, including IIV for household members who are 6 months or older. Household members may receive IIV or LAIV, if the member otherwise fulfills criteria for receipt of LAIV. Exceptions to the latter are that LAIV should not be used in a household member (or contact should be avoided for 7 days if LAIV is administered) when the immunocompromised household contact has SCID or received an HSCT within 2 months or has GVHD requiring therapy. For the 2016–2017 and 2017–2018 influenza seasons, LAIV was not recommended for use in any population because of issues with vaccine effectiveness. For current recommendations on use of LAIV, please refer to the current AAP influenza policy statement, which is updated annually and published in August or September each year.[1]

Healthy immunocompetent members of a household living with immunocompromised patients of all degrees of severity can and should receive the following live vaccines, as indicated on the annual immunization schedule: MMR, varicella-containing vaccines (Varivax [Merck & Co, Whitehouse Station, NJ], MMRV, and Zostavax [Merck & Co]), rotavirus vaccine for infants 2 through 7 months of age, and yellow fever and oral typhoid vaccines for travel. OPV, which still is available in many countries outside the United States, should not be administered to individuals who live in a household with immunocompromised patients. Immunocompromised patients should avoid contact with people who develop skin lesions after receipt of varicella or

---

[1]American Academy of Pediatrics, Committee on Infectious Diseases. Recommendations for prevention and control of influenza in children, 2017–2018. *Pediatrics.* 2017; 140(4):e20172550

zoster vaccines until lesions clear. If contact occurs inadvertently, risk of transmission is low. When transmission of vaccine-strain varicella virus has occurred, the virus is expected to maintain its attenuated characteristics. Therefore, administration of Varicella-Zoster Immune Globulin (VariZIG) or IGIV after exposure to a person with skin lesions following varicella immunization is not indicated.

SPECIAL SITUATIONS/HOSTS

CORTICOSTEROIDS

Inactivated vaccines, including IIV, and live-virus vaccines should be administered to patients well in advance of commencement of corticosteroid therapy for inflammatory or autoimmune diseases, when feasible, as for immunocompetent people and indicated on the annual immunization schedule. Inactivated vaccines should be administered at least 2 weeks before, and live-virus vaccines should be administered at least 4 weeks before, commencement of corticosteroid therapy.

Guidance for Administration of Inactivated Vaccines During Corticosteroid Therapy

Inactivated vaccines ideally are administered prior to initiation of prolonged corticosteroid therapy, but if that is not possible, they still should be administered to patients while receiving therapy long-term. Inactivated vaccine administration can be deferred temporarily until corticosteroids are discontinued if the hiatus is expected to be brief and adherence to return appointment is likely. Inactivated vaccines should not be avoided because of concern for exacerbation of an inflammatory or immune-mediated condition.

Guidance for Administration of Live-Virus Vaccines During Corticosteroid Therapy

Recommendations depend on potency, route of administration, and duration of corticosteroid therapy:

- **Topical therapy, local injections, or aerosol use of corticosteroids.** Application of low-potency topical corticosteroids to localized areas on the skin; administration by aerosolization; application on conjunctiva; or intraarticular, bursal, or tendon injections of corticosteroids usually do not result in immunosuppression that would contraindicate administration of live-virus vaccines.
- **Physiologic maintenance doses of corticosteroids.** Children who are receiving only maintenance physiologic doses of corticosteroids can receive live-virus vaccines.
- **Low or moderate doses of systemic corticosteroids given daily or on alternate days.** Children receiving <2 mg/kg per day of prednisone or its equivalent, or <20 mg/day if they weigh more than 10 kg, can receive live-virus vaccines during corticosteroid treatment.
- **High doses of systemic corticosteroids given daily or on alternate days for fewer than 14 days.** Children receiving ≥2 mg/kg per day of prednisone or its equivalent, or ≥20 mg/day if they weigh more than 10 kg, can receive live-virus vaccines immediately after discontinuation of treatment. Some experts, however, would delay immunization with live-virus vaccines until 2 weeks after discontinuation.
- **High doses of systemic corticosteroids given daily for 14 days or more.**

Children receiving ≥ 2 mg/kg per day of prednisone or its equivalent, or ≥ 20 mg/day if they weigh more than 10 kg, for 14 days or more should not receive live-virus vaccines until 4 weeks after discontinuation.

- **Low or moderate doses of systemic corticosteroids or locally administered corticosteroids in children who have a disease (eg, systemic lupus erythematosus) that, in itself, is considered to suppress the immune response or who are receiving immunosuppressant medication other than corticosteroids.** These children should not receive live-virus vaccines during therapy, except in special circumstances.

BIOLOGIC RESPONSE MODIFYING DRUGS USED TO DECREASE INFLAMMATION

Biologic response modifiers, also known as cytokine inhibitors, are drugs used to treat immune-mediated conditions, including juvenile idiopathic arthritis, rheumatoid arthritis, and inflammatory bowel disease. These drugs are antibodies to proinflammatory cytokines or proteins that bind to cytokine receptors. Their purpose is to block the action of cytokines involved in inflammation. Their immune-modulating effects can last for weeks to months after discontinuation. TNF-α inhibitors (adalimumab, certolizumab, etanercept, golimumab, infliximab) are the prototype agents, but newer biologic response modifiers in this class target other cytokines, such as IL-1 (anakinra), IL-6 (tocilizumab), IL-12, and IL-23, or the proteins that target cytokine receptors on lymphocytes. These agents often are used in combination with other immunosuppressive drugs, such as methotrexate or corticosteroids.

Patients treated with biologic response modifiers are at increased risk of infections caused by *Mycobacterium tuberculosis*, nontuberculous mycobacterium, molds (eg, *Aspergillus* species and endemic fungi (eg, *Histoplasma capsulatum* and *Candida* species), *Legionella* species, *Listeria* species, and other intracellular pathogens, and are at risk of developing lymphomas and other cancers.[1] Inhibition of the inflammatory immune response also can permit reactivation of infections that have been controlled previously and can lead to an inadequate response to new pathogens requiring cell-mediated immunity for control. Adverse events related to use of biologic response modifying drugs should be reported to the US Food and Drug Administration (FDA) MedWatch Program (**www.fda.gov/Safety/MedWatch/HowToReport/ucm053087.htm**). Table 1.20 (p 86) provides preventive strategies that should be considered in patients who are receiving or will receive immune-modifying agents. Vaccination status should be assessed pretreatment, and recommended vaccines should be administered with timing as for planned corticosteroid use. Recommended vaccines include PPSV23 for patients 2 years or older (after PCV13 doses on the routine schedule are completed, or after PCV13 for patients 6 years or older who previously did not receive PCV13).

Biologic response modifiers are considered highly immunosuppressive, and live-virus vaccines are contraindicated during therapy; inactivated vaccines, including IIV, should be administered as per the immunization schedule and should not be withheld because of concern for an exaggerated inflammatory response. The interval following therapy until live-virus vaccines can be administered safely has not been established and is likely to vary by agent.

---

[1] Davies HD; American Academy of Pediatrics, Committee on Infectious Diseases. Infectious complications with the use of biologic response modifiers in infants and children. *Pediatrics*. 2016;138(2):e20161209

Table 1.20. Recommendations for Evaluation Prior to Initiation of Biologic Response Modifying Drugs

- Perform tuberculin skin test (TST) or interferon-gamma release assay (IGRA) (see Tuberculosis, p 829)
- Consider chest radiograph on the basis of clinical and epidemiologic findings
- Document vaccination status and, if required, administer:
  - ◆ inactivated vaccines (including annual IIV) a minimum of 2 weeks before initiation of biologic response modifying drug
  - ◆ live-virus vaccines a minimum 4 weeks before initiation of biologic response modifier therapy, unless contraindicated by condition or other therapies
- Counsel household members regarding risk of infection and ensure vaccination (see Household Members of Immunosuppressed Patients, p 83)
- Consider serologic testing for *Histoplasma* species, *Toxoplasma* species, and other intracellular pathogens depending on risk of past exposure
- Perform serologic testing for hepatitis B virus and vaccinate/revaccinate if HBsAb is <10 mIU/mL.
- Consider testing for varicella-zoster virus and Epstein-Barr virus
- Counsel regarding:
  - ◆ food safety (**www.cdc.gov/foodsafety**)
  - ◆ maintenance of dental hygiene
  - ◆ risks of exposure to garden soil, pets, and other animals
  - ◆ avoiding high-risk activities (eg, excavation sites or spelunking because of risk of *Histoplasma capsulatum*)
  - ◆ avoiding travel to areas with endemic pathogenic fungi (eg, certain areas of southwestern United States for risk of *Coccidioides* species) or to areas where tuberculosis is endemic

IIV indicates inactivated influenza vaccine; HBsAb, hepatitis B surface antibody.

Modified from Le Saux N; Canadian Paediatric Society, Infectious Diseases and Immunization Committee. *Paediatric and Child Health.* Ottawa, Ontario: Canadian Paediatric Society; 2012;17(3):147–150.

Infants exposed in utero to maternally administered biologic response modifiers can have detectable drug concentrations for many months following delivery, resulting in concern for immunosuppression among infants in the 12 months after the last maternal dose during pregnancy. Some of the biologic response modifiers are more efficiently passaged transplacentally in the second and third trimesters compared with the first trimester. Until further data are available, and considering that rotavirus disease is rarely life threatening in the United States, rotavirus vaccines should be avoided in US infants for the first 12 months after the final in utero exposure to a biologic response modifier. Catch-up rotavirus vaccination is not recommended once this 12-month interval is reached, because the maximum age for first dose of rotavirus vaccine is 14 weeks, 6 days (see Rotavirus Infections, p 700). Because MMR, varicella, and measles-mumps-rubella-varicella (MMRV) vaccines are recommended routinely at 12 months of age, previous receipt of biologic response modifiers during pregnancy does not preclude the infant from receiving these live vaccines at the recommended time. For measles prevention in infants younger than 12 months following exposure during outbreak settings, IGIV is preferred over MMR during the 12 months following the last maternal dose during pregnancy. International travel for infants who were exposed to biologic response modifiers in utero should be discouraged for the 12 months following the last maternal dose during pregnancy. These recommendations may not apply to management of infants born in other countries, where risks of wild type infection may differ from the United States and where additional live vaccines may be administered in early infancy (eg, bacille Calmette-Guérin, oral poliovirus).

HEMATOPOIETIC STEM CELL TRANSPLANTATION

Patients for whom HSCT is planned should receive all routinely recommended inactivated vaccines (including IIV) well in advance and at least 2 weeks before the start of the conditioning period. Routinely recommended live-virus vaccines should be administered if the patient is not already immunosuppressed and the interval to the start of the conditioning period is at least 4 weeks. By vaccinating the nonimmune patient before HSCT, it is likely that some protection will persist in the months after transplant. The HSCT donor also should be current with routinely recommended vaccines, but if he or she is not, vaccination of the donor for benefit of the recipient is not recommended. Administration of MMR, MMRV, varicella, and zoster vaccines should be avoided within 4 weeks of hematopoietic stem cell harvest.

Household members should be counseled regarding risks of infection and should be fully immunized, with certain restrictions for use of LAIV (see Household Members of Immunocompromised Patients). Timing of immune reconstitution of HSCT recipients varies greatly depending on type of transplantation, interval since transplantation, receipt of immunosuppressive medications, and presence or absence of GVHD and other complications. Vaccinations (both routine and additional) are an important part of management and are considered according to specific guidelines and in collaboration with the patient's hematologist.

SOLID ORGAN TRANSPLANTATION

Children and adolescents with chronic or end-stage kidney, liver, heart, or lung disease or intestinal failure, including SOT candidates, should receive all vaccinations as appropriate for age, exposure history, and immune status based on the annual immunization schedule for immunocompetent people. Patients 2 years or older with these conditions also should have received, or should receive as a candidate for SOT, a dose of PPSV23, if not previously received within 5 years. No more than 2 doses of PPSV23 should be administered before 65 years of age. PCV13 is administered if not previously received, even for those 6 years or older. When PCV13 and PPSV23 both are indicated, PCV13 dose(s) should be administered first, with at least an 8-week lapse before giving PPSV23. SOT candidates who are hepatitis B surface antibody (anti-HBs) negative should receive the hepatitis B vaccine (HepB) series, followed by serologic testing and further doses if serologic test results are negative (as indicated for an immunocompetent vaccine recipient who remains seronegative). Patients 12 months or older who have not received hepatitis A vaccine (HepA), did not complete the vaccination series, or are seronegative should complete the HepA vaccine series. MMR vaccine can be administered to infants 6 through 11 months of age who are SOT candidates and who are not immunocompromised, repeating the dose at ≥12 months if still awaiting a transplant that will not occur within 4 weeks of vaccination. Living SOT donors should have up-to-date vaccination status, with considerations for required vaccines the same as for HSCT donors (see Hematopoietic Stem Cell Transplantation). Donors should avoid receiving live-virus vaccines within 4 weeks before donation. Household members of these patients should be counseled about risks of infection and should have vaccination status made current, with use of live-virus and inactivated vaccines, as indicated.

HIV INFECTION (ALSO SEE HUMAN IMMUNODEFICIENCY VIRUS INFECTION, P 459)

HIV-infected children and adolescents should receive all inactivated vaccines, including annual IIV, as indicated on the annual immunization schedule. PPSV23 should be administered to people 2 years or older, at least 8 weeks after the last required PCV13 dose. HIV-exposed or HIV-infected infants may receive rotavirus vaccine, irrespective of CD4+ T-lymphocyte percentage or count, according to the schedule for uninfected infants. MMR and varicella vaccines should be administered to children 12 months or older who are stable clinically and who have low level of immunosuppression (see General Principles, p 73).

For those receiving varicella vaccine between 1 and 8 years of age, the second dose (usually administered at 4–6 years of age) should be administered to HIV-infected children 3 months after the first dose. A varicella vaccine 2-dose series is also indicated for previously unimmunized nonimmune children or adolescents 9 years or older who do not have more than low-level immunosuppression. HIV-infected children should not receive MMRV or LAIV vaccines.

In the United States, BCG vaccine is contraindicated for HIV-infected patients. In areas of the world with a high incidence of tuberculosis, the World Health Organization (WHO) recommends administering BCG vaccine to HIV-infected children who are asymptomatic.

ASPLENIA AND FUNCTIONAL ASPLENIA

The asplenic state results from the following: (1) surgical removal of the spleen (eg, after trauma, for treatment of hemolytic conditions); (2) functional asplenia (eg, from sickle cell disease or thalassemia); or (3) congenital asplenia or polysplenia. Special recommendations for patients with asplenia apply to all 3 categories (absence and dysfunction). All infants, children, adolescents, and adults with asplenia, regardless of the reason for the asplenic state, have an increased risk of fulminant septicemia, especially associated with encapsulated bacteria, which is associated with a high mortality rate. In comparison with immunocompetent children who have not undergone splenectomy, the incidence of and mortality rate from septicemia are increased in children who have had splenectomy after trauma and in children with sickle cell disease by as much as 350-fold, and the rate may be even higher in children who have had splenectomy for thalassemia. The risk of invasive bacterial infection is higher in younger children than in older children, and the risk may be greater during the years immediately after surgical splenectomy. Fulminant septicemia, however, has been reported in adults as long as 25 years after splenectomy.

Streptococcus pneumoniae is the most common pathogen causing septicemia in children with asplenia. Less common causes include *Haemophilus influenzae* type b, *Neisseria meningitidis*, other streptococci, *Escherichia coli*, *Staphylococcus aureus*, and gram-negative bacilli, such as *Salmonella* species, *Klebsiella* species, and *Pseudomonas aeruginosa*. Those with functional or anatomic asplenia are at increased risk of severe babesiosis and may be at increased risk of fatal malaria; no vaccines currently are available to prevent these 2 infections.

Immunization

Pneumococcal conjugate and polysaccharide vaccines are vital for all children with asplenia (see Pneumococcal Infections, p 639). Following administration of an appropriate number of doses of PCV13, PPSV23 should be administered to children 24 months or older a minimum of 8 weeks after the last PCV13 dose. A second PPSV23 dose should be administered 5 years later (see Pneumococcal Infections, p 639). For children 2 through 18 years of age who have not received PCV13, even if they completed a PCV7 series or already received PPSV23 or both, 1 supplemental dose of PCV13 should be administered. When splenectomy is planned for a patient 2 years or older who is PPSV23 naïve, PPSV23 should be administered well in advance and at least 8 weeks after indicated dose(s) of PCV13 and at least 2 weeks before surgery.

Hib immunization should be initiated at 2 months of age, as recommended for otherwise healthy young children on the annual immunization schedule. Previously unimmunized children with asplenia younger than 5 years should receive Hib vaccine according to the catch-up schedule. Unimmunized children 5 years or older should receive a single dose of Hib vaccine.

Meningococcal conjugate vaccine should be administered to all children with asplenia who are 2 months or older, as recommended for those with primary complement deficiencies (see Primary Immunodeficiencies, p 82), with one important restriction to type/brand of MenACWY. MenACWY-D (Menactra [Sanofi Pasteur, Swiftwater, PA]) should not be used before 2 years of age and sooner than 4 weeks after completion of the 4-dose series of PCV13 series because of interference with antibody response to some serotypes contained in PCV13 when vaccines are administered concurrently. MenACWY-CRM (Menveo [Novartis, Cambridge, MA]) should be used in infants and toddlers as approved by age, without concern for significant interference with PCV13. Revaccination using either MenACWY conjugate vaccine is recommended 3 years after the primary series and then every 5 years for patients with asplenia who are younger than 7 years; for asplenic patients who are 7 years and older, the initial booster dose following the primary series should be at 5 years (instead of 3 years) and then every 5 years thereafter. Use of MenACWY vaccine (beginning in infancy) and MenB vaccine (beginning at 10 years of age) can be considered on a case-by-case basis for children with other primary or secondary deficiencies in whom splenic dysfunction is likely to be substantial and in whom response to vaccine is likely.

When surgical splenectomy is planned, immunization status for Hib, pneumococcal, and meningococcal vaccines should be ascertained, and all indicated vaccines should be administered well in advance and at least 2 weeks before surgery. If splenectomy is performed on an emergency basis, or if vaccination was not performed before splenectomy, indicated vaccines should be initiated as soon as possible 2 weeks or more after surgery. Vaccination(s) in the more immediate postoperative period should be considered if return after 14 days is uncertain. Whenever possible, alternatives to splenectomy should be considered. Management options include postponement of splenectomy for as long as possible in people with congenital hemolytic anemia, preservation of accessory spleens, performance of partial splenectomy for benign tumors of the spleen, conservative (nonoperative) management of splenic trauma, or when feasible, repair rather than removal. Splenectomy should be avoided if possible, especially when immunodeficiency is present (eg, Wiskott-Aldrich syndrome or autoimmune lymphoproliferative syndrome [ALPS]).

Antimicrobial Agents

Daily antimicrobial prophylaxis against pneumococcal infections is recommended for many children with asplenia, regardless of immunization status. For infants with sickle cell anemia, oral penicillin prophylaxis against invasive pneumococcal disease should be initiated as soon as the diagnosis is established and preferably by 2 months of age. Although the efficacy of antimicrobial prophylaxis has been proven only in patients with sickle cell anemia, other children with asplenia at particularly high risk, such as children with malignant neoplasms or thalassemia, also should receive daily chemoprophylaxis. Less agreement exists about the need for prophylaxis for children who have had splenectomy after trauma. In general, antimicrobial prophylaxis (in addition to immunization) should be considered for all children with asplenia younger than 5 years and for at least 1 year after splenectomy at any age.

The age at which chemoprophylaxis is discontinued often is an empiric decision. On the basis of a multicenter study, prophylactic penicillin can be discontinued at 5 years of age in children with sickle cell disease who are receiving regular medical attention, are fully immunized, and have not had a severe pneumococcal infection or surgical splenectomy. The appropriate duration of prophylaxis for children with asplenia attributable to other causes is unknown. Some experts continue prophylaxis throughout childhood and into adulthood for particularly high-risk patients with asplenia.

For antimicrobial prophylaxis, oral penicillin V (125 mg, twice a day, for children younger than 3 years; and 250 mg, twice a day, for children 3 years or older) is recommended. Some experts recommend amoxicillin (20 mg/kg per day). For children with anaphylactic allergy to penicillin, erythromycin can be given (250 mg, twice daily). A substantial percentage of pneumococcal isolates have intermediate- or high-level resistance to penicillin, resistance to macrolides and azalides, or both. When antimicrobial prophylaxis is used, these limitations must be stressed to parents and patients, who should be made aware that all febrile illnesses potentially are serious in children with asplenia and that immediate medical attention should be sought because the initial signs and symptoms of fulminant septicemia can be subtle. Likewise, medical attention should be sought for asplenic patients who suffer animal bites. When bacteremia or septicemia is a possibility, health care professionals should obtain specimens for blood and other cultures as indicated and begin treatment immediately with an antimicrobial regimen effective against *S pneumoniae*, *H influenzae* type b, and *N meningitidis* and should consider hospitalizing the child. In some clinical situations, other antimicrobial agents, such as aminoglycosides, may be indicated. If a child with asplenia travels to or resides in an area where medical care is not accessible, an appropriate antimicrobial agent should be readily available and the child's caregiver should be instructed in appropriate use.

CENTRAL NERVOUS SYSTEM ANATOMIC BARRIER DEFECTS

Patients of all ages scheduled to receive a cochlear implant as well as patients with congenital dysplasias of the inner ear or persistent cerebrospinal fluid (CSF) communication with the naso-oropharynx should receive all vaccines recommended routinely on the annual immunization schedule for immunocompetent people. No vaccine is contraindicated. Patients with a cochlear implant, those scheduled to receive a cochlear implant, and those with persistent communication between the CSF and naso-oropharynx should receive PCV13 as per the standard schedule and as recommended for children with asplenia. At 24 months or older, these patients should receive PPSV23 ($\geq$8 weeks after receipt of PCV13, if indicated). Indicated doses of PCV13 and PPSV23 should be administered well in advance and at least 2 weeks before cochlear implant surgery, when feasible.

There is no well-established evidence for use of antimicrobial prophylaxis for patients with CSF communication with the naso-oropharynx or middle ear. Risk of bacterial meningitis is highest in the first 7 to 10 days following acute traumatic breach. Some physicians recommend empiric parenteral antimicrobial therapy in the immediate post-traumatic period. Parenteral antimicrobial therapy also is given in the perioperative period for cochlear implantation and reparative neurosurgical procedures. Chronic antimicrobial prophylaxis is not indicated for persistent CSF communications or following cochlear implantation.

Immunization in Children With a Personal or Family History of Seizures

Studies have demonstrated a short-term increased risk of a febrile seizure (ie, generalized, brief, self-limited seizure) following receipt of several vaccines (eg, DTwP, MMR, MMRV, PCV13, and influenza). Infants and children with a personal or family history of seizures of any etiology might be at greater risk of having a febrile seizure after receipt of one of these vaccines compared with children without such histories. No evidence indicates that febrile seizures cause permanent brain damage or epilepsy, aggravate neurologic disorders, or affect the prognosis for children with underlying disorders.

An increased incidence of seizures has not been found with the currently recommended DTaP vaccines that have replaced the whole-cell DTwP vaccines in the United States. In the case of pertussis immunization during infancy, vaccine administration could coincide with or hasten the recognition of a disorder associated with seizures, such as infantile spasms or severe myoclonic epilepsy of infancy, which could cause confusion about the role of pertussis immunization. Hence, pertussis immunization in infants with a history of recent seizures generally is deferred until the course of the neurologic disorder is clarified. DTaP should be administered to infants and children with a stable neurologic condition, including well-controlled seizures. The nature of seizures and related neurologic status are more likely to have been established in children by the age of 12 months. This difference by age is the basis for the recommendation that measles (MMR) and varicella vaccines should not be deferred for children with a history of seizures. Similarly, although reports of febrile seizures have been associated with inactivated influenza vaccines, mainly whole-cell formulations, influenza vaccination should not be deferred in children with a personal or family history of seizures.

A family history of a seizure disorder is not a contraindication or a reason to defer any immunization. Postimmunization seizures in these children are uncommon, and if they occur, they usually are febrile in origin, have a benign outcome, and are not likely to be confused with manifestations of a previously unrecognized neurologic disorder.

Immunization in Children With Chronic Diseases

Chronic disease in children may be defined as requiring 3 components: (1) diagnosis on the basis of medical knowledge; (2) not curable currently; and (3) has been present for at least 3 months, will likely last longer than 3 months, or has occurred at least 3 times in the past year and likely will recur. Chronic diseases may make children more susceptible to the severe manifestations and complications of common infections. Unless specifically contraindicated, immunizations recommended for healthy children should be administered to children with chronic diseases. For considerations for children with chronic and immunocompromising conditions or therapies, see Immunization and Additional Considerations in Immunocompromised Children (p 72) and "Vaccines That Might Be Indicated for Persons Aged 0 Through 18 Years Based on Medical Conditions" (Figure 3 and footnotes in the Recommended Immunization Schedule for Children and Adolescents Aged 18 Years or Younger, United States, 2017; **https://redbook. solutions.aap.org/SS/Immunization_Schedules.aspx**). Children with certain chronic diseases (eg, allergic, cardiorespiratory, hematologic, metabolic, and renal disorders; cystic fibrosis; and diabetes mellitus) are at increased risk of complications of influenza, varicella, and pneumococcal infection and should be targeted to receive IIV, varicella vaccine, and pneumococcal (PCV13, polysaccharide vaccine, or both), as recommended for age and immunization status and condition (see Influenza, p 476, Varicella-Zoster Infections, p 869, and Pneumococcal Infections, p 639). All children with chronic liver disease are at risk of severe clinical manifestations of acute infection with hepatitis viruses and should receive hepatitis A (HepA) and hepatitis B (HepB) vaccines on a catch-up schedule if they have not received vaccines routinely (see Hepatitis A, p 392, and Hepatitis B, p 401). MCV4 (MenACWY) is recommended for children as young as 2 months with certain immune deficiencies, including HIV, or those who will travel to or reside in areas with high risk of exposure (see Meningococcal Infections, p 550). Meningococcal B vaccine can be administered to children with risk factors for meningococcal B disease. Siblings of children with chronic diseases and children in households of adults with chronic diseases should receive recommended vaccines, including both live and inactivated vaccines (**https://redbook.solutions.aap.org/ SS/Immunization_Schedules.aspx**).

The Institute of Medicine (IOM [now called the National Academy of Medicine, or NAM]) assessed whether vaccines (MMR, acellular pertussis-containing diphtheria and tetanus, tetanus toxoid, influenza, hepatitis A, hepatitis B, and HPV vaccines) were a potential trigger for a flare or the onset of chronic inflammatory diseases. Evidence was inadequate to establish or refute a causal relationship between each vaccine and onset or exacerbation of multiple sclerosis, systemic lupus erythematosus, vasculitis, rheumatoid arthritis, or juvenile idiopathic arthritis.[1] The IOM review concluded that overall, the preponderance of clinical evidence indicates that vaccines are not important triggers of disease or flares and should not be withheld because of this concern.

---

[1]Stratton K, Andrew F, Rusch E, Clayton E. *Adverse Effects of Vaccines: Evidence and Causality.* Washington, DC: National Academies Press; 2012

Immunization in American Indian/Alaska Native Children and Adolescents

Indigenous populations worldwide have high morbidity and mortality from infectious diseases, including vaccine-preventable infections (**wwwnc.cdc.gov/eid/article/7/7/pdfs/01-7732.pdf**). This chapter focuses on the US population of American Indian and Alaska Native (AI/AN) people and considerations for use of vaccines and biologic products that are special to these populations. For AI/AN people who live on or near reservation communities, geographic isolation and socioeconomic factors such as poverty, household crowding, substandard housing, poor indoor air quality, and lack of indoor plumbing are the major drivers of the persistence of elevated rates of infectious diseases. Currently, more than half of AI/AN people do not reside on reservation lands or in Alaska Native villages; the little data available indicate relative risk of vaccine-preventable and other infectious diseases for this subset of AI/AN people are lower compared with AI/AN living on reservations.

Historically, compared with children from other racial groups, AI/AN children living on reservation lands or in Alaska Native villages have higher rates of certain vaccine-preventable diseases, such as *Haemophilus influenzae* type b, *Streptococcus pneumoniae*, hepatitis A, and hepatitis B. Although the rate of mortality from pneumonia and influenza among AI/AN infants has steadily declined over recent decades, disparities persist, and the AI/AN infant death rate is still 5 times higher than the rate reported for white infants in the United States. The rate of diarrhea-associated hospitalizations was significantly higher in AI/AN infants than in other US infants but has declined since introduction of rotavirus vaccine. In 2013, AI/AN people ranked fifth in estimated rates of HIV diagnoses compared with other racial/ethnic groups. However, the overall statistics of new HIV infections and diagnoses among AI/AN people show several disparities; for instance, AI/AN people have poorer survival rates after an HIV diagnosis compared with other races/ethnicities (**wwwnc.cdc.gov/eid/article/7/7/pdfs/01-7732.pdf**; **www.cdc.gov/hiv/group/racialethnic/aian/index.html**).

During the past 2 decades, childhood immunizations for hepatitis A and hepatitis B in the United States have eliminated disease disparities for these pathogens in most populations of AI/AN children. Significant decreases have been documented *in* varicella hospitalizations and invasive disease caused by *H influenzae* type b and *S pneumoniae*. Disparities for some vaccine-preventable diseases persist, however. The historically high rates of infection and ongoing disparities highlight the importance of ensuring that recommendations for universal childhood immunization be implemented for all AI/AN children. Children in AI/AN communities should receive immunizations on time and should receive the full schedule of immunizations. Specific vulnerabilities are as follows.

- ***Haemophilus influenzae* type b (Hib).** There are important differences among the currently available Hib vaccines that should be considered by physicians caring for AI/AN children. Before availability and routine use of Hib conjugate vaccines, the incidence of invasive Hib disease was approximately 10 times higher among young AI/AN children compared with non-AI/AN children. Because of the historically high risk of invasive Hib disease within the first 6 months of life in many AI/AN infant populations, the Indian Health Service (IHS) and the AAP recommend that the first dose of Hib conjugate vaccine contain polyribosylribitol phosphate-meningococcal outer membrane protein (PRP-OMP; PedvaxHIB; Merck and Co Inc, Whitehouse

Station, NJ). The administration of a PRP-OMP–containing vaccine leads to more rapid development of protective concentrations of antibody compared with other Hib vaccines, and failure to use vaccine containing PRP-OMP has been associated with excess cases of Hib disease in Alaska Native infants. If the first vaccination dose is delayed by >1 month, the recommended catch-up schedule (available at **https://redbook.solutions.aap.org/SS/Immunization_Schedules.aspx**) should be followed. A booster dose (dose 3) in PRP-OMP schedule or dose 4 in other Hib conjugate vaccine schedules is recommended at age 12 through 15 months; regardless of vaccine used in the primary series, there is no preferred vaccine formulation for the booster dose (ie, any approved Hib conjugate vaccine is acceptable **[www.cdc.gov/mmwr/preview/mmwrhtml/rr6301a1.htm]**). Availability of more than one Hib vaccine product in a clinic, however, has been shown to lead to errors in vaccine administration. To avoid confusion for health care professionals who serve AI/AN children predominantly, it may be prudent to use only PRP-OMP–containing Hib vaccines, if feasible.

- *Streptococcus pneumoniae.* Recommendations for PCV13 for AI/AN children are the same as for other US children. Prior to introduction of PCV7, the incidence of invasive pneumococcal disease (IPD) in certain AI/AN children (Alaska Native, Navajo, and White Mountain Apache) was 5 to 24 times higher than the incidence among other US children. Use of PCV7 in AI/AN infants resulted in near-elimination of disease caused by vaccine serotypes and decreased incidence of overall IPD. Use of PCV13 has further reduced the incidence of IPD in AI/AN children. However, AI/AN children continue to have a three- to fourfold increased risk of IPD compared with non-AI/AN children, which largely is attributable to serotypes not targeted by the vaccine (**www.cdc.gov/mmwr/preview/mmwrhtml/rr5911a1.htm**).

- **Hepatitis viruses.** Before the introduction of hepatitis vaccines, rates of hepatitis A and hepatitis B in the AI/AN population exceeded those of the general US population. In 1970, Alaska Native people had an overall prevalence of hepatitis B surface antigen (HBsAg) of >6%, leading to high rates of hepatocellular carcinoma in Alaska Native people younger than 30 years. Universal infant immunization and population-wide screening and vaccination eliminated symptomatic hepatitis B infection and hepatocellular carcinoma in Alaska Native people younger than 20 years. Similarly, after initiation of universal childhood hepatitis A vaccination, hepatitis A infection rates among AI/AN people declined 20-fold during 1997–2001 to a rate similar to that of the general US population. Special efforts should be made to ensure catch-up hepatitis A and hepatitis B immunization of previously unimmunized adolescents.

- **Human papillomavirus (HPV).** In 1999–2009, AI/AN women in IHS Contract Health Service Delivery Areas had a death rate from cervical cancer nearly twice the rate in white women. Rates of HPV vaccination in US teenagers are lower than for other adolescent vaccines; however, HPV vaccination coverage among AI/AN teenagers is similar to or higher than that among teenagers of other races and ethnicities.

- **Influenza virus.** The disparity in influenza-related mortality rates in the AI/AN population compared with the general US population was confirmed during the 2009 H1N1 epidemic; the H1N1 death rate among AI/AN people in 12 states (representing 50% of the AI/AN population in the United States) was 4 times higher than the H1N1 death rate for all other racial and ethnic populations combined. For this reason, the AI/AN population is listed among the groups at risk of severe complications from influenza. Therefore, when vaccine or antiviral medication supplies are limited or delayed, AI/AN people are considered a high-risk priority group. Studies also have documented the value of maternal immunization to protect both the mother and infants too young to be vaccinated. Given the elevated risk of influenza in the AI/AN population, maternal influenza immunization is an important strategy.

- **Respiratory syncytial virus (RSV).** The rates of hospitalization for RSV have been much higher for AI/AN infants in rural Alaska and southwest IHS regions (113 and 91 RSV hospitalizations per 1000 births, respectively) than for other US infants (27 per 1000 births). Hospitalization rates for AI/AN infants in these areas are similar to rates among medically high-risk and preterm infants in the overall US population. RSV hospitalization rates in Alaska Native children are related, in part, to household crowding and lack of plumbed water. Improvements in these risk factors and changes in RSV epidemiology contributed to a decline in the RSV hospitalization rate among Alaska Native children during 1994–2012; however, current RSV hospitalization rates in rural Alaska Native infants and Navajo/White Mountain Apache infants still are at least threefold higher than rates in other US children. Use of RSV-specific monoclonal antibody prophylaxis (palivizumab), as recommended by the AAP, should be optimized among high-risk AI/AN infants (see Respiratory Syncytial Virus, p 682). The RSV season may be different in northern latitudes, including Alaska, and RSV prophylaxis should reflect local seasonality and risk factors in this population.
- **Rotavirus.** In the 1990s, diarrhea-associated hospitalization rates in AI/AN infants were nearly twice those of the general US infant population. Following introduction of rotavirus vaccination, diarrhea-associated hospitalization rates in AI/AN children younger than 5 years during 2008, 2009, and 2010 were 24%, 37%, and 44%, respectively, lower than expected. These numbers suggest that rotavirus played a significant role in AI/AN infant hospitalizations and reinforces the importance of this vaccine for AI/AN infants.

Immunization in Adolescent and College Populations

Immunization recommendations for adolescents and college students have expanded significantly as vaccines have been developed to protect against pertussis, meningococcal disease, and human papillomavirus infections and as this age group was included in the recommendation for annual influenza vaccination. The adolescent immunization schedule is published annually (**www.cdc.gov/vaccines/schedules/index.html** and **www.vaccines.gov/who_and_when/college/index.html**).

The adolescent population presents many immunization challenges, including less frequent visits for preventive care, scheduling conflicts because of age-appropriate activities, lack of a single age for recommended vaccines in middle or late adolescence, and providers missing opportunities to immunize. In addition, minors in some states can consent to immunization of their children but not themselves. The Society for Adolescent Health and Medicine has a position paper on adolescents consenting for vaccination and the potential impact on immunization rates (**www.adolescenthealth.org/SAHM_Main/media/Advocacy/Positions/Oct-13-Consent-Vaccination.pdf**).

To ensure age-appropriate immunization, all youth should have a routine appointment at 11 through 12 years of age for administration of appropriate vaccines and to provide comprehensive preventive health care.[1] During all adolescent visits, immunization status should be reviewed, and deficiencies should be corrected according to the recommended immunization schedule. The use of patient reminder-recall systems, provider reminders, and standing orders have been shown to increase immunization rates. Lapses in the immunization schedule do not necessitate reinitiation of a vaccine series or extra doses. Influenza vaccine should be administered annually before the start of the influenza season.

Tdap, MenACWY, and HPV vaccine should be administered at the 11- through 12-year-old visit. For people initiating HPV vaccination before their 15th birthday, the recommended schedule is 2 doses of HPV vaccine, with the second dose given 6 to 12 months after the first dose (minimum interval 5 months). For people initiating vaccination on or after their 15th birthday, the recommended schedule is 3 doses of HPV vaccine. In a 3-dose schedule, the second dose should be administered at least 1 to 2 months after the first dose (minimum interval 4 weeks), and the third dose 6 months after the first dose (minimum interval 5 months after first dose, and 12 weeks after second dose). Appointments for subsequent doses of HPV vaccine should be made at initiation to enhance completion. Providers can choose to begin HPV vaccine series as early as 9 years of age if they deem this the optimal age to attain acceptance and completion prior to the risk of acquisition of HPV. When HPV vaccine is begun at 9 or 10 years, other adolescent vaccines (eg, MenACWY and Tdap) still are recommended to be administered only at 11 to 12 years.

VACCINATION OF COLLEGE-AGED PEOPLE

A MenACWY booster dose is recommended at 16 years of age. In contrast to the other serogroups, the incidence of serogroup B meningococcal disease is not increased in college students compared with age-matched individuals not attending college. MenB vaccine is not a standard recommendation for adolescents in the absence of an outbreak or an underlying high-risk condition (eg, complement deficiency or asplenia) (see Meningococcal Infections, p 550).

A history should be obtained to assess risk factors that would require consideration for administration of additional vaccines, such as HepA, MenB, Hib, and PCV13 and PPSV23 vaccines. These vaccines should be administered as soon as the risk condition is identified. Specific indications for each of these vaccines are provided in the respective disease-specific chapters in Section 3.

Residential schools, colleges, and universities should establish a system to ensure that all students are protected against vaccine-preventable diseases and also to be able to identify unimmunized students in the event of an outbreak. Because outbreaks of vaccine-preventable diseases, including measles, mumps, and meningococcal disease, have occurred at colleges and universities, the American College Health Association encourages a comprehensive institutional prematriculation immunization policy consistent with recommendations from the CDC Advisory Committee on Immunization Practices (**www.acha.org/ACHA/Resources/Topics/Vaccine.aspx**). Many

---

[1] American Academy of Pediatrics, Committee on Practice and Ambulatory Medicine and Bright Futures Periodicity Schedule Workgroup. 2017 recommendations for pediatric preventive health care. *Pediatrics.* *2017;39*(3):e20170254

colleges and universities are mandated by state law to require vaccination against meningococcal disease and/or hepatitis B, either for all matriculating students or only those living in campus housing. Information regarding state laws requiring prematriculation immunization is available **(www.immunize.org/laws)**.

The suspected occurrence of illness attributable to a vaccine-preventable disease in a school or college should be reported promptly to local health officials for aid in management, for assessment of public health implications, and to comply with state law (see Appendix IV, p 1069).

Immunization in Health Care Personnel[1]

Adults whose occupations place them in contact with patients with contagious diseases are at increased risk of contracting vaccine-preventable diseases and, if infected, transmitting them to their coworkers and patients. For the purposes of this section, health care personnel (HCP) are defined as those who have face-to-face contact with patients, or anyone who works in a building where patient care is delivered or is employed by a health care facility (eg, laboratory workers). The definition of HCP includes trainees and volunteers. All HCP should protect themselves and susceptible patients by receiving appropriate immunizations. Physicians, health care facilities, and schools for health care professionals should play an active role in implementing policies to maximize immunization of HCP. Vaccine-preventable diseases of special concern to people involved in the health care of children are as follows (see the disease-specific chapters in Section 3 for further recommendations).

- **Pertussis.** Pertussis outbreaks involving adults occur in the community and the workplace. HCP frequently are exposed to *Bordetella pertussis*, have substantial risk of illness, and can be sources for spread of infection to patients, colleagues, families, and the community. HCP of all ages who work in hospitals or ambulatory-care settings should receive *a single dose* of tetanus toxoid, reduced diphtheria toxoid, and acellular pertussis vaccine (Tdap) as soon as is feasible if they previously have not received Tdap. Hospitals and ambulatory-care facilities should provide Tdap for HCP using approaches that maximize immunization rates.[2]

  In certain cases, if there is an increased risk of pertussis in a health care setting, as evidenced by documented or suspected health care-associated transmission of pertussis, revaccination of HCP with Tdap vaccine may be considered. **(www.cdc.gov/vaccines/vpd/pertussis/tdap-revac-hcp.html)**. In these cases, it is important to consider that vaccinating HCP with Tdap is not a substitute for infection prevention and control measures, including postexposure antimicrobial prophylaxis, and therefore that revaccinated HCP still should receive postexposure antimicrobial prophylaxis when applicable. If implemented, HCP who work with infants or pregnant women should be prioritized for revaccination. Health care facilities considering repeat Tdap doses for HCP are encouraged to consult with their

---

[1]Centers for Disease Control and Prevention. Immunization of health-care providers: recommendations of the Advisory Committee on Immunization Practices (ACIP) and the Hospital Infection Control Practices Advisory Committee (HICPAC). *MMWR Recomm Rep.* 2011;60(RR-7):1–45

[2]Centers for Disease Control and Prevention. Immunization of health-care personnel: recommendations of the Advisory Committee on Immunization Practices (ACIP) and the Hospital Infection Control Practices Advisory Committee (HICPAC). *MMWR Recomm Rep.* 2011;60(RR-7):1–45

state and local public health departments, because the effectiveness of revaccination to interrupt pertussis transmission or curtail a pertussis outbreak in a health care setting is unproven.

- **Hepatitis B.** Hepatitis B vaccine (HepB) is recommended for all HCP whose work- and training-related activities involve reasonably anticipated risk of exposure to blood or other infectious body fluids. The Occupational Safety and Health Administration of the US Department of Labor issued a regulation requiring employers of personnel at risk of occupational exposure to hepatitis B to offer HepB immunization to personnel at the employer's expense. The employer shall ensure that employees who decline to accept HepB immunization offered by the employer sign the declination statement. To determine the need for revaccination and to guide postexposure prophylaxis, postvaccination serologic testing should be performed for all recently vaccinated HCP at risk of occupational percutaneous or mucosal exposure to blood or body fluids. Postvaccination serologic testing is performed 1 to 2 months after administration of the last dose of the vaccine series using a method that allows detection of the protective concentration of hepatitis B surface antibody (anti-HBs [≥10 mIU/mL]). People determined to have anti-HBs concentrations of ≥10 mIU/mL after receipt of the primary vaccine series are considered immune, and the result should be documented.

  Although vaccine-induced anti-HBs wanes over time, protection persists for immunocompetent vaccine responders (eg, those with anti-HBs ≥10 mIU/mL at their postvaccination serologic testing). Therefore, testing HCP for anti-HBs years after vaccination (eg, when HepB vaccination was received as part of routine infant immunization) might not distinguish vaccine responders from nonresponders. Preexposure assessment of anti-HBs results at the time of hiring or matriculation, followed by one or more additional doses of HepB vaccine for HCP with anti-HBs <10 mIU/mL helps to ensure that remotely vaccinated HCP will be protected.

  In some cases, susceptible HCP immunized appropriately with HepB vaccines fail to develop serologic evidence of immunity. HCP with anti-HBs <10 mIU/mL should be reimmunized with a single dose of vaccine and retested for anti-HBs within 1 to 2 months after that dose. HCP whose anti-HBs remains <10 mIU/mL should receive 2 additional doses of vaccine (usually 6 doses total), followed by repeat anti-HBs testing 1 to 2 months after the last dose. Alternatively, it might be more practical for very recently vaccinated HCP with anti-HBs <10 mIU/mL to receive 3 consecutive additional doses of HepB vaccine (usually 6 doses total), followed by anti-HBs testing 1 to 2 months after the last dose. People who do not respond to the second series and remain hepatitis B surface antigen (HBsAg) negative should be considered susceptible to hepatitis B virus infection and will need to receive Hepatitis B Immune Globulin (HBIG) prophylaxis after any known or probable exposure to blood or body fluids infected with hepatitis B virus.[1]

- **Influenza.** Because HCP can transmit influenza to patients and because health care-associated outbreaks of influenza do occur, annual influenza immunization should be considered a patient safety responsibility and a requirement for employment in a health care facility unless an individual has a recognized medical contraindication to

[1]Centers for Disease Control and Prevention. CDC guidance for evaluating health-care personnel for hepatitis B virus protection and for administering post-exposure management. *MMWR Recomm Rep.* 2013;62(RR-10):1–19.

immunization.[1] HCP should be educated about the benefits of influenza immunization and the potential health consequences of influenza illness for themselves and their patients. Influenza vaccine should be offered at no cost annually to all eligible people, and efforts should be made to ensure that vaccine is readily available to HCP on all shifts, such as through use of mobile immunization carts. A signed declination form should be obtained from personnel who decline for reasons other than medical contraindications in any facility that does not have a formal mandatory vaccine policy. Mandatory education about the benefits of vaccination should be required for all people who decline influenza immunization. The utility of mandatory masking for unimmunized HCP is not clear (**www.cdc.gov/flu/professionals/vaccination/index.htm#ACIP**). Either inactivated vaccine or recombinant influenza vaccine is appropriate as otherwise indicated. Live attenuated vaccine should not be used for personnel who will have direct contact with hematopoietic stem cell transplant recipients prior to immune reconstitution in the 7 days following vaccine administration. For the 2016–2017 and 2017–2018 influenza seasons, LAIV was not recommended for use in any population because of issues with vaccine effectiveness. For current recommendations on use of LAIV, please refer to the current AAP influenza policy statement, which is updated annually and published in August or September each year.[2]

- **Measles.** Because measles in HCP has contributed to spread of this disease during outbreaks, evidence of immunity to measles should be required for HCP. Evidence of immunity is established by laboratory confirmation of infection, laboratory evidence of immunity (positive serologic test result for measles antibody), or documented receipt of 2 appropriately spaced doses of live virus-containing measles vaccine, the first of which was administered on or after the first birthday. HCP born before 1957 generally have been considered immune to measles. However, because measles cases have occurred in HCP in this age group, health care facilities should consider offering 2 doses of measles-containing vaccine to HCP who lack proof of immunity to measles. In communities with documented measles outbreaks, 2 doses of MMR vaccine are recommended for unvaccinated HCP born before 1957 unless evidence of serologic immunity is demonstrated.

- **Mumps.** Transmission of mumps in health care facilities can be disruptive and costly. All people who work in health care facilities should be immune to mumps. Evidence of immunity is established by laboratory confirmation of infection, laboratory evidence of immunity (positive serologic test result for mumps antibody), documented receipt of 2 appropriately spaced doses of live virus-containing mumps vaccine, the first of which was administered on or after the first birthday, or birth before 1957.[3] During an outbreak, a second dose of MMR vaccine should be offered

---

[1]American Academy of Pediatrics, Committee on Infectious Diseases. Recommendation for mandatory influenza immunization of all health care personnel. *Pediatrics.* 2010;126(4):809–815 (Reaffirmed September 2015)

[2]American Academy of Pediatrics, Committee on Infectious Diseases. Recommendations for prevention and control of influenza in children, 2017–2018. *Pediatrics.* 2017; 140(4):e20172550

[3]Centers for Disease Control and Prevention. Immunization of health-care personnel: recommendations of the Advisory Committee on Immunization Practices (ACIP) and the Hospital Infection Control Practices Advisory Committee (HICPAC). *MMWR Recomm Rep.* 2011;60(RR-7):1–45

to HCP born during or after 1957 who have only received 1 dose of MMR vaccine. HCP born before 1957 without a history of MMR immunization should obtain a mumps antibody titer to document their immune status and, if negative, should receive 2 appropriately spaced doses of MMR vaccine.

- **Rubella.** Transmission of rubella from HCP to pregnant women has been reported. Although the disease is mild in adults, the risk to a fetus necessitates documentation of rubella immunity in HCP of both genders. People should be considered immune on the basis of a positive serologic test result for rubella antibody or documented proof of 1 dose of rubella-containing vaccine. A history of rubella disease is unreliable and should not be used in determining immune status. All susceptible HCP who may be exposed to patients with rubella or who take care of pregnant women, as well as people who work in educational institutions or provide child care, should be immunized with 1 dose of MMR to prevent infection for themselves and to prevent transmission of rubella to pregnant patients.

- **Varicella.** Evidence of varicella immunity is recommended for all HCP. Evidence of immunity to varicella in HCP includes any of the following: (1) documentation of 2 doses of varicella vaccine at least 28 days apart, the first of which was administered on or after the first birthday; (2) history of varicella diagnosed or verified by a physician (for a patient reporting a history of or presenting with an atypical case, a mild case, or both, the physician should seek either an epidemiologic link with a typical varicella case or evidence of laboratory confirmation, if it was performed at the time of acute disease); (3) history of herpes zoster diagnosed by a physician; or (4) laboratory evidence of immunity or laboratory confirmation of disease. Birth in the United States before 1980 should not be considered as evidence of immunity for HCP, pregnant women, or immunocompromised people (**www.cdc.gov/chickenpox/hcp/ immunity.html**). The CDC Advisory Committee on Immunization Practices and Health Infection Control Practices Advisory Committee (HICPAC) do not recommend serologic testing of HCP for immunity to varicella after receiving varicella-zoster virus vaccine. Commercially available serologic assays may not be sufficiently sensitive to detect immunization-induced antibody.

- **Meningococcus.** Meningococcal vaccination is not recommended for HCP performing direct patient care. However, clinical microbiologists routinely exposed to isolates of *Neisseria meningitidis* are at increased risk of severe meningococcal disease if exposed to a clinical isolate and should be vaccinated with MenACWY and MenB vaccines.

Children Who Received Immunizations Outside the United States or Whose Immunization Status is Unknown or Uncertain

IMMUNIZATIONS RECEIVED OUTSIDE THE UNITED STATES

People immunized in other countries, including exchange students, internationally adopted children, refugees, and other immigrants, should be immunized according to recommended schedules (including minimal ages and intervals) in the United States for healthy infants, children, and adolescents (**http://redbook.solutions.aap.org/ SS/Immunization_Schedules.aspx**). The Immigration and Nationality Act (INA) of 1996 requires all people immigrating to the United States as legal permanent residents (ie, green card holders) to provide "proof of vaccination" with vaccines recommended by the CDC Advisory Committee on Immunization Practices (ACIP) before entry into the United States (**www.cdc.gov/immigrantrefugeehealth/exams/ti/panel/ vaccination-panel-technical-instructions.html**). Specific vaccines required for immigration must fulfill the following criteria: (1) must be an age-appropriate vaccine as recommended by the ACIP for the general US population; and (2) either must protect against a disease that has the potential to cause an outbreak or protects against a disease that has been eliminated or is in the process of being eliminated in the United States. For example, human papillomavirus (HPV) vaccine is not required. Information about immunization requirements for immigrants is available on the CDC Web site (**www.cdc.gov/immigrantrefugeehealth/**). Internationally adopted children who are 10 years and younger may obtain a waiver of exemption from the INA regulations pertaining to immunization of immigrants before arrival in the United States. Children adopted from countries that are not part of the Hague Convention can receive waivers to have their immunizations delayed until arrival in the United States (**www.adoption. state.gov**). When an exemption is granted, adoptive parents are required to sign a waiver indicating their intention to comply with ACIP-recommended immunizations within 30 days after the child arrives in the United States.

Refugees are not required to meet immunization requirements of the INA at the time of initial entry into the United States but must show proof of immunization when they apply for permanent residency, typically 1 year after arrival. However, selected refugees bound for the United States are immunized in their country of origin before arrival in the United States. Clinicians should review the CDC Refugee Health Web site (**www.cdc. gov/immigrantrefugeehealth/guidelines/overseas/interventions/ immunizations-schedules.html**) for information about which refugee populations currently are receiving immunization outside the United States. Refugee children, however, almost universally are immunized incompletely and may not have immunization records. Additional guidance about the management of refugees after arrival in the United States is available at **www.cdc.gov/immigrantrefugeehealth/ guidelines/domestic/immunizations-guidelines.html.**

In general, only written documentation should be accepted as evidence of previous immunization. BCG, DTwP or DTaP, poliovirus, measles, and hepatitis B vaccines are administered routinely and may be documented in an immunization record. Refugee and immigrant children should meet ACIP recommendations for poliovirus vaccination, which require protection against all 3 poliovirus types by age-appropriate vaccination with IPV or trivalent OPV (tOPV). Some countries may have provided monovalent or bivalent OPV during polio vaccination campaigns after April 1, 2016. Only written documentation of receipt of IPV or tOPV constitutes proof of vaccination, according to US polio vaccination recommendations. If OPV was administered before Aril 1, 2016, OPV can be counted as tOPV. If OPV was administered after April 1, 2016, it may not be counted as tOPV unless the written documentation denotes that it is tOPV. In the absence of adequate written vaccination records, vaccination or revaccination in accordance with the age-appropriate US IPV schedule is recommended (see Poliovirus Infections, p 647, for further recommendations). Immunizations to prevent infection caused by agents such as Hib, *S pneumoniae*, mumps, rubella, hepatitis A, and varicella often are administered less frequently or are not part of the routine immunization schedule in other countries, and therefore, there may not be written documentation for these vaccines. Increasingly, more of these vaccines are being incorporated into the immunization schedules in countries outside the United States. In general, written documentation of immunizations can be accepted as evidence of adequacy of previous immunization if the vaccines, dates of administration, number of doses, intervals between doses, and age of the child at the time of immunization are consistent internally and are comparable to current US or World Health Organization schedules (**http://apps. who.int/immunization_monitoring/en/globalsummary/ countryprofileselect.cfm**). Inaccuracies, fraudulent data, or other problems, such as recording MMR vaccine but giving a product that did not contain one or more of the components (eg, mumps and/or rubella) should be considered during review of records. Any vaccination documented on the official Department of State health immigration form (DS 3025) should be accepted. Studies performed in internationally adopted children have demonstrated that the majority of children with documentation of immunizations have antibodies consistent with those immunizations. Limited country-specific data are available regarding serologic verification of immunization records for other categories of immigrant children. Evaluation of concentrations of antibody to vaccine-preventable diseases is useful to ensure that vaccines were administered and were immunogenic, as well as to document immunity from past infection (see Serologic Testing to Document Immunization Status, p 102). If serologic testing is not available or is too costly, or if a positive result would not mitigate need for further immunization, the prudent course is to repeat administration of the immunizations in question.

UNKNOWN OR UNCERTAIN IMMUNIZATION STATUS IN US CHILDREN

There are circumstances in which the immunization status for a child born in the United States is uncertain or unknown because of lack of paper or electronic documentation of immunizations, an incomplete or inaccurate record, or a recording inconsistent with a recommended product or schedule. For US-born children, serologic testing can be performed to determine whether antibody concentrations are present for some of the vaccine-preventable diseases (see Serologic Testing to Document Immunization Status). A combined strategy of serologic testing for antibodies to some vaccine antigens and immunization for others may be used. If serologic testing is not available or is too costly or if a positive result would not mitigate need for further immunization, the prudent course is to repeat administration of the immunizations in question.

SEROLOGIC TESTING TO DOCUMENT IMMUNIZATION STATUS

The usefulness, validity, and interpretation of serologic testing to guide management of vaccinations can be complex and varies by age. The cost of testing versus the cost of administering a given immunization series, as well as the likelihood of adherence for completing the immunization series, also should be considered in these decisions. In most situations, a record verifying the administration of a complete vaccine series would be more reliable than serologic testing. In children older than 6 months with or without written documentation of immunization, serologic testing to document antibodies to diphtheria and tetanus toxoids (ie, ≥ 0.1 IU/mL), or Hib for a child younger than 60 months (ie, ≥ 0.15 U/mL), may be considered to determine whether the child likely has received and responded to dose(s) of the vaccine in question. If the child has "protective" antibodies, the immunization series should be completed as appropriate for that child's age. If a child does not have "protective" antibodies, the series should be restarted, with the understanding that for some vaccine-preventable diseases, fewer doses of vaccine are needed to complete the series as a child ages. The immunization record, plus presence of antibody to diphtheria and tetanus toxoids, can be used as proxy for receipt of pertussis-containing vaccine dose(s). No commercial serologic kit for pertussis is cleared by the FDA for diagnostic use, and little is understood about the clinical accuracy of these kits. No serologic test is available to assess immunity to rotavirus. In children older than 12 months, hepatitis A, measles, mumps, and rubella antibody concentrations could be measured to determine whether the child is immune; these antibody tests should not be performed in children younger than 12 months because of the potential presence of maternal antibody. Usefulness of measuring measles antibody is limited, because the majority of foreign-born children will need mumps and rubella vaccines, available in the United States only as MMR vaccine, because mumps and rubella vaccines are administered infrequently in resource-limited countries. Two doses of MMR vaccine should be administered for mumps coverage, even if measles antibodies are present. Rubella coverage is achieved following 1 dose of a rubella-containing vaccine. The documented receipt of 2 doses of varicella vaccine or positive varicella titers is the best indication of immunity to varicella. For immunocompetent children 5 years or older, Hib vaccine is not indicated even if none was administered previously; serologic testing should not be performed, because children in this age group frequently have antibody concentrations <0.15 U/mL yet are not susceptible to *H influenzae* type b infection. Only written documentation of receipt of IPV or OPV constitutes proof of poliovirus vaccination, according to ACIP recommendations; serologic testing to assess immunity no longer is available and therefore no longer is recommended by the CDC. Age-appropriate pneumococcal vaccine dose(s) should be administered if a completed series is not documented; serologic testing should not be performed for validation or evidence of immunity.

For immigrants, serologic testing for HBsAg should be performed for all children to identify chronic hepatitis B virus infection. When the HBsAg test result is negative, the results of the anti-HBs and core antibody (anti-HBc) tests will determine whether the child is immune (from immunization or disease, respectively). Refugee children who are receiving vaccinations overseas as part of the Refugee Vaccination Program also are tested for HBsAg before vaccination. The result of this test is documented on the Department of State official health immigration forms. Transient HBsAg antigenemia can occur following receipt of HepB vaccine, with HBsAg being detected as early as 24 hours after and up to 2 to 3 weeks following administration of the vaccine, so prevaccination assessment is important. Some immigrant or refugee children may have had previous hepatitis A infection; presence of immunoglobulin (Ig) G-specific antibody to hepatitis A virus would preclude need for hepatitis A vaccine.

International Travel

Approximately 60% of children traveling internationally will become ill during their travels, and up to 19% will require medical care. At particular risk are US-born children of immigrants visiting friends and relatives abroad. Additionally, adolescents and young adults are at risk during international travel either for school or between school years. Visiting a health care provider who specializes in travel medicine can mitigate this risk but requires advance planning, preferably at least 6 to 8 weeks, at minimum, prior to travel to allow time to complete necessary pretravel vaccinations. Parents should be made aware that there is increased risk of exposure to vaccine-preventable diseases overseas, even in many countries in Europe. Routinely recommended immunizations should be up-to-date before international travel, and some routinely recommended immunizations should be administered early or on an accelerated schedule to optimize protection prior to travel. Additional vaccines to prevent cholera, yellow fever, meningococcal disease, typhoid fever, rabies, and Japanese encephalitis may be indicated depending on the destination and duration and type of international travel (see disease-specific chapters in Section 3). Planning ahead is essential, because yellow fever vaccine is only available at certified centers in the United States, Japanese encephalitis virus immunization requires 28 days to complete, and catch-up immunization for routine pediatric vaccines may require more time.

In addition to exposure to vaccine-preventable illness, travelers to tropical and subtropical areas often risk exposure to malaria, dengue, chikungunya, Zika virus, tuberculosis, diarrhea, and skin diseases for which vaccines are not available. For travelers to areas with endemic malaria, antimalarial chemoprophylaxis and insect precautions are vitally important (see Malaria, p 527). Attending to hand hygiene, choosing safer foods, avoiding insect bites, and limiting exposure to contaminated sand, soil, and water reduce travelers' risk of acquiring other communicable diseases. Travelers should avoid prolonged exposure to people who have chronic cough, which may be a sign of active pulmonary tuberculosis. If meaningful exposure does occur in a country with high prevalence of tuberculosis, tuberculosis testing should be considered 8 to 10 weeks after return to the United States.

Up-to-date information, including alerts about current disease outbreaks that may affect international travelers, is available on the CDC Travelers' Health Web site (**wwwnc.cdc.gov/travel/**) or the WHO Web site (**www.who.int/ith/**). *Health Information for International Travel* (the "Yellow Book," **wwwnc.cdc.gov/travel/page/yellowbook-home**) is revised every 2 years by the CDC and is an excellent reference for travelers and for practitioners who advise international travelers of health risks. Travel information and recommendations can be obtained from the CDC (800-CDC-INFO). Local and state health departments and travel clinics[1] also can provide updated information. Many colleges have travel clinics where appropriate immunizations can be obtained. Information about cruise ship sanitation inspection scores and reports can be found on the CDC Web site (**www.cdc.gov/nceh/vsp/default.htm**). In June 2007, federal agencies developed a public health Do Not Board (DNB) list, enabling domestic and international public health officials to request that people with communicable diseases who meet specific criteria and pose a serious threat to the public be restricted

---

[1]Sources for travel clinics: Center for Disease Control and Prevention (**wwwnc.cdc.gov/travel/page/find-clinic**); American Society of Tropical Medicine and Hygiene (**www.astmh.org/for-astmh-members/clinical-consultants-directory**); International Society for Travel Medicine (**www.istm.org/AF_CstmClinicDirectory.asp**)

from boarding commercial aircraft from or arriving in the United States.[1]

RECOMMENDED IMMUNIZATIONS

Transmission of pathogens prevented by the US childhood and adolescent immunization schedule continues in other areas of the world, including some industrialized nations. Infants and children embarking on international travel should be up-to-date on receipt of immunizations recommended for their age. To optimize immunity before departure, vaccines may need to be administered on an accelerated schedule.

HEPATITIS A. Hepatitis A vaccine (HepA) is recommended routinely in a 2-dose series ≥6 months apart for all children at 12 through 23 months of age in the United States. HepA should be considered for all people who are unimmunized or underimmunized and traveling to areas with intermediate or high rates of hepatitis A infection. These include all areas of the world except Australia, Canada, Japan, New Zealand, and Western Europe. Inactivated HepA is used for postexposure immunoprophylaxis for people 12 months through 40 years of age. Immune Globulin Intramuscular (IGIM) should be used for postexposure immunoprophylaxis in children younger than 12 months, immunocompromised people, people with chronic liver disease, and people for whom HepA vaccine is contraindicated. The dose of IGIM administered for preexposure prophylaxis of hepatitis A infection may interfere with the immune response to varicella and MMR vaccines for up to 3 months (Table 1.13, p 40). A combination HepA-HepB vaccine is available for people 18 years and older.

HEPATITIS B. Hepatitis B vaccine (HepB) is recommended routinely for all children in the United States and should be considered for susceptible travelers of all ages (ie, those born before universal recommendations) visiting areas where hepatitis B infection is endemic, such as countries in Asia, Africa, and some parts of South America (see Hepatitis B, p 401). An accelerated dosing schedule is approved for 1 hepatitis B vaccine (Engerix-B [GlaxoSmithKline Biologicals, Research Triangle Park, NC]), during which the first 3 doses are administered at 0, 1, and 2 months. In another accelerated schedule, adults receive doses on days 0, 7, and 21. This schedule may benefit travelers who have insufficient time to complete a standard schedule before departure. If the accelerated schedule is used, a fourth dose should be administered at 12 months (see Hepatitis B, p 401). A combination HepA-HepB vaccine is available for people 18 years and older. This vaccine can be administered on a 3-dose schedule (0, 1, and 6 months) or on an alternate accelerated schedule administered at 0, 7, and 21 to 30 days, followed by a fourth dose at 12 months. The adult formulation of Recombivax HB (Merck & Co Inc, Whitehouse Station, NJ) is licensed as a 2-dose schedule (0 and 4–6 months) for adolescents 11 through 15 years of age (see Table 3.26, p 423).

MEASLES. People traveling abroad should be immune to measles to provide personal protection and minimize importation of the infection. Importation of measles remains an important source for measles cases in the United States.[2] People should be considered immune to measles if they have laboratory confirmation of prior infection, laboratory evidence of immunity (positive serologic test result for measles antibody), documented

---

[1] Centers for Disease Control and Prevention. Federal air travel restrictions for public health purposes—United States, June 2007–May 2008. *MMWR Morb Mortal Wkly Rep.* 2008;57(37):1009–1012

[2] Centers for Disease Control and Prevention. Measles—United States, January 4-April 2, 2015. *MMWR Morb Mortal Wkly Rep.* 2015;64(14):373–376.

receipt of 2 appropriately spaced doses of live virus-containing measles vaccine, the first of which was administered on or after the first birthday, or were born in the United States before 1957 (see Measles, p 537). Children who travel or live abroad should be vaccinated at an earlier age than recommended for children remaining in the United States. MMR vaccine is safe to use in children as young as 6 months. Children 6 through 11 months of age should receive 1 dose of MMR vaccine before departure; these children still will require 2 valid doses of MMR at 12 months or older, separated by at least 28 days, to complete the schedule. Children 12 months of age and older at the time of departure from the United States should have received 2 doses of MMR vaccine separated by at least 28 days, with the first dose administered on or after the first birthday. MMR should not be administered to a pregnant woman but should be given to household contacts when indicated. Providers should be aware of interaction among parenteral live-virus vaccines, including MMR, varicella and yellow fever vaccine, and consider this prior to updating routine immunizations prior to travel. Live-virus vaccines generally should be administered either on the same day or separated by at least 4 weeks (see Simultaneous Administration of Multiple Vaccines, p 35).

POLIOVIRUS. Polio remains endemic in a few countries in Asia and Africa; an up-to-date listing of polio cases can be found at **www.polioeradication.org.** The Western Hemisphere was declared free of wild-type poliovirus in 1994, and the Western Pacific Region was declared free in 2000. The finding of vaccine-derived poliovirus in stool samples from several asymptomatic unimmunized people in a United States community raises concerns about the risk of transmission of polio within other communities with low levels of immunization.[1] The ACIP recommends the following[2] (see Poliovirus Infections, p 647):

- The 4-dose IPV series should be administered at 2 months, 4 months, 6 through 18 months, and 4 through 6 years of age.
- The final dose in the IPV series should be administered at 4 years or older, regardless of the number of previous doses.
- The minimum interval from dose 3 to dose 4 is 6 months.
- The minimum interval from dose 1 to dose 2, and from dose 2 to dose 3, is 4 weeks.
- The minimum age for dose 1 is 6 weeks.

Travelers 18 years or older visiting regions identified on the CDC travel Web site as polio vulnerable should receive a booster dose of IPV. Some countries (Pakistan, Afghanistan) may require long-term visitors (>4 weeks) to show evidence of polio vaccination (OPV or IPV) in the previous 4 weeks to 12 months. This vaccination needs to be documented on an International Certificate of Vaccination. Current recommendations should be verified prior to departure.

REQUIRED OR RECOMMENDED TRAVEL-RELATED IMMUNIZATIONS

Depending on the destination, planned activity, and length of stay, other immunizations

---

[1] Centers for Disease Control and Prevention. Poliovirus infections in four unvaccinated children—Minnesota, Agust–October 2005. *MMWR Morb Mortal Wkly Rep.* 2005;54(41):1053–1055

[2] Centers for Disease Control and Prevention. Updated recommendations of the Advisory Committee on Immunization Practices (ACIP) regarding routine poliovirus vaccination. *MMWR Morb Mortal Wkly Rep.* 2009;58(30):829–830

may be required or recommended (see **wwwnc.cdc.gov/travel/** and disease-specific chapters in Section 3).

CHOLERA. The whole-cell inactivated cholera vaccine no longer is produced in the United States. An oral cholera vaccine (Vaxchora [PaxVax Bermuda Ltd, Redwood City, CA]) recently was approved in the United States for use in people 18 through 64 years of age. Although historically, some countries required cholera vaccination for entry, this no longer is the case (**wwwnc.cdc.gov/travel/yellowbook/2016/infectious-diseases-related-to-travel/cholera**).

JAPANESE ENCEPHALITIS.[1] Japanese encephalitis (JE) virus, a mosquito-borne Flavivirus, is the most common cause of encephalitis in Asia. The risk of JE for most travelers to Asia is low but varies on the basis of destination, duration, season, and activities (**wwwnc.cdc.gov/travel/yellowbook/2016/infectious-diseases-related-to-travel/japanese-encephalitis**). All travelers to countries with endemic JE should be informed of the risks and should use personal protective measures to reduce the risk of mosquito bites. For some travelers who will be in high-risk settings, JE vaccine can further reduce the risk for infection. JE vaccine is recommended for travelers who plan to spend a month or longer in areas with endemic infection during the JE virus transmission season. JE vaccine also should be considered for shorter-term travelers if they plan to travel outside of an urban area and have an itinerary or activities that will increase their risk of mosquito exposure in an endemic area.

An inactivated Vero cell culture-derived JE virus vaccine (Ixiaro [Valneva Scotland Ltd, Livingston, United Kingdom]) is approved and available in the United States for use in adults and children 2 months and older. The primary vaccination series is 2 doses administered 28 days apart. For adults, a booster dose may be administered at 1 year or longer after the primary series if ongoing exposure or reexposure is expected. In one small study among children from countries without endemic JE, 89% (17/19) of children were seroprotected at 3 years following a primary 2-dose series of Ixiaro. Data are not yet available on the need for a booster dose in children.

INFLUENZA. In addition to recommended annual influenza immunization, influenza vaccine may be warranted at other times for international travelers depending on the destination, duration of travel, risk of acquisition of disease (in part based on the season of the year), and the travelers' underlying health status. Because the influenza season is different in the northern and southern hemispheres and epidemic strains may differ, the antigenic composition of influenza vaccines used in North America may be different from those used in the southern hemisphere, and timing of administration may vary (see Influenza, p 476).

MENINGOCOCCUS. Three meningococcal conjugate vaccines (MCVs) can be considered for use in infants traveling to areas where meningococcal disease is hyperendemic, such as serogroups A and W in sub-Saharan Africa or other areas with current meningococcal epidemics. Saudi Arabia requires a certificate of immunization for pilgrims to Mecca or Medina during the Hajj. MCVs vary in serogroups covered, conjugating protein, ages of approved use, and dosing schedules. The following MCVs are approved for traveling infants and older people for protection against serogroups contained in the vaccines: MenACWY-CRM (Menveo, GlaxoSmithKline, Research Triangle Park, NC; for people

[1]Centers for Disease Control and Prevention. Inactivated Japanese encephalitis vaccines: Recommendations of the Advisory Committee on Immunization Practices (ACIP). *MMWR Recomm Rep.* 2010;59(RR-1):1–27

2 months to 55 years of age), and MenACWY-D (Menactra, Sanofi Pasteur, Swiftwater, PA; for people 9 months to 55 years of age). Completion of the entire series is preferred prior to travel. Vaccination for travelers against meningococcal serogroups A, C, W, and Y is as follows:

- For children younger than 7 months, MenACWY-CRM is administered at 2, 4, and 6 months (with booster at 12–18 months of age).
- For children 7 months through 23 months of age, 2 doses of MenACWY-CRM should be administered, separated by at least 3 months and with the second dose given in the second year of life.
- For children 24 months or older without persistent complement deficiencies, functional or anatomic asplenia, or HIV infection, a single dose of either MenACWY-CRM or MenACWY-D) is administered; if MenACWY-D is used, it should be administered at least 4 weeks after completion of all PCV doses. For patients with complement deficiencies, asplenia, or HIV infection, see Table 3.44 (p 559).

Revaccination with a conjugate vaccine is recommended for people who are at continuous or repeated increased risk of meningococcal infection (see Meningococcal Infections, p 550). The MenB vaccine (Trumenba [Wyeth Pharmaceuticals, Philadelphia, PA], Bexsero [Novartis Vaccines and Diagnostics, Sovicille, Italy]) series may be indicated for individuals 10 years and older traveling to areas with outbreaks of serogroup B meningococcal disease.

RABIES. Rabies immunization should be considered for children who will be traveling to areas with endemic rabies where they may encounter wild or domestic animals (particularly dogs). The preexposure series is administered in 3 doses given on days 0, 7, and 21 or 28 by intramuscular injection (see Rabies, p 673). In the event of a bite by a potentially rabid animal, all travelers (whether they have received preexposure rabies vaccine or not) should be counseled to clean the wound thoroughly with soap and water and then promptly receive postexposure prophylaxis (PEP; see Rabies, p 673). In previously unvaccinated individuals, PEP consists of Rabies Immune Globulin (RIG) plus 4 doses of rabies vaccine. In contrast, prior receipt of preexposure vaccination avoids the need for RIG, but requires 2 additional doses of rabies vaccine in the event of a potential exposure, with the first dose administered ideally on the day of exposure and the second dose given 3 days later. Travelers who have completed a 3-dose preexposure series or have received the full PEP series do not require routine boosters, except after a likely rabies exposure. Periodic serum testing for rabies virus-neutralizing antibody is not necessary for routine international travelers.

TUBERCULOSIS. The risk of being infected with *Mycobacterium tuberculosis* during international travel depends on the activities of the traveler and the epidemiology of tuberculosis in the areas in which travel occurs. In general, the risk of acquiring infection during usual tourist activities appears to be low, and no pre- or post-travel testing is recommended routinely. When travelers live or work among the general population of a country with a high prevalence of tuberculosis, the risk may be appreciably higher. In most high-prevalence countries, contact investigation of tuberculosis cases is not performed, and diagnosis and treatment of latent tuberculosis infection (LTBI) is uncommon or is restricted to high-risk people. Children returning to the United States who have signs or symptoms compatible with tuberculosis should be evaluated immediately for tuberculosis disease. It is advisable to perform a tuberculin skin test or interferon-gamma release assay 8 to 10 weeks after return for children who spent 1 month or longer in a country with high prevalence of tuberculosis and as soon as possible for children who had a known tuberculosis exposure, regardless of time abroad or countries visited. Pretravel administration of bacille Calmette-Guérin vaccine generally is not recommended.

TYPHOID. Typhoid vaccine is recommended for travelers who may be exposed to contaminated food or water. Two typhoid vaccines are available in the United States: an oral vaccine containing live attenuated *Salmonella* Typhi (Ty21a strain) approved for people 6 years and older and a parenteral Vi capsular polysaccharide (ViCPS) vaccine approved for people 2 years and older. Travelers should be reminded that typhoid immunization is not 100% effective, and typhoid fever still can occur; both vaccines protect 50% to 80% of recipients. Revaccination is required every 5 years for oral and every 2 years for inactivated vaccine if continued or renewed exposure to *Salmonella* serovar Typhi is expected. For specific recommendations, see *Salmonella* Infections (p 711). The oral vaccine capsules should be refrigerated and should not be administered during use of any antimicrobial agent other than the antimalarial agents mefloquine, chloroquine, and atovaquone/proguanil when used in prophylactic doses (**www.cdc.gov/mmwr/preview/mmwrhtml/mm6411a4.htm**). Because the vaccine is not completely efficacious, typhoid immunization is not a substitute for careful selection of food and beverages.

YELLOW FEVER. Yellow fever (YF) occurs in sub-Saharan Africa and tropical South America. Although rare, YF continues to be reported among unimmunized travelers and may be fatal. Prevention measures against YF should include protection against mosquito bites (see Prevention of Mosquitoborne and Tickborne Infections, p 195) and immunization. YF vaccine, a live attenuated virus vaccine, is available in the United States only in centers designated by state health departments. Current requirements and recommendations for YF immunization on the basis of travel destination can be obtained from the CDC Travelers' Health Web site (**wwwnc.cdc.gov/travel/**). Travelers should verify entry requirements for their countries of travel. When required, YF vaccine should be completed at least 10 days before travel.

Administration of YF vaccine is recommended for people 9 months and older who are traveling to or living in areas of South America and Africa in which risk exists for YF virus transmission. In 2015, the ACIP updated recommendations for YF vaccine, requiring only a single dose for most travelers, eliminating the recommendation for booster doses.[1] Additional doses of YF vaccine are recommended for certain populations (ie, women initially vaccinated when they were pregnant, hematopoietic stem cell transplant recipients, and HIV-infected people) who might not have a robust or sustained immune response to YF vaccine compared with other recipients. Furthermore, additional doses may be administered to certain groups believed to be at increased risk for YF because of their location and duration of travel.

Because serious adverse events can follow YF vaccine administration, only people at risk of exposure to YF or who require proof of vaccination for country entry should be immunized. Contraindications and precautions to immunization should be followed (Table 1.21). YF vaccine rarely has been found to be associated with a risk of viscerotropic disease (multiple-organ system failure) and neurologic disease (postvaccinal

---

[1] Staples JE, Bocchini JA, Rubin L, Fischer M. Yellow fever vaccine booster doses: recommendations of the Advisory Committee on Immunization Practices, 2015. *MMWR Morb Mortal Wkly Rep.* 2015;64(23):647–650

Table 1.21. Contraindications and Precautions to Yellow Fever Vaccine Administration

Contraindications	Precautions
Allergy to vaccine component	Age 6 through 8 mo
Age younger than 6 mo	Age ≥60 y
Symptomatic HIV infection or CD4+ T-lymphocyte count <200/mm³ (or <15% of total in children younger than 6 y)[a]	Asymptomatic HIV infection and CD4+ T-lymphocyte count 200–499/mm³ (or 15%–24% of total in children younger than 6 y)
Thymus disorder associated with abnormal immune function	Pregnancy
	Breastfeeding
Primary immunodeficiencies	
Malignant neoplasms	
Transplantation	
Immunosuppressive and immunomodulatory therapies	

[a]Symptoms of HIV have been classified (Panel on Antiretroviral Guidelines for Adults and Adolescents. Guidelines for the use of antiretroviral agents in HIV-1-infected adults and adolescents; US Department of Health and Human Services; 2008. Available at: **http://aidsinfo.nih.gov/Guidelines/html/1/adult-and-adolescent-treatment-guidelines/0/**; and Panel on Antiretroviral Therapy and Medical Management of HIV-Infected Children. Guidelines for the Use of Antiretroviral Agents in Pediatric HIV Infection; 2016. Available at: **http://aidsinfo.nih.gov/contentfiles/lvguidelines/pediatricguidelines.pdf.**

encephalitis). There is increased risk of adverse events in children with thymic dysfunction. YF vaccine, like all live-virus vaccines, should be avoided during pregnancy. Meningoencephalitis has been reported in several infants <1 month of age exposed to vaccine virus through breastfeeding.

YF vaccine is contraindicated before 6 months of age, and whenever possible, immunization should be delayed until 9 months of age to minimize the risk of vaccine-associated encephalitis. Administration of YF vaccine to women who are breastfeeding should be delayed until infants are at least 9 months of age unless travel is unavoidable. Consultation with a travel medicine expert or the CDC Division of Vector-Borne Infectious Diseases (970-221-6400) or the Division of Global Migration and Quarantine (404-498-1600) to weigh risks and benefits is advised. People who cannot receive YF vaccine because of contraindications should consider alternative itineraries or destinations.

OTHER CONSIDERATIONS. In addition to vaccine-preventable diseases, travelers to the tropics will be exposed to other diseases, such as malaria, which can be life threatening. Prevention strategies for malaria are twofold: prevention of mosquito bites and use of antimalarial chemoprophylaxis. For recommendations on appropriate use of chemoprophylaxis, including recommendations for pregnant women, infants, and breastfeeding mothers, see Malaria (p 527). Prevention of mosquito bites will decrease the risk of malaria, dengue, chikungunya, Zika, and other mosquito-transmitted diseases (see Prevention of Mosquitoborne and Tickborne Infections, p 195).

Travelers' diarrhea affects up to 60% of travelers but may be mitigated by attention to foods and beverages ingested (including ice). Chemoprophylaxis generally is not recommended. Educating families about self-treatment, particularly oral rehydration, is critical. Packets of oral rehydration salts can be obtained before travel and are available in most pharmacies throughout the world, including in resource-limited countries, where diarrheal diseases are most common. During international travel, families may want to carry an antimicrobial agent (eg, fluoroquinolone for older adolescents and adults and azithromycin for younger children) for treatment of moderate to severe diarrhea. The choice of agent should be determined by the resistance pattern within the particular region to be visited. Parents must be made aware that administering these antimicrobial agents puts their child at increased risk of becoming colonized with highly resistant bacteria. Antimotility agents may be considered for older children and adolescents (see *Escherichia coli* Diarrhea, p 338) for mild to moderate diarrhea (and may be used along with an antimicrobial agent); however, antimotility agents generally should be avoided in cases of bloody diarrhea or diarrhea associated with fever. Bismuth subsalicylate has been approved by the FDA for use in children ≥12 years old and has been shown to reduce the severity of travelers' diarrhea (**www.cdc.gov/travel**).

Travelers should be aware of potential acquisition of respiratory tract viruses, including novel strains of influenza. They should be counseled on hand hygiene and avoidance of close contact with animals (dead or live). Swimming, water sports, and ecotourism around freshwater carry risks of acquisition of infections from environmental contamination (notably schistosomiasis and leptospirosis from lakes, streams, or rivers). Pyogenic skin infections and cutaneous larva migrans are common. Travelers should avoid direct skin contact with sand, soil, and animals.

In addition to infectious risks incurred while traveling abroad, travelers should be counseled about the risk of motor vehicle crashes, which are the leading cause of death among travelers, resulting in an estimated 25 000 fatalities per year among tourists (**wwwnc.cdc.gov/travel/page/road-safety**).

Recommendations for Care of Children in Special Circumstances

HUMAN MILK

Breastfeeding provides numerous health benefits to infants, including protection against morbidity and mortality from infectious diseases of bacterial, viral, and parasitic (eg, *Trypanosoma cruzi*, *Strongyloides* species) origin. In addition to providing an optimal source of infant nutrition, human milk contains immune-modulating factors, including secretory antibodies, glycoconjugates, anti-inflammatory components, prebiotics, probiotics, and antimicrobial compounds such as lysozyme and lactoferrin, which contribute to the formation of a health-promoting microbiota and an optimally functioning immune system. Breastfed infants have high concentrations of protective bifidobacteria and lactobacilli in their gastrointestinal tracts, which diminish the risk of colonization and infection with pathogenic organisms. Protection by human milk is established most clearly for pathogens causing gastrointestinal tract infection. In addition, human milk likely provides protection against otitis media and upper and lower respiratory tract infections. Human milk decreases the severity of upper and lower respiratory tract respiratory infections, including bronchiolitis, resulting in more than a 70% reduction in hospitalizations. Evidence indicates that human milk may modulate the development of the immune system of infants. Maternal milk and pasteurized donor human milk are clearly superior to formula for preterm and very low birth weight infants as they are associated with decreased rates of serious infections and necrotizing enterocolitis and better feeding tolerance, growth, and neurodevelopmental outcomes.[1,2,3]

The American Academy of Pediatrics (AAP) publishes policy statements and a manual on infant feeding[4] that provide further information about the benefits of breastfeeding, recommended feeding practices, and potential contaminants of human milk. In the *Pediatric Nutrition Handbook*[5] and in the AAP policy statements on human milk

---

[1]World Health Organization. *Guidelines on Optimal Feeding of Low Birth-Weight Infants in Low- and Middle-Income Countries*. Geneva, Switzerland: World Health Organization; 2011. Available at: **www.who.int/ maternal_child_adolescent/documents/infant_feeding_low_bw/en/**

[2]American Academy of Pediatrics, Section on Breastfeeding. Breastfeeding and the use of human milk. *Pediatrics*. 2012;129(3):e827-e841

[3]American Academy of Pediatrics, Committee on Nutrition, Section on Breastfeeding, Committee on Fetus and Newborn. Donor human milk for the high-risk infant: preparation, safety, and usage options in the United States. *Pediatrics*. 2017;139(1):e20163440

[4]American Academy of Pediatrics. *Breastfeeding Handbook for Physicians. 2nd ed*. Schanler RJ, Krebs NF, Mass SB, eds. Elk Grove Village, IL: American Academy of Pediatrics; 2013

[5]American Academy of Pediatrics, Committee on Nutrition. *Pediatric Nutrition Handbook*. Kleinman RE, Greer FR, eds. 7th ed. Elk Grove Village, IL: American Academy of Pediatrics; 2014

and pasteurized donor human milk,[1,2] issues regarding immunization of lactating mothers and breastfeeding infants, transmission of infectious agents via human milk, and potential effects on breastfed infants of antimicrobial agents administered to lactating mothers are addressed.

Immunization of Mothers and Infants

EFFECT OF MATERNAL IMMUNIZATION

Women who have not received recommended immunizations before or during pregnancy may be immunized during the postpartum period, regardless of lactation status. With the exception of yellow fever vaccine,[3] no evidence exists to validate any clinical concern about the presence of other live vaccine viruses in maternal milk if the mother is immunized during lactation. Lactating women may be immunized as recommended for adults and adolescents (**www.cdc.gov/vaccines**). If previously unimmunized or if traveling to an area with endemic poliovirus circulation, a lactating mother may receive inactivated poliovirus vaccine (IPV). Women known to be pregnant or attempting to become pregnant should not receive measles-mumps-rubella (MMR) vaccine. Rubella-seronegative mothers should be immunized with MMR vaccine during the early postpartum period. Attenuated rubella virus can be detected in human milk and transmitted to breastfed infants, with subsequent seroconversion and subclinical infection in the infant. In lactating women who receive live attenuated varicella vaccine, neither varicella DNA in human milk (by polymerase chain reaction assay) nor varicella antibody in the infant can be detected. Women should receive a dose of tetanus toxoid, reduced diphtheria toxoid, and acellular pertussis (Tdap) vaccine during each pregnancy,[4] preferably between 27 and 36 weeks' gestation. If not administered during pregnancy, Tdap should be administered immediately postpartum. If not already vaccinated, pregnant women should receive their annual inactivated influenza vaccine for the current influenza season during pregnancy. Nonimmunized breastfeeding women should receive influenza vaccine.[5,6] Inactivated or live attenuated influenza vaccine may be administered during the postpartum period, although the live attenuated influenza vaccine has not

---

[1] American Academy of Pediatrics, Section on Breastfeeding. Breastfeeding and the use of human milk. *Pediatrics*. 2012;129(3):e827-e841

[2] American Academy of Pediatrics, Committee on Nutrition, Section on Breastfeeding, Committee on Fetus and Newborn. Donor human milk for the high-risk infant: preparation, safety, and usage options in the United States. *Pediatrics*. 2017;139(1):e20163440

[3] Centers for Disease Control and Prevention. Yellow fever vaccine. Recommendations of the Advisory Committee on Immunization Practices (ACIP). *MMWR Recomm Rep*. 2010;59(RR-7):1-27

[4] Centers for Disease Control and Prevention. Updated recommendations for use of tetanus toxoid, reduced diphtheria toxoid, and acellular pertussis vaccine (Tdap) in pregnant women—Advisory Committee on Immunization Practices (ACIP), 2012. *MMWR Morb Mortal Wkly Rep*. 2013;62(7):131-135

[5] Centers for Disease Control and Prevention. Prevention and control of influenza with vaccines. Recommendations of the Advisory Committee on Immunization Practices (ACIP), 2011. *MMWR Morb Mortal Wkly Rep*. 2011;60(33):1128-1132. For annual updates, see **www.cdc.gov/vaccines**

[6] American Academy of Pediatrics, Committee on Infectious Diseases. Recommendations for prevention and control of influenza, 2017-2018. *Pediatrics*. 2017;140(4):e20172550. For updates, see **https://redbook. solutions.aap.org/ss/influenza-resources.aspx**

been recommended for use in any population for the 2016-2017 or the 2017-2018 influenza seasons; recommendations for future seasons will be addressed in upcoming influenza policy statements (**https://redbook.solutions.aap.org/ss/influenza-resources.aspx**).

Breastfeeding is a precaution for yellow fever vaccine administration. Three serious adverse events have been reported in exclusively breastfed infants younger than 1 month whose mothers received yellow fever vaccine while lactating.[1] The risk for potential yellow fever vaccine virus exposure through breastfeeding is unknown. Until more information is available, yellow fever vaccine should be avoided in breastfeeding women. However, when travel of nursing mothers to an area with endemic yellow fever cannot be avoided or postponed, these women should be vaccinated. Pregnancy is a precaution to yellow fever vaccine administration, because rare cases of in utero transmission of the vaccine virus have been documented. Pregnant and breastfeeding mothers should avoid areas with yellow fever. If a pregnant or breastfeeding woman is residing in an area with a yellow fever outbreak, despite the concern about the live yellow fever vaccine virus being transmitted to her offspring, the woman should receive the yellow fever vaccine.

EFFICACY AND SAFETY OF IMMUNIZATION IN BREASTFED INFANTS

Infants should be immunized according to the recommended childhood and adolescent immunization schedule (**https://redbook.solutions.aap.org/SS/Immunization_Schedules.aspx**), regardless of the mode of infant feeding. The immunogenicity of some recommended vaccines is enhanced by breastfeeding, but data are limited as to whether this correlates with an increase in vaccine efficacy. Theoretically, high concentrations of poliovirus antibody in human milk could interfere with the immunogenicity of oral poliovirus vaccine; this is not a concern with IPV, which is the only poliovirus vaccine used in the United States. There is in vitro evidence that human milk from women who live in areas with endemic rotavirus contains antibodies that can neutralize live rotavirus vaccine virus. However, in licensing trials, the effectiveness of rotavirus vaccine in breastfed infants was comparable to that in nonbreastfed infants. Furthermore, breastfeeding reduced the likelihood of rotavirus disease in infancy.

Transmission of Infectious Agents via Human Milk

BACTERIA

Postpartum mastitis occurs in one third of breastfeeding women in the United States and leads to breast abscesses in up to 10% of cases. Both mastitis and breast abscesses have been associated with the presence of bacterial pathogens in human milk. Breast abscesses have the potential to rupture into the ductal system, releasing large numbers of organisms into milk. Although an increase in mastitis attributable to community-associated methicillin-resistant *Staphylococcus aureus* (MRSA) has been noted, cases of infant infection with MRSA were not increased in a single-center cohort study from 1998–2005.

---

[1]Centers for Disease Control and Prevention. Yellow fever vaccine. Recommendations of the Advisory Committee on Immunization Practices (ACIP). *MMWR Recomm Rep.* 2010;59(RR-7):1-27

Risk factors for postpartum breast abscess attributable to *S aureus* do not seem to have changed with the increased prevalence of community-associated MRSA. In cases of breast abscess or cellulitis, breastfeeding on the affected breast should continue, even if a drain is present, as long as the infant's mouth is not in direct contact with purulent drainage or infected tissue. In general, infectious mastitis resolves with continued lactation during appropriate antimicrobial therapy and does not pose a significant risk for the healthy term infant. Breastfeeding on the affected side in cases of mastitis generally is recommended; however, even when breastfeeding is interrupted on the affected breast, breastfeeding may continue on the unaffected breast.

Women with tuberculosis who have been treated appropriately for 2 or more weeks and who are not considered contagious (negative sputum) may breastfeed. Women with tuberculosis disease suspected of being contagious should refrain from breastfeeding and from other close contact with the infant because of potential spread of *Mycobacterium tuberculosis* through respiratory tract droplets or airborne transmission (see Tuberculosis, p 829). However, expressed human milk can be fed to the infant, as long as there is no evidence of tuberculosis mastitis, which is rare. *M tuberculosis* rarely causes mastitis or a breast abscess, but if a breast abscess caused by *M tuberculosis* is present, breastfeeding should be discontinued until the mother has received treatment and no longer is considered to be contagious.

Expressed human milk can become contaminated with a variety of bacterial pathogens, including *Staphylococcus* species and gram-negative bacilli. Outbreaks of gram-negative bacterial infections in neonatal intensive care units occasionally have been attributed to contaminated human milk specimens that have been improperly collected or stored. Expressed human milk may be a reservoir for multidrug-resistant *S aureus* and other pathogens. Liquid human milk fortifiers are preferred, because powdered human milk fortifiers and powdered infant formula receipt has been associated with invasive bacteremia and meningitis attributable to *Cronobacter* species (formerly *Enterobacter sakazakii*), resulting in death in approximately 40% of cases. Consequently, the AAP has advised against the use of powdered infant formulas/human milk fortifiers in preterm or immunocompromised infants. Routine culturing or heat treatment of a mother's milk fed to her infant has not been demonstrated to be necessary or cost-effective (see Human Milk Banks, p 120). Because of the immune-protective factors in human milk, there is a hierarchical preference for the mother's freshly expressed milk, followed by the mother's previously refrigerated or frozen milk, followed by pasteurized donor milk as the third best option for feeding of sick and/or preterm infants.[1]

VIRUSES

CYTOMEGALOVIRUS. Cytomegalovirus (CMV) may be shed intermittently in human milk. Although CMV has been found in human milk of women who delivered preterm infants, case reviews of preterm infants acquiring CMV postnatally have not demonstrated long-term clinical sequelae over several years of follow-up after infants were discharged from the neonatal intensive care unit (NICU). Very low birth weight preterm infants, however, are at greater potential risk of developing symptomatic disease shortly

[1]American Academy of Pediatrics, Committee on Nutrition, Section on Breastfeeding, Committee on Fetus and Newborn. Donor human milk for the high-risk infant: preparation, safety, and usage options in the United States. *Pediatrics.* 2017;139(1):e20163440

after postnatal acquisition of CMV, including through human milk. Decisions about breastfeeding of preterm infants by mothers known to be CMV seropositive should include consideration of the potential benefits of human milk and the risk of CMV transmission. Mothers who deliver infants at <32 weeks' gestation can be screened for CMV. Consideration should be given to holder pasteurization (62.5°C [144.5°F] for 30 minutes) and short-term pasteurization (72°C [161.6°F] for 5 seconds) of human milk from CMV-positive mothers of very low birth weight infants, because these procedures seem to inactivate CMV; short-term pasteurization may be less harmful to the beneficial constituents of human milk. Freezing milk at –20°C (–4°F) for 24 to 72 hours will decrease viral titers but does not inactivate CMV reliably.

HEPATITIS B VIRUS. Hepatitis B surface antigen (HBsAg) has been detected in milk from HBsAg-positive women. However, studies from Taiwan and England have indicated that breastfeeding by HBsAg-positive women does not significantly increase the risk of infection among their infants. In the United States, infants born to known HBsAg-positive women should receive the initial dose of hepatitis B vaccine within 12 hours of birth, and Hepatitis B Immune Globulin should be administered concurrently but at a different anatomic site. This effectively will eliminate any theoretical risk of transmission through breastfeeding (see Hepatitis B, p 401). There is no need to delay initiation of breastfeeding until after the infant is immunized.

HEPATITIS C VIRUS. Hepatitis C virus (HCV) RNA and antibody to HCV have been detected in milk from mothers infected with HCV, but transmission of HCV via breastfeeding has not been documented in mothers who have positive test results for anti-HCV antibody but negative test results for human immunodeficiency virus (HIV) antibody. Mothers infected with HCV should be counseled that transmission of HCV by breastfeeding theoretically is possible but has not been documented. According to current guidelines of the US Public Health Service, maternal HCV infection is not a contraindication to breastfeeding. The decision to breastfeed should be based on an informed discussion between a mother and her health care professional. Mothers infected with HCV should consider abstaining from breastfeeding from a breast with cracked or bleeding nipples.

HUMAN IMMUNODEFICIENCY VIRUS. All pregnant women in the United States should be screened for HIV infection as part of a prenatal testing panel (see Human Immunodeficiency Virus Infection, p 459). All women found to have HIV infection should receive appropriate antiretroviral therapy for their own health and for prevention of vertical transmission. All HIV-infected women should be counseled regarding breastfeeding.[1] HIV has been isolated from human milk and can be transmitted through breastfeeding. The risk of transmission is higher for women who acquire HIV infection during pregnancy and lactation (ie, postpartum) than for women with preexisting infection. In the absence of antiretroviral therapy, the transmission risk appears to be higher in the first few months of life and during weaning; however, transmission can occur throughout lactation. In resource-limited settings, replacement feeding and/or short-course breastfeeding (4 to 6 months) has been associated with very high rates of infant morbidity and mortality. Multiple African studies have revealed that exclusive breastfeeding for the 4 to 6 months after birth lowers, but does not eliminate, the risk of

[1]Centers for Disease Control and Prevention. Revised recommendations for HIV testing of adults, adolescents, and pregnant women in health-care settings. *MMWR Recomm Rep.* 2006;55(RR-14):1–17

HIV transmission through human milk compared with infants who received mixed feedings (breastfeeding and other foods or milks).

Randomized clinical trials have demonstrated that both maternal triple antiretroviral therapy and daily infant prophylaxis (nevirapine or nevirapine/zidovudine) during breastfeeding significantly decreases the risk of postnatal transmission via human milk. However, neither maternal nor infant postpartum antiretroviral therapy is sufficient to eliminate completely the risk of HIV transmission through breastfeeding.[1] Penetration of antiretroviral agents into human milk also raises potential concerns regarding infant toxicity as well as the selection of antiretroviral-resistant virus within human milk. Thus, decisions related to breastfeeding must balance the risks of HIV transmission against the risk of non-HIV morbidity and mortality. In settings like the United States, where the risk of infant morbidity and mortality from infectious diseases and malnutrition is low and alternative sources of feeding are available, HIV-infected women should be counseled to avoid breastfeeding and donating human milk. If HIV-infected women in the United States choose to breastfeed, consultation with a pediatric HIV expert is recommended so that HIV transmission risk is minimized.[2]

In resource-limited settings, the World Health Organization, UNICEF, and UNAIDS have recommended that countries adopt national or subnational guidelines based on local rates of HIV infection, access to health care, and rates of infant morbidity and mortality from infectious diseases and malnutrition.[3] The most appropriate feeding option for an HIV-infected mother in a resource-limited setting needs to be based on her individual circumstances (eg, access to safe alternative replacement feeding, access to antiretroviral medications, and HIV viral load) and should consider the benefits of breastfeeding and the risk of transmission of HIV by breastfeeding. HIV-infected women who breastfeed should do so exclusively for the first 6 months, and breastfeeding should be extended through 12 months as complementary foods are introduced. Weaning should occur gradually over a month. Antiretroviral prophylaxis (maternal triple antiretroviral therapy or extended infant prophylaxis) should be provided throughout the breastfeeding and weaning periods.

HUMAN T-LYMPHOTROPIC VIRUS TYPE 1. Human T-lymphotropic virus type 1 (HTLV-1), which is endemic in Japan, the Caribbean, and parts of South America, is associated with development of malignant neoplasms and neurologic disorders among adults. Epidemiologic and laboratory studies suggest that mother-to-infant transmission of human HTLV-1 occurs primarily through breastfeeding, although freezing/thawing of expressed human milk may decrease infectivity of human milk. Women in the United States who are HTLV-1 seropositive should be advised not to breastfeed and not to donate to human milk banks.

HUMAN T-LYMPHOTROPIC VIRUS TYPE 2. Human T-lymphotropic virus type 2

---

[1]Panel on Treatment of HIV-Infected Pregnant Women and Prevention of Perinatal Transmission. *Recommendations for Use of Antiretroviral Drugs in Pregnant HIV-1-Infected Women for Maternal Health and Interventions to Reduce Perinatal HIV Transmission in the United States.* August 6, 2015:1-264. Available at: **http://aidsinfo.nih. gov/contentfiles/lvguidelines/PerinatalGL.pdf**

[2]American Academy of Pediatrics, Committee on Pediatric AIDS. Infant feeding and transmission of human immunodeficiency virus in the United States. *Pediatrics.* 2013;131(2):391-396 (Reaffirmed April 2016)

[3]World Health Organization. *Guidelines on HIV and Infant Feeding: Principles and Recommendations for Infant Feeding in the Context of HIV and a Summary of Evidence.* Geneva, Switzerland: World Health Organization; 2010

(HTLV-2) is a retrovirus that has been detected among American and European injection drug users and some American Indian/Alaska Native groups. Although apparent maternal-infant transmission has been reported, the rate and timing of transmission have not been established. Until additional data about possible transmission through breastfeeding become available, women in the United States who are HTLV-2 seropositive should be advised not to breastfeed and not to donate to human milk banks. Routine screening for both HTLV-1 or HTLV-2 during pregnancy is not recommended.

HERPES SIMPLEX VIRUS TYPE 1. Women with herpetic lesions may transmit herpes simplex virus (HSV) to their infants by direct contact with the lesions. Transmission may be reduced with hand hygiene and covering of lesions with which the infant might come into contact. Women with herpetic lesions on a breast or nipple should refrain from breastfeeding an infant from the affected breast until lesions have resolved but may breastfeed from the unaffected breast when lesions on the affected breast are covered completely to avoid transmission. In addition, a woman with an active herpes lesions on her breast can feed expressed milk from that breast to her infant, as there is no concern of herpes transmission through the milk. However, no part of the breast pump should come in contact with the lesions during expression, if the milk will be fed to the infant. If the pump does come in contact with the herpetic lesions, the mother should still express to maintain her milk supply and prevent mastitis, but the milk should be discarded.

RUBELLA. Wild and vaccine strains of rubella virus have been isolated from human milk. However, the presence of rubella virus in human milk has not been associated with significant disease in infants, and transmission is more likely to occur via other routes. Women with rubella or women who have been immunized recently with a live attenuated rubella virus-containing vaccine may continue to breastfeed.

VARICELLA. Secretion of attenuated varicella vaccine virus in human milk has not been documented. Varicella vaccine may be considered for a susceptible breastfeeding mother if the risk of exposure to natural varicella-zoster virus is high. Recommendations for use of passive immunization and varicella vaccine for breastfeeding mothers who have had contact with people in whom varicella has developed, or for contacts of a breastfeeding mother in whom varicella has developed, are available (see Varicella-Zoster Infections, p 869).

WEST NILE VIRUS. West Nile virus RNA has been detected in human milk collected from a woman with disease attributable to West Nile virus. Her breastfed infant developed West Nile virus immunoglobulin M antibodies but remained asymptomatic. Such transmission appears to be rare, and no adverse effects on infants have been described. The degree to which West Nile virus is transmitted in human milk and the extent to which breastfeeding infants become infected are unknown. Because the health benefits of breastfeeding have been established and the risk of West Nile virus transmission through breastfeeding is unknown, women who reside in an area with endemic West Nile virus infection should continue to breastfeed.

ZIKA VIRUS. Although Zika virus has been detected in human milk, to date, there are no reports of infants acquiring Zika virus through breastfeeding. Although this situation may change, current evidence suggests that the benefits of breastfeeding outweigh the theoretical risks of Zika virus transmission through human milk. Infants born to women with suspected, probable, or confirmed Zika virus infection, or to women who live in or have traveled to areas with Zika virus, should be fed according to infant feeding guidelines. Because of the benefits of breastfeeding, mothers are encouraged to breastfeed even in areas where Zika virus is found.

HUMAN MILK BANKS

Some circumstances, such as preterm delivery, may preclude direct breastfeeding, but infants in these circumstances still may be fed human milk collected from their own mothers or from individual donors. The potential for transmission of infectious agents through donor human milk requires appropriate selection and screening of donors and careful collection, processing, and storage of human milk.[1] Currently, US donor milk banks that belong to the Human Milk Banking Association of North America (**www.hmbana.org/**) voluntarily follow pasteurization guidelines drafted in consultation with the US Food and Drug Administration and the Centers for Disease Control and Prevention. Other pasteurization methods also are acceptable, but use of nonpasteurized donor milk should not be recommended by health care professionals. These guidelines include screening of all donors for HBsAg and antibodies to HIV-1, HIV-2, HTLV-1, HTLV-2, hepatitis C virus, and syphilis. Donor milk is dispensed only by prescription after it is heat treated at 62.5°C (144.5°F) for 30 minutes (holder pasteurization) and prepasteurization bacterial cultures reveal no growth of pathogenic organisms (*S aureus*, group B *Streptococcus*, and lactose-fermenting coliforms) and no more than 100 000 colony-forming units/mL of normal skin bacteria, and no viable bacteria are present after pasteurization.

Increasingly, the Internet is being used for the sale and/or sharing of donor milk. Parents should be informed of the safety risks of milk obtained from unscreened donors and milk that has not been safely collected processed, handled, and stored. In addition to the infectious risks listed previously, there are risks of contamination with chemicals and prescription and/or illicit drugs and even adulteration with cow milk.

INADVERTENT HUMAN MILK EXPOSURE

Policies have been developed to deal with occasions when an infant inadvertently is fed expressed human milk not obtained from his or her mother. These policies require documentation, counseling, and observation of the affected infant for signs of infection and potential testing of the source mother for infections that could be transmitted via human milk. Recommendations for management of a situation involving an accidental exposure may be found on the CDC Web site (**www.cdc.gov/breastfeeding/ recommendations/other_mothers_milk.htm**). A summary of the recommendations includes the following:

1. For a child who has been mistakenly fed expressed human milk not from his or her mother, consider the possible exposure to HIV or other infectious diseases as if an accidental exposure to other body fluids had occurred.
2. Inform the donor mother about the inadvertent exposure, and ask:
   - When the milk was expressed and how it was handled?
   - Whether she has had a recent HIV test and, if so, would she agree to have the results shared anonymously with the parent(s) of the infant given her milk?

---

[1]American Academy of Pediatrics, Committee on Nutrition, Section on Breastfeeding, Committee on Fetus and Newborn. Donor human milk for the high-risk infant: preparation, safety, and usage options in the United States. *Pediatrics*. 2017;139(1):e20163440

- If the donor mother does not know whether she been tested for HIV, would she be willing to contact her physician to find out?
- If the donor mother has never been tested for HIV, would she be willing to be tested and have the results shared anonymously with parent(s) of the recipient infant?

3. Discuss inadvertent administration of the donor milk with the parent(s) of the recipient infant.
   - Inform the parent(s) of the recipient infant that the risk of transmission of HIV infection via this exposure is low.
   - Encourage the parents to notify the child's physician of the exposure.
   - Provide the parents with information on when the milk was expressed and how the milk was handled so that the parents may inform their own physician.
   - Recommend that a baseline HIV antibody test be performed from blood of the recipient infant.
   - Inform the parent(s) of the recipient infant that the risk of transmission with other pathogens usually considered following other blood and body fluid exposures (eg, hepatitis B or hepatitis C) via exposure to human milk is extremely low.

Antimicrobial Agents and Other Drugs in Human Milk

Antimicrobial agents often are prescribed for lactating women. Although these drugs may be detected in milk, the potential risk to an infant must be weighed against the known benefits of continued breastfeeding. As a general guideline, an antimicrobial agent is safe to administer to a lactating woman if the drug is safe to administer to an infant. Only in rare cases will interruption of breastfeeding be necessary because of maternal antimicrobial use.

The amount of drug an infant receives from a lactating mother depends on a number of factors, including maternal dose, frequency and duration of administration, absorption, timing of medication administration and breastfeeding, and distribution characteristics of the drug. When a lactating woman receives appropriate doses of an antimicrobial agent, the concentration of the compound in her milk usually is less than the equivalent of a therapeutic dose for the infant. A breastfed infant who requires antimicrobial therapy should receive the recommended doses, independent of administration of the agent to the mother.

Current information about drugs and lactation can be found on the Toxicology Data Network Web site (**www.toxnet.nlm.nih.gov/help/LactMedRecordFormat. htm**). Data for drugs, including antimicrobial agents, administered to lactating women are provided in several categories, including maternal and infant drug concentrations, effects in breastfed infants, possible effects on lactation, the category in which the drug has been placed by the AAP, alternative drugs to consider, and references. Information on potential risks for drugs and vaccines administered during lactation, including potential effects on the breastfed child, can be found in US Food and Drug Administration-approved labeling.

Biologic Response Modifiers in Human Milk

Available evidence supports a lack of any significant transfer of anti-tumor necrosis factor (anti-TNF) drugs to human milk. Women receiving treatment with anti-TNF drugs should be advised to continue breastfeeding. Breastfed infants whose mothers are receiving anti-TNF drugs should receive recommended vaccines, including live virus vaccines, as indicated and according to the recommended schedule unless vaccination is being withheld because of in utero exposure to the biologic response modifier (see Biologic Response Modifying Drugs Used to Decrease Inflammation, p 85).

CHILDREN IN OUT-OF-HOME CHILD CARE[1]

Infants and young children who are cared for in group child care settings have an increased rate of communicable infectious diseases, including infections from antimicrobial-resistant organisms. This risk applies to other group settings, such as residential treatment facilities, group homes, and substitute care (eg, foster care) settings. The illnesses transmitted in out-of-home care settings reflect what is prevalent in the community. Transmission of infections occurs among the young children in the child care setting, but then spreads to their families. Respiratory infections are nearly 9 times more common than gastrointestinal tract infections. Children in child care are more likely to experience infections requiring antimicrobial agents; hence, they may also be colonized or infected with antimicrobial-resistant organisms. Infectious diseases that can cause outbreaks or affect the health of adult caregivers working in out-of-home child care settings are discussed later in this chapter. Although younger age, more time in group child care settings, and exposure to larger group size (6 children or more) all are associated strongly with more frequent infections, as children get older and increase their time in group care, they develop lasting immunity to common infections earlier compared with peers with less exposure.[2]

Modes of Spread of Infectious Diseases

RESPIRATORY TRACT DISEASES

Young children efficiently spread respiratory pathogens because of lack of social distancing and respiratory etiquette (Table 2.1). Organisms spread by the respiratory route include viruses causing acute upper respiratory tract infections and bacterial organisms associated with invasive infections. Possible modes of spread of respiratory tract viruses include aerosols, respiratory droplets, and direct contact with secretions or indirect contact with contaminated fomites. The viral pathogens responsible for respiratory tract disease in child care settings mirror those that cause disease in the community, including respiratory syncytial virus (RSV), parainfluenza virus, influenza virus, human metapneumovirus, adenovirus, and rhinovirus. The incidence of viral infections of the respiratory tract is increased in child care settings.

Seasonal outbreaks of common respiratory infections, such as hand-foot-and-mouth disease (enterovirus), bronchiolitis, and influenza, are expected and amplified in out-of-

---

[1] American Academy of Pediatrics. *Managing Infectious Diseases in Child Care and Schools: A Quick Reference Guide, 4th Edition.* Aronson SS, Shope TR, eds. Elk Grove Village, IL: American Academy of Pediatrics; 2016

[2] Shope TR. Infectious diseases in early education and child care programs. *Pediatr Rev.* 2014;35(5):182-193

home group child care settings. Other respiratory pathogens that can cause sporadic outbreaks include group A streptococcal pharyngitis, *Neisseria meningitidis,* and some vaccine-preventable diseases such as measles, mumps, rubella, varicella, pertussis, and rarely, *Haemophilus influenzae* type b. The incidence of vaccine-preventable diseases has markedly decreased since routine immunizations were implemented, although communities with low vaccination rates continue to be at increased risk for outbreaks. More detailed recommendations for management and exclusion and return to care for these conditions are available in the relevant disease-specific chapters in Section 3 or other AAP resources.[1,2]

ENTERIC DISEASES

Young children and adult caregivers spread enteric diseases in child care settings primarily by contact with pathogens during diapering and toileting procedures. Organisms spread by the fecal-oral route include common viruses, bacterial pathogens, and parasites. Seasonal enteric pathogens include noroviruses, enteric adenoviruses, and astroviruses (see Table 2.1). Rotavirus vaccination has dramatically decreased seasonal outbreaks attributable to this virus. Hepatitis A virus can cause outbreaks in child care settings but similarly is much less common since routine implementation of hepatitis A immunization. Bacterial enteropathogens such as *Shigella* species and *Escherichia coli* O157:H7 can cause significant outbreaks in group child care settings and require a very small infective dose of organisms. *Salmonella* species, *Clostridium difficile,* and *Campylobacter* species are less common causes of outbreaks. Parasites like *Giardia intestinalis* and *Cryptosporidium* species can cause outbreaks in child care settings, in particular where shared pools are used in water play activities, because their spores are resistant to chlorination in water sources and to alcohol-based hand sanitizers (see Prevention of Illnesses Associated With Recreational Water Use, p 201). More detailed recommendations for management and exclusion and return to care for these conditions are available in the relevant disease-specific chapters in Section 3 or other references.[1,2]

OTHER INFECTIONS

Other common infections (Table 2.1) among children in child care may occur by direct contact with infected lesions, such as *Staphylococcus aureus,* group A streptococcus, herpes simplex virus, and varicella zoster virus. Pediculosis and scabies infestations and tinea

[1]American Academy of Pediatrics. *Managing Infectious Diseases in Child Care and Schools: A Quick Reference Guide, 4*th *Edition.* Aronson SS, Shope TR, eds. Elk Grove Village, IL: American Academy of Pediatrics; 2016

[2]American Academy of Pediatrics, American Public Health Association, National Resource Center for Health and Safety in Child Care and Early Education. *Caring for Our Children: National Health and Safety Performance Standards: Guidelines for Out-of-Home Child Care.* 3rd ed. Elk Grove Village, IL: American Academy of Pediatrics; and Washington, DC: American Public Health Association; 2011

Table 2.1. Modes of Transmission of Organisms in Child Care Settings

Usual Route of Transmission[a]	Bacteria	Viruses	Other[b]
Fecal-oral	*Campylobacter* species; *Clostridium difficile;* Shiga toxin-producing *Escherichia coli,* including *E coli* O157:H7; *Salmonella* species; *Shigella* species	Astrovirus, norovirus, enteric adenovirus, enteroviruses, hepatitis A virus, rotaviruses	*Cryptosporidium* species, *Enterobius vermicularis, Giardia intestinalis*
Respiratory	*Bordetella pertussis, Haemophilus influenzae* type b, *Mycobacterium tuberculosis* (children ≥10 years and adults), *Neisseria meningitidis, Streptococcus pneumoniae,* group A streptococcus, *Kingella kingae*	Adenovirus, influenza virus, human metapneumovirus, measles virus, mumps virus, parainfluenza virus, parvovirus B19, respiratory syncytial virus, rhinovirus, coronavirus, rubella virus, varicella-zoster virus	...
Person-to-person contact	Group A streptococcus, *Staphylococcus aureus*	Herpes simplex virus, varicella-zoster virus	Agents causing pediculosis, scabies, and ringworm[c]
Contact with blood, urine, and/or saliva	...	Cytomegalovirus, herpes simplex virus, hepatitis C virus	...
Bloodborne	...	Hepatitis B virus, hepatitis C virus, HIV	...

[a]The potential for transmission of microorganisms in the child care setting by food and animals also exists (see Appendix VII, Clinical Syndromes Associated With Foodborne Diseases, p 1086, and Appendix VIII, Diseases Transmitted by Animals (Zoonoses), p 1093.
[b]Parasites, fungi, mites, and lice.
[c]Transmission also may occur from contact with objects in the environment.

infections also are spread by direct contact. Cytomegalovirus (CMV) is common in children in child care settings and spreads via contact with infected bodily secretions; it is estimated that up to 70% of children 1 to 3 years of age who attend child care may shed virus in saliva or urine. CMV and parvovirus infections may have effects on the fetus of a pregnant child care worker, and those employed in child care should discuss this occupational risk with their health care providers. Bloodborne infections are a potential concern in child care settings. Hepatitis B transmission from an infected child biting a susceptible child has occurred in child care, but this is rare, especially given high hepatitis B immunization rates. Human immunodeficiency virus (HIV) transmission in a child care setting has never been documented. Finally, human-animal contact involving family and classroom pets, animal displays, and petting zoos exposes children to pathogens harbored by these animals. Such animals are commonly colonized with *Salmonella* species, *Campylobacter* species, Shiga toxin-producing *E coli*, lymphocytic choriomeningitis virus, and other viruses that may be transmitted to children via contact (see Appendix VIII, Diseases Transmitted by Animals [Zoonoses], p 1093). Detailed recommendations for management and exclusion and return to care for these conditions are available in the relevant disease-specific chapters in Section 3 or other references.[1,2]

Management and Prevention of Infectious Diseases

There are 3 primary methods for reducing the transmission of infectious diseases in group child care settings: immunization, infection control and prevention, and exclusion and return-to-care policies and practices.

IMMUNIZATION

Immunizations are by far the most effective means of preventing childhood infectious diseases. Child care programs should require that all enrollees and staff members receive age-appropriate immunizations as recommended by the American Academy of Pediatrics (AAP) and the Advisory Committee on Immunization Practices (ACIP) of the Centers for Disease Control and Prevention (CDC). Parents should be required to report their child's immunization status, programs should keep a record, and these should be reviewed by child care program personnel. Unless contraindications exist or children have received medical, religious, or philosophic exemptions (depending on state immunization laws), immunization records should demonstrate complete immunization for age as shown in the recommended childhood and adolescent immunization schedules and be adherent with state vaccine mandates (**https://redbook.solutions.aap.org/SS/ Immunization_Schedules.aspx**). The AAP views nonmedical exemptions to child care- and school-required immunizations as inappropriate for individual, public health, and ethical reasons and advocates for their elimination.[1] The immunization mandates for children in child care vary by state and can be found online (**www.immunize.org/ laws**). State requirements often lag behind the AAP and ACIP recommendations.

Children who have not received recommended age-appropriate immunizations

---

[1]American Academy of Pediatrics, Committee on Practice and Ambulatory Medicine, Committee on Infectious Diseases, Committee on State Government Affairs, Council on School Health, Section on Administration and Practice Management. Medical versus nonmedical immunization exemptions for child care and school attendance. *Pediatrics*. 2016;138(3):e20162145

before enrollment should be immunized as soon as possible, and the series should be completed according to the recommended childhood and adolescent immunization catch-up schedule as appropriate (**https://redbook.solutions.aap.org/SS/ Immunization_Schedules.aspx**). In the interim, permitting unimmunized or inadequately immunized children to attend child care should depend on state and local public health guidance regarding how to handle the risk and whether to inform parents of enrolled infants and children about potential exposure to this risk. Unimmunized or underimmunized children place appropriately immunized children and children with vaccine contraindications at risk of contracting a vaccine-preventable disease. If a vaccine-preventable disease occurs in the child care program, all unimmunized and underimmunized children should be excluded for the duration of possible exposure or until they have completed their immunizations.

All adults who work in a child care facility should receive all vaccines routinely recommended for adults (see adult immunization schedule at **www.cdc.gov/ vaccines/schedules/hcp/adult.html**). By being fully immunized, child care providers protect not only themselves but also children who have medical contraindications to immunizations and infants who are too young to receive immunizations for diseases such as influenza and pertussis, yet have the highest morbidity and mortality to these infections. More detailed information about adult child care provider immunization requirements can be found in other references.[1,2]

INFECTION CONTROL AND PREVENTION

Group child care settings are rich environments for pathogens. Young children are in close contact with each other, touching and sharing; they cough and sneeze without proper respiratory etiquette; and they need to be supervised or assisted with toileting and hand hygiene. As a result, viral, bacterial, fungal, and parasitic pathogens can be present in the air, on surfaces, in bodily secretions, and on the skin. Efforts to control the transmission of infectious diseases are important but also difficult to implement effectively. Infection control and prevention in group child care settings requires a multifaceted approach. Programs should have written policies and training for staff to be sure they properly implement the best methods. These policies should include procedures for food preparation; diaper changing; cleaning, sanitizing, and disinfecting surfaces; hand hygiene, respiratory etiquette; and other Standard Precautions.

It is difficult to decrease the spread of respiratory pathogens in group child care settings. Studies show only modest reductions in incidence of respiratory illness even with intensive education and infection control measures,[3] probably because respiratory pathogens are primarily spread by droplets expelled by sneezing and coughing. Young children have difficulty anticipating sneezing and coughing and do not effectively practice respiratory etiquette and hand hygiene. In addition, their social nature causes them to

---

[1]American Academy of Pediatrics. *Managing Infectious Diseases in Child Care and Schools: A Quick Reference Guide, 4th Edition.* Aronson SS, Shope TR, eds. Elk Grove Village, IL: American Academy of Pediatrics; 2016

[2]American Academy of Pediatrics, American Public Health Association, National Resource Center for Health and Safety in Child Care and Early Education. *Caring for Our Children: National Health and Safety Performance Standards: Guidelines for Out-of-Home Child Care.* 3rd ed. Elk Grove Village, IL: American Academy of Pediatrics; and Washington, DC: American Public Health Association; 2011

[3]Shope TR. Infectious diseases in early education and child care programs. *Pediatr Rev.* 2014;35(5):182-193

play in close proximity to each other, within the 3-foot radius most contaminated large droplets may travel before contacting another child's mucous membranes. Nevertheless, immunization, hand hygiene, and respiratory etiquette are essential elements of infection control in child care settings, and it is important that staff practice these measures for themselves as well as educate and assist young children to properly do so. Aerosolized droplets that land on surfaces may contain microorganisms capable of causing infections. Therefore, surface cleaning, disinfecting, and sanitizing are important to prevent the spread of respiratory illness.

Studies show that infection control procedures in group child care settings more effectively reduce diarrheal illness than respiratory illness.[1] Surface cleaning, sanitizing, and disinfecting are especially important for reducing gastrointestinal tract illnesses. Cleaning removes visible soil to increase the effectiveness of sanitizing or disinfecting agents. Sanitizing reduces the amount of potential pathogens on food preparation surfaces, utensils, tables, countertops, and plastic toys. Disinfection requires stronger concentration or different agents than sanitizing and is used for areas with higher likelihood of pathogens, such as door handles, drinking fountains, and toilet and diaper changing areas. As with respiratory tract infections, hand hygiene is essential to prevent the fecal-oral spread of gastrointestinal tract pathogens. Hand hygiene should occur for staff and children on arrival; when moving from one group to another; before and after contact with food or medication administration; and after diaper changing or toileting, contact with nasal or other body secretions, animals, garbage, and playing outside. Hand washing for 20 seconds with soap and water is the preferred method for hand hygiene, should be prioritized in child care settings, and is required whenever there is visible particulate matter. However, for children older than 24 months, alcohol-based hand sanitizer, when soap and water is not available, may be substituted. Alcohol-based hand sanitizers have high alcohol content (60%–95%), which can be ingested or aerosolized; therefore, adult supervision is required. Hand hygiene using soap and water is indicated for *Cryptosporidium* species, norovirus, and *Clostridium difficile,* because alcohol-based hand sanitizers are not as effective against these pathogens.

Other important environmental infection control and prevention measures include ensuring adequate air flow in the building; providing enough physical space in the facility and between cots for naps (which may increase social distancing and reduce droplet spread); ensuring physical separation and separate personnel (if possible) involved in food preparation and diaper changing; requiring appropriate handling of animals (and excluding reptiles, turtles, amphibians, birds, primates, live poultry, ferrets, or rodents in the facility), with hand hygiene before and after contact; and adhering to recommended ratios of children to care providers. Health departments should have plans for responding to reportable and nonreportable outbreaks of communicable diseases in child care programs and should provide training, written information, and technical consultation to child care programs when requested or alerted. Collaborative efforts of public health officials, licensing agencies, child care providers, child care health consultants, physicians, nurses, parents, employers, and other members of the community are necessary to address problems of infection prevention and management in child care settings.

Other resources that can assist providers and parents with these issues include the

---

[1]Shope TR. Infectious diseases in early education and child care programs. *Pediatr Rev.* 2014;35(5):182-193

Healthy Child Care America Web site (**www.healthychildcare.org/contacts. html**). People involved with early education and child care can use the published national standards[1] related to these topics to provide specific education and implementation measures.

EXCLUSION AND RETURN TO CARE

General recommendations for exclusion of children in out-of-home care are provided in Table 2.2 (p 129). Child care exclusions can put a significant economic strain on families, and studies show that many exclusion decisions are not evidence based and are inappropriate.[2] No studies demonstrate that excluding children in group care who are ill with common infectious diseases reduces the likelihood of spread to other children. Many children are infectious before developing symptoms. Asymptomatic infection, high carriage rates, and prolonged shedding of pathogens in body secretions are common and make it difficult to curb transmission by targeting only symptomatic children. Because mild illness is common among children and most minor illnesses do not constitute a reason for excluding a child from child care, decisions about exclusion should be primarily based on the child's behavior. A mildly ill child can remain in care unless the illness prevents the child from participating in normal activities, as determined by the child care staff, or the illness requires a need for care that is greater than staff can provide. However, there are some infectious diseases for which exclusion is recommended to try to control environmental contamination and/or spread because the clinical consequences are significant.

Each day as the child enters the site and throughout the day as needed, a trained staff member should evaluate the well-being of the child and observe for signs of illness. Parents should be encouraged to share information with child care staff about their child's acute and chronic illnesses and medication use utilizing a formal care plan that is signed by the child's health care provider. Examples of illnesses and conditions that do not necessitate exclusion include:

- Common cold
- Diarrhea, as long as stools are contained in the diaper (for infants), there are no accidents using the toilet (for older children), and stool frequency is no more than 2 stools above normal for that child
- Rash without fever and without behavioral change
- Lice, ringworm, and scabies (exclusion and treatment can occur at the end of the day with return the following day)
- Thrush
- Fifth disease (parvovirus B19 infection) in an immunocompetent child
- CMV infection
- Chronic hepatitis B virus (HBV) infection
- Conjunctivitis without fever and without behavioral change
- HIV infection

---

[1]American Academy of Pediatrics, American Public Health Association, National Resource Center for Health and Safety in Child Care and Early Education. *Caring for Our Children: National Health and Safety Performance Standards: Guidelines for Out-of-Home Child Care.* 3rd ed. Elk Grove Village, IL: American Academy of Pediatrics; and Washington, DC: American Public Health Association; 2011

[2]Shope TR. Infectious diseases in early education and child care programs. *Pediatr Rev.* 2014;35(5):182-193

- Colonization with methicillin-resistant *Staphylococcus aureus* (MRSA) (in children who do not have active lesions or illness that would otherwise require exclusion)

Asymptomatic children who excrete an enteropathogen usually do not need to be excluded (exceptions include children in whom Shiga toxin-producing *E coli*, *Shigella* species, or *Salmonella* serotype Typhi or Paratyphi is confirmed).

Table 2.2. General Recommendations for Exclusion of Children in Out-of-Home Child Care

Symptom(s)	Management
Illness preventing participation in activities, as determined by child care staff	Exclusion until illness resolves and able to participate in activities
Illness that requires a need for care that is greater than staff can provide without compromising health and safety of others	Exclusion or placement in care environment where appropriate care can be provided, without compromising care of others
Severe illness suggested by fever with behavior changes, lethargy, irritability, persistent crying, difficulty breathing, progressive rash with above symptoms	Medical evaluation and exclusion until symptoms have resolved
Persistent abdominal pain (2 hours or more) or intermittent abdominal pain associated with fever, dehydration, or other systemic signs and symptoms	Medical evaluation and exclusion until symptoms have resolved
Vomiting 2 or more times in preceding 24 hours	Exclusion until symptoms have resolved, unless vomiting is determined to be caused by a noncommunicable condition and child is able to remain hydrated and participate in activities
Diarrhea if stool not contained in diaper or if fecal accidents occur in a child who is normally continent, if stool frequency exceeds 2 stools above normal for that child, or stools contain blood or mucus	Medical evaluation for stools with blood or mucus; exclusion until stools are contained in the diaper or when toilet-trained children no longer have accidents using the toilet and when stool frequency becomes no more than 2 stools above that child's normal frequency for the time the child is in the program, even if the stools remain loose
Oral lesions	Exclusion if unable to contain drool or if unable to participate because of other symptoms or until child or staff member is considered to be noninfectious (lesions smaller or resolved)
Skin lesions	Exclusion if lesions are weeping and cannot be covered with a waterproof dressing

Table 2.3. Disease- or Condition-Specific Recommendations for Exclusion of Children in Out-of-Home Child Care

Condition	Management of Case	Management of Contacts
Clostridium difficile	Exclusion until stools are contained in the diaper or child or stool frequency is no more than 2 stools above that child's normal frequency for the time the child is in the program. Stool consistency does not need to return to normal to be able to return to child care. Neither test of cure nor repeat testing should be performed for asymptomatic children in whom *C difficile* was diagnosed previously.	Symptomatic contacts should be excluded until stools are contained in the diaper or child is continent and stool frequency is no more than 2 stools above that child's normal frequency for the time the child is in the program. Testing is not required for asymptomatic contacts.
Hepatitis A virus (HAV) infection	Serologic testing to confirm HAV infection in suspected cases. Exclusion until 1 week after onset of illness.	In facilities with diapered children, if 1 or more cases confirmed in child or staff attendees or 2 or more cases in households of staff or attendees, hepatitis A vaccine (HepA) or Immune Globulin Intramuscular (IGIM) should be administered within 14 days of exposure to all unimmunized staff and attendees. In centers without diapered children, HepA or IGIM should be administered to unimmunized classroom contacts of index case. Asymptomatic IGIM recipients may return after receipt of IGIM (see Hepatitis A, p 392, for further discussion on indications for HepA vaccine or IG).
Impetigo	No exclusion if treatment has been initiated and as long as lesions on exposed skin are covered.	No intervention unless additional lesions develop.

Table 2.3. Disease- or Condition-Specific Recommendations for Exclusion of Children in Out-of-Home Child Care, continued

Condition	Management of Case	Management of Contacts
Measles	Exclusion until 4 days after beginning of rash and when the child is able to participate.	Immunize exposed children without evidence of immunity within 72 hours of exposure. Children who do not receive vaccine within 72 hours or who remain unimmunized after exposure should be excluded until at least 2 weeks after onset of rash in the last case of measles. For use of IG, see Measles (p 537).
Mumps	Exclusion until 5 days after onset of parotid gland swelling.	In outbreak setting, people without documentation of immunity should be immunized or excluded. Immediate readmission may occur following immunization. Unimmunized people should be excluded for 26 or more days following onset of parotitis in last case. A second dose of MMR vaccine (or MMRV, if age appropriate) should be offered to all students (including those in postsecondary school) and to all health care personnel born in or after 1957 who have only received 1 dose of MMR vaccine. A second dose of MMR also may be considered during outbreaks for preschool-aged children who have received 1 MMR dose. People previously vaccinated with 2 doses of a mumps-containing vaccine who are identified by public health as at increased risk for mumps because of an outbreak should receive a third dose of a mumps-containing vaccine to improve protection against mumps disease and related complications (see Mumps, p 567).

Table 2.3. Disease- or Condition-Specific Recommendations for Exclusion of Children in Out-of-Home Child Care, continued

Condition	Management of Case	Management of Contacts
Pediculosis capitis (head lice) infestation	Treatment at end of program day and readmission on completion of first treatment. Children should not be excluded or sent home early from school because of head lice, because head lice has a low contagion within classrooms.	Household and close contacts should be examined and treated if infested. No exclusion necessary.
Pertussis	Exclusion until completion of 5 days of the recommended course of antimicrobial therapy if pertussis is suspected; children and providers who refuse treatment should be excluded until 21 days have elapsed from cough onset (see Pertussis, p 620).	Immunization and chemoprophylaxis should be administered as recommended for household contacts. Symptomatic children and staff should be excluded until completion of 5 days of antimicrobial therapy. Untreated adults should be excluded until 21 days after onset of cough (see Pertussis, p 620).
Rubella	Exclusion for 7 days after onset of rash for postnatal infection.	During an outbreak, children without evidence of immunity should be immunized or excluded for 21 days after onset of rash of the last case in the outbreak. Pregnant contacts should be evaluated (see Rubella, p 705).
Infection with *Salmonella* serotypes Typhi or Paratyphi	Exclusion until 3 consecutive stool cultures obtained at least 48 hours after cessation of antimicrobial therapy are negative, stools are contained in the diaper or child is continent, and stool frequency is no more than 2 stools above that child's normal frequency for the time the child is in the program.	When *Salmonella* serotype Typhi infection is identified in a child care staff member, local or state health departments may be consulted regarding regulations for length of exclusion and testing, which may vary by jurisdiction.

Table 2.3. Disease- or Condition-Specific Recommendations for Exclusion of Children in Out-of-Home Child Care, continued

Condition	Management of Case	Management of Contacts
Infection with nontyphoidal *Salmonella* species, *Salmonella* of unknown serotype	Exclusion until stools are contained in the diaper or child is continent and stool frequency is no more than 2 stools above that child's normal frequency for the time the child is in the program. Stool consistency does not need to return to normal to be able to return to child care. Negative stool culture results are **not** required for nonserotype Typhi or Paratyphi *Salmonella* species.	Symptomatic contacts should be excluded until stools are contained in the diaper or child is continent and stool frequency is no more than 2 stools above that child's normal frequency for the time the child is in the program. Stool cultures are not required for asymptomatic contacts.
Scabies	Exclusion until after treatment given.	Close contacts with prolonged skin-to-skin contact should receive prophylactic therapy. Bedding and clothing in contact with skin of infected people should be laundered (see Scabies, p 718).
Infection with Shiga toxin-producing *Escherichia coli* (STEC), including *E coli* O157:H7	Exclusion until 2 stool cultures (obtained at least 48 hours after any antimicrobial therapy, if administered, has been discontinued) are negative, and stools are contained in the diaper or child is continent, and stool frequency is no more than 2 stools above that child's normal frequency. Some state health departments have less stringent exclusion policies for children who have recovered from less virulent STEC infection.	Meticulous hand hygiene; stool cultures should be performed for any symptomatic contacts. In outbreak situations involving virulent STEC strains, stool cultures of asymptomatic contacts may aid controlling spread. Center(s) with cases should be closed to new admissions during STEC outbreak (see *Escherichia coli* Diarrhea, p 338).

Table 2.3. Disease- or Condition-Specific Recommendations for Exclusion of Children in Out-of-Home Child Care, continued

Condition	Management of Case	Management of Contacts
Shigellosis	Exclusion until treatment complete and one or more post-treatment stool cultures are negative for *Shigella* species, and stools are contained in the diaper or child is continent, and stool frequency is no more than 2 stools above that child's normal frequency for the time the child is in the program. Some states may require >1 negative stool culture.	Meticulous hand hygiene; stool cultures should be performed for any symptomatic contacts (see *Shigella* Infections, p 723).
Staphylococcus aureus skin infections	Exclusion only if skin lesions are draining and cannot be covered with a watertight dressing.	Meticulous hand hygiene; cultures of contacts are not recommended.
Streptococcal pharyngitis	Exclusion until at least 12 hours after treatment has been initiated.	Symptomatic contacts of documented cases of group A streptococcal infection should be tested and treated if test results are positive.
Tuberculosis	Most children younger than 10 years are not considered contagious. For those with active disease, exclusion until determined to be noninfectious by physician or health department authority. No exclusion for latent tuberculosis infection (LTBI).	Local health department personnel should be informed for contact investigation (see Tuberculosis, p 829).

Table 2.3. Disease- or Condition-Specific Recommendations for Exclusion of Children in Out-of-Home Child Care, continued

Condition	Management of Case	Management of Contacts
Varicella (see Varicella-Zoster Infections, p 869)	Exclusion until all lesions have crusted or, in immunized people without crusts, until no new lesions appear within a 24-hour period.	For people without evidence of immunity, varicella vaccine should be administered ideally within 3 days but up to 5 days after exposure, or when indicated, Varicella-Zoster Immune Globulin (VariZig; see Varicella Zoster Virus, p 869) should be administered up to 10 days after exposure; if VariZIG is not available, IGIV should be considered as an alternative. If vaccine cannot be administered and VariZIG/IVIG is not indicated, preemptive oral acyclovir or valacyclovir can be considered.

Disease- or condition-specific recommendations for exclusion from out-of-home care and management of contacts are shown in Table 2.3 (p 130). Despite the existence of national recommendations for exclusion,[1,2] states have been slow to adopt these. Each state has its own regulations pertaining to exclusion and return to care, and these may not be evidence based. Programs are required to follow these state-specific guidelines, which can be found at **https://childcareta.acf.hhs.gov/resource/state-and-territory-licensing-agencies-and-regulations.**

During outbreaks of certain diseases, the responsible local and state public health authorities are helpful for determining the benefits and risks of excluding children from their usual care program. Most states have laws about reporting and isolation of people with specific communicable diseases. Local or state health departments should be contacted for information about these laws, and public health authorities in these areas should be notified about cases of nationally notifiable infectious diseases and unusual outbreaks of other illnesses involving children or adults in the child care environment (see Appendix IV, Nationally Notifiable Infectious Diseases in the United States, p 1069). For most outbreaks of vaccine-preventable illnesses, unvaccinated children should be excluded until they are vaccinated and the risk of transmission no longer exists.

SCHOOL HEALTH

The clustering of children together that occurs in a school setting provides opportunities for transmission of infectious diseases. Determining the likelihood that infection in one or more children will pose a risk for schoolmates depends on an understanding of several factors: (1) the mechanism of pathogen transmission; (2) the ease with which the organism is spread (contagion); and (3) the likelihood that classmates are immune because of vaccination or previous infection. Decisions to intervene to prevent spread of infection within a school should be made through collaboration among school officials, local public health officials, and health care professionals, considering the availability and effectiveness of specific methods of prevention and risk of serious complications from infection.

The United States relies on child care and elementary and secondary school entry vaccination requirements to achieve and sustain high levels of vaccination coverage. All states require vaccination of children at the time of entry into school, and many states require vaccination of children throughout elementary and high school and of young adults entering college. The most up-to-date information about which vaccines are required in a specific state, permissible exemptions, and a minor's consent to vaccination can be obtained from the immunization program manager of each state health department, from a number of local health departments, from **www.immunize.org/laws,** and from the National Network for Immunization Information (**www.**

[1]American Academy of Pediatrics. *Managing Infectious Diseases in Child Care and Schools: A Quick Reference Guide, 4th Edition.* Aronson SS, Shope TR, eds. Elk Grove Village, IL: American Academy of Pediatrics; 2016

[2]American Academy of Pediatrics, American Public Health Association, National Resource Center for Health and Safety in Child Care and Early Education. *Caring for Our Children: National Health and Safety Performance Standards: Guidelines for Out-of-Home Child Care.* 3rd ed. Elk Grove Village, IL: American Academy of Pediatrics; and Washington, DC: American Public Health Association; 2011

immunizationinfo.net/). The American Academy of Pediatrics (AAP) supports regulations and laws requiring certification of immunization to attend child care and school as a sound means of providing a safe environment for attendees and employees of these settings. The AAP also supports medically indicated exemptions to specific immunizations as determined for each individual child. The AAP views nonmedical exemptions to school-required immunizations as inappropriate for individual, public health, and ethical reasons and advocates for their elimination.[1]

General methods for control and prevention of spread of infection in the school setting include the following:

- Meticulous hand hygiene and environmental cleaning should be performed.
- Documentation of the vaccination status of children should be reviewed at the time of enrollment and at regularly scheduled intervals thereafter, in accordance with state requirements. Although specific laws vary by state **(www.immunize.org/laws),** most states require proof of protection against poliomyelitis, tetanus, pertussis, diphtheria, *Haemophilus influenzae* type b, measles, mumps, rubella, and varicella. Vaccinations against hepatitis B virus (HBV) and meningococcal disease are mandatory in many states, and in a few states human papillomavirus (HPV) vaccine is mandated. Hepatitis A virus (HAV) vaccination is required for school entry in some states; seasonal influenza vaccination is recommended but not required. Policies established by state health departments concerning exclusion of unvaccinated children and exemptions for children with certain underlying medical conditions and families with religious or philosophic objection to vaccination should be followed **(www.cdc. gov/vaccines/imz-managers/coverage/schoolvaxview/index.html).**
- Infected children should be excluded from school until they no longer are considered contagious (for recommendations on specific diseases, see relevant disease-specific chapters in Section 3).
- Unvaccinated or undervaccinated children place other appropriately vaccinated children at risk of contracting a vaccine-preventable disease. If a vaccine-preventable disease to which children may be susceptible occurs in the school, all unvaccinated and undervaccinated children should be excluded for the duration of possible exposure or until they have completed their vaccinations (for recommendations on specific diseases, see relevant disease-specific chapters in Section 3).
- In some instances, administration of appropriate antimicrobial therapy will limit further spread of infection (eg, streptococcal pharyngitis, pertussis).
- Antimicrobial prophylaxis administered to close contacts of children with infections caused by specific pathogens may be warranted in some circumstances (eg, meningococcal infection, pertussis). Decisions about postexposure prophylaxis after an in-school exposure are best made in conjunction with local public health authorities.
- Temporary school closings can be used in limited circumstances: (1) to prevent spread of infection; (2) when an infection is expected to affect a large number of susceptible students and available control measures are considered inadequate; or (3) when an infection is expected to have a high rate of morbidity or mortality.

---

[1]American Academy of Pediatrics, Committee on Practice and Ambulatory Medicine, Committee on Infectious Diseases, Committee on State Government Affairs, Council on School Health, Section on Administration and Practice Management. Medical versus nonmedical immunization exemptions for child care and school attendance. *Pediatrics.* 2016;138(3):e20162145

- Schools should maintain a clean environment and enforce high standards of personal hygiene, provide appropriate education for school staff, and ensure that they have a reliable process for notification and education of parents during an exposure or outbreak.[1]
- If an outbreak occurs, consultation with local public health authorities is indicated before initiating interventions.

Physicians involved with school health should be aware of current public health guidelines to prevent and control infectious diseases. Close collaboration between the school and physician is encouraged to ensure that the school receives appropriate guidance and is stocked with the necessary materials to deal with outbreaks and limit spread of infections. In all circumstances requiring intervention to prevent spread of infection within the school setting, the privacy of children who are infected should be protected.

Diseases Preventable by Routine Childhood Immunization

Children and adolescents who have been fully vaccinated according to the recommended childhood and adolescent vaccination schedule (**https://redbook.solutions.aap. org/SS/Immunization_Schedules.aspx**) should be considered to be protected against diseases for which they were vaccinated. Of great importance is the removal of children who are unvaccinated or undervaccinated from schools during an outbreak of a vaccine-preventable disease. Disease-specific chapters in Section 3 should be consulted for details.

MEASLES AND VARICELLA

Measles-containing vaccines (MMR and MMRV) and varicella-containing vaccines (varicella monovalent and MMRV) have been demonstrated to provide protection in susceptible people following exposure. Timing of administration should be within 72 hours of exposure to measles, and within 5 days of exposure to varicella. Measles or varicella vaccination should be recommended immediately for all nonimmune people attending the affected school during a measles or varicella outbreak, respectively, except for people with a medical contraindication to vaccination. Individuals without evidence of immunity may not yet have been exposed; therefore, vaccinating at any stage of an outbreak can prevent disease. During an outbreak of measles, vaccination efforts should be considered at unaffected schools within a community. Students vaccinated against measles or varicella for the first time under these outbreak circumstances should be allowed to return to school after vaccination, although wild-type disease still may occur during the interval before induction of protective immunity is afforded from vaccination (typically 2–3 weeks for live-virus vaccination). Varicella-infected patients are to remain out of school until all lesions have crusted and no new lesions have appeared for 24 hours. Patients in whom measles is diagnosed are to remain out of school until 4 days (minimum) have passed since onset of the rash.

---

[1]Aronson SS, Shope TR, eds. *Managing Infectious Diseases in Child Care and Schools, 4th Edition: A Quick Reference Guide.* Elk Grove Village, IL: American Academy of Pediatrics; 2016

MUMPS AND RUBELLA

Mumps and rubella vaccines administered after exposure have not been demonstrated to prevent infection among susceptible contacts, but unvaccinated students attending the affected school(s) should receive the vaccines to protect them from infection from subsequent exposure. People who receive mumps vaccination during an ongoing outbreak should be informed of symptoms and signs of illness and to contact their medical provider should they become sick. It is imperative that any child in whom mumps is diagnosed stay home from school for 5 days after onset of parotid gland swelling. Those with rubella should be excluded from school for 7 days after the onset of rash. During a mumps outbreak, a second dose of MMR vaccine (or MMRV, if age appropriate) should be offered to all students (including those in postsecondary school) who have only received 1 dose of MMR vaccine. People previously vaccinated with 2 doses of a mumps-containing vaccine who are identified by public health as at increased risk for mumps because of an outbreak should receive a third dose of a mumps-containing vaccine to improve protection against mumps disease and related complications (see Mumps, p 567).

PERTUSSIS

Students and staff members with pertussis confirmed by culture or polymerase chain reaction testing and symptomatic contacts of an epidemiologically confirmed case should be excluded from school and related activities until they have received at least 5 days of azithromycin. Children and staff members with documented pertussis who refuse appropriate antimicrobial treatment should be excluded for 21 days after last contact with the infected person. Chemoprophylaxis should be given to all household contacts and to school contacts who are at risk of severe illness or adverse outcomes (eg, women in the third trimester of pregnancy, people with severe asthma or cystic fibrosis) or who have close contact with such people. Unvaccinated or undervaccinated contacts should be vaccinated (see Pertussis, p 620) with tetanus toxoid, reduced diphtheria toxoid, and acellular pertussis (DTaP if <7 years, Tdap if ≥7 years) vaccine (**https://redbook. solutions.aap.org/SS/Immunization_Schedules.aspx**).

HEPATITIS A VIRUS

Susceptible children 12 months of age or older who are exposed to HAV should receive single-antigen hepatitis A vaccine (HepA) or Immune Globulin (IG) within 14 days after exposure. For healthy people 12 months through 40 years of age, HAV vaccine at the age-appropriate dose is preferred to Immune Globulin Intramuscular (IGIM) because of vaccine advantages, including long-term protection and ease of administration. For people older than 40 years, Immune Globulin Intramuscular (IGIM) currently is preferred for postexposure prophylaxis because of the absence of data regarding vaccine performance in this age group and the increased risk of severe manifestations of HAV infection with increasing age. However, HepA vaccine can be used in exposed patients older than 40 years if IGIM is unavailable. People who are immunocompromised, are younger than 12 months, or have chronic liver disease should receive IGIM (see Hepatitis A, p 392). Patients with documented HAV infection are excluded from school for 1 week following onset of illness.

MENINGOCOCCAL INFECTIONS

Bacterial meningitis in school-aged children may be caused by *Neisseria meningitidis*. Infected people are not considered contagious after 24 hours of appropriate antimicrobial therapy. After discharge from the hospital, they pose no risk to classmates and may return to school. Prophylactic antimicrobial therapy or meningococcal vaccination is not recommended for school contacts in most circumstances. Vigilant observation of close contacts is recommended, and they should be evaluated promptly if a febrile illness develops. Students who have been exposed to oral secretions of an infected student, such as through kissing or sharing of food and drink, should receive chemoprophylaxis (see Meningococcal Infections, p 550).

If an outbreak of meningococcus occurs with a serotype covered by vaccination (A, C, Y, W-135, or B), vaccination of school contacts with the appropriate meningococcal vaccine should occur in consultation with local public health authorities. For outbreaks involving serotypes A, C, Y, or W-135, a single dose of meningococcal conjugate vaccine containing the outbreak serotype may be administered to patients 2 months through 55 years of age. The HibMenCT-TT vaccine previously available for children as young as 6 weeks of age is no longer available. For outbreaks involving serotype B, meningococcal B vaccine may be administered after consultation with public health officials to patients 10 years and older. Meningococcal vaccination is not recommended for postexposure prophylaxis following exposure to a single case.

INFLUENZA

Influenza virus infection is a common cause of febrile respiratory tract disease and school absenteeism. Influenza vaccine should be administered to children 6 months and older and adults annually (see Influenza Vaccine, p 483). Antiviral medications may be useful to shorten duration of illness; the greatest impact on outcome will occur if treatment can be initiated within 48 hours of illness onset but treatment still should be considered if later in the course of illness, especially for hospitalized patients. Control of influenza outbreaks includes treatment of infected patients and age-appropriate vaccinations in all unvaccinated or undervaccinated contacts. Chemoprophylaxis of susceptible patients can be offered but should not be a substitute for vaccination. It is recommended that all children in whom an influenza-like illness is diagnosed be afebrile for 24 hours after use of fever-reducing medication before returning to school, whether or not they received antiviral therapy.

Infections Spread by the Respiratory Route

Some pathogens that cause severe lower respiratory tract disease in infants and toddlers, such as respiratory syncytial virus and metapneumovirus, are of less concern in healthy school-aged children. Respiratory tract viruses, however, are associated with exacerbations of asthma and an increase in the incidence of otitis media and can cause significant complications for children with chronic respiratory tract disease, such as cystic fibrosis, or for children who are immunocompromised. Infection-control principles of respiratory etiquette—hand hygiene and covering mouth and nose with tissue when coughing or sneezing (if no tissue is available, use the upper shoulder or elbow area rather than hands)—should be taught and implemented in schools.

Mycoplasma pneumoniae causes upper and lower respiratory tract infection in school-aged children, and outbreaks of *M pneumoniae* infection occur in communities and schools. The nonspecific symptoms and signs associated with this organism make distinguishing *M pneumoniae* infection from other causes of respiratory tract illness difficult. Antimicrobial therapy does not necessarily eradicate the organism or prevent spread. Thus, intervention to prevent secondary infection in the school setting is difficult. *Mycoplasma* outbreaks in schools should be reported to the local health department. Patients with *M pneumoniae* infection may return to school when respiratory symptoms have resolved.

Students with pharyngitis caused by group A streptococcus (GAS) may return to school as early as 12 hours after initiation of antimicrobial therapy, if they are afebrile and feeling better. Students who have negative results for GAS on a rapid antigen test but who are awaiting results of culture and not receiving antimicrobial therapy may attend school during the culture incubation period. Symptomatic contacts of students with documented GAS pharyngitis should be evaluated and treated if streptococcal infection is demonstrated. Asymptomatic contacts usually require neither evaluation nor therapy.

Before 10 years of age, children with tuberculosis generally are not contagious. An adolescent or adult with infectious tuberculosis almost always is the source of infection for young children. Thus, students who are in close contact with an older child, teacher, or other adult with infectious tuberculosis should be evaluated for infection; evaluation includes an interferon-gamma release assay or tuberculin skin testing as well as a chest radiograph (see Tuberculosis, p 829). If an adult source outside the school is identified with active tuberculosis (eg, parent or grandparent of a student), efforts should be made to determine whether other students have been exposed to the same source and whether they warrant evaluation for infection.

Children with erythema infectiosum should be allowed to attend school, because the period of contagion occurs before a rash is evident. Parvovirus B19 infection poses no risk of significant illness for healthy classmates, although aplastic crisis can develop in infected children and adults with sickle cell disease or other hemoglobinopathies. Because of the risk of poor fetal outcomes, pregnant women exposed to an infected child 4 to 14 days before rash onset or to a child with parvovirus-associated aplastic crisis should be referred to their physician for counseling and possible serologic testing.

Infections Spread by Direct Contact

Infection and infestation of skin, eyes, and hair can spread through direct contact with an infected area or through contact with contaminated hands or fomites, such as hair brushes, hats, and clothing. *Staphylococcus aureus* (including methicillin-resistant *S aureus* [MRSA]) and group A streptococcal organisms may colonize the skin, oropharynx, or nasal mucosa of asymptomatic people. Clinical disease (lesions) may develop when these organisms are passed from a person with colonized or infected skin to another person. Shared fomites, such as towels, athletic equipment, and razors, also have been implicated in the spread of MRSA within school settings. Most skin infections attributable to *S aureus* and group A streptococcal organisms are minor and require only topical or oral antimicrobial therapy; thus, person-to-person spread should be interrupted easily by appropriate treatment whenever minor skin infections are recognized. Exclusion is recommended for any child with an open or draining lesion that cannot be covered. Attention should be focused additionally on proper cleaning precautions (ie, cleaning locker rooms and sports equipment).

Herpes simplex virus (HSV) infection of the mouth and skin is common among school-aged children. Infection is spread through direct contact with herpetic lesions or via asymptomatic shedding of virus from oral or genital secretions. "Cold sore" lesions of herpes labialis represent active infection, but no evidence suggests that students with active orolabial lesions pose any greater risk to their classmates than do unidentified asymptomatic shedders. Immunocompromised children and children with open skin lesions (eg, severe eczema) exposed to another child with HSV infection may have an increased risk of HSV acquisition and of severe or disseminated infection. Because of the frequency of symptomatic and asymptomatic shedding of HSV among classmates and staff members, careful hygienic practices are the best means of preventing infection (see Herpes Simplex, p 437). Individuals do not need to be excluded from school unless they are experiencing a primary infection (with intraoral ulcers and vesicles) and they do not have control of their secretions (eg, drooling).

Infectious conjunctivitis can be caused by bacterial (eg, nontypable *Haemophilus influenzae* and *Streptococcus pneumoniae*) or viral (eg, adenoviruses, enteroviruses, and HSV) pathogens. Bacterial conjunctivitis is less common in children older than 5 years. Infection occurs through contamination of hands followed by autoinoculation or from exposure of the eye to contaminated equipment (eg, ophthalmologic examination). Respiratory tract spread from large droplets also may occur. Topical antimicrobial therapy is indicated for bacterial conjunctivitis, which usually is distinguished by a purulent exudate. HSV conjunctivitis usually is unilateral and may be accompanied by vesicles on adjacent skin and preauricular adenopathy. Evaluation of HSV conjunctivitis by an ophthalmologist and administration of specific antiviral therapy are indicated. Conjunctivitis attributable to adenoviruses or enteroviruses is self-limited and requires no specific antiviral therapy. Spread of infection is minimized by careful hand hygiene, and infected people should be presumed contagious until symptoms have resolved. Infected children should be allowed to remain in school once any indicated therapy is implemented, unless they are systemically ill or their behavior with other children or school staff increases transmission risk. The local health department should be notified of an outbreak of conjunctivitis.

Fungal infections of the skin and hair are spread by direct person-to-person contact and through contact with contaminated surfaces or objects and have a predilection to multiply in moist areas of the body. *Trichophyton tonsurans*, the predominant cause of tinea capitis, remains viable for long periods on combs, hair brushes, furniture, and fabric. The fungi that cause tinea corporis (ringworm) are transmissible by direct contact. Tinea cruris (jock itch) and tinea pedis (athlete's foot) occur in adolescents and young adults. Students with fungal infections of the skin or scalp should be encouraged to receive treatment both for their benefit and to prevent spread of infection. If discovered while at school, however, that day's attendance should not be abbreviated. See the chapters on Tinea Capitis (p 798), Tinea Corporis (p 801), and Tinea Cruris (p 804) for specific treatment recommendations. They should not be excluded from school once therapy has been instituted. Students with tinea capitis should be instructed not to share combs, hair brushes, hats, or hair ornaments with classmates until they have been treated. Swimming pools should not be used by those with active tinea pedis infection, and those with active infection should be discouraged from walking barefoot on locker room and shower floors until treatment has been initiated. Sharing of towels and shower shoes during sports activities should be discouraged.[1]

Sarcoptes scabiei (scabies) and *Pediculus capitis* (head lice) are transmitted primarily through person-to-person contact. In the school setting, transmission of scabies is unlikely without prolonged skin-to-skin contact; for lice, transmission occurs by direct head-to-head contact. Transmission of scabies and head lice through shared articles of clothing or hair accessories (combs, hair brushes, hats, and hair ornaments) is possible but uncommon. Children identified as having scabies or head lice should be referred for treatment at the end of the school day. Children with scabies may return to school once treatment is completed (usually overnight). Children with lice should not be excluded from school, because there is a low risk of contagion within classrooms. "No-nit" policies have not been effective in controlling head lice transmission and are not recommended.[2] School contacts of children with scabies or lice generally should not be treated prophylactically. Caregivers who have prolonged skin-to-skin contact with students infested with scabies may benefit from prophylactic treatment (see Scabies, p 718, and Pediculosis Capitis, p 607).

Infections Spread by the Fecal-Oral Route

Pathogens spread via the fecal-oral route constitute a risk if the infected person fails to maintain good hygiene, including hand hygiene after toilet use, or if contaminated food is shared between or among schoolmates.

Implementation of the recommended universal vaccination with HepA vaccine has resulted in a reduction in school outbreaks of disease. Schoolroom exposure generally does not pose an appreciable risk of infection, and postexposure prophylaxis is not indicated when a single case occurs and the source of infection is outside the school. However, HepA vaccine or IGIM could be used for unimmunized people who have close contact with the index patient if transmission within the school setting is documented (see Hepatitis A, p 392).

School outbreaks of gastroenteritis have occurred from viral, bacterial, and parasitic pathogens. Transmission is via the fecal-oral route and may also be foodborne. Enteroviruses and noroviruses can be difficult to control. Noroviruses currently are the most common cause of foodborne illness and foodborne disease outbreaks in the United States. Person-to-person spread of bacterial and parasitic enteropathogens within school settings occurs infrequently, but foodborne outbreaks attributable to enteric pathogens can occur. People with gastroenteritis attributable to an enteric pathogen should be excluded from school settings until symptoms resolve (at a minimum). Pathogen-specific chapters and local health department rules and regulations should be consulted for other criteria allowing reentry into school.

Children in diapers constitute a far greater risk of spread of enteric pathogens compared with fully continent children. Guidelines for control of these infections in child care settings should be applied for diapered school-aged students with developmental

[1]Davies HD, Jackson MA, Rice SG; American Academy of Pediatrics, Committee on Infectious Diseases, Council on Sports Medicine and Fitness. Infectious diseases associated with organized sports and outbreak control. *Pediatrics.* 2017;140(4):e20172477

[2]Devore CD, Schutz GE; American Academy of Pediatrics, Council on School Health, Committee on Infectious Diseases. Head lice. *Pediatrics.* 2015;135(5):e1355-e1365

disabilities (see Children in Out-of-Home Child Care, p 122).[1]

Infections Spread by Blood and Body Fluids

Contact with blood or body fluids from another person requires more intimate exposure than usually occurs in the school setting. However, care required for children with developmental disabilities may expose caregivers to urine, saliva, and in some cases, blood. Cytomegalovirus (CMV) may be chronically shed in saliva or urine; however, children who are shedding CMV do not require exclusion or isolation. The application of Standard Precautions and use of hand hygiene, as recommended for children in out-of-home child care,[1] is the optimal means to prevent spread of infection from these exposures (see Children in Out-of-Home Child Care, p 122). Students infected with CMV do not need to be identified to school personnel.

School staff members should be educated on proper procedures for handling blood or body fluid that may be contaminated with blood. For children with epistaxis or bleeding from injury, staff should wear disposable gloves and use appropriate hand hygiene measures immediately after glove removal for protection from bloodborne pathogens. Staff members at the scene of an injury or bleeding incident who do not have access to gloves should use a barrier, preferably nonpermeable such as a plastic baggie, to avoid exposure to blood or blood-containing materials, use appropriate hand hygiene measures, and adhere to proper protocols for handling contaminated material, including feminine hygiene products.

Students infected with HIV, HBV, or HCV do not need to be identified to school personnel. Rather, policies and procedures to manage all potential exposures to blood or blood-containing materials should be established and universally implemented. Parents and students should be educated about the types of exposure that present a risk for school contacts. Although a student's right to privacy should be maintained, decisions about activities at school should be made by parents or guardians together with the child's physician, on a case-by-case basis, keeping the health needs of the infected student and the student's classmates in mind.

Although no prospective studies have been conducted to determine the risk of transmission of HIV, HBV, or HCV during contact sports among high school students, available evidence indicates that the transmission risk is low. Guidelines for management of bleeding injuries have been developed for college and professional athletes in recognition of the possibility of unidentified HIV, HBV, or HCV infection in any competitor. The American Academy of Pediatrics (AAP) has published recommendations for prevention of transmission of HIV and other bloodborne pathogens in the athletic setting.[2,3]

- Athletes infected with HIV, HBV, or HCV should be allowed to participate in

[1]American Academy of Pediatrics. *Managing Infectious Diseases in Child Care and Schools: A Quick Reference Guide, 4th Edition.* Aronson SS, Shope TR, eds. Elk Grove Village, IL: American Academy of Pediatrics; 2016

[2]American Academy of Pediatrics, Committee on Sports Medicine and Fitness. Human immunodeficiency virus and other blood-borne viral pathogens in the athletic setting. *Pediatrics.* 1999;104(6):1400–1403 (Reaffirmed February 2015)

[3]Rice SG; American Academy of Pediatrics, Council on Sports Medicine and Fitness. Medical conditions affecting sports participation. *Pediatrics.* 2008;121(4):841–848 (Reaffirmed June 2014)

competitive sports.

- Physicians should respect the rights of infected athletes to confidentiality. The infection status of patients should not be disclosed to other participants or the staff of athletic programs.
- Testing for bloodborne pathogens should not be mandatory for athletes or sports participants.
- Pediatricians are encouraged to counsel athletes who are infected with HIV, HBV, or HCV and assure them that they have a low risk of infecting other competitors. Infected athletes should consider choosing a sport in which this transmission risk is minimal. This may be protective for other participants and for infected athletes themselves, decreasing their possible exposure to bloodborne pathogens other than the one(s) with which they are infected. Wrestling and boxing have the greatest potential for contamination of injured skin by blood. The AAP opposes boxing as a sport for youth for other reasons.[1]
- Athletic programs should inform athletes and their parents that the program is operating under the policies of the aforementioned recommendations and that the athletes have a low risk of becoming infected with a bloodborne pathogen.
- Athletic programs should promote HBV immunization among all athletes, coaches, athletic trainers, equipment handlers, laundry personnel, janitorial staff, and other people who may be exposed to blood as an occupational hazard.
- Each coach and athletic trainer must receive training in first aid and emergency care and be well versed with the AAP recommendations to prevent transmission of bloodborne pathogens in the athletic setting. These staff members then can help implement the AAP recommendations.
- Coaches and members of the health care team should educate athletes about precautions described in the AAP recommendations. Such education should include that, unlike the assumed low risk of transmission during athletics, there are greater risks of transmission of HIV and other bloodborne pathogens through sexual activity and needle sharing during the use of injection drugs, including anabolic steroids. Athletes should be told not to share personal items, such as razors, toothbrushes, and nail clippers, that might be contaminated with blood.
- Depending on the law in some states, schools may need to comply with Occupational Safety and Health Administration (OSHA) regulations (**www.osha.gov**) for prevention of bloodborne pathogens. The athletic program must determine which OSHA rules are applicable for their enterprise. Compliance with OSHA regulations is a reasonable and recommended precaution even if this is not required specifically by the state.
- The following precautions should be adopted in sports with direct body contact and other sports in which an athlete's blood or other body fluids visibly tinged with blood may contaminate the skin or mucous membranes of other participants or staff members of the athletic program. These precautions will not eliminate the risk that a participant or staff member may become infected with a bloodborne pathogen in the athletic setting but will reduce the risk substantially.

---

[1]American Academy of Pediatrics, Council on Sports Medicine and Fitness; Canadian Paediatric Society, Healthy Active Living and Sports Medicine Committee. Boxing participation by children and adolescents. *Pediatrics*. 2011;128(3):617–623 (Reaffirmed February 2015)

♦ Athletes must cover existing cuts, abrasions, wounds, or other areas of broken skin with an occlusive dressing before and during participation. Caregivers should cover their own damaged skin to prevent transmission of infection to or from an injured athlete.

♦ Disposable, waterproof vinyl or latex gloves should be worn to avoid contact with blood or other body fluids visibly tinged with blood and any objects, such as equipment, bandages, or uniforms, contaminated with these fluids. Hands should be cleaned with soap and water or an alcohol-based antiseptic agent as soon as possible after gloves are removed.

♦ Athletes with active bleeding should be removed from competition as soon as possible. Wounds should be cleaned with soap and water. Skin antiseptic agents may be used if soap and water are not available. Athletes may return to competition once bleeding has stopped, and cleansed wounds are covered with an occlusive dressing that will remain intact and not become soaked through during further play.

♦ Athletes should be advised to report injuries and wounds in a timely fashion before or during competition.

♦ Minor cuts or abrasions that are not bleeding do not require interruption of play but can be cleaned and covered during scheduled breaks. During these breaks, if an athlete's equipment or uniform fabric is wet with blood, the equipment should be cleaned and disinfected (see next bullet), or the uniform should be replaced.

♦ Equipment and playing areas contaminated with blood must be cleaned using gloves and disposable absorbent material until all visible blood is gone and then disinfected with a product registered with the Environmental Protection Agency and applied in the manner and time recommended.[1] If the disinfecting product is bleach (1:100 dilution of household bleach), the decontaminated equipment or area should be in contact with the bleach solution for at least 30 seconds. The area then may be wiped with a disposable cloth after the minimum contact time or allowed to air dry.

♦ Emergency care must not be delayed because gloves or other protective equipment are not available. If the caregiver does not have appropriate protective equipment, a towel may be used to cover the wound until an off-the-field location is reached where gloves can be used during definitive treatment.

♦ Breathing bags (eg, Ambu manual resuscitators) and oropharyngeal airways should be available for use during resuscitation.

♦ Equipment handlers, laundry personnel, and janitorial staff must be educated in proper procedures for handling washable or disposable materials contaminated with blood.

♦ For guidelines on control and prevention of MRSA in athletes and other school settings, see *Staphylococcus aureus* (p 733).[2]

[1]Centers for Disease Control and Prevention. Guidelines for environmental infection control in health-care facilities. Recommendations of CDC and the Healthcare Infection Control Practices Advisory Committee (HICPAC). *MMWR Recomm Rep*. 2003;52(RR-10):1–42

[2]Davies HD, Jackson MA, Rice SG; American Academy of Pediatrics, Committee on Infectious Diseases, Council on Sports Medicine and Fitness. Infectious diseases associated with organized sports and outbreak control. *Pediatrics*. 2017;140(4):e20172477

INFECTION CONTROL AND PREVENTION FOR HOSPITALIZED CHILDREN

Health care-associated infections (HAIs) are a cause of substantial morbidity and some mortality in hospitalized children, particularly children in intensive care units. Hand hygiene before and after each patient contact remains the single most important practice in prevention and control of HAIs. A comprehensive set of guidelines for preventing and controlling HAIs, including isolation precautions, personnel health recommendations, and guidelines for prevention of postoperative and device-related infections, can be found on the Centers for Disease Control and Prevention (CDC) Web site (**www.cdc.gov/ infectioncontrol/guidelines/index.html**). Guidelines for prevention of intravascular catheter-related infections also are available.[1] Additional guidelines are available from the principal infection control societies in the United States, the Society for Healthcare Epidemiology of America (SHEA) and the Association for Professionals in Infection Control and Epidemiology (APIC), as well as subspecialty societies and regulatory agencies, such as the Occupational Safety and Health Administration (OSHA). The investigation and control of pathogen-specific outbreaks that occur in special pediatric settings (eg, hematopoietic stem cell transplant units, neurosurgical units) always should involve the infection control and prevention team in each facility. The Cystic Fibrosis Foundation published an updated evidence-based guideline for prevention of transmission of infectious agents among cystic fibrosis patients in 2013.[2] Accrediting organizations, such as The Joint Commission, have established infection control standards. Physicians and infection control professionals should be familiar with this increasingly complex array of guidelines, regulations, and standards. To accomplish this goal, infection control programs run by pediatric infectious diseases specialists increasingly are used in hospital settings; to be sustainable over time, these programs require adequate institutional support. Ongoing infection prevention and control programs should include education, implementation, reinforcement, documentation, and evaluation of recommendations on a regular basis. Such activities should include conducting surveillance for high-risk HAIs, participating in improvement projects to reduce the incidence of HAIs, sharing data describing the incidence of specifically targeted HAIs, and complying with key prevention activities, such as hand hygiene.

The CDC recently developed the Targeted Assessment for Prevention (TAP) strategy, which targets health care facilities and specific units within facilities with a disproportionate burden of HAIs so that gaps in infection prevention in the targeted locations can be addressed. The TAP report uses a metric called the cumulative attributable difference (CAD), which is the number of infections that must be prevented within a group, facility, or unit to achieve an HAI reduction goal (**www.cdc.gov/hai/ prevent/tap.html**).

---

[1]O'Grady NP, Alexander M, Burns LA, et al; Healthcare Infection Control Practices Advisory Committee. Guidelines for the prevention of intravascular catheter-related infections. *Am J Infect Control*. 2011;39(4 Suppl 1):S1-S34

[2]Saiman L, Siegel JD, LiPuma JJ, et al. Infection prevention and control guideline for cystic fibrosis: 2013 update. *Infect Control Hosp Epidemiol*. 2014;35(Suppl 1):S1-S67

Isolation Precautions

Isolation precautions are designed to protect hospitalized children, health care personnel, and visitors by limiting transmission of potential pathogens within the health care setting. The Healthcare Infection Control Practices Advisory Committee (HICPAC) in 2007 updated evidence-based isolation guidelines for preventing transmission of infectious agents in health care settings.[1] Adherence to these isolation policies, supplemented by health care facility policies and procedures for other aspects of infection and environmental control and occupational health, should result in reduced transmission and safer patient care. Adaptations should be made according to the conditions and populations served by each facility. For example, in 2014, the United States experienced its first cases of imported Ebola virus infections. Despite utilizing personal protective equipment (PPE) and following early guidance, adaptations were required to provide the safest care for health care personnel and the families of affected patients.

Routine and optimal performance of **Standard Precautions** (Table 2.4) is appropriate for care of all patients, regardless of diagnosis or suspected or confirmed infection status. In addition to Standard Precautions, **Transmission-Based Precautions** (Table 2.5) are used when caring for patients who are infected or colonized with pathogens transmitted by airborne, droplet, or contact routes.

STANDARD PRECAUTIONS

Standard Precautions are used to prevent transmission of all infectious agents through contact with nonintact skin, mucous membranes, or any body fluid except sweat (regardless of whether these fluids contain visible blood). Barrier techniques (eg, gloves or nonsterile gowns, as described below) are recommended to decrease exposure of health care personnel to body fluids. Standard Precautions are used with all patients when exposure to blood and body fluids is anticipated and are designed to decrease transmission of microorganisms from patients who are not recognized as harboring potential pathogens, such as bloodborne pathogens and antimicrobial-resistant bacteria. See Table 2.4, p 149, for elements of Standard Precautions (respiratory hygiene/cough etiquette). Standard Precautions include the following practices:

- **Hand hygiene[2] (www.cdc.gov/handhygiene/)** is necessary before and after all patient contact and after touching blood, body fluids, secretions, excretions, and contaminated items, whether gloves are worn or not. Hand hygiene should be performed either with alcohol-based agents or with soap and water before donning and immediately after removing (doffing) gloves, between patient contacts, and when otherwise indicated to avoid transfer of microorganisms to other patients and to items in the environment. When hands are visibly dirty or contaminated with proteinaceous material, such as blood or other body fluids, hands should be washed with soap and

---

[1]Centers for Disease Control and Prevention. Guideline for isolation precautions: preventing transmission of infectious agents in healthcare settings 2007. Recommendations of the Healthcare Infection Control Practices Advisory Committee. Atlanta, GA: Centers for Disease Control and Prevention; 2007. Available at: **www.cdc.gov/hicpac/pdf/isolation/Isolation2007.pdf**

[2]Centers for Disease Control and Prevention. Guideline for hand hygiene in health-care settings. Recommendations of the Healthcare Infection Control Practices Advisory Committee and the HICPAC/SHEA/APIC/IDSA Hand Hygiene Task Force. *MMWR Recomm Rep.* 2002;51(RR-16):1–45

water for at least 20 seconds. The best means of preventing transmission of spores (eg, *Clostridium difficile*) or norovirus is not clear, but handwashing with soap and water currently is preferred over alcohol-based agents.

Table 2.4. Recommendations for Application of Standard Precautions for Care of All Patients in All Health Care Settings

Component	Recommendations
Hand hygiene	Before and after each patient contact, regardless of whether gloves are used. After touching blood, body fluids, secretions, excretions, or contaminated items; immediately after removing gloves. Alcohol-containing antiseptic hand rubs preferred, except when hands are soiled visibly or if exposure to spores (eg, *Clostridium difficile, Bacillus anthracis*) or norovirus is likely to have occurred.
Personal protective equipment (PPE)	
Gloves	For touching blood, body fluids, secretions, excretions, or contaminated items; for touching mucous membranes and nonintact skin.
Gown	During procedures and patient-care activities when contact of clothing/exposed skin with blood/body fluids, secretions, and excretions is anticipated.
Mask, eye protection (goggles), face shield	During procedures and patient-care activities likely to generate splashes or sprays of blood, body fluids, or secretions, especially suctioning and endotracheal intubation, to protect health care personnel. For patient protection, use of a mask by the person inserting an epidural anesthesia needle or performing myelograms when prolonged exposure of the puncture site is likely to occur.
Soiled patient-care equipment	Handle in a manner that prevents transfer of microorganisms to others and to the environment; wear gloves if visibly contaminated; perform hand hygiene after contact with soiled items and after glove removal.
Environmental control	Develop procedures for routine care, cleaning, and disinfection of environmental surfaces, especially frequently touched surfaces in patient care areas.
Used textiles (linens) and laundry	Handle in a manner that prevents transfer of microorganisms to others and the environment.
Injection practices (use of needles and other sharps)	Do not recap, bend, break, or hand manipulate used needles; if recapping is required, use a one-handed scoop technique only; use needle-free safety devices when available; place used sharps in conveniently placed, puncture-resistant container. Use a sterile, single-use, disposable needle and syringe for each injection administered.

Table 2.4. Recommendations for Application of Standard Precautions for Care of All Patients in All Health Care Settings, continued

Component	Recommendations
Patient resuscitation	Use mouthpiece, resuscitation bag, or other ventilation devices to prevent contact with mouth and oral secretions.
Patient placement	Prioritize for single-patient room if patient is at increased risk of transmission, is likely to contaminate the environment, does not maintain appropriate hygiene, or is at increased risk of acquiring infection or developing adverse outcome following infection.
Respiratory hygiene/cough etiquette (source containment of infectious respiratory tract secretions in symptomatic patients) beginning at the initial point of encounter (eg, triage and reception areas in emergency departments and physician offices)	Instruct symptomatic people to cover mouth/nose when sneezing/coughing; use tissues and dispose in no-touch receptacle; observe hand hygiene after soiling of hands with respiratory tract secretions; wear surgical mask if tolerated or maintain spatial separation more than 3 feet, if possible.

Table 2.5. Transmission-Based Precautions for Hospitalized Patients[a]

Category of Precautions	Single-Patient Room	Respiratory Tract/Mucous Membrane Protection	Gowns	Gloves
Airborne	Yes, with negative air-pressure ventilation, 6–12 air exchanges per hour, ± HEPA filtration	Respirators: N95 or higher level[b]	No[c]	No[c]
Droplet	Yes[d]	Surgical masks[e]	No[c]	No[c]
Contact	Yes[d]	No	Yes	Yes

HEPA indicates high-efficiency particulate air.

[a]These recommendations are in addition to those for **Standard Precautions** for all patients.

[b]For tuberculosis and select emerging pathogens; otherwise, surgical mask acceptable.

[c]Gowns and gloves may be required as a component of **Standard Precautions** (eg, for blood collection or during procedures likely to cause blood splashes or if there are skin lesions containing transmissible infectious agents).

[d]Preferred. Cohorting of children infected with the same pathogen is acceptable if a single-patient room is not available, a distance of more than 3 to 6 feet between patients can be maintained, and precautions are observed between all contacts with different patients in the room.

[e]Masks should be donned for all health care contact within 3 to 6 feet of the patient.

- **Gloves** (clean, nonsterile) should be worn when touching blood, body fluids, secretions, excretions, and items contaminated with these fluids, except for wiping a child's tears or nose or for routine wet diaper changing in the well child. Hand hygiene should be performed before donning gloves. Clean gloves should be used by health care providers before touching mucous membranes and nonintact skin or if contact with body fluids is possible. Gloves should be changed after contact with potentially infectious material (eg, purulent drainage) and between tasks and procedures on the same patient. Hand hygiene also should be performed after removal of gloves, even if visible soiling did not occur.
- **Masks, eye protection, and face shields** should be worn to protect mucous membranes of the eyes, nose, and mouth during procedures and patient care activities likely to generate splashes or sprays of blood, body fluids, secretions, or excretions. Surgical masks should be worn when placing a catheter or injecting material into the spinal canal or subdural space (eg, during myelograms and spinal or epidural anesthesia).
- **Nonsterile gowns** that are fluid-resistant will protect skin and prevent soiling of clothing during procedures and patient care activities likely to generate splashes or sprays of blood, body fluids, secretions, or excretions. Soiled gowns should be removed promptly and carefully to avoid contamination of clothing.
- **Patient care equipment** that has been used should be handled in a manner that prevents skin or mucous membrane exposures and contamination of clothing or the environment and should be cleaned according to manufacturer's recommendations.
- **All used textiles (linens)** are considered to be contaminated and should be handled, transported, and processed in a manner that prevents aerosolization of microorganisms, skin and mucous membrane exposure, and contamination of clothing.
- **Care of the environment,** which includes shared toys and high-touch surfaces, requires that policies and procedures are established for routine and targeted cleaning of environmental surfaces as indicated by the level of patient contact and degree of soiling. A product registered by the Environmental Protection Agency that has activity against the organisms most likely present in the environment should be used.
- **Safer injection practices should be followed.** Bloodborne pathogen exposure of health care personnel should be avoided by taking precautions to prevent injuries caused by needles, scalpels, and other sharp instruments or devices during procedures; when handling sharp instruments after procedures; when cleaning used instruments; and during disposal of used needles. To prevent needlestick injuries, safety devices should be used whenever they are available. Needles should not be recapped, purposely bent or broken by hand, removed from disposable syringes, or otherwise manipulated by hand. After use, disposable syringes and needles, scalpel blades, and other sharp items should be placed in puncture-resistant containers for disposal; puncture-resistant containers should be located as close as practical to the use area. Large-bore reusable needles should be placed in a puncture-resistant container located close to the site of use for transport to the reprocessing area to ensure maximal patient safety. Sharp devices with safety features are preferred whenever such devices have equivalent function to conventional sharp devices. Single-dose vials of medication are preferred and should never be used for more than one patient.

- **Mouthpieces, resuscitation bags, and other ventilation devices** should be available in all patient care areas and used instead of mouth-to-mouth resuscitation.
- **Point-of-use equipment cleaning (eg, stethoscopes, otoscopes)** should be performed.

TRANSMISSION-BASED PRECAUTIONS

Transmission-Based Precautions are designed for patients documented or suspected to have colonization or infection with pathogens for which additional precautions beyond **Standard Precautions** are recommended to prevent transmission. The 3 types of transmission routes on which these precautions are based are airborne, droplet, and contact.

- **Airborne transmission** occurs by dissemination of airborne droplet nuclei (small-particle residue [≤5 μm in size] of evaporated droplets containing microorganisms that remain suspended in the air for long periods) or small respirable particles containing the infectious agent or spores. Microorganisms transmitted by the airborne route can be dispersed widely by air currents and can be inhaled by a susceptible host within the same room or a long distance from the source patient, depending on environmental factors. Special air handling and ventilation are required to prevent airborne transmission. Examples of microorganisms transmitted by airborne droplet nuclei are *Mycobacterium tuberculosis*, rubeola (measles) virus, and varicella-zoster virus. Specific recommendations for **Airborne Precautions** are as follows:
  - ◆ Patients with infection or colonization should be provided with a single-patient room (if unavailable, consult an infection control professional), and the door should be kept closed at all times.
  - ◆ Special ventilation should be used, including 6 to 12 air changes per hour, air flow direction from the surrounding area to the room, and room air exhausted directly to the outside or recirculated through a high-efficiency particulate air (HEPA) filter.
  - ◆ If infectious pulmonary tuberculosis is suspected or proven, respiratory protective devices (ie, National Institute for Occupational Safety and Health-certified personally "fitted" and "sealing" respirator, such as N95 or N100 respirators, or powered air-purifying respirators) should be worn while inside the patient's room.
  - ◆ Susceptible health care personnel should not enter rooms of patients with measles or varicella-zoster virus infections. If susceptible people must enter the room of a patient with measles or varicella infection or an immunocompromised patient with local or disseminated zoster infection, a respiratory protective device, such as an N95 (fit-tested) or a powered air-purifying respirator, should be worn. People with proven immunity to varicella need not wear a mask, but in caring for patients with measles, all health care personnel, including those immunized, must wear respiratory protective devices.
  - ◆ Patients suspected of having Middle East respiratory syndrome coronavirus (MERS-CoV) should be placed on airborne and contact precautions because of the severity of disease and unclear mode of transmission (**www.cdc.gov/coronavirus/mers/infection-prevention-control.html**).

- **Droplet transmission** occurs when respiratory droplets containing microorganisms are generated from an infected person, primarily during coughing, sneezing, or talking, and during the performance of certain procedures, such as suctioning and bronchoscopy, and are propelled a short distance (3–6 feet or less) and deposited into conjunctivae, nasal mucosa, or the mouth of a susceptible person. Because these relatively large droplets do not remain suspended in air, special air handling and ventilation are not required to prevent droplet transmission. Droplet transmission should not be confused with airborne transmission via droplet nuclei, which are much smaller. Specific recommendations for **Droplet Precautions** are as follows:
  - The patient should be provided with a single-patient room, if possible. If unavailable, the facility may consider cohorting patients infected with the same organism. Spatial separation of more than 3 to 6 feet should be maintained between the bed of the infected patient and the beds of the other patients in multiple-bed rooms. Standard precautions plus a mask should be used.
  - A mask should be worn on entry into the room or into the cubical space, and droplet precautions should be maintained when within 3 to 6 feet of the patient.
  - Masks and other PPE should be removed before leaving the room or caring for another patient in the same room. Hand hygiene should be performed after PPE removal.
  - Older children being transported within the health care facility should wear a mask; no mask is need for people transporting the patient.

  Specific illnesses and infections requiring **Droplet Precautions** include the following:
  - Adenovirus pneumonia
  - Diphtheria (pharyngeal)
  - *Haemophilus influenzae* type b (invasive)
  - Influenza
  - Mumps
  - *Mycoplasma pneumoniae*
  - *Neisseria meningitidis* (invasive)
  - Parvovirus B19 during the phase of illness before onset of rash in immunocompetent patients
  - Pertussis
  - Plague (pneumonic)
  - Rhinovirus
  - Rubella
  - Severe acute respiratory syndrome (SARS) (in addition to airborne and contact)
  - Group A streptococcal pharyngitis or pneumonia
- **Contact Transmission** is the most common route of transmission of HAIs. *Direct contact* transmission involves the physical transfer of microorganisms between a person with infection or colonization and a susceptible host through direct and indirect contact with infectious agents, such as occurs when a health care professional examines a patient, turns a patient, gives a patient a bath, or performs other patient care activities that require direct personal contact. Direct contact transmission also can occur between 2 patients when one serves as the source of the infectious microorganisms and the other serves as a susceptible host. *Indirect contact* transmission involves contact of a susceptible host with a contaminated intermediate object, usually

inanimate, such as contaminated instruments, needles, dressings, toys, or contaminated hands that are not cleansed or gloves that are not changed between patients.

Specific recommendations for **Contact Precautions** are as follows:

◆ The patient should be provided with a single-patient room if possible. If unavailable, cohorting patients likely to be infected with the same organism and use of Standard Precautions and Contact Precautions are permissible.

◆ Gloves (clean, nonsterile) should be used at all times.

◆ Hand hygiene should be performed before and after glove removal.

◆ Gown and gloves should be used on entry into a patient room and during direct contact with a patient, environmental surfaces, or items in the patient room and should be removed before leaving the patient's room or area.

◆ When transport or movement in any health care facility is necessary, infected or colonized areas of the patient's body should be contained and covered.

◆ Disposable noncritical patient-care equipment (eg, blood pressure cuffs) should be used, or patient-dedicated use of such equipment should be implemented. If common use of equipment for multiple patients is unavoidable, such equipment should be cleaned and disinfected per manufacturer's recommendations before use on another patient.

Specific illnesses and infections with organisms requiring **Contact Precautions** include the following:

◆ Colonization or infection with multidrug-resistant bacteria judged by the infection control practitioner on the basis of current state, regional, or national recommendations to be of special clinical and epidemiologic significance (eg, vancomycin-resistant enterococci, methicillin-resistant *Staphylococcus aureus*, multidrug-resistant gram-negative bacilli) or other epidemiologically important susceptible bacteria

◆ *C difficile*

◆ Conjunctivitis, viral and hemorrhagic

◆ Diphtheria (cutaneous)

◆ Draining abscess, decubitus ulcer

◆ Enteroviruses

◆ *Escherichia coli* O157:H7 and other Shiga toxin-producing *E coli*

◆ Hepatitis A virus

◆ Herpes simplex virus (neonatal, mucocutaneous, or cutaneous)

◆ Herpes zoster (localized with no evidence of dissemination)

◆ Human metapneumovirus

◆ Impetigo

◆ Norovirus

◆ Parainfluenza virus

◆ *Pediculosis capitis*, *Pediculosis corporis*, and *Pediculosis pubis* (lice)

◆ Respiratory syncytial virus

◆ Rotavirus

◆ *Salmonella* species

◆ Scabies

◆ *Shigella* species

♦ *S aureus* (cutaneous or draining wounds, regardless of susceptibility to methicillin)
♦ Viral hemorrhagic fevers (eg, Ebola, Lassa, Marburg)

Airborne, Droplet, and **Contact Precautions** should be combined for diseases caused by organisms that have multiple routes of transmission. When used alone or in combination, these **Transmission-Based Precautions** always are to be used in addition to **Standard Precautions,** which are recommended for all patients.

The specifications for these categories of isolation precautions are summarized in Table 2.5 (p 150), and Table 2.6 (p 156) lists syndromes and conditions that are suggestive of contagious infection and require empiric isolation precautions pending identification of a specific pathogen. When the specific pathogen is known, isolation recommendations and duration of isolation are provided in the pathogen- or disease-specific chapters in Section 3.

PEDIATRIC CONSIDERATIONS

Unique differences in pediatric care necessitate modifications of these guidelines, including the following: (1) diaper changing and wiping a child's tears or nose; (2) use of single-patient room isolation; and (3) use of common areas, such as hospital waiting rooms, playrooms, and schoolrooms. More patients and their sibling visitors with transmissible infections may be present in pediatric health care settings, especially during seasonal epidemics.

Because diapering or wiping a child's nose or tears does not soil hands routinely, wearing gloves is not mandatory except when gloves are required as part of **Transmission-Based Precautions**. If gloves are worn for diaper changing—for example, in cases in which soiling of hands is considered likely—hand hygiene should be performed before and after the diaper changing.

Single-patient rooms are recommended for all patients for **Transmission-Based Precautions** (ie, **Airborne, Droplet,** and **Contact**). Patients placed on **Transmission-Based Precautions** should not leave their rooms to use common areas, such as child life playrooms, schoolrooms, or waiting areas, except under special circumstances as defined by the facility infection control personnel. The guidelines for **Standard Precautions** state that patients who cannot control body excretions should be in single-patient rooms. Because most young children are incontinent, this recommendation does not apply to routine care of uninfected children.

CDC isolation guidelines were developed for preventing transmission of infection in hospitals and other settings in which health care is delivered. These recommendations do not apply to schools, out-of-home child care centers, and other settings in which healthy children congregate in shared space, including ambulatory care settings.

Table 2.6. Clinical Syndromes or Conditions Warranting Precautions in Addition to Standard Precautions to Prevent Transmission of Epidemiologically Important Pathogens Pending Confirmation of Diagnosis[a]

Clinical Syndrome or Condition[b]	Potential Pathogens[c]	Empiric Precautions[d]
Diarrhea		
Acute diarrhea with a likely infectious cause	Enteric pathogens[e]	Contact
Diarrhea in patient with a history of recent antimicrobial use	Clostridium difficile	Contact; use soap and water for handwashing
Meningitis	Neisseria meningitidis, Haemophilus influenzae type b	Droplet
	Enteroviruses	Contact
Rash or exanthems, generalized, cause unknown		
Petechial or ecchymotic with fever	N meningitidis	Droplet
	Hemorrhagic fever viruses	Contact plus Airborne
	Enteroviruses	Contact
Vesicular	Varicella-zoster virus	Airborne and Contact
Maculopapular with coryza and fever	Measles virus	Airborne
Respiratory tract infections		
Pulmonary cavitary disease	Mycobacterium tuberculosis	Airborne
Paroxysmal or severe persistent cough during periods of pertussis activity in the community	Bordetella pertussis	Droplet

Table 2.6. Clinical Syndromes or Conditions Warranting Precautions in Addition to Standard Precautions to Prevent Transmission of Epidemiologically Important Pathogens Pending Confirmation of Diagnosis[a], continued

Clinical Syndrome or Condition[b]	Potential Pathogens[c]	Empiric Precautions[d]
Viral infections, particularly bronchiolitis and croup, in infants and young children	Respiratory viral pathogens	Contact and Droplet
Risk of multidrug-resistant microorganisms[f]		
History of infection or colonization with multidrug-resistant organisms	Resistant bacteria	Contact
Skin, wound, or urinary tract infection in a patient with a recent stay in a hospital or chronic care facility	Resistant bacteria	Contact until resistant organism is excluded by cultures
Skin or wound infection		
Abscess or draining wound that cannot be covered	*Staphylococcus aureus*, group A streptococcus	Contact

[a]Infection control professionals are encouraged to modify or adapt this table according to local conditions. To ensure that appropriate empiric precautions are implemented, hospitals must have systems in place to evaluate patients routinely according to these criteria as part of their preadmission and admission care.

[b]Patients with the syndromes or conditions listed may have atypical signs or symptoms (eg, pertussis in neonates may present with apnea; paroxysmal or severe cough may be absent in pertussis in adults). The clinician's index of suspicion should be guided by the prevalence of specific conditions in the community and clinical judgment.

[c]The organisms listed in this column are not intended to represent the complete or even most likely diagnoses but, rather, possible causative agents that require additional precautions beyond **Standard Precautions** until a causative agent can be excluded.

[d]Duration of isolation varies by agent and the antimicrobial treatment administered.

[e]These pathogens include Shiga toxin-producing *Escherichia coli* including *E coli* O157:H7, *Shigella* organisms, *Salmonella* organisms, *Campylobacter* organisms, hepatitis A virus, enteric viruses including rotavirus, *Cryptosporidium* organisms, and *Giardia* organisms. Use masks when cleaning vomitus or stool during norovirus outbreak.

[f]Resistant bacteria judged by the infection control program on the basis of current state, regional, or national recommendations to be of special clinical or epidemiologic significance.

Strategies to Prevent Health Care-Associated Infections

HAIs in patients in acute care hospitals are associated with substantial morbidity and some mortality. Important infections include central line-associated bloodstream infections, central nervous system shunt infections, surgical site infections, urinary catheter-associated urinary tract infections, ventilator-associated pneumonias, infections caused by viruses (eg, respiratory syncytial virus, rotavirus), and colitis attributable to *C difficile*. Infection prevention strategies exist for each of these infections. Evidence-based protocols have been shown to reduce HAIs by using "bundled strategies" (when multiple prevention activities are implemented simultaneously) and with multidisciplinary participation and collaboration with members of the health care team, including administrators, physicians, nurses, therapists, and housekeeping services. Most studies documenting a favorable effect of implementation of infection prevention "bundles" have been performed in adult populations, and studies of infection prevention strategies in pediatric patients are limited. Although there are no agreed on components of an effective bundle, best-practice bundles in pediatrics have been developed to target reducing central line-associated bloodstream infections and ventilator-associated pneumonias.

   Reduction of surgical site infections (eg, spinal fusion, central nervous system shunt placement, cardiothoracic) and central line-associated bloodstream infections in neonatal and pediatric intensive care units have been demonstrated in large multicenter quality improvement collaboratives.[1] These collaboratives used bundles and their reliable implementation to prevent such infections. The bundle to prevent surgical site infections may include preoperative bathing, appropriate use of skin antisepsis, appropriate timing of intraoperative antibiotic prophylaxis and redosing, and elimination of razors. The bundle to prevent a central line-associated bloodstream infection may include the following elements (**www.cdc.gov/infectioncontrol/guidelines/BSI/index. html**):

- Educate health care personnel in central venous catheter insertion and maintenance techniques relevant to infection prevention, typically with a course or video.
- Insertion practices:
   - Perform hand hygiene before the procedure.
   - Use maximal sterile barrier precautions, including a large sterile drape to fully cover the patient and a mask and cap and sterile gown and gloves for the person inserting the catheter.
   - Use chlorhexidine-based antiseptic scrub at the insertion site (2-minute scrub at groin; 30-second scrub at all other sites) and air drying. Although chlorhexidine is not approved for use in children younger than 2 months because of absence of safety data, a growing number of institutions are using it routinely on neonates and young infants; use of chlorhexidine in preterm infants is controversial. For neonates weighing less than 1500 g at birth, an iodine-based antiseptic is recommended.

---

[1]Miller MR, Niedner MF, Huskins C, et al. Reducing PICU central line-associated bloodstream infections: 3-year results. *Pediatrics*. 2011;128(5):e1077-e1083

- ◆ Use a catheter insertion checklist and a trained observer who is empowered to halt the procedure if there is a break in the sterile technique protocol.
- Maintenance practices:
  - ◆ Catheter site care:
    - Use a chlorhexidine gluconate scrub for dressing changes (scrub for 30 seconds, air dry for 30 seconds); an iodine-based antiseptic is recommended for smaller infants.
    - Use a semipermeable, transparent dressing over the catheter insertion site.
    - Change clear dressings every 7 days or more frequently if soiled, dampened, or loosened.
    - Perform sterile tubing changes.
    - Use a prepackaged dressing-change kit or gather supplies into a cart that can be positioned adjacent to the patient at the time a dressing is to be changed.
    - If gauze dressings must be used because of bleeding, change every 2 days or more frequently if soiled, dampened, or loosened.
  - ◆ Disinfect catheter hubs, injection ports, and needleless connectors by vigorous rubbing with an alcohol swab or pad for at least 15 seconds before accessing the catheter, a procedure sometimes called "scrub the hub"; allow hub to air dry fully before accessing.
- Evaluate patients daily to determine whether there is a continued need for the central venous catheter and remove catheter if not needed.
- Monitor infection rates and adherence to infection prevention measures.
- Participate in multicenter quality improvement learning collaboratives.

Occupational Health

Transmission of infectious agents within health care settings is facilitated by close contact between patients and health care personnel and by lack of hygienic practices by infants and young children. **Standard Precautions** and **Transmission-Based Precautions** are designed to prevent transmission of infectious agents in health care settings among patients and health care personnel. To further limit risks of transmission of organisms between children and health care personnel, health care facilities should have established personnel health policies and services. Specifically, personnel should be protected against vaccine-preventable diseases by establishing appropriate screening and immunization policies (see adult immunization schedule at **www.cdc.gov/vaccines/ schedules/hcp/adult.html**). Guidelines for immunization of health care personnel have been published.[1]

For infections that are not vaccine preventable, personnel should be counseled about exposures and the possible need for leave from work if they are exposed to, ill with, or a carrier of a specific pathogen, whether the exposure occurs in the home, community, or health care setting.

The frequency and need for screening of health care personnel for tuberculosis should be determined by local epidemiologic data, as described in the CDC guideline for

---

[1]Centers for Disease Control and Prevention. Immunization of health-care personnel: recommendations of the Advisory Committee on Immunization Practices (ACIP). *MMWR Recomm Rep*. 2011;60(RR-7):1-44

prevention of transmission of tuberculosis in health care settings.[1] People with commonly occurring infections, such as gastroenteritis, dermatitis, herpes simplex virus lesions on exposed skin, or upper respiratory tract infections, should be evaluated to determine the resulting risk of transmission to patients or to other health care personnel.

Health care personnel education, including understanding of hospital policies, is of paramount importance in infection control. Pediatric health care personnel should be knowledgeable about the modes of transmission of infectious agents, proper hand hygiene techniques, and serious risks to children from certain mild infections in adults. Frequent educational sessions will reinforce safe techniques and the importance of infection control policies. Written policies and procedures relating to needlestick or sharp injuries are mandated by OSHA.[2] Recommendations for postinjury prophylaxis are available (see Human Immunodeficiency Virus Infection, p 459, and Table 3.31, p 465).[3,4]

Pregnant health care personnel who follow recommended precautions should not be at increased risk of infections that have possible adverse effects on the fetus (eg, parvovirus B19, cytomegalovirus, rubella, and varicella). Pregnant personnel should not care for immunocompromised patients with chronic parvovirus B19 infection or for those with parvovirus B19-associated aplastic crisis, because both groups are likely to be contagious. Pregnant personnel should avoid caring for those receiving aerosolized ribavirin therapy (risk of teratogenicity). The risk of severe influenza infection for pregnant health care personnel can be reduced by influenza immunization and adherence to appropriate infection control precautions.

Personnel who are immunocompromised and at increased risk of severe infection (eg, *M tuberculosis*, measles virus, herpes simplex virus, and varicella-zoster virus) should seek advice from their primary health care professional.

The consequences to pediatric patients of acquiring infections from adults can be significant. Mild illnesses in adults, such as viral gastroenteritis, upper respiratory tract viral infection, pertusis, or herpes simplex virus infection, can cause life-threatening disease in infants and children. People at greatest risk are preterm infants, children who have heart disease or chronic pulmonary disease, and people who are immunocompromised.

Sibling Visitation

Sibling visits to birthing centers, postpartum rooms, pediatric wards, and intensive care units are encouraged, although some institutions are choosing to restrict visitation of young children during times of peak respiratory viral activity because of their relatively high frequency of asymptomatic viral shedding and difficulties adhering to basic respiratory etiquette and hand hygiene practices. Neonatal intensive care often results in

---

[1]Centers for Disease Control and Prevention. Guidelines for preventing the transmission of *Mycobacterium tuberculosis* in health-care settings, 2005. *MMWR Recomm Rep.* 2005;54(RR-17):1–141

[2]Occupational Safety and Health Administration (**www.osha.gov**)

[3]Centers for Disease Control and Prevention. Updated US Public Health Service guidelines for the management of occupational exposures to HIV and recommendations for postexposure prophylaxis. *MMWR Recomm Rep.* 2005;54(RR-9):1–17

[4]Centers for Disease Control and Prevention. Guidance for evaluating health-care personnel for hepatitis B virus protection and for administering postexposure management. *MMWR Recomm Rep.* 2013;62(RR10):1–19

long hospital stays for the preterm or sick newborn, making family visits important. Sibling visits may benefit hospitalized children. Guidelines for sibling visits should be established to maximize opportunities for visiting and to minimize the risks of transmission of pathogens brought into the hospital setting by young visitors. Guidelines may need to be modified by local nursing, pediatric, obstetric, and infectious diseases staff members to address specific issues in their hospital settings. Basic guidelines for sibling visits to pediatric patients are as follows:

- Before the visit, a trained health care professional should interview the parents at a site outside the unit to assess the health of each sibling visitor. These interviews should be documented, and approval for each sibling visit should be noted. No child with fever or symptoms of an acute infection, including upper respiratory tract infection, gastroenteritis, or cellulitis, should be allowed to visit. Siblings who recently have been exposed to a person with a known communicable disease and are susceptible should not be allowed to visit.
- Siblings who are visiting should have received all recommended immunizations for their age. Before and during influenza season, siblings who visit should have received influenza vaccine.
- Asymptomatic siblings who recently have been exposed to varicella but have been immunized previously can be assumed to be immune.
- The visiting sibling should visit only his or her sibling and not be allowed in playrooms with groups of patients.
- Children should perform recommended hand hygiene before entry into the health care setting and before and after any patient contact.
- Throughout the visit, sibling activity should be supervised by parents or a responsible adult and limited to the mother's or patient's room or other designated areas where other patients are not present.

Adult Visitation

Guidelines should be established for visits by other relatives and close friends. Anyone with fever or contagious illnesses ideally should not visit. Medical and nursing staff members should be vigilant about potential communicable diseases in parents and other adult visitors (eg, a relative with a cough who may have pertussis or tuberculosis; a parent with a cold visiting a highly immunosuppressed child). Before and during influenza season, all visitors should be encouraged to have received the influenza vaccine. Adherence to these guidelines is especially important for oncology, hematopoietic stem cell transplant, and neonatal intensive care units.

Pet Visitation

Pet visitation in the health care setting includes visits by a child's personal pet and pet visitation as a part of child life therapeutic programs. Guidelines for pet visitation should be established to minimize risks of transmission of pathogens from pets to humans or injury from animals. The specific health care setting and the level of concern for zoonotic disease will influence establishment of pet visitation policies. The pet visitation policy should be developed in consultation with pediatricians, infection control professionals, nursing staff, the hospital epidemiologist, and veterinarians. Basic principles for pet visitation policies in health care settings are as follows[1]:

- Personal pets other than cats and dogs should be excluded from the hospital. No reptiles (eg, iguanas, turtles, snakes), amphibians, birds, poultry, primates, ferrets, or rodents should be allowed to visit. Exceptions may be made for end-of-life patients who are in single-patient rooms.
- Visiting pets should have a certificate of immunization from a licensed veterinarian and verification that the pet is healthy. Some institutions require an assessment of temperament (eg, Canine Good Citizen certificate).
- The pet should be bathed and groomed for the visit.
- Pet visitation should be discouraged in an intensive care unit or hematology-oncology unit, but individual circumstances can be considered and programmatic involvement with the infection control and prevention team is recommended.
- The visit of a pet should be approved by an appropriate personnel member (eg, the director of the child life therapy program), who should observe the pet for temperament and general health at the time of visit. The pet should be free of obvious bacterial skin infections, infections caused by superficial dermatophytes, and ectoparasites (fleas and ticks).
- Pet visitation should be confined to designated areas. Contact should be confined to the petting and holding of animals, as appropriate. All contact should be supervised throughout the visit by appropriate personnel and should be followed by hand hygiene performed by the patient and all who had contact with the pet. Supervisors should be familiar with institutional policies for managing animal bites and cleaning pet urine, feces, or vomitus.
- Patients having contact with pets must have approval from a physician or physician representative before animal contact. Documented allergy to dogs or cats should be considered before approving contact. For patients who are immunodeficient or for people receiving immunosuppressive therapy, the risks of exposure to the microflora of pets may outweigh the benefits of contact. Contact of children with pets should be approved on a case-by-case basis.
- Care should be taken to protect indwelling catheter sites (eg, central venous catheters, peritoneal dialysis catheters) and other medical devices. These sites should have dressings that provide an effective barrier to pet contact, including licking, and be covered with clothing or gown. Concern for contamination of other body sites should be considered on a case-by-case basis.

The pet policy should not apply to professionally trained service animals. These animals are not pets, and separate policies should govern their uses and presence in the hospital, according to the requirements of the Americans with Disabilities Act.

[1]Writing Panel of Working Group; Lefebvre SL, Golab GC, Christensen E, et al. Guidelines for animal-assisted interventions in health care facilities. *Am J Infect Control.* 2008;36(2):78-85

INFECTION CONTROL AND PREVENTION IN AMBULATORY SETTINGS

Infection prevention and control is an integral part of pediatric practice in ambulatory care settings as well as in inpatient settings.[1] All health care personnel should be aware of the routes of transmission and techniques to prevent transmission of infectious agents. Written policies and procedures for infection prevention and control should be readily available, implemented, updated annually, and enforced. Facilities should have ready access to an individual with training in infection prevention. **Standard Precautions,** as outlined for the hospitalized child (see Infection Control and Prevention for Hospitalized Children, p 147) and by the Centers for Disease Control and Prevention (CDC),[2] with a modification by the American Academy of Pediatrics exempting the use of gloves for routine diaper changes and wiping a child's nose or eyes,[1] are appropriate for most patient encounters. The CDC has created a guideline and a checklist (**www.cdc.gov/ infectioncontrol/pdf/outpatient/guide.pdf** and **www.cdc.gov/ infectioncontrol/pdf/outpatient/guidechecklist.pdf**) that health care professionals can use to ensure that appropriate infection-control practices are being followed and, thus, reduce ambulatory health care-associated infections. Key principles of infection prevention and control in an outpatient setting are as follows:

- Infection prevention and control should begin when the child's appointment is scheduled (eg, triage questions may guide additional precautions for when the patient arrives) and initiated when the child enters the office or clinic.
- **Standard Precautions** (Table 2.4, p 149) should be used when caring for all patients. Standard Precautions are supplemented by **Transmission-Based Precautions** (Table 2.5, p 150) and should include instructions to health care personnel on the proper donning and removal (doffing) of personal protective equipment (gloves, gowns, masks, and protective eyewear). Contact between contagious children and uninfected children should be minimized. Policies for children who are suspected of having contagious infections, such as varicella or measles, should be implemented promptly. Immunocompromised children and neonates should be kept away from people with potentially contagious infections.
- In waiting rooms of ambulatory care facilities, respiratory hygiene/cough etiquette and use of masks should be implemented for patients and accompanying people with suspected respiratory tract infection.[3]

---

[1]Rathore MH, Jackson MA; American Academy of Pediatrics, Committee on Infectious Diseases. Infection prevention and control in pediatric ambulatory settings. *Pediatrics.* 2017;140(5):e20172857

[2]Centers for Disease Control and Prevention. Guideline for isolation precautions: preventing transmission of infectious agents in health care settings 2007. Recommendations of the Healthcare Infection Control Practices Advisory Committee. Atlanta, GA: Centers for Disease Control and Prevention; 2007. Available at: **www.cdc.gov/hicpac/2007IP/2007isolationPrecautions.html**

[3]Centers for Disease Control and Prevention. Respiratory Hygiene/Cough Etiquette in Healthcare Settings. Available at: **www.cdc.gov/flu/professionals/infectioncontrol/resphygiene.htm**

- ♦ If it is not feasible to use waiting areas to separate patients with cystic fibrosis with the minimum recommended distance of 6 feet from other patients, it is recommended that patients with cystic fibrosis should be taken directly to an examination room after arrival.
- All health care personnel should perform hand hygiene before and after each patient contact. In health care settings, alcohol-based hand products are preferred for decontaminating hands routinely. Soap and water are preferred when hands are visibly dirty or contaminated with proteinaceous material, such as blood or other body fluids, and after caring for a patient with known or suspected infectious diarrhea (eg, *Clostridium difficile* or norovirus). Parents and children should be taught the importance of hand hygiene. Guidelines on hand hygiene can be found on the CDC Web site (**www.cdc.gov/handhygiene/providers/guideline.html**).
- Health care personnel should receive influenza vaccination annually as well as vaccinations against other vaccine-preventable infections that can be transmitted in an ambulatory setting to patients or to other health care personnel. Recommended vaccines include tetanus toxoid, reduced diphtheria toxoid, and acellular pertussis (Tdap), measles-mumps-rubella (MMR), varicella, and hepatitis B.[1]
- Health care personnel should be familiar with aseptic technique, particularly regarding insertion or manipulation of intravascular catheters, performance of other invasive procedures, and preparation and administration of parenteral medications. This includes selection and use of appropriate skin antiseptics. The preferred skin-preparation agent for immunization and venipuncture for routine blood collection is 70% isopropyl alcohol. Skin preparation for incision, suture, or collection of blood for culture requires 70% isopropyl alcohol, alcohol tinctures of iodine (10%), alcoholic chlorhexidine (containing 2% chlorhexidine) preparations, or povidone iodine.
- Needles and sharps should be handled with great care. Medical devices designed to reduce the risk of needle sticks should be used. Sharps disposal containers that are impermeable and puncture resistant should be available adjacent to the areas where sharps are used (eg, areas where injections or venipunctures are performed). Sharps containers should be replaced before they become overfilled and should be kept out of reach of young children. Policies should be established for removal and the disposal of sharps containers consistent with state and local regulations. Guidance on safe injection practices is available on the CDC Web site (**www.cdc.gov/injectionsafety/**).
- Appropriate handling of medical waste should be outlined (**www.cdc.gov/infectioncontrol/pdf/outpatient/guide.pdf**).
- A written bloodborne pathogen exposure control plan that includes policies for management of exposures to blood and body fluids, such as through needlesticks and exposures of nonintact skin and mucous membranes, should be developed, readily available to all staff, and updated and reviewed with staff regularly (at least annually) (see Hepatitis B, p 401; Hepatitis C, p 428; and Human Immunodeficiency Virus Infection, p 459).

[1]Centers for Disease Control and Prevention. Immunization of healthcare personnel. Recommendations of the Advisory Committee on Immunization Practices (ACIP). *MMWR Recomm Rep.* 2011;60(RR-7):1–45

- Standard guidelines for processing of medical devices and equipment, including decontamination, disinfection, and sterilization, should be followed meticulously.
- Appropriate use of antimicrobial agents is essential to limit the emergence and spread of drug-resistant bacteria (see Antimicrobial Stewardship, p 909; **www.cdc.gov/ features/AntibioticResistanceThreats/index.html**).
- Policies and procedures should be developed for communication with local and state health authorities about reportable diseases and suspected outbreaks (**www.cdc.gov/ hai/outbreaks/**).
- Educational programs for health care personnel that encompass appropriate aspects of infection control should be implemented, reinforced, documented, and evaluated on a regular basis.
- Outpatient facilities should employ or have access to an individual with training in infection prevention who manages the infection prevention program.
- Physicians should be aware of requirements of government agencies, such as the Occupational Safety and Health Administration (OSHA), as well as state and federal regulations that may apply to the operation of physicians' offices.

SEXUALLY TRANSMITTED INFECTIONS IN ADOLESCENTS AND CHILDREN

Physicians and other health care professionals perform a critical role in preventing and treating sexually transmitted infections (STIs) in the pediatric population. STIs are a major problem for adolescents; an estimated 25% of adolescent females will acquire an STI by 19 years of age. Although an STI in an infant or child early in life can be the result of vertical transmission or autoinoculation, certain STIs (eg, gonorrhea, syphilis, chlamydia, genital herpes, or anogenital warts) should raise suspicion of sexual abuse if acquired after the neonatal period. The detection of *any* STI in an infant, child, or adolescent should lead the health care professional to consider the possibility of sexual abuse. Whenever sexual abuse is suspected, appropriate social service and law enforcement agencies must be involved to evaluate the situation further, to ensure the child or adolescent's protection, and to provide appropriate counseling. When available, consultation with a child abuse pediatrician can help guide further evaluation, aid in decision making on reporting suspected abuse, and assist with rendering an opinion on the etiology of the STI after collaborating with investigators.

STIs in Adolescents

EPIDEMIOLOGY OF STIs IN ADOLESCENTS

Adolescents and young adults have the highest rates of several STIs when compared with any other age group. Adolescents are at greater risk of STIs because of their high rate of unprotected intercourse and increased biologic susceptibility. Furthermore, they may engage in multiple sequential monogamous partnerships of varying durations and face several potential obstacles in accessing reproductive health education and confidential health care services.[1]

Public health officials and medical professional organizations recommend routine screening of sexually active adolescent and young adult females for certain STIs, such as chlamydia and gonorrhea, but routine STI screening recommendations for heterosexual males do not exist. Hence, the rates of these reported STIs are higher in adolescent females, for whom routine testing is recommended, compared with adolescent males. Screening should be considered in clinical settings serving populations of young males with a high prevalence of STIs, such as adolescent health clinics, correctional facilities, and STI clinics.

Care must be taken when interpreting reported STI rates among adolescents, because *all* adolescents, including those who have never had sexual intercourse, are included in the denominators used to calculate age-specific STI rates. Rates among sexually experienced adolescents are higher because the denominators are lower. Furthermore, many sexually active adolescents are not tested for STIs, so infections often are not diagnosed or reported.

EVALUATION OF STIs IN ADOLESCENTS

Despite the high prevalence of STIs among adolescents and young adults, health care professionals frequently fail to confidentially inquire about sexual behaviors, assess for STI risks, counsel about risk reduction, and screen for STIs. At each well-child and sick visit, the health care provider may allow some private time, apart from the parent(s) or guardian(s), to speak with the adolescent confidentially.[2] Health care professionals can prepare patients and families by educating both parents and preadolescents about the need for confidentiality as adolescence approaches. Pediatricians should screen for STI risk by *routinely* asking all adolescent and young adult patients—apart from their parents— whether they ever have had sexual intercourse, currently are sexually active, or are planning to be sexually active in the near future. Pediatricians must be sure to define the terms "sexual intercourse" and "sexually active," because these terms can have different meanings for adolescents. If a patient indicates a history of sexual activity, the health care provider must further ascertain the type of sex (vaginal, oral, or anal) and partner gender to determine what type(s) of STI testing to perform. It is important that adolescents and young adults are educated to recognize that oral and anal intercourse, as well as vaginal intercourse, put them at risk of STIs. All adolescents and young adults should be fully immunized, screened for risk factors, and appropriately tested and treated as indicated. More detailed recommendations for preventive health care for adolescents and young adults are available from the American Academy of Pediatrics (AAP)[3] and Centers for

---

[1]Centers for Disease Control and Prevention. *Sexually Transmitted Disease Surveillance 2015*. Atlanta, GA: US Department of Health and Human Services; 2016

[2]The Society for Adolescent Health and Medicine and the American Academy of Pediatrics. Position paper: confidentiality protections for adolescents and young adults in the health care billing and insurance claims process. *J Adolesc Health*. 2016;58(3):374-377

[3]American Academy of Pediatrics, Committee on Adolescence; Society for Adolescent Health and Medicine. Screening for nonviral sexually transmitted infections in adolescents and young adults. *Pediatrics*. 2014;134(1):e302-e311

Disease Control and Prevention (CDC).[1]

In the evaluation of the postpubertal adolescent or young adult sexual assault victim, if a decision to perform STI testing is made, gonorrhea and chlamydia diagnostic evaluation from any sites of penetration or attempted penetration should be performed, per CDC guidance. Because children and adolescents may not always fully disclose all details of the assault, evaluation of sites other than those disclosed should be considered. Testing for relevant STIs is outlined in Table 2.8 (p 171). The CDC recommends nucleic acid amplification tests (NAATs) for *Chlamydia trachomatis* and *Neisseria gonorrhoeae* from specimens at the sites of penetration as the preferred diagnostic evaluation of adolescent or young adult sexual assault victims. In addition, the CDC recommends NAAT of a urine or vaginal swab specimen or point-of-care testing of a vaginal swab specimen for *Trichomonas vaginalis*. Especially if vaginal discharge, malodor, or itching is present, point-of-care testing or a wet mount of a vaginal swab specimen should be performed to evaluate for bacterial vaginosis. Baseline and follow-up serum samples for evaluation for human immunodeficiency virus (HIV) infection, hepatitis B, and syphilis should be obtained. Prophylactic treatment for STIs in cases of sexual assault is discussed later in this chapter (see Prophylaxis of Children and Adolescents After Sexual Victimization, p 173).

MANAGEMENT OF STIs IN ADOLESCENTS

All 50 states allow minors to give their own consent for confidential STI testing, diagnosis, and treatment. Pediatricians should consult their own state laws for further guidance. For treatment recommendations for specific STIs, see the disease-specific chapters in Section 3 and Tables 4.4 (p 933) and 4.5 (p 936). Single-dose therapies are available for many STIs, offering the advantage of high patient adherence; directly observed therapy should be provided where feasible. Patients and their partners treated for *N gonorrhoeae*, *C trachomatis*, pelvic inflammatory disease, and trichomoniasis should be advised to refrain from sexual intercourse for 1 week after completion of appropriate treatment.

Partner treatment is essential, both from a public health perspective and to protect the index patient from reinfection. Sexual partners during the past 60 days should be informed of the infection and encouraged to seek comprehensive STI evaluation and treatment. If it appears unlikely that partners of patients treated for gonococcal or chlamydial infections will seek care, pediatricians may consider providing expedited partner therapy (EPT) to patients.[1] EPT is the clinical practice of treating the sex partners of patients with diagnosed chlamydia or gonorrhea by providing prescriptions or medications to the patient to take to his or her partner without the health care professional first examining the partner. Information should be provided warning about the low risk of potential adverse events and allergic reactions to EPT, with instructions to seek medical attention in the event that an adverse reaction occurs. The legality of prescribing EPT varies by state. Guidance on the legal status of EPT by jurisdiction is available from the CDC (**www.cdc.gov/std/ept**).

---

[1]Centers for Disease Control and Prevention. 2015 Sexually transmitted diseases treatment guidelines. *MMWR Recomm Rep*. 2015;64(RR-3): 1-137. Available at: **www.cdc.gov/std/treatment**

PREVENTION OF STIs IN ADOLESCENTS

Pediatricians and other health care professionals can contribute to primary prevention of STIs by encouraging and supporting a teenager's decision to postpone initiating sexual intercourse. For teenagers who become sexually active, pediatricians should discuss methods of protecting against STIs and unwanted pregnancies, including the correct and consistent use of condoms with all forms of sexual intercourse (vaginal, oral, and anal). Teenagers need to be counseled to consider the possible association between alcohol or drug use and failure to appropriately use barrier methods correctly when either partner is impaired. Health care professionals should discuss other ways to decrease risk of acquiring STIs, including limiting the number of partners and choosing to abstain even if initiation of sexual intercourse already has occurred.

Adolescents who have not previously been vaccinated against human papillomavirus (HPV) or hepatitis B should complete both immunization series.

Pediatricians should counsel their adolescent patients at substantial risk for sexually transmitted HIV infection about preexposure prophylaxis (PrEP) as a potential strategy to prevent HIV infection. When used consistently, PrEP has been shown to greatly reduce the risk of HIV infection in people who are at substantial risk.[1] For sexual transmission, those at substantial risk include gay or bisexual males or heterosexual males or females whose sexual partner(s) are either HIV positive or at high risk of being infected with HIV, such as people who inject drugs or have bisexual male partners. The combination pill of 2 antiretroviral drugs, tenofovir and emtricitabine (brand name Truvada), taken in a single pill daily, was approved by the US Food and Drug Administration for use as PrEP in July 2012. In 2014, the US Public Health Service issued comprehensive guidance for the use of daily PrEP that can be found at **www.cdc.gov/hiv/pdf/guidelines/PrEPguidelines2014.pdf.** The data on the efficacy and safety of PrEP for adolescents are insufficient. Therefore, pediatricians should be familiar with state minor consent laws and discuss risks and benefits of PrEP with their adolescent patients at risk.

STIs in Children

SOCIAL IMPLICATIONS OF STIs IN CHILDREN

This section is limited in scope to management of STIs in children, with full guidance on child abuse and neglect available at **http://pediatrics.aappublications.org/content/132/2/e558.**[2] Evaluation for the possibility of sexual abuse solely on the basis of suspicion of an STI should not proceed until the STI diagnosis has been confirmed. Confirmation of an STI in a child requires repeat testing to ensure the initial test result was not a false positive. Treatment of the patient should not occur until repeat testing has been performed. It is recommended that an alternative test be used for confirmation (see

---

[1]US Public Health Service. Preexposure Prophylaxis for the Prevention of HIV Infection in the United States — 2014: A Clinical Practice Guideline. Available at: **www.cdc.gov/hiv/pdf/guidelines/PrEPguidelines2014.pdf**

[2]Kellogg N; American Academy of Pediatrics, Committee on Child Abuse and Neglect. The evaluation of sexual abuse in children. *Pediatrics.* 2005;116(2):506–512. Updated 2013 clinical report available at **http://pediatrics.aappublications.org/content/132/2/e558**

Evaluation of STIs in Children, p 172). Factors to be considered in assessing the likelihood of sexual abuse in a child with an STI include the biological characteristics of the STI in question, the age of the child, and whether the child reports a history of sexual victimization (see Table 2.7, p 170). When victimization is reported by a child or adolescent, the risk factors for STIs in a possible assailant (when available), as well as the history of type of sexual contact, may also guide testing and treatment. When possible, children who are suspected to have been sexually abused or thought to have an STI should be evaluated at child advocacy centers or hospital-based child protection programs. If these resources are unavailable, then the general pediatrician should conduct the evaluation.

Anogenital gonorrhea in a prepubertal child is indicative of sexual abuse. All confirmed cases of gonorrhea in prepubertal children beyond the neonatal period should be reported to the local child protective services agency for investigation.

First-episode symptomatic genital herpes simplex virus (HSV) infection has a short incubation period. HSV can be transmitted by sexual or nonsexual contact with another person or by self-inoculation. In an infant or toddler in diapers, genital herpes may result through any of these mechanisms. Viral typing of the isolate (if obtained by culture) or amplicon (if obtained by PCR) for HSV-1 and HSV-2 will yield additional helpful information. In a prepubertal child, the new occurrence of genital herpes should prompt a careful evaluation for possible sexual abuse. However, HSV infection alone is not diagnostic of sexual abuse.

Trichomoniasis is transmitted perinatally or by sexual contact. In a perinatally infected infant, vaginal discharge can persist for several weeks; accordingly, intense social investigation may not be warranted. However, a new diagnosis of trichomoniasis in an older infant or prepubertal child should prompt a careful investigation, including a child protective services investigation, for suspected sexual abuse. It is important to note that *T vaginalis* identified in the urine must be differentiated from *Trichomonas hominis*, a nonpathogenic contaminant found in the gastrointestinal tract.

Infections that have long incubation periods and that can be asymptomatic for a period of time after vertical transmission (eg, syphilis, HIV infection, and *C trachomatis* infection) are more problematic. The possibility of vertical transmission should be considered in these cases, but an evaluation of the patient's circumstances by the local child protective services agency usually is warranted. HPV infection has a long incubation period and can be transmitted vertically, by sexual contact, by nonsexual contact with others, or by autoinoculation. Identification of genital warts should prompt a careful evaluation for sexual abuse; however, as with HSV infection, HPV infection alone is not diagnostic of sexual abuse.

Although hepatitis B virus, hepatitis C virus, and scabies may be transmitted sexually, other modes of transmission can occur. The discovery of any of these conditions in a prepubertal child does not warrant child protective services involvement unless the health care professional finds additional information that suggests that sexual abuse might have occurred.

Table 2.7. Implications of Commonly Encountered Sexually Transmitted (ST) or Sexually Associated (SA) Infections for Diagnosis and Reporting of Sexual Abuse Among Infants and Prepubertal Children

ST/SA Confirmed	Evidence for Sexual Abuse	Suggested Action
Neisseria gonorrhoeae[a]	Diagnostic	Report[b]
Syphilis[a]	Diagnostic	Report[b]
Human immunodeficiency virus[c]	Diagnostic	Report[b]
Chlamydia trachomatis[a]	Diagnostic	Report[b]
Trichomonas vaginalis[a]	Highly suspicious	Report[b]
Genital herpes	Highly suspicious (HSV-2 especially)	Report[b,d,e]
Condylomata acuminata (anogenital warts)[a]	Suspicious	Consider report[b,d,e]
Bacterial vaginosis	Inconclusive	Medical follow-up

[a]If not likely to be perinatally acquired and rare nonsexual, vertical transmission is excluded.
[b]Reports should be made to the agency in the community mandated to receive reports of suspected child abuse or neglect.
[c]If not likely to be acquired perinatally or through transfusion.
[d]Unless there is a clear history of autoinoculation.
[e]Report if there is additional evidence to suspect abuse, including history, physical examination or other infections identified.
Table adapted from Kellogg N; American Academy of Pediatrics, Committee on Child Abuse and Neglect. The evaluation of sexual abuse in children. *Pediatrics*. 2005;116(2):506–512. Updated 2013 clinical report available at
http://pediatrics.aappublications.org/content/132/2/e558.

SCREENING SEXUALLY VICTIMIZED CHILDREN FOR STIs

Child sexual abuse has been defined as the exploitation of a child, either by physical contact or by other interactions, for the sexual gratification of an adult or a minor who is in a position of power over the child. Physicians are required by law to report known or suspected abuse to their local or state child protective services agency. Approximately 5% of sexually abused children acquire an STI as a result of victimization. The lack of identification of an STI in a child who is tested does not rule out victimization.

Factors that influence the likelihood that a sexually victimized child will acquire an STI include the regional prevalence of STIs in the adult population, the number of assailants, the type and frequency of physical contact between the perpetrator(s) and the child, the infectivity of various microorganisms, the child's susceptibility to infection, and whether the child has received postexposure antimicrobial treatment. The time interval between a child's physical contact with an assailant and the medical evaluation influences the likelihood that an exposed child will demonstrate signs or symptoms of an STI or have a positive screening test result.

The decision to obtain specimens from genital or other areas to conduct an STI evaluation of a child who has been victimized sexually must be made on an individual basis. Collaboration with a child abuse pediatrician can help guide the evaluation of a child who is suspected to have been sexually abused. The following situations involve a high risk of STIs and constitute a strong indication for physical examination and testing:

- There is disclosure of penetration or suspected penetration of the mouth, vagina, and/or anus.
- The child has or has had signs or symptoms of an STI or an infection that can be transmitted sexually, even in the absence of suspicion of sexual abuse.
- A sibling, another child, or an adult in the household or child's immediate environment has an STI.
- A suspected assailant is known to have an STI or to be at high risk of STIs (eg, has had multiple sexual partners or a history of STIs) or has an unknown history.
- The patient or family requests testing.
- Evidence of genital, oral, or anal penetration or ejaculation is present.
- The child discloses sexual abuse.

See Table 2.8 if STI testing of a child is to be performed.

Table 2.8. Sexually Transmitted Infection (STI) Testing in a Child[a] When Sexual Abuse Is Suspected

Organism/Syndrome	Specimens
Neisseria gonorrhoeae[b]	Rectal, throat, urethral (male), and/or vaginal cultures[c]
Chlamydia trachomatis[b]	Rectal, urethral (male), and vaginal cultures[c]
Syphilis	Darkfield examination (if available) of chancre fluid; blood for serologic tests at time of abuse and 4–6 weeks and 3 months later
Human immunodeficiency virus	Serologic testing of abuser (if possible); serologic testing of child at time of abuse and 4–6 weeks, 3 months, and 6 months later
Hepatitis B virus	Serum hepatitis B surface antigen testing of abuser or hepatitis B surface antibody testing of child, unless the child has received 3 doses of hepatitis B vaccine
Herpes simplex virus (HSV)	Culture of lesion specimen; in addition, polymerase chain reaction assay of lesion specimen if lesion crusted; all virologic specimens should be typed (HSV-1 vs HSV-2)
Bacterial vaginosis	Wet mount, pH, and potassium hydroxide testing of vaginal discharge or Gram stain in pubertal and postmenarcheal girls
Human papillomavirus	Clinical examination, with biopsy of lesion specimen if diagnosis unclear
Trichomonas vaginalis	Wet mount and culture of vaginal discharge[b]
Pediculosis pubis	Identification of eggs, nymphs, and lice with naked eye or using hand lens

[a]See text for examples of indications for testing for STIs.
[b]Nucleic acid amplification tests with vaginal swab specimens or urine from girls can be used as an alternative to culture.
[c]Cervical swab specimens are not recommended or necessary for prepubertal girls, but cervical or vaginal swab specimens must be obtained in pubertal premenarchal and pubertal postmenarcheal girls.

When STI screening is performed, it should focus on likely anatomic sites of infection as determined by the patient's history and physical examination or by epidemiologic considerations. In a primary care setting, a chaperone should be present at the time of evaluation, if possible. To preserve the "chain of custody" for information that may later constitute legal evidence, specimens for laboratory analysis obtained from sexually victimized patients should be labeled carefully, and standard hospital procedures for transferring specimens from site to site should be followed meticulously. A follow-up visit approximately 4 to 6 weeks after the most recent sexual exposure may include a repeat physical examination and collection of additional specimens. Another follow-up visit at 3 and 6 months after the most recent sexual exposure may be necessary to obtain convalescent sera to test for hepatitis B (if indicated), hepatitis C (if indicated), syphilis, and HIV infection.

EVALUATION OF STIs IN CHILDREN

Because of social and legal implications of a positive STI test result, STIs in children must be diagnosed using tests with high specificity. Tests that allow for isolation of the organism and have the highest specificities should be used whenever possible, but there is increasing evidence that NAATs may be used for this purpose.

In the evaluation of prepubescent children for possible sexual assault, the CDC offers the following recommendations[1]:

- Physical examination: Visually inspect the genital, perianal, and oral areas for genital discharge, odor, bleeding, irritation, warts, and ulcerative lesions.
- *C trachomatis* testing: Collect specimens for *C trachomatis* cultures from the rectum in both boys and girls and the vagina in girls. It is important to recognize that culturing of *C trachomatis* is not regulated in any way, and sensitivity may vary from laboratory to laboratory. Obtain a meatal specimen from boys for chlamydia testing if urethral discharge is present. The likelihood of recovering chlamydia from the urethra of an asymptomatic, prepubertal boy is too low to justify the trauma. Testing of pharyngeal specimens for chlamydia is not recommended for children of either sex. NAATs can be used for detection of chlamydia in vaginal swab specimens or urine from girls, but no data are available regarding NAAT use for detection of chlamydia in boys.
- *N gonorrhoeae* testing: Collect specimens for *N gonorrhoeae* from the pharynx and rectum in boys and girls, the vagina in girls, and the urethra in boys. If urethral discharge is present, a meatal specimen is an adequate substitute for an intraurethral swab specimen. The CDC indicates that NAATs can be used as an alternative to gonorrhea culture with vaginal swab or urine specimens from girls only, although consultation with an expert is necessary before using NAATs for prepubertal girls to minimize the possibility of positive reactions with nongonococcal *Neisseria* species and other commensals. All specimens should be retained for additional testing.
- *T vaginalis* testing: Test for *T vaginalis* infection, regardless of symptoms, with culture or wet mount of a vaginal swab specimen. Data on use of NAATs for *T vaginalis* detection in children are limited.[1]
- Bacterial vaginosis (BV) testing: Evaluate for BV with a wet mount of a vaginal swab

---

[1]Centers for Disease Control and Prevention. 2015 Sexually transmitted diseases treatment guidelines. *MMWR Recomm Rep.* 2015;64(RR-3): 1-137. Available at: **www.cdc.gov/std/treatment**

specimen.

- Serum sample testing: Obtain serum samples that can be tested for *T pallidum*, HIV, hepatitis C, and hepatitis B virus antibodies. Decisions regarding the pathogens for which to perform serologic tests immediately, specimens preserved for subsequent analysis, and specimens used as a baseline for comparison with follow-up serologic tests should be made on a case-by-case basis.

Unfortunately, culture-based tests for *C trachomatis* and *N gonorrhoeae* are not very sensitive, and specimens for culture can be difficult to obtain from prepubertal children. Additionally, many laboratories no longer perform culture-based tests. NAATs provide highly sensitive detection of organisms, and their specificity approaches that of culture. Therefore, the AAP recommends the use of NAATs when evaluating children and adolescents for genital infections with *C trachomatis* and *N gonorrhoeae*. Positive test results should be confirmed using additional testing. Centers should have a protocol developed for confirming positive results in populations with a low prevalence of infection when a false-positive test could have serious implications. NAATs of extragenital specimens have not been researched enough yet to be recommended for screening for pharyngeal and rectal gonorrhea and chlamydia. These tests should be interpreted with caution if used.[1]

Because of the serious implications an STI diagnosis in a child suspected of being the victim of sexual abuse, antimicrobial therapy should be withheld until the STI diagnostic testing has been performed. For more detailed diagnosis and treatment recommendations for specific STIs, see the disease-specific chapters in Section 3 and Tables 4.4 (p 933) and 4.5 (p 936). Completion of the HPV immunization series for children 9 years and older should be documented.

PROPHYLAXIS OF CHILDREN AND ADOLESCENTS AFTER SEXUAL VICTIMIZATION

Presumptive treatment for children who have been sexually assaulted or abused is not recommended, because their incidence of STIs is low, the risk of spread to the upper genital tract in prepubertal girls is low, and follow-up usually can be ensured. If the result of an STI test is positive and confirmed with additional testing, treatment then should be given. Factors that may increase the likelihood of infection or that constitute an indication for prophylaxis are the same as those listed under Screening Sexually Victimized Children for STIs (p 170).

Many experts believe that prophylaxis is warranted for **postpubertal** female patients who seek care after an episode of sexual victimization because of the possibility of a preexisting asymptomatic infection, the potential risk for acquisition of new infections with the assault, the substantial risk of pelvic inflammatory disease in females of this age group, and poor compliance with follow-up visits for sexual assault.[2] If testing is to be performed, patients who receive prophylaxis should be tested for relevant STIs (see Table 2.8, p 171) before treatment. The decision regarding which specimens and tests to obtain can be made on an individual basis depending on local STI prevalence, prior risk

[1]Jenny C, Crawford, JE; American Academy of Pediatrics, Committee on Child Abuse and Neglect. The evaluation of children in the primary care setting when sexual abuse is suspected. *Pediatrics.* 2013;132(2):e558-e567

[2]Crawford-Jakubiak JE, Alderman EM, Leventhal JM; American Academy of Pediatrics, Committee on Adolescence. Care of the adolescent after an acute sexual assault. *Pediatrics.* 2017;139(3):e20164243

factors, the nature of the sexual assault (ie, sexual abuse over time or one-time assault), the type of sexual exposure (ie, oral, vaginal, or anal exposure), and the victim's preference. Postmenarcheal patients should be tested for pregnancy before antimicrobial treatment or emergency contraception is provided. Regimens for prophylaxis are presented in Table 2.9.

HIV infection has been reported in children and adolescents for whom sexual abuse was the only known risk factor. Because of the demonstrated effectiveness of nonoccupational postexposure prophylaxis (nPEP) to prevent HIV infection, the question arises whether HIV prophylaxis is warranted for children and adolescents after sexual assault (see Figure 2.1, p 176). The risk of HIV transmission from a single sexual assault that involves transfer of secretions and/or blood is low. Prophylaxis may be considered for patients who seek care within 72 hours after an assault if the assault involved mucosal exposure to secretions; repeated abuse; multiple assailants; and oral, vaginal, and/or anal trauma and particularly if the alleged perpetrator(s) is known to have or is at high risk of having HIV infection (see Human Immunodeficiency Virus Infection, p 459).[1]

The following are recommendations for postexposure assessment within 72 hours of sexual assault:

- Review HIV/acquired immunodeficiency syndrome (AIDS) local epidemiology and assess risk of HIV infection in the assailant; the local health department may be helpful in assessing epidemiology and risk.
- Evaluate circumstances of assault that may affect risk of HIV transmission.
- Consult with a specialist in treating HIV-infected children if nPEP is considered.
- If the patient appears to be at risk of HIV transmission from the assault, discuss nPEP with the caregiver(s), including toxicity and unknown efficacy, as well as the importance of close follow-up with a medical provider knowledgeable in HIV testing and treatment.
- Baseline creatinine should be determined before administering nPEP. Health care professionals should monitor liver function, renal function, and hematologic parameters when indicated by the prescribing information for the antiretrovirals prescribed. Drug-specific recommendations are available at the online AIDS Info Drugs Database at **http://aidsinfo.nih.gov/drugs** or the antiretroviral treatment guidelines.
- If the adolescent patient or the child's caregivers choose to receive antiretroviral nPEP, enough medication should be provided until the return visit at 3 to 7 days after initial assessment to reevaluate and to assess tolerance of medication; dosages should not exceed those for adults.
- HIV antibody test should be performed at original assessment, at 4 to 6 weeks, and at 3 months and 6 months.

[1]Centers for Disease Control and Prevention. Updated Guidelines for Antiretroviral Postexposure Prophylaxis after Sexual, Injection Drug Use, or Other Nonoccupational Exposure to HIV—United States, 2016. Atlanta, GA: Centers for Disease Control and Prevention; 2016. Available at: **www.cdc.gov/hiv/pdf/ programresources/cdc-hiv-npep-guidelines.pdf**

Table 2.9. Prophylaxis After Sexual Victimization: Postpubertal Adolescents

Antimicrobial prophylaxis[a] is recommended to include an empiric regimen to prevent chlamydia, gonorrhea, and trichomoniasis. Vaccination against hepatitis B and HPV is recommended if not fully immunized.

For chlamydia, gonorrhea, and trichomoniasis	Ceftriaxone, 250 mg, intramuscularly, in a single dose **PLUS** Azithromycin, 1 g, orally, in a single dose **PLUS EITHER** Metronidazole, 2 g, orally, in a single dose,[b] **OR** Tinidazole, 2 g, orally, in a single dose[b]
For hepatitis B virus infection[c]	If assailant's hepatitis status is unknown and the survivor has not been previously vaccinated, hepatitis B vaccination without HBIG
	If assailant's hepatitis status is unknown and the survivor has been previously vaccinated, no treatment is indicated
	If the assailant is known to be HBsAg-positive and the survivor has not been previously vaccinated, both hepatitis B vaccine and HBIG should be administered at initial examination. Follow-up doses of vaccine should be administered 1–2 and 4–6 mo after the first dose.
	If the assailant is known to be HBsAg-positive and the survivor has been previously vaccinated, he or she should receive a single vaccine booster dose.
For human immunodeficiency virus (HIV) infection[a]	Consider offering prophylaxis for HIV, depending on circumstances (see Figure 2.1, p 176).
For HPV	HPV vaccine series should be initiated at ≥9 y if not already begun or completed if not fully immunized (3 doses)

Emergency contraception[d]

Levonorgestrel, 1.5 mg, orally, in a single dose[e]
OR
Ulipristal acetate, 30 mg, orally, in a single dose

HPV indicates human papillomavirus.

Source: Centers for Disease Control and Prevention. 2015 Sexually transmitted diseases treatment guidelines. *MMWR Recomm Rep.* 2015; 64(RR-3):1-137 (**www.cdc.gov/std/treatment**)

[a]See text for discussion of prophylaxis for human immunodeficiency virus (HIV) infection after sexual abuse or assault.

[b]Metronidazole or tinidazole can be taken by the patient at home rather than as directly observed therapy to minimize potential adverse effects and drug interactions, especially if emergency contraception is provided or alcohol has been ingested recently. Abstain from alcohol for 1 day with metronidazole and 3 days for tinidazole.

[c]See Table 3.23, p 416.

[d]The patient should have a negative pregnancy test result before emergency contraception is given. Although levonorgestrel emergency contraception is most effective if taken within 72 hours of event, data suggest it is effective up to 120 hours. Ulipristal acetate is effective up to 120 hours after unprotected intercourse.

[e]Levonorgestrel emergency contraception has reduced or absent efficacy for people with a body mass index >30 kg/m^2.

FIG 2.1. ALGORITHM FOR EVALUATION AND TREATMENT OF POSSIBLE NONOCCUPATIONAL HIV EXPOSURES

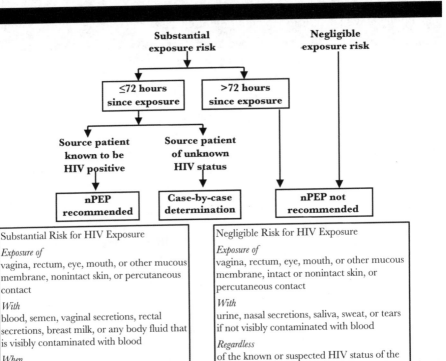

Reproduced from Centers for Disease Control and Prevention. Antiretroviral postexposure prophylaxis after sexual, injection-drug use, or other nonoccupational exposure to HIV in the United States. *MMWR Recomm Rep.* 2005;54(RR-2):1–20. nPEP indicates nonoccupational postexposure prophylaxis.

MEDICAL EVALUATION FOR INFECTIOUS DISEASES FOR INTERNATIONALLY ADOPTED, REFUGEE, AND IMMIGRANT CHILDREN[1,2]

Every year, thousands of children arrive in the United States from other countries. They arrive as immigrants (documented or undocumented), as refugees or asylum seekers, or as

[1]For additional information, see Canadian Paediatric Society (**www.kidsnewtocanada.ca**), the Centers for Disease Control and Prevention (**www.cdc.gov/travel/default.aspx**), and World Health Organization (**www.who.int**) Web sites.

[2]Information for parents can be found at **www.cdc.gov/immigrantrefugeehealth/adoption/index.html/**

adoptees. The medical evaluation of these children is a challenging and important task and is influenced by multiple factors, including the child's country of origin, socioeconomic status, and health history; availability of reliable health care in the country of origin; and the migration route, including type of travel (eg, by foot or by air), countries passed through, and the conditions during the journey.

Children arriving in the United States should be evaluated as soon as possible after arrival to begin medical assessment and preventive health services, including immunizations. In particular, screening for infectious diseases is important to identify infections with a long latency period that may not be prevalent in children born in the United States. Each of the groups mentioned previously has its own characteristics and special needs.

INTERNATIONALLY ADOPTED CHILDREN. The group of children adopted internationally has been studied extensively, and there is a great deal of information available to guide management. Some health concerns may be addressed before adoption, although some are apparent to the adoptive family only after arrival. In general, children adopted internationally have health insurance, and many adoptive families interact with the health care system before arrival of the child. This interaction provides an opportunity to provide advice to the family and to optimize immunizations that the family may need before traveling to pick up the child and for family members and caregivers who will interact with the child after arrival. These immunizations serve to protect the child from diseases that might be transmitted from family members (eg, pertussis, influenza) and to protect the family from diseases that might be transmitted by the child (eg, hepatitis). Access to and quality of medical care for international adoptees before arrival in the United States can be variable. Internationally adopted children are considered legally as a type of immigrant and are required to have a medical examination performed by a physician designated by the US Department of State in their country of origin. This examination usually is limited to completing legal requirements for screening for certain communicable diseases and to examination for serious physical or mental disorders that would prevent the issue of an immigrant visa. Information about this required health assessment is available at **www.cdc.gov/immigrantrefugeehealth/**. Such an evaluation is not a comprehensive assessment of the child's health. During preadoption visits, pediatricians can stress to prospective parents the importance of acquiring immunization and other health records. Parents who have not met with a physician before adoption should notify their physician when their child arrives so that a timely medical evaluation can be arranged. A list of pediatricians with special interest in adoption and foster care medicine is available on the American Academy of Pediatrics (AAP) Web site (**www2.aap.org/sections/adoption/directory/map-adoption. cfm**). Guidance on comprehensive assessment of a newly adopted child is available from the AAP.[1]

REFUGEES AND ASYLEES. Refugees and asylees have legal status in the United States, and various states have different protocols for the initial evaluation of a refugee. The Centers for Disease Control and Prevention (CDC) has issued recommendations for

---

[1]American Academy of Pediatrics, Committee on Early Childhood, Adoption, and Dependent Care. Comprehensive health evaluation of the newly adopted child. *Pediatrics*. 2012;129(1):e214-e223 (Reaffirmed September 2015)

screening of refugees (**www.cdc.gov/immigrantrefugeehealth/guidelines/
domestic/domestic-guidelines.html**).

IMMIGRANTS. In recent years, the number of immigrant children has increased to
represent the largest and most diverse group of new arrivals to the United States. Most
pediatricians will encounter immigrant children in their practice. Evaluation is individual
to each case, depending on whether the child is documented or has insurance coverage,
the circumstances of immigration, country of origin, medical history, and socioeconomic
status. Recommendations for refugees and internationally adopted children should guide
the pediatrician in evaluating the new immigrants. The AAP has developed a toolkit for
the evaluation of the health of immigrant children (**www.aap.org/en-us/
Documents/cocp_toolkit_full.pdf**).

Most immigrant children have received some immunizations but may have received
them on schedules different from those used in the United States or may have missed
essential immunizations. Written documentation of immunizations that includes month
and year of administration is accepted as valid if they conform to the US schedule. See
Children Who Received Immunizations Outside the United States or Whose
Immunization Status is Unknown or Uncertain (p 100) for recommendations regarding
immunizations.

Consideration for Testing for Infectious Agents

Infectious diseases are among the most common medical diagnoses identified in
immigrant children after arrival in the United States. Children may be asymptomatic,
and the diagnoses must be made by laboratory or other tests in addition to history and
physical examination. Because of inconsistent use of the birth dose of hepatitis B (HepB)
vaccine; inconsistent perinatal screening for hepatitis B virus (HBV), syphilis, and human
immunodeficiency virus (HIV); and the high prevalence of certain intestinal parasites and
tuberculosis (TB), screening for these diseases should be considered for all immigrant
children. Screening for other diseases can be considered on an individual basis, as
discussed in the following paragraphs and in the disease-specific chapters in Section 3.

HEPATITIS A

Hepatitis A virus (HAV) is endemic in most countries of origin of internationally adopted,
refugee and immigrant children. Some children may have acquired HAV infection early
in life in their country of origin and may be immune, but others may be incubating HAV
or remain susceptible at the time of entry into the United States. Serologic testing for
acute infection (hepatitis A immunoglobulin [Ig] M) and immunity (total hepatitis A IgG
and IgM antibody) can be considered at the initial visit to determine whether the child is
susceptible to HAV, has current HAV infection, or is immune. Children incubating HAV
infection could transmit the virus to others on arrival in the United States. In the case of
adoption, in which health care is planned in advance, hepatitis A (HepA) vaccine should
be administered, ideally 2 or more weeks before the arrival of the adoptee, to all
previously unvaccinated people who anticipate having close personal contact (eg,
household contact or other regular caregiver) with the child adopted internationally from
a country with high or intermediate HAV prevalence. In addition, if traveling to adopt
the child, adoptive parents and any accompanying family members should ensure that

they are immunized or otherwise immune to HAV infection before traveling to a country of high or intermediate prevalence. Children without HAV immunity who are 12 months and older should receive HepA vaccine according to the routine immunization schedule (**https://redbook.solutions.aap.org/SS/Immunization_Schedules.aspx**).

HEPATITIS B

More studies evaluating the prevalence of hepatitis B are conducted in internationally adopted and refugee children than in immigrant children. In studies conducted primarily during the 1990s, prevalence of hepatitis B surface antigen (HBsAg) ranged from 1% to 5% in internationally adopted children and from 4% to 7% in refugee children, depending on the country of origin and the year studied. Hepatitis B virus (HBV) infection was associated with country of origin and was most common in children from Asia and Africa, some countries of central and eastern Europe (eg, Romania and Bulgaria), and states of the former Soviet Union (eg, Russia and the Ukraine). Over the past 5 to 10 years, the number of countries with routine infant hepatitis B (HepB) immunization programs has increased markedly. By the end of 2014, HepB vaccine had been introduced nationwide in 184 countries, and 96 countries had introduced the birth dose (**www.who.int/mediacentre/factsheets/fs204/en/**).

Despite the number of countries that have added the birth dose, HepB vaccination coverage among infants can be suboptimal. Even when a birth dose of HepB is administered, efficacy of postexposure prophylaxis is lower among infants born to pregnant women with high HBV viral load and hepatitis B e antigen (HBeAg)-positivity. Therefore, all children should be tested for HBsAg to identify cases of chronic infection, regardless of immunization status (see Hepatitis B, p 401). Although HBV serologic tests may be performed in the country of origin, testing is not required for the immigration examination, testing may be incomplete, and children may become infected after testing. Unimmunized children with negative HBsAg and negative hepatitis B surface antibody (HBsAb) test results should be immunized according to the recommended childhood and adolescent immunization schedules (**https://redbook.solutions.aap.org/SS/ Immunization_Schedules.aspx;** also see Children Who Received Immunizations Outside the United States or Whose Immunization Status is Unknown or Uncertain, p 100).

Children with a positive HBsAg test result should be reported to the local or state health department. To distinguish between acute and chronic HBV infection, HBsAg-positive children should be evaluated further. Absence of IgM antibody to hepatitis B core antigen (IgM anti-HBc) or persistence of HBsAg for at least 6 months indicates chronic HBV infection (see Hepatitis B, p 401). Children with chronic HBV infection should be tested for biochemical evidence of liver disease and followed by a specialist who cares for patients with chronic HBV infection (see Hepatitis B, p 401). All unimmunized household contacts of children with chronic HBV infection should be immunized (see Hepatitis B, p 401).

HEPATITIS C

Testing for hepatitis C virus (HCV) infection is recommended for all internationally adopted children, given that most international adoptees in recent years have been adopted from countries with elevated rates of prevalence (eg, China, Russia, southeast

Asia) and because risk factors for infection are rarely known. HCV screening for refugee and immigrant children is not recommended routinely during the new arrival medical examination unless individuals have risk factors, including an HCV-positive mother, overseas surgery, transfusion, major dental work, intravenous drug use, tattoos, sexual activity/abuse, female genital cutting, and other traditional cutting (see "toolkit screening checklist" at **aap.org/en-us/about-the-aap/Committees-Councils-Sections/Council-on-Community-Pediatrics/Pages/Section-1-Clinical-Care.aspx#q3,** and **www.cdc.gov/immigrantrefugeehealth/guidelines/domestic/hepatitis-screening-guidelines.html).** A serum immunoglobulin (Ig) G antibody enzyme immunoassay (EIA) should be used as the initial screening test for children ≥18 months. A positive EIA result may indicate prior HCV infection and should be confirmed with a nucleic acid amplification test (NAAT) for HCV RNA. A positive NAAT result confirms current HCV infection and indicates chronic infection if positive for more than 6 months. Anti-HCV IgG can be detected in >97% of infected people by 6 months after exposure.

Passively transferred maternal antibody can remain detectable by EIA for up to 18 months (see Hepatitis C, p 428); therefore, assessment of perinatally acquired HCV infection may rely on serologic testing at 18 months of age. Prior to the serologic testing, liver enzyme testing can be performed approximately every 6 months to detect the rare HCV perinatally infected infant that has significant liver injury prior to 18 months of age. In situations in which there may be concerns about the ability to maintain contact with an HCV-perinatally exposed infant until 18 months of age, if the family is not willing to wait until 18 months of age to determine their child's HCV infection status, or if antiviral therapy becomes available to younger infants, quantitative RNA tests can be performed at as early as 1 to 2 months of age. If the initial quantitative HCV RNA result is negative, serologic testing should be performed at 18 months of age (see Hepatitis C, p 428).

INTESTINAL PATHOGENS

Serial fecal examinations for ova and parasites tested in a laboratory experienced in parasitology will identify a pathogen in 15% to 35% of internationally adopted and refugee children. Presence or absence of symptoms is not predictive of parasitosis. Prevalence of intestinal parasites varies by age of the child and by country of origin. For refugees, guidelines differ depending on whether the child received presumptive therapy overseas (**www.cdc.gov/immigrantrefugeehealth/guidelines/overseas/interventions/interventions.html).** The most common pathogens identified are *Giardia intestinalis, Dientamoeba fragilis, Hymenolepis* species, *Ascaris lumbricoides,* and *Trichuris trichiura. Strongyloides stercoralis, Entamoeba histolytica, Cryptosporidium* species, and hookworm are recovered less commonly.[1] Regardless of nutritional status or presence of symptoms, 1 to 3 stool specimens collected on separate days may be examined for ova and parasites, and direct fluorescent antibody testing or EIA may be performed for *Giardia* species and *Cryptosporidium* species. Some clinicians prefer to administer presumptive therapy with albendazole. Therapy for intestinal parasites generally is successful, but complete

---

[1] Kotloff KL, Nataro JP, Blackwelder WC, et al. Burden and aetiology of diarrhoeal disease in infants and young children in developing countries (the Global Enteric Multicenter Study, GEMS): a prospective, case-control study. *Lancet.* 2013;382(9888):209–222

eradication may not occur. Proof of eradication is not recommended for individuals who are asymptomatic following therapy. If symptoms persist after treatment, however, ova and parasite testing should be repeated to ensure successful elimination of parasites. Children who fail to demonstrate adequate catch-up growth, who have unexplained anemia, or who have gastrointestinal tract symptoms or signs that occur or recur months or even years after arrival in the United States should be reevaluated for intestinal parasites. In addition, when newly arrived children have acute onset of bloody diarrhea, stool specimens should be tested for *Salmonella* species, *Shigella* species, *Campylobacter* species, and Shiga toxin-producing *Escherichia coli*, including *E coli* O157:H7. If a bacterial pathogen is detected by a nonculture method, culture and antimicrobial susceptibility testing should be performed to inform decisions regarding possible treatment and public health measures.

TISSUE PARASITES/EOSINOPHILIA

Eosinophilia is commonly but not universally present in people with tissue parasites. Refugee children may have received presumptive treatment of intestinal helminths overseas before departure to the United States (**www.cdc.gov/ immigrantrefugeehealth/guidelines/overseas/intestinal-parasites- overseas.html**). In children who did not receive albendazole or ivermectin for presumptive therapy of intestinal helminths, who have negative stool ova and parasite test results, and in whom eosinophilia (absolute eosinophil count exceeding 450 cells/ mm^3) is found on review of complete blood cell count, serologic testing for *Toxocara canis*, strongyloidiasis, schistosomiasis, and lymphatic filariasis should be considered. Although logistically attractive to perform all tests at first encounter, predictive values of many serologic tests for parasites are suboptimal; common treatable causes of eosinophilia usually should be considered first. Because *T canis* is prevalent worldwide, screening is warranted in children who have no identified cause of eosinophilia. For all immigrant children with eosinophilia and no identified pathogen commonly associated with an increased eosinophil count, serologic testing for *Strongyloides stercoralis* is reasonable regardless of country of origin, and testing for *Schistosoma* species should be performed for all children who are from Sub-Saharan Africa, southeast Asia, or areas of the Caribbean and South America, where schistosomiasis is endemic. Serologic testing for lymphatic filariasis should be considered in children older than 2 years with eosinophilia who are from countries with endemic lymphatic filariasis (**www.cdc.gov/parasites/ lymphaticfilariasis/index.html**). A positive serologic result should be confirmed by testing in a reference laboratory (CDC or National Institutes of Health) for release of drugs for treatment of lymphatic filariasis.

SYPHILIS

Congenital syphilis, especially with involvement of the central nervous system, may not have been diagnosed or may have been treated inadequately in children from some resource-limited countries. Children 15 years and older should have had serologic testing for syphilis as part of the required overseas medical assessment, if such an assessment had been performed. Children who had positive test results are required to complete treatment before arrival in the United States. After arrival in the United States, health care professionals should screen children for syphilis by reliable nontreponemal and treponemal serologic tests, regardless of history or a report of treatment (see Syphilis, p 773). Children with positive nontreponemal or treponemal serologic test results should be evaluated by a health care professional with specific expertise to assess the differential diagnosis of pinta, yaws, and syphilis and to determine the stage of infection so that appropriate treatment can be administered (see Syphilis, p 773).

TUBERCULOSIS

Infection with an organism of the *Mycobacterium tuberculosis* complex commonly is encountered in immigrant children, although incidence rates of tuberculosis (TB) vary by country and by age within countries. Predeparture screening requirements for immigrants for TB underwent a major revision in 2007 and have been fully implemented as of October 2013. Requirements include: chest radiograph for all people 15 years and older; sputum smears and cultures for people with an abnormal chest radiograph; drug susceptibility testing for people with positive cultures; and completion of directly observed treatment before immigration for people with pulmonary disease. Refugees and immigrant children 2 to 14 years of age from countries with TB prevalence ≥20 cases per 100 000 population also must have a tuberculin skin test (TST) or interferon-gamma release assay (IGRA) performed. Children with a positive TST or IGRA result should have undergone chest radiography prior to arrival. Children younger than 2 years are not tested unless it is brought to attention of screening physicians outside the United States that they are a known contact of an active case, have known HIV infection, or have signs or symptoms suggestive of TB disease. Information about the screening and implementation requirements is available at **www.cdc.gov/ immigrantrefugeehealth/exams/ti/panel/tuberculosis-panel-technical-instructions.html.**

Because TB can be more severe in young children and can reactivate in later years, testing for latent *M tuberculosis* infection (LTBI) in this high-risk population of immigrants, adoptees, and refugees is important. Presence or absence of a bacille Calmette-Guérin (BCG) vaccine scar should be noted, but approximately 10% of children who received a BCG vaccine as infants will not have a scar. BCG coverage in most countries where the vaccine is used is very high, and health care professionals should be prepared to discuss the limitations of BCG vaccine. The efficacy of BCG vaccine against lethal forms of TB (eg, meningitis) in children is approximately 80%, but its efficacy against pulmonary TB or LTBI is much lower. Receipt of BCG vaccine is not a contraindication to a TST. Either TST or IGRA can be used for children 2 years or older, but IGRA is preferred to avoid a false-positive TST result caused by a previous vaccination with BCG (see Tuberculosis, p 829, for further guidance).[1] In BCG-vaccinated children 2 years and older, IGRA can be performed to help determine whether a "positive" TST result is attributable to LTBI or to the previous BCG vaccine.[1] Some immigrants may be anergic initially because of malnutrition, stress, or untreated HIV infection and, thus, have falsely negative TST or IGRA test results and, therefore, may require repeat testing. Routine chest radiography is not indicated in asymptomatic children in whom the TST or IGRA result is negative. In children with a positive TST or IGRA, further investigation,

[1]Starke JR; American Academy of Pediatrics, Committee on Infectious Diseases. Technical report: interferon-g release assays for diagnosis of tuberculosis infection and disease in children. *Pediatrics.* 2014;134(6):e1763-e1773

including chest radiography and a complete physical examination, is necessary to determine whether tuberculosis disease is present (see Tuberculosis, p 829). When tuberculosis disease is suspected in an immigrant child, efforts to isolate and test the organism for drug susceptibilities are imperative because of the high prevalence of drug resistance in many countries. Physicians who are experts in the management of TB should be consulted when therapy for TB infection or disease is indicated for children from countries with prevalent isoniazid resistance.

HIV INFECTION

The risk of HIV infection in newly arrived children depends on the country of origin and on individual risk factors. Because adoptees may come from populations at high risk of infection, screening for HIV should be performed for all internationally adopted children. Although some children will have HIV test results documented in their referral information, test results from the child's country of origin may not be reliable. Since 2010, refugees and immigrants no longer are required to have HIV testing routinely as part of the immigration medical assessment. HIV testing still is recommended for people who are diagnosed with tuberculosis disease as part of the overseas medical assessment. HIV testing after arrival in the United States is recommended for refugees 13 through 64 years of age and is encouraged for refugees 12 years or younger and older than 64 years of age (**www.cdc.gov/immigrantrefugeehealth/guidelines/domestic/ screening-hiv-infection-domestic.html**). The decision to screen immigrant children for HIV after arrival in the United States should depend on history and risk factors (eg, receipt of blood products, maternal drug use), physical examination findings, and prevalence of HIV infection in the child's country of origin. If there is a suspicion of HIV infection, testing should be performed before administration of live-antigen vaccines. Some experts believe HIV testing may be appropriate for most immigrant children (**http://aidsinfo.nih.gov/contentfiles/lvguidelines/oi_guidelines_ pediatrics.pdf**).

CHAGAS DISEASE (AMERICAN TRYPANOSOMIASIS)

Chagas disease is endemic throughout much of Mexico and Central and South America (see American Trypanosomiasis, p 826). The risk of Chagas disease varies by region within countries but is low in immigrant children from countries with endemic infection. Treatment of children with Chagas disease is highly effective. Countries with endemic Chagas disease include Argentina, Belize, Bolivia, Brazil, Chile, Colombia, Costa Rica, Ecuador, El Salvador, French Guiana, Guatemala, Guyana, Honduras, Mexico, Nicaragua, Panama, Paraguay, Peru, Suriname, Uruguay, and Venezuela. Transmission within countries with endemic infection is focal, but if a child comes from a country with endemic Chagas disease or has received a blood transfusion in a country with endemic disease, testing for *Trypanosoma cruzi* should be considered. Screening using serologic testing should be performed only in children 12 months or older because of the potential presence of maternal antibody.

Table 2.10. Suggested Screening Tests for Infectious Diseases in International Adoptees, Refugees, and Immigrants[a]

Hepatitis B virus serologic testing:
Hepatitis B surface antigen (HBsAg); some experts include hepatitis B surface antibody (anti-HBs) and hepatitis B core antibody (anti-HBc)[b]

Hepatitis C virus serologic testing when indicated (see text)

Syphilis serologic testing:
Nontreponemal test (eg, RPR, VDRL, or ART)
Treponemal test (eg, MHA-TP, FTA-ABS, EIA, CIA, or TPPA)

Human immunodeficiency virus (HIV) 1 and 2 serologic testing; consider combination rapid antigen/antibody testing

Complete blood cell count with red blood cell indices and differential

Stool examination for ova and parasites (1–3 specimens)[c] with specific request for *Giardia intestinalis* and *Cryptosporidium* species testing by direct fluorescent antibody or EIA testing

Tuberculin skin test[c] or interferon-gamma release assay

In children from countries with endemic infection[c]:
Trypanosoma cruzi serologic testing

In children with eosinophilia (absolute eosinophil count exceeding 450 cells/mm³) and negative stool ova and parasite examinations,[d] can consider:
Toxocara canis serologic testing
Strongyloides species serologic testing
Schistosoma species serologic testing for children from sub-Saharan African, Southeast Asian, and certain Latin American countries

Lymphatic filariasis serologic testing for children older than 2 years from countries with endemic infection[c]

RPR indicates rapid plasma reagin; VDRL, Venereal Disease Research Laboratories; ART, automated reagin test; MHA-TP, microhemagglutination test for *Treponema pallidum;* FTA-ABS, fluorescent treponemal antibody absorption; EIA, enzyme immunoassay; CIA, chemiluminescence assay; TPPA, *T pallidum* particle agglutination.
[a]For evaluation of noninfectious disease conditions, see American Academy of Pediatrics, Council on Community Pediatrics. Providing care for immigrant, migrant, and border children. *Pediatrics.* 2013;131(6):e2028-e2034.
[b]Passively acquired maternal anti-HBc may be detected in infant born to HBV-infected mothers up to age 24 months.
[c]See text.
[d]Some experts would perform serologic tests for schistosomiasis in children from areas with high endemicity regardless of eosinophil count because of its poor positive- and negative-predictive values.

OTHER INFECTIOUS DISEASES

Skin infections that occur commonly in immigrant children include bacterial (eg, impetigo) and fungal (eg, candidiasis) infections and ectoparasitic infestations (eg, scabies and pediculosis). New adoptive parents may need to be instructed on how to examine their child for signs of scabies, pediculosis, and tinea so that treatment can be initiated and transmission to others can be prevented (see Scabies, p 718, and Pediculosis chapters, p 607–613).

Diseases such as typhoid fever, leprosy, or melioidosis are encountered infrequently in immigrant children; therefore, routine screening for these diseases is not recommended. Findings of fever, splenomegaly, respiratory tract infection, anemia, or eosinophilia should prompt an appropriate evaluation on the basis of the epidemiology of infectious diseases that occur in the child's country of origin. Refugee children from sub-Saharan Africa may have received presumptive treatment for malaria before departure to the United States (**www.cdc.gov/immigrantrefugeehealth/guidelines/overseas/malaria-guidelines-overseas.html;** see Malaria, p 527).

In the United States, multiple outbreaks of measles have been reported in children adopted from China and in their US contacts. Measles elimination has been achieved only in the Americas; transmission continues in other parts of the world. Prospective parents who are traveling internationally to adopt children, as well as their household contacts, should ensure that they have a history of natural disease or have been immunized adequately for measles according to US recommendations. If these people were born after 1957, and in the absence of documented measles infection or contraindication to the vaccine, they should receive 2 doses of measles-containing vaccine after the age of 12 months and separated by at least 28 days (see Measles, p 537).

Health care professionals should be aware of potential diseases in immigrant children and their clinical manifestations. Although one of the major purposes of screening is to identify asymptomatic diseases with long latency, screening will not be performed for all such diseases; an example is neurocysticercosis, which may not be clinically apparent for many years. In most cases, the longer the interval from arrival to development of a clinical syndrome, the less likely the syndrome can be attributed to a pathogen acquired in the country of origin.

For all immigrant children, establishing a medical home with a primary care provider is of prime importance. The child's country of birth and migration history will remain an important health determinant throughout his or her life.

···

INJURIES FROM DISCARDED NEEDLES IN THE COMMUNITY

Contact with and injuries from hypodermic needles and syringes discarded in public places may pose a risk of transmission of bloodborne pathogens, including human immunodeficiency virus (HIV), hepatitis B virus (HBV), and hepatitis C virus (HCV). However, an epidemiologic study of 274 children (mean age, 7.4 years) identified with a community-acquired needlestick injury over a 19-year period observed no seroconversions, confirming that the risk of transmission of bloodborne viruses in these events is low.[1] Infection risks and options for postexposure prophylaxis (PEP) vary depending on the virus and type of injury and exposure. Although nonoccupational needlestick injuries may pose a lower risk of infection transmission than do occupational needlestick injuries, a person injured by a needle in a nonoccupational setting needs

[1] Papenburg J, Blais D, Moore D, et al. Pediatric injuries from needles discarded in the community: epidemiology and risk of seroconversion. *Pediatrics.* 2008;122(2):e487-e487

evaluation, counseling, and in some cases, PEP. Even if the potential for the discarded syringe to contain a specific bloodborne pathogen can be estimated from the background prevalence rates of these infections in the local community, the need to test the injured or exposed person usually is not influenced significantly by this assessment.

Wound Care and Tetanus Prophylaxis

Management of people with needlestick injuries includes acute wound care and consideration of the need for antimicrobial prophylaxis. Standard wound cleansing and care is indicated; such wounds rarely require closure. A tetanus toxoid-containing vaccine, with or without Tetanus Immune Globulin, should be considered as appropriate for the age, the severity of the injury, the immunization status of the exposed person, and the potential for dirt or soil contamination of the needle (see Tetanus, p 793). Tetanus and diphtheria toxoids (Td) vaccine should be used if the patient has already received all necessary doses of pertussis-containing vaccine. DTaP or Tdap should be administered if pertussis vaccine is needed (see Pertussis, p 620).

Bloodborne Pathogens

Consideration of the need for prophylaxis for HBV and HIV is the next step in exposure management; currently, there is no recommended PEP for HCV. Risk of acquisition of various pathogens depends on the nature of the wound, the ability of the pathogens to survive on environmental surfaces, the volume of source material, the concentration of virus in the source material, prevalence rates among local injection drug users, the probability that the syringe and needle were used by a local injection drug user, and the immunization status of the exposed person. Unlike an occupational blood or body fluid exposure, in which the status of the exposure source for HBV, HCV, and HIV often is known, these data usually are not available to help in the decision-making process in a nonoccupational exposure.[1,2]

HEPATITIS B VIRUS

HBV is the hardiest of the major bloodborne pathogens and can survive on environmental surfaces at room temperature for at least 7 days. Transmission occurs at a rate of 23% to 62% during needlestick injury between health care personnel and hepatitis B surface antigen (HBsAg)-positive sources. Prompt and appropriate PEP intervention reduces this risk. The effectiveness of PEP diminishes the longer after exposure it is initiated.

If the source is known to be HBsAg positive, the unimmunized person who suffered the needlestick should receive both Hepatitis B Immune Globulin (HBIG) and hepatitis B (HepB) vaccine as soon as possible after exposure, preferably within 24 hours (see Table 3.23, Guidelines for Postexposure Prophylaxis of People With Nonoccupational

[1]Centers for Disease Control and Prevention. Updated US Public Health Service guidelines for the management of occupational exposures to HBV, HCV, and HIV and recommendations for postexposure prophylaxis. *MMWR Recomm Rep*. 2001;50(RR-11):1–52

[2]US Department of Health and Human Services. Antiretroviral postexposure prophylaxis after sexual, injection-drug use, or other nonoccupational exposure to HIV in the United States: recommendations from the US Department of Health and Human Services. *MMWR Recomm Rep*. 2005;54(RR-2):1–20

Exposures to Blood or Body Fluids That Contain Blood, by Exposure Type and Vaccination Status, p 416). The vaccine series should be completed using an age-appropriate dose and schedule. People who are in the process of being immunized but who have not completed the vaccine series should receive the appropriate dose of HBIG and should complete the vaccine series. Children and adolescents who have written documentation of a complete HepB vaccine series and who did not receive postimmunization testing should receive a single vaccine booster dose (Table 3.23, p 416).

If the HBsAg status of the source is unknown, the unimmunized person who suffered the needlestick should begin the HepB vaccine series with the first dose initiated as soon as possible after exposure, preferably within 24 hours (see Table 3.23, p 416). The vaccine series should be completed using an age-appropriate dose and schedule. Children and adolescents with written documentation of a complete HepB vaccine series require no further treatment (Table 3.23, p 416).

HUMAN IMMUNODEFICIENCY VIRUS

Infection with HIV usually is the greatest concern of the victim and family. The risk of HIV transmission from a needle discarded in public is very low. To date, no cases in which HIV was transmitted by needlestick injury outside a health care setting have been reported to the Centers for Disease Control and Prevention. Risk of HIV transmission from a puncture wound caused by a needle found in the community is lower than the 0.3% risk of HIV transmission to a health care professional from a needlestick injury from a person with known HIV infection. In most reports of occupational HIV transmission by percutaneous injury, needlestick injury occurred shortly after needle withdrawal from the vein or artery of the source patient with HIV infection. HIV RNA was detected in only 3 (3.8%) of 80 discarded disposable syringes that had been used by health care professionals for intramuscular or subcutaneous injection of patients with HIV infection, indicating that most syringes will not contain transmissible HIV even after being used to draw blood from a person with HIV infection.[1] HIV is susceptible to drying, and when HIV is placed on a surface exposed to air, the 50% tissue culture infective dose decreases by approximately 1 log every 9 hours.[2]

Despite the low risk, there may be rare situations (eg, large-bore needle with fresh blood) in which HIV testing in the child who suffered the needlestick is appropriate. HIV antigen/antibody testing (or antibody testing if Ag/Ab test is unavailable) should be performed at baseline, and follow-up testing should be performed at 4 to 6 weeks and 12 weeks after injury. Because concurrent acquisition of HCV and HIV infection may be associated with delayed HIV seroconversion,[3] a child whose HCV antibody test is negative at baseline but seroconverts to positive at 4 to 6 weeks after exposure should undergo HIV follow-up testing at 3 and 6 months to rule out delayed seroconversion. Testing also is indicated if an illness consistent with acute HIV-related syndrome develops

[1] Rich JD, Dickinson BP, Carney JM, Fisher A, Heimer R. Detection of HIV-1 nucleic acid and HIV-1 antibodies in needles and syringes used for non-intravenous injection. *AIDS*. 1998;12(17):2345–2350

[2] Resnick L, Veren K, Salahuddin SZ, Tondreau S, Markham PD. Stability and inactivation of HTLV-III/LAV under clinical and laboratory environments. *JAMA*. 1986;255(14):1887–1891

[3] Terzi R, Niero F, Iemoli E, Capetti A, Coen M, Rizzardini G. Late HIV seroconversion after non-occupational postexposure prophylaxis against HIV with concomitant hepatitis C virus seroconversion. *AIDS*. 2007;21(2):262-263

before the 6-week testing and should include HIV RNA (viral load) testing and HIV antibody testing. Negative results from these initial tests support the conclusion that any subsequent positive test result likely reflects infection acquired from the needlestick. A positive initial test result in a pediatric patient requires further investigation of the cause, such as perinatal transmission, sexual abuse or activity, or drug use. An alternative option is to obtain and save a baseline serum specimen for later testing for HIV antibody or HIV PCR in the unlikely event that a subsequent test result is positive. Counseling is necessary before and after testing (see Human Immunodeficiency Virus Infection, p 459).

A local specialist in HIV infection or the CDC PEP hotline should be consulted before deciding whether to initiate PEP (PEP Hotline 888-448-4911). Antiretroviral therapy is not without risk and may or may not be associated with significant adverse effects, depending on the regimen administered (see Human Immunodeficiency Virus Infection, p 459). In the rare event that the needle user is known to be HIV positive, PEP should be started immediately. If the needle user is known and has a low risk of being HIV infected, most experts agree that PEP does not need to be administered pending test results for HIV antibody of the user.

In most situations, the needle user is not known. Data are not available on the efficacy of PEP with antiretroviral drugs in these circumstances for adults or children, and as a result, the US Public Health Service is unable to recommend for or against PEP in this circumstance.[1] PEP should be considered on a case-by-case basis, taking into consideration type of exposure and HIV prevalence in the geographic area. Some experts recommend that antiretroviral chemoprophylaxis be considered if the needle and/or syringe are available and found to contain visible blood; testing the syringe for HIV is not practical or reliable and is not recommended. If the decision to begin prophylaxis is made, any delay before starting the medications should be minimized (see Human Immunodeficiency Virus Infection, p 459). Medication should begin within 72 hours and should continue for 28 days as a combination of 3 antiretroviral drugs. The suggested medication options for children of any age will be similar for any age-appropriate antiretroviral drugs used to treat HIV-infected children (see Human Immunodeficiency Virus Infection, p 459).

HEPATITIS C VIRUS

The third bloodborne pathogen of concern is HCV, which can survive in the environment for 16 to 23 hours. The prevalence of chronic HCV infection in the United States varies by race/ethnicity, age group, geographic location, and individual history of risk behaviors. Although transmission by sharing syringes among injection drug users is efficient, the risk of transmission from a discarded syringe is likely to be low. Testing for HCV is not recommended routinely in the absence of a risk factor for infection or a known exposure to a HCV-positive source. If performed, antibody to HCV can be detected in 80% of newly infected patients within 15 weeks after exposure and in 97% of newly infected patients by 6 months after exposure. If earlier diagnosis is desired, testing for HCV RNA may be performed at 4 to 6 weeks after exposure. Positive test results should be confirmed by supplemental confirmatory laboratory tests, but a negative test

---

[1]Centers for Disease Control and Prevention. Antiretroviral postexposure prophylaxis after sexual injection-drug-use, or other nonoccupational exposure to HIV in the United States: recommendations from the US Department of Health and Human Services. *MMWR Recomm Rep.* 2005;54(RR-2):1–20

result should be followed with additional serologic testing in subsequent weeks (see Hepatitis C, p 428). There is no recommended PEP for HCV using antiviral drugs or Immune Globulin preparations, because any HCV antibody-positive donor is excluded from the pool from which Immune Globulin products are prepared.

Preventing Needlestick Injuries

Needlestick injuries of both children and adults can be minimized by implementing public health programs on safe needle disposal and programs for exchange of used syringes and needles from injection drug users for sterile needles. Syringe and needle exchanges decrease both improper needle disposal and spread of bloodborne pathogens without increasing the rate of injection drug use. The American Academy of Pediatrics supports needle-exchange programs in conjunction with drug treatment and within the context of continuing research to assess their effectiveness. In addition, children should be educated to avoid playing in areas known to be frequented by injecting drug users and to avoid playing with discarded needles and syringes.

....
BITE WOUNDS

As many as 1% of all pediatric visits to emergency departments during summer months are for treatment of human or animal bite wounds. An estimated 5 million bites occur annually in the United States; dog bites account for approximately 90% of those wounds. The rate of infection after cat bites is as high as 50%; rates of infection after dog or human bites are 5% to 15%. Although postinjury rates of infection can be minimized through early administration of proper wound care principles, the bites of humans, wild animals, or nontraditional pets are potential sources of serious morbidity. Parents should teach children to avoid contact with wild animals and secure garbage containers so that raccoons and other animals will not be attracted to the home and places where children play. Nontraditional pets, including ferrets, iguanas and other reptiles, and wild animals also pose an infection as well as an injury risk for children, and their ownership should be discouraged in households with young children. Health care professionals should be knowledgeable about and offer counseling to parents whose children will have wild animal contact at petting zoos and exotic animal summer camps. Potential transmission of rabies is increased when a bite is from a wild animal (especially a bat or a carnivore) or from a domestic animal with uncertain immunization status that cannot be captured for adequate quarantine (see Rabies, p 673). Dead animals should be avoided, because they can be infested with arthropods (fleas or ticks) infected with a variety of bacterial, rickettsial, protozoan, or viral agents. Saliva from recently deceased mammals infected with rabies can contain active rabies virus, which can be transmitted via physical contact with the virus-containing saliva.

Recommendations for bite wound management are provided in Table 2.11 (p 190). Current guidelines from the Infectious Diseases Society of America (IDSA) state that primary wound closure is not recommended for animal bite wounds, with the exception

Table 2.11. Management of Human or Animal Bite Wounds

Category of Management	Management
Cleansing	Remove visible foreign material. Cleanse the wound surface with clean water or saline. Cleansers such as 1% povidone–iodine or 1% benzalkonium chloride can be used for particularly soiled wounds. Irrigate open wounds with a copious volume of sterile water or saline solution by moderate-pressure irrigation.[a] Avoid blind high-pressure irrigation of puncture wounds. Standard Precautions should be used.
Wound culture	No, for fresh wounds,[b] unless signs of infection exist. Yes, for wounds that appear infected.[c]
Diagnostic imaging	Indicated for penetrating injuries overlying bones or joints, for suspected fracture, or to assess foreign body inoculation.
Débridement	Remove superficial devitalized tissue and foreign material.
Operative débridement and exploration	Yes, if any of the following: • Extensive wounds with devitalized tissue or mechanical dysfunction. • Penetration of joints (eg, clenched fist injury) or cranium. • Plastic or other repairs requiring general anesthesia.
Assess mechanical function	Assess and address mechanical function of injured structures.
Wound closure	Yes, for selected fresh,[b] nonpuncture bite wounds (see text).
Assess tetanus immunization status[d]	Yes, for all wounds.
Assess risk of rabies	Yes, if bite by any rabies-prone, unobservable wild or domestic animal with unknown immunization status.[e]
Assess risk of hepatitis B virus infection	Yes, for human bite wounds.[f]
Assess risk of human immunodeficiency virus	Yes, for human bite wounds.[g]
Initiate antimicrobial therapy[h]	Yes, for: • Moderate or severe bite wounds, especially if edema or crush injury is present. • Puncture wounds, especially if penetration of bone, tendon sheath, or joint has occurred. • Deep or surgically closed facial bite wounds.

Table 2.11. Management of Human or Animal Bite Wounds, continued

Category of Management	Management
	• Hand and foot bite wounds. • Genital area bite wounds. • Wounds in immunocompromised and asplenic people. • Wounds with signs of infection. • Cat bite wounds.
Follow-up	Inspect wound for signs of infection within 48 hours.

[a]Use of an 18-gauge needle with a large-volume syringe is effective. Antimicrobial or anti-infective solutions offer no advantage and may increase tissue irritation.
[b]Wounds less than 12 hours old.
[c]Both aerobic and anaerobic bacterial culture should be performed.
[d]See Tetanus, p 793.
[e]See Rabies, p 673.
[f]See Hepatitis B, p 401.
[g]See Human Immunodeficiency Virus Infection, p 459.
[h]See Table 2.12 (p 192) for suggested drug choices.

of those to the face, which should be managed with copious irrigation, cautious débridement, and preemptive antibiotics; other wounds may be approximated.[1] Bite wounds on the face carry a relatively low rate of secondary infection, perhaps because of the generous vascular supply to the area or because these wounds likely receive prompt medical attention; an exception is an injury that causes crushed tissue. The IDSA guidelines note that the anecdotal reports of infection following primary closure on regions other than the face have major limitations including lack of a control group and their anecdotal nature and lack of standardization of the type, severity, and location of the wound and circumstances surrounding the injury. In addition, thorough wound cleansing before surgical closure has brought the rate of secondary infection of these wounds to well below 10%, no matter the species of animal that inflicted the wound. These factors combine to suggest that, following thoughtful deliberation, primary closure of nonfacial wounds can be considered in some cases. Approximation of margins and closure by delayed primary or secondary intention is prudent for infected non-facial wounds. When surgical closures are required, they can be performed at the time of initial management (primary) or delayed until the patient has received a brief course of antibiotic therapy (delayed primary closure). High-pressure irrigation is conjectured to possibly drive infectious agents into deeper tissue locations and should be avoided. Use of local anesthesia can facilitate cleansing and surgical repair. Sedation can be helpful in certain circumstances. Smaller, cosmetically unimportant wounds can be cleansed and allowed to heal by secondary intention. Hand and foot wounds have a higher risk of infection. This is especially true of deeper wounds that penetrate multiple tissue planes and are more difficult to clean effectively. More-complicated injuries should be managed

---

[1]Stevens DL, Bisno AL, Chambers HF, et al. Practice guidelines for the diagnosis and management of skin and soft tissue infections: 2014 update by the Infectious Diseases Society of America. *Clin Infect Dis.* 2014;59(2):e10–e52

Table 2.12. Antimicrobial Agents for Human or Animal Bite Wounds

Source of Bite[g]	Organism(s) Likely to Cause Infection	Antimicrobial Agent			
		Oral Route	Oral Alternatives for Penicillin-Allergic Patients[a]	Intravenous Route[b,c]	Intravenous Alternatives for Penicillin-Allergic Patients[a,b,c]
Dog, cat, or mammal[d]	*Pasteurella* species, *Staphylococcus aureus*, streptococci, anaerobes, *Capnocytophaga* species, *Moraxella* species, *Corynebacterium* species, *Neisseria* species	Amoxicillin-clavulanate	Extended-spectrum cephalosporin or trimethoprim-sulfamethoxazole[e] **PLUS** Clindamycin	Ampicillin-sulbactam[f]	Extended-spectrum cephalosporin or trimethoprim-sulfamethoxazole **PLUS** Clindamycin **OR** Carbapenem
Reptile[g]	Enteric gram-negative bacteria, anaerobes	Amoxicillin-clavulanate	Extended-spectrum cephalosporin or trimethoprim-sulfamethoxazole[e] **PLUS** Clindamycin	Ampicillin-sulbactam[f] **PLUS** Gentamicin	Clindamycin **PLUS** Extended spectrum cephalosporin or gentamicin or aztreonam or quinolone **OR** Carbapenem

Table 2.12. Antimicrobial Agents for Human or Animal Bite Wounds, continued

Source of Bite	Organism(s) Likely to Cause Infection	Antimicrobial Agent			
		Oral Route	Oral Alternatives for Penicillin-Allergic Patients[a]	Intravenous Route[b,c]	Intravenous Alternatives for Penicillin-Allergic Patients[a,b,c]
Human	Streptococci, S aureus, Eikenella corrodens, Haemophilus species, anaerobes	Amoxicillin-clavulanate	Extended-spectrum cephalosporin or trimethoprim-sulfamethoxazole[e] **PLUS** Clindamycin	Ampicillin-sulbactam[f]	Extended spectrum cephalosporin or trimethoprim-sulfamethoxazole **PLUS** Clindamycin **OR** Carbapenem

[a]For patients with history of allergy to penicillin or one of its congeners, alternative drugs are recommended. In patients without a history of anaphylaxis, wheezing, angioedema, or urticaria, an extended-spectrum cephalosporin or other beta-lactam–class drug may be acceptable. For example, cefriaxone, rather than trimethoprim-sulfamethoxazole, could be used intravenously.

[b]Coverage for methicillin-resistant S aureus with vancomycin should be considered for severe bite wounds.

[c]Note that use of ampicillin-sulbactam or carbapenem monotherapy will not include activity against methicillin-resistant S aureus isolates.

[d]Data are lacking to guide antimicrobial use for bites that are not overtly infected from small mammals, such as guinea pigs and hamsters.

[e]Doxycycline is alternative coverage for Pasteurella multocida.

[f]Piperacillin-tazobactam can be used as an alternative.

[g]The role of empirical antimicrobial use for noninfected snake bite wounds is not well-defined. Therapy should be chosen on the basis of results of cultures from infected wounds.

in consultation with an appropriate surgical specialist. To minimize risk of infection, bite wounds should not be sealed with a tissue adhesive, no matter their age or appearance. Elevation of injured areas to minimize swelling will enhance wound healing.

Published evidence indicates that most infected mammalian bite wounds are polymicrobial in nature, often involving a mixture of mouth flora from the biting animal and, likely, skin flora from the victim. Specimens for both aerobic and anaerobic culture should be obtained from wounds that appear infected. Limited data exist to guide short-term antimicrobial therapy for patients with wounds that do not appear infected. Preemptive early antimicrobial therapy for 3 to 5 days is recommended for patients who (a) are immunocompromised; (b) are asplenic; (c) have advanced liver disease; (d) have preexisting or resultant edema of the affected area; (e) have moderate to severe injuries, especially to the hand or face; or (f) have injuries that may have penetrated the periosteum or joint capsule.[1]

It takes at least 12 hours for signs of infection to manifest clinically. Patients with mild injuries in which the skin is abraded do not need to be treated with antimicrobial agents. For those injuries, cleansing is sufficient.

Guidelines for initial choice of antimicrobial therapy for human and animal bites are provided in Table 2.12 (p 192). In the child with a confirmed bite wound-associated infection, initial therapy should be modified when culture results become available. Methicillin-resistant *Staphylococcus aureus* (MRSA) is a potential but uncommon bite wound pathogen; empiric therapy may require modification if MRSA is isolated from an infected wound (see *Staphylococcus aureus*, p 733). Coverage for MRSA should be considered in severe bite wound infections while cultures are pending. Likewise, MRSA should be considered in a fresh or otherwise uninfected-appearing wound of a patient known to be colonized with that agent.

The treatment of choice following most bite wounds for which therapy is provided is amoxicillin-clavulanic acid (Table 2.12, p 192). For a child with a serious allergy to penicillin, oral or parenteral treatment with trimethoprim-sulfamethoxazole, which is effective against *S aureus* (including MRSA), *Pasteurella multocida*, and *Eikenella corrodens*, in conjunction with clindamycin, which is active in vitro against anaerobic bacteria, streptococci, and many strains of *S aureus*, may be effective for preventing or treating bite wound infections. Extended-spectrum cephalosporins, such as cefotaxime or ceftriaxone parenterally or cefpodoxime orally, do not have good anaerobic activity but can be used in conjunction with clindamycin as alternative therapy for penicillin-allergic patients who can tolerate cephalosporins. Doxycycline is an alternative agent that has activity against *P multocida*, and can be used for short durations (ie, 21 days or less) without regard to patient age (see Antimicrobial Agents and Related Therapy, p 903). Azithromycin and fluoroquinolones display good in vitro activity against organisms that commonly cause bite wound infections, but clinical trial data are lacking, and fluoroquinolones are not approved for this indication in children. Carbapenems are an option for children with penicillin allergy, but cross-reactions with penicillins can occur infrequently. If a carbapenem is used as monotherapy, it should be noted that carbapenems do not have activity against MRSA. A 5-day course usually is sufficient for soft tissue infections.

---

[1]Stevens DL, Bisno AL, Chambers HF, et al. Practice guidelines for the diagnosis and management of skin and soft tissue infections: 2014 update by the Infectious Diseases Society of America. *Clin Infect Dis*. 2014;59(2):e10–e52

Longer courses of treatment may be indicated, depending on severity of infection, feasibility of draining abscesses if they occur, and patient's clinical responses. The duration of treatment for bite wound-associated bone infections is based on location, severity, and pathogens isolated.

PREVENTION OF MOSQUITOBORNE AND TICKBORNE INFECTIONS

Mosquitoborne infectious diseases in the United States are caused by arboviruses (eg, West Nile, La Crosse, Jamestown Canyon, St. Louis encephalitis, eastern equine encephalitis, and western equine encephalitis viruses [see Arboviruses, p 220]). Local transmission of other mosquitoborne viruses (eg, dengue, chikungunya, and Zika viruses) also occurs in US territories (eg, Puerto Rico, US Virgin Islands, American Samoa) and occasionally in the states. International travelers may encounter similar or different arboviruses (eg, yellow fever, dengue, chikungunya, Japanese encephalitis, or Zika virus) or other mosquitoborne infections (eg, malaria) during travel (also see disease-specific chapters in Section 3).

Tickborne infectious diseases in the United States include diseases caused by spirochetes, rickettsiae, other bacteria, protozoa, and viruses. Different species of ticks transmit different infectious agents. *Dermacentor variabilis* (American dog tick), *Dermacentor andersoni* (Rocky Mountain wood tick), and *Rhipicephalus sanguineus* (Brown dog tick) are the primary vectors of *Rickettsia rickettsii* (Rocky Mountain spotted fever). *Dermacentor andersoni* also transmits Colorado tick fever virus. *Ixodes scapularis* (deer or blacklegged tick) and *Ixodes pacificus* (western blacklegged tick) transmit *Borrelia burgdorferi* (Lyme disease) and *Anaplasma phagocytophilum* (anaplasmosis). *Ixodes* ticks also transmit *Babesia microti* (babesiosis), *Borrelia miyamotoi*, *Borrelia mayonii*, *Ehrlichia muris eauclairensis*, and Powassan virus. *Amblyomma americanum* (lone star tick) transmits *Ehrlichia chaffeensis*, *Ehrlichia ewingii*, Heartland virus, and southern tick-associated rash illness (STARI). *Francisella tularensis* (tularemia) can be transmitted by *Dermacentor andersoni*, *Dermacentor variabilis*, or *Amblyomma americanum*. Soft-bodied ticks (*Ornithodoros* species) transmit *Borrelia hermsii* and other causes of tickborne relapsing fever.

Travel health practitioners should advise travelers to use repellents and other general protective measures against biting arthropods (eg, mosquitoes and ticks). In addition, vaccines or chemoprophylactic drugs are available to protect against some vectorborne diseases such as yellow fever, Japanese encephalitis, and malaria. The effectiveness of malaria chemoprophylaxis is variable, depending on patterns of drug resistance, bioavailability, and compliance with medication. No similar chemoprophylactic agents are approved in the United States for other mosquitoborne or tickborne diseases. Prevention of infection in these instances depends on avoiding known foci of disease, reducing arthropod habitats, using personal protective measures, and for ticks, limiting the time of attachment to the skin. In areas with vector transmission, protection of children is recommended during outdoor activities, including activities related to school, child care, or camping. Education of families and other caregivers is an important component of prevention.

General Protective Measures

Avoiding exposure to mosquitoes and ticks and avoiding areas with outbreaks of mosquitoborne infections are the first steps in protection. Physicians should be aware of the burden of arthropod-related infections in their local areas. Travelers, to the extent possible, should avoid known foci of disease transmission. The Centers for Disease Control and Prevention (CDC) Travelers' Health Web site provides updates on regional disease transmission patterns and outbreaks (**wwwnc.cdc.gov/travel/**).

The following measures should be taken to reduce exposures to vectorborne diseases:

- **Eliminate local mosquito breeding sites.** Mosquitoes develop in standing water, and large numbers of mosquitoes can arise from sources at or near the home. Measures to limit mosquito breeding sites around the home include drainage or removal of receptacles for standing water (eg, tires, toys, flower pots, cans, buckets, barrels, other containers that collect rain water); keeping swimming pools, decorative pools, children's wading pools, and bird baths clean; and clearing clogged rain gutters. Under certain circumstances, large-scale mosquito-control measures may be conducted by community or public health officials. These efforts include drainage of standing water, use of larvicides in waters that are sources of mosquitoes, and use of adulticides to control biting adult mosquitoes.

- **Reduce exposure to mosquitoes**. Although mosquitoes may bite at any time, limiting outdoor activities at times of peak mosquito biting activity can help reduce exposure. Peak biting activities for vectors of some diseases (such as West Nile) are during the evening and nighttime. For others (such as malaria), peak times are during dawn and dusk or in the evening after dark, and for others (such as dengue, chikungunya, and Zika), peak time is during the day (from dawn through dusk). Bed nets, screens, and nets tucked around strollers and other confined spaces where young children are placed are important barriers against mosquitoes. Mosquito traps, electrocutors (bug zappers), ultrasonic repellers, and other devices marketed to prevent mosquitoes from biting people are not effective and should not be relied on to reduce mosquito bites.

- **Reduce exposure to ticks.** Although outdoor activity should be encouraged for general wellness, tick-infested areas should be avoided whenever possible (eg, by hiking in the center of trails). Certain ticks prefer dense woods with thick growth of shrubs and small trees. Others are found along the edges of the woods, where the woods abut lawns or fields. Other species may be located in grassy areas. Importantly, the residential backyard is a primary environment where people in the Northeast are bitten by ticks that transmit *B burgdorferi* (Lyme disease). All ticks require humidity to survive, and drier areas usually are less infested. For homes located in tick-prone areas, risk of exposure can be reduced by locating play equipment in sunny, dry areas away from forest edges, by creating a barrier of dry wood chips or gravel between recreation areas and forest, by regular mowing of vegetation, and by keeping leaves raked and underbrush cleared. The brown dog tick can survive in more arid environments and can be introduced indoors. This species may be found in cracks and crevices of housing; on walls, carpet, and furniture; or in animal housing or bedding. Control of tick populations in the wider environment often is not practical but can be effective in more defined areas, such as around places where children reside or play. Using acaricides (pesticides targeting ticks) on a property or pets can reduce tick populations and possibly the risk of tickborne disease.

- **Wear appropriate protective clothing.** Whenever possible when entering mosquito or tick habitats, clothing should be worn that covers the arms, legs, head, and other exposed skin areas. Tucking in shirts, tucking pants into socks, and wearing closed shoes instead of sandals may reduce risks.

- **Consider treatment of clothing and gear.** Permethrin (a synthetic pyrethroid) is both a pesticide and a repellent that can be sprayed onto clothes and gear. Permethrin repels both mosquitoes and ticks. Permethrin should not be sprayed directly onto skin, and treated clothing should be dried before wearing. The US Environmental Protection Agency (EPA) has approved commercial sale of permethrin-treated outdoor clothing, hats, bed nets, and camping gear, which is safe for children of all ages and for pregnant women. Purchased permethrin-treated clothing remains effective through multiple launderings. Permethrin or repellents should not be used on clothing or mosquito nets where children may chew or suck.

Repellents for Use on Skin

The EPA regulates repellent products in the United States. The CDC, US Food and Drug Administration (FDA), and American Academy of Pediatrics (AAP) recommend that people use repellent products that have been registered by the EPA. EPA registration indicates that the materials have been reviewed for both efficacy and human safety when applied according to the instructions on the label. The EPA is allowing companies to apply for permission to include the new repellency awareness graphic on product labels of skin-applied insect repellents (see Fig 2.2). This graphic is intended to help consumers easily identify the repellency time for mosquitos and ticks.

Arthropods are attracted to people by odors on the skin and by carbon dioxide and other volatile chemicals from the breath. The active ingredients in repellents make the user unattractive for feeding, but they do not kill the mosquito or tick. Repellents should be used during outdoor activities when mosquitoes or ticks are present, and should always be used according to the label instructions. Protection times listed below generally are against mosquitoes. Protection times vary against mosquitoes versus ticks (generally being shorter against ticks) and by type and concentration of active ingredient, product formulation, ambient temperatures, and personal activity (eg, protection time is reduced by perspiration, washing of skin, and involvement in water recreation). Product labels should be followed for application and reapplication. Repellent should not be reapplied more frequently than recommended on the label. Web-based guidelines are available from the EPA (**www.epa.gov/insect-repellents/find-insect-repellent-right-you**).

EPA-REGISTERED REPELLENTS

The CDC has evaluated information published in peer-reviewed scientific literature and data available from the EPA to identify several types of EPA-registered products that provide repellent activity sufficient to help people reduce the bites of disease-carrying mosquitoes and ticks (**wwwnc.cdc.gov/travel/yellowbook/2016/the-pre-travel-consultation/protection-against-mosquitoes-ticks-other-arthropods**). Products containing the following active ingredients typically provide reasonably long-lasting protection:

FIG 2.2. EXAMPLE OF A REPELLENCY AWARENESS GRAPHIC.

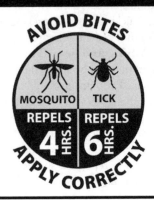

DEET. Chemical name: N,N-diethyl-meta-toluamide or N,N-diethyl-3-methyl-benzamide. Commercial products registered for direct application to human skin contain from 4% to 99.9% DEET. DEET repels both mosquitoes and ticks. The CDC recommends using products with ≥20% DEET on exposed skin. Use of products with the lowest effective DEET concentrations (ie, between 20% and 30%) seems most prudent for infants and young children, for whom it should be applied sparingly. In general, higher concentrations of active ingredient provide longer duration of protection. Protection times for DEET against mosquitoes range from 1 to 2 hours for products containing 5% concentrations (which may not protect against ticks) to 10 hours or more for products containing 40% or more DEET. There does not appear to be a meaningful increase in protection time for products containing >50% DEET. A DEET concentration of approximately 24% provides an average of 5 hours of protection. Time-released DEET formulations are available that provide 11 to 12 hours of protection with concentrations of 20% to 30% DEET.

If used appropriately, DEET does not present a health problem. Adverse effects related to DEET are rare; most often are associated with ingestions, chronic use, or excessive use; and do not appear to be related to DEET concentration used. Urticaria and contact dermatitis have been reported in a small number of people. Although rare, adverse systemic effects including encephalopathy have been reported after excessive skin application in children and after unintentional ingestion. DEET is irritating to eyes and mucous membranes. Highly concentrated formulations can damage plastic and certain fabrics.

PICARIDIN (KBR 3023). Chemical name: 2-(2-hydroxyethyl)-1-piperidinecarboxylic acid 1-methylpropyl ester. Picaridin has concentration-related efficacy and ages for use similar to DEET. Products containing 5% picaridin provide 3 to 4 hours of protection, and products with 20% picaridin can provide protection for 8 to 12 hours. Although experience is less extensive than with DEET, no serious toxicity has been reported. Picaridin-containing compounds have been used as repellents for 2 decades in Europe and Australia as a 20% formulation with no serious toxicity reported.

OIL OF LEMON EUCALYPTUS OR PMD. Para-menthane-3,8-diol (PMD) is the chemical name for the synthesized version of oil of lemon eucalyptus (OLE). Recommended use is only for EPA-registered repellent products containing the active ingredient OLE or PMD. These products are not recommended for skin application on children younger than 3 years. Products with 8% to 10% PMD protect for up to 2 hours, and products containing 30% to 40% OLE provide 6 hours of protection. The plant-based products generally do not provide protection times as long as synthetic products. "Pure" oil of lemon eucalyptus (essential oil not formulated as a repellent) is not recommended; it has not undergone similar validated testing for safety and efficacy and is not registered with the EPA as an insect repellent.

IR3535. Chemical name: 3-(N-butyl-N-acetyl)-aminopropionic acid, ethyl ester. IR3535 is available in formulations ranging from 7.5% to 20%, with estimated protection times ranging from 2 hours for the lower concentrations to up to 10 hours with the higher concentrations.

2-UNDECANONE. Chemical name: methyl nonyl ketone. 2-undecanone is a synthetic version of a molecule extracted from oil of rue or wild grown tomatoes. It contains 7.75% active ingredient and provides an estimated protection time of up to 5 hours for mosquitoes and up to 2 hours for ticks.

NONREGISTERED PRODUCTS

Products based on citronella, catnip oil, and other essential plant oils provide minimal protection and are not recommended. Ingestion of garlic or vitamin B_1, wearing devices that emit sounds, and impregnated wristbands are ineffective measures.

APPLICATION OF REPELLENTS

The following are recommended precautions for use of repellents:

- Apply repellents only to exposed skin or clothing, as directed on the product label. Do not apply repellents under clothing.
- Never use repellents over cuts, wounds, or irritated skin.
- When using sprays, do not spray directly on face – spray on hands first and then apply to face. Do not apply repellents to eyes or mouth, and apply sparingly around ears.
- Children should not handle repellents. Adults should apply repellents to their own hands first, and then gently spread on the child's exposed skin. Adults should avoid applying directly to children's hands, because children frequently put fingers and hands into their mouths.
- Use just enough repellent to cover exposed skin or clothing.
- Sprays should not be used in enclosed areas or near food.
- Hands should be washed after application to avoid accidental exposure to eyes or ingestion.

REPELLENTS AND SUNSCREEN. Repellents that are applied according to label instructions may be used with sunscreen with no reduction in repellent activity; however, limited data show a one-third decrease in the sun protection factor (SPF) of sunscreens when DEET-containing insect repellents are used after a sunscreen is applied. Products that combine sunscreen and repellent are not recommended, because sunscreen may need to be reapplied more often and in larger amounts than are needed for the repellent component. In general, it is recommended to apply sunscreen first and then apply the repellent. It may be necessary to reapply sunscreen more frequently.

Tick Inspection and Removal

Parents or caregivers should inspect, in a timely manner, themselves and their children's bodies, clothing, and equipment used both during and after possible tick exposure (known as a "tick check"). When conducting tick checks, special attention should be given to the exposed regions of the body where ticks often attach, including the head, neck, and behind the ears. Ticks also may attach at areas of tight clothing (eg, sock line, belt line, axillae, groin). Several hours might elapse before ticks attach and transmit pathogens; therefore, timely tick checks increase the likelihood of finding and removing ticks before they can transmit an infectious agent. Removing a tick as soon as possible is critical, because longer periods of attachment considerably increase the probability of transmission of tickborne pathogens. As soon as possible after potential tick exposure, it is important to remove clothes, because they may still harbor crawling ticks. Bathing or showering after coming indoors (preferably within 2 hours) can be an effective method of locating attached or crawling ticks and has been shown to be an important personal protective measure for several tickborne diseases. Unattached ticks can enter the home by hiding in or on clothing. Placing dry clothing in a dryer on high heat for at least 10 min (damp clothes can take up to 1 hour) to remove humidity has been used effectively to kill unattached ticks on clothes.

TICK REMOVAL. Ticks should be removed from skin as soon as they are discovered. For removal, it is most important to grasp the tick close to the skin. Fine-tipped forceps or tweezers are recommended; grasp close to the skin and gently pull straight out without twisting motions. Care must be taken not to break mouthparts as the tick is removed. Tweezers should be cleaned of any potential tick body tissue or fluids that may have been left after pulling on the attached tick. Tweezers then can be used to remove mouthparts or cement left on the skin. Methods such as cutting or digging to remove small remnants should be avoided. If fingers are used to remove ticks, they should be protected with a barrier, such as tissue or plastic gloves, and washed after removal of the tick. The bite site should be washed with soap and water to reduce the risk of secondary skin infections.

TESTING TICKS. Testing ticks removed from animals or humans for infectious pathogens is discouraged, as it is not diagnostically informative and may be expensive.

Other Preventive Measures

PETS. Maintaining tick-free pets also will decrease tick exposure in and around the home. Daily inspection of pets and removal of ticks are indicated, as is the routine use of appropriate veterinary products to prevent ticks on pets. Consult a veterinarian for information on suitable effective products. Products must be applied as instructed so that maximal effect can be achieved. Compliance is key for owner-applied products.

CHEMOPROPHYLAXIS. Chemoprophylaxis to prevent Lyme disease may be considered under certain circumstances and certain age groups in areas with highly endemic Lyme disease (see Lyme Disease, p 515); however, chemoprophylaxis is not recommended for other tickborne diseases, including rickettsiae.

PREVENTION OF ILLNESSES ASSOCIATED WITH RECREATIONAL WATER USE

Pathogen transmission via recreational water (eg, swimming pools, water playgrounds, lakes, oceans) is an increasingly recognized source of illness in the United States. Since the mid-1980s, the number of outbreaks associated with recreational water activities—particularly treated aquatic venues (eg, swimming pools)—has increased significantly.[1] Therefore, preventing recreational water–associated illness (RWI) and promoting healthy swimming is becoming increasingly important for children and adults. RWIs are caused by infectious pathogens transmitted by ingesting, inhaling aerosols of, or having contact with contaminated water from swimming pools, water playgrounds, hot tubs/spas, lakes, rivers, or oceans. RWIs also can be caused by chemicals in the water or chemicals that volatilize from the water and cause indoor air quality problems. Illnesses associated with recreational water can involve the gastrointestinal tract, respiratory tract, central nervous system, skin, ears, or eyes. In 2011–2012, 90 outbreaks of RWIs were reported to the Centers for Disease Control and Prevention (CDC).[1] These outbreaks resulted in at least 1788 cases of illness, 95 hospitalizations, and 1 death. Among 69 (77%) outbreaks associated with treated aquatic venues, 36 (52%) were associated with *Cryptosporidium* species. Cryptosporidiosis can cause life-threatening infection in immunocompromised children and adolescents (see Cryptosporidiosis, p 304). Among 21 (23%) outbreaks associated with untreated recreational water venues (eg, lakes), 7 (33%) were caused by *Escherichia coli* O157:H7 or *E coli* O111.

Swimming is a communal bathing activity by which the same water is shared by a few individuals to thousands of people each day, depending on venue size (eg, from inflatable or plastic kiddie pools to pools in water parks). Fecal contamination of recreational water venues is a common occurrence because of the high prevalence of diarrhea and fecal incontinence (particularly in young children) and the presence of residual fecal material on bodies of swimmers (up to 10 g on young children). Recreational water–associated outbreaks tend to affect children younger than 5 years, usually occur during the summer months, and typically manifest as gastroenteritis.

To protect swimmers from infectious pathogens, water in public treated aquatic venues is chlorinated. Maintaining pH and disinfectant concentration as recommended by the CDC[2] is sufficient to inactivate most infectious pathogens within minutes; however, some infectious pathogens are moderately to highly tolerant of halogen (chlorine or bromine) and can survive for extended periods of time, even in properly chlorinated pools. *Giardia intestinalis* has been shown to survive for up to 45 minutes and is documented to be a leading cause of recreational water-associated outbreaks. *Cryptosporidium* oocysts can survive for 7 to more than 10 days, thus contributing to the role of *Cryptosporidium* species as the leading cause of recreational water–associated

---

[1]Hlavsa MC, Roberts VA, Kahler AM, et al. Outbreaks of illness associated with recreational water—United States, 2011–2012. *MMWR Morb Mortal Wkly Rep.* 2015;64(24):668-672. Available at: **www.cdc.gov/mmwr/pdf/wk/mm6424.pdf**

[2]CDC recommends pH 7.2–7.8. The free chlorine concentration should be at least 1 ppm in pools and water playgrounds. The free bromine concentration should be at least 3 ppm in pools and water playgrounds.

outbreaks. Additional water treatments (eg, ultraviolet light, ozone, or filtration) can more efficiently inactivate *Cryptosporidium* oocysts.

Recreational water use is an ideal means for *Cryptosporidium* transmission to be amplified within a community because of the organism's extreme chlorine tolerance, low infectious dose, and high pathogen excretion concentration in addition to poor swimmer hygiene (eg, swimming when ill with diarrhea and ingesting recreational water). One or more swimmers who are ill with diarrhea can contaminate large volumes of water and expose large numbers of swimmers to *Cryptosporidium* and other pathogens, particularly if pool disinfection is inadequate. Outbreaks associated with treated aquatic venues generally can be prevented and controlled through a combination of proper pH, adequate disinfectant concentration, and improved swimmer hygiene and behavior.

CONTROL MEASURES

Swimming continues to be a safe and effective means of physical activity. Transmission of infectious pathogens that cause RWIs can be prevented by reducing contamination of swimming venues and exposure to contaminated water. Pediatricians should counsel families as follows:

- Regularly test home pools to ensure that the water's pH and free chlorine or bromine concentration are correct and safe:
    - pH should be 7.2–7.8.
    - Free chlorine concentration should be at least 1 ppm.
    - Free bromine concentration should be at least 3 ppm.
- Do not go into recreational water (eg, swim) when ill with diarrhea.
    - After cessation of symptoms, people who had diarrhea attributable to *Cryptosporidium* species also should avoid recreational water activities for an additional 2 weeks. This is because of prolonged excretion of infectious *Cryptosporidium* oocysts after cessation of symptoms, the potential for intermittent exacerbations of diarrhea, and the increased transmission potential in treated aquatic venues (eg, swimming pools) because of the organism's high chlorine tolerance.
    - After cessation of symptoms, children who had diarrhea attributable to other potential waterborne pathogens (eg, *Shigella* species) and who are incontinent should avoid recreational water activities for 1 additional week.
- Do not go into recreational water (eg, swim) with open wounds (eg, from surgery or a piercing), because these can serve as portals of entry for pathogens.
- Avoid ingestion of recreational water.
- Practice good swimmer hygiene by:
    - Showering with soap and water for at least 1 minute before entering recreational water, with particular focus on cleansing the perianal area of children.
    - Instructing children not to urinate or stool in the water.
    - Taking children to the bathroom every hour.
    - Checking diapered children every 30 to 60 minutes and changing them in a bathroom or diaper changing area—not poolside—to keep infectious agents away from the water. Swim diapers and swim pants, although able to hold in some solid feces, do not prevent leakage of pathogens such as *Cryptosporidium* species into the water.

♦ Washing hands with soap and water after using the bathroom, changing diapers, or before consumption of food and drink.

Free Healthy Swimming brochures, in English and Spanish, are available at **wwwn. cdc.gov/pubs/cdcInfoOnDemand.aspx?ProgramID=93.** More information on healthy swimming and inflatable and plastic kiddie pools is available at **http://www. cdc.gov/healthywater/swimming/swimmers/inflatable-plastic-pools. html.**

"SWIMMER'S EAR"/ACUTE OTITIS EXTERNA

Participation in recreational water activities can predispose children to infections of the external auditory canal. Acute otitis externa (AOE) or "swimmer's ear" is diffuse inflammation of the external auditory canal and usually is attributable to bacterial infection. Recreational water activities, showering, and bathing can introduce water into the ear canal, wash away protective ear wax, and cause maceration of the thin skin of the ear canal, thus predisposing the ear canal to bacterial infection. AOE is most common among children 5 to 14 years of age but can occur in all age groups, including adults. A marked seasonality is observed, with cases peaking during the summer months. Warm, humid environments and frequent submersion of the head while swimming are risk factors for AOE.

The 2 bacteria that most commonly cause AOE are *Pseudomonas aeruginosa* and *Staphylococcus aureus*. Many cases are polymicrobial. *Aspergillus* species and *Candida* species have been isolated rarely in AOE. Cultures of swab specimens taken from the external ear canal in AOE may not be entirely diagnostic, as these can reflect normal ear canal flora or pathogenic organisms.

AOE readily responds to treatment with topical antimicrobial agents with or without a topical steroid. Unless the infection has spread to surrounding tissues or the patient has complicating factors (eg, diabetes or immunocompromise), topical treatment alone should be sufficient, and systemic antimicrobials usually are not required. Polymyxin B sulfate/neomycin sulfate, gentamicin sulfate, and ciprofloxacin for 7 to 10 days are topical antibiotic agents used commonly. If clinical improvement is not noted by 48 to 72 hours, the patient should be reevaluated for possible foreign body obstruction of the canal, noncompliance with therapy, or alternate diagnoses, such as contact dermatitis or traumatic cellulitis. If delivery of topical antibiotics is being impeded by drainage obstructing the external auditory canal, placement of a cellulose wick or referral to an otolaryngologist for aural toilet should be considered. Topical agents that have the potential for ototoxicity (eg, gentamicin, neomycin, agents with a low pH, hydrocortisone-neomycin-polymyxin) should not be used in children with tympanostomy tubes or a perforated tympanic membrane. Patients with AOE should avoid submerging their head in water for 7 to 10 days, but competitive swimmers might be able to return to the pool if pain has resolved and they use well-fitting ear plugs.

All swimmers should be instructed to keep their ear canals as dry as possible. This can be accomplished by covering the opening of the external auditory canal with a bathing cap or by using ear plugs or molds. Following swimming or showering, the ears should be dried thoroughly.

If a person experiences recurring episodes of AOE, consideration can be given to use of antimicrobial otic drops after recreational water exposure as an additional preventive measure. Commercial ear-drying agents are available for use as directed, or a 1:1 mixture of acetic acid (white vinegar) and isopropanol (rubbing alcohol) may be placed in the external ear canal after swimming or showering to restore the proper acidic pH to the ear canal and to dry residual water. Otic drying agents should not be used in the presence of tympanostomy tubes, tympanic membrane perforation, AOE infection, or ear drainage.

Additional information on prevention of otitis externa is available at **www.cdc.gov/healthywater/swimming/swimmers/rwi/ear-infections.html.**

Summaries of Infectious Diseases

Actinomycosis

CLINICAL MANIFESTATIONS: Actinomycosis results from pathogen introduction following a breakdown in mucocutaneous protective barriers. Spread within the host is by direct invasion of adjacent tissues, typically forming sinus tracts that cross tissue planes. The most common species causing human disease is *Actinomyces israelii*.

There are 3 common anatomic sites of infection. **Cervicofacial** is most common, often occurring after tooth extraction, oral surgery, or other oral/facial trauma or even from carious teeth. Localized pain and induration may progress to cervical abscess and "woody hard" nodular lesions ("lumpy jaw"), which can develop draining sinus tracts, usually at the angle of the jaw or in the submandibular region. Infection may contribute to chronic tonsillar airway obstruction. **Thoracic** disease most commonly is secondary to aspiration of oropharyngeal secretions but may be an extension of cervicofacial infection. It occurs rarely after esophageal disruption secondary to surgery or nonpenetrating trauma. Thoracic presentation includes pneumonia, which can be complicated by abscesses, empyema, and rarely, pleurodermal sinuses. Focal or multifocal mediastinal and pulmonary masses may be mistaken for tumors. **Abdominal** actinomycosis usually is attributable to penetrating trauma or intestinal perforation. The appendix and cecum are the most common sites; symptoms are similar to appendicitis. Slowly developing masses may simulate abdominal or retroperitoneal neoplasms. Intra-abdominal abscesses and peritoneal-dermal draining sinuses occur eventually. Chronic localized disease often forms draining sinus tracts with purulent discharge. **Other sites** of infection include the liver, pelvis (which, in some cases, has been linked to use of intrauterine devices), heart, testicles, and brain (which usually is associated with a primary pulmonary focus). Noninvasive primary cutaneous actinomycosis has occurred.

ETIOLOGY: *A israelii* and at least 5 other *Actinomyces* species cause human disease. All are slow-growing, microaerophilic or facultative anaerobic, gram-positive, filamentous branching bacilli. They can be part of normal oral, gastrointestinal tract, or vaginal flora. *Actinomyces* species frequently are copathogens in tissues harboring multiple other anaerobic and/or aerobic species. Isolation of *Aggregatibacter (Actinobacillus) actinomycetemcomitans*, frequently detected with *Actinomyces* species, may predict the presence of actinomycosis.

EPIDEMIOLOGY: *Actinomyces* species occur worldwide, being components of endogenous oral and gastrointestinal tract flora. *Actinomyces* species are opportunistic pathogens (reported in patients with human immunodeficiency virus [HIV] and with chronic granulomatous disease), with disease usually following penetrating (including human bite wounds) and nonpenetrating trauma. Infection is uncommon in infants and children, with 80% of cases occurring in adults. The male-to-female ratio in children is 1.5:1. Overt, microbiologically confirmed, monomicrobial disease caused by *Actinomyces* species has become rare in the era of antimicrobial agents.

The **incubation period** varies from several days to several years.

DIAGNOSTIC TESTS: Microscopic demonstration of beaded, branched, gram-positive bacilli in purulent material or tissue specimens suggests the diagnosis. Only specimens from normally sterile sites should be submitted for culture. Specimens must be obtained, transported, and cultured anaerobically on semiselective (kanamycin/vancomycin) media such as the modified Thayer-Martin agar or Buffered charcoal yeast extract (BCYE) agar. Acid-fast testing can distinguish *Actinomyces* species, which are acid-fast negative, from *Nocardia* species, which are variably acid-fast positive staining. Yellow "sulfur granules" visualized microscopically or macroscopically in drainage or loculations of purulent material suggest the diagnosis. A Gram stain of "sulfur granules" discloses a dense aggregate of bacterial filaments mixed with inflammatory debris. *A israelii* forms "spiderlike" microcolonies on culture medium after 48 hours. *Actinomyces* species can be identified in tissue specimens using polymerase chain reaction assay and sequencing of the 16s rRNA.

TREATMENT: Initial therapy should include intravenous penicillin G or ampicillin for 4 to 6 weeks followed by high doses of oral penicillin (up to 2 g/day for adults), usually for a total of 6 to 12 months. Treatment for some cases of cervicofacial disease can be initiated with oral therapy. Amoxicillin, erythromycin, clindamycin, doxycycline, and tetracycline are alternative antimicrobial choices. Amoxicillin/clavulanate, piperacillin/tazobactam, ceftriaxone, clarithromycin, linezolid, and meropenem also show high activity in vitro. All *Actinomyces* species appear to be resistant to ciprofloxacin and metronidazole. Doxycycline can be used for short durations (ie, 21 days or less) without regard to patient age, but for the longer treatment duration required in actinomycosis, for which alternative treatments exist, doxycycline is not recommended for children younger than 8 years (see Tetracyclines, p 905).

Surgical drainage often is a necessary adjunct to medical management and may allow for a shorter duration of antimicrobial treatment.

ISOLATION OF THE HOSPITALIZED PATIENT: Standard precautions are recommended. There is no person-to-person spread.

CONTROL MEASURES: Appropriate oral hygiene, regular dental care, and careful cleansing of wounds, including human bite wounds, can prevent infection.

Adenovirus Infections

CLINICAL MANIFESTATIONS: Adenovirus infections of the upper respiratory tract are common and often subclinical but may cause common cold symptoms, pharyngitis, tonsillitis, otitis media, and pharyngoconjunctival fever. Life-threatening disseminated infection, lower respiratory infection (eg, severe pneumonia), hepatitis, meningitis, and encephalitis occur occasionally, especially among young infants and the immunocompromised. Adenoviruses occasionally cause a pertussis-like syndrome, croup, bronchiolitis, exudative tonsillitis, and hemorrhagic cystitis. Ocular adenovirus infections may present as follicular conjunctivitis or as epidemic keratoconjunctivitis. Enteric adenoviruses are an important cause of childhood gastroenteritis.

ETIOLOGY: Adenoviruses are double-stranded, nonenveloped DNA viruses of the *Adenoviridae* family and *Mastadenovirus* genus, with more than 50 recognized types and multiple genetic variants divided into 7 species (A–G) that infect humans. Some adenovirus types are associated primarily with respiratory tract disease (types 1–5, 7, 14, and 21), keratoconjunctivitis (types 5, 8, 19, and 37), and gastroenteritis (types 31, 40, and 41).

EPIDEMIOLOGY: Infection in children can occur at any age. Adenoviruses causing respiratory tract infections usually are transmitted by respiratory tract secretions through person-to-person contact, airborne droplets, and fomites. The conjunctiva can provide a portal of entry. Adenoviruses are hardy viruses, can survive on environmental surfaces for long periods, and are not inactivated by many disinfectants. Outbreaks of febrile respiratory tract illness attributable to adenoviruses can be a significant problem in military trainees, although less so since vaccination was reinstituted. Community outbreaks of adenovirus-associated pharyngoconjunctival fever have been attributed to water exposure from contaminated swimming pools and fomites, such as shared towels. Health care-associated transmission of adenoviral respiratory tract, conjunctival, and gastrointestinal tract infections can occur in hospitals, residential institutions, and nursing homes from exposures to infected health care personnel, patients, or contaminated equipment. Adenovirus infections in transplant recipients can occur from donor tissues. Epidemic keratoconjunctivitis commonly occurs by direct contact and has been associated with equipment used during eye examinations. Enteric strains of adenoviruses are transmitted by the fecal-oral route. Adenoviruses do not demonstrate the marked seasonality of other respiratory tract viruses and instead circulate throughout the year. Whether individual adenovirus serotypes demonstrate seasonality is not clear. Enteric disease occurs year-round and primarily affects children younger than 4 years. Adenovirus infections are most communicable during the first few days of an acute illness, but persistent and intermittent shedding for longer periods, even months, is common. In healthy people, infection with one adenovirus type should confer type-specific immunity or at least lessen symptoms associated with reinfection, which forms the basis of adenovirus vaccines used in new military recruits (see Control Measures).

The **incubation period** for respiratory tract infection varies from 2 to 14 days; for gastroenteritis, the **incubation period** is 3 to 10 days.

DIAGNOSTIC TESTS: Methods for diagnosis of adenovirus infection include molecular detection, isolation in cell culture, and antigen detection. Polymerase chain reaction assays are the preferred diagnostic method for detection of adenoviruses, and these assays are now widely available commercially. However, the persistent and intermittent shedding that commonly follows an acute adenoviral infection can complicate the clinical interpretation of a positive molecular test result. Quantitative adenovirus assays are useful for management of immunocompromised patients, such as bone marrow and solid organ transplant recipients. Adenoviruses associated with respiratory tract and ocular disease can be isolated by culture from respiratory specimens (eg, nasopharyngeal swab, oropharyngeal swab, nasal wash, sputum) and eye secretions in standard susceptible cell lines. Enteric adenoviruses types 40 and 41 usually require specialized cell lines for successful isolation. Rapid antigen-detection techniques, including immunofluorescence and enzyme immunoassay, have been used to detect virus in respiratory tract secretions, conjunctival swab specimens, and stool, but these methods lack sensitivity. Adenovirus typing by molecular methods is available from some reference laboratories. Although its clinical utility is limited, typing can help establish an etiologic association with disease. Serodiagnosis is used primarily for epidemiologic studies.

TREATMENT: Treatment of adenovirus infection is supportive. Randomized clinical trials evaluating specific antiviral therapy have not been performed. However, case reports of the successful use of cidofovir in immunocompromised patients with severe adenoviral disease have been published, albeit without a uniform dose or dosing strategy.

ISOLATION OF THE HOSPITALIZED PATIENT: In addition to standard precautions for young children with respiratory tract infections, contact and droplet precautions are indicated for the duration of hospitalization. In immunocompromised patients, contact and droplet precautions should be extended because of possible prolonged shedding of the virus. For patients with conjunctivitis and for diapered and incontinent children with adenoviral gastroenteritis, contact precautions are indicated for the duration of illness.

CONTROL MEASURES: Appropriate hand hygiene, respiratory hygiene, and cough etiquette should be followed. Children who are in group child care, particularly children from 6 months through 2 years of age, are at increased risk of adenoviral respiratory tract infections and gastroenteritis. Effective measures for preventing spread of adenovirus infection in group child care settings have not been determined, but frequent hand hygiene is recommended. If 2 or more children in a group child care setting develop conjunctivitis in the same period of time, advice should be sought from the health consultant of the program or the state health department.

Adequate chlorination of swimming pools is recommended to prevent pharyngoconjunctival fever. Epidemic keratoconjunctivitis associated with ophthalmologic practice can be difficult to control and requires use of single-dose medication dispensing and strict attention to hand hygiene and instrument sterilization procedures. Health care professionals with known or suspected adenoviral conjunctivitis should avoid direct patient contact for 14 days after onset of disease in the most recently involved eye. Adenoviruses are difficult to inactivate with alcohol-based gels, because they lack an envelope and may remain viable on skin, fomites, and environmental surfaces for extended periods. Thus, assiduous adherence to hand hygiene and use of disposable gloves when caring for infected patients are recommended.

A live, nonattenuated, oral adenovirus vaccine for types 4 and 7 (2 oral tablets, 1 for each of the 2 strains) has been licensed by the US Food and Drug Administration for prevention of febrile acute respiratory tract disease. This vaccine is approved in military populations 17 through 50 years of age who do not have contraindications. Tablets should be swallowed whole and not chewed.

Amebiasis

CLINICAL MANIFESTATIONS: The majority of individuals with *Entamoeba histolytica* have asymptomatic noninvasive intestinal tract infection. When present, symptoms associated with *E histolytica* infection generally include cramps, watery or bloody diarrhea, and weight loss. Occasionally, the parasite may spread to other organs, most commonly the liver (liver abscess), and cause fever and right upper quadrant pain. Disease is more severe in very young people, elderly people, malnourished people, and pregnant women. People with symptomatic intestinal amebiasis generally have a gradual onset of symptoms over 1 to 3 weeks. The mildest form of intestinal tract disease is nondysenteric colitis. Amebic dysentery is the most common clinical manifestation of amebiasis and generally includes diarrhea with either gross or microscopic blood in the stool, lower abdominal pain, and tenesmus. Weight loss is common because of the gradual onset, but fever occurs only in a minority of patients (8%–38%). Symptoms may be chronic, are characterized by the presence of periods of diarrhea and intestinal spasms alternating with periods of constipation, and may mimic those of inflammatory bowel disease. Progressive involvement of the colon may produce toxic megacolon, fulminant colitis, ulceration of the colon and perianal area, and rarely, perforation. Colonic progression may occur at multiples sites and has a high fatality rate. Progression may occur in patients inappropriately treated with corticosteroids or antimotility drugs. An ameboma may occur as an annular lesion of the colon and may present as a palpable mass on physical examination. Amebomas can occur in any area of the colon but are most common in the cecum. They may be mistaken for colonic carcinoma. Amebomas usually resolve with antiamebic therapy and do not require surgery.

In a small proportion of patients, extraintestinal disease may occur. The liver is the most common extraintestinal site, and infection may spread from there to the pleural space, lungs, and pericardium. Liver abscess may be acute, with fever, abdominal pain, tachypnea, liver tenderness, and hepatomegaly, or may be chronic, with weight loss, vague abdominal symptoms, and irritability. Rupture of abscesses into the abdomen or chest may lead to death. Evidence of recent intestinal tract infection usually is absent in extraintestinal disease. Infection may spread from the colon to the genitourinary tract and the skin. The organism may spread hematogenously to the brain and other areas of the body.

ETIOLOGY: The genus *Entamoeba* includes 6 species that live in the human intestine. Four of these species are identical morphologically: *E histolytica, Entamoeba dispar, Entamoeba moshkovskii,* and *Entamoeba bangladeshi.* Not all *Entamoeba* species are virulent. *E dispar* generally is recognized as a commensal, and although *E moshkovskii* generally was believed to be nonpathogenic, it may be associated with diarrhea in infants and with diarrhea and colitis in mice. *Entamoeba* species are excreted as cysts or trophozoites in stool of infected people.

EPIDEMIOLOGY: *E histolytica* can be found worldwide but is more prevalent in people of lower socioeconomic status who live in resource-limited countries, where the prevalence of amebic infection may be as high as 50% in some communities. Groups at increased risk of infection in industrialized countries include immigrants from or long-term visitors to areas with endemic infection, institutionalized people, and men who have sex with men. *E histolytica* is transmitted via amebic cysts by the fecal-oral route. Ingested cysts, which are unaffected by gastric acid, undergo excystation in the alkaline small intestine and produce trophozoites that infect the colon. Cysts that develop subsequently are the source of transmission, especially from asymptomatic cyst excreters. Infected patients excrete cysts intermittently, sometimes for years if untreated. Transmission has been associated with contaminated food or water. Fecal-oral transmission can occur in the setting of anal sexual practices or direct rectal inoculation through colonic irrigation devices.

The **incubation period** is variable, ranging from a few days to months or years, but commonly is 2 to 4 weeks.

DIAGNOSTIC TESTS: A definitive diagnosis of intestinal tract infection depends on identifying trophozoites or cysts in stool specimens. Examination of serial specimens may be necessary. Specimens of stool may be examined microscopically by wet mount within 30 minutes of collection or may be fixed in formalin or polyvinyl alcohol (available in kits) for concentration, permanent staining, and subsequent microscopic examination. Microscopy does not differentiate between *E histolytica* and less pathogenic strains, although trophozoites containing ingested red blood cells are more likely to be *E histolytica.* Antigen test kits are available in some clinical laboratories for testing of *E histolytica* directly from stool specimens. The utility of examining biopsy specimens and endoscopy scrapings (not swabs) using similar methods is not well established. Polymerase chain reaction assay and isoenzyme analysis can differentiate *E histolytica* from *E dispar, E moshkovskii,* and other *Entamoeba* species; some monoclonal antibody-based antigen detection assays also can differentiate *E histolytica* from *E dispar.*

The indirect hemagglutination (IHA) test has been replaced by commercially available enzyme immunoassay (EIA) kits for routine serodiagnosis of amebiasis. The EIA detects antibody specific for *E histolytica* in approximately 95% or more of patients with extraintestinal amebiasis, 70% of patients with active intestinal tract infection, and 10% of asymptomatic people who are passing cysts of *E histolytica.* Patients may continue to have positive serologic test results even after adequate therapy. Diagnosis of an *E histolytica* liver abscess and other extraintestinal infections is aided by serologic testing, because stool tests and abscess aspirates frequently are not revealing.

Ultrasonography, computed tomography, and magnetic resonance imaging can identify liver abscesses and other extraintestinal sites of infection. Aspirates from a liver abscess usually show neither trophozoites nor leukocytes.

TREATMENT: Treatment should be prioritized for all patients with *E histolytica,* including those who are asymptomatic, given the propensity of this organism to cause invasive infection and to spread among family members. A treatment plan should include antibiotics to eliminate invading trophozoites as well as organisms carried in the intestinal lumen. Corticosteroids and antimotility drugs administered to people with amebiasis can worsen symptoms and the disease process. In settings where tests to distinguish species are not available, treatment should be administered to symptomatic people on the basis of positive results of microscopic examination. The following regimens are recommended:

- **Asymptomatic cyst excreters (intraluminal infections):** treat with an intraluminal amebicide alone (paromomycin or diiodohydroxyquinoline/iodoquinol, or diloxanide furoate [the latter not currently available in the United States]). Metronidazole is not effective against cysts.
- **Patients with invasive colitis manifest as mild to moderate or severe intestinal tract symptoms or extraintestinal disease (including liver abscess):** treat with metronidazole (35–50 mg/kg/day in 3 divided doses for 7–10 days) or tinidazole (50 mg/kg [up to 2 g] orally once a day with food for 3 to 5 days), followed by an intraluminal amebicide (diiodohydroxyquinoline/iodoquinol 30–40 mg/kg/day in 3 divided doses for 20 days; 650 mg maximum per dose) or diloxanide furoate (20 mg/kg/day in 3 divided doses for 10 days; 500 mg maximum per dose) or, in absence of intestinal obstruction, paromomycin (25–35 mg/kg/day in 3 divided doses for 7 days). Nitazoxanide may be effective for mild to moderate intestinal amebiasis, although it is not approved by the US Food and Drug Administration for this indication.
- **Percutaneous or surgical aspiration of large liver abscesses occasionally may be required** when response of the abscess to medical therapy is unsatisfactory or there is risk of rupture. In most cases of liver abscess, however, drainage is not required and does not speed recovery. For patients who have peritonitis, broad-spectrum agent therapy should be used. In cases with toxic megacolon, colectomy may be necessary.

Follow-up stool examination is recommended after completion of therapy, because no pharmacologic regimen is completely effective in eradicating intestinal tract infection. Household members and other suspected contacts should have adequate stool examinations performed and should be treated if results are positive for *E histolytica.*

E dispar generally is considered to be nonpathogenic and does not necessarily require treatment. The pathogenic significance of finding *E moshkovskii* is unclear; treatment of symptomatic infection is reasonable.

ISOLATION OF THE HOSPITALIZED PATIENT: In addition to standard precautions, contact precautions are recommended for the duration of illness.

CONTROL MEASURES: Careful hand hygiene after defecation, sanitary disposal of fecal material, and treatment of drinking water will control spread of infection. Sexual transmission may be controlled by use of condoms and avoidance of sexual practices that may permit fecal-oral transmission. Because of the risk of shedding infectious cysts, people diagnosed with amebiasis should refrain from using recreational water venues (eg, swimming pools, water parks) until after their course of luminal chemotherapy is completed and any diarrhea they might have been experiencing has resolved.

Amebic Meningoencephalitis and Keratitis

(*Naegleria fowleri, Acanthamoeba* species, *Sappinia* species, and *Balamuthia mandrillaris*)

CLINICAL MANIFESTATIONS: *Naegleria fowleri* can cause a rapidly progressive, almost always fatal, primary amebic meningoencephalitis (PAM). Early symptoms include fever, headache, vomiting, and sometimes disturbances of smell and taste. The illness progresses rapidly to signs of meningoencephalitis, including nuchal rigidity, lethargy, confusion, personality changes, and altered level of consciousness. Seizures are common, and death generally occurs within a week of onset of symptoms. No distinct clinical features differentiate this disease from fulminant bacterial meningitis.

Granulomatous amebic encephalitis (GAE) caused by *Acanthamoeba* species and *Balamuthia mandrillaris* has a more insidious onset and develops as a subacute or chronic disease. In general, GAE progresses more slowly than PAM, leading to death several weeks to months after onset of symptoms. Signs and symptoms may include personality changes, seizures, headaches, ataxia, cranial nerve palsies, hemiparesis, and other focal neurologic deficits. Fever often is low grade and intermittent. The course may resemble that of a bacterial brain abscess or a brain tumor. Chronic granulomatous skin lesions (pustules, nodules, ulcers) may be present without central nervous system (CNS) involvement, particularly in patients with acquired immunodeficiency syndrome, and lesions may be present for months before brain involvement in immunocompetent hosts.

The most common symptoms of amebic keratitis, a vision-threatening infection usually caused by *Acanthamoeba* species, are pain (often out of proportion to clinical signs), photophobia, tearing, and foreign body sensation. Characteristic clinical findings include radial keratoneuritis and stromal ring infiltrate. *Acanthamoeba* keratitis generally follows an indolent course and initially may resemble herpes simplex or bacterial keratitis; delay in diagnosis is associated with worse outcomes.

Sappinia infection is a rare cause of encephalitis, with only 1 case reported.

ETIOLOGY: *N fowleri, Acanthamoeba* species, *Sappinia* species (only 2 species: *Sappinia diploidea* and *Sappinia pedata*), and *B mandrillaris* are free-living amebae that exist as motile, infectious trophozoites and environmentally hardy cysts.

EPIDEMIOLOGY: *N fowleri* is found in warm fresh water and moist soil. Most infections with *N fowleri* have been associated with swimming in natural bodies of warm fresh water, such as ponds, lakes, and hot springs, but other sources have included tap water from geothermal sources and contaminated and poorly chlorinated swimming pools. Disease has been reported worldwide but is uncommon. In the United States, infection occurs primarily in the summer and usually affects children and young adults. Disease has followed use of tap water for sinus rinses or exposures related to recreational activities (tap water used for backyard waterslide). The trophozoites of the parasite invade the brain directly from the nose along the olfactory nerves via the cribiform plate. In infections with *N fowleri*, trophozoites, but not cysts, can be visualized in sections of brain or in cerebrospinal fluid (CSF).

The **incubation period** for *N fowleri* infection typically is 3 to 7 days.

Acanthamoeba species are distributed worldwide and are found in soil; dust; cooling towers of electric and nuclear power plants; heating, ventilating, and air conditioning units; fresh and brackish water; whirlpool baths; and physiotherapy pools. The environmental niche of *B mandrillaris* is not delineated clearly, although it has been isolated from soil. CNS infection attributable to *Acanthamoeba* occurs primarily in debilitated and immunocompromised people. However, some patients infected with *B mandrillaris* have had no demonstrable underlying disease or defect. CNS infection by both amebae probably occurs most commonly by inhalation or direct contact with contaminated soil or water. The primary foci of these infections most likely are skin or respiratory tract, followed by hematogenous spread to the brain. Fatal encephalitis caused by *Balamuthia* species and transmitted by the donated organ has been reported in recipients of organ transplants. *Acanthamoeba* keratitis occurs primarily in people who wear contact lenses,[1] although it also has been associated with corneal trauma. Poor contact lens hygiene and/or disinfection practices as well as swimming with contact lenses are risk factors.

The **incubation periods** for *Acanthamoeba* and *Balamuthia* GAE are unknown. It is thought to take several weeks or months to develop the first symptoms of CNS disease following exposure to the amebae. Patients exposed to *Balamuthia* through solid organ transplantation can develop symptoms of *Balamuthia* GAE more quickly—within a few weeks. The **incubation period** for *Acanthamoeba* keratitis is unknown but thought to range from several days to several weeks.

DIAGNOSTIC TESTS: In *N fowleri* infection, computed tomography scans of the head without contrast are unremarkable or show only cerebral edema but with contrast might show meningeal enhancement of the basilar cisterns and sulci. These changes, however, are not specific for amebic infection. CSF pressure usually is elevated (300 to >600 mm water), and CSF indices may show a polymorphonuclear pleocytosis, an increased protein concentration, and a normal to very low glucose concentration; Gram stains are negative for bacteria. *N fowleri* infection can be documented by microscopic demonstration of the motile trophozoites on a wet mount of centrifuged CSF. Smears of CSF should be stained with Giemsa, Trichome, or Wright stains to identify the trophozoites, if present; Gram stain is not useful in ruling in *N fowleri* CNS infection. The organism can be cultured on nonnutrient agar plates layered with *Escherichia coli* or on monolayers of E6 and human lung fibroblast cells. Trophozoites can be visualized in sections of the brain. Immunofluorescence and polymerase chain reaction (PCR) assays performed on CSF and biopsy material to identify the organism are available through the Centers for Disease Control and

---

[1]Centers for Disease Control and Prevention. Contact lens–related corneal infections—United States, 2005–2015. *MMWR Morb Mortal Wkly Rep.* 2016;65(32):817–820

Prevention (CDC). The CDC also will provide consultation services for diagnosis and management (770-488-7100).

In infection with *Acanthamoeba* species and *B mandrillaris*, trophozoites and cysts can be visualized in sections of brain, lungs, and skin; in cases of *Acanthamoeba* keratitis, they also can be visualized in corneal scrapings and by confocal microscopy in vivo in the cornea. In GAE infections, CSF indices typically reveal a lymphocytic pleocytosis and an increased protein concentration, with normal or low glucose but no organisms. Computed tomography and magnetic resonance imaging of the head may show single or multiple space-occupying, ring-enhancing lesions that can mimic brain abscesses, tumors, cerebrovascular accidents, or other diseases. *Acanthamoeba* species, but not *B mandrillaris*, can be cultured by the same method used for *N fowleri*. *B mandrillaris* can be grown using mammalian cell culture. Like *N fowleri*, immunofluorescence and PCR assays can be performed on clinical specimens to identify *Acanthamoeba* species and *Balamuthia* species; these tests are available through the CDC.

TREATMENT: The most up-to-date guidance for treatment of PAM can be found on the CDC Web site (**www.cdc.gov/naegleria**). Early diagnosis and institution of combination high-dose drug therapy is thought to be important for optimizing outcome. If meningoencephalitis possibly caused by *N fowleri* is suspected, treatment should not be withheld pending confirmation. Presence of amebic organisms in CSF is valuable for probable diagnosis; however, confirmatory diagnostic tests still should be performed. Although an effective treatment regimen for PAM has not been identified, amphotericin B is the drug of choice in combination with other agents. In vitro testing indicates that *N fowleri* is highly susceptible to amphotericin B. Miltefosine, which is approved for treatment of leishmaniasis, is available through the CDC (770-488-7100) and has been used successfully to treat PAM caused by *N fowleri*. Two survivors recovered after treatment with amphotericin B in combination with an azole drug (either miconazole or fluconazole) plus rifampin, although rifampin probably had no additional effect; these patients also received dexamethasone to control cerebral edema. Although these 2 patients did not receive azithromycin, this drug has both in vitro and in vivo efficacy against *Naegleria* species and also may be considered as an adjunct with amphotericin B.

Effective treatment for infections caused by *Acanthamoeba* species and *B mandrillaris* has not been established. Several patients with *Acanthamoeba* GAE and *Acanthamoeba* cutaneous infections without CNS involvement have been treated successfully with a multidrug regimen consisting of various combinations of pentamidine, sulfadiazine, flucytosine, either fluconazole or itraconazole (voriconazole is not active against *Balamuthia* species), trimethoprim-sulfamethoxazole, and topical application of chlorhexidine gluconate and ketoconazole for skin lesions. Voriconazole, miltefosine, and azithromycin also might be of some value in treating *Acanthamoeba* infections. For patients with *B mandrillaris* infection, pentamidine, sulfadiazine, fluconazole, and either azithromycin or clarithromycin and flucytosine, in addition to surgical resection of the CNS lesions, has been reported to be successful in treatment.

Patients with *Acanthamoeba* keratitis should be evaluated by an ophthalmologist. Early diagnosis and therapy are important for a good outcome.

ISOLATION OF THE HOSPITALIZED PATIENT: Standard precautions are recommended.

CONTROL MEASURES: People should assume that there is always a slight risk of developing PAM caused by *N fowleri* when entering warm fresh water. Only avoidance of such water-related activities can prevent *Naegleria* infection, although the risk might be reduced by taking measures to limit water exposure through known routes of entry, such as getting water up the nose. Water for sinus rinses generally is discouraged, but when used should be either previously boiled or properly filtered or labeled as sterile or distilled (additional information available at **www.cdc.gov/naegleria**). Presently, no clearly defined recommendations are available to prevent GAE attributable to *Acanthamoeba* species or *B mandrillaris*. To prevent *Acanthamoeba* keratitis, steps should be taken to avoid corneal trauma, such as the use of protective eyewear during high-risk activities, and contact lens users should maintain good contact lens hygiene and disinfection practices, use only sterile solutions as applicable, change lens cases frequently, and avoid swimming and showering while wearing contact lenses. Advice for people who wear contact lenses can be found on the CDC Web site (**www.cdc.gov/contactlenses**).[1]

Anthrax[2]

CLINICAL MANIFESTATIONS: Anthrax resulting from natural infection or secondary to a bioterror event can occur in multiple forms, depending on the route of infection: cutaneous, inhalation, gastrointestinal, or injection.

Cutaneous anthrax accounts for 95% of all human infection and begins as a pruritic papule or vesicle after an incubation period of 5 to 7 days (range of 1 to 17 days) and progresses over 2 to 6 days to an ulcerated lesion with subsequent formation of a central black eschar. The lesion is characteristically painless, with surrounding edema, hyperemia, and painful regional lymphadenopathy. Patients may have associated fever, lymphangitis, and extensive edema.

Inhalation anthrax is a frequently lethal form of the disease and is a medical emergency. The initial presentation is nonspecific and may include fever, sweats, nonproductive cough, chest pain, headache, myalgia, malaise, nausea, and vomiting. Illness progresses to the fulminant phase 2 to 5 days later. In some cases, the illness is biphasic with a period of improvement between prodromal symptoms and overwhelming illness. Fulminant manifestations include hypotension, dyspnea, hypoxia, cyanosis, and shock occurring as a result of hemorrhagic mediastinal lymphadenitis, hemorrhagic pneumonia, hemorrhagic pleural effusions, bacteremia, and toxemia. A widened mediastinum is the classic finding on imaging of the chest. Chest radiography also may show pleural effusions and/or infiltrates, both of which may be hemorrhagic.

Gastrointestinal tract disease can present as one of 2 distinct clinical syndromes—intestinal or oropharyngeal. Patients with the intestinal form have symptoms of nausea, anorexia, vomiting, and fever progressing to severe abdominal pain, massive ascites, hematemesis, and bloody diarrhea related to edema and ulceration of the bowel, primarily in the ileum and cecum. Patients with oropharyngeal anthrax may have dysphagia with posterior oropharyngeal necrotic ulcers, which may be associated with marked, often unilateral neck swelling, regional lymphadenopathy, fever, and sepsis.

---

[1]Centers for Disease Control and Prevention. Estimated burden of keratitis—United States, 2010. *MMWR Morb Mortal Wkly Rep*. 2014;63(45):1027–1030

[2]Bradley JS, Peacock G, Krug SE, et al; American Academy of Pediatrics, Committee on Infectious Diseases, Disaster Preparedness Advisory Council. Clinical report: Pediatric anthrax clinical management. *Pediatrics*. 2014;133(5):e1411–e1436

Injection anthrax has not been reported to date in children. It occurs primarily among injecting drug users; however, smoking and snorting heroin also have been identified as exposure routes.

Systemic illness can result from hematogenous and lymphatic dissemination with any form of anthrax. Most patients with inhalation, gastrointestinal, and injection anthrax have systemic illness. Patients with cutaneous anthrax should be considered to have systemic illness if they have tachycardia, tachypnea, hypotension, hyperthermia, hypothermia, or leukocytosis or have lesions that involve the head, neck, or upper torso or that are large, bullous, multiple, or surrounded by edema. Anthrax meningitis or hemorrhagic meningoencephalitis can occur in any patient with systemic illness and in patients without other apparent clinical presentation. Therefore, lumbar puncture should be performed to rule out meningitis whenever clinically indicated. The case fatality rate for patients with appropriately treated cutaneous anthrax usually is less than 2%. Even with antimicrobial treatment and supportive care, the case fatality rate for inhalation or gastrointestinal tract disease is between 40% and 45% and exceeds 90% for meningitis.

ETIOLOGY: *Bacillus anthracis* is an aerobic, gram-positive, encapsulated, spore-forming, nonhemolytic, nonmotile rod. *B anthracis* has 3 major virulence factors: an antiphagocytic capsule and 2 exotoxins, called lethal and edema toxins. The toxins are responsible for the substantial morbidity and clinical manifestations of hemorrhage, edema, and necrosis.

EPIDEMIOLOGY: Anthrax is a zoonotic disease most commonly affecting domestic and wild herbivores that occurs in many rural regions of the world. *B anthracis* spores can remain viable in the soil for decades, representing a potential source of infection for livestock or wildlife through ingestion of spore-contaminated vegetation or water. In susceptible hosts, the spores germinate to become viable bacteria. Natural infection of humans occurs through contact with infected animals or contaminated animal products, including carcasses, hides, hair, wool, meat, and bone meal. Outbreaks of gastrointestinal tract anthrax have occurred after ingestion of undercooked or raw meat from infected animals. Historically, more than 95% of anthrax cases in the United States were cutaneous infections among animal handlers or mill workers. The incidence of naturally occurring human anthrax decreased in the United States from an estimated 130 cases annually in the early 1900s to 0 to 2 cases per year from 1979 through 2013. Recent cases of inhalation, cutaneous, and gastrointestinal tract anthrax have occurred in drum makers working with animal hides contaminated with *B anthracis* spores and in people participating in events where spore-contaminated drums were played. Severe soft tissue infections among heroin users, including cases with disseminated systemic infection, have been reported in Europe.

B anthracis is one of the most likely agents to be used as a biological weapon, because (1) its spores are highly stable; (2) spores can infect via the respiratory route; and (3) the resulting inhalation anthrax has a high mortality rate. In 1979, an accidental release of *B anthracis* spores from a military microbiology facility in the former Soviet Union resulted in at least 68 deaths. In 2001, 22 cases of anthrax (11 inhalation, 11 cutaneous) were identified in the United States after intentional contamination of the mail; 5 (45%) of the inhalation anthrax cases were fatal. In addition to aerosolization, there is a theoretical health risk associated with *B anthracis* spores being introduced into food products or water supplies. Use of *B anthracis* in a biological attack would require immediate response and mobilization of public health resources.[1] Anthrax meets the definition of a nationally and immediately notifiable condition, as specified by the US Council of State and Territorial Epidemiologists; therefore, every suspected case should be reported immediately to the local or state health department.

The **incubation period** typically is 1 week or less for cutaneous or gastrointestinal tract anthrax. However, because of spore dormancy and slow clearance of spores from the lungs, the **incubation period** for inhalation anthrax may be prolonged and has been reported to range from 2 to 43 days in humans and up to 2 months in experimental nonhuman primates. Discharge from cutaneous lesions is potentially infectious, but person-to-person transmission rarely has been reported, and other forms of anthrax are not associated with person-to person transmission. Both inhalation and cutaneous anthrax have occurred in laboratory workers.

DIAGNOSTIC TESTS: Depending on the clinical presentation, Gram stain, culture, and polymerase chain reaction (PCR) testing for *B anthracis* should be performed with the assistance of local health departments on specimens of blood, pleural fluid, cerebrospinal fluid (CSF), and tissue biopsy specimens and on swabs of vesicular fluid or eschar material from cutaneous or oropharyngeal lesions, rectal swabs, or stool. Acute sera may be tested for lethal factor (one of the 2 exotoxins of anthrax). Whenever possible, specimens for these tests should be obtained before initiating antimicrobial therapy, because previous treatment with antimicrobial agents makes isolation by culture unlikely. Gram-positive bacilli detected on unspun peripheral blood smears or in vesicular fluid or CSF can be an important initial finding, and polychrome methylene blue-stained smears showing bacilli stained blue with the capsule visualized in red (M'Fadyean reaction) are considered a presumptive identification of *B anthracis*. Traditional microbiologic methods can presumptively identify *B anthracis* isolated readily on routine agar media (blood and chocolate) used in clinical laboratories. Definitive identification of suspect *B anthracis* isolates can be performed via the Laboratory Response Network (LRN) in each state, accessed through local health departments. Additional diagnostic tests for anthrax are available through state health departments and the Centers for Disease Control and Prevention (CDC), including bacterial DNA detection in specimens by PCR assay, tissue immunohistochemistry, an enzyme immunoassay that measures immunoglobulin G antibodies against *B anthracis* protective antigen in paired sera, and a MALDI-TOF (matrix-assisted laser desorption/ionization–time-of-flight) mass spectrometry assay measuring lethal factor activity in sera. The sensitivity of DNA and antigen detection methods may decline after antimicrobial treatment has been initiated. A commercially available enzyme-linked immunosorbent assay (QuickELISA Anthrax-PA kit [Immunetics Inc, Boston, MA]) can be used for screening. This assay detects antibodies to protective antigen protein of *B anthracis* in human serum from individuals with clinical history or symptoms consistent with anthrax infection. Clinical evaluation of patients with suspected inhalation anthrax should include a chest radiograph and/or computed tomography scan to evaluate for widened mediastinum, pleural effusion, and/or pulmonary infiltrates. Lumbar punctures should be performed whenever feasible to rule out meningitis and to guide therapy.

---

[1]Centers for Disease Control and Prevention. Clinical framework and medical countermeasure use during an anthrax mass-casualty incident: CDC recommendations. *MMWR Recomm Rep*. 2015;64(RR-4):1–22

TREATMENT[1,2]: A high index of suspicion and rapid administration of appropriate anti-microbial therapy to people suspected of being infected, along with access to critical care support, are essential for effective treatment of anthrax. No controlled trials in humans have been performed to validate current treatment recommendations for anthrax, and there is limited clinical experience. Case reports suggest that naturally occurring localized or uncomplicated cutaneous disease can be treated effectively with 7 to 10 days of a single oral antimicrobial agent. First-line agents include ciprofloxacin (or an equivalent fluoro-quinolone) or doxycycline; clindamycin is an alternative, as are penicillins, if the isolate is known to be penicillin susceptible, which is likely to occur with environmental isolates. For bioterrorism-associated cutaneous disease in adults or children lacking signs and symptoms of systemic illness, either ciprofloxacin (30 mg/kg per day, orally, divided 2 times/day for children, not to exceed 1000 mg every 24 hours) or doxycycline (100 mg, orally, 2 times/day for children aged ≥8 years, with a maximum of 100 mg/dose; or 4.4 mg/kg per day, orally, divided 2 times/day for children aged <8 years) are recommended for initial treatment until antimicrobial susceptibility data are available. Doxycycline can be used regardless of patient age (see Tetracyclines, p 905). Because of the risk of concomitant inhalational exposure and subsequent spore dormancy in the lungs, the antimicrobial regimen in cases of bioterrorism-associated cutaneous anthrax or that were exposed to other sources of aerosolized spores should be continued for a total of 60 days to provide postexposure prophylaxis (PEP), in conjunction with administration of vaccine if available (see Control Measures).

On the basis of in vitro data and animal studies, ciprofloxacin (30 mg/kg/day, intra-venously, divided every 8 hours, not to exceed 400 mg/dose) is recommended as the primary antimicrobial component of an initial multidrug regimen for treatment of all forms of systemic anthrax until results of antimicrobial susceptibility testing are known.[1,2] Levofloxacin and moxifloxacin are considered equivalent alternatives to ciprofloxacin. Meningeal involvement should be suspected in all cases of inhalation anthrax and other systemic anthrax infections; thus, until meningitis has been ruled out, treatment of systemic anthrax should include at least 2 other agents with known central nervous system (CNS) penetration in conjunction with ciprofloxacin. There appears to be benefit to the use of a bactericidal agent and a theoretical benefit to the use of protein synthesis-inhibiting agent as the additional drugs in this combination. Meropenem is recommended as the second bactericidal antimicrobial, and if meropenem is not available, doripenem and imipenem/cilastatin are considered alternatives; if the strain is known to be susceptible, penicillin G or ampicillin are equivalent alternatives. Linezolid is recommended as the preferred protein synthesis inhibitor if central nervous system involvement is suspected.

If CNS penetration is less important because meningitis has been ruled out, treatment may consist of 2 antimicrobial agents, including a bactericidal and a protein synthesis-in-

[1]Bradley JS, Peacock G, Krug SE, et al; American Academy of Pediatrics, Committee on Infectious Diseases, Disaster Preparedness Advisory Council. Clinical report: Pediatric anthrax clinical management. *Pediatrics.* 2014;133(5):e1411–e1436

[2]Hendricks KA, Wright ME, Shadomy SV, et al. Centers for Disease Control and Prevention expert panel meetings on prevention and treatment of anthrax in adults. *Emerg Infect Dis.* 2014;20(2). Available at: **wwwnc.cdc.gov/eid/article/20/2/13-0687_intro**

hibiting agent. In such an instance, clindamycin is the preferred protein synthesis inhibitor, and linezolid, doxycycline, and rifampin are acceptable alternatives. Ciprofloxacin is the preferred bactericidal agent, with meropenem, levofloxacin, imipenem/cilastatin, and vancomycin being acceptable alternatives; if the strain is known to be susceptible, penicillin G or ampicillin are equivalent alternatives. Because of intrinsic resistance, cephalosporins and trimethoprim-sulfamethoxazole should not be used.

Treatment should continue for at least 14 days or longer, depending on patient condition. Intravenous therapy can be changed to oral therapy when progression of symptoms ceases and clinical symptoms are improving. There is the risk of spore dormancy in the lungs in people with bioterrorism-associated cutaneous or systemic anthrax or people who were exposed to other sources of aerosolized spores. In these cases, the antimicrobial regimen should be continued for a total of 60 days to provide PEP, in conjunction with administration of vaccine (see Control Measures); antimicrobial drug options are the same as those for PEP.

For patients with anthrax and evidence of systemic illness, including fever, shock, and dissemination to other organs, Anthrax Immune Globulin, or obiltoxaximab or raxibacumab, both monoclonal antibodies against *B anthracis*, should be considered in consultation with the CDC. Supportive symptomatic (intensive care) treatment is important. Aggressive pleural fluid or ascites drainage is critical if effusions exist, because drainage appears to be associated with improved survival. Obstructive airway disease resulting from associated edema may complicate cutaneous anthrax of the face or neck and can require aggressive monitoring for airway compromise.

ISOLATION OF THE HOSPITALIZED PATIENT: Standard precautions are recommended. In addition, contact precautions should be implemented when draining cutaneous lesions are present. Cutaneous lesions become sterile within 24 hours of starting appropriate antimicrobial therapy. Patient care does not appear to be a risk for transmission. Contaminated dressings and bedclothes should be incinerated or steam sterilized (121°C for 30 minutes) to destroy spores. Terminal cleaning of the patient's room can be accomplished with an Environmental Protection Agency-registered hospital-grade disinfectant and should follow standard facility practices typically used for all patients. Autopsies performed on patients with systemic anthrax require special precautions.

CONTROL MEASURES: BioThrax (anthrax vaccine adsorbed [AVA]), the only anthrax vaccine licensed in the United States for use in humans, is prepared from a cell-free culture filtrate. The vaccine's efficacy for prevention of anthrax is based on animal studies, a single placebo-controlled human trial of the alum-precipitated precursor of the current AVA, observational data from humans, and immunogenicity data from humans and other mammals. In the human trial in adult mill workers, the alum-precipitated precursor to AVA had a demonstrated 93% efficacy for preventing cutaneous and inhalation anthrax. Multiple reviews and publications evaluating AVA safety have found adverse events usually are local injection site reactions, with rare systemic symptoms, including fever, chills, muscle aches, and hypersensitivity.

The CDC updated its recommendations on exposure to anthrax through bioterrorism in 2014. In the event of a bioterrorism event, information for health care professionals and the public will be posted on the CDC anthrax Web site (**https://emergency.cdc.gov/agent/anthrax/index.asp**). Within 48 hours of exposure to *B anthracis* spores, public health authorities plan to provide a 10-day course of antimicrobial prophylaxis to the local population, including children likely to have been exposed to spores.

Within 10 days of exposure, public health authorities plan to further define those who have had a clear and significant exposure and will require an additional 50 days of antimicrobial PEP and a 3-dose anthrax vaccine (AVA) series.

The general procedure for AVA vaccination in the preevent or preexposure setting is a primary series of three 0.5-mL intramuscular (IM) injections at 0, 1, and 6 months, with boosters at 12 and 18 months and annually thereafter for those at continued risk of infection. People with medical contraindications to IM administration (eg, people with coagulation disorders) may receive the vaccine by subcutaneous administration. Preevent immunization is recommended for people at risk of repeated exposures to aerosolized B anthracis spores, including selected laboratory workers, environmental investigators and remediation workers, military personnel, and some emergency and other responders.

Postexposure management for previously unvaccinated people older than 18 years who have been exposed to aerosolized *B anthracis* spores consists of 60 days of appropriate antimicrobial prophylaxis combined with 3 subcutaneous doses of AVA (administered at 0, 2, and 4 weeks postexposure). AVA is not licensed for use in pregnant women; however, in a postevent setting that poses a high risk of exposure to aerosolized *B anthracis* spores, pregnancy is neither a precaution nor a contraindication to its use in PEP. There is no evidence to suggest an increased risk for serious adverse events associated with the use of AVA in pediatric populations. However, AVA is not licensed for use in pediatric populations and has not been studied in children. Until there are sufficient data to support FDA approval, AVA is likely to be made available for children at the time of an event as an investigational vaccine under an appropriate regulatory mechanism that will require institutional review board approval, including the use of appropriate informed consent documents. Information on the process required for use of AVA in children will be available on the CDC Web site at the time of an event (**www.cdc.gov/anthrax**), as well as through the American Academy of Pediatrics (AAP)[1] and the FDA. All exposed children 6 weeks and older should receive 3 doses of AVA at 0, 2, and 4 weeks in addition to 60 days of antimicrobial chemoprophylaxis. The recommended route of vaccine administration in children is subcutaneous. Children younger than 6 weeks should immediately begin antimicrobial prophylaxis, but initiation of the vaccine series should be delayed until they reach 6 weeks of age.

When no information is available about antimicrobial susceptibility of the implicated strain of *B anthracis*, ciprofloxacin and doxycycline are equivalent first-line antimicrobial agents for initial PEP for adults or children (see Tetracyclines, p 905). Levofloxacin and clindamycin are second-line antimicrobial agents for PEP. Safety data on extended use of levofloxacin in any population for longer than 28 days are limited; therefore, levofloxacin should only be used when the benefit outweighs the risk. When the antimicrobial susceptibility profile demonstrates appropriate sensitivity to amoxicillin (minimum inhibitory concentration $\leq$0.125 µg/mL), public health authorities may recommend changing PEP antimicrobial therapy for children to oral amoxicillin. Because of the lack of data on amoxicillin dosages for treating anthrax (and the associated high mortality rate), the AAP recommends a higher-than-usual dosage of oral amoxicillin, 80 mg/kg per day, divided into 3 daily doses administered every 8 hours (each dose not to exceed 500 mg). Because

---

[1]Bradley JS, Peacock G, Krug SE, et al; American Academy of Pediatrics, Committee on Infectious Diseases, Disaster Preparedness Advisory Council. Clinical report: Pediatric anthrax clinical management. *Pediatrics*. 2014;133(5):e1411–e1436

of intrinsic resistance, cephalosporins and trimethoprim-sulfamethoxazole should not be used for prophylaxis.

Arboviruses (also see Chikungunya, p 271, Dengue, p 317, West Nile Virus, p 888 and Zika Virus, p 894)

(Including California serogroup, Colorado tick fever, Eastern equine encephalitis, Japanese encephalitis, Powassan, St. Louis encephalitis, tickborne encephalitis, Venezuelan equine encephalitis, Western equine encephalitis, and yellow fever viruses)

CLINICAL MANIFESTATIONS: More than 100 arthropodborne viruses (arboviruses) are known to cause human disease. Although most infections are subclinical, symptomatic illness usually manifests as 1 of 3 primary clinical syndromes: generalized febrile illness, neuroinvasive disease, or hemorrhagic fever (Table 3.1).

Table 3.1. Clinical Manifestations for Select Domestic and International Arboviral Diseases

Virus	Systemic Febrile Illness	Neuroinvasive Disease[a]	Hemorrhagic Fever
Domestic			
Chikungunya	Yes[b]	Rare	No
Colorado tick fever	Yes	Rare	No
Dengue	Yes	Rare	Yes
Eastern equine encephalitis	Yes	Yes	No
Jamestown Canyon	Yes	Yes	No
La Crosse	Yes	Yes	No
Powassan	Yes	Yes	No
St. Louis encephalitis	Yes	Yes	No
Western equine encephalitis	Yes	Yes	No
West Nile	Yes	Yes	No
Zika	Yes	Yes	No
International			
Japanese encephalitis	Yes	Yes	No
Mayaro	Yes	No	No
Tickborne encephalitis	Yes	Yes	No
Venezuelan equine encephalitis	Yes	Yes	No
Yellow fever	Yes	No	Yes
Toscana virus	Yes	Yes	No

[a]Aseptic meningitis, encephalitis, or acute flaccid myelitis.
[b]Most often characterized by sudden onset of high fever and severe joint pain.

- **Generalized febrile illness.** Most arboviruses are capable of causing a systemic febrile illness that often includes headache, arthralgia, myalgia, and rash. Some viruses can cause more characteristic clinical manifestations, such as focal neurologic defects (see West Nile Virus, p 888), severe polyarthralgia (see Chikungunya Virus, p 271), or jaundice (eg, yellow fever virus). With some arboviruses, fatigue, malaise, and weakness can linger for weeks following the initial infection.
- **Neuroinvasive disease.** Many arboviruses cause neuroinvasive disease, including aseptic meningitis, encephalitis, or acute flaccid myelitis. Illness usually presents with a prodrome similar to the systemic febrile illness followed by neurologic symptoms. The specific symptoms vary by virus but can include vomiting, stiff neck, mental status changes, seizures, or focal neurologic deficits. West Nile virus can cause a syndrome of acute flaccid myelitis, either in conjunction with meningoencephalitis or as an isolated finding (see West Nile Virus, p 888). The full range of neurologic manifestations of Zika virus is, as yet, unclear (see Zika, p 894). The severity and long-term outcome of the illness vary by etiologic agent and the underlying characteristics of the host, such as age, immune status, and preexisting medical condition. The Centers for Disease Control and Prevention has developed a comprehensive Web site for assessing and managing patients with acute flaccid myelitis as part of its emerging infection surveillance efforts (eg, West Nile virus, enterovirus D68) and in preparation for the final efforts to eradicate polioviruses worldwide **(www.cdc.gov/acute-flaccid-myelitis/hcp/index.html).**
- **Hemorrhagic fever.** Hemorrhagic fevers can be caused by dengue (see Dengue, p 317) or yellow fever viruses. After several days of nonspecific febrile illness, the patient may develop overt signs of hemorrhage (eg, petechiae, ecchymoses, bleeding from the nose and gums, hematemesis, and melena) and shock (eg, decreased peripheral circulation, azotemia, tachycardia, and hypotension). Hemorrhagic fever and shock caused by yellow fever viruses has a high mortality rate and may be confused with hemorrhagic fevers transmitted by rodents (eg, Argentine hemorrhagic fever, Bolivian hemorrhagic fever, and Lassa fever) or those caused by Ebola or Marburg viruses. Although dengue may be associated with severe hemorrhage, the shock is primarily attributable to a capillary leak syndrome, which, if properly treated with fluids, can result in a high recovery rate. For information on other potential infections causing hemorrhagic manifestations, see Dengue (p 317), Hemorrhagic Fevers Caused by Arenaviruses (p 381), Hemorrhagic Fevers and Related Syndromes Caused by Bunyaviruses (p 384), and Hemorrhagic Fevers Caused by Filoviruses: Ebola and Marburg (p 387).

ETIOLOGY: Arboviruses are RNA viruses that are transmitted to humans primarily through bites of infected arthropods (mosquitoes, ticks, sand flies, and biting midges). The viral families responsible for most arboviral infections in humans are Flaviviridae (genus *Flavivirus*), Togaviridae (genus *Alphavirus*), and Bunyaviridae (genus *Orthobunyavirus* and *Phlebovirus*). Reoviridae (genus *Coltivirus*) also are responsible for a smaller number of human arboviral infections (eg, Colorado tick fever) (Table 3.2).

EPIDEMIOLOGY: Most arboviruses maintain cycles of transmission between birds or small mammals and arthropod vectors. Humans and domestic animals usually are infected incidentally as "dead-end" hosts (Table 3.2). Important exceptions are dengue, yellow fever, chikungunya, and Zika virus, which can be spread from person-to-arthropod-to-person (anthroponotic transmission). For other arboviruses, humans usually do not develop a

Table 3.2. Genus, Geographic Location, Vectors, and Average Number of Annual Cases Reported in the United States for Selected Domestic and International Arboviral Diseases

Virus	Genus	Predominant Geographic Locations		Vectors	Number of US Cases/ Year (Range)[a]
		United States	Non-United States		
Domestic					
Chikungunya	Alphavirus	Imported, and peri-odic local transmission	Asia, Africa, Indian Ocean, Western Pacific, Caribbean, South America, North America	Mosquitoes	2006–2013: 28 (5–65) 2014: 2811 2015: 896
Colorado tick fever	Coltivirus	Rocky Mountain states	Western Canada	Ticks	5 (4–14)
Dengue	Flavivirus	Puerto Rico, Florida, Texas, and Hawaii	Worldwide in tropical areas	Mosquitoes	725 (254–821)[b]
Eastern equine encephalitis	Alphavirus	Eastern and gulf states	Canada, Central and South America	Mosquitoes	7 (4–21)
Jamestown Canyon	Orthobunya-virus	Widespread	Canada	Mosquitoes	1 (0–25)
La Crosse	Orthobunya-virus	Midwest and Appala-chia	Canada	Mosquitoes	78 (50–130)
Powassan	Flavivirus	Northeast and Mid-west	Canada, Russia	Ticks	7 (0–16)
St. Louis encephalitis	Flavivirus	Widespread	Canada, Caribbean, Mexico, Central and South America	Mosquitoes	10 (1–49)
Western equine encephalitis	Alphavirus	Central and West	Central and South America	Mosquitoes	Less than 1

Table 3.2. Genus, Geographic Location, Vectors, and Average Number of Annual Cases Reported in the United States for Selected Domestic and International Arboviral Diseases, continued

| Virus | Genus | Predominant Geographic Locations | | Vectors | Number of US Cases/ Year (Range)[a] |
		United States	Non-United States		
West Nile	Flavivirus	Widespread	Canada, Europe, Africa, Asia, South America	Mosquitoes	2469 (712–9862)
Zika	Flavivirus	Imported, and periodic local transmission	Asia, Africa, Indian Ocean, Western Pacific, Caribbean, South America, North America	Mosquitoes	2010–2014: 11 2015: 54 2016: >2500[c]
International					
Japanese encephalitis	Flavivirus	Imported only	Asia	Mosquitoes	Less than 1
Mayaro	Alphavirus	Imported only	South America	Mosquitoes	Less than 1
Tickborne encephalitis	Flavivirus	Imported only	Europe, northern Asia	Ticks	Less than 1
Venezuelan equine encephalitis	Alphavirus	Imported only	Mexico, Central and South America	Mosquitoes	Less than 1
Yellow fever	Flavivirus	Imported only	South America, Africa	Mosquitoes	Less than 1

[a] Average annual number of domestic and/or imported cases reported from 2003 through 2015, unless otherwise noted.

[b] Data from 2010 through 2015, when dengue was nationally notifiable, includes domestic and imported cases reported to the CDC, excluding local transmission in Puerto Rico and the US Virgin Islands.

[c] Updated information on Zika virus in the Americas can be found at www.cdc.gov/zika/geo/united-states.html and www.paho.org/hq/index.php?option=com_content&view=article&id=11585&Itemid=41688&lang=en.

sustained or high enough level of viremia to infect biting arthropod vectors. Direct person-to-person spread of arboviruses can occur through blood transfusion, organ transplantation, sexual transmission, intrauterine transmission, perinatal transmission, and human milk (see Human Milk, p 113). Transmission through percutaneous, mucosal, or aerosol exposure to some arboviruses has occurred rarely in laboratory and occupational settings.

In the United States, arboviral infections primarily occur from late spring through early fall, when mosquitoes and ticks are most active. The number of domestic or imported arboviral disease cases reported in the United States varies greatly by specific etiology and year (Table 3.2). Underreporting and underdiagnosis of milder disease makes a true determination of the number of cases difficult.

Overall, the risk of severe clinical disease for most arboviral infections in the United States is higher among adults than among children. One notable exception is La Crosse virus infection, for which children are at highest risk of severe neurologic disease and possible long-term sequelae. Eastern equine encephalitis virus causes a low incidence of disease but high case fatality rate (40%) across all age groups.

The **incubation periods** for arboviral diseases typically range between 2 and 15 days. Longer incubation periods can occur in immunocompromised people and for tickborne viruses, such as tickborne encephalitis and Powassan viruses.

DIAGNOSTIC TESTS: Arboviral infections are confirmed most frequently by detection of virus-specific antibody in serum or cerebrospinal fluid (CSF). Acute-phase serum specimens should be tested for virus-specific immunoglobulin (Ig) M antibody. With clinical and epidemiologic correlation, a positive IgM test result has good diagnostic predictive value, but cross-reaction with related arboviruses from the same viral family can occur (eg, West Nile and St. Louis encephalitis viruses, which both are flaviviruses). For most arboviral infections, IgM is detectable 3 to 8 days after onset of illness and persists for 30 to 90 days, but longer persistence has been documented, especially with West Nile virus. Therefore, a positive serum IgM test result occasionally may reflect a prior infection. Serum collected within 10 days of illness onset may not have detectable IgM, and the test should be repeated on a convalescent sample. IgG antibody generally is detectable in serum shortly after IgM and persists for years. A plaque-reduction neutralization test can be performed to measure virus-specific neutralizing antibodies and to discriminate between cross-reacting antibodies in primary arboviral infections. Either seroconversion or a fourfold or greater increase in virus-specific neutralizing antibodies between acute- and convalescent-phase serum specimens collected 2 to 3 weeks apart may be used to confirm recent infection. In patients who have been immunized against or infected with another arbovirus from the same virus family in the past (ie, secondary infection), cross-reactive antibodies in both the IgM and neutralizing antibody assays may make it difficult to identify which arbovirus is causing the patient's illness. For some arboviral infections (eg, Colorado tick fever), the immune response may be delayed, with IgM antibodies not appearing until 2 to 3 weeks after onset of illness and neutralizing antibodies taking up to a month to develop. Patients with significant immunosuppression (eg, patients who have received a solid organ transplant or recent chemotherapy) may have a delayed or blunted serologic response. Immunization and travel history, date of symptom onset, and information regarding other arboviruses known to circulate in the geographic area that may cross-react in serologic assays should be considered when interpreting results.

Viral culture and nucleic acid amplification tests (NAATs) for RNA can be performed on acute-phase serum, CSF, or tissue specimens. Arboviruses that are more likely to be detected using culture or NAATs early in the illness include Colorado tick fever, dengue, yellow fever, and Zika viruses. For other arboviruses, results of these tests often are negative even early in the clinical course because of the relatively short duration of viremia. Immunohistochemical staining (IHC) can detect specific viral antigen in fixed tissue.

Antibody testing for common domestic arboviral diseases is performed in most state public health laboratories and many commercial laboratories. Confirmatory plaque-reduction neutralization tests, viral culture, NAATs, immunohistochemical staining, and testing for less common domestic and international arboviruses are performed at the Centers for Disease Control and Prevention (CDC; telephone: 970-221-6400) and selected other reference laboratories. Confirmatory testing typically is arranged through local and state health departments.

TREATMENT: The primary treatment for all arboviral disease is supportive. Although various antiviral and immunologic therapies have been evaluated for several arboviral diseases, none have shown clear benefit.

ISOLATION OF THE HOSPITALIZED PATIENT: Standard precautions are recommended.

CONTROL MEASURES: Reduction of vectors in areas with endemic transmission is important to reduce risk of infection. Use of certain personal protective strategies can help decrease the risk of human infection. These strategies include using insect repellent, wearing long pants and long-sleeved shirts while outdoors, conducting a full-body check for ticks after outdoor activities, staying in screened or air-conditioned dwellings, and limiting outdoor activities during peak vector feeding times (see Prevention of Mosquitoborne and Tickborne Infections, p 194). Select arboviral infections also can be prevented through screening of blood and organ donations and through immunization. The blood supply in the United States is routinely screened for West Nile and Zika viruses. Although some arboviruses can be transmitted through human milk, transmission appears rare. Because the benefits of breastfeeding seem to outweigh the low risk of illness in breastfeeding infants, mothers should be encouraged to breastfeed even in areas of active arboviral transmission. Because Zika virus can be transmitted by sex, the CDC has issued guidance for prevention of sexual transmission (see Zika, p 894).

Vaccines are available in the United States to protect against travel-related yellow fever and Japanese encephalitis.

Yellow Fever Vaccine.[1] Live attenuated (17D strain) yellow fever vaccine is available at state-approved immunization centers. A single dose provides long-term protection for most individuals. Unless contraindicated, yellow fever immunization is recommended for all people 9 months or older living in or traveling to areas with endemic disease and is required by international regulations for travel to and from certain countries (**wwwnc.cdc.gov/travel/**). Infants younger than 6 months should not be immunized with yellow fever vaccine, because they have an increased risk of vaccine-associated encephalitis. The decision to immunize infants between 6 and 9 months of age must balance the infant's risk of exposure with the risk of vaccine-associated encephalitis.

Booster doses of yellow fever vaccine are no longer recommended for most travelers,

---

[1]Centers for Disease Control and Prevention. Yellow fever vaccine: recommendations of the Advisory Committee on Immunization Practices (ACIP). *MMWR Recomm Rep.* 2010;59(RR-7):1–27

because a single dose of yellow fever vaccine provides long-lasting protection.[1] However, additional doses of yellow fever vaccine are recommended for certain populations (ie, women initially vaccinated when they were pregnant, hematopoietic stem cell transplant recipients, and people infected with human immunodeficiency virus [HIV]) who might not have a robust or sustained immune response to yellow fever vaccine compared with other recipients. Furthermore, additional doses may be administered to certain groups believed to be at increased risk for yellow fever disease because of their location and duration of travel or because of more consistent exposure to virulent virus (ie, laboratory workers).

Yellow fever vaccine is a live-virus vaccine produced in embryonic chicken eggs and, thus, is contraindicated in people who have a history of acute hypersensitivity to eggs or egg products and in people who are immunocompromised. Procedures for immunizing people with severe egg allergy are described in the vaccine package insert. Generally, people who are able to eat eggs or egg products may receive the vaccine. Pregnancy and breastfeeding are precautions to yellow fever vaccine administration, because rare cases of transmission of the vaccine virus in utero or through breastfeeding have been documented. Whenever possible, pregnant and breastfeeding women should defer travel to areas where yellow fever is endemic. If travel to an area with endemic disease is unavoidable and the risks for yellow fever virus exposure are believed to outweigh the vaccination risks, a pregnant or breastfeeding woman should be vaccinated. If the risks of vaccination are believed to outweigh the risks for yellow fever virus exposure, a pregnant or breastfeeding woman should be excused from immunization and issued a medical waiver letter to fulfill health regulations. For more detailed information on the yellow fever vaccine, including adverse events, precautions, and contraindications, visit **wwwnc.cdc.gov/travel/** or see Required or Recommended Travel-Related Immunizations (p 106).

As of early 2018, the yellow fever vaccine (YF-VAX) is in shortage in the United States. A new manufacturing facility is anticipated to open in 2018 and should alleviate this production problem. In the interim, the manufacturer of YF-VAX, Sanofi Pasteur, has worked with the FDA to import its Stamaril yellow fever vaccine under an investigational new drug (IND) application and distribute it in the United States in an Expanded Access Program. Stamaril is manufactured by Sanofi Pasteur in France and uses the 17D-204 strain of yellow fever virus, which is the same strain as in YF-VAX. More than 430 million doses have been distributed worldwide, and its safety and efficacy profile is comparable to YF-VAX vaccine. During this period of shortage of YF-VAX, health care providers of yellow fever vaccine can direct their patients to Stamaril vaccine sites (**wwwnc.cdc.gov/travel/page/search-for-stamaril-clinics**).

Japanese Encephalitis Vaccine.[2] The risk of Japanese encephalitis for most travelers to Asia is low but varies on the basis of destination, duration, season, and activities. All travelers to countries with endemic Japanese encephalitis should be informed of the risks and should use personal protective measures to reduce the risk of mosquito bites. For some travelers who will be in high-risk settings, Japanese encephalitis vaccine can further reduce the risk for infection. The CDC recommends Japanese encephalitis vaccine for travelers who plan

[1]Staples JE, Bocchini JA, Rubin L, Fischer M. Yellow fever vaccine booster doses: recommendations of the Advisory Committee on Immunization Practices, 2015. *MMWR Morb Mortal Wkly Rep.* 2015;64(23):647–650

[2]Centers for Disease Control and Prevention. Inactivated Japanese encephalitis vaccines: recommendations of the Advisory Committee on Immunization Practices (ACIP). *MMWR Recomm Rep.* 2010;59(RR-1):1–27

to spend a month or longer in areas with endemic infection during the Japanese encephalitis virus transmission season. Japanese encephalitis vaccine also should be considered for shorter-term travelers if they plan to travel outside of an urban area and have an itinerary or activities that will increase their risk of mosquito exposure in an endemic area. Information on the location of Japanese encephalitis virus transmission and detailed information on vaccine recommendations and adverse events can be obtained from the CDC (**wwwnc.cdc.gov/travel/**).

An inactivated Vero cell culture-derived Japanese encephalitis vaccine (Ixiaro [JE-VC]) is licensed and available in the United States for use in adults and children 2 months and older.[1] The primary vaccination series is 2 doses administered 28 days apart. The dose is 0.25 mL for children 2 months through 2 years of age and 0.5 mL for adults and children 3 years and older. For adults, a booster dose may be administered at 1 year or longer after the primary series if ongoing exposure or reexposure is expected.[2] From the one available observational study, most adults were still seroprotected approximately 6 years after receiving a booster dose. Data are not yet available on the need for a booster dose in children. In one pediatric long-term duration of protection study conducted among children from countries without endemic Japanese encephalitis, 89% of children were seroprotected at 3 years following a primary 2-dose series of JE-VC.

No efficacy data exist for JE-VC. The vaccine was licensed on the basis of its ability to induce Japanese encephalitis virus-neutralizing antibodies as a surrogate for protection and because of its safety profile. No safety concerns have been identified in passive post-marketing surveillance of more than 400 000 doses distributed in the United States.

Other Arboviral Vaccines. An inactivated vaccine for tickborne encephalitis virus is licensed in some countries in Europe where the disease is endemic, but this vaccine is not available in the United States. A live attenuated tetravalent dengue vaccine has been licensed in several countries in Latin America and Asia but is not yet licensed in the United States. Chikungunya and Zika virus vaccines are under development.

REPORTING: Most arboviral diseases are nationally notifiable conditions and should be reported to the appropriate local and state health authorities. For select arboviruses (eg, chikungunya, dengue, and yellow fever viruses), patients may remain viremic during their acute illness. Such patients pose a risk for further person-to-mosquito-to-person transmission, increasing the importance of timely reporting.

Arcanobacterium haemolyticum Infections

CLINICAL MANIFESTATIONS: Acute pharyngitis attributable to *Arcanobacterium haemolyticum* often is indistinguishable from group A streptococcal pharyngitis. Fever, erythema and exudates, cervical lymphadenopathy, and rash are common, but palatal petechiae and strawberry tongue are absent. A morbilliform or scarlatiniform exanthem is present in half of cases, beginning on extensor surfaces of the distal extremities, spreading

---

[1]Centers for Disease Control and Prevention. Use of Japanese encephalitis vaccine in children: recommendations of the Advisory Committee on Immunization Practices, 2013. *MMWR Morb Mortal Wkly Rep.* 2013;62(45):898–910

[2]Centers for Disease Control and Prevention. Recommendations for use of a booster dose of inactivated Vero cell culture-derived Japanese encephalitis vaccine— Advisory Committee on Immunization Practices, 2011. *MMWR Morb Mortal Wkly Rep.* 2011;60(20):661–663

centripetally, sparing the face, palms, and soles. Rash typically develops 1 to 4 days after onset of sore throat, although rash preceding pharyngitis can occur. Respiratory tract infections that mimic diphtheria, including membranous pharyngitis, peritonsillar and pharyngeal abscesses, and skin and soft tissue infections, including chronic ulcers, cellulitis, paronychia, and wound infection, have been attributed to *A haemolyticum*. Invasive infections may include peritonsillar abscess, Lemierre syndrome, bacteremia, sepsis, endocarditis, brain abscess, orbital cellulitis, pyogenic arthritis, or rarely, other infections. No nonsuppurative sequelae have been reported.

ETIOLOGY: *A haemolyticum* is a catalase-negative, weakly acid-fast, facultative, hemolytic, anaerobic, gram-positive to gram-variable, slender, sometimes club-shaped bacillus formerly classified as *Corynebacterium haemolyticum*.

EPIDEMIOLOGY: Humans are the primary reservoir of *A haemolyticum*, and spread is person to person, presumably via droplet respiratory secretions. Severe disease occurs almost exclusively among immunocompromised people. *Arcanobacterium* pharyngitis occurs primarily in adolescents and young adults and only rarely in young children. *A haemolyticum* accounts for approximately 0.5% of pharyngeal infections overall and 2.5% of pharyngeal infections in 15- to 25-year-olds. Isolation of the bacterium from the nasopharynx of asymptomatic people is rare. *A haemolyticum* can be isolated with other pathogens. Person-to-person spread is inferred from family studies.

The **incubation period** is unknown.

DIAGNOSTIC TESTS: *A haemolyticum* grows on blood-enriched agar, but colonies are small, have narrow bands of hemolysis, and may not be visible for 48 to 72 hours. The organism is not detected by rapid antigen tests for group A streptococci. Detection is enhanced by culture on rabbit or human blood agar rather than on sheep blood agar, which yields larger colony size and wider zones of hemolysis. Presence of 5% carbon dioxide enhances growth. *A haemolyticum* is missed in routine throat cultures on sheep blood agar if laboratory personnel are not trained specifically to identify the organism. Pits characteristically form under colonies on blood agar plates. Two biotypes of *A haemolyticum* have been identified: a rough colonial biotype predominates in respiratory tract infections, and a smooth biotype typically in skin and soft-tissue infections.

TREATMENT: Erythromycin and azithromycin are drugs of choice for *A haemolyticum* tonsillopharyngitis, but no prospective trials have been performed. *A haemolyticum* generally is susceptible in vitro to azithromycin, erythromycin, clindamycin, ciprofloxacin, vancomycin, and tetracycline. Treatment failures with penicillin despite predicted susceptibility from in vitro testing have been described, which likely is attributable to the organism's intracellular survival. Resistance to trimethoprim-sulfamethoxazole is common. In rare cases of disseminated infection, susceptibility tests should be performed. While awaiting results, initial empiric combination therapy can be initiated using a parenteral beta lactam agent, with or without a macrolide, and with consideration of metronidazole if *Fusobacterium* infection is possible.

ISOLATION OF THE HOSPITALIZED PATIENT: Standard precautions are recommended.

CONTROL MEASURES: None.

Ascaris lumbricoides Infections

CLINICAL MANIFESTATIONS: Most infections with *Ascaris lumbricoides* are asymptomatic, although moderate to heavy infections may lead to nonspecific gastrointestinal tract symptoms, malnutrition, and growth delay. During the larval migratory phase, an acute transient pneumonitis (Löffler syndrome) associated with cough, substernal discomfort, fever, and marked eosinophilia may occur. Acute intestinal obstruction has been associated with heavy infections. Children are prone to this complication because of the small diameter of the intestinal lumen and their propensity to acquire large worm burdens. Worm migration can cause peritonitis secondary to intestinal wall perforation, as well as appendicitis or common bile duct obstruction resulting in biliary colic, cholangitis, or pancreatitis. Adult worms can be stimulated to migrate by stressful conditions (eg, fever, illness, or anesthesia) and by some anthelmintic drugs.

ETIOLOGY: Following ingestion of embryonated eggs, usually from contaminated soil, larvae hatch in the small intestine, penetrate the mucosa, and are transported passively by portal blood to the liver and lungs. After migrating into the airways, larvae ascend through the tracheobronchial tree to the pharynx, are swallowed, and mature into adults in the small intestine. Female worms produce approximately 200 000 eggs per day, which are excreted in stool and must incubate in soil for 2 to 3 weeks to become infectious. Adult worms can live in the lumen of the small intestine for 12 to 18 months. Female worms are longer than male worms and can measure 40 cm in length and 6 mm in diameter.

EPIDEMIOLOGY: *A lumbricoides* is the most prevalent of all human intestinal nematodes (roundworms), with approximately 1 billion people infected worldwide. Infection with *A lumbricoides* is most common in resource-limited countries, including rural and urban communities characterized by poor sanitation. Direct person-to-person transmission does not occur.

The **incubation period** (interval between ingestion of eggs and development of egg-laying adults) is approximately 9 to 11 weeks.

DIAGNOSTIC TESTS: Ascariasis is diagnosed by examining a fresh or preserved stool specimen for eggs using light microscopy. Adult worms also may be passed from the rectum, through the nares, or from the mouth, usually in vomitus. Imaging of the gastrointestinal tract or biliary tree using computed tomography or ultrasonography may detect adult *Ascaris* worms, which can cause filling defects following administration of oral contrast.

TREATMENT: Albendazole (taken with food in a single dose), mebendazole (a single dose or once daily for 3 days), and pyrantel pamoate are first-line agents for treatment of ascariasis. Ivermectin (taken on an empty stomach in a single dose) and nitazoxanide are alternative therapies. Cure rates range from 90% with pyrantel pamoate to 100% with albendazole (see Drugs for Parasitic Infections, p 985). Albendazole, pyrantel pamoate, and ivermectin are not approved by the US Food and Drug Administration for treatment of ascariasis, although albendazole has become the drug of choice for most soil-transmitted nematode infections, including *Ascaris*. Studies in children as young as 1 year suggest that albendazole can be administered safely to this population. Safety of ivermectin in children weighing less than 15 kg and in pregnant women has not been established. Reexamination of stool specimens may be performed 2 to 3 months after therapy and patients who remain infected can be retreated.

Conservative management of small bowel obstruction, including nasogastric suction and intravenous fluids, may alleviate symptoms before administration of anthelmintic therapy. Use of mineral oil or diatrizoate meglumine and diatrizoate sodium solution (Gastrografin), either orally or by nasogastric tube, also may cause relaxation of a bolus of worms. Although not available in the United States, treatment with piperazine has been recommended for relief of intestinal obstruction caused by high-intensity infection with *A lumbricoides*. Endoscopic retrograde cholangiopancreatography has been used successfully for extraction of worms from the biliary tree. Surgical intervention (eg, laparotomy) is indicated for intestinal or biliary tract obstruction that does not resolve with conservative therapy or for patients with volvulus or peritonitis secondary to perforation.

ISOLATION OF THE HOSPITALIZED PATIENT: Standard precautions are recommended.

CONTROL MEASURES: Sanitary disposal of human feces prevents transmission. Vegetables cultivated in areas where uncomposted human feces are used as fertilizer must be washed thoroughly and cooked before eating.

Preventive chemotherapy (once or twice annually with albendazole [400 mg] or mebendazole [500 mg]) targeting high-risk groups, most notably preschool or school-aged children, is recommended by the World Health Organization for control of *A lumbricoides* and other soil-transmitted nematodes in communities with >20% prevalence of infection. Reinfection is common in high-prevalence areas, and additional public health measures, including improved sanitation, safe drinking water, and health education, will be required to eliminate these infections.

Aspergillosis

CLINICAL MANIFESTATIONS: Aspergillosis manifests as 5 principal clinical entities: invasive aspergillosis, pulmonary aspergilloma, allergic bronchopulmonary aspergillosis, allergic sinusitis, and chronic aspergillosis. Colonization of the respiratory tract is common. The clinical manifestations and severity depend on the immune status (either immunocompromised or atopic) of the host.

- Invasive aspergillosis occurs almost exclusively in immunocompromised patients with prolonged neutropenia, graft-versus-host disease, or impaired phagocyte function (eg, chronic granulomatous disease) or those who have received T-lymphocyte immunosuppressive therapy (eg, corticosteroids, calcineurin inhibitors, tumor necrosis factor [TNF]-alpha inhibitors). Children at highest risk include those with new-onset acute myelogenous leukemia, relapse of hematologic malignancy, aplastic anemia, chronic granulomatous disease, and recipients of allogeneic hematopoietic stem cell and certain types (eg, heart, lung) of solid organ transplants. Invasive infection usually involves pulmonary, sinus, cerebral, or cutaneous sites. Rarely, endocarditis, osteomyelitis, meningitis, peritonitis, infection of the eye or orbit, and esophagitis occur. The hallmark of invasive aspergillosis is angioinvasion with resulting thrombosis, dissemination to other organs, and occasionally erosion of the blood vessel wall with catastrophic hemorrhage. Invasive aspergillosis in patients with chronic granulomatous disease is unique in that it is more indolent and displays a general lack of angioinvasion.
- Aspergillomas and otomycosis are 2 syndromes of nonallergic colonization by *Aspergillus* species in immunocompetent children. Aspergillomas ("fungal balls") grow in preexisting pulmonary cavities or bronchogenic cysts without invading pulmonary tissue; almost all patients have underlying lung disease, such as cystic fibrosis or tuberculosis. Patients with otomycosis have chronic otitis media with colonization of the external auditory canal by a fungal mat that produces a dark discharge.
- Allergic bronchopulmonary aspergillosis is a hypersensitivity lung disease that manifests as episodic wheezing, expectoration of brown mucus plugs, low-grade fever,

eosinophilia, and transient pulmonary infiltrates. This form of aspergillosis occurs most commonly in immunocompetent children with asthma or cystic fibrosis and can be a trigger for asthmatic flares.

- Allergic sinusitis is a far less common allergic response to colonization by *Aspergillus* species than is allergic bronchopulmonary aspergillosis. Allergic sinusitis occurs in children with nasal polyps or previous episodes of sinusitis or in children who have undergone sinus surgery. Allergic sinusitis is characterized by symptoms of chronic sinusitis with dark plugs of nasal discharge and is different from invasive *Aspergillus* sinusitis.

- Chronic aspergillosis typically affects patients who are not immunocompromised or are less immunocompromised, although exposure to corticosteroids is common, and patients often have underlying pulmonary conditions. Diagnosis of chronic aspergillosis requires at least 3 months of chronic pulmonary symptoms or chronic illness or progressive radiologic abnormalities along with an elevated *Aspergillus* immunoglobulin (Ig) G concentration or other microbiological evidence. Because of the ubiquitous nature of *Aspergillus* species, a positive sputum culture alone is not diagnostic.

ETIOLOGY: *Aspergillus* species are ubiquitous molds that grow on decaying vegetation and in soil. *Aspergillus fumigatus* is the most common (>75%) cause of invasive aspergillosis, with *Aspergillus flavus* being the next most common. Several other major species, including *Aspergillus terreus*, *Aspergillus nidulans*, and *Aspergillus niger*, also cause invasive human infections. Of increasing concern are emerging *Aspergillus* species that are resistant to antifungals, such as *Aspergillus calidoustus* (azole resistant).

EPIDEMIOLOGY: The principal route of transmission is inhalation of conidia (spores) originating from multiple environmental sources (eg, plants, vegetables, dust from construction or demolition), soil, and water supplies (eg, shower heads). Incidence of disease in hematopoietic stem cell transplant recipients is highest during periods of neutropenia or during treatment for graft-versus-host disease. In solid organ transplant recipients, the risk is highest approximately 6 months after transplantation or during periods of increased immunosuppression. Disease has followed use of contaminated marijuana in the immunocompromised host. Health care-associated outbreaks of invasive pulmonary aspergillosis in susceptible hosts have occurred in which the probable source of the fungus was a nearby construction site or faulty ventilation system; however, the source of health care-associated aspergillosis frequently is not known. Cutaneous aspergillosis occurs less frequently and usually involves sites of skin injury, such as intravenous catheter sites (including in neonates), sites of traumatic inoculation, and sites associated with occlusive dressings, burns, or surgery. Transmission by direct inoculation of skin abrasions or wounds is less likely. Person-to-person spread does not occur.

The **incubation period** is unknown and may be variable.

DIAGNOSTIC TESTS: Dichotomously branched and septate hyphae, identified by microscopic examination of 10% potassium hydroxide wet preparations or of Gomori methenamine-silver nitrate stain of tissue or bronchoalveolar lavage specimens, are suggestive of the diagnosis. Isolation of *Aspergillus* species or molecular testing with specific reagents is required for definitive diagnosis. The organism usually is not recoverable from blood (except *A terreus*) but is isolated readily from lung, sinus, and skin biopsy specimens when cultured on Sabouraud dextrose agar or brain-heart infusion media (without cycloheximide). *Aspergillus* species can be a laboratory contaminant, but when evaluating results from immunocompromised patients, recovery of this organism frequently indicates infection. Biopsy is required to confirm the diagnosis, and care should be taken to distinguish aspergillosis from mucormycosis, which appears similar by diagnostic imaging studies but is pauci-septate (few septa) and requires a different treatment regimen.

An enzyme immunosorbent assay for detection of galactomannan, a molecule found in the cell wall of *Aspergillus* species, from serum or bronchoalveolar lavage (BAL) fluid is available commercially and has been found to be useful in children and adults. A test result of ≥0.5 from the serum or ≥1.0 from BAL fluid supports a diagnosis of invasive aspergillosis, and monitoring of serum antigen concentrations twice weekly in periods of highest risk (eg, neutropenia and active graft-versus-host disease) may be useful for early detection of invasive aspergillosis in at-risk patients. False-positive test results have been reported and can be related to consumption of food products containing galactomannan (eg, rice and pasta), other invasive fungal infections (eg, *Fusarium*), and colonization of the gut of neonates with *Bifidobacterium* species. Previous cross-reactivity with antimicrobial agents derived from fungi (especially piperacillin-tazobactam) no longer occurs because of manufacturing changes. A negative galactomannan test result does not exclude diagnosis of invasive aspergillosis, and the greatest utility may be in monitoring response to disease rather than in its use as a diagnostic marker. False-negative galactomannan test results consistently occur in patients with chronic granulomatous disease, so the test should not be used in these patients. Galactomannan is not recommended for routine screening in patients receiving mold-active antifungal therapy or prophylaxis (see Table 4.7, p 942). Galactomannan is not recommended for screening in solid organ transplant recipients because of poor sensitivity.

Limited data suggest that other nonspecific fungal biomarkers, such as 1,3-β-D glucan testing, may be useful in the diagnosis of aspergillosis. *Aspergillus* polymerase chain reaction testing is promising but not yet recommended for routine clinical use. Unlike adults, children frequently do not manifest cavitation or the air crescent or halo signs on chest radiography, and lack of these characteristic signs does not exclude the diagnosis of invasive aspergillosis.

In allergic aspergillosis, diagnosis is suggested by a typical clinical syndrome with elevated total concentrations of IgE (≥1000 ng/mL) and *Aspergillus*-specific serum IgE, eosinophilia, and a positive result from a skin test for *Aspergillus* antigens. In people with cystic fibrosis, the diagnosis is more difficult, because wheezing, eosinophilia, and a positive skin test result not associated with allergic bronchopulmonary aspergillosis often are present.

TREATMENT[1]: Voriconazole is the drug of choice for all clinical forms of invasive aspergillosis, except in neonates, for whom amphotericin B deoxycholate in high doses is recommended (see Antifungal Drugs for Systemic Fungal Infections, p 938). Voriconazole has been shown to be superior to amphotericin B in a large, randomized trial in adults. Immune reconstitution is paramount; decreasing immunosuppression, if possible (specifically corticosteroid dose), is critical to disease control. The diagnostic workup needs to be aggressive to confirm disease, but it should never delay antifungal therapy in the setting of true concern for invasive aspergillosis. Therapy is continued for a minimum of 6 to 12 weeks, but treatment duration should be individualized on the basis of degree and duration of immunosuppression. Monitoring of serum galactomannan concentrations in those with significant elevation at onset may be useful to assess response to therapy concomitant with clinical and radiologic evaluation. Voriconazole is metabolized in a linear fashion in

[1]Patterson TF, Thompson GR 3rd, Denning DW. Practice guidelines for the diagnosis and management of aspergillosis: 2016 update by the Infectious Diseases Society of America. *Clin Infect Dis.* 2016;63(4):e1–e60

children (nonlinear in adults), so the recommended adult dosing (per kg) is too low for children, especially the youngest children. The optimal dose for children 2 to 12 years of age is to load with 9 mg/kg, intravenously, every 12 hours, for 1 day and then continue with 8 mg/kg/dose, intravenously, every 12 hours. Children 12 years and older who weigh ≥50 kg should receive the adult dose of 6 mg/kg, intravenously, every 12 hours, for 1 day and then continue with 4 mg/kg/dose, intravenously, every 12 hours. Conversion to oral voriconazole requires a dose increase to 9 mg/kg, orally, every 12 hours, because the bioavailability of oral voriconazole in children is only approximately 50% (versus >90% in adults). Close monitoring of voriconazole serum trough concentrations is critical for both efficacy and safety, and most experts agree that for children, voriconazole trough concentrations should be between 2 μg/mL and 6 μg/mL.[1,2] It is important to individualize dosing in patients following initiation of voriconazole therapy, because there is high interpatient variability in metabolism. Certain *Aspergillus* species (*A calidoustus*) are inherently resistant to azoles, and isolation of azole-resistant *A fumigatus* is increasing and may be related to environmental acquisition through use of agricultural pesticides.

Alternative therapies include liposomal amphotericin B, isavuconazole, or other lipid formulations of amphotericin B. Primary therapy with an echinocandin alone (caspofungin, micafungin) is not recommended, but an echinocandin can be used in settings in which an azole or amphotericin B are contraindicated.

Caspofungin has been studied in pediatric patients older than 3 months as salvage therapy for invasive aspergillosis. The pharmacokinetics of caspofungin in adults differ from those in children, in whom a body-surface area dosing scheme is preferred to a weight-based dosing regimen. Limited data from a predominantly adult population are available but suggest that micafungin and caspofungin have similar efficacy in treatment of refractory aspergillosis. Caspofungin is FDA approved for children 3 months and older, with a loading dose of 70 mg/m^2, followed by daily maintenance dosing of 50 mg/m^2 (not to exceed 70 mg).[3] In refractory disease, treatment may include posaconazole. The pharmacokinetics and safety of posaconazole have not been evaluated in younger children. Posaconazole absorption is significantly improved with use of the extended-release tablet than the oral suspension. Isavuconazole is an alternative therapy in adults but has not been studied in children.

Combination antifungal therapy with voriconazole and an echinocandin may be considered in select patients with documented invasive aspergillosis.

If primary antifungal therapy fails, general strategies for salvage therapy include (a) changing the class of antifungal; (b) tapering or reversal of underlying immunosuppression when feasible; (c) susceptibility testing of any *Aspergillus* isolates recovered; and (d) surgical resection of necrotic lesions in selected cases. In pulmonary disease, surgery is indicated only when a mass is impinging on a great vessel.

Allergic bronchopulmonary aspergillosis is treated with corticosteroids, and adjunctive antifungal therapy is recommended. Allergic sinus aspergillosis also is treated with

[1]Chen J, Chan C, Colantonio D, et al. Therapeutic drug monitoring of voriconazole in children. *Ther Drug Monit*. 2012;34(1):77–84

[2]Choi SH, Lee SY, Hwang JY, et al. Importance of voriconazole therapeutic drug monitoring in pediatric cancer patients with invasive aspergillosis. *Pediatr Blood Cancer*. 2013;60(1):82–87

[3]Patterson TF, Thompson GR 3rd, Denning DW. Practice guidelines for the diagnosis and management of aspergillosis: 2016 update by the Infectious Diseases Society of America. *Clin Infect Dis*. 2016;63(4):e1–e60

corticosteroids, and surgery has been reported to be beneficial in many cases. Antifungal therapy has not been found to be useful, but there may be an emerging role for immunotherapy.

ISOLATION OF THE HOSPITALIZED PATIENT: Standard precautions are recommended.

CONTROL MEASURES: Outbreaks of invasive aspergillosis and *Aspergillus* colonization have occurred among hospitalized patients during construction in hospitals or at nearby sites. Environmental measures reported to be effective include erecting suitable barriers between patient care areas and construction sites, routine cleaning of air-handling systems, repair of faulty air flow, and replacement of contaminated air filters. High-efficiency particulate air filters and laminar flow rooms markedly decrease the risk of exposure to conidia in patient care areas. These latter measures may be expensive and difficult for patients to tolerate.

Posaconazole has been shown to be effective in 2 randomized controlled trials as prophylaxis against invasive aspergillosis for patients 13 years and older who have undergone hematopoietic stem cell transplantation and have graft-versus-host disease and in patients with hematologic malignancies with prolonged neutropenia, although breakthrough disease has been reported in those with gastrointestinal tract issues (eg, graft-versus-host disease) affecting drug bioavailability. Low-dose amphotericin B, itraconazole, voriconazole, or posaconazole prophylaxis have been reported for other high-risk patients, but controlled trials have not been completed in pediatric patients.

Patients at risk of invasive infection should avoid high environmental exposure (eg, gardening) following discharge from the hospital. People with allergic aspergillosis should take measures to reduce exposure to *Aspergillus* species in the home.

Astrovirus Infections

CLINICAL MANIFESTATIONS: Astrovirus illness is characterized by acute diarrhea accompanied by low-grade fever, malaise, and nausea, and less commonly, vomiting and mild dehydration. Illness in an immunocompetent host is self-limited, lasting a median of 5 to 6 days. Asymptomatic infections are common. Recently, astrovirus infections associated with encephalitis and meningitis have been reported, particularly in immunocompromised individuals.

ETIOLOGY: Astroviruses are nonenveloped, single-stranded RNA viruses with a characteristic starlike appearance when visualized by electron microscopy. Genetically, astroviruses can be classified in the genus *Mamastrovirus* (MAstV), which infect humans, and *Avastrovirus*, which infect poultry. Four distinct astroviruses have been identified in humans: MAstV 1, MAstV 3, MAstV 8, and MAstV 9. MAstV 1 include the 8 antigenic types of classic human astroviruses, whereas MAstV 3, MAstV 8, and MAstV 9 are novel astroviruses that have been identified in recent years.

EPIDEMIOLOGY: Human astroviruses have a worldwide distribution. Multiple antigenic types cocirculate in the same region. MAstV 1 astroviruses have been detected in as many as 5% to 17% of sporadic cases of nonbacterial gastroenteritis among young children in the community but appear to cause a lower proportion of cases of more severe childhood gastroenteritis requiring hospitalization (2.5% to 9%). MAstV 1 infections occur predominantly in children younger than 4 years and have a seasonal peak during the late winter and spring in the United States. Transmission is via the fecal-oral route through contaminated food or water, person-to-person contact, or contaminated surfaces. Outbreaks tend to occur in closed populations of the young and the elderly, particularly among hospitalized children (health care-associated infections) and children in child care centers. Excretion lasts a median of 5 days after onset of symptoms, but asymptomatic excretion after illness can last for several weeks in healthy children. Persistent excretion may occur in immunocompromised hosts. Astroviruses have been detected sporadically in stool samples, blood, cerebrospinal fluid, and brain tissue of immunocompromised patients with acute encephalitis.

The **incubation period** is 3 to 4 days.

DIAGNOSTIC TESTS: Commercial tests for diagnosis have not been available in the United States until recently, although enzyme immunoassays are available in many other countries. Two multiplex nucleic acid-based assays for the detection of gastrointestinal tract pathogens, one of which includes astrovirus (MAstV 1), are approved by the US Food and Drug Administration (FDA). These multiplex tests are more sensitive and are replacing traditional tests to detect fecal viral pathogens. Interpretation of assay results may be complicated by the frequent detection of viruses in fecal samples from asymptomatic children and the detection of multiple viruses in a single sample. A few research and reference laboratories perform enzyme immunoassay for detection of viral antigen in stool and real-time reverse transcriptase-polymerase chain reaction (RT-PCR) assay for detection of viral RNA in stool. Of these tests, RT-PCR assay is the most sensitive.

TREATMENT: No specific antiviral therapy is available. Oral or parenteral fluids and electrolytes are given to prevent and correct dehydration.

ISOLATION OF THE HOSPITALIZED PATIENT: In addition to standard precautions, contact precautions are recommended for diapered or incontinent children for the duration of illness.

CONTROL MEASURES: No specific control measures are available. The spread of infection in child care settings can be decreased by using general measures for control of diarrhea, such as training care providers in infection-control procedures, maintaining cleanliness of surfaces, keeping food preparation duties and areas separate from child care activities, exercising adequate hand hygiene, cohorting ill children, and excluding ill child care providers, food handlers, and children (see Children in Out-of-Home Child Care, p 122).

Babesiosis

CLINICAL MANIFESTATIONS: *Babesia* infection often is asymptomatic or associated with mild, nonspecific symptoms. The infection can be severe and life threatening, particularly in people who are asplenic, immunocompromised, or elderly. In general, babesiosis, like malaria, is characterized by the presence of fever and hemolytic anemia; however, some infected people who are immunocompromised or at the extremes of age (eg, preterm infants) are afebrile. Infected people may have a prodromal illness, with gradual onset of symptoms, such as malaise, anorexia, and fatigue, followed by development of fever and other influenza-like symptoms (eg, chills, sweats, myalgia, arthralgia, headache, anorexia, nausea). Less common findings include sore throat, nonproductive cough, abdominal pain, vomiting, weight loss, conjunctival injection, photophobia, emotional lability, and hyperesthesia. Congenital infection with nonspecific manifestations suggestive of sepsis has been reported.

Clinical signs generally are minimal, often consisting only of fever and tachycardia, although hypotension, respiratory distress, mild hepatosplenomegaly, jaundice, and dark urine may be noted. Thrombocytopenia is common; disseminated intravascular coagulation can be a complication of severe babesiosis. If untreated, the infection can last for several weeks or months; even asymptomatic people can have persistent low-level parasitemia, sometimes for longer than 1 year.

ETIOLOGY: *Babesia* species are intraerythrocytic protozoa. The etiologic agents of babesiosis in the United States include *Babesia microti*, which is the cause of most reported cases, and several other genetically and antigenically distinct organisms, such as *Babesia duncani* (formerly the WA1-type parasite).

EPIDEMIOLOGY: Babesiosis predominantly is a tickborne zoonosis. *Babesia* parasites also can be transmitted via blood transfusion and congenital/perinatal routes. In the United States, the primary reservoir host for *B microti* is the white-footed mouse *(Peromyscus leucopus),* and the tick vector is *Ixodes scapularis,* which can transmit other pathogens, such as *Borrelia burgdorferi,* the causative agent of Lyme disease, and *Anaplasma phagocytophilum,* the causative agent of human granulocytic anaplasmosis. The tick bite often is not noticed, in part because the nymphal stage of the tick is about the size of a poppy seed. White-tailed deer *(Odocoileus virginianus)* serve as hosts for blood meals by the tick but are not reservoir hosts of *B microti.* An increase in the deer population in some geographic regions, including in some suburban areas, during the past few decades is thought to be a major factor in the spread of *I scapularis.* The reported vectorborne cases of *B microti* infection have been acquired in the Northeast (particularly, in parts of Connecticut, Massachusetts, New Jersey, New York, and Rhode Island, as well as other states, including Maine and Pennsylvania) and in the upper Midwest (Wisconsin and Minnesota). Occasional human cases of babesiosis caused by other species have been described in various regions of the United States; tick vectors and reservoir hosts for these agents typically have not yet been identified. Whereas most US vectorborne cases of babesiosis occur during late spring, summer, or fall, transfusion-associated cases can occur year round. There were 1804 confirmed cases of babesiosis in 2015, with the majority in the New England and Mid-Atlantic regions.

The **incubation period** typically ranges from approximately 1 week to 5 weeks following a tick bite. The median **incubation period** following a contaminated blood transfusion is 37 days (range, 11 to 176 days) but occasionally is longer (eg, latent infection might become symptomatic after splenectomy).

DIAGNOSTIC TESTS: Acute, symptomatic cases of babesiosis typically are diagnosed by microscopic identification of *Babesia* parasites on Giemsa- or Wright-stained blood smears. If the diagnosis of babesiosis is being considered, manual (nonautomated) review of blood smears for parasites should be requested explicitly. If seen, the tetrad (Maltese-cross) form is pathognomonic. *B microti* and other *Babesia* species can be difficult to distinguish from *Plasmodium falciparum;* examination of blood smears by a reference laboratory should be considered for confirmation of the diagnosis.

Molecular (eg, polymerase chain reaction) and serologic testing are available at some clinical and public health laboratories as well as at the Centers for Disease Control and Prevention. Several real-time polymerase chain reaction (PCR) assays are available and have been useful in detecting low-grade *B microti* parasitemia, with increased sensitivity compared with blood smear microscopy. PCR assay is particularly recommended for use in early infection, when parasites are more difficult to visualize on blood smear. However, PCR assay should be used with caution when monitoring response to therapy, because

B microti can be detected for weeks and months after parasites no longer are visualized on blood smear.

Antibody detection tests are useful for detecting infected individuals with very low levels of parasitemia (such as asymptomatic blood donors in transfusion-associated cases), for diagnosis after infection is cleared by therapy, and for discrimination between *Plasmodium falciparum* and *Babesia* infection in patients whose blood smear examinations are inconclusive and whose travel histories cannot exclude either parasite. (**www.cdc.gov/dpdx/babesiosis/dx.html**).

If indicated, the possibility of concurrent *B burgdorferi* or *Anaplasmataceae* infection should be considered. In one study, the seroprevalence of *B microti* infection in individuals who were seropositive for Lyme disease was 29%, suggesting possible coinfections. When a coinfection is documented, patients should receive therapies appropriate for each infection.

TREATMENT: For mild disease in children, atovaquone plus azithromycin orally for 7 to 10 days is the regimen of choice (see Drugs for Parasitic Infections, p 985). Recommended therapy for severely ill children and adults is combination therapy using clindamycin plus quinine, intravenously. Exchange transfusions should be considered for patients who are critically ill (eg, with hemodynamic instability, severe hemolysis, or pulmonary, renal, or hepatic compromise), especially, but not necessarily exclusively, in patients with parasitemia levels of approximately 10% or higher. In severely immunocompromised patients, treatment for at least 6 weeks or longer, with negative blood smears for 2 weeks or longer prior to discontinuing therapy, is recommended. In addition, higher doses of azithromycin (600 to 1000 mg per day, orally, in adolescents/adults) should be considered when treating a highly immunocompromised patient.

ISOLATION OF THE HOSPITALIZED PATIENT: Standard precautions are recommended.

CONTROL MEASURES: Babesiosis is a nationally notifiable disease and is a reportable disease in many states. Recommendations for prevention of tick bites are similar to those for prevention of Lyme disease and other tickborne infections (see Prevention of Mosquitoborne and Tickborne Infections, p 194). People with a known history of *Babesia* infection are deferred indefinitely from donating blood. In 2015, the Blood Products Advisory Committee (BPAC) of the US Food and Drug Administration met to discuss *B microti* screening for blood donations, and recommended year-round antibody screening for *B microti* nationally, with the addition of nucleic acid testing in the 5 states with highest endemicity (**www.fda.gov/downloads/advisorycommittees/committeesmeetingmaterials/bloodvaccinesandotherbiologics/bloodproductsadvisorycommittee/ucm446274.pdf**).

Bacillus cereus Infections and Intoxications

CLINICAL MANIFESTATIONS: *Bacillus cereus* is associated primarily with 2 toxin-mediated foodborne illnesses, emetic and diarrheal, but it also can cause invasive extraintestinal infection. The emetic syndrome develops after a short incubation period, similar to staphylococcal foodborne illness. It is characterized by nausea, vomiting, and abdominal cramps, and diarrhea may follow in up to one third of patients. The diarrheal syndrome has a longer incubation period, is more severe, and resembles *Clostridium perfringens* foodborne illness. It is characterized by moderate to severe abdominal cramps and watery diarrhea, vomiting in approximately 25% of patients, and occasionally low-grade fever.

Both illnesses usually are short-lived, but the emetic toxin is occasionally associated with fulminant liver failure.

Invasive extraintestinal infection can be severe and includes wound and soft tissue infections; sepsis and bacteremia, including central line-associated bloodstream infection; endocarditis; osteomyelitis; purulent meningitis and ventricular shunt infection; pneumonia; and ocular infections (ie, endophthalmitis and keratitis). Infection can be acquired through use of contaminated blood products, especially platelets. *B cereus* is a leading cause of bacterial endophthalmitis following penetrating ocular trauma. Endogenous endophthalmitis can result from bacteremic seeding. Other ocular manifestations include an indolent keratitis related to corneal abrasions and may be seen in contact lens users or those who have undergone cataract surgery.

Rare infections that clinically resemble anthrax attributable to *B cereus* strains that express anthrax toxin genes, have been reported.

ETIOLOGY: *B cereus* is an aerobic and facultative anaerobic, spore-forming, Gram-positive or Gram-variable bacillus.

EPIDEMIOLOGY: *B cereus* is ubiquitous in the environment because of the high resistance of their endospores to extreme conditions, including heat, cold, desiccation, salinity, and radiation, and commonly is present in small numbers in raw, dried, and processed foods and in the feces of healthy people. The organism is a common cause of foodborne illness in the United States but may be underrecognized, because few people seek care for mild illness and physicians and clinical laboratories do not routinely test for *B cereus*. Several confirmed outbreaks were reported to the Centers for Disease Control and Prevention (CDC) in recent years. A wide variety of food vehicles has been implicated.

Spores of *B cereus* are heat resistant and can survive pasteurization, brief cooking, boiling, and high saline concentrations. They germinate to vegetative forms that produce enterotoxins over a wide range of temperatures, both in foods and in the gastrointestinal tract. The diarrheal syndrome is caused by at least 3 distinct toxins that are ingested preformed or are produced after spores germinate in the gastrointestinal tract. The diarrheal toxins are heat labile and can be destroyed by heating. The emetic syndrome occurs after eating contaminated food containing a preformed toxin called cereulide. The best known association of the emetic syndrome is with ingestion of fried rice made from boiled rice stored at room temperature overnight, but a wide variety of foods, especially starchy foods, has been implicated. The toxin is elaborated by vegetative forms that germinate from spores upon reheating the food; it is heat stable and gastric acid resistant. Foodborne illness caused by *B cereus* is not transmissible from person to person.

Risk factors for invasive disease attributable to *B cereus* include history of injection drug use, presence of indwelling intravascular catheters or implanted devices, neutropenia or immunosuppression, and preterm birth. *B cereus* endophthalmitis has occurred after penetrating ocular trauma and injection drug use. Hospital outbreaks have been associated with contaminated medical equipment, but pseudoepidemics are more common and refer to sharp increases in contamination rates of clinical specimens associated with common source contamination, for example ethanol pads or solutions, linen and blood culture media.

The **incubation period** for foodborne illness is 0.5 to 6 hours for the emetic syndrome and 6 to 15 hours for the diarrheal syndrome.

DIAGNOSTIC TESTS: Diagnostic testing is not recommended for sporadic cases. For foodborne outbreaks, isolation of *B cereus* from the stool or vomitus of 2 or more ill people and not from control patients, or isolation of 10^5 colony-forming units/g or greater from epidemiologically implicated food, suggests that *B cereus* is the cause of the outbreak. Because the organism can be recovered from stool specimens from some well people, the presence of *B cereus* in feces or vomitus of ill people is not definitive evidence of infection. Food samples must be tested for both types of diarrheal enterotoxins, because either alone can cause illness. Although there is currently no commercial kit that detects the cereulide emetic toxin, *B cereus* colonies isolated from food or specimens of ill individuals may be tested by polymerase chain reaction assay for the emetic toxin gene in diagnostic laboratories.

In patients with risk factors for invasive disease (eg, preterm infants, people with immunosuppressing conditions), isolation of *B cereus* from wounds or from blood or other sterile body fluids is significant. The common perception of *Bacillus* species as "contaminants" may delay recognition and treatment of serious *B cereus* infections.

TREATMENT: *B cereus* foodborne illness usually requires only supportive treatment, including rehydration. Antimicrobial therapy is indicated for patients with invasive disease. Prompt removal of any potentially infected foreign bodies, such as central lines or implants, is essential. For intraocular infections, an ophthalmologist should be consulted regarding use of intravitreal vancomycin therapy in addition to systemic therapy. *B cereus* usually is resistant to beta-lactam antibiotics and clindamycin but is susceptible to vancomycin, which is the drug of choice. Alternative drugs, including linezolid, clindamycin, aminoglycosides, erythromycin, tetracyclines, and fluoroquinolones, may be considered depending on susceptibility results.

ISOLATION OF THE HOSPITALIZED PATIENT: Standard precautions are recommended.

CONTROL MEASURES: Proper cooking and appropriate storage of foods, particularly rice cooked for later use, will help prevent foodborne outbreaks. Information on recommended safe food handling practices, including time and temperature requirements during cooking, storage, and reheating, can be found at **www.foodsafety.gov.** Hand hygiene and strict aseptic technique in caring for immunocompromised patients or patients with indwelling intravascular catheters are important to minimize the risk of invasive disease. The organism can survive in high concentrations of ethanol, but hand washing and use of 2% chlorhexidine are effective preventive measures.

Bacterial Vaginosis

CLINICAL MANIFESTATIONS: Bacterial vaginosis (BV) is a polymicrobial clinical syndrome characterized by changes in vaginal flora, with replacement of normally abundant *Lactobacillus* species by high concentrations of anaerobic bacteria. BV is diagnosed primarily in sexually active postpubertal females, but females who have never been sexually active can be affected rarely. BV is asymptomatic in 50% to 75% of females with microbiologic evidence of infection. Symptoms include vaginal discharge and/or vaginal odor. Classic signs, when present, include a thin white or grey, homogenous, adherent vaginal discharge with a fishy odor after intercourse or during menses. Symptoms of vulvovaginal irritation, pruritus, dysuria, or abdominal pain are not associated with BV but are suggestive of mixed vaginitis. In pregnant females, BV has been associated with adverse outcomes, including chorioamnionitis, premature rupture of membranes, preterm delivery, and postpartum endometritis.

Vaginitis and vulvitis in prepubertal girls rarely, if ever, are manifestations of BV.

Vaginitis in prepubertal girls frequently is nonspecific, but possible causes include foreign bodies and infections attributable to group A streptococci, *Escherichia coli*, herpes simplex virus, *Neisseria gonorrhoeae*, *Chlamydia trachomatis*, *Trichomonas vaginalis*, or enteric bacteria, including *Shigella* species. In any prepubertal girl who has symptoms of bacterial vaginitis, a full history and work up needs to be performed to rule out sexual abuse and/or a sexually transmitted infection (STI [see STIs in Children, p 168]). If sexual abuse is suspected, those who are mandated to report need to follow their state's regulations for immediate reporting.

ETIOLOGY: The microbiologic cause of BV has not been delineated fully. Hydrogen peroxide-producing *Lactobacillus* species predominate among vaginal flora and play a protective role. In females with BV, these species largely are replaced by commensal anaerobes. Increased concentrations of *Gardnerella vaginalis*, *Mycoplasma hominis*, *Prevotella* species, *Mobiluncus* species, and *Ureaplasma* species are typical microbiologic findings on vaginal swab specimens. Numerous other fastidious organisms have been associated with BV. These organisms are collectively referred to as BV-associated bacteria.

EPIDEMIOLOGY: BV is the most common cause of vaginal discharge in sexually active adolescent and adult females. Having multiple partners and not using or incorrectly using condoms puts the adolescent population at higher risk. In this population, BV may be the sole cause of the symptoms, or it may accompany other conditions associated with vaginal discharge, such as trichomoniasis or cervicitis secondary to other STIs. BV occurs more frequently in females with a new sexual partner or a higher number of sexual partners and in those who engage in douching. Although evidence of sexual transmission of BV is inconclusive, BV can influence the acquisition of other STIs, including human immunodeficiency virus (HIV), herpes simplex virus-2, *N gonorrhoeae*, and *C trachomatis*, and increase the risk of infectious complications following gynecologic surgery and pregnancy complications. Because BV is a polymicrobial infection, an **incubation period** has not been defined. Recurrence is common.

DIAGNOSTIC TESTS: BV most commonly is diagnosed clinically using the Amsel criteria, requiring that 3 or more of the following symptoms or signs are present:

- Homogenous, thin grey or white vaginal discharge that smoothly coats the vaginal walls;
- Vaginal fluid pH greater than 4.5;
- A fishy (amine) odor of vaginal discharge before or after addition of 10% potassium hydroxide (ie, the "whiff test"); or
- Presence of clue cells (squamous vaginal epithelial cells covered with bacteria, which cause a stippled or granular appearance and ragged "moth-eaten" borders) representing at least 20% of the total vaginal epithelial cells seen on microscopic evaluation of vaginal fluid.

An alternative method for diagnosing BV is the Nugent score, which is used widely as the gold standard for making the diagnosis in the research setting. A Gram stain of the vaginal fluid is evaluated, and a numerical score is generated on the basis of the apparent quantity of lactobacilli relative to BV-associated bacteria. The score is interpreted as normal (0–3), intermediate (4–6), or BV (7–10). Douching, recent intercourse, menstruation, and coexisting infection can alter findings on Gram stain.

The Affirm VPIII (Becton Dickinson, Sparks, MD) is a DNA hybridization probe test that detects *G vaginalis* as well as *Trichomonas vaginalis* and *Candida albicans* and can be used in the evaluation of vaginitis. Clinical Laboratory Improvement Amendments (CLIA)-

waived rapid tests for BV that measure the activity of sialidase, an enzyme generated by several BV-associated bacteria, such as OSOM BVBlue Test (Sekisui Diagnostics, Framingham, MA), have acceptable performance criteria compared with the Nugent criteria. Culture for *G vaginalis* is not recommended as a diagnostic tool, because it is not specific. Although a proline aminopeptidase card test is available for the detection of elevated pH and trimethylamine, it has low sensitivity and specificity and, therefore, is not recommended. Papanicolaou (Pap) testing is not recommended for the diagnosis of BV because of its low sensitivity.

Sexually active females with BV should be evaluated for coinfection with other STIs, including syphilis, gonorrhea, chlamydia, trichomoniasis, and HIV infection. If the hepatitis B and human papillomavirus vaccine series have not been completed, these immunizations should be offered if appropriate for age.

TREATMENT[1]: Symptomatic patients should be treated. The goals of treatment are to relieve the symptoms and signs of infection and potentially to decrease the risk of acquiring other STIs. Treatment considerations should include patient preference for oral versus intravaginal treatment, possible adverse effects, and the presence of coinfections.

Nonpregnant females may be treated orally with metronidazole (500 mg, twice daily for 7 days) or topically with metronidazole gel 0.75% (one full 5-g applicator, intravaginally for 5 days), metronidazole gel 1.3% (administered intravaginally once daily at bedtime for 5 days), or clindamycin cream 2% (one full 5-g applicator, intravaginally at bedtime for 7 days). Alternative regimens include oral tinidazole (2 g, orally, once daily for 2 days, or 1 g, orally, once daily for 5 days), oral clindamycin (300 mg, orally, twice daily for 7 days), or clindamycin intravaginal ovules (100 mg, intravaginally, once at bedtime for 3 days) (see Table 4.4, p 933, and Table 4.5, p 936). Patients who are treated with metronidazole or tinidazole should not consume alcohol during therapy and for 72 hours after completion of therapy. Patients should refrain from sexual intercourse or use condoms appropriately during treatment, keeping in mind that clindamycin cream is oil-based and can weaken latex condoms and diaphragms for up to 5 days after completion of therapy. There is no evidence that treatment of sexual partners effects treatment response or risk of recurrence. Follow-up is not necessary if symptoms resolve.

Pregnant females with symptoms of BV should be treated. Pregnant women with BV are at high risk of having preterm or low birth weight infants, premature rupture of membranes, intra-amniotic infections, and postpartum endometriosis. Metronidazole crosses the placenta. However, there are no studies showing any teratogenic evidence. Because oral therapy has not been shown to be superior to topical therapy for treating symptomatic BV in effecting cure or preventing adverse outcomes of pregnancy, symptomatic pregnant females can be treated with either of the oral or vaginal metronidazole or clindamycin regimens recommended for nonpregnant females. Tinidazole should be avoided during pregnancy; animal studies have shown teratogenic effects.

Breastfeeding females with symptoms of BV should be treated. Metronidazole is secreted in human milk, so topical metronidazole is preferred for treating breastfeeding mothers. Some clinicians advise deferring breastfeeding for 12 to 24 hours following oral maternal treatment with a single 2-g dose of metronidazole. Because information on safety of tinidazole in breastfeeding mothers is limited, it should only be used to treat

[1]Centers for Disease Control and Prevention. Sexually transmitted diseases treatment guidelines, 2015. *MMWR Recomm Rep.* 2015;64(RR-3):1–137

proven drug-resistant strains.

Approximately 30% of appropriately treated females have a recurrence within 3 months. Retreatment with the same regimen or an alternative regimen are both reasonable options for treating persistent or recurrent BV after the first occurrence. For females with multiple recurrences, metronidazole gel 0.75%, twice weekly for 4 to 6 months, has been shown to reduce recurrences, although this benefit might not persist when suppressive therapy is discontinued. Limited data suggest that metronidazole or tinidazole, 500 mg, twice daily for 7 days, followed by intravaginal boric acid, 600 mg, daily for 21 days, and then suppressive metronidazole gel 0.75%, twice weekly for 4 to 6 months, might be an option for recurrent BV. Monthly oral metronidazole (2 g), administered with fluconazole (150 mg), has been evaluated as suppressive therapy. Studies do not support currently available lactobacillus formulations or probiotics as an adjunctive or replacement therapy for BV management.

ISOLATION OF THE HOSPITALIZED PATIENT: Standard precautions are recommended.
CONTROL MEASURES: None.

Bacteroides, Prevotella, and Other Anaerobic Gram-Negative Bacilli Infections

CLINICAL MANIFESTATIONS: *Bacteroides* and *Prevotella* and other anaerobic gram-negative bacilli (AGNB) organisms from the oral cavity can cause chronic sinusitis, chronic otitis media, parotitis, dental infection, peritonsillar abscess, cervical adenitis, retropharyngeal space infection, aspiration pneumonia, lung abscess, pleural empyema, or necrotizing pneumonia. Species from the gastrointestinal tract are recovered in patients with peritonitis, intra-abdominal abscess, pelvic inflammatory disease, Bartholin cyst abscess, tubo-ovarian abscess, endometritis, acute and chronic prostatitis, prostatic and scrotal abscesses, scrotal gangrene, postoperative wound infection, and vulvovaginal and perianal infections. Invasion of the bloodstream from the oral cavity or intestinal tract can lead to brain abscess, meningitis, endocarditis, arthritis, or osteomyelitis. Skin and soft tissue infections include bacterial gangrene and necrotizing fasciitis; omphalitis in newborn infants; cellulitis at the site of fetal monitors, human bite wounds, or burns; infections adjacent to the mouth or rectum; and infected decubitus ulcers. Neonatal infections, including conjunctivitis, pneumonia, bacteremia, or meningitis, rarely occur. In most cases in which *Bacteroides, Prevotella,* and other AGNB are implicated, the infections are polymicrobial, with between 5 and 10 different organisms being present.

ETIOLOGY: Most *Bacteroides, Prevotella, Porphyromonas, Fusobacterium, Peptostreptococcus,* and *Propionibacterium* organisms associated with human disease are pleomorphic, non-spore–forming, facultatively anaerobic, gram-negative bacilli.

EPIDEMIOLOGY: *Bacteroides, Prevotella,* and other AGNB are part of the normal flora of the mouth, gastrointestinal tract, and female and male genital tracts. Members of the *Bacteroides fragilis* group predominate in the gastrointestinal tract flora; enterotoxigenic *B fragilis* may be a cause of diarrhea. Members of the *Prevotella melaninogenica* (formerly *Bacteroides melaninogenicus*) and *Prevotella oralis* (formerly *Bacteroides oralis*) groups are more common in the oral cavity. These species cause infection as opportunists, usually after an alteration in skin or mucosal membranes in conjunction with other endogenous species, and often are associated with chronic injury. Rates of upper respiratory tract, head, and neck infections associated with AGNB are higher in children. Endogenous infection results from aspiration, bowel perforation, or damage to mucosal surfaces from trauma, surgery, or chemotherapy. Mucosal injury or granulocytopenia predispose to infection. Except in infections resulting from human bites, no evidence of person-to-person transmission exists.

The **incubation period** is variable and depends on the inoculum and the site of involvement but usually is 1 to 5 days.

DIAGNOSTIC TESTS: Anaerobic culture media are necessary for recovery of *Bacteroides*, *Prevotella*, and other AGNB species. Because infections usually are polymicrobial, aerobic and anaerobic cultures should be obtained. A putrid odor, with or without gas in the infected site, suggests anaerobic infection. Use of an anaerobic transport tube or a sealed syringe is recommended for collection of clinical specimens.

TREATMENT: Abscesses should be drained when feasible; abscesses involving the brain, liver, and lungs may resolve with effective antimicrobial therapy. Necrotizing soft tissue lesions should be débrided surgically.

The choice of antimicrobial agent(s) is based on anticipated or known in vitro susceptibility testing and local antimicrobial resistance patterns. *Bacteroides* infections of the mouth and respiratory tract generally are susceptible to penicillin G, ampicillin, and extended-spectrum penicillins, such as ticarcillin or piperacillin. However, some species of *Bacteroides* and almost 50% of *Prevotella* species produce beta-lactamase, and penicillin treatment failure has emerged as a consequence, so penicillin is not recommended for empirical coverage or for treatment of severe oropharyngeal or pleuropulmonary infections or for any abdominopelvic infections. A beta-lactam penicillin active against *Bacteroides* species combined with a beta-lactamase inhibitor (ampicillin-sulbactam, amoxicillin-clavulanate, or piperacillin-tazobactam) can be useful to treat these infections. *Bacteroides* species of the gastrointestinal tract usually are resistant to penicillin G but are susceptible predictably to metronidazole, beta-lactam plus beta-lactamase inhibitors, chloramphenicol, and sometimes clindamycin. More than 80% of isolates are susceptible to cefoxitin, ceftizoxime, linezolid, imipenem, and meropenem. Tigecycline has demonstrated in vitro activity against *Prevotella* and *Bacteroides* species but is not approved by the US Food and Drug Administration for use in people younger than 18 years, because pediatric trials with this agent have not been conducted. Cefuroxime, cefotaxime, and ceftriaxone are not reliably effective.

ISOLATION OF THE HOSPITALIZED PATIENT: Standard precautions are recommended.

CONTROL MEASURES: None.

Balantidium coli Infections
(Balantidiasis)

CLINICAL MANIFESTATIONS: Most human infections are asymptomatic. Acute symptomatic infection is characterized by rapid onset of nausea, vomiting, abdominal discomfort or pain, and bloody or watery mucoid diarrhea. In some patients, the course is chronic with intermittent episodes of diarrhea, anorexia, and weight loss. Rarely, organisms spread to mesenteric nodes, pleura, lung, liver, or genitourinary sites. Inflammation of the gastrointestinal tract and local lymphatic vessels can result in bowel dilation, ulceration, perforation, and secondary bacterial invasion. Colitis produced by *Balantidium coli* often is indistinguishable from colitis produced by *Entamoeba histolytica*. Fulminant disease can occur in malnourished or otherwise debilitated or immunocompromised patients.

ETIOLOGY: *B coli*, a ciliated protozoan, is the largest pathogenic protozoan known to infect humans.

EPIDEMIOLOGY: Pigs are the primary host reservoir of *B coli*, but other sources of infection have been reported. Infections have been reported in most areas of the world but are rare in industrialized countries. Cysts excreted in feces can be transmitted directly from hand to mouth or indirectly through fecally contaminated water or food. Excysted trophozoites infect the colon. A person is infectious as long as cysts are excreted in stool. Cysts may remain viable in the environment for months.

The **incubation period** is not established but may be several days.

DIAGNOSTIC TESTS: Diagnosis of infection is established by scraping lesions via sigmoidoscopy or colonoscopy, histologic examination of intestinal biopsy specimens, or ova and parasite examination of stool. The diagnosis usually is established by demonstrating trophozoites (or less frequently, cysts) in stool or tissue specimens. Stool examination is less sensitive, and repeated stool examination may be necessary to diagnose infection, because shedding of organisms can be intermittent. Microscopic examination of fresh diarrheal stools must be performed promptly, because trophozoites degenerate rapidly.

TREATMENT: The drug of choice is a tetracycline (see Drugs for Parasitic Infections, p 985). Alternative drugs are metronidazole, iodoquinol, and doxycycline. Successful use of nitazoxanide has been reported.

ISOLATION OF THE HOSPITALIZED PATIENT: In addition to standard precautions, contact precautions are recommended, because human-to-human transmission can occur rarely.

CONTROL MEASURES: Control measures include sanitary disposal of human feces, avoidance of contamination of food and water with porcine feces, and handwashing with soap and clean water after toilet use and before eating or handling food. Travelers should avoid ingestion of potentially contaminated food or water. Despite chlorination of water, waterborne outbreaks of disease have occurred.

Bartonella henselae (Cat-Scratch Disease)

CLINICAL MANIFESTATIONS: The predominant clinical manifestation of *Bartonella henselae* infection (in an immunocompetent person) is regional lymphadenopathy/lymphadenitis (cat-scratch disease [CSD]). Most people with CSD are afebrile or have low grade fever with mild systemic symptoms, such as malaise, anorexia, fatigue, and headache. Fever and mild systemic symptoms occur in approximately 30% of patients.

A skin papule or pustule often is found at the presumed site of inoculation and usually precedes development of lymphadenopathy by approximately 1 to 2 weeks (range, 5–50 days). Lymphadenopathy involves nodes that drain the site of inoculation, typically axillary, but cervical, submental, epitrochlear, or inguinal nodes can be involved. The skin overlying affected lymph nodes is often tender, warm, erythematous, and indurated, and approximately 10% to 25% of affected nodes suppurate spontaneously. Typically, lymphadenopathy will resolve spontaneously within 2 to 4 months.

Less common manifestations of *B henselae* infection likely reflect bloodborne disseminated disease and include culture-negative endocarditis, encephalopathy, osteolytic lesions, granulomata in the liver and spleen, glomerulonephritis, pneumonia, thrombocytopenic purpura, and erythema nodosum. CSD may present with fevers for 1 to 3 weeks (ie, fever of unknown origin) and may be associated with nonspecific symptoms, such as malaise, abdominal pain, headache, and myalgia.

Ocular manifestations occur in 5% to 10% of patients. The most classic and frequent presentation of ocular *Bartonella* infection is neuroretinitis, characterized by unilateral painless vision impairment, granulomatous optic disc swelling, and macular edema, with lipid exudates (macular star); simultaneous bilateral involvement has been reported but is less common. Inoculation of the periocular tissue can result in Parinaud oculoglandular syndrome, which consists of follicular conjunctivitis and ipsilateral preauricular lymphadenopathy. Additional rare ocular manifestations include retinochoroiditis, anterior uveitis, vitritis, pars planitis, retinal vasculitis, retinitis, branch retinal arteriolar or venular occlusions, macular hole, or serous retinal detachments (extraordinarily rare).

ETIOLOGY: *B henselae*, the causative organism of CSD, is a fastidious, slow-growing, gram-negative bacillus that also is the causative agent of bacillary angiomatosis (vascular proliferative lesions of skin and subcutaneous tissue) and bacillary peliosis (reticuloendothelial lesions in visceral organs, primarily the liver). The latter 2 manifestations of infection are reported among immunocompromised patients, primarily those with human immunodeficiency virus infection. Additional species, such as *Bartonella clarridgeiae*, also have been found to cause CSD. *B henselae* is related closely to *Bartonella quintana*, the agent of louse-borne trench fever that caused significant illness and disease among troops during World War I, and also is a causative agent of bacillary angiomatosis. *B quintana* can cause endocarditis.

EPIDEMIOLOGY: *B henselae* is a common cause of regional lymphadenopathy/lymphadenitis in children. The highest incidence is found in children 5 to 9 years of age; infection occurs more often during the fall and winter. Children 14 years or younger account for 32.5% of all reported cases. Cats are the natural reservoir for *B henselae*, with a seroprevalence of 13% to 90% in domestic and stray cats in the United States. Other animals, including dogs, can be infected and occasionally are associated with human infection. Cat-to-cat transmission occurs via the cat flea (*Ctenocephalides felis*), with feline infection resulting in bacteremia that usually is asymptomatic and lasts weeks to months. Fleas acquire the organism when feeding on a bacteremic cat and then shed infectious organisms in their feces. The bacteria are transmitted to humans by inoculation through a scratch, lick, or bite from a bacteremic cat or by hands contaminated by flea feces touching an open wound or the eye. Most patients have a history of recent contact with apparently healthy cats, typically kittens. Kittens (more often than cats) and animals from shelters or adopted as strays are more likely to be bacteremic. There is no convincing evidence to date that ticks are a competent vector for transmission of *Bartonella* organisms to humans. No evidence of person-to-person transmission exists.

The **incubation period** from the time of the scratch to appearance of the primary cutaneous lesion is 7 to 12 days; the period from the appearance of the primary lesion to the appearance of lymphadenopathy is 5 to 50 days (median, 12 days).

DIAGNOSTIC TESTS: The indirect immunofluorescent antibody (IFA) assay for detection of serum antibodies to antigens of *Bartonella* species is useful for diagnosis of CSD. The IFA test is available at many commercial laboratories and through the Centers for Disease Control and Prevention (CDC), but because of cross-reactivity with other infections, clinical correlation is essential. Enzyme immunoassays for detection of antibodies to

B henselae have been developed; however, further investigation is required to determine whether they are more sensitive or specific than the IFA test. Immunoglobulin (Ig) M production is brief and could be missed, yielding low testing sensitivity. Generally speaking, if an IFA IgG titer is <1:64, the patient does not have acute infection. Titers between 1:64 and 1:256 may represent past or acute infection, and follow-up titers in 2 weeks should be considered. An IgG titer of >1:256 is consistent with acute infection. Recent studies report highly specific IgM enzyme-linked immunosorbent assays for *B henselae* using refined N-lauroyl-sarcosine-insoluble proteins.

Polymerase chain reaction (PCR) assays are available in some commercial and research laboratories for testing of tissue or body fluids. Health care professionals are cautioned against using newly developed diagnostic tests that have not been independently validated or cleared by the US Food and Drug Administration (eg, preenrichment culture, then PCR assay).

B henselae is a fastidious organism; recovery by routine culture rarely is successful. Specialized laboratories experienced in isolating *Bartonella* organisms are recommended for processing of cultures. Lysis centrifugation tubes or automated blood culture systems can be attempted to grow *Bartonella* species, followed by culture on solid media. Generally, yield on blood culture is poor and delayed. Acridine orange staining or blind subculture of negative blood culture bottles may improve detection.

If tissue (eg, lymph node) specimens are available, bacilli occasionally may be visualized using a silver stain (eg, Warthin-Starry or Steiner stain); however, this test is not specific for *B henselae*. Early histologic changes in lymph node specimens consist of lymphocytic infiltration with epithelioid granuloma formation. Later changes consist of polymorphonuclear leukocyte infiltration with granulomas that become necrotic and resemble granulomas from patients with tularemia, brucellosis, and mycobacterial infections.

TREATMENT: Management of localized uncomplicated CSD primarily is aimed at relief of symptoms, because the disease usually is self-limited, resolving spontaneously in 2 to 4 months. Azithromycin has been shown to have a modest clinical benefit in treating localized CSD (lymphadenopathy/lymphadenitis), with a significantly greater decrease in lymph node volume after 1 month of therapy compared with placebo; however, no other differences in clinical outcome were demonstrated. Painful suppurative nodes can be treated with needle aspiration for relief of symptoms; incision and drainage should be avoided, because this may facilitate fistula formation, and surgical excision generally is unnecessary.

Many experts recommend antimicrobial therapy in acutely or severely ill immunocompetent patients with systemic symptoms, particularly people with retinitis, hepatic or splenic involvement, or painful adenitis. Reports suggest that several oral antimicrobial agents (azithromycin, clarithromycin, ciprofloxacin, doxycycline, trimethoprim-sulfamethoxazole, and rifampin) and parenteral gentamicin are effective. The optimal duration of therapy is not known but may be several months for systemic disease.

Although evidence is lacking, neuroretinitis often is treated with both systemic antimicrobial agents and corticosteroids to decrease the optic disc swelling and promote a more rapid return of vision. Doxycycline plus rifampin is preferred for patients with neuroretinitis, in whom doxycycline should be used regardless of patient age (see Tetracyclines, p 905). Reports in the literature note that a large majority of such patients experience significant visual recovery to 20/40 or better.

Antimicrobial therapy is recommended for all immunocompromised people, because treatment of bacillary angiomatosis and bacillary peliosis has been shown to be beneficial. Erythromycin or doxycycline is effective for treatment of these conditions; therapy should be administered for several months to prevent relapse in immunocompromised people. In these patients, doxycycline can be used for short durations (ie, 21 days or less) without regard to patient age; for the longer treatment durations required for treatment of *Bartonella* in immunocompromised people, for whom the alternative treatment of erythromycin exists, doxycycline is not recommended in children younger than 8 years (see Tetracyclines, p 905).

For patients with unusual manifestations of *Bartonella* infection (eg, culture-negative endocarditis, neuroretinitis, disease in immunocompromised patients), consultation with a pediatric infectious diseases expert is recommended.

ISOLATION OF THE HOSPITALIZED PATIENT: Standard precautions are recommended.

CONTROL MEASURES: Effort should be undertaken to avoid scratches and bites from cats or kittens. Immunocompromised people should avoid contact with cats younger than 1 year, stray cats, and cats that scratch or bite. Sites of cat scratches or bites should be washed immediately. Care of cats should include flea control. Testing or treatment of cats for *Bartonella* infection is not recommended, nor is declawing or removal of the cat from the household.

Baylisascaris Infections

CLINICAL MANIFESTATIONS: Infection with *Baylisascaris procyonis*, a raccoon roundworm, can present with nausea and fatigue. It is a rare cause of acute eosinophilic meningoencephalitis. In a young child, acute central nervous system (CNS) disease (eg, altered mental status and seizures) accompanied by peripheral and/or cerebrospinal fluid (CSF) eosinophilia can occur 2 to 4 weeks after infection. Severe neurologic sequelae or death are usual outcomes. *B procyonis* is a rare cause of extraneural disease in older children and adults. Ocular larva migrans can result in diffuse unilateral subacute neuroretinitis; direct visualization of larvae in the retina sometimes is possible. Visceral larval migrans can present with nonspecific signs, such as macular rash, pneumonitis, and hepatomegaly. Similar to visceral larva migrans caused by *Toxocara* species, subclinical or asymptomatic infection is thought to be the most common outcome of infection.

ETIOLOGY: *B procyonis* is a 10- to 25-cm long roundworm (nematode) with a direct life cycle usually limited to its definitive host, the raccoon. Domestic dogs and some less commonly owned pets, such as kinkajous and ringtails, can serve as definitive hosts and a potential source of human disease.[1]

EPIDEMIOLOGY: *B procyonis* is distributed focally throughout the United States; in areas where disease is endemic, 22% to 80% of raccoons can harbor the parasite in their intestines. Reports of infections in dogs raise concern that infected dogs may be able to spread the disease. Embryonated eggs containing infective larvae are ingested from the soil by raccoons, rodents, and birds. When infective eggs or an infected host is eaten by a raccoon, the larvae grow to maturity in the small intestine, where adult female worms shed millions of eggs per day. Eggs become infective after 2 to 4 weeks in the environment and may persist long-term in the soil. Cases of raccoon infection have been reported in many

---

[1]Centers for Disease Control and Prevention. Raccoon roundworms in pet kinkajous—three states, 1999 and 2010. *MMWR Morb Mortal Wkly Rep.* 2011;60(10):302–305

parts of the United States. Risk of human infection is greatest in areas where significant raccoon populations live in peridomestic settings. Fewer than 30 cases of *Baylisascaris* CNS disease have been documented in the United States, although cases may be undiagnosed or underreported.

Risk factors for *Baylisascaris* infection include contact with raccoon latrines (communal defecation sites often found at or on the base of trees, raised flat surfaces such as tree stumps, logs, rocks, decks, and rooftops, or unsealed attics or garages), geophagia/pica, age younger than 4 years, and in older children, developmental delay. Most reported cases of CNS disease have been in males.

DIAGNOSTIC TESTS: *Baylisascaris* infection is confirmed by identification of larvae in biopsy specimens. A presumptive diagnosis can be made on the basis of clinical (meningoencephalitis, diffuse unilateral subacute neuroretinitis, pseudotumor), epidemiologic (raccoon exposure), and laboratory (blood and CSF eosinophilia) findings. Serologic testing (serum, CSF) for patients with clinical symptoms is available at the Centers for Disease Control and Prevention. Neuroimaging results can be normal initially, but as larvae grow and migrate through CNS tissue, focal abnormalities are found in periventricular white matter and elsewhere. In ocular disease, ophthalmologic examination can reveal characteristic chorioretinal lesions or rarely larvae. Because eggs are not shed in human feces, stool examination is not helpful. The disease is not transmitted from person to person.

TREATMENT: On the basis of CNS and CSF penetration and in vitro activity, albendazole, in conjunction with high-dose corticosteroids, has been advocated most widely (see Drugs for Parasitic Infections, p 985). Treatment with anthelmintic agents and corticosteroids may not affect clinical outcome once severe CNS disease manifestations are evident. If the infection is suspected, treatment should be initiated while the diagnostic evaluation is being completed. Limited data are available regarding safety and efficacy of alternate anthelmintic therapies in children. Preventive therapy with albendazole should be considered for children with a history of ingestion of soil potentially contaminated with raccoon feces; however, no definitive preventive dosing regimen has been established. Larvae localized to the retina may be killed by direct photocoagulation.

ISOLATION OF THE HOSPITALIZED PATIENT: Standard precautions are recommended.

CONTROL MEASURES: *Baylisascaris* infections are prevented by avoiding ingestion of soil contaminated with stool of infected animal reservoirs, primarily raccoons; avoiding raccoon defecation sites (latrines); washing hands after contact with soil or with pets or other animals; discouraging raccoon presence by limiting access to human or pet food sources; and decontaminating raccoon latrines (especially if located near homes) by treating the area with boiling water or a propane torch, in keeping with local fire safety regulations, or through proper removal if located within the home (eg, attic).

Infections With *Blastocystis hominis* and Other Subtypes

CLINICAL MANIFESTATIONS: The importance of *Blastocystis* species as a cause of gastrointestinal tract disease is controversial. The asymptomatic carrier state is well documented. Clinical symptoms reported include bloating, flatulence, mild to moderate diarrhea without fecal leukocytes or blood, abdominal pain, nausea, and poor growth. Some case series and reports have noted an association between infection with *Blastocystis hominis* and chronic urticaria and irritable bowel syndrome. When *B hominis* is identified in stool from symptomatic patients, other causes of this symptom complex, particularly *Giardia intestinalis* and *Cryptosporidium parvum,* should be investigated before assuming that *B hominis* is the cause of the signs and symptoms. Polymerase chain reaction fingerprinting suggests that some *B hominis* organisms are disease associated, but others are not.

ETIOLOGY: *B hominis* previously has been classified as a protozoan, but molecular studies have characterized it as a stramenopile (a eukaryote). Multiple forms have been described: vacuolar, which is observed most commonly in clinical specimens; granular; which is seen rarely in fresh stools; ameboid; and cystic.

EPIDEMIOLOGY: *Blastocystis* species are recovered from 1% to 20% of stool specimens examined for ova and parasites. Because transmission is believed to be via the fecal-oral route, presence of the organism may be a marker for presence of other pathogens spread by fecal contamination. Transmission from animals occurs.

The **incubation period** has not been established.

DIAGNOSTIC TESTS: Stool specimens should be preserved in polyvinyl alcohol and stained with trichrome or iron-hematoxylin before microscopic examination. The trophozoite stage of the parasite is very difficult to identify and rarely is seen. Small round cysts, the most common form, are characterized by a large central body (similar to large vacuole) surrounded by multiple nuclei. The parasite may be present in varying numbers, and infections may be reported as light to heavy. The presence of 5 or more organisms per high-power (x400 magnification) field can indicate heavy infection, which to some experts suggests causation when other enteropathogens are absent. Other experts consider the presence of 10 or more organisms per 10 oil immersion fields (x1000 magnification) to represent heavy infection.

TREATMENT: Indications for treatment are not established. Some experts recommend that treatment should be reserved for patients who have persistent symptoms and in whom no other pathogen or process is found to explain the gastrointestinal tract symptoms. Randomized controlled treatment trials with both nitazoxanide and metronidazole have demonstrated benefit in symptomatic patients. Tinidazole is an alternative that may be tolerated better than metronidazole. Trimethoprim-sulfamethoxazole, paromomycin, and iodoquinol have been used with limited success (see Drugs for Parasitic Infections, p 985). Notably, other experts believe that *B hominis* does not cause symptomatic disease and recommend only a careful search for other causes of symptoms.

ISOLATION OF THE HOSPITALIZED PATIENT: In addition to standard precautions, contact precautions are recommended for diapered or incontinent children.

CONTROL MEASURES: Personal hygiene measures, including hand washing with soap and warm water after using the toilet, after changing diapers, and before preparing food, should be practiced.

Blastomycosis

CLINICAL MANIFESTATIONS: Infections can be acute, chronic, or fulminant but are asymptomatic in up to 50% of infected people. The most common clinical manifestation of blastomycosis in children is cough (often productive) accompanying pulmonary disease, with fever, chest pain, and nonspecific symptoms such as fatigue and myalgia. Rarely, patients may develop acute respiratory distress syndrome (ARDS). Typical radiographic patterns include consolidation, patchy pneumonitis, a mass-like infiltrate, or nodules. Blastomycosis can be misdiagnosed as bacterial pneumonia, tuberculosis, sarcoidosis, or malignant neoplasm. Disseminated blastomycosis, which can occur in up to 25% of symptomatic cases, most commonly involves the skin, osteoarticular structures, and the genitourinary tract. Cutaneous manifestations can be verrucous, nodular, ulcerative, or pustular. Abscesses usually are subcutaneous but can involve any organ. Erythema nodosum, which is common in patients with histoplasmosis and coccidioidomycosis, is rare in blastomycosis. Central nervous system infection is less common, and intrauterine or congenital infection is rare.

ETIOLOGY: Blastomycosis is caused by *Blastomyces* species *(Blastomyces dermatitidis* and *Blastomyces gilchristii)*, thermally dimorphic fungi existing in the yeast form at 37°C (98°F) in infected tissues and in a mycelial form at room temperature and in soil. Conidia, produced from hyphae of the mycelial form, are infectious.

EPIDEMIOLOGY: Infection is acquired through inhalation of conidia from soil. Increased mortality rates for patients with pulmonary blastomycosis have been associated with advanced age, chronic obstructive pulmonary disease, cancer, and African American race. Person-to-person transmission does not occur. In the United States, blastomycosis is endemic in the central states, with most cases occurring in the Ohio and Mississippi river valleys, the southeastern states, and states that border the Great Lakes; however, sporadic cases have occurred outside these areas. Similar to *Histoplasma capsulatum, Blastomyces* species can grow in bird and animal excreta. Occupational and recreational activities associated with infection involve disruption of soil and include construction of homes or roads, boating and canoeing, tubing on a river, fishing, exploration of beaver dams and underground forts, and use of a community compost pile.

The **incubation period** ranges from 2 weeks to 3 months.

DIAGNOSTIC TESTS: Definitive diagnosis of blastomycosis is based on microscopic identification of characteristic thick-walled, broad-based, single budding yeast cells either by culture at 37°C or in histopathologic specimens. The organism may be seen in sputum, tracheal aspirates, cerebrospinal fluid, urine, or histopathologic specimens from lesions processed with 10% potassium hydroxide or a silver stain. Children with pneumonia who are unable to produce sputum may require bronchoalveolar lavage or open biopsy to establish the diagnosis. Bronchoalveolar lavage is high yield, even in patients with bone or skin manifestations. Organisms can be cultured on brain-heart infusion media and Sabouraud dextrose agar at 25°C to 30°C as a mold; identification can be confirmed by conversion to yeast phase at 37°C. Chemiluminescent DNA probes are available for identification of *B dermatitidis;* rare false-positive identification attributable to cross-reactivity with other endemic fungi has been reported. Because serologic tests (immunodiffusion and complement fixation) lack adequate sensitivity, effort should be made to obtain appropriate specimens for culture. Sensitivity is low for localized infection and higher in disseminated disease. Negative serum reaction testing during the acute phase may be repeated 3 to 4 weeks later. An enzyme immunoassay that detects *Blastomyces* antigen in urine has replaced classic serologic studies and performs well for the diagnosis of disseminated and pulmonary disease as well as monitoring response to antifungal therapy. Antigen testing in urine performs better than antigen testing of serum. Significant cross-reactivity occurs in patients with other endemic mycoses (specifically, *H capsulatum, Paracoccidioides brasiliensis,* and *Penicillium marneffei*); clinical and epidemiologic considerations often aid with interpretation.

TREATMENT[1]: Because of the high risk of dissemination, some experts recommend that all cases of blastomycosis in children should be treated. Amphotericin B deoxycholate or an amphotericin B lipid formulation is recommended for initial therapy of severe pulmonary disease for 1 to 2 weeks or until improvement, followed by 6 to 12 months of itraconazole therapy. Oral itraconazole is recommended for 6 to 12 months for mild to moderate infection. Some experts suggest 12 months of therapy for patients with osteoarticular disease. For central nervous system infection, a lipid formulation of amphotericin B is recommended for 4 to 6 weeks, followed by an azole for at least 12 months and until resolution of all cerebrospinal fluid abnormalities. The preferred azole for prolonged central nervous system infection treatment is fluconazole, but voriconazole and itraconazole are alternatives (see Antifungal Drugs for Systemic Fungal Infections, p 938). Itraconazole is indicated for treatment of non–life-threatening infection outside the central nervous system in adults and is recommended in children.[1] Serum trough concentrations of itraconazole should be 1 to 2 µg/mL. Concentrations should be checked after 1 to 2 weeks of therapy to ensure adequate drug exposure. When measured by high-pressure liquid chromatography, both itraconazole and its bioactive hydroxyitraconazole metabolite are reported, the sum of which should be considered in assessing drug levels. The itraconazole oral solution formulation is preferred because of improved absorption.

ISOLATION OF THE HOSPITALIZED PATIENT: Standard precautions are recommended.

CONTROL MEASURES: None.

Bocavirus

CLINICAL MANIFESTATIONS: Human bocavirus (HBoV) first was identified in 2005 from a cohort of children with acute respiratory tract symptoms. Cough, rhinorrhea, wheezing, and fever have been attributed to HBoV. HBoV has been identified in 5% to 33% of all children with acute respiratory tract infections in various settings (eg, inpatient facilities, outpatient facilities, child care centers). High rates of HBoV subclinical infections have been documented in children of similar age, complicating etiologic association with disease. The role of HBoV as a pathogen in human infection is further confounded by simultaneous detection of other viral pathogens in patients in whom HBoV is identified, with coinfection rates ranging from 20% to as high as 80%. However, a number of lines of evidence support the role of HBoV as a pathogen, at least during primary infection. These include longitudinal cohort studies showing an association of primary infection with symptomatic illness and case-control studies showing associations of illness with monoinfection, high viral load, and detection of mRNA.

HBoV has been detected in stool samples from children with acute gastroenteritis; however, further studies are needed to better understand the role of HBoV in gastroenteritis. Infection with HBoV appears to be ubiquitous, because nearly all children develop serologic evidence of previous HBoV infection by 5 years of age.

ETIOLOGY: HBoV is a nonenveloped, single-stranded DNA virus classified in the family *Parvoviridae*, subfamily *Parvovirinae*, genus *Bocaparvovirus*, on the basis of its genetic similarity to the closely related **bo**vine parvovirus 1 and **ca**nine minute virus, from which the name "**boca**virus" was derived. Four distinct genotypes have been described (HBoV types 1–4),

---

[1]Chapman SW, Dismukes WE, Proia LA, et al. Clinical guidelines for the management of blastomycosis: 2008 update by the Infectious Diseases Society of America. *Clin Infect Dis.* 2008;46(12):1801–1812

although there are no data regarding antigenic variation or distinct serotypes. HBoV1 replicates primarily in the respiratory tract and has been associated with upper and lower respiratory tract illness. HBoV2, HBoV3, and HBoV4 have been found predominantly in stool, without clear association with any clinical illness, except a few reports that have associated HBoV2 with gastroenteritis.

EPIDEMIOLOGY: Detection of HBoV has been described only in humans. Transmission is presumed to be from respiratory tract secretions, although fecal-oral transmission may be possible on the basis of the finding of HBoV in stool specimens from children, including symptomatic children with diarrhea.

The frequent codetection of other viral pathogens of the respiratory tract in association with HBoV has led to speculation about the role played by HBoV; it may be a true pathogen or copathogen, and emerging evidence seems to support both roles. Codetection of HBoV with other respiratory viruses is more common when HBoV is present at lower viral loads ($\leq 10^4$ copies/mL). Extended and intermittent shedding of HBoV has been reported for up to 12 weeks after initial detection. Because HBoV may be shed for long periods after primary infection and because of the possibility of reactivation during subsequent viral infections and the high rate of detection in healthy people, clinical interpretation of HBoV detection is difficult.

HBoV circulates worldwide and throughout the year. In temperate climates, seasonal clustering in the spring associated with increased transmission of other respiratory tract viruses has been reported.

DIAGNOSTIC TESTS: Commercial molecular diagnostic assays for HBoV are available. HBoV polymerase chain reaction and detection of HBoV-specific antibody also are used by research laboratories to detect the presence of virus and infection, respectively.

TREATMENT: No specific therapy is available.

ISOLATION OF THE HOSPITALIZED PATIENT: The presence of virus in respiratory tract secretions and stool suggests that, in addition to standard precautions, contact precautions should be initiated to limit the spread of infection for the duration of the symptomatic illness in infants and young children. Prolonged shedding of virus in respiratory tract secretions and in stool may occur after resolution of symptoms, particularly in immunocompromised hosts; therefore, the duration of contact precautions should be extended in these situations.

CONTROL MEASURES: Appropriate respiratory hygiene and cough etiquette should be followed. Although possible health care-associated transmission of HBoV has been described, investigations of transmissibility of HBoV in the community or health care settings have not been published. Appropriate hand hygiene, particularly when handling respiratory tract secretions or diapers of ill children, is recommended. The presence of HBoV DNA in serum also raises the possibility of transmission by transfusion, although this mode of transmission has not been documented.

Borrelia Infections Other Than Lyme Disease
(Relapsing Fever)

CLINICAL MANIFESTATIONS: Two types of relapsing fever occur in humans: tickborne and louseborne. Both are characterized by sudden onset of high fever, shaking chills, sweats, headache, muscle and joint pain, altered sensorium, nausea, and diarrhea. A fleeting macular rash of the trunk and petechiae of the skin and mucous membranes sometimes occur. Findings and complications can differ between types of relapsing fever and include hepatosplenomegaly, jaundice, thrombocytopenia, iridocyclitis, cough with pleuritic pain, pneumonitis, meningitis, and myocarditis. Mortality rates can exceed 30% in untreated louseborne relapsing fever (possibly related to comorbidities in refugee-type settings, where this disease typically is found) and 4% to 10% in untreated tickborne relapsing fever. Death occurs predominantly in people with underlying illnesses, infants, and elderly people. Early treatment reduces mortality to less than 5%. Untreated, an initial febrile period of 2 to 7 days terminates spontaneously, and is followed by an afebrile period of several days to weeks, then by 1 relapse or more (0–13 for tickborne, 1–5 for louseborne). Relapses typically become shorter and progressively milder as afebrile periods lengthen. Relapse is associated with expression of new borrelial antigens, and resolution of symptoms is associated with production of antibody specific to those new antigenic determinants. Infection during pregnancy often is severe and can result in spontaneous abortion, preterm birth, stillbirth, or neonatal infection.

ETIOLOGY: Relapsing fever is caused by certain spirochetes of the genus *Borrelia*. Worldwide, at least 14 *Borrelia* species cause tickborne (endemic) relapsing fever, including *Borrelia hermsii, Borrelia turicatae, Borrelia parkeri*, and *Borrelia miyamotoi* in North America. Louseborne (epidemic) relapsing fever is cause by *Borrelia recurrentis*. Lyme disease, caused by the more distantly related *Borrelia burgdorferi* and *Borrelia mayonii*, is discussed in the Lyme Disease chapter (p 515).

EPIDEMIOLOGY: Endemic tickborne relapsing fever is distributed widely throughout the world. Most species, including *B hermsii, B turicatae,* and *B parkeri*, are transmitted by soft-bodied ticks (*Ornithodoros* species). *B miyamotoi*, which has only recently been recognized as a cause of human illness, is transmitted by hard-bodied ticks (*Ixodes* species). Vector ticks become infected by feeding on rodents or other small mammals and transmit infection via their saliva during subsequent blood meals. Ticks may serve as reservoirs of infection through transovarial and trans-stadial transmission. Because of differences in the distribution, life cycle, and feeding habits of soft- and hard-bodied ticks, the epidemiology of tickborne relapsing fever differs somewhat for infections transmitted by these 2 classes of ticks.

Soft-bodied ticks typically live within rodent nests. They inflict painless bites and feed briefly (15–90 minutes), usually at night, so that people often are unaware of having been bitten. In the United States, vector soft-bodied ticks are found in mountainous areas of the West. Human infection typically results from sleeping in rustic, rodent-infested cabins, although cases have been associated with primary residences and luxurious rental properties. Cases occur sporadically or in small clusters among families or cohabiting groups and may be seen in residents of other states following trips to the Rocky Mountains or Sierra Nevada Mountains. *B hermsii* is the most common cause of these infections. *B turicatae* infections occur less frequently; most cases have been reported from Texas and are associated with tick exposures in rodent-infested caves. A single human infection has been reported with *B parkeri*; the tick infected with this *Borrelia* species is associated with arid areas or grasslands in the western United States.

The hard-bodied ticks *Ixodes scapularis* and *Ixodes pacificus* transmit *B miyamotoi* in North America. These ticks are better known as vectors of Lyme disease, anaplasmosis, and babesiosis. They are common in areas of the northeastern, Mid-Atlantic, and upper Midwest regions as well as focal areas along the Pacific coast. They live in grassy and wooded areas and must remain attached for approximately 72 hours to obtain a full blood meal.

Reported rates of infection with *B miyamotoi* typically are 1% to 2% across all areas studied. The epidemiology of human infection is poorly defined at present; to date, most human cases in the United States have been reported from the Northeast.

Louseborne epidemic relapsing fever has been reported in Ethiopia, Eritrea, Somalia, and the Sudan, especially in refugee and displaced populations. Epidemic transmission occurs when body lice *(Pediculus humanus)* become infected by feeding on humans with spirochetemia; infection is transmitted when infected lice are crushed and their body fluids contaminate a bite wound or skin abraded by scratching.

Infected body lice and ticks may remain alive and infectious for several years without feeding. Relapsing fever is not transmitted between individual humans, but perinatal transmission from an infected mother to her infant occurs and can result in preterm birth, stillbirth, and neonatal death.

The **incubation period** is 2 to 18 days, with a mean of 7 days.

DIAGNOSTIC TESTS: Spirochetes can be observed by dark-field microscopy and in Wright-, Giemsa-, or acridine orange-stained preparations of thin or dehemoglobinized thick smears of peripheral blood or in stained buffy-coat preparations. Organisms often can be visualized in blood obtained while the person is febrile, particularly during initial febrile episodes; organisms are less likely to be recovered from subsequent relapses. Spirochetes can be cultured from blood in Barbour-Stoenner-Kelly medium or by intraperitoneal inoculation of immature laboratory mice, although these tests are not widely available. Serum antibodies to *Borrelia* species can be detected by enzyme immunoassay and Western immunoblot analysis at some reference and commercial specialty laboratories; a fourfold increase in titer is considered confirmatory. These antibody tests are not standardized and are affected by antigenic variations among and within *Borrelia* species and strains. Serologic cross-reactions occur with other spirochetes, including *B burgdorferi*, *Treponema pallidum*, and *Leptospira* species. Biological specimens for laboratory testing can be sent to the Division of Vector-Borne Diseases, Centers for Disease Control and Prevention, 3156 Rampart Rd, Fort Collins, CO 80521 (telephone: 970-221-6400).

B miyamotoi polymerase chain reaction (PCR) and antibody-based tests are under development and not widely commercially available but can be ordered from a limited number of laboratories approved under the Clinical Laboratory Improvement Amendments (CLIA).

TREATMENT: Treatment of tickborne relapsing fever with a 5- to 10-day course of doxycycline produces prompt clearance of spirochetes and remission of symptoms; doxycycline can be used regardless of patient age (see Tetracyclines, p 905). For pregnant women, penicillin and erythromycin are the preferred drugs. Penicillin G procaine or intravenous penicillin G is recommended as initial therapy for people who cannot tolerate oral therapy, although low-dose penicillin G has been associated with a higher frequency of relapse. A Jarisch-Herxheimer reaction (an acute febrile reaction accompanied by headache, myalgia, respiratory distress in some cases, and an aggravated clinical picture lasting less than 24 hours) commonly is observed during the first few hours after initiating antimicrobial therapy. Because this reaction sometimes is associated with transient hypotension attributable to decreased effective circulating blood volume (especially in louseborne relapsing fever), patients should be hospitalized and monitored closely, particularly during the first 4 hours of treatment. However, the Jarisch-Herxheimer reaction in children typically is mild and usually can be managed with antipyretic agents alone.

Physicians have successfully treated patients infected with *B miyamotoi* with a 2- to 4-week course of doxycycline. Amoxicillin and ceftriaxone also have been used.

For louseborne relapsing fever, single-dose treatment using doxycycline, penicillin, or erythromycin is effective therapy.

ISOLATION OF THE HOSPITALIZED PATIENT: Standard precautions are recommended. If louse infestation is present, contact precautions are indicated until delousing (see Pediculosis, p 607–613).

CONTROL MEASURES: Soft ticks often can be found in rodent nests; exposure is reduced most effectively by preventing rodent infestations of homes or cabins by blocking rodent access to foundations and attics and other forms of rodent control. Dwellings infested with soft ticks should be rodent-proofed and treated professionally with chemical agents. When in a louse-infested environment, body lice can be controlled by bathing, washing clothing at frequent intervals, and use of pediculicides (see Pediculosis, p 607–613). Reporting of suspected cases of relapsing fever to health authorities is required in most western states and is important for initiation of prompt investigation and institution of control measures.

Brucellosis

CLINICAL MANIFESTATIONS: Onset of brucellosis in children can be acute or insidious. Manifestations are nonspecific and include fever, night sweats, weakness, malaise, anorexia, weight loss, arthralgia, myalgia, back pain, abdominal pain, and headache. Physical findings may include lymphadenopathy, hepatosplenomegaly, and arthritis. Abdominal pain and peripheral arthritis are reported more frequently in children than in adults. Neurologic deficits, ocular involvement, epididymo-orchitis, and liver or spleen abscesses are reported. Anemia, leukopenia, thrombocytopenia, or less frequently, pancytopenia are hematologic findings that might suggest the diagnosis. Serious complications include meningitis, endocarditis, and osteomyelitis and, less frequently, pneumonitis and aortic involvement. A detailed history including travel, exposure to animals, and food habits, including ingestion of unpasteurized milk or cheese, and occupational history should be obtained if brucellosis is considered. Chronic disease is less common among children than among adults, although the rate of relapse has been found to be similar. Brucellosis in pregnancy is associated with risk of spontaneous abortion, preterm delivery, miscarriage, and intrauterine infection with fetal death.

ETIOLOGY: *Brucella* bacteria are small, nonmotile, gram-negative coccobacilli. The species that are known to infect humans are *Brucella abortus*, *Brucella melitensis*, *Brucella suis*, and rarely, *Brucella canis*. Three recently identified species, *Brucella ceti*, *Brucella pinnipedialis*, and *Brucella inopinata*, are potential human pathogens.

EPIDEMIOLOGY: Brucellosis is a zoonotic disease of wild and domestic animals. It is transmissible to humans by direct or indirect exposure to aborted fetuses or tissues or fluids of infected animals. Transmission occurs by inoculation through mucous membranes or cuts and abrasions in the skin, inhalation of contaminated aerosols, or ingestion of undercooked meat or unpasteurized dairy products.[1] People in occupations such as farming, ranching, and veterinary medicine, as well as abattoir workers, meat inspectors,

---

[1]American Academy of Pediatrics, Committee on Infectious Diseases, Committee on Nutrition. Consumption of raw or unpasteurized milk and milk products by pregnant women and children. *Pediatrics*. 2014;133(1):175–179

and laboratory personnel, are at increased risk. Clinicians should alert the laboratory if they anticipate *Brucella* might grow from microbiologic specimens so that appropriate laboratory precautions can be taken. In the United States, approximately 100 to 200 cases of brucellosis are reported annually, and 3% to 10% of cases occur in people younger than 19 years. The majority of pediatric cases reported in the United States result from ingestion of unpasteurized dairy products. Human-to-human transmission is rare, but sexual transmission has been reported, in utero transmission has been reported, and infected mothers can transmit *Brucella* to their infants through breastfeeding.

The **incubation period** varies from less than 1 week to several months, but most people become ill within 3 to 4 weeks of exposure.

DIAGNOSTIC TESTS: A definitive diagnosis is established by recovery of *Brucella* species from blood, bone marrow, or other tissue specimens. A variety of media will support growth of *Brucella* species, but the physician should contact laboratory personnel and ask them to incubate cultures for a minimum of 4 weeks. Newer BACTEC systems have greater reliability and can detect *Brucella* species within 7 days with no need to prolong incubation. Caution should be taken with culture manipulation of this organism because of the high risk of laboratory-acquired infection.

In patients with a clinically compatible illness, serologic testing using the serum agglutination test can confirm the diagnosis with a fourfold or greater increase in antibody titers between acute and convalescent serum specimens collected at least 2 weeks apart. The serum agglutination test, the gold standard test for serologic diagnosis, will detect antibodies against *B abortus, B suis,* and *B melitensis* but not *B canis,* which requires use of *B canis*-specific antigen. Although a single titer is not diagnostic, most patients with active infection in an area without endemic infection will have a titer of 1:160 or greater within 2 to 4 weeks of clinical disease onset. Lower titers may be found early in the course of infection. Immunoglobulin (Ig) M antibodies are produced within the first week, followed by a gradual increase in IgG synthesis. Low IgM titers may persist for months or years after initial infection. Increased concentrations of IgG agglutinins are found in acute infection, chronic infection, and relapse. When interpreting serum agglutination test results, the possibility of cross-reactions of *Brucella* antibodies with antibodies against other gram-negative bacteria, such as *Yersinia enterocolitica* serotype 09, *Francisella tularensis, Escherichia coli* O116 and O157, *Salmonella urbana, Vibrio cholerae, Xanthomonas maltophilia,* and *Afipia clevelandensis,* should be considered. Enzyme immunoassay is a sensitive method for determining IgG, IgA, and IgM anti-*Brucella* antibody titers. Until better standardization is established, enzyme immunoassay should be used only for suspected cases with negative serum agglutination test results or for evaluation of patients with suspected chronic brucellosis, reinfection, or complicated cases.

Polymerase chain reaction tests that can be performed in blood and body tissue samples have been developed but are not yet available in most clinical laboratories, as improved standardization and better understanding of their clinical applicability are needed. If a laboratory is not available to perform diagnostic testing for *Brucella* species, the physician should contact the state health department for assistance.

TREATMENT: Prolonged antimicrobial therapy is imperative for achieving a cure. Relapses generally are not associated with development of *Brucella* resistance but rather with premature discontinuation of therapy or localized infection. Because monotherapy is associated with a high rate of relapse, combination therapy is recommended as standard treatment. Most combination regimens include oral doxycycline or trimethoprim-sulfa-methoxazole plus rifampin.

Oral doxycycline (4.4 mg/kg per day, maximum 200 mg/day, in 2 divided doses) is the drug of choice and should be administered for a minimum of 6 weeks. Because of this prolonged duration of therapy, doxycycline is not recommended for children younger than 8 years (see Tetracyclines, p 905). These younger children (under 8 years) should receive oral trimethoprim-sulfamethoxazole (trimethoprim, 10 mg/kg per day, maximum 480 mg/day; and sulfamethoxazole, 50 mg/kg per day, maximum 2.4 g/day), divided in 2 doses for at least 6 weeks. Rifampin (15–20 mg/kg per day, maximum 600–900 mg/day, in 1 or 2 divided doses) should be added to doxycycline or trimethoprim-sulfamethoxazole. Because of the potential emergence of rifampin resistance, rifampin monotherapy is not recommended. Failure to complete the full 6-week course of therapy may result in relapse.

For treatment of serious infections or complications, including endocarditis, meningitis, spondylitis, and osteomyelitis, a 3-drug regimen should be used, with gentamicin included for the first 7 to 14 days of therapy, in addition to doxycycline (or trimethoprim-sulfamethoxazole, if doxycycline is not used) and rifampin for a minimum of 6 weeks. For life-threatening complications of brucellosis, such as meningitis or endocarditis, the duration of therapy often is extended for 4 to 6 months. Surgical intervention should be considered in patients with complications, such as deep tissue abscesses, endocarditis, mycotic aneurysm, and foreign body infections.

The benefit of corticosteroids for people with neurobrucellosis is unproven. Occasionally, a Jarisch-Herxheimer-like reaction (an acute febrile reaction accompanied by headache, myalgia, and an aggravated clinical picture lasting less than 24 hours) occurs shortly after initiation of antimicrobial therapy, but this reaction rarely is severe enough to require corticosteroids.

ISOLATION OF THE HOSPITALIZED PATIENT: In addition to standard precautions, contact precautions are indicated for patients with draining wounds.

CONTROL MEASURES: The control of human brucellosis depends on control of *Brucella* species from cattle, goats, swine, and other animals. Vaccination of cattle, sheep, and goats can be effective but needs to be sustained over several years. Contact with infected animals should be avoided, especially female animals that have aborted or are giving birth. Pasteurization of dairy products for human consumption is important to prevent disease, especially in children.[1] The certification of raw milk does not eliminate the risk of transmission of *Brucella* organisms. Mothers with active brucellosis should not breastfeed their infants until their infection is eradicated. People who have consumed raw milk or raw milk products that are potentially contaminated with the bovine *Brucella* vaccine strain RB51 are at high risk for brucellosis infection. For these people, postexposure prophylaxis with doxycycline plus either trimethoprim-sulfamethoxazole or another suitable antimicrobial agent is recommended for 21 days. Patients should be monitored for fever for 4 weeks following the last exposure and for 6 months for symptoms of brucellosis (see **https://emergency.cdc.gov/han/han00407.asp** for additional information).

---

[1] American Academy of Pediatrics, Committee on Infectious Diseases, Committee on Nutrition. Consumption of raw or unpasteurized milk and milk products by pregnant women and children. *Pediatrics.* 2014;133(1):175–179

Burkholderia Infections

CLINICAL MANIFESTATIONS: Species within the *Burkholderia cepacia* complex have been associated with infections in individuals with cystic fibrosis, chronic granulomatous disease, hemoglobinopathies, or malignant neoplasms and in preterm infants. Airway infections in people with cystic fibrosis usually occur later in the course of disease, after respiratory epithelial damage and bronchiectasis have occurred. Patients with cystic fibrosis can become chronically infected with little change in the rate of pulmonary decompensation or can experience an accelerated decline in pulmonary function or an unexpectedly rapid deterioration in clinical status that results in death. In patients with chronic granulomatous disease, pneumonia is the most common manifestation of *B cepacia* complex infection; lymphadenitis also occurs. Disease onset is insidious, with low-grade fever early in the course and systemic effects occurring 3 to 4 weeks later. Pleural effusions are common, and lung abscesses can occur. Health care-associated infections including wound and urinary tract infections and pneumonia have been reported, and clusters of disease have been associated with contaminated pharmaceutical products, including nasal sprays, mouthwash, sublingual probes, prefilled saline flush syringes, and oral docusate sodium.

   Burkholderia pseudomallei is the cause of melioidosis. Its geographic range is expanding, and disease now is known to be endemic in Southeast Asia, northern Australia, areas of the Indian Subcontinent, southern China, Hong Kong, Taiwan, several Pacific and Indian Ocean Islands, and some areas of South and Central America. Melioidosis can occur in the United States, usually among travelers returning from areas with endemic disease. Melioidosis can be asymptomatic or can manifest as a localized infection or as fulminant septicemia. Approximately 40% to 60% of adults with melioidosis are bacteremic on admission; bacteremia is less common in children. Pneumonia is the most commonly reported clinical manifestation of melioidosis in adults. A recent report from Australia found that localized cutaneous disease was the most common presentation in immunocompetent children. Genitourinary infections including prostatic abscesses, septic arthritis and osteomyelitis, and central nervous system involvement, including brain abscesses, also occur. Acute suppurative parotitis is a manifestation that occurs frequently in children in Thailand and Cambodia but is less commonly seen in other areas with endemic infection. Localized infection usually is nonfatal. In severe cutaneous infection, necrotizing fasciitis has been reported. In disseminated infection, hepatic and splenic abscesses can occur, and relapses are common without prolonged therapy.

ETIOLOGY: The *Burkholderia* genus comprises more than 90 species that are nutritionally diverse, oxidase- and catalase-producing, non–lactose-fermenting, gram-negative bacilli. *B cepacia* complex comprises at least 20 species. Additional members of the complex continue to be identified but are rare human pathogens. Other clinically important species of *Burkholderia* include *Burkholderia pseudomallei*, *Burkholderia gladioli*, and *Burkholderia mallei* (the agent responsible for glanders). *Burkholderia thailandensis* and *Burkholderia oklahomensis* are rare human pathogens.

EPIDEMIOLOGY: *Burkholderia* species are environmentally derived waterborne and soilborne organisms that can survive for prolonged periods in a moist environment. Depending on the species, transmission may occur from other people (person to person), from contact with contaminated fomites, and from exposure to environmental sources. Epidemiologic studies of recreational camps and social events attended by people with cystic fibrosis from different geographic areas have documented person-to-person spread of *B* *cepacia* complex. The source of acquisition of *B cepacia* complex by patients with chronic granulomatous disease has not been clearly identified, although environmental sources seem likely. Health care-associated spread of *B cepacia* complex most often is associated with contamination of disinfectant solutions used to clean reusable patient equipment, such as bronchoscopes and pressure transducers, or to disinfect skin. Contaminated medical products, including mouthwash and inhaled medications, have been identified as a cause of multistate outbreaks of colonization and infection. *B gladioli* has been isolated from sputum of people with cystic fibrosis and may be mistaken for *B cepacia*. *B gladioli* may be associated with transient or more prolonged, chronic infection in patients with cystic fibrosis; poor outcomes have been noted in lung transplant recipients who have *B gladioli* infection.

In areas with highly endemic infection, *B pseudomallei* is acquired early in life, with the highest seroconversion rates between 6 months and 4 years of age. Melioidosis is seasonal, with more than 75% of cases occurring during the rainy season. Disease can be acquired by direct inhalation of aerosolized organisms or dust particles containing organisms, by percutaneous or wound inoculation with contaminated soil or water, or by ingestion of contaminated soil, water, or food. People also can become infected as a result of laboratory exposures when proper techniques and/or proper personal protective equipment guidelines are not followed. Symptomatic infection can occur in children 1 year or younger, with pneumonia and parotitis reported in infants as young as 8 months; in addition, 2 cases of human milk transmission from mothers with mastitis have been reported. Risk factors for melioidosis include frequent contact with soil and water as well as underlying chronic disease, such as diabetes mellitus, renal insufficiency, chronic pulmonary disease, thalassemia, and immunosuppression not related to human immunodeficiency virus (HIV) infection. *B pseudomallei* also has been reported to cause pulmonary infection in people with cystic fibrosis and septicemia in children with chronic granulomatous disease.

The **incubation period** for melioidosis is 1 to 21 days, with a median of 9 days, but can be prolonged (years).

DIAGNOSTIC TESTS: Culture is the appropriate method to diagnose *B cepacia* complex infection. In cystic fibrosis airway infection, culture of sputum on selective agar is recommended to decrease the potential for overgrowth by mucoid *Pseudomonas aeruginosa*. Confirmation of identification of *B cepacia* complex species by polymerase chain reaction assay (investigational use only) or mass spectroscopy (approved for use) is recommended.

Definitive diagnosis of melioidosis is made by isolation of *B pseudomallei* from blood or other infected sites. The likelihood of successfully isolating the organism is increased by culture of sputum, throat, rectum, and ulcer or skin lesion specimens. A direct polymerase chain reaction assay, available at the Centers for Disease Control and Prevention, may provide a more rapid result than culture but is less sensitive, especially when performed on blood, and is not recommended for routine use as a diagnostic assay. Serologic testing is not adequate for diagnosis in areas with endemic infection because of high background seropositivity. However, a positive result by the indirect hemagglutination assay for a traveler who has returned from an area with endemic infection may support the diagnosis of melioidosis; definitive diagnosis still requires isolation of *B pseudomallei* from an infected site. Other rapid assays are being developed for diagnosis of melioidosis but are not yet commercially available.

Suspected isolates of *B mallei* and *B pseudomallei* should be referred to State Public

Health Laboratory Response Network Laboratories. If confirmed, laboratory procedures to evaluate for occupational exposure should be reviewed.

TREATMENT: Meropenem is the agent most active against the majority of *B cepacia* complex isolates, although other drugs that may be effective include imipenem, trimethoprim-sulfamethoxazole, ceftazidime, doxycycline, and chloramphenicol. Some experts recommend combinations of antimicrobial agents that provide synergistic activity against *B cepacia* complex in vitro. The majority of *B cepacia* complex isolates are intrinsically resistant to aminoglycosides and polymyxins.

The drugs of choice for initial treatment of melioidosis depend on the type of clinical infection, susceptibility testing, and presence of comorbidities in the patient (eg, diabetes, liver or renal disease, cancer, hemoglobinopathies, cystic fibrosis). Treatment of severe invasive infection should include meropenem or ceftazidime (rare resistance) for a minimum of 10 to 14 days. After acute therapy is completed, oral eradication therapy with trimethoprim-sulfamethoxazole for 3 to 6 months is recommended to reduce recurrence. Amoxicillin clavulanate and doxycycline are considered second-line oral agents and may be associated with a higher rate of relapse.

ISOLATION OF THE HOSPITALIZED PATIENT: In addition to standard precautions, contact and droplet precautions are recommended for all cystic fibrosis patients regardless of infection status. Human-to-human transmission is extremely rare for *B pseudomallei*, and standard precautions are recommended.

CONTROL MEASURES: Because some strains of *B cepacia* complex cause a highly virulent course in some patients with new acquisition, the Cystic Fibrosis Foundation recommends that all cystic fibrosis care centers limit contact between patients. This includes inpatient, outpatient, and social settings. When in a health care setting, patients with cystic fibrosis should wear a mask while outside of a clinic examination room or a hospital room. Education of patients and families about hand hygiene and appropriate personal hygiene is recommended.

Prevention of infection with *B pseudomallei* in areas with endemic disease can be difficult, because contact with contaminated water and soil is common. People with diabetes mellitus, renal insufficiency, or skin lesions should avoid contact with soil and standing water in these areas, and it is recommended that they stay inside during weather that could result in aerosolization of the organism. Wearing boots and gloves during agricultural work in areas with endemic disease is recommended. Patients with cystic fibrosis should be educated regarding their risk of infection when traveling to regions where *B pseudomallei* is endemic. A human vaccine is not available, but research is ongoing. Cases of melioidosis are notifiable in many states, and reporting cases to local or state health departments is prudent.

Campylobacter Infections

CLINICAL MANIFESTATIONS: Predominant symptoms of *Campylobacter* infections include diarrhea, abdominal pain, malaise, and fever. Stools can contain visible or occult blood. In neonates and young infants, bloody diarrhea without fever can be the only manifestation of infection. Pronounced fevers in children can result in febrile seizures that can occur before gastrointestinal tract symptoms. Abdominal pain can mimic that produced by appendicitis or intussusception. Mild infection lasts 1 or 2 days and resembles viral gastroenteritis. Most patients recover in less than 1 week, but 10% to 20% have a relapse or a prolonged or severe illness. Severe or persistent infection can mimic acute inflammatory bowel disease. Bacteremia is uncommon but can occur in elderly patients and in patients with underlying conditions. Immunocompromised hosts can have prolonged, relapsing, or extraintestinal infections, especially with *Campylobacter fetus* and other *Campylobacter* species. Immunoreactive complications, such as Guillain-Barré syndrome (occurring in 1:1000), Miller Fisher variant of Guillain-Barré syndrome (ophthalmoplegia, areflexia, ataxia), reactive arthritis (with the classic triad, formerly known as Reiter syndrome, consisting of arthritis, urethritis, and bilateral conjunctivitis), myocarditis, pericarditis, and erythema nodosum, can occur during convalescence.

ETIOLOGY: *Campylobacter* species are motile, comma-shaped, gram-negative bacilli that cause gastroenteritis. There are 25 species within the genus *Campylobacter*, but *Campylobacter jejuni* and *Campylobacter coli* are the species isolated most commonly from patients with diarrhea. *C fetus* predominantly causes systemic illness in neonates and debilitated hosts. Other *Campylobacter* species, including *Campylobacter upsaliensis*, *Campylobacter lari*, and *Campylobacter hyointestinalis,* can cause similar diarrheal or systemic illnesses in children.

EPIDEMIOLOGY: Although incidence decreased in the early 2000s, data from the Foodborne Diseases Active Surveillance Network (**www.cdc.gov/foodnet**) indicate that the 2012 incidence of culture-confirmed cases of 14.3 per 100 000 population represented a 14% increase over a 2006–2008 baseline. Disease incidence has remained stable since 2010–2012, with 13.8 cases per 100 000 population in 2013.[1] The highest rates of infection occur in children younger than 5 years (24.08 per 100 000 in 2009). The majority of *Campylobacter* infections are acquired domestically, but it is also a very common cause of laboratory-confirmed diarrhea in returning international travelers. In susceptible people, as few as 500 *Campylobacter* organisms can cause infection.

The gastrointestinal tracts of domestic and wild birds and animals are reservoirs of the bacteria. *C jejuni* and *C coli* have been isolated from feces of 30% to 100% of healthy chickens, turkeys, and water fowl. Poultry carcasses commonly are contaminated. Many farm animals, pets, and meat sources can harbor the organism and are potential sources of infection. Transmission of *C jejuni* and *C coli* occurs by ingestion of contaminated food or water or by direct contact with fecal material from infected animals or people. Improperly cooked poultry, untreated water, and unpasteurized milk have been the main vehicles of transmission. *Campylobacter* infections usually are sporadic; outbreaks are rare but have occurred among school children who drank unpasteurized milk,[2] including children who participated in field trips to dairy farms. Person-to-person spread occurs occasionally, particularly among very young children, and risk is greatest during the acute phase of illness. Uncommonly, outbreaks of diarrhea in child care centers have been reported. Person-to-person transmission has occurred in neonates of infected mothers and has resulted in health care-associated outbreaks in nurseries. In perinatal infection, *C jejuni* and *C coli* usually cause neonatal gastroenteritis, whereas *C fetus* often causes neonatal septicemia or

---

[1] Centers for Disease Control and Prevention. Incidence and trends of infection with pathogens transmitted commonly through food—Foodborne Diseases Active Surveillance Network, 10 U.S. Sites, 2006–2013. *MMWR Morb Mortal Wkly Rep.* 2014;63(15):328–332

[2] American Academy of Pediatrics, Committee on Infectious Diseases and Committee on Nutrition. Consumption of raw or unpasteurized milk and milk products by pregnant women and children. *Pediatrics.* 2014;133(1):175–179 (Reaffirmed October 2017)

meningitis. Enteritis occurs in people of all ages. Excretion of *Campylobacter* organisms typically lasts 2 to 3 weeks without antimicrobial treatment and can be as long as 7 weeks.

The **incubation period** usually is 2 to 5 days but can be longer.

DIAGNOSTIC TESTS: *C jejuni* and *C coli* can be recovered from feces, and *Campylobacter* species, including *C fetus*, can be recovered from blood. Isolation of *C jejuni* and *C coli* from stool specimens requires selective media, microaerobic conditions, and an incubation temperature of 42°C. Although other *Campylobacter* species occasionally are isolated using routine culture methods, additional methods that use nonselective isolation techniques and increased hydrogen microaerobic conditions usually are required for isolation of species other than *C jejuni* and *C coli*. *C upsaliensis, C hyointestinalis, C lara,* and *C fetus* may not be isolated because of susceptibility to antimicrobial agents present in the *Campylobacter*-selective media used routinely to isolate *C jejuni* and *C coli*. Direct-examination, culture-independent methods are available, in addition to culture, but all have the major drawback of not providing an opportunity to determine antibiotic susceptibilities for the infecting organism. *C jejuni* and *C coli* can be detected directly (but not differentiated) by commercially available enzyme immunoassays. These immunologic assays provide rapid diagnosis of enteric infection with *C jejuni* and *C coli* but have variable performance. False-positive results from these non–culture-based techniques have been reported, and given that *Campylobacter* infection is a low-incidence disease, raise concern regarding the specificity of these tests. A number of multiplex nucleic acid amplification tests (NAATs) that detect select *Campylobacter* species and other bacterial, viral, or parasitic gastrointestinal pathogens were recently cleared by the US Food and Drug Administration. These assays cannot always distinguish between *Campylobacter* species. Clinical interpretation and experience with these new molecular tests is limited at this time. For serious infection, isolation of the organism is preferred to confirm diagnosis, and the isolate should be retained for antimicrobial susceptibility testing.

TREATMENT: Rehydration is the mainstay of treatment for all children with diarrhea. Azithromycin and erythromycin shorten the duration of illness and excretion of susceptible organisms (2% of *C jejuni* isolates are resistant to erythromycin and azithromycin and 17% and 18% of *C coli* are resistant to erythromycin and azithromycin, respectively) and prevent relapse when administered early in gastrointestinal tract infection. Treatment with azithromycin (10 mg/kg/day, for 3 days) or erythromycin (40 mg/kg/day, in 4 divided doses, for 5 days) usually eradicates the organism from stool within 2 or 3 days. A fluoroquinolone, such as ciprofloxacin, may be effective, but resistance to ciprofloxacin is common (34% of *C coli* isolates and 22% of *C jejuni* isolates in the United States in 2013 **[www.cdc.gov/NARMS]**) (see Fluoroquinolones, p 904). If antimicrobial therapy is administered for treatment of gastroenteritis, the recommended duration is 3 to 5 days. Antimicrobial agents for bacteremia should be selected on the basis of antimicrobial susceptibility tests. *C fetus* generally is susceptible to aminoglycosides, extended-spectrum cephalosporins, meropenem, imipenem, ampicillin, and erythromycin. Antimotility agents should not be used, because they have been shown to prolong symptomatology and may be associated with an increased risk of death.

ISOLATION OF THE HOSPITALIZED PATIENT: In addition to standard precautions, contact precautions are recommended for diapered and incontinent children for the duration of illness.

CONTROL MEASURES:

- Hand hygiene should be performed after handling raw poultry, cutting boards and utensils should be washed with soap and water after contact with raw poultry, and contact of fruits and vegetables with juices of raw poultry should be avoided.

- Poultry should be cooked thoroughly.
- Hand hygiene should be performed after contact with feces of dogs and cats, particularly stool of puppies and kittens with diarrhea.
- People should not drink raw milk.[1] The certification of raw milk does not eliminate the risk of transmission of *Campylobacter* organisms.
- Chlorination of water supplies is important.
- People with diarrhea should be excluded from food handling, care of patients in hospitals, and care of people in custodial care and child care centers.
- Infected food handlers and hospital employees who are asymptomatic need not be excluded from work if proper personal hygiene measures, including hand hygiene, are maintained.
- Outbreaks are uncommon in child care centers. General measures for interrupting enteric transmission in child care centers are recommended (see Children in Out-of-Home Child Care, p 122). Infants and children should be excluded from child care centers until stools are contained in the diaper or when toilet-trained children no longer have accidents using the toilet and when stool frequency becomes no more than 2 stools above that child's normal frequency for the time the child is in the program, even if the stools remain loose. Azithromycin or erythromycin treatment may further limit the potential for transmission.
- Stool cultures of asymptomatic exposed children are not recommended.

Candidiasis

CLINICAL MANIFESTATIONS: Mucocutaneous infection results in oral-pharyngeal (thrush) or vaginal or cervical candidiasis; intertriginous lesions of the gluteal folds, buttocks, neck, groin, and axilla; paronychia; and onychia. Dysfunction of T lymphocytes, other immunologic disorders, and endocrinologic diseases are associated with chronic mucocutaneous candidiasis. Chronic or recurrent oral candidiasis can be the presenting sign of human immunodeficiency virus (HIV) infection or primary immunodeficiency. Esophageal and laryngeal candidiasis can occur in immunocompromised patients. Disseminated candidiasis has a predilection for extremely preterm infants and immunocompromised or debilitated hosts, can involve virtually any organ or anatomic site, and can be rapidly fatal. Candidemia can occur with or without associated end-organ disease in patients with indwelling central vascular catheters, especially in patients receiving prolonged intravenous infusions with parenteral alimentation or lipids. Peritonitis can occur in patients undergoing peritoneal dialysis, especially in patients receiving prolonged broad-spectrum antimicrobial therapy. Candiduria can occur in patients with indwelling urinary catheters, focal renal infection, or disseminated disease.

ETIOLOGY: *Candida* species are yeasts that reproduce by budding. *Candida albicans* and several other species form long chains of elongated yeast forms called pseudohyphae. *C albicans* causes most infections, but in some regions and patient populations, non-albicans

---

[1]American Academy of Pediatrics, Committee on Infectious Diseases, Committee on Nutrition. Consumption of raw or unpasteurized milk and milk products by pregnant women and children. *Pediatrics.* 2014;133(1):175–179

Candida species now account for more than half of invasive infections. Other species, including *Candida tropicalis, Candida parapsilosis, Candida glabrata, Candida krusei, Candida guilliermondii, Candida lusitaniae,* and *Candida dubliniensis,* can cause serious infections, especially in immunocompromised and debilitated hosts. *C parapsilosis* is second only to *C albicans* as a cause of systemic candidiasis. *Candida auris* is a drug-resistant *Candida* species that recently has emerged, virtually is always found in immunocompromised hosts, and often is acquired in health care settings.

EPIDEMIOLOGY: Like other *Candida* species, *C albicans* is present on skin and in the mouth, intestinal tract, and vagina of immunocompetent people. Vulvovaginal candidiasis is associated with pregnancy, and newborn infants can acquire the organism in utero, during passage through the vagina, or postnatally. Mild mucocutaneous infection is common in healthy infants. Person-to-person transmission occurs rarely. Invasive disease typically occurs in those with impaired immunity, with infection usually arising endogenously from colonized sites. Factors such as extreme prematurity, neutropenia, or treatment with corticosteroids or cytotoxic chemotherapy increase the risk of invasive infection. People with diabetes mellitus generally have localized mucocutaneous lesions. People with neutrophil defects, such as chronic granulomatous disease or myeloperoxidase deficiency, are at increased risk. People undergoing intravenous alimentation or receiving broad-spectrum antimicrobial agents, especially extended-spectrum cephalosporins, carbapenems, and vancomycin, or requiring long-term indwelling central venous or peritoneal dialysis catheters have increased susceptibility to infection. Postsurgical patients can be at risk, particularly after cardiothoracic or abdominal procedures.

The **incubation period** is unknown.

DIAGNOSTIC TESTS: The presumptive diagnosis of mucocutaneous candidiasis or thrush usually can be made clinically, but other organisms or trauma can cause clinically similar lesions. Yeast cells and pseudohyphae can be found in *C albicans*-infected tissue and are identifiable by microscopic examination of scrapings prepared with Gram, calcofluor white, or fluorescent antibody stains or in a 10% to 20% potassium hydroxide suspension. Endoscopy is useful for diagnosis of esophagitis. Although ophthalmologic examination can reveal typical retinal lesions attributable to hematogenous dissemination, the yield of routine ophthalmologic evaluation in affected patients is low. Lesions in the brain, kidney, liver, heart, or spleen can be detected by ultrasonography, computed tomography (CT), or magnetic resonance imaging; however, these lesions typically are not detected by imaging until late in the course of disease or after neutropenia has resolved.

A definitive diagnosis of invasive candidiasis requires isolation of the organism from a normally sterile body site (eg, blood, cerebrospinal fluid, bone marrow) or demonstration of organisms in a tissue biopsy specimen. Negative results of culture for *Candida* species do not exclude invasive infection in immunocompromised hosts; in some settings, blood culture is <50% sensitive. Special fungal culture media are not needed to grow *Candida* species. A presumptive species identification of *C albicans* can be made by demonstrating germ tube formation, and molecular fluorescence in situ hybridization testing rapidly can distinguish *C albicans* from non-albicans *Candida* species. *Candida auris,* a recently emerging pathogen, may be misidentified as another *Candida* species. Recovery of the organism is expedited using automated blood culture systems or a lysis-centrifugation method. The peptide nucleic acid fluorescent in situ hybridization (PNA FISH) probes cleared by the US Food and Drug Administration (FDA) and multiplex polymerase chain reaction (PCR) assays have been developed for rapid detection of *Candida* species directly from positive blood culture bottles.

A new FDA-cleared molecular assay (T2Candida [T2 Biosystems, Lexington, MA]), which uses magnetic resonance technology, can identify 5 different *Candida* species directly from patient's whole blood in 3 to 5 hours.

Patient serum can be tested using the assay for (1,3)-beta-D-glucan from fungal cell walls, which does not distinguish *Candida* species from other fungi. Data on use of this assay for children are more limited than for adult patients, and there are a significant number of false-positive results.

Testing for azole susceptibility is recommended for all bloodstream and other clinically relevant *Candida* isolates. Testing for echinocandin susceptibility should be considered in patients who have had prior treatment with an echinocandin and among those who have infection with *C glabrata* or *C parapsilosis*.

TREATMENT[1]:

Mucous Membrane and Skin Infections. Oral candidiasis in immunocompetent hosts is treated with oral nystatin suspension, clotrimazole troches applied to lesions, or miconazole mucoadhesive buccal tablets. Troches should not be used in infants. Fluconazole may be more effective than oral nystatin or clotrimazole troches and may be considered if other treatments fail. Fluconazole can be beneficial for immunocompromised patients with oropharyngeal candidiasis. For fluconazole-refractory disease, itraconazole, voriconazole, posaconazole, amphotericin B deoxycholate oral suspension, or intravenous echinocandins (caspofungin, micafungin) are alternatives.

Esophagitis caused by *Candida* species generally is treated with oral fluconazole. Intravenous fluconazole, an echinocandin, or amphotericin B should be used for patients who cannot tolerate oral therapy. For disease refractory to fluconazole, itraconazole solution, voriconazole, posaconazole, or an echinocandin is recommended. The recommended duration of therapy is 14 to 21 days. However, the duration of treatment depends on severity of illness and patient factors, such as age and degree of immunocompromise. Deescalating to oral therapy with fluconazole is recommended when the patient is able to tolerate oral intake. Suppressive therapy with fluconazole (3 times weekly) is recommended for recurrent infections.

Skin infections are treated with topical nystatin, miconazole, clotrimazole, naftifine, ketoconazole, econazole, or ciclopirox (see Topical Drugs for Superficial Fungal Infections, p 956). Nystatin usually is effective and is the least expensive of these drugs.

Vulvovaginal candidiasis is treated effectively with many topical formulations, including clotrimazole or miconazole (available over the counter). Such topically applied azole drugs are more effective than nystatin. Oral azole agents also are effective and should be considered for recurrent or refractory cases (see Recommended Doses of Parenteral and Oral Antifungal Drugs, p 945). Azole treatment of *C glabrata* vulvovaginal candidiasis is not effective; nystatin intravaginal suppositories have been effective.

For chronic mucocutaneous candidiasis, fluconazole, itraconazole, and voriconazole are effective drugs. Low-dose amphotericin B administered intravenously is effective in severe cases. Relapses are common with any of these agents once therapy is terminated, and treatment should be viewed as a lifelong process that generally requires intermittent pulses of antifungal agents. Invasive infections in patients with this condition are rare.

---

[1]Pappas PG, Kauffman CA, Andes DR, et al. Clinical practice guideline for the management of candidiasis: 2016 update by the Infectious Diseases Society of America. *Clin Infect Dis*. 2016;62(4):e1–e50

For asymptomatic candiduria, elimination of predisposing factors, such as indwelling bladder catheters, is strongly recommended whenever feasible. Antifungal treatment is not recommended unless patients are at high risk of candidemia, such as neutropenic patients, very low birth weight infants (<1500 g), and patients who will undergo urologic manipulation. If candiduria occurs in a very low birth weight infant, evaluation should be performed (blood cultures, cerebrospinal fluid evaluation, ophthalmologic examination, brain imaging, and abdominal ultrasonography) and treatment should be initiated. For patients with symptomatic *Candida* cystitis, elimination of predisposing factors, such as indwelling bladder catheters, is strongly recommended, as well as fluconazole for 2 weeks. An alternative is a short course (7 days) of low-dose amphotericin B intravenously (0.3 mg/kg per day). Repeated bladder irrigations with amphotericin B (50 μg/mL of sterile water) have been used to treat patients with candidal cystitis, but this does not treat disease beyond the bladder and is not recommended routinely. A urinary catheter in a patient with candidiasis should be removed or replaced promptly. Echinocandins have poor urinary concentration.

Keratomycosis is treated with corneal baths of voriconazole (1%) and always in conjunction with systemic therapy. Vision-threatening infections (near the macula or into the vitreous) require intravitreal injection of antifungal agents, usually amphotericin B deoxycholate or voriconazole, with or without vitrectomy, in addition to systemic antifungal agents.

Invasive Disease

General Recommendations. Most *Candida* species are susceptible to amphotericin B, although *C lusitaniae* and some strains of *C glabrata* and *C krusei* exhibit decreased susceptibility or resistance (see Table 4.7, p 942). *C auris* has been described as often drug resistant, and therapy must be targeted as indicated by susceptibility testing. Among patients with persistent candidemia despite appropriate therapy, investigation for a deep focus of infection should be conducted. Lipid-associated preparations of amphotericin B can be used as an alternative to amphotericin B deoxycholate in patients who experience significant toxicity during therapy.

C krusei is resistant to fluconazole, and more than 50% of *C glabrata* isolates can be resistant. Although voriconazole is effective against *C krusei*, it often is ineffective against *C glabrata*. The echinocandins (caspofungin, micafungin, and anidulafungin) all are active in vitro against most *Candida* species and are appropriate first-line drugs for *Candida* infections in severely ill or neutropenic patients (see Antifungal Drugs for Systemic Fungal Infections, p 938). The echinocandins should be used with caution against *C parapsilosis* infection, because some decreased in vitro susceptibility has been reported. If an echinocandin is initiated empirically and *C parapsilosis* is isolated in a patient who is recovering, then the echinocandin can be continued.

Removal of infected devices (eg, ventriculostomy drains, shunts, nerve stimulators, prosthetic reconstructive devices) in addition to antifungal treatment is necessary.

Neonatal Candidiasis. Infants are more likely than older children and adults to have meningitis as a manifestation of candidiasis. Although meningitis can occur in association with candidemia, approximately half of infants with *Candida* meningitis do not have a positive blood culture. Central nervous system disease in the infant typically manifests as meningoencephalitis and should be assumed to be present in the infant with candidemia and signs and symptoms of meningoencephalitis because of the high incidence of this complication. A lumbar puncture, brain imaging, and dilated retinal examination are recommended for all neonates with cultures positive for *Candida* in the blood and/or urine. CT or ultrasonography of genitourinary tract, liver, and spleen also should be performed.

Amphotericin B deoxycholate (first choice for neonates), fluconazole (for infants who have not been on fluconazole prophylaxis), or an echinocandin (generally reserved for salvage therapy) can be used in infants with systemic candidiasis. For initial treatment of meningitis, amphotericin deoxycholate, 1 mg/kg, intravenously, daily, is recommended; for step-down treatment after the patient has responded to initial treatment, fluconazole, 12 mg/kg daily, may be used for isolates that are susceptible to fluconazole. Therapy for candidemia without metastatic disease should continue for 2 weeks after documented clearance of *Candida* species from the bloodstream and resolution of signs attributable to candidemia. Therapy for central nervous system infection is at least 3 weeks and should be continued until all signs, symptoms, and CSF and radiological abnormalities, if present, have resolved. CT or ultrasonography of the genitourinary tract, liver, heart and spleen should be performed or repeated if blood cultures are persistently positive for *Candida* species.

Lipid formulations of amphotericin B should be used with caution in infants, particularly in patients with urinary tract involvement. Recent evidence suggests that treatment of infants with lipid formulations of amphotericin may be associated with worse outcomes when compared with amphotericin B deoxycholate or fluconazole. Published reports in adults and anecdotal reports in preterm infants indicate that lipid-associated amphotericin B preparations have failed to eradicate renal candidiasis, because these large-molecule drugs may not penetrate well into the renal parenchyma. It is unclear whether this is the reason for the inferior outcomes reported with the lipid formulations. Flucytosine in neonates with meningitis is not routinely recommended because of concerns regarding toxicity.

Older Children and Adolescents. In nonneutropenic children and adults, an echinocandin (caspofungin, micafungin, anidulafungin) is preferred, but fluconazole may be considered in those who are considered clinically stable and also unlikely to have a fluconazole-resistant isolate. Transition from an echinocandin to fluconazole (usually in 5 to 7 days) is indicated in patients who are clinically stable, have isolates that are susceptible to fluconazole, and have negative blood cultures since initiation of antifungal therapy. Amphotericin B deoxycholate or lipid formulations are alternative therapies (see Antifungal Drugs for Systemic Fungal Infections, p 938). In nonneutropenic patients with candidemia and no metastatic complications, treatment should continue for 2 weeks after documented clearance of *Candida* organisms from the bloodstream and resolution of clinical manifestations associated with candidemia.

In critically ill neutropenic patients, an echinocandin is recommended because of the fungicidal nature of these agents when compared with fluconazole, which is fungistatic. A lipid formulation of amphotericin B is an effective yet less attractive alternative. In neutropenic patients who are not critically ill, fluconazole is the alternative treatment for patients who have not had recent azole exposure, but voriconazole can be considered in situations in which additional mold coverage is desired. The duration of treatment for candidemia without metastatic complications is 2 weeks after documented clearance of *Candida* organisms from the bloodstream and resolution of symptoms attributable to candidemia. Avoidance or reduction of systemic immunosuppression is advised when feasible.

For chronic disseminated candidiasis (hepatosplenic infection), initial therapy with lipid formulation amphotericin B or an echinocandin for several weeks is recommended, followed by oral fluconazole (only for patients who are unlikely to have a fluconazole-resistant isolate). Discontinuation of therapy is recommended once lesions have resolved on repeated imaging.

Management of Indwelling Catheters. Prompt removal of any infected vascular or peritoneal catheters is strongly recommended. For neutropenic children, catheter removal should be considered. The recommendation in this population is weaker, because the source of candidemia in the neutropenic child is more likely to be gastrointestinal, and it is difficult to determine the relative contribution of the catheter. Immediate replacement of a catheter over a wire in the same catheter site is not recommended. Replacement can be attempted once the infection is controlled.

Additional Assessments. In neutropenic patients, ophthalmologic findings of choroidal and vitreal infection are minimal until recovery from neutropenia; therefore, dilated fundoscopic examinations should be performed within the first week after recovery from neutropenia. All nonneutropenic patients with candidemia should have a dilated ophthalmologic examination within the first week after diagnosis.

Chemoprophylaxis. Invasive candidiasis in infants is associated with prolonged hospitalization and neurodevelopmental impairment or death in almost 75% of affected infants with extremely low birth weight (less than 1000 g). The poor outcomes, despite prompt diagnosis and therapy, make prevention of invasive candidiasis in this population desirable. A number of randomized controlled trials of fungal prophylaxis in extremely preterm infants have demonstrated significant reduction of invasive candidiasis in nurseries with a moderate or high incidence of invasive candidiasis. In addition to birth weight, other risk factors for invasive candidiasis in infants include inadequate infection prevention practices and prolonged exposure to broad-spectrum antibiotic agents. Adherence to optimal infection control practices, including "bundles" for intravascular catheter insertion and maintenance and antimicrobial stewardship, can diminish infection rates and should be optimized before implementation of chemoprophylaxis as standard practice in a neonatal intensive care unit. On the basis of current data, fluconazole is the preferred agent for prophylaxis, because it has been shown to be effective and safe. Fluconazole prophylaxis is recommended for extremely low birth weight infants (<1000 g) cared for in neonatal intensive care units with high (≥10%) rates of invasive candidiasis. The recommended regimen for extremely low birth weight infants is to initiate fluconazole treatment intravenously during the first 48 to 72 hours after birth at a dose of 3 to 6 mg/kg and then to administer it twice a week for up to 6 weeks or until intravenous access no longer is required for care. For infants who tolerate enteral feeds, fluconazole oral absorption is good, even in preterm infants. This chemoprophylaxis dosage, dosing interval, and duration has not been associated with emergence of fluconazole-resistant *Candida* species in randomized trials.

Fluconazole prophylaxis can decrease the risk of mucosal (eg, oropharyngeal and esophageal) candidiasis in patients with advanced HIV disease. Adults undergoing allogeneic hematopoietic stem cell transplantation have significantly fewer *Candida* infections when receiving fluconazole, but limited data are available for children. Micafungin has been used for prophylaxis. Among patients without HIV infection receiving prophylaxis with fluconazole, an increased incidence of infections attributable to *C krusei* (which intrinsically is resistant to fluconazole) has been reported. Prophylaxis should be considered for children undergoing allogenic hematopoietic stem cell transplantation and other highly myelosuppressive chemotherapy during the period of neutropenia. Prophylaxis is not recommended routinely for other immunocompromised children, including children with HIV infection.

ISOLATION OF THE HOSPITALIZED PATIENT: Standard precautions are recommended.

CONTROL MEASURES: Prolonged broad-spectrum antimicrobial therapy and use of systemic corticosteroids in susceptible patients promote overgrowth of *Candida* and predispose to invasive infection. Meticulous care of central intravascular catheters is recommended for any patient requiring long-term intravenous access.

Chancroid and Cutaneous Ulcers

CLINICAL MANIFESTATIONS: Chancroid is an acute ulcerative disease of the genitalia that occurs primarily in sexually active adolescents and adults. An ulcer begins as an erythematous papule that becomes pustular and erodes over several days, forming a sharply demarcated, somewhat superficial lesion with a serpiginous border. The base of the ulcer is friable and can be covered with a gray or yellow, purulent exudate. Single or multiple ulcers can be present. Unlike a syphilitic chancre, which is painless and indurated, the chancroid ulcer often is painful and nonindurated and can be associated with a painful, unilateral inguinal suppurative adenitis (bubo). Without treatment, ulcer(s) can spontaneously resolve, cause extensive erosion of the genitalia, or lead to scarring and phimosis, a painful inability to retract the foreskin.

In most males, chancroid manifests as a genital ulcer with or without inguinal tenderness; edema of the prepuce is common. In females, most lesions are at the vaginal introitus, and symptoms include dysuria, dyspareunia, vaginal discharge, pain on defecation, or anal bleeding. Constitutional symptoms are unusual.

In the tropics, cutaneous ulcers in children have long been attributed to *Treponema pallidum* subspecies *pertenue*, or yaws. Recently, the organism that causes chancroid was identified as a major cause of cutaneous ulcers in multiple countries with endemic yaws in equatorial Africa and the South Pacific. The vast majority of these cutaneous ulcers are on the legs. Ulcers attributable to yaws tend to be round and deep with indurated edges, a uniform color, and a granulating ulcer bed; those attributable to *Haemophilus ducreyi* are superficial with ragged edges and tend to be more painful. However, mixed infections are common, and the clinical presentations overlap.

ETIOLOGY: Chancroid and cutaneous ulcers are caused by *H ducreyi,* which is a gram-negative coccobacillus.

EPIDEMIOLOGY: Chancroid is a sexually transmitted infection associated with poverty, commercial sex work, and illicit drug use. Chancroid is endemic in Africa and the tropics but is rare in the United States, and when it does occur, it usually is associated with sporadic outbreaks. Coinfection with syphilis or herpes simplex virus (HSV) occurs in as many as 17% of patients. Chancroid is a well-established cofactor for transmission of human immunodeficiency virus (HIV). Because sexual contact is the major primary route of transmission, the diagnosis of chancroid ulcers, especially in the genital region or buttocks, in infants and young children is strong evidence of sexual abuse.

Cutaneous ulcers caused by *H ducreyi*, especially on the legs, in children in the tropics are not sexually transmitted and seem to be facilitated by poor hygiene, the practice of bed sharing, and close contact between infected individuals. Recent studies suggest that asymptomatic colonization, contaminated bed linens, and flies are environmental sources of *H ducreyi*. In some cases, *T pallidum* subspecies *pertenue* may initiate the ulcers, allowing *H ducreyi* to infect the skin. The acquisition of a leg ulcer attributable to *H ducreyi* in a child who visits a country with endemic infection should not be considered evidence of sexual abuse.

The **incubation period** is 1 to 10 days.

DIAGNOSTIC TESTS: Chancroid usually is diagnosed on the basis of clinical findings (1 or more painful genital ulcers with tender suppurative inguinal adenopathy) and by excluding other genital ulcerative diseases, such as syphilis, HSV infection, or lymphogranuloma venereum. Cutaneous ulcers can be diagnosed on the basis of clinical findings described, but clinical overlap and mixed infections with *H ducreyi* and *T pallidum* subspecies *pertenue* are common. Confirmation is made by isolation of *H ducreyi* from an ulcer or lymph node aspirate, although sensitivity is less than 80%. Because special culture media and conditions are required for isolation, laboratory personnel should be informed of the suspicion of *H ducreyi*. Approximately 30% to 40% of lymph node aspirates are culture positive. Polymerase chain reaction assays can provide a specific diagnosis but are not available in most clinical laboratories.

TREATMENT: Genital strains of *H ducreyi* have been uniformly susceptible only to third-generation cephalosporins, macrolides, doxycycline, and quinolones. The prevalence of antibiotic resistance is unknown because of syndromic management of genital ulcers and the lack of diagnostic testing. Recommended regimens include azithromycin (1 g, orally, in a single dose), ceftriaxone (250 mg, intramuscularly, in a single dose), erythromycin (500 mg, orally, 3 times a day for 7 days), or ciprofloxacin (500 mg, orally, twice a day for 3 days) (see Table 4.4, p 933, and Table 4.5, p 936). Patients with HIV infection may need prolonged therapy. Syndromic management for genital ulcers usually includes treatment for syphilis.

Penicillin has long been used as empiric therapy for cutaneous ulcers in the tropics, but at least one beta-lactamase–producing cutaneous *H ducreyi* strain has been recovered. Cutaneous ulcers, therefore, should be treated with single-dose azithromycin to cover both *T pallidum* subspecies *pertenue* and *H ducreyi*.

Clinical improvement occurs 3 to 7 days after initiation of therapy, and healing is complete in approximately 2 weeks. Adenitis often is slow to resolve and can require needle aspiration or surgical incision. Patients should be reexamined 3 to 7 days after initiating therapy to verify healing. If healing has not begun, the diagnosis may be incorrect or the patient may have an additional sexually transmitted infection, both of which necessitate further testing. Slow clinical improvement and relapses can occur after therapy, especially in HIV-infected people. Close clinical follow-up is recommended; retreatment with the original regimen usually is effective in patients who experience a relapse.

Patients with chancroid should be evaluated for other sexually transmitted infections, including syphilis, herpes simplex virus, chlamydia, gonorrhea, and HIV infection, at the time of diagnosis. Because chancroid is a risk factor for HIV infection and facilitates HIV transmission, if the initial HIV test result is negative, it should be repeated 3 months later. If the hepatitis B and human papillomavirus vaccine series have not been completed, these immunizations should be offered if appropriate for age. Because syphilis and *H ducreyi* frequently are cotransmitted, serologic testing for syphilis also should be repeated if the result initially is negative. All people having sexual contact with patients with chancroid within 10 days before onset of the patient's symptoms need to be examined and treated, even if they are asymptomatic.

Cutaneous ulcers attributable to *H ducreyi* respond to single-dose azithromycin. Given the environmental sources, there is no evidence that contacts of people with leg ulcers should be treated.

ISOLATION OF THE HOSPITALIZED PATIENT: Standard precautions are recommended.

CONTROL MEASURES: Identification, examination, and treatment of sexual partners of patients with chancroid are important control measures. Regular condom use may decrease transmission, and male circumcision is thought to be partially protective. Whether improvement in hygiene and control of flies will help control cutaneous ulcers needs to be studied.

Chikungunya

CLINICAL MANIFESTATIONS: The majority of people (72%–97%) infected with chikungunya virus become symptomatic. The disease most often is characterized by acute onset of high fever (typically >39°C [102°F]) and polyarthralgia. Other symptoms may include headache, myalgia, arthritis, conjunctivitis, nausea, vomiting, or maculopapular rash. Fever typically lasts for several days to a week and can be biphasic. Rash usually occurs after onset of fever and typically involves the trunk and extremities, but the palms, soles, and face may be affected. Joint symptoms are often severe and debilitating, usually are bilateral and symmetric, and occur most commonly in the hands and feet but can affect more proximal joints. Clinical laboratory findings can include lymphopenia, thrombocytopenia, elevated creatinine, and elevated hepatic transaminases. Acute symptoms typically resolve within 7 to 10 days. Rare complications include uveitis, retinitis, myocarditis, hepatitis, nephritis, bullous skin lesions, hemorrhage, meningoencephalitis, myelitis, Guillain-Barré syndrome, and cranial nerve palsies. In infants, acrocyanosis without hemodynamic instability, symmetrical vesicobullous lesions, and edema of the lower extremities may occur. People at risk for severe disease include neonates exposed perinatally, older adults (eg, >65 years), and people with underlying medical conditions (eg, hypertension, diabetes, cardiovascular disease). Some patients might have relapse of rheumatologic symptoms (polyarthralgia, polyarthritis, and tenosynovitis) in the months following acute illness. Studies report variable proportions of patients with persistent joint pains for months to years. Mortality is rare.

ETIOLOGY: Chikungunya virus is a single-stranded RNA virus in the genus *Alphavirus* and *Togaviridae* family.

EPIDEMIOLOGY: Chikungunya virus primarily is transmitted to humans through the bites of infected mosquitoes, predominantly *Aedes aegypti* and *Aedes albopictus*. Humans are the primary host of chikungunya virus during epidemic periods. Bloodborne transmission is possible; cases have been documented among laboratory personnel handling infected blood and a health care worker drawing blood from an infected patient. Rare in utero transmission has been documented, mostly during the second trimester. Intrapartum transmission also has been documented when the mother was viremic around the time of delivery.

Prior to 2013, outbreaks of chikungunya infection were reported from countries in Africa, Asia, Europe, and the Indian and Pacific Oceans. In late 2013, chikungunya virus was found for the first time in the Americas on islands in the Caribbean. The virus then spread rapidly throughout the Americas, with local transmission reported from 44 countries and territories and more than 1 million suspected cases reported by the end of 2014. In the United States, widespread outbreaks occurred in Puerto Rico and the US Virgin Islands in 2014. Eleven locally transmitted cases were reported in Florida in 2014 and one locally transmitted case was reported in Texas in 2015. Updated reports of cases in the Americas can be found at **www.cdc.gov/chikungunya/** and **www.paho.org/hq/index.php?Itemid=40931.**

The **incubation period** typically is between 3 and 7 days (range, 1 to 12 days). **DIAGNOSTIC TESTS:** Preliminary diagnosis is based on the patient's clinical features, places and dates of travel, and activities. Laboratory diagnosis generally is accomplished by testing serum to detect virus, viral nucleic acid, or virus-specific immunoglobulin (Ig) M and neutralizing antibodies. During the first week after onset of symptoms, chikungunya virus infection often can be diagnosed by performing reverse transcriptase-polymerase chain reaction (RT-PCR) on serum. Chikungunya virus-specific IgM and neutralizing antibodies normally develop toward the end of the first week of illness. A plaque-reduction neutralization test can be performed to measure virus-specific neutralizing antibodies and to discriminate between cross-reacting antibodies (eg, Mayaro and O'nyong nyong viruses). IgM antibodies usually persist for 30 to 90 days, but longer persistence has been documented. Therefore, a positive IgM test result on serum occasionally may reflect a past infection. Immunohistochemical staining can detect specific viral antigen in fixed tissue.

Routine molecular and serologic testing for chikungunya virus is performed at state health departments and the Centers for Disease Control and Prevention (CDC). Plaque-reduction neutralization tests and immunohistochemical staining are performed at CDC and selected other reference laboratories.

TREATMENT: There is no antiviral treatment available for chikungunya. The primary treatment is supportive care and includes rest, fluids, analgesics, and antipyretics. In areas where dengue is endemic, acetaminophen is the preferred treatment for fever and joint pain until a dengue diagnosis is ruled out to reduce the risk of hemorrhagic complications. Patients with persistent joint pain may benefit from the use of nonsteroidal anti-inflammatory drugs, corticosteroids, and physiotherapy.

ISOLATION OF THE HOSPITALIZED PATIENT: Standard precautions are recommended.

CONTROL MEASURES: No vaccines or preventive drugs are available. Reduction of vectors in areas with endemic transmission is important to reduce risk of infection. Symptomatic febrile patients should be protected from mosquito bites to reduce further spread. Use of certain personal protective measures can help decrease the risk of human infection, including using insect repellent, wearing long pants and long-sleeved shirts while outdoors, staying in screened or air-conditioned dwellings, and limiting outdoor activities during peak vector feeding times (see Prevention of Mosquitoborne and Tickborne Infections, p 194). Chikungunya also can be prevented through screening of blood and organ donations.

Breastfeeding. Studies have not found chikungunya virus in human milk.

REPORTING: Health care professionals should report suspected chikungunya cases to their state or local health departments to facilitate diagnosis and mitigate the risk of local transmission. As a nationally notifiable disease, state health departments should report laboratory-confirmed cases to the CDC through ArboNET, the national surveillance system for arboviral diseases.

CHLAMYDIAL INFECTIONS

Chlamydia pneumoniae

CLINICAL MANIFESTATIONS: Patients may be asymptomatic or mildly to moderately ill with a variety of respiratory tract diseases caused by *Chlamydia pneumoniae*, including pneumonia, acute bronchitis, prolonged cough, and less commonly, pharyngitis, laryngitis, otitis media, and sinusitis. In some patients, a sore throat precedes the onset of cough by a week or more. The clinical course can be biphasic, culminating in atypical pneumonia. *C pneumoniae* can present as severe community-acquired pneumonia in immunocompromised hosts and has been associated with acute exacerbation of respiratory symptoms in patients with asthma, cystic fibrosis, and acute chest syndrome in children with sickle cell disease.

Physical examination may reveal nonexudative pharyngitis, pulmonary rales, and bronchospasm. Chest radiography may reveal a variety of findings ranging from pleural effusion and bilateral infiltrates to a single patchy subsegmental infiltrate. Illness can be prolonged and cough can persist for 2 to 6 weeks or longer.

ETIOLOGY: *C pneumoniae* is an obligate intracellular bacterium for which entry into mucosal epithelial cells is necessary for intracellular survival and growth. It exists in both an infectious nonreplicating extracellular form called an elementary body and a replicating intracellular form called a reticulate body. Reticulate bodies replicate within a protective intracellular membrane-bound vesicle called an inclusion.

EPIDEMIOLOGY: *C pneumoniae* infection is presumed to be transmitted from person to person via infected respiratory tract secretions. It is unknown whether there is an animal reservoir. The disease occurs worldwide, but in tropical and less developed areas, disease occurs earlier in life than in industrialized countries in temperate climates. The timing of initial infection peaks between 5 and 15 years of age; however, studies have shown that the prevalence rate of infection in children beyond early infancy is similar to that in adults. In the United States, approximately 50% of adults have *C pneumoniae*-specific serum antibody by 20 years of age, indicating previous infection by the organism. Recurrent infection is common, especially in adults. Clusters of infection have been reported in groups of children and adults. There is no evidence of seasonality.

The mean **incubation period** is 21 days.

DIAGNOSTIC TESTS: Serologic testing has been the primary laboratory means of diagnosis of *C pneumoniae* infection but is problematic in many respects. The microimmunofluorescent antibody test is the most sensitive and specific serologic test for acute infection; however, it may be less sensitive in children. A fourfold increase in immunoglobulin (Ig) G titer between acute and convalescent sera or an IgM titer of 1:16 or greater are evidence of acute infection; use of acute and convalescent titers is preferred to a single elevated IgM titer. Use of a single IgG titer in diagnosis of acute infection is not recommended, because during primary infection, IgG antibody may not appear until 6 to 8 weeks after onset of illness during primary infection and increases within 1 to 2 weeks with reinfection. In primary infection, IgM antibody appears approximately 2 to 3 weeks after onset of illness, but caution is advised when interpreting a single IgM antibody titer for diagnosis, because a single result can be either falsely positive because of cross-reactivity with other *Chlamydia* species or falsely negative in cases of reinfection, when IgM may not appear. Early antimicrobial therapy may suppress antibody response. Past exposure is indicated by a stable IgG titer of 1:16 or greater.

C pneumoniae is difficult to culture but can be isolated from swab specimens obtained from the nasopharynx or oropharynx or from sputum, bronchoalveolar lavage, or tissue biopsy specimens. Specimens should be placed into appropriate transport media and stored at 4°C until inoculation into cell culture; specimens that cannot be processed within 24 hours should be frozen and stored at −70°C. A positive culture is confirmed by propagation of the isolate or a positive polymerase chain reaction (PCR) assay result. Nasopharyngeal shedding can occur for months after acute disease, even with treatment. Immunohistochemistry, used to detect *C pneumoniae* in tissue specimens, requires control antibodies and tissues in addition to skill in recognizing staining artifacts to avoid false-positive results.

Because of the difficulty of accurately detecting *C pneumoniae* via culture, serologic testing, or immunohistochemistry testing, several types of PCR assays, including multiplex, hybridization probe methods, and fluorescent probe-based method, have been developed. Sensitivity and specificity of these different PCR techniques remain largely unknown, and reliability of results has been reported to vary widely between laboratories using the same PCR assay. Multiplex PCR assays have been cleared by the US Food and Drug Administration for the diagnosis of *C pneumoniae* using nasopharyngeal swab samples. The tests appear to have high sensitivity and specificity.

TREATMENT: Most respiratory tract infections thought to be caused by *C pneumoniae* are treated empirically. For suspected *C pneumoniae* infections, treatment with macrolides (eg, azithromycin, erythromycin, or clarithromycin) is recommended. Doxycycline can be used for short durations (ie, 21 days or less) without regard to patient age. Tetracycline may be used but should not be administered routinely to children younger than 8 years (see Tetracyclines, p 905). Newer fluoroquinolones (levofloxacin and moxifloxacin) are alternative drugs for patients who are unable to tolerate macrolide antibiotic agents but should not be used as first-line treatment. In vitro data suggest that *C pneumoniae* is not susceptible to sulfonamides.

Duration of therapy typically is 10 to 14 days for erythromycin, clarithromycin, tetracycline, or doxycycline. With azithromycin, the treatment duration typically is 5 days. Duration of therapy for levofloxacin is 7 to 14 days and for moxifloxacin is 10 days. However, with all these antimicrobial agents, the optimal duration of therapy has not been established.

ISOLATION OF THE HOSPITALIZED PATIENT: In addition to standard precautions, droplet precautions are recommended for the duration of symptomatic illness.

CONTROL MEASURES: Recommended prevention measures include minimizing crowding, employing respiratory hygiene (or cough etiquette), and frequent hand hygiene.

Chlamydia psittaci
(Psittacosis, Ornithosis, Parrot Fever)

CLINICAL MANIFESTATIONS: Psittacosis (ornithosis) is an acute respiratory tract infection with systemic symptoms and signs that often include fever, nonproductive cough, dyspnea, headache, myalgia, chills, and malaise. Less common symptoms include pharyngitis, diarrhea, constipation, nausea and vomiting, abdominal pain, arthralgia, rash, and altered mental status. Extensive interstitial pneumonia can occur, with radiographic changes characteristically more severe than would be expected from physical examination findings. Rarely, infection with *Chlamydia psittaci* has been reported to affect organ systems other than the respiratory tract, resulting in conditions including endocarditis, myocarditis, pericarditis, dilated cardiomyopathy, thrombophlebitis, nephritis, hepatitis, cranial nerve palsy (including sensorineural hearing loss), transverse myelitis, meningitis, and encephalitis. Infection in pregnancy may be life-threatening to the mother and cause fetal loss. There are conflicting reports regarding an association of psittacosis with ocular adnexal marginal zone lymphomas involving orbital soft tissue, lacrimal glands, and conjunctiva.

ETIOLOGY: *C psittaci* is an obligate intracellular bacterial pathogen that exists in 2 forms. The extracellular form is called an elementary body (EB) and is infectious. The EB invades the epithelial host cell and transforms to a replicating reticulate body (RB) within a membrane-bound vesicle called an inclusion. Reticulate bodies use host cell nutrients to multiply and later revert to infectious EBs that are released from the host cell to infect neighboring cells.

EPIDEMIOLOGY: Birds are the major reservoir of *C psittaci*. The term psittacosis commonly is used, although the term ornithosis more accurately describes the potential for nearly all domestic and wild birds to spread this infection, not just psittacine birds (eg, parakeets, parrots, macaws, cockatoos). In the United States, psittacine birds and turkeys have been reported as sources of human disease. Importation and illegal trafficking of exotic birds may be associated with disease in humans, because shipping, crowding, and other stress factors may increase shedding of the organism among birds with latent infection. Infected birds, whether they appear healthy or are obviously ill, may transmit the organism. Infection usually is acquired by direct contact or inhaling aerosolized excrement or respiratory secretions from the eyes or beaks of infected birds. Handling of plumage and mouth-to-beak contact are the modes of exposure described most frequently, although transmission has been reported through exposure to aviaries, bird exhibits, and lawn mowing. Excretion of *C psittaci* from birds may be intermittent or continuous for weeks or months. Pet owners and workers at poultry slaughter plants, poultry farms, and pet shops may be at increased risk of infection. Laboratory personnel working with *C psittaci* also are at risk. Psittacosis is worldwide in distribution and tends to occur sporadically in any season.

The **incubation period** usually is 5 to 15 days but may be longer.

DIAGNOSTIC TESTS: The diagnosis of *C psittaci* disease historically has been based on clinical presentation and a positive serologic test result using microimmunofluorescence (MIF) with paired sera. Although the MIF generally is more sensitive and specific than complement fixation (CF) tests, MIF still displays cross-reactivity with other *Chlamydia* species in some instances. Because of this, a titer less than 1:128 should be interpreted with caution. Paired acute- and convalescent-phase serum specimens obtained at least 2 to 4 weeks apart should be obtained and performed simultaneously within a single laboratory to ensure consistency of results.[1] Treatment with antimicrobial agents may suppress the antibody response, and in such cases, a third serum sample obtained 4 to 6 weeks after the acute-phase sample may be useful in confirming the diagnosis. Although serologic testing is more commonly used and available than molecular testing, results can often be

---

[1]National Association of State Public Health Veterinarians. Compendium of measures to control *Chlamydia psittaci* infection among humans (psittacosis) and pet birds (avian chlamydiosis). *J Avian Med Surg.* 2017;31(3). Available at: **www.nasphv.org/Documents/PsittacosisCompendium.pdf**

ambiguous, subjective in their interpretation, and misleading because of the inherent limitations of this approach. If possible, serologic testing should be considered a supportive test that augments the findings of other more reliable assays, such as nucleic acid-based tests.

Nucleic acid amplification tests (NAATs) have been developed that can distinguish *C psittaci* from other chlamydial species. Real-time PCR assays are now available within specialized laboratories (**www.cdc.gov/laboratory/specimen-submission/detail.html?CDCTestCode=CDC-10153**). Currently, there are no NAATs cleared by the US Food and Drug Administration for detection of *C psittaci* in clinical specimens. Because the organism is difficult to recover in culture and laboratory-acquired cases have been reported, culture generally is not recommended and should be attempted only by experienced personnel in laboratories in which strict containment measures to prevent spread of the organism are used. *C psittaci* currently is classified as an organism requiring biological safety level-3 biocontainment precautions.

TREATMENT: Doxycycline is the drug of choice and can be used for short durations (ie, 21 days or less) without regard to patient age. Erythromycin and azithromycin are alternative agents and are recommended for pregnant women. Therapy should continue for 10 to 14 days after fever abates. Most *C psittaci* infections are responsive to antimicrobial agents within 1 to 2 days. In patients with severe infection, intravenous doxycycline may be considered (4.4 mg/kg/day, divided into 2 infusions, maximum 100 mg/dose).

ISOLATION OF THE HOSPITALIZED PATIENT: Standard precautions are recommended. Person-to-person transmission is thought to be rare but has been reported (**www.eurosurveillance.org/ViewArticle.aspx?ArticleId=20937**).

CONTROL MEASURES: Human psittacosis is a nationally notifiable disease and should be reported to public health authorities. All birds suspected to be the source of human infection should be seen by a veterinarian for evaluation and management. Birds with *C psittaci* infection should be isolated and treated with appropriate antimicrobial agents.[1] Birds suspected of dying from *C psittaci* infection should be transported to an animal diagnostic laboratory for testing as directed by the laboratory. All potentially contaminated caging and housing areas should be disinfected thoroughly before reuse to eliminate any infectious organisms. People cleaning cages, handling birds confirmed with *C psittaci*, or handling birds exposed to those confirmed with *C psittaci* should wear personal protective equipment including gloves, eyewear, a disposable hat, and disposable particulate respirator (ie, a preshaped mask that molds firmly around the mouth and nose). *C psittaci* is susceptible to many but not all household disinfectants and detergents. Effective disinfectants include 1:1000 dilutions of quaternary ammonium compounds and freshly prepared 1:32 dilutions of household bleach (1/2 cup per gallon). People exposed to common sources of infection should be observed for development of fever or respiratory tract symptoms; early diagnostic tests should be performed, and therapy should be initiated if symptoms appear.

Chlamydia trachomatis

CLINICAL MANIFESTATIONS: *Chlamydia trachomatis* is associated with a range of clinical

---

[1]National Association of State Public Health Veterinarians. Compendium of measures to control *Chlamydia psittaci* infection among humans (psittacosis) and pet birds (avian chlamydiosis). *J Avian Med Surg.* 2017;31(3). Available at: **www.nasphv.org/Documents/PsittacosisCompendium.pdf**

manifestations, including neonatal conjunctivitis, nasopharyngitis, and pneumonia in young infants as well as genital tract infection, lymphogranuloma venereum (LGV), and trachoma in children and adolescents.

- **Neonatal chlamydial conjunctivitis** is characterized by ocular congestion, edema, and discharge developing a few days to several weeks after birth and lasting for 1 to 2 weeks and sometimes longer. In contrast to trachoma, scars and pannus formation are rare.
- **Pneumonia** in young infants usually is an afebrile illness of insidious onset occurring between 2 and 19 weeks after birth. A repetitive staccato cough, tachypnea, and rales in an afebrile 1-month-old infant are characteristic but not always present. Wheezing is uncommon. Hyperinflation usually accompanies infiltrates seen on chest radiographs. Nasal stuffiness and otitis media may occur. Untreated disease can linger or recur. Severe chlamydial pneumonia has occurred in infants and some immunocompromised adults.
- **Genitourinary tract** manifestations, such as vaginitis in prepubertal girls; urethritis, cervicitis, endometritis, salpingitis, proctitis, and perihepatitis (Fitz-Hugh-Curtis syndrome) in postpubertal females; urethritis, epididymitis, and proctitis in males; and reactive arthritis (with the classic triad, formerly known as Reiter syndrome, consisting of arthritis, urethritis, and bilateral conjunctivitis) can occur. Infection can persist for months to years. Reinfection is common. In postpubertal females, chlamydial infection can progress to pelvic inflammatory disease and can result in ectopic pregnancy, infertility, or chronic pelvic pain.
- **LGV** classically is an invasive lymphatic infection with an initial ulcerative lesion on the genitalia accompanied by tender, suppurative inguinal and/or femoral lymphadenopathy that typically is unilateral. The ulcerative lesion often has resolved by the time the patient seeks care. Proctocolitis may occur in women or men who engage in receptive anal intercourse. Symptoms can resemble those of inflammatory bowel disease, including mucoid or hemorrhagic rectal discharge, constipation, tenesmus, and/or anorectal pain. Stricture or fistula formation can follow severe or inadequately treated infection.
- **Trachoma** is a chronic follicular keratoconjunctivitis with neovascularization of the cornea that results from repeated and chronic infection. Blindness secondary to extensive local scarring and inflammation occurs in 1% to 15% of people with trachoma.

ETIOLOGY: *C trachomatis* is an obligate intracellular bacterial agent with at least 18 serologic variants (serovars) divided between the following biologic variants (biovars): oculogenital (serovars A–K) and LGV (serovars L1, L2, and L3). Trachoma usually is caused by serovars A through C, and genital and perinatal infections are caused by B and D through K.

EPIDEMIOLOGY: *C trachomatis* is the most common reportable sexually transmitted infection (STI) in the United States, with high rates among sexually active adolescents and young adult females. A significant proportion of patients are asymptomatic, providing an ongoing reservoir for infection. Prevalence of the organism consistently is highest among adolescent and young adult females. Among sexually active 14- to 24-year-old females participating in the 2007–2012 National Health and Nutrition Examination Survey, the estimated prevalence was 4.7%. Racial disparities are significant. Among sexually active females 14 to 24 years of age, the estimated prevalence among non-Hispanic black females (13.5%) was higher than the estimated prevalence among Mexican American females (4.5%) and non-Hispanic white females (1.8%).[1] Among men who have sex with men (MSM) screened for rectal chlamydial infection, positivity ranges from 11% to 20%.[2] Oculogenital serovars of *C trachomatis* can be transmitted from the genital tract of infected mothers to their infants during birth. Acquisition occurs in approximately 50% of infants born vaginally to infected mothers and in some infants born by cesarean delivery with membranes intact. The risk of conjunctivitis is 25% to 50%, and the risk of pneumonia is 5% to 30% in infants who contract *C trachomatis*. The nasopharynx is the anatomic site most commonly infected.

Genital tract infection in adolescents and adults is sexually transmitted. The possibility of sexual abuse always should be considered in prepubertal children beyond infancy who have vaginal, urethral, or rectal chlamydial infection. Sexual abuse is not limited to prepubertal children, and chlamydial infections can result from sexual abuse/assault in postpubertal adolescents as well. Health care professionals are required to report suspected sexual abuse to their state child protective services agency.

Asymptomatic infection of the nasopharynx, conjunctivae, vagina, and rectum can be acquired at birth. Nasopharyngeal cultures have been observed to remain positive for as long as 28 months, and vaginal and rectal cultures have remained positive for more than 1 year from infants with infection acquired at birth. Infection is not known to be communicable among infants and children. The degree of contagiousness of pulmonary disease is unknown but seems to be low.

LGV biovars are worldwide in distribution but particularly are prevalent in tropical and subtropical areas. Although disease occurs rarely in the United States, outbreaks of LGV proctocolitis have been reported among MSM. Infection often is asymptomatic in females. Perinatal transmission is rare. LGV is infectious during active disease. Little is known about the prevalence or duration of asymptomatic carriage.

Although rarely observed in the United States since the 1950s, trachoma is the leading infectious cause of blindness worldwide, causing up to 3% of the world's blindness. Trachoma is transmitted by transfer of ocular discharge and it generally is confined to poor populations in resource-limited nations in Africa, the Middle East, Asia, and Latin America; the Pacific Islands; and remote aboriginal communities in Australia. Predictors of scarring and blindness for trachoma include increasing age and constant, severe trachoma.

The **incubation period** of chlamydial illness is variable, depending on the type of infection, but usually is at least 1 week.

DIAGNOSTIC TESTS[3]: Among **postpubescent individuals,** nucleic acid amplification

[1]Centers for Disease Control and Prevention. Prevalence of *Chlamydia trachomatis* genital infection among persons aged 14–39 years — United States, 2007–2012. *MMWR Morb Mortal Wkly Rep.* 2014;63(38):834–838

[2]Patton ME, Kidd S, Llata E, Stenger M, Braxton J, et al. Extragenital gonorrhea and chlamydia testing and infection among men who have sex with men—STD Surveillance Network, United States, 2010–2012. *Clin Infect Dis.* 2014;58(11):1564–1570

[3]American Academy of Pediatrics, Committee on Adolescence; Society for Adolescent Health and Medicine. Screening for nonviral sexually transmitted infections in adolescents and young adults. *Pediatrics.* 2014;134(1):e302–e311

tests (NAATs) are the most sensitive *C trachomatis* tests and are recommended for laboratory diagnosis.[1] Older, culture-independent methods including DNA probe, direct fluorescent antibody (DFA) assay, or enzyme immunoassay have inferior sensitivity and specificity characteristics and are not recommended for *C trachomatis* testing.[1] Commercial NAATs have been FDA-cleared for testing vaginal (provider or patient collected), endocervical, and male intraurethral swabs; male and female first-catch urine specimens placed in appropriate transport devices; and liquid cytology specimens. Most of these assays are designed to detect *C trachomatis* and *N gonorrhoeae*. Package inserts for individual NAAT products must be reviewed, however, because the particular specimens approved for use with each test may vary. The Centers for Disease Control and Prevention (CDC) recommends a vaginal swab as the preferred means of screening females and urine as the preferred means for screening males for *C trachomatis* infection by NAAT. Female urine also is an acceptable NAAT specimen but may have slightly reduced performance when compared with cervical or vaginal swab specimens. NAATs have not been FDA-cleared for use with rectal, pharyngeal, or conjunctival swab specimens, but clinical laboratories that have met Clinical Laboratory Improvement Amendments (CLIA) and other regulatory requirements and have validated test performance on such specimens may offer this testing. NAATs performed on self-collected rectal swab specimens yield comparable results to those performed on rectal swab specimens collected by health care professionals. The performance of a NAAT on a rectal swab specimen is the preferred approach for testing MSM presenting with proctocolitis. *C trachomatis* testing of pharyngeal specimens from asymptomatic postpubescent individuals generally is not recommended, because the clinical significance of oropharyngeal *C trachomatis* infection is unclear. NAATs permit dual testing of specimens for *C trachomatis* and *N gonorrhoeae*.

Sensitive and specific methods used to diagnose **neonatal chlamydial ophthalmia** include both cell culture-independent methods and nonculture tests (eg, DFA and NAAT). DFA is the only culture-independent method that is FDA approved for the detection of chlamydia from conjunctival swab specimens; NAATs are not FDA cleared for the detection of chlamydia from conjunctival swab specimens, but clinical laboratories may offer such testing once they have verified the use of such specimens according to CLIA regulations.

For diagnosing **infant pneumonia** caused by *C trachomatis*, specimens for chlamydial testing should be collected from the posterior nasopharynx. Isolation of the organism in cell culture is the definitive standard diagnostic test for chlamydial pneumonia. Culture-independent tests (eg, DFA and NAAT) can be used. DFA is the only culture-independent FDA-approved test for the detection of *C trachomatis* from nasopharyngeal specimens. DFA testing of nasopharyngeal specimens has a lower sensitivity and specificity than culture. If NAATs are to be used for the detection of chlamydia from nasopharyngeal specimens, the clinical laboratories must verify the procedure according to CLIA regulations. Tracheal aspirates and lung biopsy specimens, if collected, should be tested for *C trachomatis* by cell culture.

In the **evaluation of prepubescent children for possible sexual assault,** the CDC recommends culture for *C trachomatis* of a swab specimen collected from the rectum

[1]Centers for Disease Control and Prevention. Recommendations for the laboratory-based detection of *Chlamydia trachomatis* and *Neisseria gonorrhoeae*—2014. *MMWR Recomm Rep.* 2014;63(RR-2):1–19

in both boys and girls and from the vagina in girls. A meatal swab specimen should be obtained from boys for chlamydia testing if urethral discharge is present. NAATs are not FDA cleared for this indication but are available more widely and are more sensitive than culture in limited published evaluations. Test specificity, which is of critical concern because of the potential legal consequences of positive test results, has been high in limited published evaluations of NAATs for this indication. CDC recommends that NAATs can be used for detection of *C trachomatis* either alone or in addition to culture in vaginal specimens or urine from prepubescent girls. Culture remains the method of choice for meatal swab specimens from boys and from nonurogenital sites for both boys and girls. Thus, it is important that clinical laboratories maintain the capability to culture for *C trachomatis* to comply with these recommendations. All specimens should be retained for additional testing. Some have suggested that an initial positive NAAT in this setting should be tested with a second NAAT targeting an alternative gene sequence especially when culture confirmation is unavailable.

Serologic testing has little, if any, value in diagnosing uncomplicated genital *C trachomatis* infection. In **children with pneumonia,** an acute microimmunofluorescent serum titer of *C trachomatis*-specific immunoglobulin (Ig) M of 1:32 or greater is diagnostic. Diagnosis of **LGV** can be supported but not confirmed by a positive result (ie, titer >1:64) on a complement-fixation test for *Chlamydia* or a high titer (typically >1:256, but this can vary by laboratory) on a microimmunofluorescent antibody test for *C trachomatis*. However, serologic test interpretation for LGV is not standardized, tests have not been validated for clinical proctitis presentations, and *C trachomatis* serovar-specific serologic tests are not widely available.

Diagnosis of genitourinary tract chlamydial disease in a child should prompt examination for **other STIs,** including syphilis, gonorrhea, trichomoniasis, and human immunodeficiency virus (HIV) infection, and investigation of sexual abuse/assault. In the case of an infant, because cultures can be positive for at least 12 months after infection acquired at birth, evaluation of the mother also is advisable.

Diagnosis of **ocular trachoma** usually is made clinically in countries with endemic infection.

TREATMENT[1]:

- **Infants with chlamydial conjunctivitis or pneumonia** are treated with oral erythromycin base or ethylsuccinate (50 mg/kg/day in 4 divided doses daily) for 14 days or with azithromycin (20 mg/kg as a single daily dose) for 3 days. Follow-up of infants treated with either drug is recommended to determine whether initial treatment was effective. A diagnosis of *C trachomatis* infection in an infant should prompt treatment of the mother and her sexual partner(s). The need for treatment of infants can be avoided by screening pregnant females to detect and treat *C trachomatis* infection before delivery. Neonates with documented chlamydial infection should be evaluated for possible gonococcal infection but should not be treated with ceftriaxone unless the diagnostic assessment is positive for *N gonorrhoeae*. An association between orally administered erythromycin and azithromycin and infantile hypertrophic pyloric stenosis (IHPS) has been reported in infants younger than 6 weeks. Infants treated with either of these antimicrobial agents should be followed for signs and symptoms of IHPS.

---

[1]Centers for Disease Control and Prevention. Sexually transmitted diseases treatment guidelines, 2015. *MMWR Recomm Rep.* 2015;64(RR-3):1–137

- Infants born to mothers known to have untreated chlamydial infection are at high risk of infection; however, prophylactic antimicrobial treatment is not indicated, because the efficacy of such treatment is unknown. Infants should be monitored clinically to ensure appropriate treatment if infection develops. If adequate follow-up cannot be ensured, preemptive therapy should be considered.

- For uncomplicated *C trachomatis* **anogenital tract infection in adolescents or adults,** oral doxycycline (100 mg, twice daily) for 7 days or azithromycin in a single 1-g oral dose is recommended. Alternatives include oral erythromycin base (500 mg, 4 times/day) for 7 days, erythromycin ethylsuccinate (800 mg orally, 4 times/day) for 7 days, ofloxacin (300 mg orally, twice daily) for 7 days, or levofloxacin (500 mg orally, once daily) for 7 days. Doxycycline delayed-release (200-mg tablet, once daily) for 7 days, although more costly, might be an alternative regimen to doxycycline, 100 mg, twice daily for 7 days. Erythromycin may be less efficacious than azithromycin or doxycycline because of gastrointestinal tract adverse effects and frequent dosing that can lead to treatment nonadherence. Levofloxacin and ofloxacin are more expensive and offer no advantage in the dosage regimen. **For children who weigh <45 kg,** the recommended regimen is oral erythromycin base or ethylsuccinate, 50 mg/kg/day, divided into 4 doses daily for 14 days. Data are limited on the effectiveness and optimal dose of azithromycin for treatment of chlamydial infections in infants and children who weigh <45 kg. **For children who weigh ≥45 kg but who are younger than 8 years,** the recommended regimen is azithromycin, 1 g, orally, in a single dose. **For children 8 years and older,** the recommended regimen is azithromycin, 1 g, orally, in a single dose, or doxycycline, 100 mg, orally, twice a day for 7 days. **For pregnant females,** the recommended treatment is azithromycin (1 g, orally, as a single dose). Amoxicillin (500 mg, orally, 3 times/day for 7 days), erythromycin base (500 mg, orally, 4 times/day for 7 days or 250 mg, orally, 4 times/day for 14 days), and erythromycin ethylsuccinate (800 mg, orally, 4 times/day for 7 days or 400 mg, orally, 4 times/day for 14 days) are alternative regimens. Doxycycline, ofloxacin, and levofloxacin are contraindicated during pregnancy.

  Follow-up Testing. Test of cure is not recommended for nonpregnant adult or adolescent patients treated for uncomplicated chlamydial infection unless compliance is in question, symptoms persist, or reinfection is suspected. Reinfection is common after initial infection and treatment, and all infected adolescents and adults should be tested for *C trachomatis* in the next 3 months following initial treatment. If retesting at 3 months is not possible, patients should be retested when they next present for health care in the 12 months after initial treatment, regardless of whether patients believe their sexual partners were treated.

- For **LGV,** doxycycline (100 mg, orally, twice daily for 21 days) is the preferred treatment, and can be used for short durations (ie, 21 days or less) without regard to patient age. Erythromycin (500 mg, orally, 4 times daily for 21 days) is an alternative regimen. Azithromycin (1 g, once weekly for 3 weeks) probably is effective but has not been as well studied. Fluoroquinolone-based treatment also might be effective, but the optimal duration of treatment has not been evaluated.

- Treatment of **trachoma** is azithromycin, orally, as a single dose of 20 mg/kg (maximum dose of 1000 mg), as recommended by the World Health Organization for all people diagnosed with trachoma as well as for all of their household contacts.

ISOLATION OF THE HOSPITALIZED PATIENT: Standard precautions are recommended.

CONTROL MEASURES:

Pregnancy. Identification and treatment of females with *C trachomatis* genital tract infection during pregnancy can prevent disease in the infant. The CDC recommends routine screening of pregnant women younger than 25 years and older women at increased risk of chlamydia (eg, those who have a new sex partner, more than one sex partner, a sex partner with concurrent sex partners, or a sex partner who has a sexually transmitted infection) at the first prenatal visit, and advises retesting of all pregnant females younger than 25 years and those at increased risk during the third trimester to prevent perinatal complications. Test of cure (preferably by NAAT) is recommended 3 to 4 weeks after treatment of pregnant females. In addition, all pregnant females who have chlamydia diagnosed should be retested 3 months after treatment.

Neonatal Chlamydial Conjunctivitis. Recommended topical prophylaxis with erythromycin or tetracycline for all newborn infants for prevention of gonococcal ophthalmia will not prevent neonatal chlamydial conjunctivitis or extraocular infection (see Prevention of Neonatal Ophthalmia, p 1046).

Contacts of Infants With C trachomatis *Conjunctivitis or Pneumonia.* Mothers of infected infants and mothers' sexual partners should be treated for *C trachomatis*.

Routine Screening Tests.[1] All sexually experienced adolescent and young adult females (25 years or younger) should be tested at least annually for *Chlamydia* infection, even if no symptoms are present or barrier contraception is reported. Sexually experienced adolescent and adult MSM should be screened routinely for rectal and urethral chlamydia annually if they engaged in receptive or insertive anal intercourse, respectively. MSM should be screened every 3 to 6 months if at high risk because of multiple or anonymous sex partners, sex in conjunction with illicit drug use, or sex with partners who participate in these activities. Annual screening may be considered for sexually active young males who have sex with females in settings with high prevalence rates, such as jails or juvenile corrections facilities, national job training programs, STI clinics, high school clinics, and adolescent clinics for patients who have a history of multiple partners.

Management of Sex Partners. All people with sexual contact in the 60 days preceding diagnosis or onset of symptoms of patients with *C trachomatis* infection (whether symptomatic or asymptomatic), nongonococcal urethritis, mucopurulent cervicitis, epididymitis, or pelvic inflammatory disease should be evaluated and treated for *C trachomatis* infection. The patient's last sex partner should be treated even if last sexual contact was more than 60 days before diagnosis in the index case. Among females or heterosexual male patients, if concerns exist that sex partners who are referred for evaluation and treatment will not seek care, expedited partner therapy (EPT, which is the practice of treating the sex partners of patients with chlamydia or gonorrhea by providing prescriptions or medications to the index patient to take to his or her partner without the health care provider first examining the partner) can be considered. To clarify the legal status of EPT in each state, refer to the CDC Web site (**www.cdc.gov/std/ept/**). EPT should include efforts to educate partners about symptoms of chlamydia and gonorrhea and to encourage partners to seek clinical evaluation. EPT should not be considered a routine partner management

---

[1]American Academy of Pediatrics, Committee on Adolescence; Society for Adolescent Health and Medicine. Screening for nonviral sexually transmitted infections in adolescents and young adults. *Pediatrics.* 2014;134(1):e302–e311

strategy in MSM because of the high risk of coexisting undiagnosed STIs or HIV infection.

LGV. Nonspecific preventive measures for LGV are the same as measures for STIs in general and include education, case reporting, condom use, and avoidance of sexual contact with infected people. Partners exposed to an LGV-infected person within the 60 days before the patient's symptom onset should be tested and presumptively treated.

Trachoma. Although rarely observed in the United States since the 1950s, trachoma is the leading infectious cause of blindness worldwide. Prevention methods recommended by the World Health Organization for global elimination of blindness attributable to trachoma by 2020 include surgery, antimicrobial agents, face washing, and environmental improvement (SAFE). Azithromycin (20 mg/kg, maximum 1 g), once a year as a single oral dose, is used in mass drug administration campaigns for trachoma control. Azithromycin typically is administered to children up to 14 years of age to decrease the reservoir of active trachoma.[1]

CLOSTRIDIAL INFECTIONS

Botulism and Infant Botulism
(Clostridium botulinum)

CLINICAL MANIFESTATIONS: Botulism is a neuroparalytic disorder characterized by an acute, afebrile, symmetric, descending, flaccid paralysis. Paralysis is caused by blockade of neurotransmitter release at the voluntary motor and autonomic neuromuscular junctions. Four naturally occurring forms of human botulism exist: infant, foodborne, wound, and adult intestinal colonization. Cases of iatrogenic botulism, which result from injection of excess therapeutic botulinum toxin, have been reported, and botulinum neurotoxins are considered a potential agent of bioterrorism. Symptoms of botulism can occur abruptly, within hours of exposure, or evolve gradually over several days and include diplopia, dysphagia, dysphonia, and dysarthria. Cranial nerve palsies are followed by symmetric, descending, flaccid paralysis of somatic musculature in patients who remain fully alert. Infant botulism, which occurs predominantly in infants younger than 6 months (range, 1 day to 12 months), is preceded by or begins with constipation and manifests as decreased movement, loss of facial expression, poor feeding, weak cry, diminished gag reflex, ocular palsies, loss of head control, and progressive descending generalized weakness and hypotonia. Some reports suggest that sudden infant death could result from rapidly progressing infant botulism.

ETIOLOGY: Botulism occurs after absorption of botulinum toxin into the circulation from a mucosal or wound surface. Seven antigenic toxin types (A–G) of *Clostridium botulinum* are known. An eighth toxin type (H) has been reported, but its identity as a distinct serotype remains controversial. Non-*botulinum* species of *Clostridium* rarely may produce these neurotoxins and cause disease. The most common botulinum toxin serotypes associated with

---

[1]Northern Territory Government, Centre for Disease Control. *Guidelines for Management of Trachoma in the Northern Territory 2008*. Alice Springs, Northern Territory, Australia: Department of Health and Families; 2008. Available at: **www.k4health.org/sites/default/files/Guidelines%20for%20Management%20of%20Trachoma%20-%20CDC.pdf**

naturally occurring illness are types A, B, E, and rarely, F. Most cases of infant botulism result from toxin types A and B, but a few cases of types E and F have been caused by *Clostridium butyricum* (type E), *Clostridium botulinum* (type E), and *Clostridium baratii* (type F) (especially in very young infants). *C botulinum* spores are ubiquitous in soils and dust world-wide and have been isolated from the home environment and vacuum cleaner dust of infant botulism cases.

EPIDEMIOLOGY: Infant botulism (annual average, 125 laboratory-confirmed cases in 2011–2015; age range, 1 to 73 weeks; median age, 17.6 weeks) results after ingested spores of *C botulinum* or related neurotoxigenic clostridial species germinate, multiply, and produce botulinum toxin in the large intestine through transient colonization of the intestinal microflora. Cases may occur in breastfed infants at the time of first introduction of nonhuman milk substances; the source of spores usually is not identified. Honey has been identified as an avoidable source of spores. No case of infant botulism has been proven to be attributable to consumption of corn syrup. Rarely, intestinal botulism can occur in older children and adults, usually after intestinal surgery and exposure to antimicrobial agents.

Foodborne botulism (annual average, 15 cases per year in 2011–2014; age range, 8–87 years; median age, 40 years) results when food that carries spores of *C botulinum* is preserved or stored improperly under anaerobic conditions that permit germination, multiplication, and toxin production. Illness follows ingestion of the food containing preformed botulinum toxin. Home processing of foods is the most common cause of foodborne botulism in the United States, followed by rare outbreaks associated with commercially processed foods, restaurant-associated foods, and wine produced in prisons ("pruno" and "hooch").

Wound botulism (annual average, 13 laboratory-confirmed cases in 2011–2014; age range, 5–66 years; median age, 46 years) results when *C botulinum* contaminates traumatized tissue, germinates, multiplies, and produces toxin. Gross trauma or crush injury can be a predisposing event. During the last decade, self-injection of contaminated black tar heroin has been associated with most cases.

Immunity to botulinum toxin does not develop in botulism. Botulism is not transmitted from person to person. The usual **incubation period** for foodborne botulism is 12 to 48 hours (range, 6 hours–8 days). In infant botulism, the **incubation period** is estimated at 3 to 30 days from the time of ingestion of spores. For wound botulism, the **incubation period** is 4 to 14 days from time of injury until onset of symptoms.

DIAGNOSTIC TESTS: A toxin neutralization bioassay in mice[1] is used to detect botulinum toxin in serum, stool, enema fluid, gastric aspirate, or suspect foods. Enriched selective media is required to isolate *C botulinum* from stool and foods. The diagnosis of infant botulism is made by demonstrating botulinum toxin or botulinum toxin-producing organisms in feces or enema fluid or toxin in serum. Wound botulism is confirmed by demonstrating organisms in the wound or tissue or toxin in the serum. To increase the likelihood of diagnosis in foodborne botulism, all suspect foods should be collected, and serum and stool or enema specimens should be obtained from all people with suspected illness. In foodborne cases, serum specimens may be positive for toxin as long as 10 days after illness onset. Although toxin can be demonstrated in serum in some infants with botulism (13% in one

---

[1]For information, consult your state health department.

large study), stool is the best specimen for diagnosis; enema effluent also can be useful. If constipation makes obtaining a stool specimen difficult, an enema of sterile, nonbacteriostatic water should be administered promptly. Because results of laboratory bioassay testing may require several days, treatment with antitoxin should be initiated urgently for all forms of botulism on the basis of clinical suspicion. The most prominent electromyographic finding is an incremental increase of evoked muscle potentials at high-frequency nerve stimulation (20–50 Hz). In addition, a characteristic pattern of brief, small-amplitude, overly abundant motor action potentials may be seen after stimulation of muscle, but its absence does not exclude the diagnosis; this test sometimes is needed to assist with diagnosis.

TREATMENT:

Meticulous Supportive Care. Meticulous supportive care, in particular respiratory and nutritional support, constitutes a fundamental aspect of therapy in all forms of botulism. Recovery from botulism may take weeks to months.

Antitoxin for Infant Botulism. Human-derived antitoxin should be administered immediately. Human Botulism Immune Globulin for intravenous use (BIG-IV; BabyBIG) is licensed by the US Food and Drug Administration (FDA) for treatment of infant botulism caused by *C botulinum* type A or type B. BabyBIG is produced and distributed by the California Department of Public Health (24-hour telephone number: 510-231-7600; **www. infantbotulism.org**). BabyBIG significantly decreases days of mechanical ventilation, days of intensive care unit stay, and total length of hospital stay by almost 1 month and is cost saving. BabyBIG is first-line therapy for naturally occurring infant botulism. Equine-derived heptavalent botulinum antitoxin (BAT; see below) was licensed by the FDA in 2013 for treatment of adult and pediatric botulism and is available through the Centers for Disease Control and Prevention (CDC). BAT has been used to treat type F infant botulism patients, where the antitoxin is not contained in BabyBIG, on a case-by-case basis.

As with other Immune Globulin Intravenous preparations, routine live-virus vaccines should be delayed for 6 months after receipt of BabyBIG because of potential interference with immune responses (see Table 1.13, p 40).

Antitoxin for Noninfant Forms of Botulism. Immediate administration of antitoxin is the key to successful therapy, because antitoxin treatment ends the toxemia and stops further uptake of toxin. However, because botulinum neurotoxin becomes internalized in the nerve ending, administration of antitoxin does not reverse paralysis. If foodborne botulism is suspected, the state health department should be contacted immediately to discuss and report the case; all states maintain a 24-hour telephone service. If contact cannot be made with the state health department, the CDC Emergency Operations Center should be contacted at 770-488-7100 for botulism case consultation and antitoxin. Since 2010, BAT is the only botulinum antitoxin released in the United States for treatment of noninfant botulism. BAT contains antitoxin against all 7 (A–G) botulinum toxin types and has been "despeciated" by enzymatic removal of the Fc immunoglobulin fragment, resulting in a product that is >90% Fab and F(ab')$_2$ immunoglobulin fragments. BAT is provided by the CDC with the product information that includes specific, detailed instructions for intravenous administration of antitoxin. Additional information may be found on the CDC Web site (**www.cdc.gov/botulism/**).

Antimicrobial Agents. Antimicrobial therapy is not prescribed in infant botulism unless clearly indicated for a concurrent infection. Aminoglycoside agents can potentiate the paralytic effects of the toxin and should be avoided. Given theoretical concerns of toxin release from antibiotic-induced bacterial cell death, providers may consider delaying the use of antibiotics in wound botulism until after antitoxin is administered, depending on the clinical situation. The role for antimicrobial therapy in the adult intestinal colonization form of botulism, if any, has not been established.

ISOLATION OF THE HOSPITALIZED PATIENT: Standard precautions are recommended.

CONTROL MEASURES:

- Any case of suspected botulism is a nationally notifiable disease and is required by law to be reported immediately to local and state health departments. Immediate reporting of suspected cases is particularly important, because a single case could be the harbinger of many more cases, as with foodborne botulism, and because of possible use of botulinum toxin as a bioterrorism weapon.
- Honey should not be given to children younger than 12 months because of the possibility of contaminating spores. Many foods and commercial products contain honey, and the honey is included in a variety of ways. Because the details of each manufacturing process vary, the California Department of Public Health is unable to comment on the likelihood that the honey-containing food product may contain viable *C botulinum* spores (**www.infantbotulism.org/general/faq.php**). Prudence would dictate that these types of foods also should be avoided during the first 12 months of life.
- Prophylactic antitoxin is not recommended for asymptomatic people who have ingested a food known to contain botulinum toxin. Physicians treating a patient who has been exposed to toxin or is suspected of having any type of botulism should contact their state health department immediately. People exposed to toxin who are asymptomatic should have close medical observation in nonsolitary settings.
- Education regarding safe practices in food preparation and home-canning methods should be promoted. Use of a pressure cooker (at 116°C [240.8°F]) is necessary to kill spores of *C botulinum*. Bringing the internal temperature of foods to 85°C (185°F) for 10 minutes will destroy the toxin. Time, temperature, and pressure requirements vary with altitude and the product being heated. Food containers that appear to bulge may contain gas produced by *C botulinum* and should be discarded. Other foods that appear to have spoiled should not be eaten or tasted (**https://nchfp.uga.edu/publications/publications_usda.html**).
- The investigational pentavalent botulinum toxoid vaccine (types A, B, C, D, and E) has been discontinued by the CDC for immunization of laboratory workers at high risk of exposure to botulinum toxin and no longer is available.[1]

Clostridial Myonecrosis
(Gas Gangrene)

CLINICAL MANIFESTATIONS: Disease onset is heralded by acute and progressive pain at the site of the wound, followed by edema, increasing exquisite tenderness, and exudate. Systemic findings initially include tachycardia disproportionate to the degree of fever, pallor, and diaphoresis. Crepitus is suggestive but not pathognomonic of *Clostridium* infection

---

[1]Centers for Disease Control and Prevention. Notice of CDC's discontinuation of investigational pentavalent (ABCDE) botulinum toxoid vaccine for workers at high risk for occupational exposure to botulinum toxins. *MMWR Morb Mortal Wkly Rep.* 2011;60(42):1454–1455

and is not always present. Tense bullae containing thin, serosanguineous or dark fluid develop in the overlying skin and areas of green-black cutaneous necrosis appear. Fluid in the bullae has a foul odor. Disease can progress rapidly with development of hypotension, renal failure, and alterations in mental status. Diagnosis is based on clinical manifestations, including the characteristic appearance of necrotic muscle at surgery. Untreated gas gangrene can lead to disseminated myonecrosis, suppurative visceral infection, septicemia, and death within hours.

Nontraumatic gas gangrene usually is caused by *Clostridium septicum* and is a complication of bacteremia, which is the result of an occult gastrointestinal mucosal lesion (most commonly colon cancer) or a complication of neutropenic colitis, leukemia, or diabetes mellitus.

ETIOLOGY: Clostridial myonecrosis is caused by *Clostridium* species, most often *Clostridium perfringens*. These organisms are large, gram-positive, spore-forming, anaerobic bacilli with blunt ends. Disease manifestations are caused by potent clostridial exotoxins (eg, *Clostridium sordellii* with medical abortion and *C septicum* with malignancy). Other *Clostridium* species (eg, *Clostridium sordellii*, *C septicum*, *Clostridium novyi*) also have been associated with myonecrosis. Mixed infection with other gram-positive and gram-negative bacteria is common.

EPIDEMIOLOGY: Clostridial myonecrosis usually results from contamination of deep open wounds. The sources of *Clostridium* species are soil, contaminated foreign bodies, and human and animal feces. Dirty surgical or traumatic wounds, particularly those with retained foreign bodies or significant amounts of devitalized tissue, predispose to disease. Rarely, nontraumatic gas gangrene occurs in immunocompromised people, most frequently in those with underlying malignancy, neutrophil dysfunction, or diseases associated with bowel ischemia.

The **incubation period** from the time of injury is 6 hours to 4 days.

DIAGNOSTIC TESTS: Anaerobic cultures of wound exudate, involved soft tissue and muscle, and blood should be performed. Both matrix-assisted laser desorption/ionization–time-of-flight (MALDI-TOF) devices approved by the US Food and Drug Administration have an approved indication to identify *C perfringens*. Because *Clostridium* species are ubiquitous, their recovery from a wound is not diagnostic unless typical clinical manifestations are present. A Gram-stained smear of wound discharge demonstrating characteristic gram-positive bacilli and few, if any, polymorphonuclear leukocytes suggests clostridial infection. Tissue specimens (not swab specimens) for anaerobic culture must be obtained to confirm the diagnosis. Because some pathogenic *Clostridium* species are exquisitely sensitive to oxygen, care should be taken to optimize anaerobic growth conditions. A radiograph of the affected site might demonstrate gas in the tissue, but this is a nonspecific finding that is not always present. Occasionally, blood cultures are positive and are considered diagnostic.

TREATMENT:

- Prompt and complete surgical excision of necrotic tissue and removal of foreign material is essential. Repeated surgical débridement may be required to ensure complete removal of all infected tissue. Vacuum-assisted wound closure can be used following multiple débridements.
- Management of shock, fluid and electrolyte imbalance, hemolytic anemia, and other complications is crucial.

- High-dose penicillin G (250 000–400 000 U/kg per day; maximum daily dose: 24 million units) should be administered intravenously. Clindamycin, metronidazole, meropenem, ertapenem, and chloramphenicol can be considered as alternative drugs for patients with a serious penicillin allergy or for treatment of polymicrobial infections. The combination of penicillin G and clindamycin may be superior to penicillin alone because of the theoretical benefit of clindamycin inhibiting toxin synthesis.
- Hyperbaric oxygen may be beneficial, but efficacy data from adequately controlled clinical studies are not available.

ISOLATION OF THE HOSPITALIZED PATIENT: Standard precautions are recommended.

CONTROL MEASURES: Prompt and careful débridement, flushing of contaminated wounds, and removal of foreign material should be performed.

Penicillin G (50 000 U/kg per day) or clindamycin (20–30 mg/kg per day) has been used for prophylaxis in patients with grossly contaminated wounds, but efficacy is unknown.

Clostridium difficile

CLINICAL MANIFESTATIONS: *Clostridium difficile* is associated with a spectrum of gastrointestinal illness, as well as with asymptomatic colonization that is common, especially in young infants. Mild to moderate illness is characterized by watery diarrhea, low-grade fever, and mild abdominal pain. Symptoms often begin while the child is hospitalized receiving antimicrobial therapy but can occur up to 10 weeks after therapy cessation. Pseudomembranous colitis is characterized by diarrhea with mucus in feces, abdominal cramps and pain, fever, and systemic toxicity. Toxic megacolon (acute dilatation of the colon) should be considered in children who develop marked abdominal tenderness and distension with minimal diarrhea and may be associated with hemodynamic instability. Other complications of *C difficile* disease include intestinal perforation, hypotension, shock, and death. Complicated infections are less common in children than adults. Severe or fatal disease is more likely to occur in neutropenic children with leukemia, infants with Hirschsprung disease, and patients with inflammatory bowel disease. Clinical illness attributable to *C difficile* is rare in children younger than 12 months. Extraintestinal manifestations of *C difficile* infection can include bacteremia, wound infections, and reactive arthritis.

ETIOLOGY: *C difficile* is a spore-forming, obligate anaerobic, gram-positive bacillus. Some strains produce exotoxins (toxins A and B), which are responsible for the clinical manifestations of disease when there is overgrowth of *C difficile* in the large intestine.

EPIDEMIOLOGY: *C difficile* is shed in feces. People can acquire infection from the stool of other colonized or infected people through the fecal-oral route. Any surface (including hands), device, or material that has become contaminated with feces may also transmit *C difficile* spores. Hospitals, nursing homes, and child care facilities are major reservoirs for *C difficile*. Risk factors for acquisition of the bacterium include prolonged hospitalization and exposure to an infected person either in the hospital or the community. Risk factors for *C difficile* disease include antimicrobial therapy, repeated enemas, proton pump inhibitor therapy, prolonged nasogastric tube placement, gastrostomy and jejunostomy tube placement, underlying bowel disease, gastrointestinal tract surgery, renal insufficiency, and immunocompromised state. *C difficile* colitis has been associated with exposure to almost every antimicrobial agent; cephalosporins and fluoroquinolones are considered to be the highest-risk antibiotic agents, particularly for recurrent *C difficile* disease and infections with epidemic strains. The NAP-1 strain is a virulent strain of *C difficile* because of increased toxin production and is associated with an increased risk of severe disease. NAP-1 strains of *C difficile* have emerged as a cause of outbreaks among adults and are reported sporadically in children.

Community-associated *C difficile* disease is occurring with increasing frequency in recent years. Although the rates of both community- and health care-associated *C difficile* disease are increasing in children, recent data suggest the incidence of pediatric community-associated *C difficile* disease may be twice as frequent as health care-associated disease.

Asymptomatic intestinal colonization with *C difficile* (including toxin-producing strains) is common in children younger than 5 years and is most common in infants younger than 1 year. Epidemiologic studies show that up to 50% of healthy infants have colonization. Colonization rates drop to less than 5% in healthy children older than 5 years and adults. Asymptomatic colonization with *C difficile* is common in recently hospitalized patients, with rates upward of 20%.

The **incubation period** is unknown; colitis usually develops 5 to 10 days after initiation of antimicrobial therapy but can occur on the first day of treatment and up to 10 weeks after therapy cessation.

DIAGNOSTIC TESTS: Endoscopic findings of pseudomembranes (2- to 5-mm, raised yellowish plaques) and hyperemic, friable rectal mucosa suggesting pseudomembranous colitis is highly correlated with *C difficile* disease. More commonly, the diagnosis of *C difficile* disease is based on laboratory methods including the detection of *C difficile* toxin(s) or toxin gene(s) in a diarrheal stool specimen. In general, laboratory tests for *C difficile* should not be ordered on a patient who is having formed stools unless ileus or toxic megacolon is suspected. Notwithstanding the availability of several test methods, there presently is no generally agreed on gold standard laboratory test method for the diagnosis of *C difficile* disease.

Molecular assays using nucleic acid amplification tests (NAATs) now are commonly used testing methods for toxigenic strains of *C difficile* toxins in both adult and pediatric hospitals. NAATs detect genes responsible for the production of toxins A and B, rather than free toxins A and B in the stool that are detected by enzyme immunoassay (EIA). EIAs are rapid, performed easily, and highly specific for diagnosis of *C difficile* infection, but their sensitivity is relatively low. The cell culture cytotoxicity assay, which also tests for toxin in stool, is more sensitive than the EIA but is labor intensive and has a long turnaround time, limiting its usefulness in the clinical setting. NAATs combine excellent sensitivity and analytic specificity, and provide results to clinicians in times comparable to EIAs. However, detecting toxin gene(s) in patients who are only colonized by *C difficile* is common and likely contributes to misdiagnosis of *C difficile* infection in children with other causes of diarrhea, leading to unnecessary antibiotic treatment for *C difficile*. Several steps can be taken to reduce the likelihood of misdiagnosis of *C difficile* infection related to use of highly sensitive NAATs. For example, because colonization with *C difficile* in infants is common and symptomatic infection in this age group is not thought to occur, *C difficile* diagnostic testing on samples from children under 12 months of age should be discouraged. Because sensitivity is nearly 100%, repeat NAAT testing for the same episode of diarrhea is discouraged because it is more likely to result in subsequent false positive tests. Furthermore, testing should be avoided or deferred in children with other more likely causes of diarrhea, such as concomitant laxative use and in children with symptoms more consistent of viral or noninfectious etiologies. Finally, because shedding of *C difficile* in the stool can persist for several months after symptoms resolution, tests of cure are impractical and should not be performed.

TREATMENT: A central tenet to control *C difficile* infection is the discontinuation of precipitating antimicrobial therapy; stopping these agents will allow competing gut flora to reemerge and, thus, crowd out *C difficile* within the intestine. A variety of therapies are available; use of a particular treatment modality is dependent on severity of illness, the number of recurrences of infection, tolerability of adverse effects, and cost. Recommended therapies for first occurrence, first recurrence, and second recurrence are provided in Table 3.3 (p 482). Drugs that decrease intestinal motility should not be administered. Follow-up testing for toxin is not recommended. Asymptomatic patients should not be treated.

When vancomycin is being used orally, as a cost-saving measure, vancomycin for intravenous use can be administered orally. The intravenous formulation is less expensive than the product available for oral use. Intravenously administered vancomycin is not effective for *C difficile* infection.

Fidaxomicin is approved for treatment of *C difficile*-associated diarrhea in adults. Studies have demonstrated equivalent efficacy to oral vancomycin, although subjects with life-threatening and fulminant infection, hypotension, septic shock, peritoneal signs, significant dehydration, or toxic megacolon were excluded. No comparative data of fidaxomicin to metronidazole are available. There are anecdotal reports of fidaxomicin use in children, although it is not approved for use in patients younger than 18 years.

There are limited data on the use of nitazoxanide in the treatment of recurrent *C difficile* infection in adults, but it has not been approved for this indication and no pediatric data are available.

Up to 20% of patients experience a recurrence after discontinuing therapy, but infection usually responds to a second course of the same treatment. Metronidazole should not be used for treatment of a second recurrence or for prolonged therapy, because neurotoxicity is possible. Tapered or pulse regimens of vancomycin may be considered for recurrent disease, often as 3 times a day for several days followed by twice a day for several days. Data are limited for the following vancomycin regimens:

- Vancomycin, orally, 10 mg/kg/dose (maximum 125 mg/dose), 4 times a day for 7 days, then 3 times a day for 7 days, then twice a day for 7 days, then once daily for 7 days, then once every other day for 7 days, then every 72 h for 7 days.
- Vancomycin, orally, 10 mg/kg/dose (maximum 125 mg/dose) 4 times a day for 14 days, then twice a day for 7 to 14 days, then once daily for 7 to 14 days, then every 2 to 3 days for 2 to 8 weeks.
- Vancomycin, orally, 10 mg/kg/dose (maximum 125 mg/dose) 4 times a day for 14 days, then either:
  - ♦ Rifaximin, orally, 400 mg, 3 times a day for 14 days (note that rifaximin dosing in pediatric patients is not well described, but it is poorly water-soluble and minimally absorbed; it should be avoided if the patient recently has received rifaximin for *C difficile* infection or another indication).
    OR
  - ♦ Nitazoxanide, orally, 100 mg, twice a day (1–3 years of age), 200 mg, twice a day (4–11 years of age), or 500 mg, twice a day (≥12 years of age) for 10 days.

Table 3.3. Treatments for *Clostridium difficile* Infection

Severity	Recommendation
	First Occurrence
Mild-moderate	Metronidazole, 30 mg/kg/day, PO, every 6 h (preferred), or IV, every 6 h for 10 days (maximum 500 mg/dose)
	If failure to respond in 5–7 days: Consider switch to vancomycin, 40 mg/kg/day, PO, every 6 h for 10 days (maximum 125 mg/dose)
	For pregnant/breastfeeding or metronidazole-intolerant patients: Vancomycin, 40 mg/kg/day, PO, every 6 h for 10 days (maximum 125 mg/dose)
	In patients for whom oral therapy cannot reach colon: To above regimen, **ADD** vancomycin, 500 mg/100 mL normal saline, enema, as needed every 8 h until improvement
Severe[a]	Vancomycin, 40 mg/kg/day, PO, every 6 h for 10 days (maximum 125 mg/dose)
Severe and complicated[b]	If no abdominal distension (use both for 10 days): Vancomycin, 40 mg/kg/day, PO, every 6 h (maximum 125 mg/dose) **PLUS** metronidazole, 30 mg/kg/day, IV, every 6 h (maximum 500 mg/dose)
	If complicated with ileus or toxic colitis and/or significant abdominal distension (use all for 10 days): Vancomycin, 40 mg/kg/day, PO, every 6 h (maximum 500 mg/dose) **PLUS** metronidazole, 30 mg/kg/day, IV, every 6h (maximum 500 mg/dose) **PLUS** vancomycin, 500 mg/100 mL normal saline enema, as needed every 8 h until improvement
Severity	**Recommendation**
	First Recurrence
Mild-moderate	Same regimen as for first occurrence (see above)
Severe	Vancomycin, 40 mg/kg/day, PO, every 6 h (maximum 125 mg/dose)
	Second Recurrence
All	DO NOT USE METRONIDAZOLE Vancomycin, PO, as pulsed or prolonged tapered dose (see text for options)

PO indicates orally; IV, intravenously.

[a]Severe: not well defined in children, but should be considered in the presence of leukocytosis, leukopenia, or worsening renal function.

[b]Severe and complicated: intensive care unit admission, hypotension or shock, pseudomembranous colitis by endoscopy, ileus, toxic megacolon.

Fecal transplant (intestinal microbiota transplantation) appears to be effective in adults, but there are limited data in pediatrics. No pediatric data are available evaluating use of human monoclonal antibodies (against toxin A and B); a lower rate of recurrent disease in adult patients receiving antibiotic therapy for primary or recurrent *C difficile* infection is reported in those receiving human monoclonal antibodies. Cholestyramine is not recommended. Other potential adjunctive therapies of unclear efficacy include Immune Globulin therapy and probiotics (particularly *Saccharomyces boulardii* and kefir).

ISOLATION OF THE HOSPITALIZED PATIENT: In addition to standard precautions, contact precautions and a private room (if feasible) are recommended at the time that disease is suspected through resolution of diarrhea.

CONTROL MEASURES: Exercising meticulous hand hygiene, properly handling contaminated waste (including diapers), disinfecting fomites, and limiting use of antimicrobial agents are the best available methods for control of *C difficile* infection. Gloves should be worn for all in-room care to prevent hand contamination and hand hygiene should be performed immediately after glove removal. Alcohol-based hand hygiene products do not inactivate *C difficile* spores. Washing hands with soap and water is considered to be more effective in removing *C difficile* spores from contaminated hands. There is disagreement among experts about when and whether soap-and-water hand hygiene should be used preferentially over alcohol hand gel in nonoutbreak settings. However, in outbreak settings or an increased *C difficile* infection rate,[1] washing hands with soap and water is the preferred method of hand hygiene after each contact with a *C difficile*-infected patient.

Thorough cleaning of hospital rooms and bathrooms of patients with *C difficile* disease, as well as reusable equipment with which infected patients had contact, is essential. Because *C difficile* spores are difficult to kill with standard hospital disinfectants approved by the US Environmental Protection Agency, many health care facilities have instituted the use of disinfectants with sporicidal activity (eg, hypochlorite).

Children with *C difficile* diarrhea should be excluded from child care settings until stools are contained in the diaper or the child is continent, and stool frequency is no more than 2 stools above that child's normal frequency for the time the child is in the program, and infection-control measures should be enforced (see Children in Out-of-Home Child Care, p 122).

Clostridium perfringens Food Poisoning

CLINICAL MANIFESTATIONS: *Clostridium perfringens* foodborne illness is characterized by a sudden onset of watery diarrhea and moderate-to-severe crampy, mid-epigastric pain. Symptoms usually resolve within 24 hours. The shorter incubation period, shorter duration of illness, and absence of fever in most patients differentiate *C perfringens* foodborne disease from shigellosis and salmonellosis. As compared with foodborne illnesses associated with heavy metals, *Staphylococcus aureus* enterotoxins, *Bacillus cereus* emetic toxin, and fish and shellfish toxins, *C perfringens* foodborne illness is infrequently associated with vomiting. Diarrheal illness caused by *B cereus* diarrheal enterotoxins can be indistinguishable from that caused by *C perfringens* (see Appendix VII, Clinical Syndromes Associated with Foodborne Diseases, p 1086). Necrotizing colitis and death have been described in patients with disease attributable to type A *C perfringens* who received antidiarrheal

---

[1]McDonald LC, Gerding DN, Johnson S, et al. Clinical practice guidelines for *Clostridium difficile* infection in adults and children: 2017 update by the Infectious Diseases Society of America (IDSA) and Society for Healthcare Epidemiology of America (SHEA). *Clin Infect Dis*. Published online February 15, 2018. Available at: **https://doi.org/10.1093/cid/cix1085**

medications resulting in constipation. Enteritis necroticans (also known as pigbel) results from hemorrhagic necrosis of the midgut and is a cause of severe illness and death attributable to *C perfringens* food poisoning caused by contamination with *Clostridium* strains carrying a β toxin. Rare cases have been reported in the Highlands of Papua New Guinea and in Thailand; protein malnutrition is an important risk factor. Additionally, enteritis necroticans has been reported in a child with poorly controlled diabetes in the United States who consumed chitterlings (pig intestine).

ETIOLOGY: Typical food poisoning is caused by a heat-labile *C perfringens* enterotoxin, produced during sporulation in the small intestine. *C perfringens* type A, which produces α toxin and enterotoxin, commonly causes foodborne illness. Enteritis necroticans is caused by *C perfringens* type C, which produces a β toxin that causes necrotizing small bowel inflammation.

EPIDEMIOLOGY: *C perfringens* is a gram-positive, spore-forming bacillus that is ubiquitous in the environment, the intestinal tracts of humans and animals, and commonly present in raw meat and poultry. Spores of *C perfringens* that survive cooking can germinate and multiply rapidly during slow cooling, when stored at temperatures from 20°C to 60°C (68°F–140°F), and during inadequate reheating. At an optimum temperature, *C perfringens* has one of the fastest rates of growth of any bacterium. Illness results from consumption of food containing high numbers of vegetative organisms ($>10^5$ colony forming units/g) that produce enterotoxin in the intestine.

Ingestion of the organism is most commonly associated with foods prepared by restaurants or caterers or in institutional settings (eg, schools and camps) where food is prepared in large quantities, cooled slowly, and stored inappropriately for prolonged periods. Beef, poultry, gravies, and dried or precooked foods are the most commonly implicated sources. Illness is not transmissible from person to person.

The **incubation period** is 6 to 24 hours, usually 8 to 12 hours.

DIAGNOSTIC TESTS: Because the fecal flora of healthy people commonly includes *C perfringens,* counts of *C perfringens* of 10^6 colony forming units (CFU)/g of feces or greater obtained within 48 hours of onset of illness are required to support the diagnosis in ill people. The diagnosis also can be supported by detection of enterotoxin in stool. *C perfringens* can be confirmed as the cause of an outbreak if 10^6 CFU/g are isolated from stool or enterotoxin is demonstrated in the stool of 2 or more ill people or when the concentration of organisms is at least 10^5 CFU/g in the implicated food. Although *C perfringens* is an anaerobe, special transport conditions are unnecessary. Stool specimens, rather than rectal swab specimens, should be obtained, transported in ice packs, and tested within 24 hours. For enumeration and enterotoxin testing, obtaining stool specimens in bulk without added transport media is required.

TREATMENT: Oral rehydration or, occasionally, intravenous fluid and electrolyte replacement may be indicated to prevent or treat dehydration. Antimicrobial agents are not indicated.

ISOLATION OF THE HOSPITALIZED PATIENT: Standard precautions are recommended.

CONTROL MEASURES: Preventive measures depend on limiting proliferation of *C perfringens* in foods by cooking foods thoroughly and maintaining food at warmer than 60°C (140°F) or cooler than 7°C (45°F). Meat dishes should be served hot shortly after cooking. Foods should never be held at room temperature to cool; they should be refrigerated in shallow containers after removal from warming devices or serving tables as soon as possible and within 2 hours of preparation. Information on recommended safe food handling practices, including time and temperature requirements during cooking, storage, and reheating, can be found at **www.foodsafety.gov.**

Coccidioidomycosis

CLINICAL MANIFESTATIONS: Primary pulmonary infection is acquired by inhaling fungal conidia and is asymptomatic or self-limited in 60% to 65% of infected children and adults. Constitutional symptoms, including extreme fatigue and weight loss, are common and can persist for weeks or months. Symptomatic disease can resemble influenza or community-acquired pneumonia, with malaise, fever, cough, myalgia, arthralgia, headache, and chest pain. Pleural effusion, empyema, and mediastinal involvement are more common in children.

Acute infection may be associated only with cutaneous abnormalities, such as erythema multiforme, an erythematous maculopapular rash, or erythema nodosum manifesting as bilateral symmetrical violaceous nodules usually overlying the shins. Chronic pulmonary lesions are rare, but approximately 5% of infected people develop asymptomatic pulmonary radiographic residua (eg, cysts, nodules, cavitary lesions, coin lesions).

Nonpulmonary primary infection is rare and usually follows trauma associated with contamination of wounds by arthroconidia. Cutaneous lesions and soft tissue infections often are accompanied by regional lymphadenitis.

Disseminated (extrapulmonary) infection occurs in less than 0.5% of infected people; common sites of dissemination include skin, bones and joints, and the central nervous system (CNS). Meningitis invariably is fatal if untreated. Congenital infection is rare.

ETIOLOGY: *Coccidioides* species are dimorphic fungi. In soil, *Coccidioides* organisms exist in the mycelial phase as mold growing as branching, septate hyphae. Infectious arthroconidia (ie, spores) produced from hyphae become airborne, infecting the host after inhalation or, rarely, inoculation. In tissues, arthroconidia enlarge to form spherules; mature spherules release hundreds to thousands of endospores that develop into new spherules and continue the tissue cycle. Molecular studies have divided the genus *Coccidioides* into 2 species: *Coccidioides immitis*, confined mainly to California, and *Coccidioides posadasii*, encompassing the remaining areas of distribution of the fungus within certain deserts of the southwestern United States, northern Mexico, and areas of Central and South America.

EPIDEMIOLOGY: *Coccidioides* species are found mostly in soil in areas of the southwestern United States with endemic infection, including California, Arizona, New Mexico, west and south Texas, southern Nevada, and Utah; northern Mexico; and throughout certain parts of Central and South America. In areas with endemic coccidioidomycosis, clusters of cases can follow dust-generating events, such as storms, seismic events, archaeologic digging, and recreational and construction activities, including building of solar farms. The majority of cases occur without a known preceding event. The incidence of reported coccidioidomycosis cases in areas of endemicity (Arizona, California, Nevada, New Mexico, and Utah) has increased substantially over the past decade and a half, rising from 5.3 per 100 000 population in 1998 to 42.6 per 100 000 in 2011.[1] As locally acquired infections have been reported from eastern Washington and Missouri, areas of endemicity

---

[1]Centers for Disease Control and Prevention. Increase in reported coccidioidomycosis—United States, 1998–2011. *MMWR Morb Mortal Wkly Rep.* 2013;62(12):217–221

may extend beyond the traditionally defined range.[1] Infection is thought to provide life-long immunity. Person-to-person transmission of coccidioidomycosis does not occur except in rare instances of cutaneous infection with actively draining lesions, donor-derived transmission via an infected organ, and congenital infection following in utero exposure. People with impairment of T-lymphocyte–mediated immunity caused by a congenital immune defect or HIV infection or those receiving immune modulating medications (eg, tumor necrosis factor [TNF] alpha antagonist) are at major risk for severe primary coccidioidomycosis, disseminated disease, or relapse of past infection. Other people at elevated risk of severe or disseminated disease include people of African or Filipino ancestry, women in the third trimester of pregnancy and those postpartum, and children younger than 1 year. Cases may occur in people who do not reside in regions with endemic infection but who previously have visited these areas. In regions without endemic infection, careful travel histories should be obtained from people with symptoms or findings compatible with coccidioidomycosis. Because the signs and symptoms of infection are nonspecific, the diagnosis is not considered, and therefore, most infections are not identified.

The **incubation period** typically is 1 to 4 weeks in primary infection; disseminated infection may develop years after primary infection.

DIAGNOSTIC TESTS: Diagnosis of coccidioidomycosis is best established using serologic, histopathologic, and culture methods. Nucleic acid amplification tests have been developed but are not widely available.

Serologic tests are useful in the diagnosis and management of infection. The immunoglobulin (Ig) M response can be detected by enzyme immunoassay (EIA) or immunodiffusion methods. In approximately 50% and 90% of primary infections, IgM is detected in the first and third weeks, respectively; however, an EIA positive result by IgM alone should be interpreted with caution because of the low specificity of this test. IgG response can be detected by immunodiffusion, EIA, or complement fixation (CF) tests. Immunodiffusion is considered more specific, whereas CF is more sensitive. A combination of both CF and immunodiffusion tests is often helpful in diagnosis; however, both immunodiffusion and especially CF are known to cross react with *Histoplasma* organisms. CF antibodies in serum usually are of low titer and are transient if the disease is asymptomatic or mild. Persistent high titers (≥1:16) occur with severe disease and are almost always seen in disseminated infection. Cerebrospinal fluid (CSF) antibodies also are detectable by immunodiffusion or CF testing. Increasing serum and CSF titers indicate progressive disease, and decreasing titers usually suggest improvement. CF titers may not be reliable in immunocompromised patients; low or nondetectable titers in immunocompromised patients should be interpreted with caution.

Spherules are as large as 80 μm in diameter and can be visualized with 100x to 400x magnification in infected body fluid specimens (eg, pleural fluid, bronchoalveolar lavage) and biopsy specimens of skin lesions or organs. For biopsy specimens, use of silver or period-acid Schiff staining is helpful. The presence of a mature spherule with endospores is pathognomonic of infection. Isolation of *Coccidioides* species in culture establishes the diagnosis, even in patients with mild symptoms. When a specimen from a patient suspected of having coccidioidomycosis is sent for culture, the diagnostic laboratory should be alerted.

---

[1]Centers for Disease Control and Prevention. Coccidioidomycosis in a state where it is not known to be endemic—Missouri, 2004–2013. *MMWR Morb Mortal Wkly Rep.* 2015;64(23):636–639

Culture of organisms is possible on a variety of artificial media but is hazardous to laboratory personnel, because spherules can convert to arthroconidia-bearing mycelia on culture plates. Suspect cultures should be sealed and handled using appropriate safety equipment and procedures. A DNA probe can identify *Coccidioides* species in cultures.

Although limited in availability, at least one commercial laboratory offers an EIA test for urine, serum, plasma, CSF, or bronchoalveolar lavage fluid for detection of *Coccidioides* antigen. Antigen may be positive in patients with more severe forms of disease (sensitivity 71%) in a study of immunosuppressed patients. Cross reactions occur in patients with histoplasmosis, blastomycosis, or paracoccidioidomycosis.

TREATMENT: Antifungal therapy for uncomplicated primary infection in people without risk factors for severe disease is controversial. Although most cases will resolve without therapy, some experts believe that treatment may reduce illness duration or risk of severe complications. Most experts recommend treatment of coccidioidomycosis for people at risk of severe disease or people with severe primary infection. Severe primary infection is manifested by complement fixation titers of 1:16 or greater, infiltrates involving more than half of one lung or portions of both lungs, weight loss of greater than 10%, marked chest pain, severe malaise, inability to work or attend school, intense night sweats, or symptoms that persist for more than 2 months. In such cases, fluconazole is recommended for 3 to 6 months. During pregnancy, amphotericin B (including lipid formulations) is the treatment of choice over fluconazole (and likely other azole antifungals), as fluconazole has been demonstrated to be a teratogen in early pregnancy. Repeated patient encounters every 1 to 3 months for up to 2 years, either to document radiographic resolution or to identify residual abnormalities or pulmonary or extrapulmonary complications, are recommended. For diffuse pneumonia, defined as bilateral reticulonodular or miliary infiltrates, a preparation of amphotericin B or high-dose fluconazole is recommended. Amphotericin B is used more frequently in the presence of severe hypoxemia or rapid clinical deterioration. The total length of therapy for diffuse pneumonia is 1 year.

Oral fluconazole or itraconazole is the recommended initial therapy for disseminated infection not involving the CNS. Amphotericin B is recommended as alternative therapy if lesions are progressing or are in critical locations, such as the vertebral column, or in fulminant infections, because it is thought to result in more rapid improvement. In patients experiencing failure of conventional amphotericin B deoxycholate therapy or experiencing drug-related toxicities, a lipid formulation of amphotericin B can be substituted.

Consultation with a specialist for treatment of patients with CNS disease caused by *Coccidioides* species is recommended. High-dose oral fluconazole (adult dose: 400 mg/day, up to 800 or 1000 mg/day) is recommended for treatment of patients with CNS infection. Patients who respond to azole therapy should continue this treatment indefinitely. For CNS infections that are unresponsive to oral azoles or are associated with severe basilar inflammation, intrathecal amphotericin B deoxycholate therapy (0.1–1.5 mg per dose) can be used to augment the azole therapy. A subcutaneous reservoir can facilitate administration into the cisternal space or lateral ventricle. Hydrocephalus is a common complication of coccidioidal meningitis and nearly always requires a shunt for decompression.

There are reports of success with voriconazole, posaconazole, and isavuconazole in treatment of coccidioidomycosis, but this has not been established in children. These newer agents may be administered in certain clinical settings, such as therapeutic failure in severe coccidioidal disease (eg, meningitis). When used, these newer azoles should be administered in consultation with experts experienced with their use in treatment of coccidioidomycosis.

The duration of antifungal therapy is variable and depends on the site(s) of involvement, clinical response, and mycologic and immunologic test results. In general, therapy is continued until clinical and laboratory evidence indicates that active infection has resolved. Treatment for disseminated coccidioidomycosis is at least 6 months but for some patients may be extended to 1 year or longer. However, on discontinuation of therapy, relapses occur in approximately one third of all patients. The role of subsequent suppressive azole therapy is uncertain, except for patients with CNS infection, osteomyelitis, or underlying human immunodeficiency virus (HIV) infection or solid organ transplant recipients. The duration of suppressive therapy may be lifelong for certain high-risk groups.[1] Women should be advised to avoid pregnancy while receiving fluconazole, which is known to be teratogenic.

Surgical débridement or excision of lesions in bone, pericardium, and lung has been advocated for localized, symptomatic, persistent, resistant, or progressive lesions. In some localized infections with sinuses, fistulae, or abscesses, amphotericin B has been instilled locally or used for irrigation of wounds. Antifungal prophylaxis for solid organ transplant recipients may be considered if they reside in areas with endemicity and have prior serologic evidence or a history of coccidioidomycosis.

ISOLATION OF THE HOSPITALIZED PATIENT: Standard precautions are recommended. Care should be taken in handling, changing, and discarding dressings, casts, and similar materials through which arthroconidial contamination could occur.

CONTROL MEASURES: Coccidioidomycosis is a reportable disease in many states and some countries. Measures to control dust are recommended in areas with endemic infection, including construction sites, archaeologic project sites, or other locations where activities cause excessive soil disturbance. Immunocompromised people residing in or traveling to areas with endemic infection should be counseled to avoid exposure to activities that may aerosolize spores in contaminated soil.

Coronaviruses, Including SARS and MERS

CLINICAL MANIFESTATIONS: Human coronaviruses (HCoVs) 229E, OC43, NL63 and HKU1 are associated most frequently with an upper respiratory tract infection characterized by rhinorrhea, nasal congestion, sore throat, sneezing, and cough that may be associated with mild fever. Symptoms are self-limited and typically peak on day 3 or 4 of illness. These HCoV infections also may be associated with acute otitis media or asthma exacerbations. Less frequently, they are associated with lower respiratory tract infections, including bronchiolitis, croup, and pneumonia, primarily in infants and immunocompromised children and adults.

SARS-CoV was responsible for the 2002–2003 global outbreak of severe acute respiratory syndrome (SARS), which was associated with more severe symptoms, although a spectrum of disease including asymptomatic infections and mild disease occurred. SARS-

---

[1]Panel on Opportunistic Infections in HIV-Exposed and HIV-Infected Children. Guidelines for the Prevention and Treatment of Opportunistic Infections in HIV-Exposed and HIV-Infected Children. Rockville, MD: US Department of Health and Human Services; 2013. Available at: **https://aidsinfo.nih.gov/contentfiles/lvguidelines/oi_guidelines_pediatrics.pdf**

CoV disproportionately affected adults, who typically presented with fever, myalgia, headache, malaise, and chills followed by a nonproductive cough and dyspnea generally 5 to 7 days later. Approximately 25% of infected adults developed watery diarrhea. Twenty percent developed respiratory distress requiring intubation and ventilation. The overall mortality rate was approximately 10%, with most deaths occurring in the third week of illness. The case-fatality rate in people older than 60 years approached 50%. Typical laboratory abnormalities include lymphopenia and increased lactate dehydrogenase (LDH) and creatine kinase concentrations. Most had progressive unilateral or bilateral ill-defined airspace infiltrates on chest imaging. Pneumothoraces and other signs of barotrauma were common in critically ill patients receiving mechanical ventilation.

During the 2002–2003 outbreak, SARS-CoV infections in children were less severe than in adults; notably, no infant or child deaths from SARS-CoV infection were documented. Infants and children younger than 12 years who develop SARS typically present with fever, cough, and rhinorrhea. Associated lymphopenia is less severe, and radiographic changes are milder and generally resolve more quickly than in adolescents and adults. Adolescents who develop SARS have clinical courses more closely resembling those of adult disease, presenting with fever, myalgia, headache, and chills. Adolescents also are more likely to develop dyspnea, hypoxemia, and worsening chest radiographic findings. Laboratory abnormalities are comparable to those in adult disease.

MERS-CoV, the HCoV associated with the Middle East respiratory syndrome (MERS), also can cause severe disease. MERS-CoV is associated with a severe respiratory illness similar to that with SARS-CoV, although a spectrum of disease, including asymptomatic infections and mild disease, may occur. The majority of cases have been identified in male adults with comorbidities. Infected children typically present with milder symptoms. Patients initially present with fever, myalgia, and chills followed by a nonproductive cough and dyspnea a few days later. Approximately 25% of patients may experience vomiting, diarrhea, or abdominal pain. Rapid deterioration of oxygenation with progressive unilateral or bilateral airspace infiltrates on chest imaging may follow, requiring mechanical ventilation and often associated with acute renal failure. The case-fatality rate is high, estimated at 36%, but may partially reflect surveillance bias for more severe disease. Laboratory abnormalities may include thrombocytopenia, lymphopenia, and increased lactate dehydrogenase (LDH), particularly among severely infected individuals.

ETIOLOGY: Coronaviruses are enveloped, nonsegmented, single-stranded, positive-sense RNA viruses named after their corona- or crown-like surface projections observed on electron microscopy that correspond to large surface spike proteins. Coronaviruses are classified in the Nidovirales order. Coronaviruses are host specific and can infect humans as well as a variety of different animals, causing diverse clinical syndromes. Four distinct genera have been described: *Alphacoronavirus, Betacoronavirus, Gammacoronavirus,* and *Deltacoronavirus.* HCoVs 229E and NL63 belong to the genus *Alphacoronavirus.* HCoVs OC43 and HKU1 belong to lineage A, SARS-CoV belongs to lineage B, and MERS-CoV belongs to lineage C of the genus *Betacoronavirus.*

EPIDEMIOLOGY: Coronaviruses were recognized as animal pathogens in the 1930s. Thirty years later, HCoVs 229E and OC43 were identified as human pathogens, along with other coronavirus strains that were not investigated further and for which little is known regarding their prevalence and associated disease syndromes. In 2003, SARS-CoV was identified as a novel virus responsible for a global outbreak that lasted for 9 months and resulted in 8096 reported cases and 774 deaths. No SARS-CoV infections have been reported worldwide since early 2004. Data suggest SARS-CoV evolved from a natural reservoir of SARS-CoV-like viruses in horseshoe bats through civet cats or intermediate animal hosts in wet markets of China. Whether or not a large-scale reemergence of SARS will occur is unknown. Finding a novel HCoV sparked a renewed interest in HCoV research, and 2 years later NL63 and HKU1 were identified as newly recognized HCoVs. Investigations have revealed that HCoV NL63 was present in archived human respiratory tract specimens as early as 1981 and HKU1 as early as 1995. In 2012, MERS-CoV was identified as a novel virus responsible for severe respiratory illness, first detected in an individual from the Kingdom of Saudi Arabia and another individual from Qatar. Data suggest MERS-CoV likely evolved from bat CoV, with dromedary camels acting as intermediate hosts. A total of 1733 cases and 678 deaths have been associated with MERS-CoV as of May 2016. Updated figures on global cases can be found on the World Health Organization Web site (**www.who.int/emergencies/ mers-cov/en/**).

HCoVs 229E, OC43, NL63, and HKU1 can be found worldwide. They cause most disease in the winter and spring months in temperate climates. Seroprevalence data for these HCoVs suggest that exposure is common in early childhood, with approximately 90% of adults being seropositive for HCoVs 229E, OC43, and NL63 and 60% being seropositive for HCoV HKU1. In contrast, SARS-CoV infection has not been detected in humans since early 2004. MERS-CoV cases continue primarily in the Middle East, primarily linked to exposure to camels or close contact with an unrecognized case. Healthcare associated transmission has occurred during care of a MERS-CoV-infected patient. In 2015, a large outbreak of MERS-CoV in South Korea, resulting in 186 cases and 36 deaths, was traced back to an individual who returned from travel in the Middle East. Limited other travel-related cases have occurred without comparable secondary transmission.

The modes of transmission for CoVs 229E, OC43, NL63, and HKU1 have not been well studied. However, on the basis of studies of other respiratory tract viruses, it is likely that transmission occurs primarily via a combination of droplet and direct and indirect contact spread. Which of these modes are most important remains to be determined, and the possible role of aerosol spread requires further study. For MERS-CoV, studies suggest that droplet and direct contact spread are likely the most common modes of transmission, although evidence of indirect contact spread and aerosol spread also exist. Fecal droplet and fecal-oral transmission also have been proposed as possible routes of MERS-CoV transmission. There is no evidence of vertical transmission of MERS-CoV. HCoVs 229E and OC43 are most likely to be transmitted during the first few days of illness, when symptoms and respiratory viral loads are at their highest. Further study is needed to confirm that this holds true for HCoVs NL63 and HKU1. SARS-CoV and MERS-CoV are most likely to be transmitted during the second week of illness, when both symptoms and respiratory viral loads peak. Supershedding events have been associated with both SARS-CoV and MERS-CoV.

The **incubation period for HCoV-229E** is 2 to 5 days (median 3 days). Further study is needed to confirm the incubation periods for HCoVs OC43, NL63, and HKU1. The **incubation period for SARS-CoV** is estimated to be 2 to 10 days (median, 4 days). The **incubation period for MERS-CoV** is estimated to be 2 to 14 days (median 5 days).

DIAGNOSTIC TESTS: Following the SARS global outbreak, some clinical laboratories started offering comprehensive respiratory molecular diagnostic testing using reverse transcriptase-polymerase chain reaction (RT-PCR) assays, some of which include HCoVs 229E, OC43, NL54, and HKU1 as targets. Public health laboratories offer RT-PCR and antibody testing for MERS-CoV. Diagnostic laboratory and clinical guidance for SARS is available on the Centers for Disease Control and Prevention (CDC) SARS Web site (**www.cdc.gov/sars/index.html**). Given the potential for false-positive test results and the associated public health implications, testing for MERS-CoV in the absence of known person-to-person transmission of MERS must be performed in consultation with regional public health departments and only when there is a high degree of suspicion. Guidance regarding testing for MERS-CoV is available on the CDC MERS Web site (**www.cdc.gov/coronavirus/MERS/index.html**).

Specimens obtained from the upper and lower respiratory tract are the most appropriate samples for HCoV detection. The yield from lower respiratory tract specimens is higher than that from upper respiratory tract specimens for SARS-CoV and MERS-CoV. Stool and serum samples also frequently test positive using RT-PCR in patients with SARS-CoV and have tested positive in some patients with MERS-CoV and HCoV HKU1. For HCoVs 229E and OC43, specimens are most likely to be positive during the first few days of illness; whether this also is true for HCoVs NL63 and HKU1 requires further study. For SARS-CoV, respiratory and stool specimens may not test positive until the second week of illness when symptoms and viral loads peak; serum samples most likely test positive in the first week of illness. Compared with adults, infants and children with SARS-CoV infections are less likely to have positive test results, consistent with the milder symptoms and presumed corresponding lower viral loads seen in this age group. For both SARS-CoV and MERS-CoV, it is recommended to collect specimens for RT-PCR from the lower respiratory and upper respiratory tract along with serum. A stool sample is recommended for patients with suspected SARS-CoV. Serologic testing is available for SARS-CoV and MERS-CoV at public health laboratories, primarily for research and surveillance purposes.

TREATMENT: Infections attributable to HCoVs generally are treated with supportive care. SARS-CoV and MERS-CoV infections are more serious. Steroids, type 1 interferons, convalescent plasma, ribavirin, and lopinavir/ritonavir all were used clinically to treat patients with SARS, albeit without benefit of controlled data and, thus, no evidence of efficacy. There are reports of patients with SARS who were treated with supportive care only who recovered uneventfully. In the event that SARS-CoV reemerges, clarification of the effectiveness of treatments through controlled clinical trials is required. In vitro data suggest type 1 interferons and lopinavir inhibit MERS-CoV replication. However, treatment efficacy of any antiviral agent for MERS-CoV has yet to be established.

ISOLATION OF THE HOSPITALIZED PATIENT: In addition to standard precautions, health care professionals should use droplet and contact precautions when examining and caring for infants and young children with signs and symptoms of a respiratory tract infection for the duration of their illness (**www.cdc.gov/hicpac/2007IP/ 2007isolationPrecautions.html**). Airborne, droplet, and contact precautions are recommended for patients with suspected SARS-CoV infection for the duration of illness plus 10 days after resolution of fever, provided respiratory symptoms are absent or improving. Airborne, droplet, and contact precautions are recommended as well for patients with suspected MERS-CoV infection. When precautions should be discontinued for MERS-CoV has not yet been established, and it is recommended that this decision be made in conjunction with public health authorities (**www.cdc.gov/coronavirus/ mers/infection-prevention-control.html**).

CONTROL MEASURES: Practicing appropriate hand and respiratory hygiene likely is the most useful and easily implemented control measure to curb spread of all respiratory tract viruses, including HCoVs. Cleaning and disinfection of high-touch environmental surfaces using standard disinfectants should decrease the potential for indirect transmission of HCoVs via fomites. For hospitalized patients, following additional infection-control practices is recommended. Public health departments should be notified of any suspected cases of SARS-CoV and MERS-CoV as soon as possible. The control of the 2002–2003 SARS global outbreak was credited to the rapid identification of cases and early implementation of infection-control and public health measures, such as contact tracing, isolation, and quarantine. If SARS-CoV reemerges, all measures should be implemented quickly to attempt to prevent a recurrent worldwide outbreak. MERS-CoV transmission within hospitals and households can be averted with case identification and the use of infection control and public health measures including contact tracing. However, preventing the transmission of MERS-CoV from camels to humans is more challenging, given the prevalent use of camels in some Middle East countries. Most experts believe that sporadic transmission will continue until an effective MERS-CoV vaccine is found.

Cryptococcus neoformans and *Cryptococcus gattii* Infections (Cryptococcosis)

CLINICAL MANIFESTATIONS: Primary pulmonary infection is acquired by inhalation of aerosolized *Cryptococcus* fungal elements found in contaminated soil or organic material (eg, trees, rotting wood, and bird guano) and often is asymptomatic or mild in degree. Pulmonary disease, when symptomatic, is characterized by cough, chest pain, and constitutional symptoms. Chest radiographs may reveal solitary or multiple masses; patchy, segmental, or lobar consolidation, which often is multifocal; or nodular or reticulonodular interstitial changes. Pulmonary cryptococcosis may present as acute respiratory distress syndrome (ARDS) and may mimic *Pneumocystis* pneumonia. Hematogenous dissemination to the central nervous system (CNS), bones, skin, and other sites can occur, is uncommon, and almost always occurs in children with defects in T-lymphocyte–mediated immunity (eg, children with leukemia or lymphoma, children taking corticosteroids, children with congenital immunodeficiency or acquired immunodeficiency syndrome [AIDS], or children who have undergone solid organ transplantation). Usually, several sites are infected, but manifestations of involvement at 1 site predominate. Cryptococcal meningitis, the most common and serious form of cryptococcal disease, often follows an indolent course. Symptoms are characteristic of meningitis, meningoencephalitis, or space-occupying lesions but sometimes manifest only as subtle, nonspecific findings such as fever, headache, or behavioral changes. Cryptococcal fungemia without apparent organ involvement occurs in patients with human immunodeficiency virus (HIV) infection but is rare in children.

ETIOLOGY: Although there are more than 30 species of *Cryptococcus*, only 2 species, *Cryptococcus neoformans* (var *neoformans* and var *grubii*) and *Cryptococcus gattii*, are regarded as human pathogens.

EPIDEMIOLOGY: *C neoformans* var *neoformans* and *C neoformans* var *grubii* are isolated primarily from soil contaminated with pigeon or other bird droppings and cause most human infections, especially infections in immunocompromised hosts. *C neoformans* infects 5% to 10% of adults with AIDS, but infection is rare in HIV-infected children. *C gattii* (formerly *C neoformans* var *gattii*) is associated with trees and surrounding soil and has emerged as a pathogen producing a respiratory syndrome with or without neurologic findings in individuals from British Columbia, Canada, the Pacific Northwest region of the United States, and occasionally other regions of the United States. A high frequency of disease also has been reported in Aboriginal people in Australia and in the central province of Papua New Guinea. *C gattii* causes disease in immunocompetent and immunocompromised people, and cases have been reported in children. Person-to-person transmission does not occur.

The **incubation period for *C neoformans*** is unknown but likely variable; dissemination often represents reactivation of latent disease acquired previously. The **incubation period for *C gattii*** is 8 weeks to 13 months.

DIAGNOSTIC TESTS: The cerebrospinal fluid (CSF) profile of cryptococcal meningoencephalitis is characterized by a lack in both cellularity and alterations in biochemical profile, especially in HIV-infected individuals. Laboratory diagnosis of cryptococcal infection is best performed using antigen detection methods or by culture. The latex agglutination test (most commonly used), lateral flow immunoassay, and enzyme immunoassay for detection of cryptococcal capsular polysaccharide antigen (galactoxylomannan) in serum or CSF specimens are excellent rapid diagnostic tests for those with suspected meningitis. India ink stain for screening of CSF in cases of suspected cryptococcal meningitis has significantly lower sensitivity and is not recommended as a stand-alone rapid test. Antigen is detected in CSF or serum specimens from more than 95% of patients with cryptococcal meningitis. In patients with cryptococcal meningitis, antigen test results can be falsely negative when antigen concentrations are very high (prozone effect), which can be addressed by dilution of samples. Although antigen detection assays are useful in diagnosis, they have limited utility in following response to therapy. A lateral flow assay, which shows good agreement with standard antigen testing, has been developed for the diagnosis of cryptococcosis, especially in resource-limited countries.

Definitive diagnosis requires isolation of the organism from body fluid or tissue specimens. Blood should be cultured by lysis-centrifugation. Media containing cycloheximide, which inhibits growth of *C neoformans*, should not be used. Most laboratories confirm the production of urease by *Cryptococcus* species, noting that virtually all other fungi are urease negative (exceptions being *Trichosporon* species and some *Candida* species). The production of melanin by *Cryptococcus* species can be confirmed using Niger seed agar or using the caffeic acid disk test. Differentiation between *C neoformans* and *C gattii* can be made by the use of the selective medium L-canavanine glycine bromothymol blue (CGB) agar. *C gattii* will grow in the presence of L-canavanine, utilizing the glycine and causing the bromothymol indicator to turn the agar blue. *C neoformans* will not grow or grows poorly in presence of L-canavanine and will not utilize glycine, so the yellow agar remains unchanged in color. Sabouraud dextrose agar is useful for isolation of *Cryptococcus* organisms from sputum, bronchopulmonary lavage, tissue, or CSF specimens. In refractory or relapse cases, susceptibility testing can be helpful, although antifungal resistance is uncommon. CSF specimens may contain only a few organisms, and a large quantity of CSF may be needed to recover the organism. Polymerase chain reaction assays are investigational. Encapsulated yeast cells can be visualized using India ink or other stains of CSF and bronchoalveolar lavage specimens, but this method has limited sensitivity. Focal pulmonary or skin lesions can be biopsied for fungal staining and culture.

TREATMENT: The Infectious Diseases Society of America, the Pediatric Infectious Diseases Society, the American Academy of Pediatrics, the National Institutes of Health, and the Centers for Disease Control and Prevention have published practice management guidelines for cryptococcal disease.[1,2] No trials dedicated to children have been performed, so optimal dosing and duration of therapy for children with cryptococcal infection have not been precisely determined. Amphotericin B deoxycholate, 1 mg/kg/day (see Antifungal Drugs for Systemic Fungal Infections, p 938), in combination with oral flucytosine, 25 mg/kg/dose, 4 times/day, is indicated as induction therapy for patients with meningeal and other serious cryptococcal infections. Monitoring of blood counts and/or serum peak flucytosine concentrations (with a target of 40 to 60 µg/mL 2 hours after the dose) is recommended to prevent neutropenia. Patients with meningitis should receive induction combination therapy for at least 2 weeks and until a repeat CSF culture is negative, followed by consolidation therapy with fluconazole (6 mg/kg [maximum dose, 400 mg] daily) for a minimum of 8 weeks. Liposomal amphotericin B (3–6 mg/kg/day) or amphotericin B lipid complex (5 mg/kg/day) can be used in children with renal impairment or those intolerant to amphotericin B deoxycholate. If flucytosine cannot be administered, amphotericin B alone has been successfully used in pediatric cryptococcosis. A lumbar puncture should be performed after 2 weeks of therapy to document microbiologic clearance. The 20% to 40% of patients in whom culture is positive after 2 weeks of therapy will require a more prolonged induction treatment course. For any relapse, induction antifungal therapy should be restarted for 4 to 10 weeks, CSF cultures should be repeated every 2 weeks until sterile, and antifungal susceptibility of the relapse isolate should be determined. Monitoring of serum cryptococcal antigen is not useful to monitor response to therapy in patients with cryptococcal meningitis.

Increased intracranial pressure occurs frequently despite microbiologic response and often is associated with clinical deterioration. Significant elevation of intracranial pressure is a major source of morbidity and should be managed with frequent repeated lumbar punctures or placement of a lumbar drain. Immune reconstitution inflammatory syndrome (IRIS) is described, and although there are no guidelines for specific management of IRIS in children, a patient should be closely monitored for signs and symptoms associated with IRIS.

Children with HIV infection who have completed initial therapy for cryptococcosis should receive long-term suppressive therapy with fluconazole (6 mg/kg daily; maximum dose 400 mg). Oral itraconazole daily (oral solution preferred over capsule because of better bioavailability and no need to take with food) or amphotericin B deoxycholate, 1 to 3 times weekly, are less effective alternatives. Discontinuing chronic suppressive therapy for cryptococcosis (after 1 year or longer of secondary prophylaxis) can be considered in asymptomatic children 6 years or older who are receiving antiretroviral therapy, have sustained (≥6 months) increases in CD4+ T-lymphocyte counts to ≥100 cells/mm³, and

---

[1] Perfect J, Dismukes WE, Dromer F, et al. Clinical practice guidelines for the management of cryptococcal disease: 2010 update by the Infectious Diseases Society of America. *Clin Infect Dis.* 2010;50(3):291–322

[2] Panel on Opportunistic Infections in HIV-Exposed and HIV-Infected Children. Guidelines for the Prevention and Treatment of Opportunistic Infections in HIV-Exposed and HIV-Infected Children. Rockville, MD: US Department of Health and Human Services; 2013. Available at: **https://aidsinfo.nih.gov/contentfiles/lvguidelines/oi_guidelines_pediatrics.pdf**

have an undetectable HIV viral load for at least 3 months. Secondary prophylaxis should be reinstituted if the CD4+ T-lymphocyte count decreases to <100/mm^3. Although screening for cryptococcal antigen has not been recommended for children, screening for antigen in adults with CD4+ T-lymphocyte ≤100 cells/mm^3 and particularly those with CD4+ T-lymphocyte ≤50 cells/mm^3 is recommended by some experts and may be considered in children. Most experts would not discontinue secondary prophylaxis for patients younger than 6 years.[1]

Patients with less severe nonmeningeal disease (pulmonary disease) can be treated with fluconazole, but data on use of fluconazole for children with *C neoformans* infection is limited; itraconazole is a potential alternative. Another potential treatment option for patients with less severe disease or patients in whom amphotericin B treatment is not possible is combination therapy with fluconazole and flucytosine. The combination of fluconazole and flucytosine has superior efficacy compared with fluconazole alone. Echinocandins are not active against cryptococcal infections and should not be used.

ISOLATION OF THE HOSPITALIZED PATIENT: Standard precautions are recommended.

CONTROL MEASURES: None.

Cryptosporidiosis

CLINICAL MANIFESTATIONS: Frequent, nonbloody, watery diarrhea is the most common manifestation of cryptosporidiosis, although infection can be asymptomatic. Other symptoms include abdominal cramps, fatigue, fever, vomiting, anorexia, and weight loss. In infected immunocompetent adults and children, diarrheal illness is self-limited, usually resolving within 2 to 3 weeks. Infected immunocompromised hosts, such as children who have received solid organ transplants or who have advanced human immunodeficiency virus (HIV) disease, can experience profuse diarrhea lasting weeks to months; this can lead to malnutrition and wasting and, as such, could be a significant contributing factor leading to death. Extraintestinal cryptosporidiosis (eg, disease in the pulmonary or biliary tract or rarely in the pancreas) has been reported in immunocompromised people.

The diagnosis of cryptosporidiosis should be considered in any solid organ transplant recipient or HIV-infected patient with diarrhea. Delay in diagnosis and treatment can be associated with prolonged diarrhea and weight loss. Elevated tacrolimus concentrations have been reported in solid organ transplant recipients, are thought to be related to altered drug metabolism in the small intestine, and are associated with acute kidney injury.

ETIOLOGY: *Cryptosporidium* species are oocyst-forming coccidian protozoa. Oocysts are excreted in feces of an infected host and are transmitted via the fecal-oral route. *Cryptosporidium hominis* (which predominantly infects people) and *Cryptosporidium parvum* (which infects people, preweaned bovine calves, and other mammals) cause more than 90% of human cryptosporidiosis.

EPIDEMIOLOGY: Extensive waterborne disease outbreaks have been associated with contamination of drinking water and recreational water (eg, swimming pools, lakes, and

---

[1]Panel on Opportunistic Infections in HIV-Exposed and HIV-Infected Children. Guidelines for the Prevention and Treatment of Opportunistic Infections in HIV-Exposed and HIV-Infected Children. Rockville, MD: US Department of Health and Human Services; 2013. Available at: **https://aidsinfo.nih.gov/contentfiles/lvguidelines/oi_guidelines_pediatrics.pdf**

water playgrounds). Since 2004, the incidence of nationally reported cryptosporidiosis increased 2 to 3 times.[1] In children, the incidence of cryptosporidiosis is greatest during summer and early fall, corresponding to the outdoor swimming season. Cases are most frequently reported in children 1 through 4 years of age, followed by those 5 through 9 years of age.

Because oocysts are extremely chlorine tolerant, multistep treatment processes often are used to remove (eg, filter) and inactivate (eg, ultraviolet treatment) oocysts to protect public drinking water supplies. Typical filtration systems used for swimming pools do not efficiently remove oocysts from contaminated water. As a result, *Cryptosporidium* species have become the leading cause of recreational water–associated illness outbreaks, responsible for 36 (68%) of 53 outbreaks linked to treated aquatic venues (eg, swimming pools) in which an infectious cause was identified.[2]

In addition to waterborne transmission, people can acquire infections from livestock and from animals found in petting zoos, particularly preweaned bovine calves and lambs, or from pets. Foodborne transmission can occur. *Cryptosporidium* organisms have been detected in raw produce and in raw or unpasteurized milk.[3] Person-to-person transmission occurs as well and can cause outbreaks in child care centers, in which up to 70% of attendees reportedly have been infected. *Cryptosporidium* species can cause travelers' diarrhea **(www.cdc.gov/parasites/crypto/audience-travelers.html).**

The **incubation period** usually is 2 to 10 days. Recurrence of symptoms has been reported frequently. In immunocompetent people, oocyst shedding usually ceases within 2 weeks after complete symptom resolution. In immunocompromised people, the period of oocyst shedding can continue for months.

DIAGNOSTIC TESTS: Routine laboratory examination of stool for ova and parasites might not include testing for *Cryptosporidium* species, so testing for the organism should be requested specifically. The direct fluorescent antibody (DFA) method for microscopic detection of oocysts in stool, as well as multiwell plate enzyme immunoassays (EIAs) targeting cryptosporidial antigens, are widely available and are recommended for diagnosis of cryptosporidiosis. Some of these assays target both *Cryptosporidium* species and *Giardia lamblia* in a single test format. Rapid lateral flow immunochromatographic tests (point-of-care rapid tests) for detecting antigen in stool are available. The detection of oocysts on microscopic examination of stool specimens may be accomplished by direct wet mount if concentration of the oocysts is high. Alternatively, the formalin ethyl acetate stool concentration method can be used followed by staining of the stool specimen with a modified Kinyoun acid-fast stain. Oocysts generally are small (4–6 μm in diameter) and can be missed in a rapid scan of a slide.

Because shedding can be intermittent, at least 3 stool specimens collected on separate days should be examined before considering test results to be negative. Organisms also

[1]Centers for Disease Control and Prevention. Cryptosporidiosis surveillance—United States, 2011–2012. *MMWR Morb Mortal Wkly Rep.* 2015;64(SS-3):1–13

[2]Centers for Disease Control and Prevention. Recreational water–associated disease outbreaks—United States, 2011–2012. *MMWR Morb Mortal Wkly Rep.* 2015;64(24):668–72

[3]American Academy of Pediatrics, Committee on Infectious Diseases, Committee on Nutrition. Consumption of raw or unpasteurized milk and milk products by pregnant women and children. *Pediatrics.* 2014;133(1):175–179 (Reaffirmed October 2017)

can be identified in intestinal biopsy tissue or sampling of intestinal fluid. Molecular methods are being used increasingly for detection of cryptosporidiosis, particularly nucleic acid amplification tests (NAATs) that target multiple gastrointestinal tract pathogens in a single assay and have received clearance from the US Food and Drug Administration (FDA).

TREATMENT: Generally, immunocompetent people may not need specific therapy. A 3-day course of nitazoxanide oral suspension has been approved by the US Food and Drug Administration (FDA) for treatment of diarrhea associated with cryptosporidiosis in patients 1 year or older. The nitazoxanide dose for healthy children not infected with HIV is age based, as follows: 1 through 3 years of age, 100 mg, orally, twice daily; 4 through 11 years of age, 200 mg, orally, twice daily; 12 years or older, 500 mg, orally, twice daily.

Courses of nitazoxanide (generally >14 days) have been recommended in children who are solid organ transplant recipients for the treatment of diarrhea caused by *Cryptosporidium*, although efficacy is questionable. Disease in children with immune dysfunction, especially solid organ transplant recipients or those with HIV infection, can be refractory to therapy.

In HIV-infected patients, improvement in CD4+ T-lymphocyte count associated with antiretroviral therapy can lead to symptom resolution and cessation of oocyst shedding. For this reason, administration of combination antiretroviral therapy (cART) is the primary treatment for cryptosporidiosis in patients with HIV infection. In vitro and observational studies suggest cART containing a protease inhibitor could be preferable because of a potential direct effect of the protease inhibitor on the parasite. Given the seriousness of this infection in immunocompromised people, use of nitazoxanide can be considered in immunocompromised HIV-infected children in conjunction with cART for immune restoration. The recommended nitazoxanide dosing duration is 3 to 14 days for HIV-infected children.[1]

ISOLATION OF THE HOSPITALIZED PATIENT: In addition to standard precautions, contact precautions are recommended for diapered or incontinent people for the duration of illness or to control institutional outbreaks. Hydrogen peroxide is preferred over bleach for environmental cleaning.

CONTROL MEASURES: In immunocompetent people, oocyst shedding usually ceases within 2 weeks after complete symptom resolution (also see Children in Out-of-Home Child Care, p 122). The following recommendations can help prevent and control cryptosporidiosis:

- Wash hands with soap and water for at least 20 seconds, rubbing hand over hand vigorously and scrubbing all surfaces:
  - Before preparing or eating food;
  - After using the toilet or assisting someone with using the toilet;
  - After changing a diaper or having a diaper changed;
  - After caring for someone with diarrhea; and
  - After handling an animal or its waste.

---

[1]Panel on Opportunistic Infections in HIV-Exposed and HIV-Infected Children. Guidelines for the Prevention and Treatment of Opportunistic Infections in HIV-Exposed and HIV-Infected Children. Department of Health and Human Services. Available at: **https://aidsinfo.nih.gov/contentfiles/lvguidelines/oi_guidelines_pediatrics.pdf**

- Do not participate in recreational water activities, such as swimming, while having diarrhea and for 2 weeks after symptoms have completely resolved because of prolonged excretion of infectious *Cryptosporidium* oocysts after cessation of symptoms, the potential for intermittent exacerbations of diarrhea, and the increased transmission potential in treated aquatic venues (eg, swimming pools) because of the organism's high chlorine tolerance.
- Avoid ingestion of recreational water. For additional information on healthy swimming habits, visit **www.cdc.gov/healthywater/swimming/swimmers/ swim-healthy.html.**
- Educate families, especially those with immunocompromised children, about risk of with exposure to recreational water.
- Do not consume inadequately treated water or ice. This includes water or ice from lakes, rivers, springs, ponds, streams, or shallow wells.
- When traveling in countries where the drinking water supply might be unsafe, do not consume inadequately treated water or ice.
  - ◆ If the safety of drinking water is questionable:
    - – Drink bottled water from an unopened, factory-sealed container.
    - – Disinfect water by heating it to a rolling boil for 1 minute and leave to cool. At elevations above 6500 feet (1981 meters), boil for 3 minutes.
    - – Use a filter that has been tested and rated by NSF Standard 53 or 58 for cyst and oocyst reduction/removal or has an absolute pore size of 1 μm or smaller; filtered water will need additional treatment to kill or inactivate bacteria and viruses.
    - – Use bottled, boiled, or filtered water (as described previously) to wash fruits and vegetables that will be eaten raw.

Cutaneous Larva Migrans

CLINICAL MANIFESTATIONS: Nematode larvae produce pruritic, reddish papules at the site of skin entry. As the larvae migrate through skin, advancing several millimeters to a few centimeters a day, intensely pruritic serpiginous tracks are formed, a condition referred to as creeping eruption. Bullae may develop later as a complication of the larval migration. This condition most often is caused by larvae of the dog and cat hookworm *Ancylostoma braziliense* but can be caused by other nematodes, including *Strongyloides* and human hookworm species. Larval activity can continue for several weeks or months, but the infection is self-limiting. The incubation period for cutaneous larva migrans typically is short, with signs and symptoms developing several days after larval penetration of the skin. However, in some cases, onset of disease may be delayed for weeks to months. Cutaneous larva migrans is a clinical diagnosis based on advancing serpiginous tracks in the skin with associated intense pruritus. Rarely, in infections with certain species of parasites, larvae may penetrate deeper tissues and cause pneumonitis (Löffler syndrome), which can be severe. Occasionally, the larvae of *Ancylostoma caninum* can reach the intestine and may cause eosinophilic enteritis.

ETIOLOGY: Infective larvae of cat and dog hookworms (ie, *Ancylostoma braziliense* and *Ancylostoma caninum*) are the usual causes. Other skin-penetrating nematodes are occasional causes.

EPIDEMIOLOGY: Cutaneous larva migrans is a disease of children, utility workers, gardeners, sunbathers, and others who come in contact with soil contaminated with cat and dog feces. In the United States, locally acquired cases are mostly in the Southeast, but the majority of identified cases are among travelers, not locally acquired, particularly those who have walked barefoot on beaches.

DIAGNOSTIC TESTS: The diagnosis is made clinically, and biopsies are not indicated. Biopsy specimens typically demonstrate an eosinophilic inflammatory infiltrate, but the migrating parasite is not visualized. Eosinophilia and increased immunoglobulin (Ig) E serum concentrations occur in some cases. Larvae have been detected in sputum and gastric washings in patients with the rare complication of pneumonitis. Enzyme immunoassay or Western blot analysis using antigens of *A caninum* have been developed in research laboratories, but these assays are not available for routine diagnostic use.

TREATMENT: The disease usually is self-limited, with spontaneous cure after several weeks or months. Orally administered ivermectin or albendazole is the recommended therapy (see Drugs for Parasitic Infections, p 985). Safety of ivermectin in young infants (<15 kg) and pregnant women remains to be established. Animal studies have shown adverse effects on the fetus. Ingestion of ivermectin with a meal increases its bioavailability. Children younger than 2 years or weighing less than 15 kg may be treated with topical preparations.

ISOLATION OF THE HOSPITALIZED PATIENT: Standard precautions are recommended.

CONTROL MEASURES: Skin contact with moist soil contaminated with animal feces should be avoided. In warm climates, beaches should be kept free of dog and cat feces.

Cyclosporiasis

CLINICAL MANIFESTATIONS: Watery diarrhea is the most common symptom of cyclosporiasis and can be profuse and protracted. Anorexia, nausea, vomiting, substantial weight loss, flatulence, abdominal cramping, myalgia, and prolonged fatigue can occur. Low-grade fever occurs in approximately 50% of patients. Biliary tract disease has been reported. Infection usually is self-limited, but untreated people may have remitting, relapsing symptoms for weeks to months. Asymptomatic infection has been documented most commonly in settings where cyclosporiasis is endemic.

ETIOLOGY: *Cyclospora cayetanensis* is a coccidian protozoan; oocysts (rather than cysts) are passed in stools.

EPIDEMIOLOGY: *C cayetanensis* is known to be endemic in many resource-limited countries and has been reported as a cause of travelers' diarrhea. Both foodborne and waterborne outbreaks have been reported. Most of the outbreaks in the United States and Canada have been associated with consumption of imported fresh produce (eg, basil, cilantro, raspberries). Humans are the only known hosts for *C cayetanensis*. Direct person-to-person transmission is unlikely, because excreted oocysts take days to weeks under favorable environmental conditions to sporulate and become infective. Oocysts are resistant to most disinfectants used in food and water processing and can remain viable for prolonged periods in cool, moist environments.

The **incubation period** typically is 1 week but can range from 2 days to 2 or more weeks.

DIAGNOSTIC TESTS: Diagnosis is made by identification of oocysts (8–10 μm in diameter) in stool, intestinal fluid/aspirates, or intestinal biopsy specimens. Oocysts may be shed at low levels, even by people with profuse diarrhea. This constraint underscores the utility of repeated stool examinations, sensitive recovery methods (eg, concentration procedures including formalin-ethyl acetate sedimentation or sucrose centrifugal flotation), and detection methods that highlight the organism. Oocysts are autofluorescent and are variably acid fast after modified acid-fast staining of stool specimens. Investigational molecular diagnostic assays (eg, polymerase chain reaction) are available at the Centers for Disease Control and Prevention and some other reference laboratories.

TREATMENT: Trimethoprim-sulfamethoxazole, typically for 7 to 10 days, is the drug of choice (see Drugs for Parasitic Infections, p 985); immunocompromised patients may need longer courses of therapy. No highly effective alternatives have been identified for people who cannot tolerate trimethoprim-sulfamethoxazole (**www.cdc.gov/ parasites/cyclosporiasis/health_professionals/tx.html**).

ISOLATION OF THE HOSPITALIZED PATIENT: In addition to standard precautions, contact precautions are recommended for diapered or incontinent children.

CONTROL MEASURES: Avoiding food or water that may be contaminated with feces is the best known way to prevent cyclosporiasis. Fresh produce always should be washed thoroughly before it is eaten or avoided entirely in high-risk settings. This precaution, however, may not eliminate the risk for transmission. Cyclosporiasis is a nationally notifiable disease and is a reportable disease in many states.

Cystoisosporiasis (formerly Isosporiasis)

CLINICAL MANIFESTATIONS: Watery diarrhea is the most common symptom of cystoisosporiasis and can be profuse and protracted, even in immunocompetent people. Manifestations are similar to those caused by other enteric protozoa (eg, *Cryptosporidium* and *Cyclospora* species) and can include abdominal pain, cramping, anorexia, nausea, vomiting, weight loss, and low-grade fever. The proportion of infected people who are asymptomatic is unknown. Severity of infection ranges from self-limiting in immunocompetent hosts to debilitating and life-threatening in immunocompromised patients, particularly people infected with human immunodeficiency virus (HIV). Infections of the biliary tract and reactive arthritis also have been reported. Peripheral eosinophilia may occur.

ETIOLOGY: *Cystoisospora belli* (formerly *Isospora belli*) is a coccidian protozoan; oocysts (rather than cysts) are passed in stools.

EPIDEMIOLOGY: Infection occurs predominantly in tropical and subtropical regions of the world and can cause traveler's diarrhea. Infection results from ingestion of sporulated oocysts (eg, in contaminated food or water). Humans are the only known host for *C belli* and shed noninfective oocysts in feces. These oocysts must mature (sporulate) outside the host in the environment to become infective. Under favorable conditions, sporulation can be completed in 1 to 2 days and perhaps more quickly in some settings. Oocysts probably are resistant to most disinfectants and can remain viable for prolonged periods in a cool, moist environment.

The **incubation period** averages 1 week but may range from several days to 2 or more weeks.

DIAGNOSTIC TESTS: Identification of oocysts in feces or in duodenal aspirates or finding developmental stages of the parasite in biopsy specimens (eg, of the small intestine) is diagnostic. Oocysts in stool are elongate and ellipsoidal (length, 25 to 30 μm). Oocysts can be shed in low numbers, even by people with profuse diarrhea. This constraint underscores the utility of repeated stool examinations, sensitive recovery methods (eg, concentration methods), and detection methods that highlight the organism (eg, oocysts stain bright red with modified acid-fast techniques and autofluoresce when viewed by ultraviolet fluorescence microscopy). The laboratory should be notified specifically when any coccidian parasite is suspected on clinical grounds so that the latter special microscopic methods are used in addition to traditional ova and parasite examination.

TREATMENT: Trimethoprim-sulfamethoxazole, typically for 7 to 10 days, is the drug of choice (see Drugs for Parasitic Infections, p 985). Immunocompromised patients may need higher doses and a longer duration of therapy. Ciprofloxacin is less effective than trimethoprim-sulfamethoxazole. Pyrimethamine (plus leucovorin, to prevent myelosuppression) is an alternative treatment for people who cannot tolerate (or whose infection does not respond to) trimethoprim-sulfamethoxazole. Nitazoxanide has been reported to be effective, but data are limited. In adolescents and adults coinfected with HIV with CD4+ T-lymphocyte counts of <200 cells/mm^3, maintenance therapy is recommended to prevent recurrent disease. In adults, secondary prophylaxis may be discontinued once the CD4+ T-lymphocyte count is >200 cells/mm^3 for >6 months after initiation of antiretroviral therapy. In children, a reasonable time to discontinue secondary prophylaxis would be after sustained improvement (for >6 months) in CD4+ T-lymphocyte count or CD4+ T-lymphocyte percentage from CDC immunologic category 3 to 1 or 2 in response to antiretroviral therapy (**https://aidsinfo.nih.gov/guidelines/html/5/pediatric-oi-prevention-and-treatment-guidelines/410/isosporiasis--cystoisosporiasis-)**.

ISOLATION OF THE HOSPITALIZED PATIENT: In addition to standard precautions, contact precautions are recommended for diapered and incontinent people.

CONTROL MEASURES: Preventive measures include avoiding fecal exposure (eg, food, water, skin, and fomites contaminated with stool), practicing hand and personal hygiene, and thorough washing of fruits and vegetables before eating.

Cytomegalovirus Infection

CLINICAL MANIFESTATIONS: Manifestations of acquired human cytomegalovirus (CMV) infection vary with the age and immunocompetence of the host. Asymptomatic infections are the most common, particularly in children. An infectious mononucleosis-like syndrome with prolonged fever and mild hepatitis, occurring in the absence of heterophile antibody production ("monospot negative"), may occur in adolescents and adults. End-organ disease, including pneumonia, colitis, retinitis, meningoencephalitis, or transverse myelitis, or a CMV syndrome characterized by fever, thrombocytopenia, leukopenia, and mild hepatitis may occur in immunocompromised hosts, including people receiving treatment for malignant neoplasms, people infected with human immunodeficiency virus (HIV), and people receiving immunosuppressive therapy for solid organ or hematopoietic stem cell transplantation. Less commonly, patients treated with biologic response modifiers (see Biologic Response Modifiers Used to Decrease Inflammation, p 85) can exhibit CMV end-organ disease, such as retinitis and hepatitis.

　　Congenital CMV infection has a spectrum of clinical manifestations but usually is not evident at birth (asymptomatic congenital CMV infection). Approximately 10% of infants with congenital CMV infection exhibit clinical findings that are evident at birth (symptomatic congenital CMV disease), with manifestations including jaundice attributable to direct hyperbilirubinemia, petechiae attributable to thrombocytopenia, purpura, hepatosplenomegaly, microcephaly, intracerebral (typically periventricular) calcifications, sensorineural hearing loss, and retinitis; developmental delays are common among affected infants in later infancy and early childhood. Death attributable to congenital CMV is estimated to occur in 3% to 10% of infants with symptomatic disease, or 0.3% to 1.0% of all infants with congenital CMV infection.

Congenital CMV infection is the leading nongenetic cause of sensorineural hearing loss (SNHL) in children in the United States. Approximately 20% of all hearing loss at birth and 25% of all hearing loss at 4 years of age is attributable to congenital CMV infection. SNHL is the most common sequela following congenital CMV infection, with SNHL occurring in up to 50% of children with congenital infections that are symptomatic at birth and up to 15% of those with asymptomatic infections. Between 55% and 75% of symptomatic and asymptomatic children, respectively, who ultimately develop congenital CMV-associated SNHL will not have hearing loss detectable within the first month of life, illustrating the increased incidence of late-onset SNHL in these populations. For this reason, targeted CMV testing of infants who fail their universal newborn hearing screen will not detect a majority of infants who are at risk of CMV-associated hearing loss, especially in infants with asymptomatic congenital CMV infection. Up to 65% of children with CMV-associated SNHL continue to have further deterioration (progression) of their hearing loss over time. As such, children with symptomatic or asymptomatic congenital CMV infection should be evaluated at regular intervals for early detection of hearing loss or progression and for implementation of appropriate interventions (eg, hearing aids).

Infection acquired during the intrapartum period from maternal cervical secretions or in the postpartum period from human milk usually is not associated with clinical illness in term infants. In preterm infants, however, postpartum infection resulting from human milk or from transfusion from CMV-seropositive donors has been associated with hepatitis, interstitial pneumonia, hematologic abnormalities including thrombocytopenia and leukopenia, and a viral sepsis syndrome. A correlation between postnatally acquired CMV in extremely low birth weight infants and chronic lung disease of prematurity has been suggested in retrospective studies, but well-designed, large-scale prospective studies addressing this have not yet been performed.

ETIOLOGY: Human CMV, also known as human herpesvirus 5, is a member of the herpesvirus family (*Herpesviridae*), the beta-herpesvirus subfamily (*Betaherpesvirinae*), and the *Cytomegalovirus* genus. The viral genome contains double-stranded DNA, and at 196 000 to 240 000 bp encoding at least 166 proteins, is the largest of the human herpesvirus genomes.

EPIDEMIOLOGY: CMV is highly species-specific, and only human CMV has been shown to infect humans and cause disease. The virus is ubiquitous, and CMV strains exhibit extensive genetic diversity. Transmission occurs horizontally (by direct person-to-person contact with virus-containing secretions), vertically (from mother to infant before, during, or after birth), and via transfusions of blood, platelets, and white blood cells from infected donors. CMV also can be transmitted with organ or hematopoietic stem cell transplantation. Infections have no seasonal predilection. CMV persists after a primary infection, with intermittent virus shedding; symptomatic infection can occur throughout the lifetime of the infected person, particularly under conditions of immunosuppression. Reinfection with other strains of CMV can occur in seropositive hosts, including pregnant women. The seroprevalence of CMV immunoglobulin (Ig) G antibody in a population is determined by many factors, including age, geographic location, race or ethnicity, cultural and socioeconomic status, and child-rearing practices. Studies have shown that in the United States, there appears to be 3 periods in life when there is an increased incidence of CMV acquisition: early childhood, adolescence, and the child-bearing years.

Horizontal transmission probably is the result of exposure to saliva, urine, and genital secretions from infected individuals. Spread of CMV in households and child care centers is well documented. Excretion rates from urine or saliva in children 1 to 3 years of age who attend child care centers usually range from 30% to 40% but can be as high as 70%. In addition, children who attend child care frequently excrete large quantities of virus for prolonged periods. Young children can transmit CMV to their parents, including mothers who may be pregnant, and other caregivers, including child care staff (see Children in Out-of-Home Child Care, p 122). In adolescents and adults, sexual transmission occurs, as evidenced by detection of virus in seminal and cervical fluids. As such, CMV is considered to be a sexually transmitted infection (STI).

CMV-seropositive healthy people have latent CMV in their leukocytes and tissues; hence, blood transfusions and organ transplantation can result in transmission. Severe CMV disease following transfusion or solid organ transplantation is more likely to occur if the recipient is immunosuppressed and CMV seronegative before transplant. In contrast, among nonautologous hematopoietic stem cell transplant recipients, CMV-seropositive recipients who receive transplants from seronegative donors are at greatest risk of disease when exposed to CMV after transplant, perhaps secondary to the failure of transplanted graft to provide immunity to the recipient. Latent CMV may reactivate in immunosuppressed individuals and result in disease if immunosuppression is severe (eg, in patients with acquired immunodeficiency syndrome [AIDS] or solid organ or hematopoietic stem cell transplant recipients).

Vertical transmission of CMV to an infant occurs in one of the following time periods: (1) in utero, by transplacental passage of maternal bloodborne virus; (2) at birth, by passage through an infected maternal genital tract; or (3) postnatally, by ingestion of CMV-positive human milk or by transfusion. Between 0.5% and 1% of all live-born infants are infected in utero and excrete CMV at birth, making this the most common congenital viral infection in the United States. In utero fetal infection can occur in women with no preexisting CMV immunity (maternal primary infection) or in women with preexisting antibody to CMV (maternal nonprimary infection) either by acquisition of a different viral strain during pregnancy or by reactivation of an existing maternal infection. Congenital infection and associated sequelae can occur irrespective of the trimester of pregnancy when the mother is infected, but severe sequelae are associated more commonly with primary maternal infection acquired during the first half of gestation. Damaging fetal infections following nonprimary maternal infection have been reported, and acquisition of a different viral strain during pregnancy in women with preexisting CMV antibody can cause symptomatic congenital infection with sequelae. It is estimated that more than three quarters of infants with congenital CMV infection in the United States are born to women with nonprimary infection, and the contribution of nonprimary maternal infection as a cause of damaging congenital CMV infection is believed to be common in populations with higher maternal CMV seroprevalence than the United States. Thus, the definition of protective immunity in congenital CMV infection remains unclear and is an active area of research.

Although disease can occur in previously uninfected infants receiving human milk containing CMV from CMV-infected mothers, most infants who acquire CMV from ingestion of human milk do not develop clinical illness or sequelae, most likely because of the presence of passively transferred maternal antibody. Among infants who acquire infection from maternal cervical secretions or human milk, preterm infants born before 32 weeks' gestation and with a birth weight less than 1500 g are at greater risk of developing CMV disease than are full-term infants.

The **incubation period** for horizontally transmitted CMV infections is highly variable. Infection usually manifests 3 to 12 weeks after blood transfusions and between 1 and 4 months after organ transplantation. Experimental models have related the variations in incubation period to the size of the virus inoculum and route of infection.

DIAGNOSTIC TESTS: The diagnosis of CMV disease is confounded by the ubiquity of the virus, the high rate of asymptomatic excretion, the frequency of reactivated infections, the development of serum immunoglobulin (Ig) M CMV-specific antibody in some episodes of reactivation, reinfection with different strains of CMV, and concurrent infection with other pathogens.

CMV can be isolated in conventional cell culture from urine, saliva, peripheral blood leukocytes, human milk, semen, cervical secretions, and other tissues and body fluids. Recovery of virus from a target organ provides strong evidence that the disease is caused by CMV infection. Standard viral cultures must be maintained for more than 28 days before considering such cultures negative. In contrast, rapid shell vial culture coupled with staining of cells using immunofluorescence antibody techniques for immediate early antigen provides results within 24 to 72 hours.

Viral DNA can be detected by polymerase chain reaction (PCR) and other nucleic acid amplification assay methods in tissues and some fluids, including cerebrospinal fluid (CSF), amniotic fluid, aqueous and vitreous humor fluids, urine, saliva and other respiratory secretions, and peripheral blood. Detection of CMV DNA by PCR in blood does not necessarily indicate acute infection or disease, especially in immunocompetent people. Detection of pp65 antigen (CMV antigenemia assay) in white blood cells or quantification of viral DNA by quantitative PCR assay in whole blood, white blood cells, plasma, or serum (whole blood or plasma is preferred) often is used to detect infection in immunocompromised hosts and for monitoring of CMV disease progression, because these tests can be correlated with active infection in that population. The antigenemia assay is labor intensive and requires timely processing of specimens to obtain accurate results. Thus, PCR is preferred by many laboratories. Several antigenemia assays have been cleared by the US Food and Drug Administration (FDA), and at least 2 quantitative PCR assays for detection of CMV have been cleared by the FDA. Nucleic acid amplification techniques are calibrated to a standard calibrator, such as the World Health Organization International Standard for Human CMV, and the specimen tested and the method used should be clearly described. The same specimen type should always be used when testing any given patient over time.

Various serologic assays, including immunofluorescence assays, latex agglutination assays, and enzyme immunoassays, are available for detecting both IgG and IgM CMV-specific antibodies. Single serum specimens for IgG antibody testing are useful in screening for past infection in individuals at risk for CMV reactivation or for screening potential organ transplant donors and recipients. For diagnosis of suspected recent infection, testing for CMV IgG in paired sera obtained at least 2 weeks apart and testing for IgM in a single serum specimen may be useful. Determination in pregnant women of low-avidity CMV IgG in the presence of CMV IgM can suggest more recent infection.

Amniocentesis has been used in several small series of patients to establish the diagnosis of intrauterine infection. Following delivery, proof of congenital infection requires detection of CMV in urine, saliva, respiratory tract secretions, blood, or CSF obtained within 3 weeks of birth. The analytical sensitivity of CMV DNA detection by PCR assay of dried blood spots is low, limiting use of this type of specimen for widespread screening for congenital CMV infection. A positive PCR assay result from a neonatal dried blood spot confirms congenital infection, but a negative result does not rule out congenital infection. In contrast, PCR assay of liquid and dried saliva specimens from infants has been shown to be >97% sensitive and specific for the identification of infants with congenital CMV infection on newborn screening. Differentiation between intrauterine and perinatal infection is difficult at later than 2 to 4 weeks of age unless clinical manifestations of the former, such as chorioretinitis or intracranial calcifications, are present. A strongly positive CMV-specific IgM during early infancy can be suggestive of congenital CMV infection; however, IgM serologic methods commonly have reduced specificity and may yield false-positive results, making serologic diagnosis of congenital CMV infection problematic.

TREATMENT: Intravenous ganciclovir (see Non-HIV Antiviral Drugs, p 966) is approved for induction and maintenance treatment of retinitis caused by acquired or recurrent CMV infection in immunocompromised adult patients, including HIV-infected patients, and for prophylaxis and treatment of CMV disease in adult transplant recipients. Valganciclovir, the oral prodrug of ganciclovir, also is approved for treatment (induction and maintenance) of CMV retinitis in immunocompromised adult patients, including HIV-infected patients, and for prevention of CMV disease in kidney, kidney-pancreas, or heart transplant recipients at high risk of CMV disease. Valganciclovir also is approved for prevention of CMV disease in pediatric kidney transplant patients 4 months and older and for pediatric heart transplant patients 1 month and older. Ganciclovir and valganciclovir are used to treat CMV infections of other sites (esophagus, colon, lungs) and for preemptive treatment of immunosuppressed adults with CMV antigenemia or viremia. Oral ganciclovir no longer is available in the United States, but oral valganciclovir is available in both tablet and powder for oral solution formulations.

Neonates with symptomatic congenital CMV disease with or without central nervous system (CNS) involvement have improved audiologic and neurodevelopmental outcomes at 2 years of age when treated with oral valganciclovir (16 mg/kg/dose, administered orally twice daily) for 6 months. The dose should be adjusted each month to account for weight gain. Therapy can be accomplished using oral valganciclovir for the entire treatment course, because drug exposure following appropriate dosing of valganciclovir is the same as that achieved with intravenous ganciclovir. If an infant is unable to absorb medications reliably from the gastrointestinal tract (eg, because of necrotizing enterocolitis or other bowel disorders), intravenous ganciclovir at 6 mg/kg/dose can be used initially. Significant neutropenia occurs in one fifth of infants treated with oral valganciclovir and in two thirds of infants treated with parenteral ganciclovir. Absolute neutrophil counts should be performed weekly for 6 weeks, then at 8 weeks, then monthly for the duration of antiviral treatment; serum alanine transaminase concentration should be measured monthly during treatment. Antiviral therapy should be limited to patients with moderate to severe symptomatic congenital CMV disease who are able to start treatment within the first month of life. Infants with asymptomatic congenital CMV infection should not receive antiviral treatment. Neonates with mild symptomatic disease or with isolated SNHL and no other disease manifestations should not routinely receive antiviral treatment because of a lack of data suggesting benefit in this less severely affected population. International consensus recommendations for congenital CMV diagnosis and management have been published.[1]

Preterm infants with perinatally acquired CMV infection can have symptomatic, end-organ disease (eg, pneumonitis, hepatitis, thrombocytopenia). Antiviral treatment has not been studied in this population. If such patients are treated with parenteral ganciclovir, a reasonable approach is to treat for 2 weeks and then reassess responsiveness to therapy. If clinical data suggest benefit of treatment, an additional 1 to 2 weeks of parenteral ganciclovir can be considered if symptoms and signs have not resolved. Valganciclovir generally is not a reasonable alternative in this setting, given the degree of illness these infants are experiencing and the corresponding effect that this potentially could have on gastrointestinal tract absorption of valganciclovir and first-pass hepatic metabolism to ganciclovir.

In hematopoietic stem cell transplant recipients, the combination of Immune Globulin Intravenous (IGIV) or CMV Immune Globulin Intravenous (CMV-IGIV) and ganciclovir, administered intravenously, has been reported to be synergistic in treatment of CMV pneumonia. Unlike CMV-IGIV, IGIV products have varying anti-CMV antibody concentrations from lot to lot, are not tested routinely for their quantities of anti-CMV antibodies, and do not have a specified titer of antibodies to CMV that have correlated with efficacy. Valganciclovir and foscarnet have been approved for treatment and maintenance of CMV retinitis in adults with acquired immunodeficiency syndrome (see Non-HIV Antiviral Drugs, p 966). Foscarnet is more toxic (with high rates of limiting nephrotoxicity) but may be advantageous for some patients with HIV infection, including people with disease caused by ganciclovir-resistant virus or people who are unable to tolerate ganciclovir. Cidofovir is efficacious for CMV retinitis in adults with AIDS, but cidofovir has not been studied in children and is associated with significant nephrotoxicity.

CMV establishes lifelong persistent infection, and as such, it is not eliminated from the body with antiviral treatment of CMV disease. Until immune reconstitution is achieved with antiretroviral therapy, chronic suppressive therapy should be administered to HIV-infected patients with a history of CMV end-organ disease (eg, retinitis, colitis, pneumonitis) to prevent recurrence. Recognizing limitations of the pediatric data but drawing on the growing experience in adult patients, discontinuing prophylaxis may be considered for pediatric patients 6 years and older with CD4+ T-lymphocyte counts of >100 cells/mm^3 for >6 consecutive months and for children younger than 6 years with CD4+ T-lymphocyte percentages of >15% for >6 consecutive months. For immunocompromised children with CMV retinitis, such decisions should be made in close consultation with an ophthalmologist and should take into account such factors as magnitude and duration of CD4+ T-lymphocyte increase, anatomic location of the retinal lesion, vision

[1]Rawlinson W, Boppana S, Fowler KB, et al. Congenital cytomegalovirus infection in pregnancy and the neonate: consensus recommendations for prevention, diagnosis, and therapy. *Lancet Infect Dis.* 2017;17(6):e177–e188

in the contralateral eye, and the feasibility of regular ophthalmologic monitoring. All patients who have had anti-CMV maintenance therapy discontinued should continue to undergo regular ophthalmologic monitoring at a minimum of 3- to 6-month intervals for early detection of CMV relapse as well as immune reconstitution uveitis.[1]

ISOLATION OF THE HOSPITALIZED PATIENT: Standard precautions are recommended.

CONTROL MEASURES:

Care of Exposed People. When caring for children, hand hygiene, particularly after changing diapers, is advised to decrease transmission of CMV. Because asymptomatic excretion of CMV is common in people of all ages, a child with congenital CMV infection should not be treated differently from other children.

Although unrecognized exposure to people who are shedding CMV likely is common, concern may arise when immunocompromised patients or nonimmune pregnant women, including health care professionals, are exposed to patients with clinically recognizable CMV infection. Standard precautions should be sufficient to interrupt transmission of CMV (see Infection Control and Prevention for Hospitalized Children, p 146).

Child Care. Female child care workers in child care centers should be aware of CMV and its potential risks and should have access to appropriate hand hygiene measures to minimize occupationally acquired infection (**www.cdc.gov/cmv/index.html**).

Immunoprophylaxis. CMV-IGIV has been developed for prophylaxis of CMV disease in seronegative kidney, lung, liver, pancreas, and heart transplant recipients. CMV-IGIV seems to be moderately effective in kidney and liver transplant recipients and has been used in combination with antiviral agents. Results of an initial study of its use in pregnant women to prevent CMV transmission to the fetus were compromised by methodologic weaknesses in the conduct of the trial, and a well-designed but relatively small second study failed to demonstrate significant benefit on decreasing the risk of congenital CMV infection or disease. Therefore, use of CMV-IGIV in pregnant women to prevent CMV transmission is not recommended at this time. The role of CMV-IGIV in the prevention of intrauterine transmission of CMV in pregnant women with primary CMV infection currently is being evaluated in a large prospective randomized clinical trial conducted by the National Institute of Child Health and Human Development Maternal and Fetal Medicine Network. Evaluation of investigational vaccines in healthy volunteers and renal transplant recipients is in progress, but to date only inconsistent evidence of efficacy has been reported.

Prevention of Transmission by Blood Transfusion. Transmission of CMV by blood transfusion to newborn infants or other immune-compromised hosts virtually has been eliminated by use of CMV antibody-negative donors, by freezing red blood cells in glycerol before administration, by removal of the buffy coat, or by filtration to remove white blood cells.

Prevention of Transmission by Human Milk. Pasteurization or freezing of donated human milk can decrease the likelihood of CMV transmission. Holder pasteurization (62.5°C [144.5°F] for 30 minutes) and short-term pasteurization (72°C [161.6°F] for 5 seconds) of

[1]Siberry GK, Abzug MJ, Nachman S, et al; Panel on Opportunistic Infections in HIV-Exposed and HIV-Infected Children. Guidelines for the prevention and treatment of opportunistic infections in HIV-exposed and HIV-infected children: recommendations from the National Institutes of Health, Centers for Disease Control and Prevention, the HIV Medicine Association of the Infectious Diseases Society of America, the Pediatric Infectious Diseases Society, and the American Academy of Pediatrics. *Pediatr Infect Dis J.* 2013;32(Suppl 2). Available at: **https://aidsinfo.nih.gov/contentfiles/lvguidelines/oi_guidelines_pediatrics.pdf**

human milk appear to inactivate CMV; short-term pasteurization may be less harmful to the beneficial constituents of human milk. Freezing human milk at −20°C (−4°F) will decrease viral titers but does not eliminate CMV transmission. If fresh donated human milk is needed for infants born to CMV antibody-negative mothers, providing these infants with milk from only CMV antibody-negative women should be considered. For infants already infected with CMV, either congenitally or postnatally, the benefits of human milk from their mothers likely outweigh any risk of additional CMV exposure. For further information on human milk banks, see Human Milk (p 113).

Prevention of Transmission in Transplant Recipients. CMV-seronegative recipients of tissue from CMV-seropositive donors are at high risk of CMV disease. If such circumstances cannot be avoided, prophylactic administration of antiviral therapy or monitoring for viremia and administering preemptive antiviral therapy have been shown to be clearly beneficial in decreasing the incidence of CMV disease in these patients.

Dengue

CLINICAL MANIFESTATIONS: Dengue infection may be asymptomatic or, if symptomatic, may have a wide range of clinical presentations. Approximately 5% of patients develop severe dengue (ie, dengue hemorrhagic fever or dengue shock syndrome), a life-threatening disease, which is more common with second or other subsequent infections. Less common clinical syndromes include myocarditis, pancreatitis, hepatitis, and neuroinvasive disease.

Dengue begins abruptly with a nonspecific, acute febrile illness lasting 2 to 7 days (**febrile phase**), often accompanied by muscle, joint, and/or bone pain, headache, retro-orbital pain, facial erythema, injected oropharynx, macular or maculopapular rash, leukopenia, and petechiae or other minor bleeding manifestations. During fever defervescence, usually on days 3 through 7 of illness, an increase in vascular permeability in parallel with increasing hematocrit (hemoconcentration) may occur. The period of clinically significant plasma leakage usually lasts 24 to 48 hours (**critical phase**), followed by a **convalescent phase** with gradual improvement and stabilization of the hemodynamic status. Warning signs of progression to severe dengue occur in the late febrile phase and include persistent vomiting, severe abdominal pain, mucosal bleeding, difficulty breathing, early signs of shock, and a rapid decline in platelet count with an increase in hematocrit. Patients with nonsevere disease begin to improve during the critical phase, but people with clinically significant plasma leakage attributable to increased vascular permeability develop severe disease that may include pleural effusions, ascites, hypovolemic shock, and hemorrhage.

ETIOLOGY: Four related RNA viruses of the genus *Flavivirus* (see Arboviruses, p 220), dengue viruses 1, 2, 3, and 4, cause symptomatic (approximately 25%) and asymptomatic (approximately 75%) infections. Infection with one dengue virus type produces lifelong immunity against that type and a period of cross-protection (often lasting 1 to 3 years) against infection with the other 3 types. After this period of cross-protection, infection with a different strain may predispose to more severe disease. A person has a lifetime risk of up to 4 dengue virus infections.

EPIDEMIOLOGY: Dengue virus primarily is transmitted to humans through the bite of infected *Aedes aegypti* (and less commonly, *Aedes albopictus* or *Aedes polynesiensis*) mosquitoes. Humans are the main amplifying host of dengue virus and the main source of virus for

Aedes mosquitoes. A sylvatic nonhuman primate dengue virus transmission cycle exists in parts of Africa and Southeast Asia but rarely crosses to humans. Because of the approximately 7 days of viremia, dengue virus can be transmitted following receipt of blood products, donor organs, or tissue; through percutaneous exposure to blood; by exposure in utero or at parturition; and via breastfeeding.

Dengue is a major public health problem in the tropics and subtropics; an estimated 50 to 100 million dengue cases occur annually in more than 100 countries, and 40% of the world's population lives in areas with dengue virus transmission. In the United States, dengue is endemic in Puerto Rico and the Virgin Islands. Periodic outbreaks occur in American Samoa. In addition, millions of US travelers, including children, are at risk, because dengue is the leading cause of febrile illness among travelers returning from the Caribbean, Latin America, and South Asia. Outbreaks with local dengue virus transmission have occurred in Texas, Hawaii, and Florida in the last decade (see Table 3.2, p 222). However, although 16 states have *A aegypti* and 35 states have *A albopictus* mosquitoes, local dengue virus transmission is uncommon because of infrequent contact between people and infected mosquitoes. Dengue occurs in both children and adults. It is most likely to cause severe disease in infants, pregnant women, and patients with chronic diseases (eg, asthma, sickle cell anemia, and diabetes mellitus).

The **incubation period** for dengue virus replication in mosquitoes is 8 to 12 days (extrinsic incubation); mosquitoes remain infectious for the remainder of their life cycle. In humans, the **incubation period** is 3 to 14 days before symptom onset (intrinsic incubation). Infected people, both symptomatic and asymptomatic, can transmit dengue virus to mosquitoes 1 to 2 days before symptoms develop and throughout the approximately 7-day viremic period.

DIAGNOSTIC TESTS: Laboratory confirmation of the clinical diagnosis of dengue can be made on a single serum specimen obtained during the febrile phase of the illness by testing for dengue virus either by detection of dengue virus RNA by reverse transcriptase-polymerase chain reaction (RT-PCR) assay or detection of dengue virus nonstructural protein 1 (NS-1) antigen by immunoassay and testing for anti-dengue virus immunoglobulin (Ig) M antibodies by enzyme immunoassay (EIA). Dengue virus is detectable by RT-PCR or NS1 antigen EIAs from the beginning of the febrile phase until day 7 to 10 after illness onset. Anti-dengue virus IgM antibodies are detectable beginning 3 to 5 days after illness onset but can cross-react with IgM antibodies against Zika virus and other closely related flaviviruses. Other tests, such as IgG anti-dengue virus EIA and hemagglutination inhibition assay, are not as specific for making the diagnosis of dengue. Anti-dengue virus IgG antibody remains elevated for life after dengue virus infection and often is falsely positive in people with previous infection with or immunization against other flaviviruses (eg, West Nile, Japanese encephalitis, yellow fever, or Zika viruses). A fourfold or greater increase in anti-dengue virus IgG antibody titers between the acute ($\leq$5 days after onset of symptoms) and convalescent (>15 days after onset of symptoms) samples confirms recent infection. Dengue diagnostic testing is available through commercial reference laboratories and some state public health laboratories; reference testing is available from the Dengue Branch of the Centers for Disease Control and Prevention (**www.cdc. gov/dengue/**).

TREATMENT: No specific antiviral therapy exists for dengue. During the febrile phase, patients should stay well hydrated and avoid use of aspirin (acetylsalicylic acid), salicylate-containing drugs, and other nonsteroidal anti-inflammatory drugs (eg, ibuprofen) to minimize the potential for bleeding. Additional supportive care is required if the patient becomes dehydrated or develops warning signs of severe disease at or around the time of fever defervescence.

Early recognition of shock and intensive supportive therapy can reduce risk of death from approximately 10% to less than 1% in severe dengue. During the critical phase, maintenance of fluid volume and hemodynamic status is crucial to management of severe cases. Patients should be monitored for early signs of shock, occult bleeding, and resolution of plasma leak to avoid prolonged shock, end organ damage, and fluid overload. Patients with refractory shock may require intravenous colloids and/or blood or blood products after an initial trial of intravenous crystalloids. Reabsorption of extravascular fluid occurs during the convalescent phase with stabilization of hemodynamic status and diuresis. It is important to watch for signs of fluid overload, which may manifest as a decrease in the patient's hematocrit as a result of the dilutional effect of reabsorbed fluid.

ISOLATION OF THE HOSPITALIZED PATIENT: Standard precautions are recommended, with attention to the potential for bloodborne transmission. When indicated, attention should be given to control of *Aedes* mosquitoes to prevent secondary transmission of dengue virus from patients to others.

CONTROL MEASURES: A recombinant live attenuated tetravalent dengue vaccine with a 3-dose schedule administered at 0, 6, and 12 months has been approved for use in 11 countries (ie, Brazil, Costa Rica, El Salvador, Guatemala, Indonesia, Mexico, Paraguay, the Philippines, Peru, Singapore, and Thailand). A number of other vaccine candidates are in clinical trials to evaluate immunogenicity, safety, and efficacy, as are innovative approaches to vector control. As noted previously, no chemoprophylaxis or antiviral medication is available to treat patients with dengue. People traveling to areas with endemic dengue (see DengueMap: **www.healthmap.org/dengue/**) are at risk of dengue and should take precautions to protect themselves from mosquito bites. Travelers should select accommodations that are air conditioned and/or have screened windows and doors. *Aedes* mosquitoes bite most often during the daytime, so bed nets are indicated for children sleeping during the day. Travelers should wear clothing that fully covers arms and legs, especially during early morning and late afternoon. Adults, including pregnant women, should use mosquito repellents containing up to 50% N,N-diethyl-meta-toluamide (DEET), and the concentration of DEET should be between 20% and 30% in infants and young children, for whom it should be applied sparingly (see Prevention of Mosquito-borne and Tickborne Infections, p 194).

Dengue, acquired locally in the United States and during travel, became a nationally notifiable disease in 2010. Suspected cases should be reported to local or state health departments.

Diphtheria

CLINICAL MANIFESTATIONS: Respiratory tract diphtheria usually presents as membranous nasopharyngitis or obstructive laryngotracheitis. Membranous pharyngitis with bloody nasal discharge suggests diphtheria. Local infections are associated with low-grade fever and gradual onset of manifestations over 1 to 2 days. Less commonly, diphtheria presents as cutaneous, vaginal, conjunctival, or otic infection. Cutaneous diphtheria is more common in tropical areas and among urban homeless. Extensive neck swelling with cervical lymphadenitis (bull neck) is a sign of severe disease. Life-threatening complications of respiratory diphtheria include upper airway obstruction caused by membrane formation; myocarditis, with heart block; and cranial and peripheral neuropathies. Palatal palsy, noted by nasal speech, frequently occurs in pharyngeal diphtheria. Case fatality rates are 5% to 10%, sometimes exceeding 20% in older adults.

ETIOLOGY: Diphtheria is caused by toxigenic strains of *Corynebacterium diphtheriae*. Toxigenic strains of *Corynebacterium ulcerans* also have emerged as an important cause of diphtheria-like illness. *C diphtheriae* is an irregularly staining, gram-positive, nonspore-forming, nonmotile, pleomorphic bacillus with 4 biotypes (*mitis, intermedius, gravis*, and *belfanti*). All biotypes of *C diphtheriae* may be toxigenic or nontoxigenic. Bacteria remain confined to superficial layers of skin or mucosal surfaces, inducing a local inflammatory reaction. Within several days of respiratory tract infection, a dense pseudomembrane forms, becoming adherent to tissue. Toxigenic strains produce an exotoxin that consists of an enzymatically active A domain and a binding B domain, which promotes the entry of A into the cell. The toxin gene, *tox*, is carried by a family of related corynebacteria phages. The toxin, an ADP-ribosylase toxin, inhibits protein synthesis in all cells, including myocardial, renal, and peripheral nerve cells, resulting in myocarditis, acute tubular necrosis, and delayed peripheral nerve conduction. Nontoxigenic strains of *C diphtheriae* can cause sore throat and, rarely, other invasive infections, including endocarditis and foreign body infections.

EPIDEMIOLOGY: Humans are the sole reservoir of *C diphtheriae*. Infection is spread by respiratory tract droplets and by contact with discharges from skin lesions. The **incubation period** usually is 2 to 5 days (range, 1–10 days). In untreated people, organisms can be present in discharges from the nose and throat and from eye and skin lesions 2 to 6 weeks after infection. Patients treated with an appropriate antimicrobial agent usually are not infectious 48 hours after treatment is initiated. Transmission results from intimate contact with patients or carriers. People traveling to areas with endemic diphtheria or people who come into contact with infected travelers from such areas are at increased risk of being infected with the organism; rarely, fomites or milk products can serve as vehicles of transmission. Severe disease occurs more often in people who are unimmunized or inadequately immunized. Fully immunized people may be asymptomatic carriers or have mild sore throat.

From 1980 through 2015, 56 cases of diphtheria were reported in the United States; only 2 cases were reported since 2004. Cases of cutaneous diphtheria still occur in the United States, but only respiratory tract cases are nationally notifiable. The incidence of respiratory diphtheria is greatest during fall and winter, but summer epidemics may occur in warm climates where skin infections are prevalent. Globally, endemic diphtheria occurs in Africa, Latin American, Asia, the Middle East, and parts of Europe where immunization coverage with diphtheria toxoid-containing vaccines is suboptimal. In 2014, 7321 global cases of diphtheria were reported by the World Health Organization, but it is probable that many more cases went unrecognized.

DIAGNOSTIC TESTS: Laboratory personnel should be notified that *C diphtheriae* is suspected. Specimens for culture should be obtained from the nasopharynx and throat or any mucosal or cutaneous lesion. Obtaining multiple samples from respiratory sites increases yield of culture. Material should be obtained for culture from beneath the membrane (if present) or a portion of the membrane. Specimens collected for culture can be placed in any transport medium (eg, Amies semisolid transport medium) or in a sterile container and transported at 4°C or in silica gel packs. Inoculation on 5% sheep blood agar plus at least 1 selective medium (eg, cystine-tellurite blood agar or modified Tinsdale agar) is required for isolation. All isolates of *C diphtheriae* should be sent through the state health department to the Centers for Disease Control and Prevention (CDC). Nonculture detection methods include matrix-assisted laser desorption/ionization (MALDI-TOF) mass spectroscopy for *C diphtheriae* and *C ulcerans* and polymerase chain reaction-based methods for detection of diphtheria toxin gene in isolates.

TREATMENT:

Antitoxin. Because patients with diphtheria can deteriorate rapidly, a single dose of equine antitoxin should be administered on the basis of clinical diagnosis before culture results are available. Antitoxin, its indications for use, suggested dosage, and instructions for administration are available through the CDC (CDC Emergency Operations Center [770-488-7100] or at **www.cdc.gov/diphtheria/dat.html).** To neutralize toxin as rapidly as possible, intravenous administration of antitoxin is preferred. Before intravenous administration of antitoxin, tests for sensitivity to horse serum should be performed according to instructions provided with the material. Allergic reactions to horse serum varying from anaphylaxis to rash can be expected in 5% to 20% of patients. The dose of antitoxin depends on the site and size of the membrane, duration of illness, and degree of toxic effects; presence of soft, diffuse cervical lymphadenitis suggests moderate to severe toxin absorption. Suggested dose ranges are: pharyngeal or laryngeal disease of 2 days' duration or less, 20 000 to 40 000 U; nasopharyngeal lesions, 40 000 to 60 000 U; extensive disease of 3 or more days' duration or diffuse swelling of the neck, 80 000 to 120 000 U. Antitoxin probably is of no value for cutaneous disease, but some experts recommend administration of 20 000 to 40 000 U if a toxigenic *C diphtheriae* strain is isolated from a cutaneous lesion and/or signs of systemic toxicity are evident.

Antimicrobial Therapy. Erythromycin administered orally or parenterally for 14 days, aqueous penicillin G administered intravenously for 14 days, or penicillin G procaine administered intramuscularly for 14 days constitute acceptable therapy (see Table 4.3, Antibacterial Drugs for Pediatric Patients Beyond the Newborn Period, p 920). Antimicrobial therapy is required to stop toxin production, eradicate *C diphtheriae* organism, and prevent transmission but is not a substitute for antitoxin. Elimination of the organisms should be documented 24 hours after completion of treatment by 2 consecutive negative cultures from specimens taken 24 hours apart.

Immunization. Active immunization against diphtheria should be undertaken during convalescence from diphtheria; disease does not necessarily confer immunity.

Cutaneous Diphtheria. Thorough cleansing of the lesion with soap and water and administration of an appropriate antimicrobial agent for 10 days are recommended.

Carriers. If not immunized, carriers should receive active immunization promptly, and measures should be taken to ensure completion of the immunization schedule. If a carrier has been immunized previously but has not received a booster of diphtheria toxoid within 5 years, a booster dose of age-appropriate vaccine containing diphtheria toxoid (DTaP, Tdap, DT, or Td) should be administered. Carriers should receive oral erythromycin for 10 to 14 days or a single intramuscular dose of penicillin G benzathine (600 000 U for children weighing <30 kg, and 1.2 million U for children weighing ≥30 kg or for adults). Two follow-up cultures should be performed after completing antimicrobial treatment to detect persistence of carriage, which occurs in as many as 20% of patients treated with erythromycin. The first culture should be performed 24 hours after completing treatment.

If results of cultures are positive, an additional 10-day course of oral erythromycin should be administered, and follow-up cultures should be performed again. Erythromycin-resistant strains have been identified, but their epidemiologic significance is undetermined. Fluoroquinolones (see Fluoroquinolones, p 904), rifampin, clarithromycin, and azithromycin have good in vitro activity and may be better tolerated than erythromycin, but these drugs have not been evaluated in clinical infection or in carriers.

ISOLATION OF THE HOSPITALIZED PATIENT: In addition to standard precautions, droplet precautions are recommended for patients and carriers with pharyngeal diphtheria until 2 cultures from both the nose and throat collected 24 hours after completing antimicrobial treatment are negative for *C diphtheriae*. Contact precautions are recommended for patients with cutaneous diphtheria until 2 cultures of skin lesions taken at least 24 hours apart and 24 hours after cessation of antimicrobial therapy are negative.

CONTROL MEASURES:

Care of Exposed People. Whenever respiratory diphtheria is suspected or proven, local public health officials should be notified promptly. Cases of cutaneous diphtheria generally are caused by infections with nontoxigenic strains of *C diphtheriae* and are not included for national notification. However, if a toxigenic *C diphtheriae* strain is isolated from a cutaneous lesion, investigation and prophylaxis of close contacts should be undertaken, as with respiratory diphtheria. If a nontoxigenic *C diphtheriae* strain is isolated from a cutaneous lesion, routine investigation or prophylaxis of contacts is not necessary. Management of exposed people is based on individual circumstances, including immunization status and likelihood of adherence to follow-up and prophylaxis. Close contacts of a person suspected to have diphtheria should be identified, and the following are recommended:

- Contact tracing usually can be limited to household members and people with direct, habitual close contact or health care personnel exposed to nasopharyngeal secretions, people sharing kitchen facilities, or people caring for infected children.
- For close contacts, *regardless of their immunization status,* the following measures should be taken: (1) surveillance for evidence of disease for 7 days from last exposure to an untreated patient; (2) culture for *C diphtheriae;* and (3) antimicrobial prophylaxis with oral erythromycin (40–50 mg/kg per day for 7 to 10 days, maximum 1 g/day) or a single intramuscular injection of penicillin G benzathine (600 000 U for children weighing <30 kg, and 1.2 million U for children weighing ≥30 kg and for adults). Follow-up cultures of pharyngeal specimens should be performed after completion of therapy for contacts proven to be carriers (see Carriers, p 321). If cultures are positive, an additional 10-day course of erythromycin should be administered, and follow-up cultures of pharyngeal specimens again should be performed.
- Asymptomatic, previously immunized close contacts should receive a booster dose of an age-appropriate diphtheria toxoid-containing vaccine (DTaP [or DT], Tdap, or Td) if they have not received a booster dose of a diphtheria toxoid-containing vaccine within 5 years.
- Asymptomatic close contacts who have had fewer than 3 doses of a diphtheria toxoid-containing vaccine, children younger than 7 years in need of their fourth dose of DTaP (or DT), or people whose immunization status is not known should be immunized with an age-appropriate diphtheria toxoid-containing vaccine (DTaP, DT, Tdap or Td, as indicated).
- Contacts who cannot be kept under surveillance should receive penicillin G ben-

zathine rather than erythromycin, and if not fully immunized or if immunization status is not known, they should be immunized with DTaP, Tdap, DT, or Td vaccine, as appropriate for age.

- Use of equine diphtheria antitoxin in unimmunized close contacts is not recommended, because there is no evidence that antitoxin provides additional benefit.

Immunization. Universal immunization with a diphtheria toxoid-containing vaccine is the only effective control measure. The schedules for immunization against diphtheria are presented in the childhood and adolescent (**http://aapredbook.aappublications. org/site/resources/izschedules.xhtml**) and adult (**www.cdc.gov/vaccines**) immunization schedules.

Immunization of children from 2 months of age through 6 years of age (to the seventh birthday) routinely consists of 5 doses of diphtheria and tetanus toxoid-containing and acellular pertussis vaccines (DTaP). Regular booster injections of diphtheria toxoid as Td (or as Tdap once) are required every 10 years after completion of the initial immunization series. Immunization against diphtheria and tetanus for children younger than 7 years in whom pertussis immunization is contraindicated (see Pertussis, p 620) should be accomplished with DT. Other recommendations for diphtheria immunization, including recommendations for older children (7 through 18 years of age) and adults, can be found in Tetanus (p 793) as well as the childhood and adolescent and adult immunization schedules. When children and adults require booster tetanus toxoid for wound management (see Tetanus, p 793), Td (or Tdap, if never received) is used. Tetanus toxoid no longer is available as a single-antigen preparation in the United States.

Travelers to countries with endemic or epidemic diphtheria should have their diphtheria immunization status reviewed and updated when necessary.

Pneumococcal and meningococcal conjugate vaccines containing inactivated diphtheria toxoid or CRM_{197} protein, a nontoxic variant of diphtheria toxin, are not substitutes for diphtheria toxoid immunization.

Precautions and Contraindications. See Pertussis (p 620) and Tetanus (p 793).

Ehrlichia, Anaplasma, and Related Infections
(Human Ehrlichiosis, Anaplasmosis, and Related Infections Attributable to Bacteria in the Family *Anaplasmataceae*)

CLINICAL MANIFESTATIONS: Infections by members of the bacterial family *Anaplasmataceae* (genera *Anaplasma, Ehrlichia, Neorickettsia,* and the proposed genus *Candidatus* Neoehrlichia) cause human illness with similar signs, symptoms, and clinical courses. All are acute febrile illnesses with common systemic manifestations including fever, headache, chills, malaise, myalgia, and nausea. More variable symptoms include arthralgia, vomiting, diarrhea, cough, and confusion. In adults, skin rash is reported more often for *Ehrlichia* infections than for *Anaplasma* infections. Rash is seen in up to 60% of *Ehrlichia chaffeensis* cases in children. Neorickettsiosis is characterized by fever, weakness, anorexia, and lymphadenopathy, which is not common in ehrlichiosis or anaplasmosis. Neoehrlichiosis is characterized by fever, chills, arthralgia, myalgia, and less specific symptoms such as cough, diarrhea, and weight loss. There is a high incidence of vascular events, including thromboembolic complications. Most reported cases of neoehrlichiosis have been in older people with underlying immunosuppressive conditions. Patients may require hospitalization, and more severe manifestations of these diseases can include acute respiratory distress syndrome, encephalopathy, meningitis, disseminated intravascular co-agulation, spontaneous hemorrhage, and renal failure.

Significant laboratory findings in *Anaplasma* and *Ehrlichia* infections may include leukopenia with neutropenia (anaplasmosis) or lymphopenia (ehrlichiosis), thrombocytopenia, hyponatremia, and elevated serum hepatic transaminase concentrations. Cerebrospinal fluid abnormalities (eg, pleocytosis with a predominance of lymphocytes and increased total protein concentration) are common. In neoehrlichiosis, leukocytosis and elevated C-reactive protein concentrations can occur, but serum hepatic transaminase concentrations usually are within normal ranges.

Without treatment, symptoms typically last 1 to 2 weeks, but empiric and prompt treatment with doxycycline shortens duration and reduces the risk of serious manifestations and sequelae. Following infection, fatigue can last several weeks; neurologic sequelae have been reported in some children after severe disease and more commonly with *Ehrlichia* infections. Severe disease and fatal outcome is more common in *E chaffeensis* infections (approximately 1%–3% case fatality) than with *Anaplasma phagocytophilum* infection (less than 1% case fatality). One fatal case has been reported for *Candidatus* Neoehrlichia infection. Secondary or opportunistic infections can occur with severe illness, resulting in a delay in recognition and administration of appropriate antimicrobial treatment. People with underlying immunosuppression are at greater risk of severe disease. Severe disease has been reported in people who initially received trimethoprim-sulfamethoxazole before a correct diagnosis was made.

Ehrlichia and *Anaplasma* species do not cause vasculitis or endothelial cell damage characteristic of some other rickettsial diseases. Because of the nonspecific presenting symptoms, Rocky Mountain spotted fever should be considered in the differential diagnosis of tickborne *Anaplasmataceae* infections in the United States. Infections with *Candidatus* Neoehrlichia mikurensis, which has been detected in ticks from several European, Asian, and African countries, have a high incidence of complicating vascular events.

The recently discovered Heartland virus infection also manifests with clinical features similar to ehrlichiosis; health care professionals should consider Heartland virus testing in patients who develop fever, leukopenia, and thrombocytopenia after a tick bite. Heartland virus should be considered in patients without a more likely explanation and who have tested negative for *Ehrlichia* and *Anaplasma* infection or have not responded to doxycycline therapy.[1]

ETIOLOGY: In the United States, human ehrlichiosis and anaplasmosis are caused by at least 4 different species of obligate intracellular bacteria: *E chaffeensis*, *Ehrlichia ewingii*, *Ehrlichia muris eauclairensis*, and *A phagocytophilum* (Table 3.4). However, most US cases are caused by *E chaffeensis* and *A phagocytophilum*. *Ehrlichia* and *Anaplasma* species are gram-negative cocci that measure 0.5 to 1.5 μm in diameter with tropisms for different white blood cell types (monocytes and granulocytes, respectively). Human *Ehrlichia canis* and *Anaplasma platys* and *Ehrlichia ruminantium* have been reported in only a few cases within or outside the United States. *Anaplasma ovis* (in Iran and Crete) and *Anaplasm capra* (in China) have been found as emerging causes of human infections. *Ehrlichia muris* is suspected to cause disease in Russia and Japan. *Neorickettsia sennetsu* causes illness in Asia, and *Candidatus* Neoehrlichia mikurensis is an increasing cause of human illness in European and Asian countries.

---

[1]Centers for Disease Control and Prevention. Notes from the field: Heartland virus disease—United States, 2012–2013. *MMWR Morb Mortal Wkly Rep.* 2014;63(12):270–271

Table 3.4. Human Ehrlichiosis, Anaplasmosis, and Related Infections

Disease	Causal Agent	Major Target Cell	Tick Vector	Geographic Distribution
Ehrlichiosis caused by *Ehrlichia chaffeensis* (also known as human monocytic ehrlichiosis)	*E chaffeensis*	Usually monocytes	Lone star tick (US) *(Amblyomma americanum)*	US: Predominantly southeast, south central, and east coast states; has been reported outside US
Anaplasmosis (also known as human granulocytic anaplasmosis)	*Anaplasma phagocytophilum*	Usually granulocytes	Blacklegged tick *(Ixodes scapularis)* or Western blacklegged tick *(Ixodes pacificus)* (US)	US: Northeastern and upper Midwestern states and northern California; Europe and Asia
Ehrlichiosis caused by *Ehrlichia ewingii*	*E ewingii*	Usually granulocytes	Lone star tick (US) *(A americanum)*	US: Southeastern, south central, and Midwestern states; Africa, Asia
Ehrlichiosis caused by *Ehrlichia muris eauclairensis*	*E muris eauclairensis*	Unknown, suspected in monocytes	*I scapularis* is identified as a likely vector	US: Minnesota, Wisconsin
Ehrlichiosis caused by *Ehrlichia muris*	*Ehrlichia muris sensu stricto*	Unknown, suspected in monocytes	*Ixodes persulcatus, Ixodes ovatus*	Asia
Ehrlichiosis caused by *Ehrlichia canis*	*E canis*	Monocytes	*Rhipicephalus sanguineus* (suspected)	Venezuela
Thrombocytic anaplasmosis	*Anaplasma platys*	Platelets	*Rhipicephalus sanguineus* (suspected)	Venezuela
Neorickettsiosis, sennetsu fever, glandular fever	*Neorickettsia sennetsu*	Monocytes	Ingestion of infected trematodes residing in fish	Japan, Malaysia, Laos
Neoehrlichiosis	*Candidatus* Neoehrlichia mikurensis	Unknown, demonstrated in endothelium of experimentally infected animals	*Ixodes ricinus, Ixodes persulcatus, Haemaphysalis flava*	Europe and Asia, possibly Africa

EPIDEMIOLOGY: In the United States, the reported incidences of *E chaffeensis* and *A phagocytophilum* infections during 2008–2012 were 3.2 and 6.3 cases per million population, respectively. Reported incidence of *E ewingii* infections during this time period were 0.04 cases per million population, but the incidence is thought to be underreported because of nonspecific illness similar to *E chaffeensis* infections.

These diseases are underrecognized, and selected active surveillance programs have shown the incidence to be substantially higher in some areas where infection is endemic.

Most cases of *E chaffeensis* and *E ewingii* infection are reported from the south central and southeastern United States as well as East Coast states. Ehrlichiosis caused by *E chaffeensis* and *E ewingii* are associated with the bite of the lone star tick *(Amblyomma americanum)* and are reported from states within its geographic range. To date, cases attributable to *E muris eauclairensis* have been reported only from Minnesota and Wisconsin and are thought to be transmitted by the blacklegged tick (*Ixodes scapularis*). Most cases of human anaplasmosis have been reported from the upper Midwest and northeast United States (eg, Wisconsin, Minnesota, Connecticut, and New York) and northern California. In most of the United States, *A phagocytophilum* is transmitted by *Ixodes scapularis*, which also is the vector for Lyme disease (*Borrelia burgdorferi*) and babesiosis (*Babesia microti*). In the western United States, the western blacklegged tick *(Ixodes pacificus)* is the main vector for *A phagocytophilum*. Various mammalian wildlife reservoirs for the agents of human ehrlichiosis and anaplasmosis have been identified, including white-tailed deer and wild rodents. In other parts of the world, other bacterial species of this family are transmitted by the endemic tick vectors for that area. An exception is *N sennetsu*, which is transmitted through ingestion of neorickettsia-infected trematodes residing in fish.

Reported cases of symptomatic ehrlichiosis and anaplasmosis are most frequent in people older than 40 years. However, seroprevalence data indicate that exposure to *E chaffeensis* may be common in children. In the United States, most human infections occur between April and September, with the peak occurrence from May through July. Coinfections of anaplasmosis with other tickborne diseases, including babesiosis and Lyme disease, can cause illness that is more severe or of longer duration than a single infection. Possible perinatal transmission of *A phagocytophilum* has been reported. Several cases of *Anaplasmataceae* infections have occurred after blood transfusion or solid organ donation from asymptomatic donors.

The **incubation period** usually is 5 to 14 days for *E chaffeensis* and 5 to 21 days for *A phagocytophilum*.

DIAGNOSTIC TESTS: The diagnosis of ehrlichiosis or anaplasmosis must be made on the basis of clinical signs and symptoms and later can be confirmed using specialized laboratory testing. Polymerase chain reaction (PCR) testing on whole blood for the organism is most sensitive for anaplasmosis, ehrlichiosis, and other *Anaplasmataceae* infections during the first week of illness. Sensitivity of PCR decreases rapidly following the administration of doxycycline. Although a positive PCR result is helpful, a negative result does not rule out the diagnosis. Both broad-based and specific PCR assays are available at many commercial laboratories, reference centers, and state public health laboratories. Sequence confirmation of the amplified product provides specific identification and often is necessary to identify infection with certain species (eg, *E ewingii* and *E muris eauclairensis* in the United States). In the case of fatal infections, PCR testing can be performed on autopsy specimens, including liver, spleen, and lung. In addition, immunohistochemistry can be used to demonstrate *Ehrlichia* or *Anaplasma* antigen in formalin-fixed, paraffin-embedded tissues.

Occasionally, *Anaplasmataceae* bacteria can be identified in Giemsa or Wright-stained peripheral blood smears or buffy coat leukocyte preparations in the first week of illness by detection of classic microcolonies of *Anaplasma* organisms known as **morulae,** but this is an insensitive method for diagnosis. Culture for isolation is not performed. Immunoglobulin (Ig) M serologic assays are prone to false-positive reactions, and IgM and can remain elevated for lengthy periods of time, reducing its diagnostic utility. Serologic testing may be used to demonstrate a fourfold change in IgG-specific antibody titer by indirect immunofluorescence antibody (IFA) assay between paired acute and convalescent specimens taken 2 to 4 weeks apart. Specific antigens are available for serologic testing of *E chaffeensis* and *A phagocytophilum* infections, although cross-reactivity between species can make interpretation difficult in areas where geographic distributions overlap. Because *E ewingii* has not been grown in culture, no antigens are available for diagnostic use; use of peptide-based assays has provided serologic tests for veterinary use. Although *E ewingii* and *E muris eauclairensis* infections are best confirmed by specific molecular PCR detection methods, these organisms share some antigens with *E chaffeensis* and sometimes can be presumptively diagnosed serologically using *E chaffeensis* serologic tests. These serologic tests are available in reference, commercial, and state public health laboratories, and at the Centers for Disease Control and Prevention (CDC).

TREATMENT: Doxycycline is the drug of choice for treatment of human ehrlichiosis and anaplasmosis and should be used regardless of patient age (see Tetracyclines, p 905). Doxycycline also has been shown to be very effective for the other *Anaplasmataceae* infections. The recommended pediatric dosage of doxycycline is 4.4 mg/kg per day, divided every 12 hours, intravenously or orally (maximum 100 mg/dose). Oral dosing is preferred for children who are able tolerate oral medication. For larger children and adults, the dose is 100 mg, every 12 hours. Ehrlichiosis and anaplasmosis can be severe or fatal in untreated patients, especially in immunocompromised patients; initiation of therapy early in the course of disease helps minimize complications of illness and should not be delayed awaiting laboratory confirmation. Most patients begin to respond within 48 hours of initiating doxycycline treatment. Treatment with trimethoprim-sulfamethoxazole has been linked to more severe outcome and is contraindicated. Treatment with doxycycline should continue for at least 3 days after defervescence; the standard course of treatment is 7 to 14 days. Treatments for neorickettsiosis and neoehrlichiosis are less defined, but similar courses have resulted in good outcomes. Rifampin may provide an alternate to doxycycline in patients with hypersensitivity to doxycycline for anaplasmosis and neoehrlichiosis.

Clinical manifestations and geographic distributions of ehrlichiosis, anaplasmosis, and Rocky Mountain spotted fever overlap in the United States. As with other rickettsial diseases, when a presumptive diagnosis of ehrlichiosis or anaplasmosis is made, clinical samples should be taken for analysis, and testing for multiple possible etiologies may be appropriate. Doxycycline should be started immediately and should not be delayed pending laboratory confirmation of infection.

ISOLATION OF THE HOSPITALIZED PATIENT: Standard precautions are recommended. Human-to-human transmission via direct contact has not been documented.

CONTROL MEASURES: Limiting exposures to ticks and tick bites is the primary means of prevention (see Prevention of Mosquitoborne and Tickborne Infections, p 194). The risk of transmission through blood transfusion or organ transplantation should be considered in areas with endemic infection. Because of its unique mode of transmission, neorickettsiosis can be prevented by proper cooking of fish. Obtaining a travel history to areas with other species of *Anaplasmataceae* is important if imported infection is suspected. Prophylactic administration of doxycycline after a tick bite is not indicated because of the low risk of infection and lack of proven efficacy. Cases of ehrlichiosis and anaplasmosis are notifiable diseases in the United States and should be reported to the local or state health department. Additional information is available on the CDC Web sites (**www.cdc.gov/ehrlichiosis**, **www.cdc.gov/anaplasmosis**, and **www.cdc.gov/ticks**), including a collaborative report providing recommendations for the diagnosis and management of tickborne rickettsial diseases.[1]

Serious Bacterial Infections Caused by *Enterobacteriaceae*
(With Emphasis on Septicemia and Meningitis in Neonates)

CLINICAL MANIFESTATIONS: Neonatal septicemia or meningitis caused by *Escherichia coli* and other gram-negative bacilli cannot be differentiated clinically from septicemia or meningitis caused by other organisms. The early signs of sepsis can be subtle and similar to signs observed in noninfectious processes. Signs of septicemia include fever, temperature instability, heart rate abnormalities, grunting respirations, apnea, cyanosis, lethargy, irritability, anorexia, vomiting, jaundice, abdominal distention, cellulitis, and diarrhea. Meningitis, especially early in the course, can occur without overt signs suggesting central nervous system involvement. Some gram-negative bacilli, such as *Citrobacter koseri*, *Cronobacter* (formerly *Enterobacter*) *sakazakii*, *Serratia marcescens*, and *Salmonella* species, are associated with brain abscesses in infants with meningitis caused by these organisms.

ETIOLOGY: *Enterobacteriaceae* are a large family of gram-negative, facultatively anaerobic, rod-shaped bacteria that include *Escherichia* species, *Klebsiella* species, *Enterobacter* species, *Proteus* species, *Providencia* species, and *Serratia* species, among many others. *E coli* strains, often those with the K1 capsular polysaccharide antigen, are the most common cause of septicemia and meningitis in neonates. Other important gram-negative bacilli causing neonatal septicemia include *Klebsiella* species, *Enterobacter* species, *Proteus* species, *Citrobacter* species, *Salmonella* species, *Pseudomonas* species, *Acinetobacter* species, and *Serratia* species. Nonencapsulated strains of *Haemophilus influenzae* and anaerobic gram-negative bacilli are rare causes. *Elizabethkingia meningosepticum* (originally known as *Flavobacterium meningosepticum* after discovery in 1959, then reclassified as *Chryseobacter meningosepticum* before being renamed in 2006) has been associated with outbreaks of neonatal meningitis, with infections in immunocompromised people or with other health care-associated outbreaks related to environmental contamination. *Elizabethkingia anophelis* has been reported as a recent cause of health care-associated infection in adults older than 65 years, with rare cases reported in neonates.

EPIDEMIOLOGY: The source of *E coli* and other gram-negative bacterial pathogens in neonatal infections during the first days of life typically is the maternal genital tract. Reservoirs for gram-negative bacilli can be present within the health care environment. Acquisition of gram-negative organisms can occur through person-to-person transmission from hospital nursery personnel as well as from nursery environmental sites such as sinks, countertops, powdered infant formula, and respiratory therapy equipment, especially among very preterm infants who require prolonged neonatal intensive care management. Predisposing factors in neonatal gram-negative bacterial infections include maternal intrapartum infection, gestation less than 37 weeks, low birth weight, and prolonged rupture of membranes. Metabolic abnormalities (eg, galactosemia), fetal hypoxia, and acidosis have

---

[1]Biggs HM, Behravesh CB, Bradley KK, et al. Diagnosis and management of tickborne rickettsial diseases: Rocky Mountain spotted fever and other spotted fever group rickettsioses, ehrlichioses, and anaplasmosis—United States. *MMWR Recomm Rep.* 2016;65(RR-2):1–44. Available at: **www.cdc.gov/mmwr/volumes/65/rr/rr6502a1.htm**

been implicated as predisposing factors. Neonates with defects in the integrity of skin or mucosa (eg, myelomeningocele) or abnormalities of gastrointestinal or genitourinary tracts are at increased risk of gram-negative bacterial infections. In neonatal intensive care units, systems for respiratory and metabolic support, invasive or surgical procedures, indwelling vascular catheters, and frequent use of broad-spectrum antimicrobial agents enable selection and proliferation of strains of gram-negative bacilli that are resistant to multiple antimicrobial agents.

Multiple mechanisms of resistance in gram-negative bacilli can be present simultaneously. Resistance resulting from production of chromosomally encoded or plasmid-derived **AmpC beta-lactamases** or from plasmid-mediated **extended-spectrum beta-lactamases (ESBLs)** occurs primarily in *E coli*, *Klebsiella* species, and *Enterobacter* species but has been reported in many other gram-negative species. Resistant gram-negative infections have been associated with nursery outbreaks, especially in very low birth weight infants. Additional risk factors associated with neonatal ESBL infection include prolonged mechanical ventilation, extended hospital stay, use of invasive devices, and use of antimicrobial agents. Infants born to mothers colonized with ESBL-producing *E coli* are themselves at an increased risk of acquiring colonization with ESBL-producing *E coli* compared with infants born to mothers without colonization. Organisms that produce ESBLs typically are resistant to penicillins, cephalosporins, and monobactams and can be resistant to aminoglycosides. **Carbapenemase-producing *Enterobacteriaceae* (CPE)** also have emerged, especially *Klebsiella pneumoniae*, *Pseudomonas aeruginosa*, and *Acinetobacter* species. ESBL- and carbapenemase-producing bacteria often carry additional plasmidborne genes that encode for high-level resistance to aminoglycosides, fluoroquinolones, and trimethoprim-sulfamethoxazole.

The **incubation period** is variable; time of onset of infection ranges from birth to several weeks after birth or longer in very low birth weight, preterm infants with prolonged hospitalizations.

DIAGNOSTIC TESTS: Diagnosis is established by growth of *E coli* or other gram-negative bacilli from blood, cerebrospinal fluid (CSF), or other usually sterile sites. Isolates may be identified by traditional biochemical tests, by a variety of commercially available biochemical test systems, by mass spectrometry of bacterial cell components, or by molecular methods. Multiplexed molecular tests capable of rapidly identifying a variety of gram-negative rods including *E coli* directly in positive blood culture bottles have been cleared by the US Food and Drug Administration. Special screening and confirmatory laboratory procedures are required to detect some multidrug-resistant gram-negative organisms. Molecular diagnostics are being used increasingly for identification of pathogens; specimens should be saved for resistance testing.

TREATMENT:

- Initial empiric treatment for suspected early-onset gram-negative septicemia in neonates should be based on local and regional antimicrobial susceptibility data. The proportion of *E coli* bloodstream infections with onset within 72 hours of life that are resistant to ampicillin is high among very low birth weight infants. These *E coli* infections almost invariably are susceptible to gentamicin, although monotherapy with an aminoglycoside is not recommended.

- Ampicillin and an aminoglycoside may be first line therapy in areas with low ampicillin resistance. An alternative regimen of ampicillin and an extended-spectrum cephalosporin (such as cefotaxime) can be used, but rapid emergence of cephalo-sporin-resistant organisms, especially *Enterobacter* species, *Klebsiella* species, and *Serratia* species, and increased risk of colonization or infection with ESBL-producing *Enterobacteriaceae* can occur when cephalosporin use is routine in a neonatal unit. Hence, routine use of an extended-spectrum cephalosporin is not recommended unless gram-negative bacterial meningitis is suspected. If cefotaxime is unavailable or if there is a concern for meningitis caused by a multidrug-resistant gram-negative organism, a carbapenem is the preferred choice for empirical therapy.

- Once the causative agent and its in vitro antimicrobial susceptibility pattern are known, nonmeningeal infections should be treated with ampicillin, an appropriate aminoglycoside, or an extended-spectrum cephalosporin (such as cefotaxime) on the basis of the susceptibility results. Some experts treat nonmeningeal infections caused by *Enterobacter* species, *Serratia* species, or *Pseudomonas* species and some other less commonly occurring gram-negative bacilli with a beta-lactam antimicrobial agent and an aminoglycoside. For ampicillin-susceptible CSF isolates of *E coli*, meningitis can be treated with ampicillin or cefotaxime; meningitis caused by an ampicillin-resistant, cefotaxime-susceptible isolate can be treated with cefotaxime. Combination therapy with cefotaxime and an aminoglycoside is used for empirical therapy and until CSF is sterile. If cefotaxime is unavailable, a carbapenem should be substituted for empirical therapy for neonates and infants younger than 91 days. Expert advice from an infectious disease specialist is helpful for management of meningitis.

- A carbapenem is the drug of choice for treatment of infections caused by ESBL-producing organisms, especially some *Klebsiella pneumoniae* isolates. Of the aminoglycosides, amikacin retains the most activity against ESBL-producing strains. An aminoglycoside or cefepime can be used if the organism is susceptible, because cefepime does not induce chromosomal AmpC enzymes. *E meningosepticum* intrinsically is resistant to most beta-lactams, including carbapenems, and has variable susceptibility to trimethoprim-sulfamethoxazole and fluoroquinolones; most are susceptible to piperacillin-tazobactam and rifampin. Expert advice from an infectious disease specialist is helpful in management of multidrug-resistant infection (eg, *E meningoseptica*) and ESBL-producing gram-negative infections in neonates.

- The treatment of infections caused by carbapenemase-producing gram-negative organisms is guided by the susceptibility profile and can include an aminoglycoside, especially amikacin; trimethoprim-sulfamethoxazole; or colistin. Isolates often are susceptible to tigecycline, fluoroquinolones, and polymyxin B, for which experience in neonates is limited. Patterns of susceptibility depend on the carbapenemase type. Some isolates may retain susceptibility to aztreonam. Combination therapy often is used. Treatment regimens utilizing carbapenems may be an option if the carbapenem minimal inhibitory concentration is 8 µg/mL or lower, and with a second antibiotic agent being added or when a prolonged infusion regimen is used. Expert advice from an infectious disease specialist is helpful in management of carbapenemase-producing gram-negative infections in neonates.

- All neonates with gram-negative meningitis should undergo repeat lumbar puncture to ensure sterility of the CSF after 24 to 48 hours of therapy. If CSF remains culture positive, choice and doses of antimicrobial agents should be reevaluated, and another lumbar puncture should be performed after another 48 to 72 hours.

- Duration of therapy is based on clinical and bacteriologic response of the patient and the site(s) of infection; the usual duration of therapy for uncomplicated bacteremia is 10 to 14 days, and for meningitis, minimum duration is 21 days.

- All infants with gram-negative meningitis should undergo careful follow-up examinations, including testing for hearing loss, neurologic abnormalities, and developmental delay.
- Immune Globulin Intravenous (IGIV) therapy for newborn infants receiving antimicrobial agents for suspected or proven serious infection has been shown to have no effect on outcomes measured and is not recommended.

ISOLATION OF THE HOSPITALIZED PATIENT: Standard precautions are recommended. Exceptions include hospital nursery epidemics, infants with *Salmonella* infection, and infants with infection caused by gram-negative bacilli that are resistant to multiple antimicrobial agents, including ESBL-producing strains and carbapenemase-producing *Enterobacteriaceae*; in these situations, contact precautions also are indicated.[1]

CONTROL MEASURES: Infection-control personnel should be aware of pathogens causing infections in infants so that clusters of infections are recognized and investigated appropriately. Several cases of infection caused by the same genus and species of bacteria occurring in infants in physical proximity or caused by an unusual pathogen indicate the need for an epidemiologic investigation (see Infection Control and Prevention for Hospitalized Children, p 146). Periodic review of in vitro antimicrobial susceptibility patterns of clinically important bacterial isolates from newborn infants, especially infants in the neonatal intensive care unit, can provide useful epidemiologic and therapeutic information.

Enterovirus (Nonpoliovirus)
(Group A and B Coxsackieviruses, Echoviruses, Numbered Enteroviruses)

CLINICAL MANIFESTATIONS: Nonpolio enteroviruses are responsible for significant and frequent illnesses in infants and children and result in protean clinical manifestations. The most common manifestation is nonspecific febrile illness, which in young infants may lead to evaluation for bacterial sepsis. Other manifestations can include the following: (1) respiratory: coryza, pharyngitis, herpangina, stomatitis, parotitis, croup, bronchiolitis, pneumonia, pleurodynia, and bronchospasm; (2) skin: hand-foot-and-mouth disease, onychomadesis (periodic shedding of nails), and nonspecific exanthems (particularly associated with echoviruses); (3) neurologic: aseptic meningitis, encephalitis, and motor paralysis (acute flaccid myelitis); (4) gastrointestinal/genitourinary: vomiting, diarrhea, abdominal pain, hepatitis, pancreatitis, and orchitis; (5) eye: acute hemorrhagic conjunctivitis and uveitis; (6) heart: myopericarditis; and (7) muscle: pleurodynia and other skeletal myositis. Neonates, especially those who acquire infection in the absence of serotype-specific maternal antibody, are at risk of severe and life-threatening disease, including viral sepsis, meningoencephalitis, myocarditis, hepatitis, coagulopathy, and pneumonitis. Infection with enterovirus 71 is associated with hand-foot-and-mouth disease, herpangina, and in a small proportion of cases, severe neurologic disease, including brainstem encephalomyelitis, paralytic disease, and other neurologic manifestations; secondary pulmonary edema/hemorrhage and cardiopulmonary collapse can occur, resulting in fatalities and

---

[1]Centers for Disease Control and Prevention. Guidance for control of infections with carbapenem-resistant or carbapenemase-producing *Enterobacteriaceae* in acute care facilities. *MMWR Morb Mortal Wkly Rep.* 2009;58(10): 256–260

sequelae. Other noteworthy but not exclusive serotype associations include coxsackieviruses A6 and A16 with hand-foot-and-mouth disease (including severe hand-foot-and-mouth disease and atypical cutaneous involvement with coxsackievirus A6), coxsackievirus A24 variant and enterovirus 70 with acute hemorrhagic conjunctivitis, and coxsackieviruses B1 through B5 with pleurodynia and myopericarditis.

Enterovirus D68 (EV-D68) is associated with mild to severe respiratory illness in infants, children, and teenagers and was responsible for a large multinational outbreak of respiratory disease in 2014. Disease was characterized by exacerbation of preexisting asthma or new-onset wheezing in children without any history of asthma, often requiring hospitalization and, in some patients, intensive supportive care. Concurrent with this outbreak, cases of a polio-like, acute neurologic syndrome were reported, often with a history of recent respiratory illness, some of which were demonstrated to have been caused by EV-D68. Neurologic illness consisted of acute onset of limb weakness accompanied by cerebrospinal fluid pleocytosis and nonenhancing lesions restricted to the gray matter on magnetic resonance imaging of the spinal cord. EV-D68 was not detectable in cerebrospinal fluid samples, precluding confirmation that it was the cause of neurologic illness, although 2 previously published reports of children with neurologic illnesses confirmed EV-D68 infection by cerebrospinal fluid testing. The full spectrum of disease caused by EV-D68 remains unknown.

Patients with humoral and combined immune deficiencies can develop persistent central nervous system infections, a dermatomyositis-like syndrome, and/or disseminated infection. Severe neurologic and/or multisystem disease is reported in hematopoietic stem cell and solid organ transplant recipients, children with malignancies, and patients treated with anti-CD20 monoclonal antibody.

ETIOLOGY: The enteroviruses comprise a genus in the *Picornaviridae* family of RNA viruses. The nonpolio enteroviruses include more than 100 distinct serotypes formerly subclassified as group A coxsackieviruses, group B coxsackieviruses, echoviruses, and newer numbered enteroviruses. A more recent classification system groups these nonpolio enteroviruses into 4 species (Enterovirus [EV] A, B, C, and D) on the basis of genetic similarity, although traditional serotype names are retained for some individual serotypes. Echoviruses 22 and 23 have been reclassified as human parechoviruses 1 and 2, respectively (see Human Parechovirus Infections, p 601).

EPIDEMIOLOGY: Humans are the only known reservoir for human enteroviruses, although some primates can become infected. Enterovirus infections are common and distributed worldwide; the majority of infections are asymptomatic. Enteroviruses are spread by fecal-oral and respiratory routes, and from mother to infant prenatally, in the peripartum period, and possibly via breastfeeding. EV-D68 is thought to be spread primarily by respiratory transmission. Enteroviruses may survive on environmental surfaces for periods long enough to allow transmission from fomites, and transmission via contaminated water and food can occur. Hospital nursery and other institutional outbreaks may occur. Infection incidence, clinical attack rates, and disease severity typically are greatest in infants and young children, and infections occur more frequently in tropical areas and where poor sanitation, poor hygiene, and high population density are present. Most enterovirus infections in temperate climates occur in the summer and fall (June through October in the northern hemisphere), but seasonal patterns are less evident in the tropics. Epidemics of enterovirus meningitis, enterovirus 71-associated hand-foot-and-mouth disease with neurologic and cardiopulmonary complications (particularly in southern and eastern

Asia), and enterovirus 70- and coxsackievirus A24-associated acute hemorrhagic conjunctivitis (characterized by viral shedding in tears and spread by contact; limited to subtropical and tropical regions) occur. Fecal viral shedding of most enteroviruses can persist for several weeks or months after onset of infection, but respiratory tract shedding usually is limited to 1 to 3 weeks or less. Fecal shedding is uncommon with EV-D68. Infection and viral shedding can occur without signs of clinical illness.

The usual **incubation period** for enterovirus infections is 3 to 6 days, except for acute hemorrhagic conjunctivitis, in which the **incubation period** is 24 to 72 hours.

DIAGNOSTIC TESTS: Enteroviruses generally can be detected by reverse transcriptase-polymerase chain reaction (RT-PCR) assay and culture from a variety of specimens, including stool, rectal swabs, throat swabs, nasopharyngeal aspirates, conjunctival swabs, tracheal aspirates, blood, urine, and tissue biopsy specimens, and from cerebrospinal fluid (CSF) when meningitis is present. RT-PCR assay is more rapid and more sensitive than isolation of enteroviruses in cell culture and can detect all enteroviruses, including serotypes that are difficult to cultivate in viral culture. Patients with enterovirus 71 neurologic disease often have negative results of RT-PCR assay and culture of CSF (even in the presence of CSF pleocytosis) and blood; RT-PCR assay and culture of throat or rectal swab and/or vesicle fluid specimens (in cases of hand-foot-and-mouth disease) more frequently are positive. RT-PCR assays for detection of enterovirus RNA are available at many reference and commercial laboratories for CSF, blood, and other specimens.

EV-D68 is demonstrated primarily in respiratory tract specimens and can be detected with multiplex respiratory RT-PCR assays, but these assays do not distinguish enteroviruses from rhinoviruses. Definitive identification of EV-D68 requires partial genomic sequencing or amplification by an EV-D68-specific RT-PCR assay.

Sensitivity of culture ranges from 0% to 80% depending on serotype and cell lines used. Many group A coxsackieviruses grow poorly or not at all in vitro. Culture usually requires 3 to 8 days to detect growth. The serotype of enterovirus may be identified either by partial genomic sequencing or by serotype-specific antibody staining or neutralization assay of a viral isolate at select reference laboratories (eg, the Centers for Disease Control and Prevention [CDC]). Serotyping may be indicated in cases of special clinical interest or for epidemiologic purposes (eg, for investigation of disease clusters or outbreaks). Acute infection with a known enterovirus serotype can be determined at reference laboratories by demonstration of a change in neutralizing or other serotype-specific antibody titer between acute and convalescent serum specimens or by detection of serotype-specific immunoglobulin (Ig) M, but serologic assays are relatively insensitive, may lack specificity, and rarely are used for diagnosis of acute infection. Antigen detection assays for enterovirus 71 have been developed but are not routinely available.

TREATMENT: No specific therapy is available for enteroviruses infections. Immune Globulin Intravenous (IGIV), administered intravenously or via intraventricular administration, may be beneficial for chronic enterovirus meningoencephalitis in immunodeficient patients. IGIV also has been used for life-threatening neonatal enterovirus infections (maternal convalescent plasma has also been used), severe enterovirus infections in transplant recipients and people with malignancies, suspected viral myocarditis, and enterovirus 71 neurologic disease, but proof of efficacy for these uses is lacking. High-titer enterovirus 71 Immune Globulin is being evaluated in areas with epidemic disease. Interferons occasionally have been used for treatment of enterovirus-associated myocarditis, without definitive proof of efficacy.

The antiviral drug pleconaril has activity against enteroviruses (but likely not parechoviruses) but is not available commercially at this time. Pocapavir is another antiviral drug being developed primarily for the treatment of polioviruses, and it has activity against at least some nonpolio enteroviruses, but it also is not commercially available.

The CDC has developed a comprehensive Web site for assessing and managing patients with acute flaccid myelitis as part of its emerging infection surveillance efforts (eg, West Nile virus, enterovirus D68) and in preparation for the final efforts to eradicate polioviruses worldwide (**www.cdc.gov/acute-flaccid-myelitis/hcp/index.html**).

ISOLATION OF THE HOSPITALIZED PATIENT: In addition to standard precautions, contact precautions are indicated for infants and young children for the duration of enterovirus illness. Droplet precautions also are indicated for EV-D68 respiratory infections. Cohorting of infected neonates has been effective in controlling hospital nursery enterovirus outbreaks.

CONTROL MEASURES: Hand hygiene, especially after diaper changing, and respiratory hygiene (particularly for EV-D68) are important in decreasing spread of enteroviruses within families and institutions. Other measures include avoidance of contaminated utensils and fomites and disinfection of surfaces. Recommended chlorination treatment of drinking water and swimming pools may help prevent transmission.

Maintenance administration of IGIV in patients with severe deficits of B-lymphocyte function (eg, severe combined immunodeficiency syndrome, X-linked agammaglobulinemia) may prevent chronic enterovirus infection of the central nervous system. Vaccines for select enterovirus serotypes associated with more severe disease are under investigation. There is one enterovirus 71 vaccine licensed in China.

Epstein-Barr Virus Infections
(Infectious Mononucleosis)

CLINICAL MANIFESTATIONS: Infectious mononucleosis is the most common presentation of primary symptomatic Epstein-Barr virus (EBV) infection. It manifests typically as fever, pharyngitis with petechiae, exudative pharyngitis, lymphadenopathy, hepatosplenomegaly, and atypical lymphocytosis. The spectrum of disease is wide, ranging from asymptomatic to fatal infection. Infections commonly are unrecognized in infants and young children. Rash can occur and is more common in patients treated with ampicillin or amoxicillin as well as with other penicillins. Central nervous system (CNS) manifestations include aseptic meningitis, encephalitis, myelitis, optic neuritis, cranial nerve palsies, transverse myelitis, Alice in Wonderland syndrome, and Guillain-Barré syndrome. Hematologic complications include splenic rupture, thrombocytopenia, agranulocytosis, hemolytic anemia, and hemophagocytic lymphohistiocytosis (HLH, or hemophagocytic syndrome). Pneumonia, orchitis, and myocarditis are observed infrequently. Early in the course of primary infection, up to 20% of circulating B lymphocytes are infected with EBV, and EBV-specific cytotoxic/suppressor T lymphocytes account for up to 30% of the CD8+ T lymphocytes in the blood. Replication of EBV in B lymphocytes results in T-lymphocyte proliferation and inhibition of B-lymphocyte proliferation by T-lymphocyte cytotoxic responses. Fatal disseminated infection or B-lymphocyte or T-lymphocyte lymphomas can occur in children with no detectable immunologic abnormality as well as in children with congenital or acquired cellular immune deficiencies.

EBV is associated with several other distinct disorders, including X-linked lymphoproliferative syndrome, post-transplantation lymphoproliferative disorders, Burkitt lymphoma, nasopharyngeal carcinoma, and undifferentiated B- or T-lymphocyte lymphomas and leiomyosarcoma. X-linked lymphoproliferative syndrome occurs in people with an inherited, maternally derived, recessive genetic defect in the SH2DIA gene, which is important in several lymphocyte signaling pathways. The syndrome is characterized by several phenotypic expressions, including occurrence of fatal infectious mononucleosis early in life among boys; nodular B-lymphocyte lymphomas, often with CNS involvement; and profound hypogammaglobinemia. Similarly, "X-linked immunodeficiency with magnesium defect, EBV infection, and neoplasia" (XMEN) disease is characterized by loss-of-function mutations in the gene encoding magnesium transporter 1 (MAGT1), chronic high-level EBV with increased EBV-infected B cells, and heightened susceptibility to EBV-associated lymphomas.

EBV-associated lymphoproliferative disorders result in a number of complex syndromes in patients who are immunocompromised, such as transplant recipients or people infected with human immunodeficiency virus (HIV). The highest incidence of these disorders occurs in liver and heart transplant recipients, in whom the proliferative states range from benign lymph node hypertrophy to monoclonal lymphomas. Other EBV syndromes are of greater importance outside the United States. EBV is present in virtually 100% of endemic Burkitt lymphoma (a B-lymphocyte tumor predominantly found in head and neck lymph nodes primarily in Central Africa) versus 20% in sporadic Burkitt lymphoma (found in abdominal lymphoid tissue predominantly in North America and Europe). EBV is found in nasopharyngeal carcinoma in Southeast Asia and the Inuit populations. EBV also has been associated with Hodgkin disease (B-lymphocyte tumor), non-Hodgkin lymphomas (B and T lymphocyte), gastric carcinoma "lymphoepitheliomas," and a variety of common epithelial malignancies.

Chronic fatigue syndrome is not related to EBV infection; however, fatigue lasting weeks to months may follow approximately 10% of cases of classic infectious mononucleosis.

ETIOLOGY: EBV (also known as human herpesvirus 4) is a gamma herpesvirus of the *Lymphocryptovirus* genus and is the most common cause of infectious mononucleosis (>90% of cases).

EPIDEMIOLOGY: Humans are the only known reservoir of EBV, and approximately 90% of US adults have been infected. Close personal contact usually is required for transmission. The virus is viable in saliva for several hours outside the body, but the role of fomites in transmission is unknown. EBV may be transmitted by blood transfusion or transplantation. Infection commonly is contracted early in life, particularly among members of lower socioeconomic groups, in which intrafamilial spread is common. Endemic infectious mononucleosis is common in group settings of adolescents, such as in educational or military institutions. No seasonal pattern has been documented. Intermittent excretion in saliva is lifelong after infection.

The **incubation period** of infectious mononucleosis is estimated to be 30 to 50 days.

DIAGNOSTIC TESTS: Routine diagnosis depends on serologic testing. Nonspecific tests for heterophile antibody, including the Paul-Bunnell test and slide agglutination reaction test, are available most commonly. The heterophile antibody response primarily is immunoglobulin (Ig) M, which appears during the first 2 weeks of illness and gradually disappears over a 6-month period. The results of heterophile antibody tests often are negative in children younger than 4 years of age with EBV infection, but heterophile antibody tests identify approximately 85% of cases of classic infectious mononucleosis in older children and adults during the second week of illness. An absolute increase in atypical lymphocytes during the second week of illness with infectious mononucleosis is a characteristic but nonspecific finding. Nevertheless, the finding of greater than 10% atypical lymphocytes together with a positive heterophile antibody test result in the classical illness pattern is considered diagnostic of acute EBV infection.

Multiple specific serologic antibody tests for EBV infection are available in diagnostic virology laboratories (see Table 3.5 and Fig 3.1). The most commonly performed test is for antibody against the viral capsid antigen (VCA). Because IgG antibodies against VCA occur in high titer early in infection and persist for life at modest levels, testing of acute and convalescent serum specimens for IgG anti-VCA alone is not useful for establishing the presence of active infection. In contrast, testing for the presence of IgM anti-VCA antibody and the absence (or very low titers of) of antibodies to Epstein-Barr nuclear antigen (EBNA) is useful for identifying active and recent infections. Because serum antibody against EBNA is not present until several weeks to months after onset of infection and rises with convalescence, a very elevated anti-EBNA antibody concentration typically excludes active primary infection. Testing for antibodies against early antigen (EA) is not required to assess EBV-associated mononucleosis. However, in selected situations, it may be beneficial if it is performed by a laboratory that is proficient with the EA test. Interpretations of EBV serologic testing classically were based on quantitative immunofluorescence antibody tests performed during various stages of mononucleosis and its resolution, although most clinical laboratories today usually perform enzyme immunoassays for detection of antibodies. Typical patterns of antibody responses to EBV infection are illustrated in Table 3.5 and Fig 3.1.

Serologic testing for EBV is useful, particularly for evaluating patients who have heterophile-negative infectious mononucleosis, are younger than 4 years, or in whom the infectious mononucleosis syndrome is not classic. Testing for other agents, especially cytomegalovirus, *Toxoplasma*, human herpesvirus 6, adenovirus, and HIV (in those with HIV risk factors), may be indicated for some patients. Diagnosis of the entire range of EBV-associated illness requires use of additional molecular and antibody techniques, particularly for patients with immune deficiencies.

Table 3.5. Serum Epstein-Barr Virus (EBV) Antibodies in EBV Infection

Infection	VCA IgG	VCA IgM	EA (D)	EBNA
No previous infection	−	−	−	−
Acute infection	+	+	+/−	−
Recent infection	+	+/−	+/−	+/−
Past infection	+	−	+/−	+

VCA IgG indicates immunoglobulin (Ig) G class antibody to viral capsid antigen; VCA IgM, IgM class antibody to VCA; EA (D), early antigen diffuse staining; and EBNA, EBV nuclear antigen.

FIG 3.1. SCHEMATIC REPRESENTATION OF THE EVOLUTION OF ANTIBODIES TO VARIOUS EPSTEIN-BARR VIRUS ANTIGENS IN PATIENTS WITH INFECTIOUS MONONUCLEOSIS.

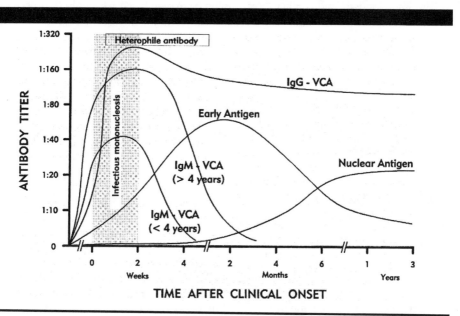

TIME AFTER CLINICAL ONSET

Source: *Manual of Clinical Laboratory Immunology*. Washington, DC: *American Society for Microbiology*; 1997:636. © 1997 American Society for Microbiology. Used with permission. No further reproduction or distribution is permitted without the prior written permission of American Society for Microbiology.

Isolation of EBV from oropharyngeal secretions by culture in cord blood cells is possible, but techniques for performing this procedure usually are not available in routine diagnostic laboratories, and virus isolation does not necessarily indicate acute infection. Polymerase chain reaction (PCR) assay for detection of EBV DNA in serum, plasma, and tissue and reverse transcriptase-PCR assay for detection of EBV RNA in lymphoid cells, tissue, and/or body fluids are available commercially and may be useful in evaluation of immunocompromised patients and in complex clinical situations.

TREATMENT: Patients suspected to have infectious mononucleosis should not receive ampicillin or amoxicillin, which may cause nonallergic morbilliform rashes in a significant proportion of patients with active EBV infection. Although therapy with short-course corticosteroids may have a beneficial effect on some acute symptoms, because of potential adverse effects their use should be considered only for patients with marked tonsillar inflammation with impending airway obstruction, massive splenomegaly, myocarditis, hemolytic anemia, or HLH. The dosage of prednisone usually is 1 mg/kg per day, orally (maximum 20 mg/day), for 7 days, in some cases followed by tapering. Life-threatening HLH has been treated with cytotoxic agents and immunomodulators, including etoposide, cyclosporine, and/or corticosteroids. Although acyclovir and valacyclovir have in vitro antiviral activity against EBV and in some small studies appear to have a virologic effect, the clinical benefit of antiviral therapy has not been established in infectious mononucleosis or in EBV lymphoproliferative syndromes. Decreasing immunosuppressive therapy often is beneficial for patients with EBV-induced post-transplant lymphoproliferative disorders.

Strenuous activity and contact sports should be avoided for 21 days after onset of symptoms of infectious mononucleosis. After 21 days, limited noncontact aerobic activity can be allowed if there are no symptoms and there is no overt splenomegaly. Clearance to participate in contact sports is appropriate after 4 to 6 weeks following the onset of symptoms if the athlete is asymptomatic and has no overt splenomegaly. Imaging modalities rarely are helpful in decisions about clearance to return to contact sports. Repeat monospot or EBV serologic testing is not useful in most clinical situations. It may take 3 to 6 months or longer following mononucleosis for an athlete to return to preillness fitness.

ISOLATION OF THE HOSPITALIZED PATIENT: Standard precautions are recommended.

CONTROL MEASURES: None in the hospital or clinic. Avoid salivary exchange or sharing food or drink with someone who recently had infectious mononucleosis.

Escherichia coli Diarrhea
(Including Hemolytic-Uremic Syndrome)

CLINICAL MANIFESTATIONS: At least 5 pathotypes of diarrhea-producing *Escherichia coli* strains have been identified. Clinical features of disease caused by each pathotype are summarized as follows (see Table 3.6):

- Shiga toxin-producing *E coli* (STEC) organisms are associated with diarrhea, hemorrhagic colitis, and hemolytic-uremic syndrome (HUS). STEC O157:H7 is the serotype most often implicated in outbreaks and consistently is a virulent STEC serotype, but other serotypes can cause illness. STEC illness typically begins with nonbloody diarrhea. Stools usually become bloody after 2 or 3 days, representing the onset of hemorrhagic colitis. Severe abdominal pain typically is short lived, and low-grade fever is present in approximately one third of cases. Diseases caused by *E coli* O157:H7 and other STEC organisms should be considered in people with presumptive diagnoses of intussusception, appendicitis, inflammatory bowel disease, or ischemic colitis. There are 2 types of Shiga toxin (Stx), Stx1 and Stx2; several variants of each type exist. In general, STEC strains that produce Stx2, especially variants Stx2a, Stx2c, and Stx2d, are more virulent than strains that only produce Stx1. However, in the clinical setting, there is limited ability to differentiate between Stx variants.

- Diarrhea caused by enteropathogenic *E coli* (EPEC) is watery. Illness occurs almost exclusively in children younger than 2 years and predominantly in resource-limited countries, either sporadically or in epidemics. Although usually mild, diarrhea can result in dehydration and even death, particularly in resource-limited countries. EPEC diarrhea can be persistent and can result in wasting or growth restriction. EPEC infection is uncommon in breastfed infants.

- Diarrhea caused by enterotoxigenic *E coli* (ETEC) is a 1- to 5-day, self-limited illness of moderate severity, typically with watery stools and abdominal cramps. ETEC is common in infants in resource-limited countries and in travelers to those countries. ETEC infection rarely has been diagnosed in the United States, because methods to detect these infections have not been available commercially until recently. However, ETEC infections may be detected more frequently as culture-independent diagnostic tests become more common. Outbreaks and studies with small numbers of patients have demonstrated that ETEC infection occurs in travelers returning from resource-limited countries and occasionally is acquired in the United States.

- Diarrhea caused by enteroinvasive *E coli* (EIEC) is similar clinically to diarrhea caused by *Shigella* species. Although dysentery can occur, diarrhea usually is watery without blood or mucus. Patients often are febrile, and stools can contain leukocytes.

- Enteroaggregative *E coli* (EAEC) organisms cause watery diarrhea and are common in people of all ages in industrialized as well as resource-limited countries. It may present as childhood diarrhea in developing countries, acute diarrhea in travelers, and persistent diarrhea in children or HIV-infected patients. EAEC has been associated with prolonged diarrhea (14 days or longer). Asymptomatic infection can be accompanied by subclinical inflammatory enteritis, which can cause growth disturbance.

Sequelae of STEC Infection. HUS is a serious sequela of STEC enteric infection. *E coli* O157 is the STEC serogroup most commonly associated with HUS, which is defined by the triad of microangiopathic hemolytic anemia, thrombocytopenia, and acute renal dysfunction. HUS occurs in approximately 15% of children younger than 5 years (children 1 through 4 years of age are at higher risk than are infants) with laboratory-confirmed *E coli* O157 infection, as compared with approximately 6% among people of all ages. HUS occurs in approximately 1% of patients of all ages with laboratory-confirmed non-O157:H7 STEC infection.

Table 3.6. Classification of *Escherichia coli* Associated With Diarrhea

Pathotype	Epidemiology	Type of Diarrhea	Mechanism of Pathogenesis
Shiga toxin-producing *E coli* (STEC)	Hemorrhagic colitis and hemolytic-uremic syndrome in all ages	Bloody or nonbloody	Shiga toxin production, large bowel adherence, coagulopathy
Enteropathogenic *E coli* (EPEC)	Acute and chronic endemic and epidemic diarrhea in infants in resource-limited countries	Watery	Small bowel adherence and effacement
Enterotoxigenic *E coli* (ETEC)	Infant diarrhea in resource-limited countries and travelers' diarrhea in all ages	Watery	Small bowel adherence, heat stable and/or heat-labile enterotoxin production
Enteroinvasive *E coli* (EIEC)	Diarrhea with fever in all ages	Bloody or nonbloody; dysentery	Mucosal invasion and inflammation of large bowel
Enteroaggregative *E coli* (EAEC)	Acute and chronic diarrhea in all ages	Watery, occasionally bloody	Small and large bowel adherence, enterotoxin and cytotoxin production

HUS typically develops 7 days (up to 2 weeks, and rarely 2–3 weeks) after onset of diarrhea. More than 50% of children with HUS require dialysis, and 3% to 5% die. Patients with HUS can develop neurologic complications (eg, seizures, coma, or cerebral vessel thrombosis). Children presenting with an increased white blood cell count (>20 x 10^9/mL) or oliguria or anuria are at higher risk of poor outcome, as are, seemingly paradoxically, children with hematocrit close to normal rather than low. Most patients who survive have a very good prognosis, which can be predicted by normal creatinine clearance and no proteinuria or hypertension 1 year or more after HUS.

ETIOLOGY: The 5 pathotypes of diarrhea-producing *E coli* have been distinguished by genetic, pathogenic, and clinical characteristics. Each pathotype is defined by the presence of virulence-related genes, and each comprises characteristic serotypes, indicated by somatic (O) and flagellar (H) antigens.

EPIDEMIOLOGY: Transmission of most diarrhea-associated *E coli* strains is from food or water contaminated with human or animal feces or from infected symptomatic people. STEC is shed in feces of cattle and, to a lesser extent, sheep, deer, and other ruminants. Human infection is acquired via contaminated food or water or via contact with an infected person, a fomite, or a carrier animal or its environment. Many foods have caused *E coli* O157 outbreaks, including undercooked ground beef, raw leafy vegetables, and unpasteurized milk and juice. Outbreak investigations have implicated petting zoos, drinking water, and ingestion of recreational water. The infectious dose is low; thus, person-to-person transmission is common in households and child care centers. Less is known about the epidemiology of STEC strains other than O157. The non-O157 STEC serogroups most commonly linked to illness in the United States are (in order of incidence) O26, O103, O111, O121, O45, and O145. In fall 2015, a 9-state outbreak of *E coli* O26 infection affecting 55 people was reported from 11 states, and a common-source restaurant food product was implicated, although a specific food was not identified. Whole-genome sequencing performed on 36 isolates showed that all were highly related. No cases of HUS were reported. A severe outbreak of bloody diarrhea and HUS occurred in Europe in 2011; the outbreak was attributed to an EAEC strain of serotype O104:H4 that had acquired the Shiga toxin 2a-encoding phage. This experience highlights the importance of considering serogroups other than O157 in outbreaks and cases of HUS.

With the exception of EAEC, non-STEC pathotypes most commonly are associated with disease in resource-limited countries, where food and water supplies commonly are contaminated and facilities and supplies for hand hygiene are suboptimal. For young children in resource-limited countries, transmission of ETEC, EPEC, and other diarrheal pathogens via contaminated weaning foods (sometimes by use of untreated drinking water in the foods) is common. ETEC diarrhea occurs in people of all ages but is especially frequent and severe in infants in resource-limited countries. ETEC is a major cause of travelers' diarrhea. EAEC increasingly is reported as a cause of diarrhea in the United States.

The **incubation period** for most *E coli* strains is 10 hours to 6 days; for *E coli* O157:H7, the **incubation period** usually is 3 to 4 days (range, 1–8 days).

DIAGNOSTIC TESTS: Diagnosis of infection caused by diarrhea-associated *E coli* other than STEC is difficult, because tests are not widely available to distinguish these pathotypes from normal *E coli* strains present in stool flora. Culture-independent tests are necessary to detect non-O157:H7 STEC infections. Several US Food and Drug Administration (FDA)-cleared multiplex polymerase chain reaction (PCR) assays can detect a variety of enteric infections, including ETEC and STEC, the latter by detection of the genes encoding Stx1 and Stx2. Several commercially available, sensitive, specific, and rapid immunologic assays for Shiga toxins in stool or broth culture of stool, including enzyme immunoassays (EIA) and immunochromatographic assays, have been approved by the FDA.[1] The assays performed on broth enriched stool specimens (usually incubated 18–24 hours) generally are more sensitive than those that test stool directly.

Ideally, all stool specimens submitted for routine culture testing from patients with acute community-acquired diarrhea (regardless of patient age, season, or presence or absence of blood in the stool) should be tested for Shiga toxin and cultured simultaneously for *E coli* O157:H7, although the yield will be low in some geographic regions, including the southern tier states.

Rapid and optimal diagnosis facilitates patient management and prompt institution of fluid rehydration to provide nephroprotection. Shiga toxin testing should be performed on growth from broth enrichments or primary isolation media, because this method is more sensitive and specific than direct testing of stool. Most *E coli* O157 isolates can be identified presumptively when grown on sorbitol-containing selective media, because they cannot ferment sorbitol within 24 hours. All presumptive *E coli* O157:H7 isolates and all Shiga toxin-positive stool specimens that did not yield a presumptive *E coli* O157 isolate should be sent to a public health laboratory for further characterization, including selective methods to identify non-O157 STEC, serotyping, pulsed-field gel electrophoresis, and/or genetic sequencing.

STEC should be sought in stool specimens from all patients diagnosed with postdiarrheal HUS. However, the absence of STEC does not preclude the diagnosis of probable STEC-associated HUS, because HUS typically is diagnosed a week or more after onset of diarrhea, when the organism may not be detectable by conventional bacteriologic methods. When low numbers of organisms are suspected, the selective enrichment of stool samples followed by immunomagnetic separation can markedly enhance the isolation of *E coli* O157 and other STEC for which immunomagnetic reagents are available. The test is available at some state public health laboratories and, through requests to state health departments, at the Centers for Disease Control and Prevention (CDC). Multiplex PCR assays increasingly are available in clinical laboratories and provide sensitive detection of Shiga toxin-encoding genes in fecal samples. DNA probes are available in reference and research laboratories. Serologic diagnosis using enzyme immunoassay to detect serum antibodies to *E coli* O157 and O111 lipopolysaccharides is available at the CDC for outbreak investigations and for patients with HUS and can be arranged through state health departments.

TREATMENT: Orally administered electrolyte-containing solutions usually are adequate to prevent or treat dehydration and electrolyte abnormalities.[2] Antimotility agents should not be administered to children with inflammatory or bloody diarrhea. Patients with proven or suspected STEC infection should be rehydrated fully but prudently as soon as clinically feasible. Many experts advocate intravenous volume expansion during the first 4 days of proven STEC infection to maintain renal perfusion and reduce the risk of HUS.

---

[1]Centers for Disease Control and Prevention. Recommendations for diagnosis of Shiga toxin-producing *Escherichia coli* infections by clinical laboratories. *MMWR Recomm Rep.* 2009;58(RR-12):1–14

[2]Centers for Disease Control and Prevention. Managing acute gastroenteritis among children: oral rehydration, maintenance, and nutritional therapy. *MMWR Recomm Rep.* 2003;52(RR-16):1–16

Careful monitoring of patients with hemorrhagic colitis (including complete blood cell count with smear, blood urea nitrogen, and creatinine concentrations) is recommended to detect changes suggestive of HUS. If patients have no laboratory evidence of hemolysis, thrombocytopenia, or nephropathy 3 days after resolution of diarrhea, their risk of developing HUS is low.

In resource-limited countries, nutritional rehabilitation, including supplemental zinc and vitamin A, should be provided as part of case management algorithms for diarrhea where feasible. Feeding, including breastfeeding, should be continued for young children with *E coli* enteric infection. Bismuth subsalicylate has been approved by the FDA for use in children 12 years and older and has been shown to reduce the severity of travelers' diarrhea.

Antimicrobial Therapy. Antimicrobial therapy in patients with STEC infection remains controversial because of its association with an increased risk of developing HUS in some studies. A recent meta-analysis did not find that children with hemorrhagic colitis caused by STEC have a greater risk of developing HUS if treated with an antimicrobial agent. However, an association was found in analyses restricted to studies with low risk of bias and using the accepted HUS definition. Moreover, a controlled trial has not been performed, and a beneficial effect of antimicrobial treatment has not been proven. The most recently published observational studies found that treatment of diarrhea with at least some classes of antimicrobial agents was associated with HUS development. Most experts advise not prescribing antimicrobial therapy for children with *E coli* O157 enteritis or a clinical or epidemiologic picture strongly suggestive of STEC infection.

Empiric self-treatment of diarrhea for travelers to a resource-limited country can slightly reduce duration of diarrhea; however, the prevalence of antimicrobial-resistant enteric pathogens in resource-limited settings is increasing. Azithromycin or a fluoroquinolone have been the most reliable agents for therapy (see Fluoroquinolones, p 904); the choice of therapy depends on the pathogen and local antibiotic resistance patterns. Rifaximin may be used for people 12 years and older.

ISOLATION OF THE HOSPITALIZED PATIENT: In addition to standard precautions, contact precautions are indicated for diapered and incontinent patients with all types of *E coli* diarrhea for the duration of illness. Prolonged shedding has been noted in children younger than 5 years. Patients with postdiarrheal HUS should be presumed to have STEC infection.

CONTROL MEASURES:
Escherichia coli O157:H7 and Other STEC Infection. All meat should be cooked thoroughly. Ground beef should be cooked thoroughly until no pink meat remains and the juices are clear or to an internal temperature of 160°F (71°C). Raw milk should not be ingested, and the certification of raw milk does not eliminate the risk of transmission of *E coli* organisms.[1] Only pasteurized apple juice and cider products should be consumed. Care should be taken to prevent cross-contamination in areas of food preparation. Hands should be washed with soap and water immediately after contact with animals, the environment around animals, and animal food or treats; adults should supervise hand washing for young children.

---

[1]American Academy of Pediatrics, Committee on Infectious Diseases, Committee on Nutrition. Consumption of raw or unpasteurized milk and milk products by pregnant women and children. *Pediatrics.* 2014;133(1):175–179 (Reaffirmed October 2017)

Outbreaks in Child Care Centers. If an outbreak of HUS or diarrhea attributable to STEC occurs in a child care center, immediate involvement of public health authorities is critical. Infection caused by STEC is notifiable, and rapid reporting of cases allows interventions to prevent further disease. Ill children with STEC O157 infection or virulent non-O157 STEC infection (such as those caused by Stx2-producing strains or in the context of an outbreak that includes HUS cases or a high frequency of bloody diarrhea) should not be permitted to reenter the child care center until 2 stool cultures (obtained at least 48 hours after any antimicrobial therapy, if administered, has been discontinued) are negative, stools are contained in the diaper or the child is continent, stool frequency is no more than 2 stools above that child's normal frequency for the time the child is in the program, and the health department agrees with the return to child care. Some state health departments have less stringent exclusion policies for children who have recovered from less virulent STEC infection. Stool cultures should be performed for any symptomatic contacts. In outbreak situations involving virulent STEC strains, stool cultures of asymptomatic contacts may aid controlling spread. Strict attention to hand hygiene is important but can be insufficient to prevent transmission. The child care center should be closed to new admissions during an outbreak, and care should be exercised to prevent transfer of exposed children to other centers.

Nursery and Other Institutional Outbreaks. Strict attention to hand hygiene is essential for limiting spread. Exposed patients should be observed closely, their stools should be cultured for the causative organism, and they should be separated from unexposed infants (see Children in Out-of-Home Child Care, p 122).

Travelers' Diarrhea. Travelers' diarrhea usually is acquired by ingestion of contaminated food or water or contact with fomites and is a significant problem for people traveling in resource-limited countries. Diarrhea commonly is caused by ETEC. Diarrhea attributable to *E coli* O157 is rare in US travelers; a much higher proportion of patients with non-O157 STEC infection have traveled internationally in the previous week. Travelers should be advised to drink only bottled or canned beverages and boiled or bottled water; travelers should avoid ice, raw produce including salads, and fruit that they have not peeled themselves. Cooked foods should be eaten steaming hot. Hands should be washed carefully before preparing or eating food or feeding another person. Rehydration is the mainstay of treatment. Packets of oral rehydration salts can be added to boiled or bottled water and ingested to help maintain fluid balance. Antimicrobial agents are not recommended for prevention of travelers' diarrhea in children. Antimicrobial therapy generally is recommended for travelers in resource-limited areas when diarrhea is moderate to severe or is associated with fever or bloody stools; however, the prevalence of antimicrobial resistance among enteric pathogens is increasing. Several antimicrobial agents, such as azithromycin, rifaximin, and ciprofloxacin, can be effective in treatment of travelers' diarrhea. The drug of first choice for children is azithromycin and for adults is azithromycin or ciprofloxacin. Treatment for no more than 3 days is advised.

Recreational Water. People should avoid ingesting recreational water. Because STEC has a low infectious dose and can be waterborne, people with proven or suspected STEC infection should not use recreational water venues (eg, swimming pools, water slides) when ill with diarrhea. Children who have diarrhea attributable to STEC and who are incontinent should continue not to use recreational water venues until 1 week after symptoms resolve. Showering before swimming, taking children to the restroom frequently, and changing diapers at designated diapering stations and then washing hands can limit transmission of diarrheal pathogens through recreational water.

Other Fungal Diseases

In addition to the mycoses discussed in individual chapters of Section 3 of the *Red Book* (eg, aspergillosis, blastomycosis, candidiasis, coccidioidomycosis, cryptococcosis, histoplasmosis, paracoccidioidomycosis, and sporotrichosis), uncommonly encountered fungi can cause infection in infants and children with immunosuppression or other underlying conditions. These include invasive mold infections, such as mucormycosis, fusariosis, scedosporiosis, and the phaeohyphomycoses (black molds), as well as invasive yeasts such as *Malazzesia, Trichosporon, Rhodotorula,* and many more. Children can acquire infection with these fungi through inhalation via the respiratory tract or through direct inoculation after traumatic disruption of cutaneous barriers. A list of some of these fungi and the pertinent underlying host conditions, reservoirs or routes of entry, clinical manifestations, diagnostic laboratory tests, and treatments can be found in Table 3.7. Taken as a group, few in vitro antifungal susceptibility data are available on which to base treatment recommendations for these uncommon invasive fungal infections, especially in children (see Antifungal Drugs for Systemic Fungal Infections, p 938, and Table 4.7, p 942). Consultation with a pediatric infectious disease specialist experienced in the diagnosis and treatment of invasive fungal infections should be considered when caring for a child infected with one of these mycoses.

Table 3.7. Additional Fungal Diseases

Disease and Agent	Underlying Host Condition(s)	Reservoir(s) or Route(s) of Entry	Common Clinical Manifestations	Diagnostic Laboratory Test(s)	Treatment
Hyalohyphomycosis					
Fusarium species	Granulocytopenia; hematopoietic stem cell transplantation; severe immunocompromise; severe neutropenia and/or T-lymphocyte immunodeficiency	Respiratory tract; sinuses; skin; ingestion	Pulmonary infiltrates; cutaneous lesions (eg, ecthyma); sinusitis; disseminated infection	Culture of blood or tissue specimen, histopathologic examination of tissue	Voriconazole, Posaconazole,[a,b] isavuconazole,[a,b] or D-AMB[c]
Pseudallescheria boydii (*Scedosporium apiospermum*) *Scedosporium prolificans*	None or trauma or immunosuppression; cystic fibrosis; chronic granulomatous disease; chronic glucocorticoid use; hematologic malignancy	Environment; respiratory tract; direct inoculation (eg, skin puncture)	Pneumonia; localized pulmonary process or disseminated infection; osteomyelitis or septic arthritis; mycetoma (immunocompetent patients); endocarditis; keratitis and endophthalmitis; brain abscesses; lesions of the skin, soft tissue, or bone	Culture and histopathologic examination of tissue	Voriconazole[d] or isavuconazole[b]

Table 3.7. Additional Fungal Diseases, continued

Disease and Agent	Underlying Host Condition(s)	Reservoir(s) or Route(s) of Entry	Common Clinical Manifestations	Diagnostic Laboratory Test(s)	Treatment
Penicilliosis					
Penicillium (Talaromyces) marneffei	Human immunodeficiency virus infection and exposure to southeast Asia	Respiratory tract	Pneumonitis; invasive dermatitis; disseminated infection	Culture of blood, bone marrow, or tissue; histopathologic examination of tissue	Amphotericin B drug of choice; alternative, voriconazole[b]
Phaeohyphomycosis					
Alternaria species	None, trauma, or immunosuppression	Respiratory tract; skin	Sinusitis; cutaneous lesions	Culture and histopathologic examination of tissue	Voriconazole[b] or high-dose D-AMB[c]
Bipolaris species	None, trauma, immunosuppression, or chronic sinusitis	Environment	Sinusitis; cerebral and disseminated infection	Culture and histopathologic examination of tissue	Voriconazole,[b] posaconazole,[b] itraconazole,[e] or D-AMB[c]; surgical excision
Cladophialophora species	None, trauma, or immunosuppression	Environment	Cerebral infection	Culture and histopathologic examination of tissue	Voriconazole,[b] posaconazole,[b] itraconazole,[e] or D-AMB[c]; surgical excision

Table 3.7. Additional Fungal Diseases, continued

Disease and Agent	Underlying Host Condition(s)	Reservoir(s) or Route(s) of Entry	Common Clinical Manifestations	Diagnostic Laboratory Test(s)	Treatment
Curvularia species	Immunosuppression; altered skin integrity; asthma or nasal polyps; chronic sinusitis	Environment	Allergic fungal sinusitis; invasive dermatitis; disseminated infection	Culture and histopathologic examination of tissue	Allergic fungal sinusitis: surgery and corticosteroids Invasive disease: voriconazole,[b] itraconazole,[b,e] or D-AMB[c]
Exophiala species, *Exserohilum* species	None, trauma, or immunosuppression	Environment	Sinusitis; cutaneous lesions; disseminated infection; meningitis associated with contaminated steroid for epidural use	Culture and histopathologic examination of tissue	Voriconazole,[b,f] itraconazole,[b,e] D-AMB, or surgical excision
Invasive Yeasts					
Trichosporon species	Immunosuppression; central venous catheter; hematologic malignancy, often with neutropenia; acquired immunodeficiency syndrome; extensive burns; glucocorticoid treatment; heart valve surgery; exposure to tropical environments	Environment; normal flora of gastrointestinal tract	Bloodstream infection; superficial skin lesions endocarditis; peritonitis; pneumonitis; disseminated infection	Blood culture; histopathologic examination of tissue or nodules; urine, sputum and cerebrospinal cultures; bronchoscopy with alveolar lavage cultures	For invasive infections, voriconazole[b,d]; For superficial infections, shaving of the hair and application of a topical azole antifungal to the affected areas

Table 3.7. Additional Fungal Diseases, continued

Disease and Agent	Underlying Host Condition(s)	Reservoir(s) or Route(s) of Entry	Common Clinical Manifestations	Diagnostic Laboratory Test(s)	Treatment
Malassezia species	Immunosuppression; preterm birth; exposure to parenteral nutrition that includes fat emulsions	Skin	Pityriasis versicolor, seborrheic dermatitis, central line-associated bloodstream infection; interstitial pneumonitis; urinary tract infection; meningitis	Culture of blood, catheter tip, or tissue specimen (requires special laboratory handling)	Removal of catheters and temporary cessation of lipid infusion; D-AMB, azole therapy
Mucormycosis (formerly Zygomycosis)					
Rhizopus; *Mucor*; *Lichtheimia* (formerly *Absidia*) species; *Rhizomucor* species; *Cunninghamella* species	Immunosuppression; hematologic malignant neoplasm; renal failure; diabetes mellitus; iron overload syndromes	Respiratory tract; skin	Rhinocerebral infection; pulmonary infection; disseminated infection; skin (traumatic wounds) and gastrointestinal tract (less commonly)	Histopathologic examination of tissue and culture	High dose of D-AMB for initial therapy and consider posaconazole[a] for maintenance therapy, with surgical excision, and débridement, as feasible; isavuconazole (voriconazole has no activity); echinocandins (eg, caspofungin) may have clinical utility when combined with AMB

D-AMB indicates deoxycholate amphotericin B; if the patient is intolerant of or refractory to D-AMB, liposomal amphotericin B can be substituted.

L-AMB indicates liposomal amphotericin B.

ABLC indicates amphotericin B lipid complex.

[a] Demonstrates activity in vitro, but few clinical data are available for children.

[b] No US Food and Drug Administration indication for this indication.

[c] Consider use of a lipid-based formulation of amphotericin B.

[d] Itraconazole may be the treatment of choice, but data on safety and effectiveness in children are limited.

[e] Itraconazole has been shown to be effective for cutaneous disease in adults, but safety and efficacy have not been established in children younger than 12 years.

[f] Voriconazole demonstrates activity in vitro, but no clinical data are available.

Fusobacterium Infections

(Including Lemierre Disease)

CLINICAL MANIFESTATIONS: *Fusobacterium* species, including *Fusobacterium necrophorum* and *Fusobacterium nucleatum*, can be isolated from oropharyngeal specimens in healthy people, are frequent components of human dental plaque, and may lead to periodontal disease. Invasive disease attributable to *Fusobacterium* species has been associated with otitis media, tonsillitis, gingivitis, and oropharyngeal trauma, including dental surgery. *Fusobacterium* species have been associated with acute appendicitis and suppurative portomesenteric vein thrombosis. Ten percent of cases of invasive *Fusobacterium* infections are associated with concomitant Epstein-Barr virus infection. Risk may be increased after use of macrolide-class antibiotic agents.

Otogenic infection is the most frequent primary source in children and can be complicated by meningitis and thrombosis of dural venous sinuses. Invasive infection following tonsillitis was described early in the 20th century and was referred to as postanginal sepsis or Lemierre syndrome. The classic syndrome starts with sore throat symptoms, which may improve or may continue to worsen. Fever and sore throat are followed by severe neck pain (anginal pain) that can be accompanied by unilateral neck swelling, trismus, and dysphagia. Patients with classic Lemierre disease have a sepsis syndrome with multiple organ dysfunction. Metastatic complications from septic embolic phenomena associated with suppurative jugular venous thrombosis (JVT) are common and may manifest as disseminated intravascular coagulation, pleural empyema, pyogenic arthritis, or osteomyelitis. Persistent headache or other neurologic signs may indicate the presence of cerebral venous sinus thrombosis (eg, cavernous sinus thrombosis), meningitis, or brain abscess. *Fusobacterium* species (most commonly *Fusobacterium necrophorum)* is isolated from blood or other normally sterile sites. Lemierre-like syndromes also have been reported following infection with *Arcanobacterium haemolyticum*, *Bacteroides* species, anaerobic *Streptococcus* species, other anaerobic bacteria, and methicillin-susceptible and resistant strains of *Staphylococcus aureus*.

JVT can be completely vaso-occlusive. Surgical débridement of necrotic tissue may be necessary for patients who do not respond to antimicrobial therapy. Some children with JVT associated with Lemierre disease have evidence of thrombophilia at diagnosis. These findings often resolve over several months and can indicate response to the inflammatory, prothrombotic process associated with infection rather than an underlying hypercoagulable state.

ETIOLOGY: *Fusobacterium* species are anaerobic, non–spore-forming, gram-negative bacilli. Human infection usually results from *F necrophorum* subspecies *funduliforme*, but infections with other species including *F nucleatum*, *Fusobacterium gonidiaformans*, *Fusobacterium naviforme*, *Fusobacterium mortiferum*, and *Fusobacterium varium* have been reported. Infection with *Fusobacterium* species, alone or in combination with other oral anaerobic bacteria, may result in Lemierre disease.

EPIDEMIOLOGY: *Fusobacterium* species commonly are found in soil and in the respiratory tracts of animals, including cattle, dogs, fowl, goats, sheep, and horses, and can be isolated from the oropharynx of healthy people. *Fusobacterium* infections are most common in adolescents and young adults, but infections, including fatal cases of Lemierre disease, have been reported in infants and young children.

DIAGNOSTIC TESTS: *Fusobacterium* species can be isolated using conventional liquid anaerobic blood culture media. However, the organism grows best on semisolid media for fastidious anaerobic organisms or blood agar supplemented with vitamin K, hemin, menadione, and a reducing agent. Colonies generally are cream to yellow colored, smooth, and round and may show a narrow zone of alpha or beta-hemolysis on blood agar, depending on the species of blood used in the medium; however, *F nucleatum* may appear as bread crumb-like colonies. Many strains fluoresce chartreuse green under ultraviolet light. Most *Fusobacterium* organisms are indole positive. On gram stain, *F nucleatum* usually exhibits spindle-shaped cells with tapered ends, while *F necrophorum* and other species may be highly pleomorphic with swollen areas. The accurate identification of anaerobes to the species level has become important with the increasing incidence of microorganisms that are resistant to multiple drugs. Conventional and commercial culture-based biochemical test systems are reasonably accurate, at least to the genus level. Sequencing of the 16S rRNA gene and phylogenetic analysis or the use of mass spectrometry of bacterial cell components can accurately identify *Fusobacterium* species to the species level.

Currently, there are no commercially available tests for diagnosing *Fusobacterium necrophorum* pharyngitis. Routine throat cultures for beta-hemolytic streptococci do not generally include screening for the presence of *Fusobacterium* species. Researchers have used special media to grow *F necrophorum* from throat swab specimens or have used polymerase chain reaction techniques to document and describe *F necrophorum* tonsillitis/pharyngitis.

One should consider Lemierre syndrome in ill-appearing febrile children and especially adolescents having a sore throat and developing exquisite neck pain and swelling over the angle of the jaw. Aerobic and anaerobic blood cultures should be performed to detect invasive *Fusobacterium* species and other possible pathogens. Computed tomography and magnetic resonance imaging are more sensitive than ultrasonography to document thrombosis and thrombophlebitis of the internal jugular vein early in the course of illness and to better identify thrombus extension.

TREATMENT: *Fusobacterium* species generally are susceptible to metronidazole, clindamycin, chloramphenicol, carbapenems (meropenem or imipenem), cefoxitin, and ceftriaxone. Antimicrobial resistance has increased in anaerobic bacteria, and susceptibility no longer is predictable. Therefore, susceptibility testing is indicated for all clinically significant anaerobic isolates, including *Fusobacterium* species. Combination therapy with metronidazole or clindamycin, in addition to a beta-lactam agent active against aerobic oral and respiratory tract pathogens (cefotaxime, ceftriaxone, or cefuroxime), is recommended for patients with invasive infection caused by *Fusobacterium* species. Alternatively, some experts use monotherapy with a penicillin-beta-lactamase inhibitor combination (ampicillin-sulbactam or piperacillin-tazobactam) or a carbapenem (meropenem, imipenem, or ertapenem). Up to 50% of *F nucleatum* and 20% of *F necrophorum* isolates produce beta-lactamases, rendering them resistant to penicillin, ampicillin, and some cephalosporins. *Fusobacterium* species intrinsically are resistant to gentamicin, fluoroquinolone agents, and typically, macrolides. Tetracyclines have limited activity.

The duration of antimicrobial therapy depends on the anatomic location and severity of infection but usually is several weeks. Surgical intervention involving débridement or incision and drainage of abscesses may be necessary. Anticoagulation therapy has been used in both adults and children with JVT and cavernous sinus thrombosis. In cases with extensive thrombosis, anticoagulation therapy may decrease the risk of clot extension and shorten recovery time.

ISOLATION OF THE HOSPITALIZED PATIENT: Standard precautions are recommended. Person-to-person transmission of *Fusobacterium* species has not been documented.

CONTROL MEASURES: Oral hygiene and dental cleanings may reduce density of oral colonization with *Fusobacterium* species, prevent gingivitis and dental caries, and reduce the risk of invasive disease.

Giardia intestinalis (formerly *Giardia lamblia* and *Giardia duodenalis*) Infections

(Giardiasis)

CLINICAL MANIFESTATIONS: Asymptomatic infection is common, with approximately 50% to 75% of people who acquire infection in outbreaks occurring in child care settings and in the community remaining asymptomatic. Symptomatic infection can manifest with acute infectious diarrhea or, more commonly, chronic diarrhea with failure to thrive or persistent gastrointestinal tract symptoms. Symptoms vary by age, with symptomatic infections more frequent in children than adults. Children can have occasional days of acute watery diarrhea with abdominal cramps, or they may experience a protracted, intermittent, often debilitating disease characterized by passage of foul-smelling stools associated with anorexia, flatulence, malaise, weakness, nausea, vomiting, low grade fever, and abdominal distention. Humoral immunodeficiencies predispose to chronic symptomatic *Giardia intestinalis* infections. Patients with cystic fibrosis have an increased prevalence of *G intestinalis* infection. Extraintestinal involvement (eg, arthritis, urticaria, retinal changes, and bile or pancreatic ducts) is unusual.

ETIOLOGY: *G intestinalis* is a flagellate protozoan that exists in trophozoite and cyst forms; the infective form is the cyst. Infection is limited to the small intestine and biliary tract. Giardia cysts are infectious immediately after being excreted in feces and remain viable for 3 months in water at 4°C. Freezing does not eliminate infectivity completely, but heating, drying, and seawater are likely to do so.

EPIDEMIOLOGY: Giardiasis is the most common intestinal parasitic infection of humans identified in the United States and globally with a worldwide distribution. The highest incidence is reported among children 1 through 9 years of age, adults 45 through 49 years of age, and residents of northern states. Peak onset of illness occurs annually during early summer through early fall.[1] Humans are the principal reservoir of infection, but *Giardia* organisms can infect dogs, cats, beavers, rodents, sheep, cattle, nonhuman primates, and other animals. *G intestinalis* assemblages are quite species-specific, such that the organisms that affect nonhumans usually are not infectious to humans. People become infected directly from an infected person, through ingestion of fecally contaminated water or food, or rarely through animal contact (eg, petting zoo, farm, reptile at long term care facility). Most community-wide epidemics have resulted from a contaminated drinking water supply; outbreaks associated with recreational water also have been reported.

Transmission of *Giardia lamblia* is common in certain high-risk groups, including (1) children and employees in child care centers; (2) travelers to areas of the world with

[1] Painter, JE, Gargano JW, Collier SA, Yoder JS. Giardiasis surveillance—United States, 2011–2012. *MMWR Surveill Summ.* 2015;64(3):15–25

endemic disease; (3) close contact with infected people; (4) people who swallow contaminated drinking water or recreational water; (5) people exposed to infected domestic and wild animals (dogs, cats, cattle, deer, and beaver); (6) people who take part in outdoor activities (eg, camping or backpacking) who consume unfiltered or untreated water; and (7) men who have sex with men. Although less common, outbreaks associated with food or food handlers have been reported. Surveys conducted in the United States have identified overall prevalence rates of *Giardia* organisms in stool specimens that range from 5% to 7%, with variations depending on age, geographic location, and seasonality. Duration of cyst excretion is variable but can range from weeks to months. Giardiasis is communicable for as long as the infected person excretes cysts.

The **incubation period** usually is 1 to 3 weeks.

DIAGNOSTIC TESTS: Commercially available, sensitive, and specific enzyme immunoassay (EIA) and direct fluorescence antibody (DFA) assays are the standard tests used for diagnosis of giardiasis in the United States. These antigen-based tests have largely replaced microscopic ova and parasite examination as first line diagnosis of giardiasis. EIA has a sensitivity of up to 95% and a specificity of 98% to 100% when compared with microscopy. DFA assay has the additional advantage that organisms are visualized. Both EIA and DFA are available as dual tests for the simultaneous detection of both *Giardia* and *Cryptosporidium* species. Laboratories can reduce reagent and personnel costs by pooling multiple specimens submitted from the same patient before evaluation either by DFA or EIA. In general, it is sufficient to diagnose giardiasis based on a single stool specimen when DFA or EIA is used. This is also true for the more multiplexed nucleic acid amplification tests recently cleared by the US Food and Drug Administration (FDA) for detection of *Giardia*, *Cryptosporidium*, and other intestinal pathogens. Only molecular testing (polymerase chain reaction assay) can be used to subtype *Giardia* species.

There are a number of advantages in use of antigen- or nucleic acid amplification-based tests for giardiasis. Traditionally, diagnosis has been based on the microscopic identification of trophozoites or cysts in stool specimens. However, sensitivity can be suboptimal if the specimen contains low numbers of organisms. When giardiasis is suspected clinically but the organism is not found on repeated stool examination, inspection of duodenal contents obtained by direct aspiration or by using a commercially available string test (Enterotest) may be diagnostic. Rarely, duodenal or intestinal biopsy is required for diagnosis in patients with characteristic clinical symptoms who have negative results of stool examinations and duodenal fluid specimen testing. Giardiasis is not associated with eosinophilia.

TREATMENT: Some infections are self-limited, and treatment is not required. Dehydration and electrolyte abnormalities can occur and should be corrected. Metronidazole, nitazoxanide, and tinidazole are the drugs of choice. Although not FDA approved for this indication, metronidazole (if used for a 5-day course) is the least expensive of these therapies; however, it generally has poor palatability when compounded into a suspension. A 5- to 7-day course of metronidazole has an efficacy of 80% to 100% in pediatric patients. A single dose of tinidazole, a nitroimidazole for children 3 years and older, has a median efficacy of 91% in pediatric patients (range, 80%–100%) and has fewer adverse effects than does metronidazole. A 3-day course of nitazoxanide oral suspension has similar efficacy to metronidazole and has the advantage(s) of treating other intestinal parasites and of being approved for use in children 1 year and older (tablets approved for pediatric patients 12 years and older). Paromomycin, a poorly absorbed aminoglycoside that is 50%

to 70% effective, is recommended for treatment of symptomatic infection in pregnant women in the second and third trimester.

Symptom recurrence after completing antimicrobial treatment can be attributable to reinfection, post-*Giardia* lactose intolerance (occurs in 20%–40% of patients), immunosuppression, insufficient treatment, or drug resistance. Detailed exposure history and repeat fecal testing is important in determining the cause of recurrence of symptoms. If reinfection is suspected, a second course of the same drug should be effective. Treatment with a different class of drug is recommended for resistant giardiasis. Other treatment options include combination of a nitroimidazole plus quinacrine for at least 2 weeks or high-dose courses of the original agent.

Patients who are immunocompromised because of hypogammaglobulinemia or lymphoproliferative disease are at higher risk of giardiasis, and it is more difficult to treat in these patients. Among human immunodeficiency virus (HIV)-infected children and adults without acquired immunodeficiency syndrome (AIDS), effective combination antiretroviral therapy (cART) and antiparasitic therapy are the major initial treatments for these infections. Especially in HIV-infected children, cART should be part of the primary initial treatment for giardiasis. Patients with AIDS often respond to standard therapy; however, in some cases, additional treatment is required. If giardiasis is refractory to standard treatment among HIV-infected patients with AIDS, longer treatment duration, or combination antiparasitic therapy (eg, metronidazole plus one of the following: paromomycin, albendazole, or quinacrine) may be appropriate.

Treatment of asymptomatic carriers is not recommended but could be considered for carriers in households of patients with hypogammaglobulinemia or cystic fibrosis.

ISOLATION OF THE HOSPITALIZED PATIENT: In addition to standard precautions, contact precautions for the duration of illness are recommended for diapered and incontinent children.

CONTROL MEASURES: Prevention of giardiasis involves good hygiene and avoidance of water and food that might be contaminated. Infected people and people at risk especially should adhere to strict hand-hygiene techniques after contact with feces.

- **Handwashing:** Wash hands with soap and water for at least 20 seconds, rubbing hands together vigorously and scrubbing all surfaces:
  - ◆ Before preparing or eating food;
  - ◆ After using the toilet or assisting someone with using the toilet;
  - ◆ After changing a diaper or having a diaper changed;
  - ◆ After caring for someone who is ill with diarrhea; and
  - ◆ After handling an animal or its waste.
- **Child care centers:** In child care centers, improved sanitation and personal hygiene should be emphasized (also see Children in Out-of-Home Child Care, p 122). Hand hygiene with soap and water by staff and children should be emphasized, especially after toilet use or handling of soiled diapers, which is a key preventive action for control of spread of giardiasis. When an outbreak is suspected, the local health department should be contacted, and an epidemiologic investigation should be undertaken to identify and treat all symptomatic children, child care providers, and family members infected with *G intestinalis*. Infected children should be excluded until stools are contained in the diaper or the child is continent, stool frequency is no more than 2 stools above that child's normal frequency for the time the child is in the program, and the health

department agrees with the return to child care. Treatment or exclusion of asymptomatic carriers is not effective for outbreak control and is not recommended; testing of asymptomatic individuals is not recommended.

- **Drinking water:** Waterborne disease can be prevented by a combination of adequate filtration of water from surface water sources (eg, lakes, rivers, streams), chlorination, and maintenance of water distribution systems.
- **Camping/hiking:** Where water might be contaminated, travelers, campers, and hikers should be advised of methods to make water safe for drinking, including boiling, chemical disinfection, and filtration. Boiling is the most reliable method to make water safe for drinking. The time of boiling depends on altitude (1 minute at sea level). Chemical disinfection with iodine is an alternative method of water treatment using either tincture of iodine or tetraglycine hydroperiodide tablets. Chlorine in various forms also can be used for chemical disinfection, but germicidal activity is dependent on several factors, including pH, temperature, and organic content of the water. Commercially available portable water filters provide various degrees of protection. Many commercially available filters are marketed as being able to remove *Giardia* and *Cryptosporidium* organisms from water. Additional information about water purification, including a traveler's guide for buying water filters, can be found at **http://www.cdc. gov/parasites/crypto/gen_info/filters.html.**
- **Recreational water:** People with diarrhea caused by *Giardia* species should not use recreational water venues (eg, swimming pools, water slides) while symptomatic. After cessation of symptoms, children who had diarrhea attributable to *Giardia* and who are incontinent should avoid recreational water activities for 1 additional week. People should avoid ingestion of recreational water. For additional information, see Prevention of Illnesses Associated With Recreational Water Use (p 200).
- **Immunosuppressed/HIV-infected people:** For immunosuppressed people, the risk of giardiasis and severity of the infection increases with the severity of immunosuppression. There is no specific preventive course, but cART is the primary method to prevent advanced immunodeficiency.[1]

Gonococcal Infections

CLINICAL MANIFESTATIONS: Gonococcal infections in children and adolescents occur in 3 distinct age groups.
- Infection in the **newborn infant** usually involves the eyes. Other possible manifestations of neonatal gonococcal infection include scalp abscess (which can be associated with fetal scalp monitoring) and disseminated disease with bacteremia, arthritis, or meningitis. Vaginitis and urethritis may occur as well.
- In children beyond the newborn period, including **prepubertal children,** gonococcal infection may occur in the genital tract and almost always is transmitted sexually. Vaginitis is the most common manifestation in prepubertal females. Progression to pelvic inflammatory disease (PID) appears to be less common in this age group than in

[1]Panel on Opportunistic Infections in HIV-Exposed and HIV-Infected Children. Guidelines for the Prevention and Treatment of Opportunistic Infections in HIV-Exposed and HIV-Infected Children. Rockville, MD: US Department of Health and Human Services; 2013. Available at: **https://aidsinfo.nih.gov/contentfiles/ lvguidelines/oi_guidelines_pediatrics.pdf**

older adolescents. Gonococcal urethritis is possible but uncommon in prepubertal males. Anorectal and tonsillopharyngeal infection can occur in prepubertal children and often is asymptomatic.

- In **sexually active adolescent and young adult females,** gonococcal infection of the genital tract often is asymptomatic. Common clinical syndromes include urethritis, endocervicitis, and salpingitis. In males, infection often is symptomatic, and the primary site is the urethra. Infection of the rectum and pharynx can occur alone or with genitourinary tract infection in either gender. Rectal and pharyngeal infections often are asymptomatic. Extension from primary genital mucosal sites in males can lead to epididymitis and in females can lead to bartholinitis, PID with resultant tubal scarring, and perihepatitis (Fitz-Hugh-Curtis syndrome). Even asymptomatic infection in females can progress to PID with tubal scarring that can result in ectopic pregnancy, infertility, or chronic pelvic pain. Infection involving other mucous membranes can produce conjunctivitis, pharyngitis, or proctitis. Hematogenous spread from mucosal sites can involve skin and joints (arthritis-dermatitis syndrome; disseminated gonococcal infection) and occurs in up to 3% of untreated people with mucosal gonorrhea. Bacteremia can result in a maculopapular rash with necrosis, tenosynovitis, and migratory arthritis. Arthritis may be reactive (sterile) or septic in nature. Meningitis and endocarditis occur rarely.

ETIOLOGY: *Neisseria gonorrhoeae* is a gram-negative, oxidase-positive diplococcus.

EPIDEMIOLOGY: Gonococcal infections occur only in humans. The source of the organism is exudate and secretions from infected mucosal surfaces; *N gonorrhoeae* is communicable as long as a person harbors the organism. Transmission results from intimate contact, such as sexual acts, parturition, and very rarely, household exposure in prepubertal children. Sexual abuse should be considered strongly when genital, rectal, or pharyngeal colonization or infection is diagnosed in prepubertal children beyond the newborn period (see STIs in Children, p 168).

N gonorrhoeae infection is the second most commonly reported sexually transmitted infection (STI) in the United States, following *Chlamydia trachomatis* infection. In 2014, a total of 350 062 cases of gonorrhea were reported in the United States, a rate of 111 cases per 100 000 population, and 53% of reported gonorrhea cases were diagnosed among 15 through 24-year-olds.[1] Among males and females, the rate is highest in those 20 through 24 years of age. Racial disparities are remarkable. In 2014, the rate of gonorrhea among black people was 11 times the rate among white people. Rates were 4 times higher among American Indian/Alaska Native people, 3 times higher among Native Hawaiian/Pacific Islander people, and 2 times higher among Hispanic people than among white people. Disparities in gonorrhea rates also are observed by sexual behavior. Surveillance networks that monitor trends in STI prevalence among men who have sex with men (MSM) have found very high proportions of positive gonorrhea pharyngeal, urethral, and rectal test results as well as coinfection with other STIs and human immunodeficiency virus (HIV).

The **incubation period** usually is 2 to 7 days.

Concurrent infection with *C trachomatis* is common. Diagnosis of genitourinary tract gonorrhea infection in a child, adolescent, or young adult should prompt investigation for other STIs, including chlamydia, trichomoniasis, syphilis, and HIV infection.

---

[1]Centers for Disease Control and Prevention. *Sexually Transmitted Disease Surveillance 2014.* Atlanta, GA: US Department of Health and Human Services; 2015

DIAGNOSTIC TESTS[1,2]: Microscopic examination of Gram-stained smears of exudate from the conjunctivae, vagina of prepubertal girls, male urethra, skin lesions, synovial fluid, and when clinically warranted, cerebrospinal fluid (CSF) may be useful in the initial evaluation. Identification of gram-negative intracellular diplococci in these smears can be helpful, particularly if the organism is not recovered in culture. However, because of low sensitivity, a negative smear result should not be considered sufficient for ruling out infection. Intracellular gram-negative diplococci identified on Gram stain of conjunctival exudate justify presumptive treatment for gonorrhea after appropriate cultures and antimicrobial susceptibility testing for *N gonorrhoeae* are performed.

N gonorrhoeae can be isolated from normally sterile sites, such as blood, CSF, or synovial fluid, using nonselective chocolate agar with incubation in 5% to 10% carbon dioxide. Selective media that inhibit normal flora and nonpathogenic *Neisseria* organisms are used for cultures from nonsterile sites, such as the cervix, vagina, rectum, urethra, and pharynx. Specimens for *N gonorrhoeae* culture from mucosal sites should be inoculated immediately onto appropriate agar, because the organism is extremely sensitive to drying and temperature changes.

Nucleic acid amplification tests (NAATs) are far superior in overall performance compared with other *N gonorrhoeae* culture and nonculture diagnostic methods to test genital and nongenital specimens.[2] Most commercially available products now are approved by the US Food and Drug Administration (FDA) for testing male urethral swab specimens, female endocervical or vaginal swab specimens (provider or patient collected), male or female urine specimens, or liquid cytology specimens. Package inserts for individual NAAT products should be reviewed, because the particular specimens approved for use with each test may vary. Many clinical laboratories have met Clinical Laboratory Improvement Amendment (CLIA) and other regulatory requirements and have validated gonorrhea NAAT performance on specimens. Providers can check with their clinical laboratory regarding gonorrhea specimen testing availability. Use of less-invasive specimens, such as urine or vaginal swab specimens, increases feasibility of routine testing of sexually active adolescents by their primary care providers and in other clinical settings. NAATs also permit dual testing of specimens for *C trachomatis* and *N gonorrhoeae*. The Centers for Disease Control and Prevention (CDC) recommends the vaginal swab specimen, including self-collected specimens, as the preferred means of screening females and urine as the preferred means of screening males for *N gonorrhoeae* infection. Female urine remains an acceptable gonorrhea NAAT specimen but may have slightly reduced performance when compared with cervical or vaginal swab specimens.

For identifying *N gonorrhoeae* from nongenital sites, culture is the most widely used test and allows for antimicrobial susceptibility testing to aid in management should infection persist following initial therapy. NAATs are not FDA cleared for *N gonorrhoeae* testing on rectal or pharyngeal swabs but are more sensitive compared with *N gonorrhoeae* culture. Some NAATs have the potential to cross-react with nongonococcal *Neisseria* species that commonly are found in the throat, leading to false-positive test results.

---

[1]American Academy of Pediatrics, Committee on Adolescence; Society for Adolescent Health and Medicine. Screening for nonviral sexually transmitted infections in adolescents and young adults. *Pediatrics.* 2014;134(1):e302–e311

[2]Centers for Disease Control and Prevention. Recommendations for the laboratory-based detection of *Chlamydia trachomatis* and *Neisseria gonorrhoeae*—2014. *MMWR Recomm Rep.* 2014;63(RR-2):1–19

Sexual Abuse.[1] In all prepubertal children beyond the newborn period and in adolescents who have gonococcal infection but report no prior sexual activity, sexual abuse must be considered to have occurred until proven otherwise (see Sexually Transmitted Infections in Adolescents and Children, p 165). Health care providers have a responsibility to report suspected sexual abuse to the state child protective services agency. This mandate does not require that the provider is certain that abuse has occurred but only that there is "reasonable cause to suspect abuse." Cultures should be performed on specimens from the pharynx and anus in boys and girls, the vagina in girls, and the urethra in boys before antimicrobial treatment is administered. Cervical specimens are not recommended for prepubertal girls. For boys with urethral discharge, a meatal discharge specimen is an adequate substitute for an intraurethral swab specimen. All gonococcal isolates from such patients should be retained for additional testing. Nonculture gonococcal tests, including Gram stain, DNA probes, enzyme immunoassays, or NAATs of oropharyngeal, rectal, or genital tract swab specimens in children may have false-positive results. NAATs can be used as alternative to culture with vaginal swab specimens or urine specimens from prepubertal girls. Culture remains the preferred method for urethral specimens from boys and extragenital specimens (pharynx and rectum) in boys and girls.

Detection of gonorrhea in a child requires an evaluation for other STIs, such as *C trachomatis* infection, syphilis, trichomoniasis, and HIV infection. If the hepatitis B and human papillomavirus vaccine series have not been completed, these immunizations should be offered if appropriate for age.

TREATMENT[2,3,4]: The rapid emergence of antimicrobial resistance has led to a limited number of approved therapies for gonococcal infections. Resistance to penicillin and tetracycline is widespread, and as of 2007, the CDC no longer recommends the use of fluoroquinolones for gonorrhea because of the increased prevalence of quinolone-resistant *N gonorrhoeae* in the United States. This leaves the cephalosporins as the only recommended antimicrobial class for the treatment of gonococcal infections. Over the past decade, the minimum inhibitory concentrations (MIC) for cefixime against *N gonorrhoeae* strains circulating in the United States and other countries has increased, suggesting that resistance to this drug is emerging. Treatment failure following the use of cefixime has been described in North America, Europe, and Asia. Therefore, as of 2012, the CDC no longer recommends the use of cefixime as a first-line treatment for gonococcal infection.

To minimize disease transmission, people treated for gonorrhea should be instructed to abstain from sexual activity for 7 days after treatment and until all sex partners are adequately treated (7 days after receiving treatment and resolution of symptoms, if present).

---

[1]Jenny C, Crawford-Jakubiak JE; American Academy of Pediatrics, Committee on Child Abuse and Neglect. The evaluation of children in the primary care setting when sexual abuse is suspected. *Pediatrics.* 2013;132(2): e558–e567

[2]Centers for Disease Control and Prevention. Sexually transmitted diseases treatment guidelines, 2015. *MMWR Recomm Rep.* 2015;64(RR-3):1–137

[3]American Academy of Pediatrics, Committee on Adolescence; Society for Adolescent Health and Medicine. Screening for nonviral sexually transmitted infections in adolescents and young adults. *Pediatrics.* 2014;134(1): e302–e311

[4]Centers for Disease Control and Prevention. *Sexually Transmitted Disease Surveillance 2015: Gonococcal Isolate Surveillance Project (GISP) Supplement and Profiles.* Atlanta: US Department of Health and Human Services; 2017. Available at: **www.cdc.gov/std/gisp/default.htm**

All patients with presumed or proven gonorrhea should be evaluated for concurrent syphilis, HIV, and *C trachomatis* infections.

Uncomplicated Gonococcal Infections of the Cervix, Urethra, and Rectum in Adolescents. Dual therapy using ceftriaxone (250 mg, intramuscularly, once) with azithromycin (1 g, orally) is the recommended treatment for all uncomplicated gonococcal infections (see Table 3.8, p 361). As dual therapy, ceftriaxone and azithromycin should be administered together on the same day, preferably simultaneously and under direct observation. Although other parenteral extended-spectrum cephalosporins, such as ceftizoxime (500 mg, intramuscularly), cefoxitin (2 g, intramuscularly, with probenecid, 1 g, orally), and cefotaxime (500 mg, intramuscularly), may be acceptable, they offer no clear advantage over ceftriaxone in most cases, and their efficacy in the treatment of pharyngeal infections has not been well documented. Oral cefixime (400 mg, orally, in a single dose, plus azithromycin, 1 g, orally) should only be considered for treatment of an anogenital infection if parenteral treatment with ceftriaxone is not available.

Pharyngeal Infection. Pharyngeal infection generally is more difficult to cure than anogenital infection. Patients with uncomplicated pharyngeal gonococcal infection should be treated with ceftriaxone (250 mg, intramuscularly, in a single dose) plus azithromycin (1 g, orally, in a single dose). See Table 3.9 (p 362).

Neonatal Disease. Infants with clinical evidence of ophthalmia neonatorum, scalp abscess, or disseminated infections attributable to *N gonorrhoeae* should be hospitalized. Cultures of blood, eye discharge, and other potential sites of infection, such as CSF, should be performed on specimens from infants to confirm the diagnosis and to determine antimicrobial susceptibility. Tests for concomitant infection with *C trachomatis*, congenital syphilis, and HIV infection should be performed; azithromycin should not be administered unless the diagnostic assessment is positive for *C trachomatis*. Results of the maternal test for hepatitis B surface antigen should be confirmed. The mother and her partner(s) need appropriate examination and treatment for *N gonorrhoeae*.

Ophthalmia Neonatorum. Recommended antimicrobial therapy for ophthalmia neonatorum caused by *N gonorrhoeae* is a single one-time dose of ceftriaxone (25 to 50 mg/kg, intravenously or intramuscularly, not to exceed 125 mg). Ceftriaxone should not be used in neonates (28 days of age and younger) receiving (or expected to receive) calcium-containing intravenous products. Infants with gonococcal ophthalmia should receive eye irrigations with saline solution immediately and at frequent intervals until discharge is eliminated. Topical antimicrobial treatment alone is inadequate as well as unnecessary when recommended systemic antimicrobial treatment is administered. Infants with gonococcal ophthalmia should be hospitalized, managed in consultation with an infectious disease specialist, and evaluated for disseminated infection (sepsis, arthritis, meningitis).

Disseminated Neonatal Infections and Scalp Abscesses. Recommended therapy for arthritis, septicemia, or abscess is ceftriaxone (25 to 50 mg/kg/day, intravenously or intramuscularly, in a single daily dose for 7 days) or cefotaxime (25 mg/kg, every 12 hours for 7 days). Cefotaxime is recommended for infants with hyperbilirubinemia. If meningitis is documented, treatment should be continued for a total of 10 to 14 days.

Gonococcal Infections in Children Beyond the Neonatal Period and Adolescents. Recommendations for treatment of gonococcal infections, by site of infection, age, and weight, are provided in Tables 3.9 (p 362) and 3.10 (p 362).

Table 3.8. Gonococcal Infection: Recommended Treatment of Children Weighing >45 kg, Adolescents, and Young Adults

Disease	Recommended Treatment	Alternative Treatment
Uncomplicated gonococcal infections of the cervix, urethra, and rectum	Ceftriaxone, 250 mg, IM, in a single dose **PLUS** Azithromycin, 1 g, orally, in a single dose	If ceftriaxone not available: Ceftizoxime, 500 mg, IM, **OR** Cefoxitin, 2 g, IM, with Probenecid, 1 g, orally, **OR** Cefotaxime, 500 mg, IM, in a single dose **PLUS** Azithromycin, 1 g, orally, in a single dose If parenteral cephalosporin treatment is not available: Cefixime, 400 mg, orally, **PLUS** Azithromycin, 1 g, orally, in a single dose If cephalosporin allergy: Gemifloxacin, 320 mg, orally, **OR** Gentamicin, 240 mg, IM, in a single dose **PLUS** Azithromycin, 2 g, orally, in a single dose If azithromycin allergy: Doxycycline, 100 mg, orally, twice a day for 7 days in place of azithromycin when used in combination with Ceftriaxone or Cefixime If using alternative treatment regimen: test of cure using either gonorrhea culture or NAAT 14 days after treatment
Uncomplicated gonococcal infections of the pharynx	Ceftriaxone, 250 mg, IM, in a single dose **PLUS** Azithromycin, 1 g, orally, in a single dose	

Table 3.8. Gonococcal Infection: Recommended Treatment of Children Weighing >45 kg, Adolescents, and Young Adults, *continued*

Disease	Recommended Treatment	Alternative Treatment
Conjunctivitis[a,b]	Ceftriaxone, 1 g, IM, in a single dose **PLUS** Azithromycin, 1 g, orally, in a single dose	
Disseminated gonococcal infection: arthritis and arthritis-dermatitis syndrome[a,c,d]	Ceftriaxone, 1 g, IM or IV, every 24 hours **PLUS** Azithromycin, 1 g, orally, in a single dose	Cefotaxime, 1 g, IV, **OR** Ceftizoxime, 1 g, IV, every 8 hours **PLUS** Azithromycin, 1 g, orally, in a single dose
Disseminated gonococcal infection: meningitis and endocarditis[a,c,e]	Ceftriaxone, 1–2 g, IV, every 12–24 hours **PLUS** Azithromycin, 1 g, orally, in a single dose	
Epididymitis	Ceftriaxone, 250 mg, IM, in a single dose **PLUS** Doxycycline, 100 mg, orally, twice daily for 10 days	
Pelvic inflammatory disease	See Table 3.50 (p 618)	

IV indicates intravenously; IM, intramuscularly; NAAT, nucleic acid amplification test.

[a]Consult infectious-disease specialist.

[b]Consider one-time lavage of the infected eye with saline solution.

[c]Hospitalization for initial therapy recommended.

[d]Can switch to oral agent guided by antimicrobial susceptibility testing 24–48 hours after substantial clinical improvement for at least 7 days of total therapy.

[e]Therapy for meningitis continued for 10–14 days; parenteral antimicrobial therapy for endocarditis should be administered for at least 28 days.

Adapted from Centers for Disease Control and Prevention. Sexually transmitted diseases treatment guidelines, 2015. *MMWR Recomm Rep.* 2015;64(RR-3):1–137.

Table 3.9. Uncomplicated Gonococcal Infection: Recommended Treatment of Infants and Children Beyond the Newborn Period[a]

Disease	Prepubertal Children Who Weigh ≤100 lb (≤45 kg)	Disease	Patients Who Weigh >100 lb (>45 kg)
Uncomplicated vulvovaginitis, cervicitis, urethritis, proctitis, or pharyngitis	Ceftriaxone, 25–50 mg/kg, IV or IM, in a single dose, not to exceed 125 mg	Uncomplicated endocervicitis, urethritis, proctitis, or pharyngitis	Treat with one of the regimens recommended f[z]or adults (see Table 3.8) Alternative regimen for patients with severe cephalosporin allergy: consult an expert in infectious diseases[b]

IV indicates intravenously; IM, intramuscularly.

[a]No data exist regarding the use of dual therapy for treating children with gonococcal infection.

[b]Because data are limited regarding alternative regimens for treating gonorrhea among children who have documented cephalosporin allergy, consultation with an expert in infectious diseases is recommended.

Adapted from Centers for Disease Control and Prevention. Sexually transmitted diseases treatment guidelines, 2015. *MMWR Recomm Rep.* 2015;64(RR-3):1–137.

Table 3.10. Complicated Gonococcal Infection: Treatment of Infants and Children Beyond the Newborn Period[a]

Disease	Prepubertal Children Who Weigh ≤100 lb (≤45 kg)
Bacteremia or arthritis[b,c]	Ceftriaxone, 50 mg/kg/day (maximum 1 g/day), IV or IM, once a day for 7 days
Meningitis or endocarditis[b,c]	Ceftriaxone, 50 mg/kg/day (maximum 2 g/day), IV or IM, administered every 12–24 h; for meningitis, duration is 10–14 days; for endocarditis, duration is at least 28 days
Conjunctivitis[b,d]	Ceftriaxone, 50 mg/kg (maximum 125 mg), IM, in a single dose

IV indicates intravenously; IM, intramuscularly.

[a]No data exist regarding the use of dual therapy for treating children with gonococcal infection.

[b]Consult infectious-disease specialist.

[c]Hospitalization for initial therapy recommended

[d]Eyes should be lavaged with saline solution to clear accumulated secretions

Adapted from Centers for Disease Control and Prevention. Sexually transmitted diseases treatment guidelines, 2015. *MMWR Recomm Rep.* 2015;64(RR-3):1–137.

Special Problems in Treatment of Children (Beyond the Neonatal Period) and Adolescents. Providers treating patients with uncomplicated infections of the vagina, endocervix, urethra, or anorectum and a history of severe **adverse reactions to cephalosporins** (eg, anaphylaxis, ceftriaxone-induced hemolysis, Stevens-Johnson syndrome, toxic epidermal necrolysis) should consult an expert in infectious diseases. In adolescents, dual treatment with a single dose of gemifloxacin (320 mg) plus oral azithromycin (2 g) or dual treatment with a single dose of intramuscular gentamicin (240 mg) plus oral azithromycin (2 g) are potential therapeutic options. However, gastrointestinal tract adverse events might limit the use of these regimens. Monotherapy with azithromycin (2 g, orally, as a single dose) no longer is recommended because of concerns about the ease with which *N gonorrhoeae* can develop resistance to macrolides and because several studies have documented azithromycin treatment failures. Spectinomycin (40 mg/kg, maximum 2 g, administered intramuscularly as a single dose) is an alternative but is not being produced in the United States. In the case of **azithromycin allergy,** doxycycline (100 mg, orally, twice a day for 7 days) can be used in place of azithromycin as an alternative second antimicrobial when used in combination with ceftriaxone or cefixime. Children or adolescents with **HIV infection** should receive the same treatment for gonococcal infection as children without HIV infection.

Acute PID. *N gonorrhoeae* and *C trachomatis* are implicated in many cases of PID; most cases have a polymicrobial etiology. No reliable clinical criteria distinguish gonococcal from nongonococcal-associated PID. Hence, broad-spectrum treatment regimens are recommended (see Pelvic Inflammatory Disease, p 614).

Acute Epididymitis. Sexually transmitted organisms, such as *N gonorrhoeae* or *C trachomatis,* can cause acute epididymitis in sexually active adolescents and young adults but rarely, if ever, cause acute epididymitis in prepubertal children. The recommended regimen for sexually transmitted epididymitis is ceftriaxone (250 mg, intramuscularly, once) plus doxycycline (100 mg, twice daily for 10 days). See Table 3.10 (p 362).

ISOLATION OF THE HOSPITALIZED PATIENT: Standard precautions are recommended, including for newborn infants with ophthalmia.

CONTROL MEASURES:

Follow-Up. A test of cure is not required for adolescents with uncomplicated urogenital or rectal gonorrhea who are asymptomatic after being treated with a recommended or alternative antimicrobial regimen. If an alternative regimen is used for treatment of pharyngeal gonorrhea infection, the CDC recommends a test of cure 14 days after treatment with culture or NAAT; if the NAAT result remains positive, every effort should be made to obtain a culture for susceptibility testing. Children treated with ceftriaxone do not require follow-up cultures unless they remain in an at-risk environment, but if treated with other regimens for pharyngeal infection, follow-up culture is indicated. Patients who have symptoms that persist after treatment or whose symptoms recur shortly after treatment should be reevaluated by culture for *N gonorrhoeae* (with or without simultaneous NAAT), and any gonococci isolated should be tested for antimicrobial susceptibility. Treatment failures should be reported to the CDC through the local or state health department.

Because patients may be reinfected by a new or untreated partner within a few months after diagnosis and treatment, providers should advise all adolescents with a diagnosis of gonorrhea to be retested approximately 3 months after treatment. Patients who do not receive a test of reinfection at 3 months should be tested whenever they are seen for care within the next 12 months. All patients with presumed or proven gonorrhea should be evaluated for concurrent syphilis, HIV, and *C trachomatis* infections.

Neonatal Ophthalmia. For routine prophylaxis of infants immediately after birth, 0.5% erythromycin ophthalmic ointment is instilled into each eye; subsequent irrigation should not be performed (see Prevention of Neonatal Ophthalmia, p 1046). Erythromycin is the only antibiotic ointment recommended in neonates. Prophylaxis may be delayed for up to 1 hour after birth to facilitate parent-infant bonding, but a monitoring system should be in place to ensure that all newborn infants receive prophylaxis no later than 1 hour after birth. Topical prophylaxis for preventing chlamydial ophthalmia is not effective, likely because colonization of the nasopharynx is not prevented.

Infants Born to Mothers With Gonococcal Infections. When prophylaxis is administered correctly, infants born to mothers with gonococcal infection rarely develop gonococcal ophthalmia. However, because gonococcal ophthalmia or disseminated infection occasionally can occur in this situation, infants born to mothers known to have gonorrhea should receive ceftriaxone as a single dose of 25 to 50 mg/kg (maximum dose, 125 mg), intravenously or intramuscularly (see Prevention of Neonatal Ophthalmia, p 1046). Ceftriaxone should not be used in neonates (28 days of age and younger) receiving (or expected to receive) calcium-containing intravenous products. When systemic ceftriaxone therapy is administered prophylactically, topical antimicrobial therapy is not necessary.

Children and Adolescents With Sexual Exposure to a Patient Known to Have Gonorrhea. Exposed people should undergo examination and culture and should receive the same treatment as do people known to have gonorrhea.

Pregnancy. All pregnant females younger than 25 years should be screened for gonorrhea at the first prenatal visit. A repeat test in the third trimester is recommended for females at continued risk of gonococcal infection, including females younger than 25 years. Pregnant females with a diagnosis of gonorrhea should be treated immediately and retested within 3 months. Pregnant females who remain at high risk for gonococcal infection should be retested during the third trimester. Health care professionals should consider the communities they serve and may choose to consult local public health authorities for guidance on identifying groups that are at increased risk. Gonococcal infection, in particular, is concentrated in specific geographic locations and communities. For pregnant females who are severely allergic to cephalosporins, consultation with an infectious diseases expert is indicated.

Routine Screening Tests.[1] All sexually active females younger than 25 years should be tested at least annually for gonorrhea infection, even if no symptoms are present or barrier contraception is reported. Sexually active adolescent and young adult MSM should be screened routinely for oral, rectal, and urethral gonorrhea at least annually if they engage in receptive oral or anal or insertive intercourse, respectively. Screening should be performed every 3 to 6 months if the person is at high risk because of multiple or anonymous partners, sex in conjunction with illicit drug use, or having sex partners who participate in these activities. Screening should be considered annually for sexually active males who have sex with females on the basis of individual and population-based risk factors, such as disparities by race and neighborhoods.

Case Reporting and Management of Sexual Partners. All cases of gonorrhea must be reported

---

[1]American Academy of Pediatrics, Committee on Adolescence, and Society for Adolescent Health and Medicine. Screening for nonviral sexually transmitted infections in adolescents and young adults. *Pediatrics.* 2014;134(1):e302–e311

to local public health officials (see Appendix IV, Nationally Notifiable Infectious Diseases in the United States, p 1069). Ensuring that sexual contacts are treated and counseled to use condoms is essential for community control, prevention of reinfection, and prevention of complications in contacts. All sexual contacts in the 60 days preceding onset of symptoms in the index case should be evaluated for *N gonorrhoeae* infection and presumptively treated. If time of the last sexual contact was more than 60 days before symptom onset or patient diagnosis, the most recent sex partner should be evaluated and treated. Recommendations for services provided to partners of people with gonorrhea are available.[1] Cases in prepubertal children must be investigated to determine the source of infection.

Among females or heterosexual male patients, if concerns exist that sex partners will not seek care, expedited partner therapy (EPT), the clinical practice of treating the sex partners of patients with a diagnosis of chlamydia or gonorrhea by providing prescriptions or medications to the patient to take to his or her partner without the health care provider first examining the partner, can be considered.[2] For EPT for gonorrhea infection, cefixime (400 mg) and azithromycin (1 g) can be delivered to the partner by the patient. EPT, especially for gonorrhea, always should be accompanied by efforts to educate partners about symptoms and to encourage partners to seek clinical evaluation. To clarify the legal status of EPT in each state, refer to the CDC Web site (**www.cdc.gov/std/ept/**). EPT should not be considered a routine partner management strategy in MSM because of the high risk of coexisting undiagnosed STIs or HIV infection.

Granuloma Inguinale
(Donovanosis)

CLINICAL MANIFESTATIONS: Initial lesions of this sexually transmitted infection are single or multiple painless subcutaneous nodules that gradually ulcerate. These nontender, granulomatous ulcers are beefy red and highly vascular and bleed readily on contact. Lesions usually involve the genitalia without regional adenopathy, but anal infections occur in 5% to 10% of patients; lesions at distant sites (eg, face, mouth, or liver) are rare. Subcutaneous extension into the inguinal area results in induration that can mimic inguinal adenopathy (ie, "pseudobubo"). Verrucous, necrotic, and fibrous lesions may occur as well. Fibrosis manifests as sinus tracts, adhesions, and lymphedema, resulting in extreme genital deformity. Urethral obstruction can occur.

ETIOLOGY: The disease, Donovanosis, is caused by *Klebsiella granulomatis* (formerly known as *Calymmatobacterium granulomatis*), an intracellular gram-negative bacillus.

EPIDEMIOLOGY: Indigenous granuloma inguinale occurs very rarely in the United States and most industrialized nations. The disease is endemic in some tropical and developing areas, including India, Papua New Guinea, the Caribbean, central Australia, and southern Africa. The incidence of infection seems to correlate with sustained high temperatures and high relative humidity. Infection usually is acquired by sexual intercourse, most commonly with a person with active infection but possibly also from a person with

---

[1]Centers for Disease Control and Prevention. Recommendations for partner services programs for HIV infection, syphilis, gonorrhea, and chlamydial infection. *MMWR Recomm Rep.* 2008;57(RR-9):1–63

[2]Society for Adolescent Health and Medicine. Expedited partner therapy for adolescents diagnosed with chlamydia or gonorrhea: a position paper of the Society for Adolescent Medicine [Endorsed by the American Academy of Pediatrics in *Pediatrics* 2009;124(4):1264]. *J Adolesc Health.* 2009;45(3):303–309

asymptomatic rectal infection. Young children can acquire infection by contact with infected secretions. The period of communicability extends throughout the duration of active lesions or rectal colonization.

The **incubation period** is 8 to 80 days.

DIAGNOSTIC TESTS: The causative organism is difficult to culture, and diagnosis requires microscopic demonstration of dark-staining intracytoplasmic Donovan bodies on Wright or Giemsa staining of a crush preparation from subsurface scrapings of a lesion or tissue. The microorganism also can be detected by histologic examination of biopsy specimens. Lesions should be cultured for *Haemophilus ducreyi* to exclude chancroid. Granuloma inguinale often is misdiagnosed as carcinoma, which can be excluded by histologic examination of tissue or by response of the lesion to antimicrobial agents. Culture of *K granulomatis* is difficult to perform and is not available routinely. No molecular tests exist that have been cleared by the US Food and Drug Administration for the detection of *K granulomatis* DNA. Diagnosis by polymerase chain reaction assay and serologic testing is only available in research laboratories.

TREATMENT[1]: The recommended treatment regimen is azithromycin (1 g, orally, once per week, or 500 mg, daily) for at least 3 weeks and until all lesions have completely healed. Alternative therapies include doxycycline (100 mg, orally, twice a day), ciprofloxacin (750 mg, orally, twice a day), erythromycin base (500 mg, orally 4 times a day), or trimethoprim-sulfamethoxazole (1 double-strength [160 mg/800 mg] tablet, orally, twice a day). All treatment regimens should continue for at least 3 weeks and until all lesions have completely healed. Doxycycline can be used for short durations (ie, 21 days or less) without regard to patient age (see Tetracyclines, p 905). The addition of another antimicrobial agent to these regimens can be considered if improvement is not evident within the first few days of therapy. Addition of an aminoglycoside, such as gentamicin (1 mg/kg, intravenously, every 8 hours), to these regimens is an option. Treatment has been shown to halt progression of lesions. Partial healing usually is noted within 7 days of initiation of therapy and typically proceeds inward from the ulcer margins. Prolonged therapy usually is required to permit granulation and re-epithelialization of the ulcers. Relapse can occur, especially if the antimicrobial agent is stopped before the primary lesion has healed completely. In addition, relapse can occur 6 to 18 months after apparently effective therapy. Complicated or long-standing infection can require surgical intervention. Pregnant and lactating females should be treated with either erythromycin base (500 mg, orally, 4 times/day) or azithromycin (1 g, orally, once per week, or 500 mg daily) for at least 3 weeks and until all lesions have completely healed, and consideration should be given to adding a parenteral aminoglycoside (eg, gentamicin).

Patients should be evaluated for other sexually transmitted infections, such as gonorrhea, syphilis, chancroid, chlamydia, hepatitis B virus, and human immunodeficiency virus infections. If the hepatitis B and human papillomavirus vaccine series have not been completed, these immunizations should be offered if appropriate for age.

ISOLATION OF THE HOSPITALIZED PATIENT: Standard precautions are recommended.

CONTROL MEASURES: Sexual partners should be examined, counseled to use condoms, and offered antimicrobial therapy. The value of treating asymptomatic sexual partners has not been demonstrated.

---

[1]Centers for Disease Control and Prevention. Sexually transmitted diseases treatment guidelines, 2015. *MMWR Recomm Rep.* 2015; 64(RR-3):1–137

Haemophilus influenzae Infections

CLINICAL MANIFESTATIONS: *Haemophilus influenzae* type b (Hib) causes pneumonia, bacteremia, meningitis, epiglottitis, septic arthritis, cellulitis, otitis media, purulent pericarditis, and less commonly, endocarditis, endophthalmitis, osteomyelitis, peritonitis, and gangrene. Non-type b–encapsulated strains present in a similar manner to type b infections. Nontypable strains more commonly cause infections of the respiratory tract (eg, otitis media, sinusitis, pneumonia, conjunctivitis), but cases of bacteremia, meningitis, chorioamnionitis, and neonatal septicemia are well described.

ETIOLOGY: *H influenzae* is a pleomorphic gram-negative coccobacillus. Encapsulated strains express 1 of 6 antigenically distinct capsular polysaccharides (a through f); nonencapsulated strains lack capsule genes and are designated nontypable.

EPIDEMIOLOGY[1]: The mode of transmission is person to person by inhalation of respiratory tract droplets or by direct contact with respiratory tract secretions. In neonates, infection is acquired intrapartum by aspiration of amniotic fluid or by contact with genital tract secretions containing the organism. Pharyngeal colonization by *H influenzae* is relatively common, especially with nontypable and non-type b capsular type strains. Similar to findings in the pre-Hib vaccine era, in resource-limited countries where Hib vaccine has not been routinely implemented, the major reservoir of Hib is young infants and toddlers, who carry the organism in the upper respiratory tract.

Before introduction of effective Hib conjugate vaccines, Hib was the most common cause of bacterial meningitis in children in the United States. The peak incidence of invasive Hib infections occurred between 6 and 18 months of age. In contrast, the peak age for Hib epiglottitis was 2 to 4 years of age.

Unimmunized children younger than 5 years are at increased risk of invasive Hib disease. Factors that predispose to invasive disease include sickle cell disease, asplenia, human immunodeficiency virus (HIV) infection, certain immunodeficiency syndromes, and malignant neoplasms. Historically, invasive Hib infection was more common in black, Alaska Native, Apache, and Navajo children; boys; child care attendees; children living in crowded conditions; and children who were not breastfed.

Since introduction of Hib conjugate vaccines in the United States, the incidence of invasive Hib disease has decreased by 99% to fewer than 1 case per 100 000 children younger than 5 years. In 2013, 31 cases of invasive type b disease were reported in children younger than 5 years. In the United States, invasive Hib disease occurs primarily in underimmunized children and among infants too young to have completed the primary immunization series. Hib remains an important pathogen in many resource-limited countries where Hib vaccines are not available routinely.

The epidemiology of invasive *H influenzae* disease in the United States has shifted in the postvaccination era. Nontypable *H influenzae* now causes the majority of invasive *H influenzae* disease in all age groups. From 2009 through 2014, the annual incidence of invasive nontypable *H influenzae* disease was 1.7/100 000 in children younger than 5 years and 5.0/100 000 in adults 65 years and older. Nontypable *H influenzae* causes approximately 50% of episodes of acute otitis media and sinusitis in children and is a common cause of

---

[1]Centers for Disease Control and Prevention. Prevention and control of *Haemophilus influenzae* type b disease: recommendations of the Advisory Committee on Immunization Practices (ACIP). *MMWR Recomm Rep.* 2014;63(RR-1):1–14

recurrent otitis media. The rate of nontypable *H influenzae* infections (eg, otitis media and sinusitis) in boys is twice that in girls and peaks in the late fall.

In some North American indigenous populations, *H influenzae* type a (Hia) has emerged as the most common encapsulated serotype causing invasive disease, with a clinical presentation similar to Hib. The 2002–2012 incidence of Hia infection in Alaska Native children younger than 5 years was 18/100 000 (vs 0.5/100 000 in nonnative children). The incidence was highest in southwestern Alaska Native children younger than 5 years (72/100 000). Similarly, Hia has emerged among northern Canadian indigenous children, who experienced an incidence of 102/100 000/year in children younger than 2 years. There is an ongoing lower level of Hia disease in Navajo children younger than 5 years (20/100 000/year). Invasive disease has also been caused by other encapsulated non-type b strains.

The **incubation period** is unknown.

DIAGNOSTIC TESTS: The diagnosis of invasive disease is established by growth of *H influenzae* from cerebrospinal fluid (CSF), blood, synovial fluid, pleural fluid, or pericardial fluid. Because occult meningitis is well reported in young children with invasive Hib disease, a lumbar puncture should be strongly considered in the presence of invasive disease, even in the absence of central nervous system signs and symptoms. Gram stain of an infected body fluid specimen can facilitate presumptive diagnosis. Antigen detection methods, which have historically been used on CSF, blood, and urine specimens, no longer are recommended because they lack sensitivity and specificity. Nucleic acid amplification tests (NAATs) have been developed to detect *H influenzae* directly in clinical specimens, including at least 1 multiplexed assay that has received US Food and Drug Administration clearance for testing of CSF to detect a variety of agents of encephalitis and meningitis. This assay detects but does not differentiate among the 6 capsular polysaccharide types. At this time, such NAATs should be used in addition to culture because of limited clinical experience. Such a practice would allow for recovery of an isolate from CSF for serotyping for epidemiologic investigations as well as monitoring antimicrobial susceptibilities.

All *H influenzae* isolates associated with invasive infection should be typed to determine the capsular polysaccharide associated with the isolate. Serotyping by slide agglutination using polyclonal antisera traditionally had been the method of choice for typing. The potential for suboptimal sensitivity and specificity exists with serotyping depending on reagents used and the experience of the technologist. Capsule typing by molecular methods, such as PCR assay of the *cap* gene locus or outer membrane protein D gene locus, have enhanced sensitivity and specificity and are acceptable methods for capsule typing. If serotyping or typing by molecular methods are not available locally, isolates should be submitted to the state health department or to a reference laboratory for testing.

Otitis media attributable to *H influenzae* is diagnosed by culture of tympanocentesis fluid; organisms isolated from other respiratory tract swab specimens (eg, throat, ear drainage) may not be the same as those from middle-ear culture.

TREATMENT:

- Initial therapy for children with *H influenzae* meningitis is cefotaxime or ceftriaxone. Ampicillin may be substituted if the isolate is susceptible. Beta-lactamase–negative, ampicillin-resistant strains of *H influenzae* have been described, and some experts recommend caution in using ampicillin when minimum inhibitory concentrations (MICs) of 1 to 2 µg/mL are found, especially in the setting of invasive infection or disease in immunocompromised hosts. Treatment of other invasive *H influenzae* infections is similar. Therapy is continued for 7 to 10 days by the intravenous route and longer in complicated infections.

- Dexamethasone is beneficial for treatment of infants and children with Hib meningitis to diminish the risk of hearing loss, if administered before or concurrently with the first dose of antimicrobial agent(s).
- Epiglottitis is a medical emergency. An airway must be established promptly via controlled intubation.
- Infected pleural or pericardial fluid should be drained.
- For empiric treatment of acute otitis media in children younger than 2 years or in children 2 years or older with severe disease, oral amoxicillin (see details in Pneumococcal Infections, p 639, and Appropriate Use of Antimicrobial Agents, p 906) is recommended, unless the child has a prior history of amoxicillin therapy within the past 30 days.[1] For those younger than 2 years, the duration of therapy is 10 days. A 7-day course is considered for children 2 through 5 years of age, and a 5-day course may be used for older children. In the United States, approximately 30% to 40% of *H influenzae* isolates produce beta-lactamase, so amoxicillin may fail, necessitating use of a beta-lactamase–resistant agent, such as amoxicillin-clavulanate; an oral cephalosporin, such as cefdinir, cefuroxime, or cefpodoxime; or azithromycin for children with beta-lactam antibiotic allergy. In vitro susceptibility testing of isolates from middle-ear fluid specimens helps guide therapy in complicated or persistent cases.

ISOLATION OF THE HOSPITALIZED PATIENT: In addition to standard precautions, in patients with invasive Hib disease, droplet precautions are recommended for 24 hours after initiation of effective antimicrobial therapy.

CONTROL MEASURES (FOR INVASIVE HIB DISEASE):

Care of Exposed People. Secondary cases of Hib disease have occurred in unimmunized or incompletely immunized children exposed in a child care or household setting to invasive Hib disease. Such children should be observed carefully for fever or other signs/symptoms of disease. Exposed young children in whom febrile illness develops should receive prompt medical evaluation.

Chemoprophylaxis.[2] The risk of invasive Hib disease is increased among unimmunized household contacts younger than 4 years. Rifampin eradicates Hib from the pharynx in approximately 95% of carriers and decreases the risk of secondary invasive illness in exposed household contacts. Child care center contacts also may be at increased risk of secondary disease, but secondary disease in child care contacts is rare when all contacts are older than 2 years. Indications and guidelines for chemoprophylaxis in different circumstances are summarized in Table 3.11.

---

[1] Lieberthal AS, Carroll AE, Chonmaitree T, et al; American Academy of Pediatrics, Subcommittee on Diagnosis and Management of Acute Otitis Media. Clinical practice guideline: the diagnosis and management of acute otitis media. *Pediatrics.* 2013;131(3):e964–e999

[2] Centers for Disease Control and Prevention. Prevention and control of *Haemophilus influenzae* type b disease: recommendations of the Advisory Committee on Immunization Practices (ACIP). *MMWR Recomm Rep.* 2014;63(RR-1):1–14

Table 3.11. Indications and Guidelines for Rifampin Chemoprophylaxis for Contacts of Index Cases of Invasive *Haemophilus influenzae* Type b (Hib) Disease

Chemoprophylaxis Recommended

- For all household contacts[a] in the following circumstances:
  - ◆ Household with at least 1 contact younger than 4 years who is unimmunized or incompletely immunized[b]
  - ◆ Household with a child younger than 12 months who has not completed the primary Hib series
  - ◆ Household with a contact who is an immunocompromised child, regardless of that child's Hib immunization status or age
- For preschool and child care center contacts when 2 or more cases of Hib invasive disease have occurred within 60 days (see text)
- For index patient, if younger than 2 years or member of a household with a susceptible contact and treated with a regimen other than cefotaxime or ceftriaxone, chemoprophylaxis at the end of therapy for invasive infection

Chemoprophylaxis Not Recommended

- For occupants of households with no children younger than 4 years other than the index patient
- For occupants of households when all household contacts are immunocompetent, all household contacts 12 through 48 months of age have completed their Hib immunization series, and when household contacts younger than 12 months have completed their primary series of Hib immunizations
- For preschool and child care contacts of 1 index case
- For pregnant women

[a]Defined as people residing with the index patient or nonresidents who spent 4 or more hours with the index patient for at least 5 of the 7 days preceding the day of hospital admission of the index case.
[b]Complete immunization is defined as having had at least 1 dose of conjugate vaccine at 15 months of age or older; 2 doses between 12 and 14 months of age; or the 2- or 3-dose primary series when younger than 12 months with a booster dose at 12 months of age or older.

Clinicians may consider prophylaxis of contacts of index cases of invasive Hia disease, using the same criteria as that recommended in Table 3.11 and below for Hib disease. Chemoprophylaxis generally is not recommended for contacts of people with invasive disease caused by non-type b, non-type a, or nontypable *H influenzae* strains, because secondary disease is rare.

- **Household.** In households with a person with invasive Hib disease and at least 1 household member who is younger than 48 months and unimmunized or incompletely immunized against Hib, rifampin prophylaxis is recommended for all household contacts, regardless of age. In households with an immunocompromised child, even if the child is older than 48 months and fully immunized, all members of the household should receive rifampin because of the possibility that immunization may not have been effective. Similarly, in households with a contact younger than 12 months who has not received the 2- or 3-dose primary series of Hib conjugate vaccine, depending on vaccine product, all household members should receive rifampin prophylaxis. Given that most secondary cases in households occur during the first week after hospitalization of the index case, when indicated, prophylaxis (see Table 3.11) should be initiated as soon as possible. Because some secondary cases occur later, initiation of prophylaxis 7 days or more after hospitalization of the index patient still may be of some benefit.

- **Child care and preschool.** When 2 or more cases of invasive Hib disease have occurred within 60 days and unimmunized or incompletely immunized children attend the child care facility or preschool, rifampin prophylaxis for all attendees (irrespective of their age and vaccine status) and child care providers should be considered. In addition to these recommendations for chemoprophylaxis, unimmunized or incompletely immunized children should receive a dose of vaccine and should be scheduled for completion of the recommended age-specific immunization schedule (**https:// redbook.solutions.aap.org/SS/Immunization_Schedules.aspx**). Data are insufficient on the risk of secondary transmission to recommend chemoprophylaxis for attendees and child care providers when a single case of invasive Hib disease occurs; the decision to provide chemoprophylaxis in this situation is at the discretion of the local health department.

- **Index case.** Treatment of Hib disease with cefotaxime or ceftriaxone eradicates Hib colonization, eliminating the need for prophylaxis of the index patient. Patients who do not receive at least 1 dose of cefotaxime or ceftriaxone and who are younger than 2 years should receive rifampin prophylaxis at the end of therapy for invasive infection.

- **Dosage.** For prophylaxis, rifampin should be administered orally, once a day for 4 days (20 mg/kg; maximum dose, 600 mg). The dose for infants younger than 1 month is not established; some experts recommend lowering the dose to 10 mg/kg. For adults, each dose is 600 mg.

Immunization.[1] Three single-antigen (monovalent) Hib conjugate vaccine products and 1 combination vaccine product that contain Hib conjugate are available in the United States (see Table 3.12). The Hib conjugate vaccine consists of the Hib capsular polysaccharide (polyribosylribotol phosphate [PRP]) covalently linked to a carrier protein. Protective antibodies are directed against PRP.

Depending on the vaccine, the recommended primary series consists of 3 doses administered at 2, 4, and 6 months of age or of 2 doses administered at 2 and 4 months of age (see Recommendations for Immunization, p 373, and Table 3.13). The regimens in Table 3.13 likely are to be equivalent in protection after completion of the recommended primary series. For American Indian/Alaska Native children, optimal immune protection is achieved by administration of PRP-OMP (outer membrane protein complex) Hib vaccine (see American Indian/Alaska Native Children and Adolescents, *Haemophilus influenzae* type b, p 93). Information on immunogenicity after dose 1 of new Hib-containing vaccines is important for assessing their suitability for use in AI/AN children.

Combination Vaccine. There is one combination vaccine that contains Hib licensed in the United States: DTaP-IPV/Hib (DTaP-IPV/PRP-T [see Table 3.12]), licensed for children 6 weeks through 4 years of age, administered as a 4-dose series at 2, 4, 6, and 15 through 18 months of age.

Vaccine Interchangeability. Hib conjugate vaccines licensed within the age range for the

[1]Centers for Disease Control and Prevention. Prevention and control of *Haemophilus influenzae* type b disease: recommendations of the Advisory Committee on Immunization Practices (ACIP). *MMWR Recomm Rep.* 2014;63(RR-1):1–14

primary vaccine series are considered interchangeable as long as recommendations for a total of 3 doses in the first year of life are followed (ie, if 2 doses of Hib-OMP are not administered, 3 doses of a Hib-containing vaccine are required).

Dosage and Route of Administration. The dose of each Hib conjugate vaccine is 0.5 mL, administered intramuscularly.

Table 3.12. *Haemophilus influenzae* Type b (Hib) Conjugate Vaccines Licensed and Available for Use in Infants and Children in the United States[a]

Vaccine	Trade Name	Components	Manufacturer
PRP-T	ActHIB	PRP conjugated to tetanus toxoid	Sanofi Pasteur
PRP-T[a]	Hiberix	PRP conjugated to tetanus toxoid	GlaxoSmithKline Biologicals
PRP-OMP	PedvaxHIB	PRP conjugated to OMP	Merck & Co, Inc
DTaP-IPV/PRP-T[b]	Pentacel	DTaP-IPV + PRP-T	Sanofi Pasteur

PRP-T indicates polyribosylribotol phosphate-tetanus toxoid; DTaP, diphtheria and tetanus toxoids and acellular pertussis; OMP, outer membrane protein complex from *Neisseria meningitidis;* HepB, hepatitis B vaccine.

[a] Hib conjugate vaccines may be administered in combination products or as reconstituted products, provided the combination or reconstituted vaccine is licensed by the US Food and Drug Administration (FDA) for the child's age and administration of the other vaccine component(s) also is justified.

[b] The DTaP-IPV liquid component is used to reconstitute a lyophilized ActHIB vaccine component to form Pentacel.

Table 3.13. Recommended Regimens for Routine *Haemophilus influenzae* Type b (Hib) Conjugate Immunization for Children Immunized at 2 Months Through 4 Years of Age[a]

Vaccine Product	Primary Series	Booster Dose	Catch-up Doses[b]
PRP-T (ActHIB, Sanofi Pasteur)	2, 4, 6 mo	12 through 15 mo	16 mo through 4 y
PRP-T (Hiberix, GlaxoSmith-Kline)	2, 4, 6 mo	12 through 15 mo	16 mo through 4 y
PRP-OMP (PedvaxHIB, Merck)[c,d]	2, 4 mo	12 through 15 mo	16 mo through 4 y
Combination vaccine			
DTaP-IPV/PRP-T (Pentacel, Sanofi Pasteur)	2, 4, 6 mo	12 through 15 mo	16 mo through 4 y

PRP-T indicates polyribosylribotol phosphate-tetanus toxoid; OMP, outer membrane protein complex from *Neisseria meningitidis.*

[a] See text and Table 3.12 (p 372) for further information about specific vaccines and Table 1.12 (p 37) for information about combination vaccines.

[b] See Catch-up Immunization Schedule (**https://redbook.solutions.aap.org/SS/Immunization_Schedules.aspx**) for additional information.

[c] If a PRP-OMP vaccine is not administered as both doses in the primary series, a third dose of Hib conjugate vaccine is needed to complete the primary series.

[d] Preferred for American Indian/Alaska Native children.

Children With Immunologic Impairment. Children at increased risk of Hib disease may have impaired anti-PRP antibody responses to conjugate vaccines. Examples include children with functional or anatomic asplenia, HIV infection, or immunoglobulin deficiency (including an isolated immunoglobulin [Ig] G2 subclass deficiency) or early component complement deficiency); recipients of hematopoietic stem cell transplants; and children undergoing chemotherapy for a malignant neoplasm. Some children with immunologic impairment may benefit from more doses of conjugate vaccine than usually indicated (see Recommendations for Immunization: Indications and Schedule).

Adverse Reactions. Adverse reactions to Hib conjugate vaccines are uncommon. Pain, redness, and swelling at the injection site occur in approximately 25% of recipients, but these symptoms typically are mild and last fewer than 24 hours.

Recommendations for Immunization:

Indications and Schedule

- All children should be immunized with a Hib conjugate vaccine beginning at approximately 2 months of age (see Table 3.13). Other general recommendations are as follows:
  - ◆ Immunization can be initiated as early as 6 weeks of age.
  - ◆ Vaccine can be administered during visits for other childhood immunizations (see Simultaneous Administration of Multiple Vaccines, p 35).
- For routine immunization of children younger than 7 months, the following guidelines are recommended:
  - ◆ **Primary series.** A 3-dose regimen of PRP-T (tetanus toxoid conjugate)-containing or a 2-dose regimen of PRP-OMP-containing vaccine should be administered (see Table 3.13). Doses are administered at approximately 2-month intervals. When sequential doses of different vaccine products are administered or uncertainty exists about which products previously were used, 3 doses of a conjugate vaccine are considered sufficient to complete the primary series, regardless of the regimen used.
  - ◆ **Booster immunization at 12 through 15 months of age.** For children who have completed a primary series, an additional dose of conjugate vaccine is recommended at 12 through 15 months of age and at least 2 months after the last dose. Any monovalent or combination Hib conjugate vaccine is acceptable for this dose.
- Children younger than 5 years who did not receive Hib conjugate vaccine during the first 6 months of life should be immunized according to the recommended catch-up immunization schedule (see **https://redbook.solutions.aap.org/SS/Immunization_Schedules.aspx** and Table 3.13). For accelerated immunization in infants younger than 12 months, a minimum of a 4-week interval between doses can be used.
- Children with invasive Hib infection younger than 24 months can remain at risk of developing a second episode of disease. These children should be immunized according to the age-appropriate schedule for unimmunized children as if they had received no previous Hib vaccine doses (see Table 3.13, and Table 1.12, p 37). Immunization should be initiated 1 month after onset of disease or as soon as possible thereafter.

Immunologic evaluation should be performed in children who experience invasive Hib disease despite 2 to 3 doses of vaccine and in children with recurrent invasive disease attributable to type b strains.

- Special circumstances are as follows (Table 3.14):
  - **Lapsed immunizations.** Recommendations for children who have had a lapse in the schedule of immunizations are based on limited data. Current recommendations are summarized in the annual immunization schedule (**https://redbook.solutions.aap.org/SS/Immunization_Schedules.aspx).
  - **Preterm infants.** For preterm infants, immunization should be based on chronologic age and should be initiated at 2 months of age according to recommendations in Table 3.13.
  - **Functional/anatomic asplenia.** Children with decreased or absent splenic function who have received a primary series of Hib immunizations and a booster dose at 12 months or older need not be immunized further. Children who have not received a primary series and a booster dose and are undergoing scheduled splenectomy (eg, for Hodgkin disease, spherocytosis, immune thrombocytopenia, or hypersplenism) may benefit from an additional dose of any licensed conjugate vaccine. This dose should be provided at least 14 days before the procedure.
  - **Recipients of chemotherapy, radiation therapy, or hematopoietic stem cell transplants.** Because of potential suboptimal antibody response, Hib vaccination during chemotherapy or radiation therapy may not be effective; children younger than 60 months who are vaccinated within 14 days before starting immunosuppressive therapy or while receiving immunosuppressive therapy should be considered unimmunized, and doses should be repeated beginning at least 3 months after completion of chemotherapy. Recipients of hematopoietic stem cell transplants should be revaccinated with a 3-dose series at least 3 months after successful transplant, regardless of vaccination history or age.
  - **Other high-risk groups.** Children with HIV infection, IgG2 subclass deficiency, or early component complement deficiency are at increased risk of invasive Hib disease. Whether these children will benefit from additional doses after completion of the primary series of immunizations and the booster dose at 12 months or older is unknown.
- **Catch-up immunization for high-risk groups (https://redbook.solutions.aap.org/SS/Immunization_Schedules.aspx)** (Table 3.14):
  - For children 12 through 59 months of age with an underlying condition predisposing to Hib disease (functional or anatomic asplenia, HIV infection, immunoglobulin deficiency, early component complement deficiency, or receipt of hematopoietic stem cell transplant or chemotherapy for a malignant neoplasm) who are not immunized or have received only 1 dose of conjugate vaccine before 12 months of age, 2 doses of any conjugate vaccine, separated by 2 months, are recommended. For children in this age group who received 2 or more doses before 12 months of age, 1 additional dose of conjugate vaccine is recommended.
  - Unimmunized children older than 59 months of age with HIV infection or functional or anatomic asplenia, including sickle cell disease, should receive 1 dose of any licensed Hib conjugate vaccine.
  - Unimmunized children ≥15 months undergoing elective splenectomy should receive 1 dose of any licensed Hib vaccine; this dose should be provided well in advance of the procedure. Patients who have not received a primary series and booster dose or at least 1 dose of Hib vaccine after 14 months of age are considered unimmunized.

Table 3.14. Use of *Haemophilus influenzae* Type b (Hib) Conjugate Immunization in Special Populations

High-Risk Group	Vaccine Recommendations
Patient <12 mo	Follow routine Hib vaccination recommendations
Patients 12 through 59 mo	If unimmunized or received 0 or 1 dose before age 12 months: 2 doses 2 months apart
	If received 2 or more doses before age 12 months: 1 dose
	If completed a primary series and received a booster dose at age 12 months or older: no additional doses
Patients undergoing chemotherapy or radiation therapy, age <60 mo	If routine Hib doses administered 14 or more days before starting therapy: revaccination not required
	If dose administered within 14 days of starting therapy or administered during therapy: repeat doses starting at least 3 months following therapy completion
Patients undergoing elective splenectomy, age ≥15 mo	If unimmunized[a]: 1 dose prior to procedure
Asplenic patients ≥60 mo and adults	If unimmunized[a]: 1 dose
HIV-infected children ≥60 mo	If unimmunized[a]: 1 dose
HIV-infected adults	Hib vaccination is not recommended
Recipients of hematopoietic stem cell transplant, all ages	Regardless of Hib vaccination history: 3 doses (at least 1 month apart) beginning 6–12 mo after transplant

[a]Patients who have not received a primary series and booster dose or at least 1 dose of Hib vaccine after 14 months of age are considered unimmunized.

Reporting. All cases of *H influenzae* invasive disease, including type b, non-type b, and non-typeable, should be reported to the local or state public health department.

Hantavirus Pulmonary Syndrome

CLINICAL MANIFESTATIONS: Hantaviruses cause 2 distinct clinical syndromes: hantavirus pulmonary syndrome (HPS) characterized by noncardiogenic pulmonary edema, which is observed in the Americas; and hemorrhagic fever with renal syndrome (HFRS), which occurs worldwide (see Hemorrhagic Fevers and Related Syndromes Caused by Bunyaviruses, p 384). After an incubation period of 1 to 6 weeks, the prodromal illness of HPS lasts 3 to 7 days and is characterized by fever, chills, headache, myalgia, nausea, vomiting, diarrhea, dizziness, and sometimes cough. Respiratory tract symptoms or signs usually do not occur during the first 3 to 7 days, but then pulmonary edema and severe hypoxemia appear abruptly and present as cough and dyspnea. The disease then progresses over hours. In severe cases, myocardial dysfunction causes hypotension, which is why the syndrome sometimes is called hantavirus cardiopulmonary syndrome.

Extensive bilateral interstitial and alveolar pulmonary edema with pleural effusions are attributable to diffuse pulmonary capillary leak. Intubation and assisted ventilation usually are required for only 2 to 4 days, with resolution heralded by onset of diuresis and rapid clinical improvement.

The severe myocardial depression is different from that of septic shock, with low cardiac indices and stroke volume index, normal pulmonary wedge pressure, and increased systemic vascular resistance. Poor prognostic indicators include persistent hypotension, marked hemoconcentration, a cardiac index of less than 2, and abrupt onset of lactic acidosis with a serum lactate concentration of >4 mmol/L (36 mg/dL).

The mortality rate for patients with HPS is between 30% and 40%; death usually occurs in the first 1 or 2 days of hospitalization. Asymptomatic and milder forms of disease have been reported. Limited information suggests that clinical manifestations and prognosis are similar in adults and children. Serious sequelae are uncommon.

ETIOLOGY: Hantaviruses are RNA viruses of the *Bunyaviridae* family. Sin Nombre virus (SNV) is the major cause of HPS in the western and central regions of the United States. Bayou virus, Black Creek Canal virus, Monongahela virus, and New York virus are responsible for sporadic cases in Louisiana, Texas, Florida, New York, and other areas of the eastern United States. Andes virus, Oran virus, Laguna Negra virus, and Choclo virus are responsible for cases in South and Central America. There are 20 to 40 cases of HPS reported annually in the United States. Cases in children younger than 10 years are exceedingly rare. Children may be less likely to become infected than adults because children are less likely to perform tasks that would place them at increased risk. Also, nonspecific immune mechanisms may reduce the risk of symptoms in children.

EPIDEMIOLOGY: Rodents are the natural hosts for hantaviruses and acquire lifelong, asymptomatic, chronic infection with prolonged viruria and virus in saliva and feces. Humans acquire infection through direct contact with infected rodents, rodent droppings, or rodent nests, or through the inhalation of aerosolized virus particles from rodent urine, droppings, or saliva. Rarely, infection may be acquired from rodent bites or contamination of broken skin with excreta. At-risk activities include handling or trapping rodents, cleaning or entering closed or rarely used rodent-infested structures, cleaning feed storage or animal shelter areas, hand plowing, and living in a home with an increased density of mice. For backpackers or campers, sleeping in a structure also inhabited by rodents has been associated with HPS, with a notable outbreak occurring in 2012 in Yosemite National Park secondary to rodent infested cabins. Exceptionally heavy rainfall improves rodent food supplies, resulting in an increase in the rodent population with more frequent contact between humans and infected rodents, resulting in more human disease. Most cases occur during the spring and summer, with the geographic location determined by the habitat of the rodent carrier.

SNV is transmitted by the deer mouse, *Peromyscus maniculatus;* Black Creek Canal virus is transmitted by the cotton rat, *Sigmodon hispidus;* Bayou virus is transmitted by the rice rat, *Oryzomys palustris;* and New York virus is transmitted by the white-footed mouse, *Peromyscus leucopus.*

DIAGNOSTIC TESTS: HPS should be considered when thrombocytopenia occurs with severe pneumonia clinically resembling acute respiratory distress syndrome in the proper epidemiologic setting. Other characteristic laboratory findings include neutrophilic leukocytosis with immature granulocytes, including more than 10% immunoblasts (basophilic cytoplasm, prominent nucleoli, and an increased nuclear-cytoplasmic ratio) and increased hematocrit.

Molecular detection of virus has been described in peripheral blood mononuclear cells and other clinical specimens from the early phase of the disease but not usually in bronchoalveolar lavage fluids. Viral culture is not useful. Hantavirus-specific immunoglobulin (Ig) M and IgG antibodies often are present at the onset of clinical disease, and serologic testing remains the method of choice for diagnosis. IgG may be negative in rapidly fatal cases.

Immunohistochemical staining of tissues (capillary endothelial cells of the lungs and almost every organ in the body) can establish the diagnosis at autopsy.

TREATMENT: Patients with suspected HPS should be transferred immediately to a tertiary care facility where supportive management of pulmonary edema, severe hypoxemia, and hypotension can occur during the first critical 24 to 48 hours.

In severe forms, early mechanical ventilation and inotropic and pressor support are necessary. Extracorporeal membrane oxygenation (ECMO) should be considered when pulmonary wedge pressure and cardiac indices have deteriorated, and may provide short-term support for the severe capillary leak syndrome in the lungs.

Ribavirin is active in vitro against hantaviruses, including SNV. However, 2 clinical studies of intravenous ribavirin (1 open-label study and 1 randomized, placebo-controlled, double-blind study) failed to show benefit in treatment of HPS in the cardiopulmonary stage. At the present time ribavirin should not be considered the standard of care.

Cytokine blocking agents for HPS theoretically may have a role, but these agents have not been evaluated in a systematic fashion. Antibacterial agents are unlikely to offer benefit. However, broad-spectrum antibiotic therapy often is administered until the diagnosis is established, because bacterial shock is far more common than shock attributable to hantavirus.

ISOLATION OF THE HOSPITALIZED PATIENT: Standard precautions are recommended. Health care-associated or person-to-person transmission has not been associated with HPS in the United States but has been reported in Chile and Argentina with the Andes virus.

CONTROL MEASURES:

Care of Exposed People. Serial clinical examinations should be used to monitor individuals at high risk of infection after exposure (see Epidemiology).

Environmental Control. Hantavirus infections of humans occur primarily in adults and are associated with domestic, occupational, or leisure activities facilitating contact with infected rodents, usually in a building in a rural setting. Eradicating the host reservoir is not feasible. Risk reduction includes practices that discourage rodents from colonizing the home and work environment and that minimize aerosolization and contact with rodent saliva and excreta. Tactics include eliminating food sources for the rodent, reducing nesting sites by sealing holes, and using "snap traps" and rodenticides. Before entering areas with potential rodent infestations, doors and windows should be opened to ventilate the enclosure.

Hantaviruses, because of their lipid envelope, are susceptible to diluted bleach solutions, detergents, and most general household disinfectants. Dusty areas or articles should be moistened with 10% bleach or other disinfectant solution before being cleaned. Brooms and vacuum cleaners should not be used to clean rodent-infested areas. Use of a 10% bleach solution to disinfect dead rodents and wearing rubber gloves before handling trapped or dead rodents is recommended. Gloves and traps should be disinfected after use. The cleanup of areas potentially infested with hantavirus-infected rodents should be conducted by knowledgeable professionals using appropriate personal protective equipment. Potentially infected material should be handled according to local regulations for infectious waste.

Chemoprophylaxis measures or vaccines are not available.

Public Health Reporting. Possible hantavirus occurrence should be reported immediately to local and state public health authorities. In addition, HPS is reportable in the United States using the guidelines of the Council of State and Territorial Epidemiologists.

Helicobacter pylori Infections

CLINICAL MANIFESTATIONS: Most infections of *Heliobacteri pylori* in patients are thought to be asymptomatic. *H pylori* may cause chronic active gastritis and may result in duodenal and, to a lesser extent, gastric ulcers. Persistent infection with *H pylori* increases the risk of gastric cancer in adults, but this is an infrequent complication in children. In children, *H pylori* infection can result in gastroduodenal inflammation that can manifest as epigastric pain, nausea, vomiting, hematemesis, and guaiac-positive stools. Symptoms can resolve within a few days or can wax and wane. Nodular gastritis associated with *H pylori* infection commonly occurs in childhood and is regarded as benign with no clinical significance. Extraintestinal conditions in children that have been associated with *H pylori* infection include iron-deficiency anemia, short stature, and chronic immune thrombocytopenia. However, there is no clear association between infection and recurrent abdominal pain in the absence of peptic ulcer disease. *H pylori* infection is not associated with secondary gastritis (eg, autoimmune or associated with nonsteroidal anti-inflammatory agents).

ETIOLOGY: *H pylori* is a gram-negative, spiral, curved, or U-shaped microaerobic bacillus that has single or multiple flagella at one end. The organism is positive for catalase, oxidase, and urease activity.

EPIDEMIOLOGY: *H pylori* organisms have been isolated from humans and other primates. An animal reservoir for human transmission has not been demonstrated. Organisms are thought to be transmitted from infected humans by the fecal-oral, gastro-oral, and oral-oral routes.

H pylori is estimated to have infected 70% of people living in resource-limited countries and 30% to 40% of people living in industrialized countries. Infection rates in children are low in resource-rich, industrialized countries, except in children from lower socioeconomic groups and those living in poor hygienic conditions. Most infections are acquired in the first 5 years of life and can reach prevalence rates of up to 80% in resource-limited countries. Approximately 70% of infected people are asymptomatic; esophagogastroduodenoscopic changes are found in 20% of people, either grossly or with microscopic findings of ulceration; and an estimated 1% have features of neoplasia. The organism can persist in the stomach for years or for life.

The **incubation period** is unknown.

DIAGNOSTIC TESTS: *H pylori* infection can be diagnosed by culture of gastric biopsy tissue on nonselective media (eg, chocolate agar, brucella agar, brain-heart infusion agar) or selective media (eg, Skirrow agar) at 37°C under microaerobic conditions (decreased oxygen, increased carbon dioxide, and increased hydrogen concentrations) for 3 to 10 days. Colonies are small, smooth, and translucent, and are positive for catalase, oxidase, and urease activity. Antimicrobial susceptibility testing of cultured isolates may be necessary to guide therapy in refractory cases. Organisms can be visualized on histologic sections with Warthin-Starry silver, Steiner, Giemsa, or Genta staining. Presence of *H pylori* can be confirmed but not excluded on the basis of hematoxylin-eosin stains. Immunohistological staining with specific *H pylori* antibodies may improve specificity. Because of production of high levels of urease by these organisms, urease testing of a gastric biopsy specimen can give a rapid and specific microbiologic diagnosis. Urease hydrolyzes urea into ammonia and carbonate; the resulting increase in pH from the production of ammonia is detected in the assay.

Noninvasive, commercially available tests include urea breath tests and stool antigen tests; these tests are designed for detection of active infection and have high sensitivity and specificity. The urea breath test detects labeled carbon dioxide in expired air after oral administration of isotope-labeled urea (^{13}C or ^{14}C). Although these tests are expensive and are not useful in young children, there is an *H pylori* breath test approved by the US Food and Drug Administration for children 3 to 17 years of age. Stool antigen tests by enzyme immunoassay monoclonal antibodies are available commercially and can be used for children of any age, especially before and after treatment.

The organism can be detected by polymerase chain reaction (PCR) or fluorescence in situ hybridization (FISH) of gastric biopsy tissue, and PCR also has been applied to detecting the organism in stool specimens; however, none of these assays currently are cleared by the FDA.

Serologic testing for *H pylori* infection by detection of immunoglobulin (Ig) G antibodies specific for *H pylori* may be useful for epidemiologic surveys but does not distinguish between active and resolved infection; therefore, serologic testing is not recommended for diagnosis or for confirming eradication.

The European Society for Paediatric Gastroenterology Hepatology and Nutrition and the North American Society for Pediatric Gastroenterology, Hepatology and Nutrition recommend against a "test and treat" strategy for *H pylori* infection in children. Instead, they recommend the following[1]:

- The diagnosis of *H pylori* infection should be based on either (a) histopathology (*H pylori*–positive gastritis) plus at least 1 other positive biopsy-based test, or (b) positive culture.
- When testing for *H pylori*, wait at least 2 weeks after stopping a proton pump inhibitor (PPI) and 4 weeks after stopping antimicrobial agents.
- Testing for *H pylori* should be performed in children with gastric or duodenal ulcers. If *H pylori* infection is identified, then treatment should be advised and eradication should be confirmed.
- Noninvasive diagnostic testing for *H pylori* infection may be considered when investigating causes of chronic immune thrombocytopenic purpura.
- Diagnostic testing for *H pylori* infection should not be performed as part of the initial investigation in children with iron-deficiency anemia. In children with refractory iron deficiency anemia in which other causes have been ruled out, testing for *H pylori* during upper endoscopy may be considered.
- Diagnostic testing for *H pylori* infection should not be performed in children with functional abdominal pain.
- Diagnostic testing for *H pylori* infection should not be performed when investigating causes of short stature.

[1]Jones NL, Koletzko S, Goodman K, et al; ESPGHAN, NASPGHAN. Joint ESPGHAN/NASPGHAN guidelines for the management of *Helicobacter pylori* in children and adolescents (update 2016). *J Pediatr Gastroenterol Nutr.* 2017;64(6):991–1003

TREATMENT[1]**:** Treatment is recommended for infected patients who have peptic ulcer disease, gastric mucosa-associated lymphoid tissue-type lymphoma, or early gastric cancer. Screening for and treatment of infection, if found, may be considered for children who have unexplained and refractory iron-deficiency anemia. Additionally, the American Society of Hematology's 2011 evidence-based practice guideline for immune thrombocytopenia recommends eradication if infection is associated with chronic immune thrombocytopenic purpura.[2] For patients with *H pylori* infection in the absence of clinical or endoscopic evidence of peptic ulcer disease, treatment is not recommended unless the patient is within a risk group or region with high incidence of gastric cancer. Compliance is critical to the success of eradication therapy.

The backbone of all recommended therapies includes a PPI and amoxicillin. Additions of metronidazole, clarithromycin, and/or bismuth are based on the patient's previous treatment experience, known susceptibilities to clarithromycin and metronidazole, and the local rates of successful eradication; the latter 2 factors may be difficult to ascertain. Reports of increasing prevalence of antibiotic-resistant strains (particularly clarithromycin resistance) as well as increasing failures of triple therapies suggest the need for quadruple therapy regimens and longer durations (14 days) for eradication of *H pylori*. A number of treatment regimens have been evaluated and are approved for use in adults; the safety and efficacy of these regimens in pediatric patients have not been firmly established. There is no current evidence to support the use of probiotics to reduce medication adverse effects or improve eradication of *H pylori*.

Initial Therapy

- In a treatment-naïve patient with *H pylori* known to be fully susceptible, initial treatment includes a PPI plus amoxicillin plus clarithromycin for 14 days; an alternate regimen uses a sequence of dual therapy with amoxicillin and a PPI for 5 days, followed by 5 days of triple therapy (a PPI plus clarithromycin and metronidazole).

- In a treatment-naïve patient with *H pylori* of unknown or reduced susceptibilities, an effective regimen is a PPI plus amoxicillin plus metronidazole (with or without bismuth).

- In all treatment-naïve patients, a breath or stool test should be performed to document organism clearance 4 to 6 weeks after completion of initial therapy; relief of clinical symptoms is not an indicator of successful eradication.

Recurrent Therapy

- Infection within the first 12 months following treatment is likely a relapse of the previous infection; illness 12 months or more after the beginning of treatment is likely attributable to reinfection with a new strain. The reinfection rate within 5 years may be as high as 50%. In contrast to adults, reduced options exist for rescue therapy for children.

- When initial triple therapy with clarithromycin fails to eradicate a fully susceptible isolate, a recommended rescue therapy is PPI plus amoxicillin plus metronidazole. Eradication failure following the other prescribed initial therapies should prompt repeat

[1] Jones NL, Koletzko S, Goodman K, et al; ESPGHAN, NASPGHAN. Joint ESPGHAN/NASPGHAN guidelines for the management of *Helicobacter pylori* in children and adolescents (update 2016). *J Pediatr Gastroenterol Nutr*. 2017;64(6):991–1003

[2] Neunert C, Lim W, Crowther M, Cohen A, Solberg L Jr, Crowther MA. The American Society of Hematology 2011 evidence-based guideline for immune thrombocytopenia. *Blood*. 2011;117(16):4190–4207

endoscopy to assess antimicrobial susceptibilities (eg, to clarithromycin and metronidazole). These results may then lead to a regimen of PPI plus amoxicillin plus bismuth with addition of clarithromycin and/or metronidazole (depending on susceptibilities of isolates recovered from repeat endoscopy).

- If the patient is unable or unwilling to undergo endoscopy, an empiric rescue regimen may include PPI plus amoxicillin plus metronidazole, with or without bismuth. A breath or stool test should be performed to document organism eradication 4 to 6 weeks after completion of rescue therapy. Limited options exist for penicillin-allergic patients.

ISOLATION OF THE HOSPITALIZED PATIENT: Standard precautions are recommended.

CONTROL MEASURES: Disinfection of gastroscopes prevents transmission of the organism between patients.

Hemorrhagic Fevers Caused by Arenaviruses[1]

CLINICAL MANIFESTATIONS: Arenaviruses are responsible for several hemorrhagic fevers (HFs): Old World arenavirus HFs include Lassa fever and Lujo virus infections in western and southern Africa. New World arenavirus HFs include Argentine, Bolivian, Brazilian, Venezuelan, and Chapare virus infection. Lymphocytic choriomeningitis virus (LCMV) is an Old World arenavirus that generally induces less severe disease, although it can cause HFs in immunosuppressed patients; LCMV is discussed in a separate chapter (p 525). Disease associated with arenaviruses ranges in severity from asymptomatic or mild, acute, febrile infections to severe illnesses in which vascular leak, shock, and multiorgan dysfunction are prominent features. Fever, headache, arthralgia, myalgia, conjunctival suffusion, retro-orbital pain, facial flushing, anorexia, vomiting, diarrhea, and abdominal pain are common early symptoms in all infections. Thrombocytopenia, leukopenia, petechiae, generalized lymphadenopathy, and encephalopathy usually are present in Argentine HF, Bolivian HF, and Venezuelan HF, and exudative pharyngitis often occurs in Lassa fever. Mucosal bleeding generally occurs in severe cases as a consequence of vascular damage, coagulopathy, thrombocytopenia, and platelet dysfunction. However, hemorrhagic manifestations occur in only one third of patients with Lassa fever. Proteinuria is common, but renal failure is unusual. Increased serum concentrations of aspartate transaminase (AST) can portend a severe or possibly fatal outcome of Lassa fever. Shock develops 7 to 9 days after onset of illness in more severely ill patients with these infections. Upper and lower respiratory tract symptoms can develop in people with Lassa fever. Encephalopathic signs, such as tremor, alterations in consciousness, and seizures, can occur in South American HFs and in severe cases of Lassa fever. Transitory or permanent deafness is reported in 30% of convalescents of Lassa fever. The mortality rate in South American HFs is 10% to 35% and in Lujo virus infection is 80% (estimated from a small number of patients). Symptoms resolve 10 to 15 days after disease onset in surviving patients.

ETIOLOGY: Mammalian arenaviruses (mammarenaviruses) are enveloped, bisegmented, single-stranded RNA viruses. The Old World complex of arenaviruses includes Lassa virus, which causes Lassa fever in western Africa, as well as Lujo virus, which caused fatal human-to-human transmission in an outbreak in southern Africa. The major New World

---

[1]Does not include lymphocytic choriomeningitis virus, which is reviewed on p 525.

arenavirus HFs occurring in the Western hemisphere are caused by the Tacaribe sero-complex of clade B arenaviruses: Argentine HF caused by Junín virus, Bolivian HF caused by Machupo virus and Chapare virus, Brazilian HF caused by Sabiá virus, and Venezuelan HF caused by Guanarito virus. Antibodies to Whitewater Arroyo and Tami-ami viruses have been detected in individuals in North America, but clinical disease has not been confirmed. Several other arenaviruses are known only from their rodent reservoirs in the Old and New World.

EPIDEMIOLOGY: Arenaviruses are maintained in nature by association with specific rodent hosts, in which they produce chronic viremia and viruria. The principal routes of infection are inhalation and contact of mucous membranes and skin (eg, through cuts, scratches, or abrasions) with urine and salivary secretions from these persistently infected rodents. Ingestion of food contaminated by rodent excrement also may cause disease transmission. Tacaribe viruses have not been associated with a rodent host; although they have reportedly been isolated in bats, mosquitoes, and ticks, transmission through these vectors has not been definitely confirmed. All arenaviruses are infectious as aerosols, and human-to-human transmission may occur in community or hospital settings following unprotected contact or through droplets. Excretion of arenaviruses in urine and semen for several weeks after infection has been documented. Arenaviruses causing HF should be considered highly hazardous to people working with any of these viruses in the laboratory. Laboratory-acquired infections have been documented with Lassa, Machupo, Junín, and Sabiá viruses. The geographic distribution and habitats of the specific rodents that serve as reservoir hosts largely determine areas with endemic infection and populations at risk. Before a vaccine became available in Argentina, several hundred cases of Argentine HF occurred annually in agricultural workers and inhabitants of the Argentine pampas. The Argentine HF vaccine is not licensed in the United States. Epidemics of Bolivian HF occurred in small towns between 1962 and 1964; sporadic disease activity in the countryside has continued since then. Venezuelan HF first was identified in 1989 and occurs in rural north-central Venezuela. Lassa fever is endemic in most of western Africa, where rodent hosts live in proximity with humans, causing thousands of infections annually. Lassa fever has been reported in the United States and Western Europe in people who have traveled to western Africa. Mammalian HF arenaviruses are classified by the Centers for Disease Control and Prevention (CDC) as category A agents because of the high risk they pose to public health and national security.

The **incubation periods** are from 6 to 17 days.

DIAGNOSTIC TESTS: Viral nucleic acid can be detected in acute disease by reverse transcriptase-polymerase chain reaction assay. These viruses may be isolated from blood of acutely ill patients as well as from various tissues obtained postmortem, but isolation should be attempted only under Biosafety level-4 (BSL-4) conditions. Virus antigen is detectable by enzyme immunoassay (EIA) in acute specimens and postmortem tissues. Virus-specific immunoglobulin (Ig) M antibodies are present in the serum during acute stages of illness by immunofluorescent antibody or enzyme-linked immunosorbent assays but may be undetectable in rapidly fatal cases. The IgG antibody response is delayed. Diagnosis can be made retrospectively by immunohistochemical staining of formalin-fixed tissues obtained from autopsy.

If a viral hemorrhagic fever is suspected, the state/local health department or CDC (Viral Special Pathogens Branch: 404-639-1115) should be contacted to assist with case investigation, diagnosis, treatment, and control measures.

TREATMENT: Intravenous ribavirin substantially decreases the mortality rate in patients with severe Lassa fever, particularly if they are treated during the first week of illness. For Argentine HF, transfusion of immune plasma in defined doses of neutralizing antibodies is the standard specific treatment when administered during the first 8 days from onset of symptoms, and reduces mortality to 1% to 2%. Intravenous ribavirin has been used with success to abort a Sabiá laboratory infection and to treat Bolivian HF patients and the only known Lujo virus infection survivor. Ribavirin did not reduce mortality when initiated 8 days or more after onset of Argentine HF symptoms. Whether ribavirin treatment initiated early in the course of the disease has a role in the treatment of Argentine HF remains to be seen. Intravenous ribavirin is available only from the manufacturer through an investigational new drug (IND) protocol. Health care providers who need to obtain intravenous ribavirin should contact the US Food and Drug Administration (FDA [301-796-1500; 24-hour emergency line: 866-300-4374]) or the manufacturer (Valeant Pharmaceuticals [800-548-5100; after hours, 510-595-9853]). Meticulous fluid balance is an important aspect of supportive care in each of the HFs.

ISOLATION OF THE HOSPITALIZED PATIENT: In addition to standard precautions, contact and droplet precautions, including careful prevention of needlestick injuries and careful handling of clinical specimens for the duration of illness, are recommended for all HFs caused by arenaviruses. A negative-pressure ventilation room is recommended for patients with prominent cough or severe disease, and people entering the room should wear personal protection respirators. A negative-pressure room should be used when aerosol-generating procedures are conducted, such as intubation or airway suctioning. The CDC infection prevention recommendations for patients under investigation for Ebola virus disease in US hospitals are applicable in the event that an HF virus is used as a weapon of bioterrorism.[1]

CONTROL MEASURES:

Care of Exposed People. No specific measures are warranted for exposed people unless direct contamination with blood, excretions, or secretions from an infected patient has occurred. If such contamination has occurred, recording body temperature twice daily for 21 days is recommended. Reporting of fever or of symptoms of infection is an indication for intravenous ribavirin treatment for Lassa fever, Bolivian HF, or Sabiá or Lujo virus infections.

Immunoprophylaxis. A live attenuated Junín vaccine protects against Argentine HF and probably against Bolivian HF. The vaccine is associated with minimal adverse effects in adults; similar findings have been obtained from limited safety studies in children 4 years and older. The vaccine is not available in the United States.

Environmental. In town-based outbreaks of Bolivian HF, rodent control has proven successful. Area rodent control is not practical for control of Argentine HF or Venezuelan HF. Intensive rodent control efforts have decreased the rate of peridomestic Lassa virus infection, but rodents eventually reinvade human dwellings, and infection still occurs in rural settings.

Public Health Reporting. Because of the risk of health care-associated transmission, state

---

[1]Centers for Disease Control and Prevention. Infection Prevention and Control Recommendations for Hospitalized Patients Under Investigation (PUIs) for Ebola Virus Disease (EVD) in U.S. Hospitals. Atlanta, GA: Centers for Disease Control and Prevention; 2015. Available at: **www.cdc.gov/vhf/ebola/healthcare-us/hospitals/infection-control.html**

health departments and the CDC should be contacted for specific advice about management and diagnosis of suspected cases. Lassa fever and New World arenavirus HFs are reportable in the United States according to guidelines of the US Council of State and Territorial Epidemiologists.

Hemorrhagic Fevers Caused by Bunyaviruses[1]

CLINICAL MANIFESTATIONS: Bunyaviruses are vectorborne infections (except for hantavirus) that often result in severe febrile disease with multisystem involvement. Human infection by bunyaviruses may be associated with high rates of morbidity and mortality. In the United States, disease attributable to a bunyavirus most likely is caused by either hantavirus or members of the California serogroup.

Hemorrhagic fever with renal syndrome (HFRS) is a complex, multiphasic disease characterized by vascular instability and varying degrees of renal insufficiency. Fever, flushing, conjunctival injection, headache, blurred vision, abdominal pain, and lumbar pain are followed by hypotension, oliguria, and subsequently, polyuria. Petechiae are frequent, but more serious bleeding manifestations are rare. Shock and acute renal insufficiency may occur. Nephropathia epidemica (attributable to Puumala virus) occurs in Europe and presents as a milder disease with acute influenza-like illness, abdominal pain, and proteinuria. Acute renal dysfunction also occurs, but hypotensive shock and requirement for dialysis are rare. However, more severe forms of HFRS (ie, attributable to Dobrava virus) occur in Europe.

Crimean-Congo hemorrhagic fever (CCHF) is a multisystem disease characterized by hepatitis and profuse bleeding. Fever, headache, and myalgia are followed by signs of a diffuse capillary leak syndrome with facial suffusion, conjunctivitis, icteric hepatitis, proteinuria, and disseminated intravascular coagulation associated with petechiae and purpura on the skin and mucous membranes. A hypotensive crisis often occurs after the appearance of frank hemorrhage from the gastrointestinal tract, nose, mouth, or uterus. Mortality rates range from 20% to 35%.

Rift Valley fever (RVF), in most cases, is a self-limited undifferentiated febrile illness. In 8% to 10% of cases, however, hemorrhagic fever with shock and icteric hepatitis, encephalitis, or retinitis develops.

ETIOLOGY: *Bunyaviridae* are segmented, single-stranded RNA viruses with different geographic distributions depending on their vector or reservoir. Hemorrhagic fever syndromes are associated with viruses from 3 genera: hantaviruses, nairoviruses (CCHF virus), and phleboviruses (RVF and Heartland virus in the United States, sandfly fever viruses in Europe, and severe fever with thrombocytopenia syndrome [SFTS] virus in China). Old World hantaviruses (Hantaan, Seoul, Dobrava, and Puumala viruses) cause HFRS, and New World hantaviruses (Sin Nombre and related viruses) cause hantavirus pulmonary syndrome (see Hantavirus Pulmonary Syndrome, p 375).

EPIDEMIOLOGY: The epidemiology of these diseases mainly is a function of the distribution and behavior of their reservoirs and vectors. All genera except hantaviruses are associated with arthropod vectors, and hantavirus infections are associated with airborne exposure to infected wild rodents, primarily via inhalation of virus-contaminated urine, droppings, or nesting materials.

---

[1]Does not include hantavirus pulmonary syndrome, which is reviewed on p 376.

Classic HFRS occurs throughout much of Asia and Eastern and Western Europe, with up to 100 000 cases per year. The most severe form of the disease is caused by the prototype Hantaan and Dobrava viruses in rural Asia and Europe, respectively; Puumala virus is associated with milder disease (nephropathia epidemica) in Western Europe. Seoul virus is distributed worldwide in association with *Rattus* species and can cause a disease of variable severity. Person-to-person transmission never has been reported with HFRS. Fatal outcome is seen in 1% to 15% of cases, depending on the species of virus and the level of care.

CCHF occurs in much of sub-Saharan Africa, the Middle East, areas in West and Central Asia, and the Balkans. CCHF virus is transmitted by hard ticks and occasionally by contact with viremic livestock and wild animals at slaughter. Health care-associated transmission of CCHF is a frequent and serious hazard. Fatal outcome is seen in 9% to 50% of hospitalized patients.

RVF occurs throughout sub-Saharan Africa and has caused large epidemics in Egypt in 1977 and 1993–1995, Mauritania in 1987, Saudi Arabia and Yemen in 2000, Kenya and Tanzania in 1997 and 2006–2007, Madagascar in 1990 and 2008, and South Africa in 2010. The virus is mosquitoborne and is transmitted from domestic livestock to humans. The virus also can be transmitted by aerosol in laboratory conditions and by direct contact with infected aborted tissues or freshly slaughtered infected animal carcasses. Person-to-person transmission has not been reported, but laboratory-acquired cases are well documented. Overall fatal outcome occurs in 1% to 2% of cases but has been reported to be up to 30% in hospitalized patients.

The **incubation periods** for CCHF and RVF range from 2 to 10 days; for HFRS, **incubation periods** usually are longer, ranging from 7 to 42 days.

DIAGNOSTIC TESTS: Viral culture of blood and/or tissue, detection of virus antigen by enzyme immunoassay (EIA), acute-phase quantitative reverse transcriptase-polymerase chain reaction (qRT-PCR) and serologic testing may facilitate diagnosis (Table 3.15). Immunoglobulin (Ig) M antibodies or increasing IgG titers in paired serum specimens, as demonstrated by EIA, are diagnostic; neutralizing antibody tests provide greater virus-strain specificity but rarely are used. Serum IgM and IgG virus-specific antibodies typically develop early in convalescence in CCHF and RVF but can be absent in rapidly fatal causes of CCHF. In HFRS, IgM and IgG antibodies usually are detectable at the time of onset of illness or within 48 hours, when it is too late for virus isolation and qRT-PCR assay. Diagnosis can be made retrospectively by immunohistochemical staining of formalin-fixed tissues.

TREATMENT: Ribavirin, administered intravenously to patients with HFRS within the first 4 days of illness, may be effective in decreasing renal dysfunction, vascular instability, and mortality. However, intravenous ribavirin is not available commercially in the United States and is available only from the manufacturer through an investigational new drug (IND) protocol. Health care providers who need to obtain intravenous ribavirin should contact the US Food and Drug Administration (FDA [24-hour emergency line: 866-300-4374 or 301-796-8240]) or the manufacturer (Valent Pharmaceuticals [800-548-5100]). Supportive therapy for HFRS should include: (1) treatment of shock; (2) monitoring of fluid balance; (3) dialysis for complications of renal failure; (4) control of hypertension during the oliguric phase; and (5) early recognition of possible myocardial failure with appropriate therapy.

Table 3.15. Diagnostic Tests To Be Performed for Hemorrhagic Fevers Caused by Bunyaviruses

Diagnostic Testing	HFRS	CCHF	RVF
Virus culture of blood or tissue	No (usually not detected at time of illness)	Yes (in Biosafety Level 4 [BSL-4] conditions, which is the highest)	Yes (in Biosafety Level 4 [BSL-4] conditions, which is the highest)
Virus antigen assay (EIA)	No (usually not detected at time of illness)	Yes	Yes
Acute phase virus qRT-PCR	Yes, but not routinely done	Yes	Yes
IgM and IgG serology	Yes (at time of illness onset or within 48 h)	Yes (detectable in early convalescence, but could be absent in fatal cases)	Yes (detectable in early convalescence)

Oral and intravenous ribavirin, when administered early in the course of CCHF, has been associated with milder disease, although no controlled studies have been performed. Ribavirin also may be efficacious as postexposure prophylaxis of CCHF.

During the RVF outbreak in Saudi Arabia in 2000, a clinical trial of ribavirin in patients with confirmed disease was halted because of an increased observation of encephalitis in patients receiving ribavirin (more than expected in RVF patients). Experimental data in hamster, mice, and rats reported the same type of observation when treatment was delayed. Therefore, ribavirin should be avoided in RVF.

ISOLATION OF THE HOSPITALIZED PATIENT: In addition to standard precautions, contact and droplet precautions, including careful prevention of needlestick injuries and management of clinical specimens, are indicated for patients with CCHF for the duration for their illness. Airborne isolation may be required in certain circumstances when patients undergo procedures that stimulate coughing and promote generation of aerosols. Standard precautions should be followed with RVF and HFRS.

CONTROL MEASURES:

Care of Exposed People. People having direct contact with blood or other secretions from patients with CCHF should be observed closely for 21 days with daily monitoring for fever. Immediate therapy with intravenous ribavirin should be considered at the first sign of disease. Ribavirin also may be efficacious as postexposure prophylaxis of CCHF.

Environmental.

Hemorrhagic Fever With Renal Syndrome. Monitoring of laboratory rat colonies and urban rodent control may be effective for ratborne HFRS.

Crimean-Congo Hemorrhagic Fever. Arachnicides for tick control generally have limited benefit but should be used in stockyard settings. Personal protective measures (eg, physical tick removal and protective clothing with permethrin sprays) may be effective for people at-risk (farmers, veterinarians, abattoir workers).

Rift Valley Fever. Regular immunization of domestic animals should have an effect on limiting or preventing RVF outbreaks and protecting humans but is not performed routinely in the United States and countries with endemic disease. However, some livestock vaccines are currently in use in areas with endemicity. Personal protective clothing (with permethrin sprays) and insect repellants may be effective for people at risk (farmers, veterinarians, abattoir workers). Mosquito control measures are difficult to implement.

Immunoprophylaxis. No vaccines currently are approved for use in humans against HFs caused by bunyaviruses.

Public Health Reporting. Because of the risk of health care-associated transmission of CCHF and diagnostic confusion with other viral hemorrhagic fevers, state health departments and the CDC (Viral Special Pathogens Branch: 404-639–1115) should be contacted about any suspected diagnosis of viral hemorrhagic fever and the management plan for the patient. CCHF is reportable in the United States, according to guidelines of the US Council of State and Territorial Epidemiologists.

Hemorrhagic Fevers Caused by Filoviruses: Ebola and Marburg

CLINICAL MANIFESTATIONS: Data on Ebola and Marburg virus infections primarily are derived from adult populations. More is known about Ebola virus disease than Marburg virus disease, although the same principles apply generally to the 2 filoviruses known to cause human disease. Asymptomatic cases of human filovirus infections have been reported, and symptomatic disease ranges from mild to severe; case fatality rates for severely affected people range from 25% to 90% (and varied significantly even during the 2014 Ebola outbreak). Data from the 2 largest outbreaks have confirmed that the lowest case fatality rates are in adolescents. After a typical incubation period of 8 to 10 days (range, 2–21 days), disease in children and adults begins with nonspecific signs and symptoms including fever, severe headache, myalgia, fatigue, abdominal pain, and weakness followed several days later by vomiting, diarrhea, and sometimes unexplained bleeding or bruising. Data from the 2014–2015 Ebola outbreak indicate that children may have shorter incubation periods than adults. Respiratory symptoms are more common and central nervous system manifestations are less common in children than in adults. A fleeting maculopapular rash on the torso or face after approximately 4 to 5 days of illness may occur. Hiccups have been reported. Conjunctival injection or subconjunctival hemorrhage may be present. Leukopenia, frequently with lymphopenia, is followed later by elevated neutrophils, a left shift, and thrombocytopenia. Hepatic dysfunction, with elevations in aspartate transaminase (AST) at markedly higher levels than alanine transaminase (ALT), and metabolic derangements, including hypokalemia, hyponatremia, hypocalcemia, and hypomagnesemia, are common. In the most severe cases, microvascular instability ensues around the end of the first week of disease. Although hemostasis is impaired, hemorrhagic manifestations develop in a minority of patients. In the 2001 Ebola virus outbreak in Uganda and Sudan, all children with laboratory-confirmed Ebola virus disease were febrile and only 16% had hemorrhage. In a study of 122 children from 5 Ebola units during the 2014–2015 outbreak, bleeding was rare at presentation (5%) and manifested subsequently in fewer than 50%. The most common hemorrhagic manifestations consist of bleeding from the gastrointestinal tract, sometimes with oozing from the mucous membranes or venipuncture sites in late stages.

Central nervous system manifestations and renal failure are frequent in end-stage disease. In fatal cases, death typically occurs around 10 to 12 days after symptom onset, usually resulting from viral- or bacterial-induced septic shock and multiorgan system failure. Factors associated with pediatric Ebola deaths in the 2014–2015 outbreak were age <5 years, bleeding at any time during hospitalization, and high viral load.

Approximately 30% of pregnant women with Ebola virus disease present with spontaneous abortion and vaginal bleeding. Maternal mortality approaches 90% when infection occurs during the third trimester. There has only been one report of survival of a neonate born to a mother with active Ebola virus disease. The exact cause of neonatal deaths is unknown, but high viral loads of Ebola virus have been documented in amniotic fluid, placental tissue, and fetal tissues of stillborn neonates. New data are emerging that survivors are at risk for reactivation of disease in immune-privileged sites, such as the eye or the central nervous system, because of persistence of Ebola virus. However, disease reactivation currently is thought to be a rare event. Long-term shedding of virus in semen has been implicated in the origin of several clusters of Ebola virus disease in West Africa.

ETIOLOGY: The *Filoviridae* (from the Latin filo meaning thread, referring to their filamentous shape) are single-stranded, negative-sense RNA viruses. Marburg and Ebola viruses are the only known members of the filovirus family. Four of the 5 species in the *Ebolavirus* genus and both of the known species in the *Marburgvirus* genus are associated with human disease. The known human pathogenic filoviruses are endemic only in Africa.

EPIDEMIOLOGY: Fruit bats are believed to be the animal reservoir for filoviruses. Human infection is believed to occur from inadvertent exposure to infected bat excreta or saliva following entry into roosting areas in caves, mines, and forests. Nonhuman primates, especially gorillas and chimpanzees, and other wild animals may become infected from bat contact and serve as intermediate hosts that transmit filoviruses to humans through contact with their blood and bodily fluids, usually associated with hunting and butchering (see Control Measures, Environmental). For unclear reasons, filovirus outbreaks tend to occur after prolonged dry seasons.

Molecular epidemiologic evidence shows that most outbreaks result from a single point introduction (or very few) into humans from wild animals, followed by human-to-human transmission, almost invariably fueled by health care-associated transmission in areas with inadequate infection-control equipment and resources. Although filoviruses are the most transmissible of all hemorrhagic fever viruses, secondary attack rates in households still generally are only 15% to 20% in African communities and are lower if proper universal and contact precautions are maintained. Human-to-human transmission usually occurs through oral, mucous membrane, or nonintact skin exposure to bodily fluids of a symptomatic person with filovirus disease, most often in the context of providing care to a sick family or community member (community transmission) or patient (health care-associated transmission). Funeral rituals that entail the touching of the corpse also have been implicated. Sexual transmission has been documented and implicated in several clusters of disease. Ebola virus has been detected in human milk; genomic analysis in a recent case of fatal Ebola in a 9-month-old strongly suggested Ebola virus transmission through human milk (see Control Measures, Breastfeeding). Infection through fomites cannot be excluded. Health care-associated transmission is highly unlikely if rigorous infection-control practices are in place in health care facilities (see Isolation of the Hospitalized Patient). Filoviruses are not spread through the air, by water, or in general by food (with the exception of bushmeat; see Control Measures, Environmental). Respiratory spread of virus does not occur.

Children may be less likely to become infected from interfamilial spread than adults when a primary case occurs in a household, possibly secondary to the fact that they are not typically primary caregivers of sick individuals and are less likely to take part in funeral rituals that involve touching and washing of the deceased person's body. Underreporting of Ebola cases in children to health officials also is possible.

The degree of viremia correlates with the clinical state. People are most infectious late in the course of severe disease, especially when copious vomiting, diarrhea, and/or bleeding are present. Transmission during the incubation period, when the person is asymptomatic, is not believed to occur. Virus may persist in a few immunologically protected sites for several weeks to months after clinical recovery, including in testicles/semen, human milk, the central nervous system, joints, and the chambers of the eye (resulting in transient uveitis and other ocular problems). Because of the risk of sexual transmission, abstinence or use of condoms is recommended for at least 9 months after recovery and possibly longer.

The 2014–2015 West Africa Ebola outbreak was the largest since the virus was first identified in 1976. Updated information on identification and current management of people traveling from areas of transmission or with contact with a person with Ebola virus infection can be found on the Centers for Disease Control and Prevention (CDC) Web site (**www.cdc.gov/vhf/ebola/**) and the AAP Web site (for pediatricians: **www. aap.org/en-us/advocacy-and-policy/aap-health-initiatives/Children-and-Disasters/Pages/Ebola.aspx** and for parents or caregivers: **www.healthychildren. org/English/health-issues/conditions/infections/Pages/Ebola.aspx** and **www.cdc.gov/vhf/ebola/pdf/how-talk-children-about-ebola.pdf**).

DIAGNOSTIC TESTS: The diagnosis of filovirus infection should be considered in a person who develops a fever within 21 days of travel to an area with endemic infection. Because initial clinical manifestations are difficult to distinguish from those of more common febrile diseases, prompt laboratory testing is imperative in a suspected case. Malaria, measles, typhoid fever, Lassa fever, and dengue should be included in the differential diagnosis of a symptomatic person returning from Africa within 21 days and are much more likely than a filovirus to be the cause of fever. Filovirus disease can be diagnosed by testing of blood by reverse transcriptase-polymerase chain reaction (RT-PCR) assay, enzyme-linked immunosorbent assay (ELISA) for viral antigens or immunoglobulin (Ig) M, and virus isolation early in the disease course, with the latter being attempted only under Biosafety level-4 conditions. Viral RNA generally is detectable by RT-PCR assay within 3 to 10 days after the onset of symptoms. IgM and IgG antibodies may be used later in disease course or after recovery. Postmortem diagnosis can be made via immunohistochemical staining of skin or liver or spleen tissue. Testing generally is not performed routinely in clinical laboratories. Local and state public health department officials must be contacted and can facilitate testing at a regional certified laboratory or at the CDC. Current information on the most appropriate diagnostic testing for Ebola is available on the CDC Web site (**www.cdc.gov/vhf/ebola/diagnosis/index.html**).

TREATMENT: People suspected of having filovirus infection should be placed in isolation immediately, and public health officials should be notified. Management of patients with filovirus disease primarily is supportive, including oral or intravenous fluids with electrolyte repletion, vasopressors, blood products, total parenteral nutrition, and antimalarial and antimicrobial medications when coinfections are suspected or confirmed (**www. cdc.gov/vhf/ebola/treatment/index.html**). Volume losses can be enormous (10 L/day in adults), and some centers in the United States report better results with repletion using lactated Ringer solution rather than normal saline solution in management of adult patients. When antimicrobial agents are used to treat sepsis, the medications should have coverage for intestinal microbiota based on limited evidence of translocation of gut bacteria into the blood of patients with filovirus disease.

There currently are no specific therapies approved by the US Food and Drug Administration (FDA) for filovirus infection. Investigational agents have been evaluated in nonhuman primates, and some candidate agents (eg, monoclonal antibody and convalescent serum products) currently are in clinical development and were used during the 2014–2015 Ebola outbreak. Because therapeutic options are likely to change following results from numerous ongoing clinical trials, it would be appropriate to consult with the CDC to determine the most current treatment guidelines (**www.cdc.gov/vhf/ebola/treatment/index.html**).

ISOLATION OF THE HOSPITALIZED PATIENT: Standard, contact, and droplet precautions are recommended for management of hospitalized patients with known or suspected Ebola virus disease. Although prudent to place the patient in a negative-pressure room as an extra precaution, availability of such a resource should not prevent care, because there is no evidence for natural aerosol transmission between humans. Access to the patient should be limited to a small number of designated staff and family members with specific instructions and training on filovirus infection control and on the use of personal protective equipment. Although experience suggests that standard universal and contact protections usually are protective, viral hemorrhagic fever precautions consisting of at least 2 pairs of gloves, fit-tested N95 or particulate respirator, impermeable or fluid-resistant gown, face shield (if using N95 respirator), protective apron, and shoe covers or rubber boots are recommended when filovirus infection is confirmed or suspected. Health care workers should have no skin exposed, and a buddy system should be used for donning and doffing personal protective equipment. All health care workers should be knowledgeable with and proficient in the donning and doffing of personnel protective equipment prior to participating in management of a patient. Particulate respirators are recommended when aerosol-generating procedures, such as endotracheal intubation, are performed. Current guidance from the CDC on personal protective equipment can be found on the CDC Web site (**www.cdc.gov/vhf/ebola/healthcare-us/ppe/guidance.html**).

The American Academy of Pediatrics has published a clinical report[1] that provides guidance to health care providers and hospitals on options to consider regarding parental presence at the bedside while caring for a child with suspected or proven Ebola virus disease or other highly consequential infections. Options are presented to help meet the needs of the patient and the family while also posing the least risk to providers and health care organizations. The optimal way to minimize risk is to limit contact between the person under investigation or being treated and family members/caregivers whenever possible while working to meet the emotional support needs of both patient and family.

CONTROL MEASURES:

Contact Tracing. Monitoring and movement of people with potential Ebola virus exposure currently is based on the degree of possible risk. Categories include high risk, some risk,

---

[1]American Academy of Pediatrics, Committee on Infectious Diseases. Parental presence during treatment of Ebola or other highly consequential infection. *Pediatrics.* 2016;138(3):e20161891. Available at: **https://pediatrics.aappublications.org/content/138/3/e20161891**

low risk, and no identifiable risk. Full descriptions of recommended management for people in these categories can be found on the CDC Web site (**www.cdc.gov/vhf/ ebola/exposure/risk-factors-when-evaluating-person-for-exposure.html**). Asymptomatic people at high, some, or low risk should have active monitoring consisting of, at a minimum, daily reporting of measured temperatures and symptoms consistent with Ebola (including severe headache, fatigue, muscle pain, weakness, diarrhea, vomiting, abdominal pain, or unexplained hemorrhage) by the individual to the public health authority. People actively being monitored should measure their temperature twice daily, monitor themselves for symptoms, report as directed to the public health authority, and immediately notify the public health authority if they develop fever or other symptoms. Restrictions on movement and activities sometimes are recommended, and the latest recommendations can be found at **www.cdc.gov/vhf/ebola/exposure/monitoring- and-movement-of-persons-with-exposure.html.** Hospitalization of asymptomatic contacts is not warranted, but contacts who develop fever or other manifestations of filovirus disease should be isolated immediately until the diagnosis can be ruled out. Despite lack of evidence for transmission during the incubation period, it usually is recommended that asymptomatic exposed people avoid close contact or activities that might result in exposure to bodily fluids, such as sharing utensils, kissing, and sexual activity.

Immunoprophylaxis. Although there currently are no FDA-approved vaccines, a number of experimental vaccines and passively transferred immunoglobulins have been shown to be efficacious in nonhuman primate models, including when administered after exposure. Several Ebola virus vaccine candidates currently are in clinical development.

Breastfeeding. It is not known whether Ebola virus can be transmitted from mothers to their infants through breastfeeding, but live virus has been cultured from human milk and at least 1 fatal case associated with breastfeeding has been reported. Given what is known about transmission of Ebola virus, regardless of breastfeeding status, infants whose mothers are acutely infected with Ebola virus already are at high risk of acquiring Ebola virus infection through close contact with the mother and are at high risk of death overall. Therefore, mothers with probable or confirmed Ebola virus infection should not have close contact with their infants (including breastfeeding). There is not enough evidence to provide guidance on when it is safe to resume breastfeeding after a mother's recovery, unless her milk can be demonstrated to be Ebola virus-free by laboratory testing.

Travelers. Nonessential travel to areas where Ebola outbreaks are occurring is not recommended. Travelers to an area affected by an Ebola outbreak should practice careful hygiene (eg, wash hands with soap and water or a 9:1 water to bleach solution, use an alcohol-based hand sanitizer, and avoid contact with blood and body fluids). Travelers should not handle items that may have come in contact with an infected person's blood or body fluids, such as clothes, bedding, needles, and medical equipment. Funeral or burial rituals that require handling the body of someone who has died from Ebola should be avoided. Travelers should avoid hospitals where Ebola patients are being treated in areas of Africa with endemic disease; the United States embassy or consulate often is able to provide advice on facilities that should be avoided. Following return to the United States, travelers should monitor their health closely for 21 days and seek medical care immediately if they develop symptoms of Ebola (see Control Measures, Environmental). State laws mandating confinement or quarantine may apply. Current travel information for countries affected by Ebola can be found on the CDC Web site (**www.cdc.gov/vhf/ebola/ travelers/index.html**).

Environmental. Avoiding contact with bats, primarily by avoiding entry into caves and mines in areas with endemic disease, is a key preventive measure for filoviruses. People also should avoid exposure to fresh blood, bodily fluids, or meat of wild animals (bushmeat), especially nonhuman primates but also bats, porcupines, duikers (a type of antelope), and other mammals, in areas with endemic filovirus disease.

Public Health Reporting. Because of the risk of health care-associated transmission, state/local health departments and the CDC should be contacted immediately for specific advice about confirmation and management of suspected cases. In the United States, Ebola and Marburg hemorrhagic fevers are reportable by guidelines of the Council of State and Territorial Epidemiologists. If a filoviral hemorrhagic fever is suspected, the state/local health department or CDC Emergency Operations Center (770-488-7100) should be contacted to assist with case investigation, diagnosis, management, and control measures.

Hepatitis A

CLINICAL MANIFESTATIONS: Hepatitis A characteristically is an acute, self-limited illness associated with fever, malaise, jaundice, anorexia, and nausea. Symptomatic hepatitis A virus (HAV) infection occurs in approximately 30% of infected children younger than 6 years; few of these children will have jaundice. Among older children and adults, infection usually is symptomatic and typically lasts several weeks, with jaundice occurring in 70% or more of cases. Signs and symptoms typically last less than 2 months, although 10% to 15% of symptomatic people have prolonged or relapsing disease lasting as long as 6 months. Fulminant hepatitis is rare but is more common in people with underlying liver disease. Chronic infection does not occur.

ETIOLOGY: HAV is a small, nonenveloped, positive-sense RNA virus with an icosahedral capsid and classified as a member of the family *Picornaviridae*, genus *Hepatovirus*.

EPIDEMIOLOGY: The most common mode of transmission is person to person, resulting from fecal contamination and oral ingestion (ie, the fecal-oral route). In resource-limited countries where infection is endemic, most people are infected during the first decade of life. Rates of HAV decreased drastically in children after universal infant vaccination was recommended. Rates of reported hepatitis A cases in the United States were 0.4/100 000 population in 2015, which has not changed significantly since 2011, when the rate of infections was at a historic low (**www.cdc.gov/hepatitis/statistics/2015surveillance/index.htm**). Vaccine coverage for children 19 to 35 months of age is high. Significant decreases in anti-HAV seroprevalence in older adults (40 years and older) have occurred because of reduced exposure to HAV earlier in life since the introduction of universal infant vaccination, which has resulted in an increasing proportion of adults in the United States being susceptible to hepatitis A. The majority of HAV cases are in adults 20 years and older. The mean age of people hospitalized for HAV infection increased significantly between 2002 and 2011 (mean age, 37.6 years in 2002–2003, compared with 45.5 years in 2010–2011).

Recognized risk factors for HAV infection include close personal contact with a person infected with HAV, international travel, household or personal contact with a newly arriving international adoptee, a recognized foodborne outbreak, men who have sex with men, and use of illegal drugs. Community-wide epidemics have been observed infrequently in recent years; however, outbreaks have been a problem in countries with low incidence of disease after food was imported from countries where HAV is endemic. Waterborne outbreaks are rare and are typically associated with sewage-contaminated or inadequately treated water. Health care-associated outbreaks have occurred through blood transfusions and liver transplantation.

Patients infected with HAV are most infectious during the 1 to 2 weeks before onset of jaundice or elevation of liver enzymes, when concentration of virus in the stool is highest. The risk of transmission subsequently diminishes and is minimal by 1 week after onset of jaundice. However, HAV can be detected in stool for longer periods, especially in neonates and young children.

The **incubation period** is 15 to 50 days, with an average of 28 days.

DIAGNOSTIC TESTS: Serologic tests for HAV-specific total antibody (ie, immunoglobulin [Ig] G plus IgM), IgG only anti-HAV, and IgM only anti-HAV are available commercially, primarily in enzyme immunoassay format. A single total or IgG anti-HAV test does not have diagnostic value for acute infection. The presence of serum IgM anti-HAV indicates current or recent infection, although false-positive results may occur.[1] IgM anti-HAV generally is included in most acute hepatitis serologic test panels offered by hospital or reference laboratories. IgM anti-HAV is detectable in up to 20% of vaccine recipients when measured 2 weeks after hepatitis A immunization. In most infected people, serum IgM anti-HAV becomes detectable 5 to 10 days before onset of symptoms and declines to undetectable concentrations within 6 months after infection. People who have positive test results for IgM anti-HAV more than 1 year after infection have been reported. IgG anti-HAV is detectable shortly after appearance of IgM. A positive total anti-HAV (ie, IgM and IgG) test result with a negative IgM anti-HAV test result indicates immunity from past infection or vaccination. Polymerase chain reaction assays for hepatitis A are available but not currently cleared by the US Food and Drug Administration (FDA). They may be considered for detection of very early acute infections and for confirmation of questionable IgM anti-HAV results.

TREATMENT: Supportive.

ISOLATION OF THE HOSPITALIZED PATIENT: In general, hospitalization is not required for patients with uncomplicated acute hepatitis A. When hospitalization is necessary, contact precautions are recommended in addition to standard precautions for diapered and incontinent patients for at least 1 week after onset of symptoms.

CONTROL MEASURES[2-4]:

General Measures. The major methods of prevention of HAV infections are improved sanitation (eg, in food preparation and of water sources) and personal hygiene (eg, hand hygiene after toileting and diaper changes in child care settings) and administration of either

---

[1]Centers for Disease Control and Prevention. Positive test results for acute hepatitis A virus infection among persons with no recent history of acute hepatitis—United States, 2002–2004. *MMWR Morb Mortal Wkly Rep.* 2005;54(18):453–456

[2]Centers for Disease Control and Prevention. Prevention of hepatitis A through active or passive immunization: recommendations of the Advisory Committee on Immunization Practices (ACIP). *MMWR Recomm Rep.* 2006;55(RR-7):1–23

[3]Centers for Disease Control and Prevention. Prevention after exposure and in international travelers. *MMWR Morb Mortal Wkly Rep.* 2007;56(41):1080–1084

[4]Centers for Disease Control and Prevention. Use of vaccine in close contacts of international adoptees. *MMWR Morb Mortal Wkly Rep.* 2009;58(36):1006–1007

hepatitis A vaccine (HepA) or Immune Globulin (IG) for postexposure prophylaxis within 14 days of last exposure.

Schools, Child Care, and Work. Children and adults with acute HAV infection who work as food handlers or attend or work in child care settings should be excluded for 1 week after onset of the illness.

Immune Globulin. Immune Globulin Intramuscular (IGIM), when administered within 2 weeks after exposure to HAV, is more than 85% effective in preventing symptomatic infection. When administered for preexposure prophylaxis, 1 dose of 0.02 mL/kg confers protection against hepatitis A for up to 3 months, and a dose of 0.06 mL/kg protects for 3 to 5 months. Recommended preexposure and postexposure IGIM doses and duration of protection are provided in Tables 3.16 and 3.17. HAV vaccine is preferred for preexposure protection in all populations (age ≥1 year) unless contraindicated and should be administered at least 2 weeks before expected exposure. Vaccine may be used for postexposure prophylaxis for most people 1 through 40 years of age (see Postexposure Prophylaxis, p 399).

Hepatitis A Vaccine. Two inactivated hepatitis A (HepA) vaccines, Havrix (GlaxoSmithKline, Research Triangle Park, NC) and Vaqta (Merck & Co Inc, Whitehouse Station, NJ), are available in the United States. The vaccines are prepared from cell culture-adapted HAV, which is propagated in human fibroblasts, purified from cell lysates, formalin inactivated, and adsorbed to an aluminum hydroxide adjuvant. Vaqta contains no preservative. Havrix contains 0.5% 2-phenoxyethanol as a preservative.

Table 3.16. Recommendations for Preexposure Immunoprophylaxis of Hepatitis A Virus (HAV) for Travelers to Countries With High or Intermediate Hepatitis A Endemicity[a]

Age	Recommended Prophylaxis	Notes
Younger than 12 mo	IGIM	0.02 mL/kg[b] protects for up to 3 mo. For trips of 3 mo or longer, 0.06 mL/kg[b] should be administered at departure and every 5 mo if exposure to HAV continues.
12 mo through 40 y	HepA vaccine[c]	
41 y or older	HepA vaccine, with or without IGIM[c]	If departure is in less than 2 wk, older adults, immunocompromised people, and people with chronic liver disease or other chronic medical conditions can receive IGIM with the initial dose of HepA vaccine to ensure optimal protection.

IGIM indicates Immune Globulin Intramuscular; HepA, hepatitis A vaccine.

[a]All people 12 months of age or older at high risk of HAV disease should be immunized routinely (see People at Increased Risk, p 397).

[b]IGIM should be administered deep into a large muscle mass. Ordinarily, no more than 5 mL should be administered in one site in an adult or large child; lesser amounts (maximum 3 mL in one site) should be administered to small children and infants.

[c]People who have a contraindication to HepA vaccine should receive IGIM.

Table 3.17. Recommendations for Postexposure Immunoprophylaxis of Hepatitis A Virus (HAV)

Time Since Exposure	Age of Patient	Recommended Prophylaxis
2 wk or less	Younger than 12 mo	IGIM, 0.02 mL/kg[a]
	12 mo through 40 y	HepA vaccine[b]
	41 y or older	IGIM, 0.02 mL/kg,[a] but HepA vaccine[b] can be used if IGIM is unavailable[a]
	People of any age who are immunocompromised, have chronic liver disease, or contraindication to vaccination	IGIM, 0.02 mL/kg[a]
More than 2 wk	Younger than 12 mo	No prophylaxis
	12 mo or older	No prophylaxis, but HepA vaccine may be indicated for ongoing exposure[b]

IGIM indicates Immune Globulin Intramuscular; HepA, hepatitis A vaccine.

[a] IGIM should be administered deep into a large muscle mass. Ordinarily, no more than 5 mL should be administered in one site in an adult or large child; lesser amounts (maximum 3 mL in one site) should be administered to small children and infants.

[b] Dosage and schedule of hepatitis A vaccine as recommended according to age in Table 3.18. Only monovalent hepatitis A vaccine (Havrix or Vaqta) should be used for postexposure prophylaxis.

Table 3.18. Recommended Doses and Schedules for Inactivated Hepatitis A Virus (HepA) Vaccines[a]

Age	Vaccine	Hepatitis A Antigen Dose	Volume per Dose, mL	No. of Doses	Schedule
12 mo through 18 y	Havrix	720 ELU	0.5	2	Initial and 6–12 mo later
12 mo through 18 y	Vaqta	25 U[b]	0.5	2	Initial and 6–18 mo later
19 y or older	Havrix	1440 ELU	1.0	2	Initial and 6–12 mo later
19 y or older	Vaqta	50 U[b]	1.0	2	Initial and 6–18 mo later
18 y or older	Twinrix[c]	720 ELU	1.0	3 or 4	Initial, 1 mo, and 6 mo later **OR** Initial, 7 days, and 21–30 days, followed by a dose at 12 mo

ELU indicates enzyme-linked immunosorbent assay units.

[a] Havrix and Twinrix are manufactured by GlaxoSmithKline Biologicals (Research Triangle Park, NC); Vaqta is manufactured and distributed by Merck & Co Inc (Whitehouse Station, NJ).

[b] Antigen units (each unit is equivalent to approximately 1 μg of viral protein).

[c] A combination of hepatitis B (Engerix-B, 20 μg) and hepatitis A (Havrix, 720 ELU) vaccine (Twinrix) is licensed for use in people 18 years and older in 3-dose and 4-dose schedules.

Administration, Dosages, and Schedules (see Table 3.18). HepA vaccines are licensed for people 12 months and older and have pediatric and adult formulations that are administered in a 2-dose schedule. The adult formulations are approved for people 19 years and older. Recommended doses and schedules for these different products and formulations are provided in Table 3.18. A combination HepA/hepatitis B vaccine (Twinrix [GlaxoSmithKline, Research Triangle Park, NC]) is licensed in the United States for people 18 years and older and can be administered in a 3-dose schedule or an accelerated 4-dose schedule (see Table 3.18). All HepA-containing vaccines are administered intramuscularly.

Immunogenicity. Available HepA vaccines are highly immunogenic when administered in their respective recommended schedules and doses. At least 95% of healthy children, adolescents, and adults have protective antibody concentrations when measured 1 month after receipt of the first dose of either single-antigen vaccine. One month after a second dose, more than 99% of healthy children, adolescents, and adults have protective antibody concentrations.

Available data on the immunogenicity of HepA vaccine in young children indicate high rates of seroconversion, but antibody concentrations are lower in infants with passively acquired maternal anti-HAV in comparison with vaccine recipients lacking anti-HAV. By 12 months of age, passively acquired maternal anti-HAV antibody no longer is detectable in most infants. HepA vaccine is highly immunogenic for children who begin immunization at 12 months or older, regardless of maternal anti-HAV status.

Efficacy. In double-blind, controlled, randomized trials, the protective efficacy in preventing clinical HAV infection was 94% to 100%.

Duration of Protection. Additional booster doses beyond the 2-dose primary immunization series are not recommended. Detectable antibody persists after a 2-dose series for at least 17 years in adults and 15 years in children. Kinetic models of antibody decline indicate that protective levels of anti-HAV could be present for 40 years or longer in adults and 14 to 20 years in children.

Vaccine in Immunocompromised Patients. The immune response in immunocompromised people, including people with human immunodeficiency virus infection, may be suboptimal based on the level of immunosuppression at the time of vaccine administration.

Vaccine Interchangeability. The 2 single-antigen HepA vaccines licensed by the FDA, when administered as recommended, seem to be similarly effective. Studies among adults have found no difference in the immunogenicity of a vaccine series that mixed the 2 currently available vaccines, compared with using the same vaccine throughout the licensed schedule. Therefore, although completion of the immunization regimen with the same product is preferable, immunization with either product is acceptable.

Administration With Other Vaccines. Data indicate that HepA vaccine may be administered simultaneously with other vaccines. Vaccines should be administered in a separate syringe and at a separate injection site (see Simultaneous Administration of Multiple Vaccines, p 35).

Adverse Events. Adverse reactions are mild and include local pain and, less commonly, induration at the injection site. No serious adverse events attributed definitively to HepA vaccine have been reported. The vaccine can be administered either in the thigh or the arm, because the site of injection does not affect the incidence of local reactions.

Precautions and Contraindications to Immunization. The vaccine should not be administered to people with hypersensitivity to any of the vaccine components. A review published in

2014 of Vaccine Adverse Event Reporting System (VAERS) results from January 1, 1996, to April 5, 2013, did not identify any concerning pattern of adverse events in pregnant women or their infants following maternal hepatitis A immunizations during pregnancy. The risk to the fetus is considered to be low or nonexistent, because the vaccine contains inactivated, purified virus particles. In pregnant women, the risk associated with vaccination should be weighed against the risk of HAV infection. Because HepA vaccine is inactivated, no special precautions need to be taken when vaccinating immunocompromised people.

Preimmunization Serologic Testing. Preimmunization testing for anti-HAV generally is not recommended for children because of their expected low prevalence of infection. Testing may be cost-effective for people who have a high likelihood of immunity from previous infection, including people whose childhood was spent in a country with high endemicity, people with a history of jaundice potentially caused by HAV, and people older than 50 years.

Postimmunization Serologic Testing. Postimmunization testing for anti-HAV is not indicated because of the high seroconversion rates in adults and children. In addition, some commercially available anti-HAV tests may not detect low but protective concentrations of antibody among immunized people.

PREVENTION MEASURES:

Preexposure Prophylaxis Against HAV Infection (see Tables 3.16, p 394, and 3.18, p 395). Immunization with HepA vaccine is recommended routinely for children 12 through 23 months of age, for people who are at increased risk of infection, for people who are at increased risk of severe manifestations of hepatitis A if infected, and for any person who wants to obtain immunity.

Children Who Routinely Should Be Immunized or Considered for Immunization. All children in the United States should receive HepA vaccine at 12 through 23 months of age, as recommended in the routine childhood immunization schedule (**https://redbook. solutions.aap.org/SS/Immunization_Schedules.aspx**). Table 3.18 (p 395) shows HepA-containing vaccines licensed by the FDA, their doses, and schedules. Children who are not immunized or have not completed the series by 2 years of age can be immunized at subsequent visits.

People at Increased Risk of HAV Infection or its Consequences Who Routinely Should Be Immunized.

- **People traveling internationally.**[1] All susceptible people traveling to or working in countries that have high or intermediate hepatitis A endemicity should be immunized or receive IGIM before departure (see Table 3.16, p 394), which includes all countries except Western Europe, Scandinavia, Australia, Canada, Japan, and New Zealand. HepA vaccine at the age-appropriate dose is preferred to IGIM. The first dose of HepA vaccine should be administered as soon as travel is considered.
  - ♦ One dose of single-antigen vaccine administered at any time before departure can provide adequate protection for most healthy people. However, no data are available for other populations or other hepatitis A vaccine formulations (eg, the combination HepA-hepatitis B vaccine).
  - ♦ Adults 40 years and older, immunocompromised people, and people with chronic

---

[1]Centers for Disease Control and Prevention. Update: prevention of hepatitis A after exposure to hepatitis A virus and in international travelers. Updated recommendations of the Advisory Committee on Immunization Practices (ACIP). *MMWR Morb Mortal Wkly Rep.* 2007;56(41):1080–1084

liver disease or other chronic medical conditions who are traveling to an area with endemic infection in 2 weeks or less should receive the initial dose of vaccine and simultaneously can receive IGIM (0.02 mL/kg) at a separate anatomic site. People whose travel period is 3 to 5 months should receive IGIM at 0.06 mL/kg. The vaccine series then should be completed according to the licensed schedule.

◆ Travelers who elect not to receive vaccine, are younger than 12 months, or are allergic to a vaccine component should receive a single dose of IGIM (0.02 mL/kg), which provides effective protection for up to 3 months.

- **Close contacts of newly arriving international adoptees.**[1,2] Data from a study conducted at 3 adoption clinics in the United States indicate that 1% to 6% of newly arrived international adoptees have acute HAV infection. The risk of HAV infection among close personal contacts of international adoptees is estimated at 106 (range, 90–819) per 100 000 household contacts of international adoptees within the first 60 days of their arrival in the United States. Therefore, HepA vaccine should be administered to all previously unvaccinated people who anticipate close personal contact (eg, household contact or regular babysitting) with an international adoptee from a country with high or intermediate endemicity during the first 60 days following arrival of the adoptee in the United States. The first dose of the 2-dose HepA vaccine series should be administered as soon as adoption is planned, ideally 2 or more weeks before the arrival of the adoptee.
- **Men who have sex with men.** Cyclic outbreaks of hepatitis A among men who have sex with men have been reported often, including in urban areas in the United States, Canada, and Australia. Therefore, men (adolescents and adults) who have sex with men should be immunized. Preimmunization serologic testing may be cost-effective for older people in this group.
- **Users of injection and noninjection drugs.** Periodic outbreaks among injection and noninjection drug users have been reported in many parts of the United States and in Europe. Adolescents and adults who use illegal drugs should be immunized. Preimmunization serologic testing may be cost-effective for older people in this group.
- **Patients with clotting-factor disorders.** Reported outbreaks of hepatitis A in patients with hemophilia receiving solvent-detergent–treated factor VIII and factor IX concentrates were identified during the 1990s, primarily in Europe, although 1 case was reported in the United States. Therefore, susceptible patients with chronic clotting disorders who receive clotting-factor concentrates should be immunized. Preimmunization testing for anti-HAV may be cost-effective for older people in this group.
- **People at risk of occupational exposure (eg, handlers of nonhuman primates and people working with HAV in a research laboratory setting).** Outbreaks of hepatitis A have been reported among people working with nonhuman primates. These infected primates were born in the wild and were not primates that had been born and raised in captivity. People working with HAV-infected primates or with HAV in a research laboratory setting should be immunized.

---

[1]Centers for Disease Control and Prevention. Updated recommendations from the Advisory Committee on Immunization Practices (ACIP) for use of hepatitis A vaccine in close contacts of newly arriving international adoptees. *MMWR Morb Mortal Wkly Rep.* 2009;58(36):1006–1007

[2]American Academy of Pediatrics, Committee on Infectious Diseases. Recommendations for administering hepatitis A vaccine to contacts of international adoptees. *Pediatrics.* 2011;128(4):803–804

- **People with chronic liver disease.** Because people with chronic liver disease are at increased risk of fulminant hepatitis A, susceptible patients with chronic liver disease should be immunized. Susceptible people who are awaiting or have received liver transplants should be immunized.

Postexposure Prophylaxis (see Table 3.17, p 395).[1] A randomized clinical trial conducted among people 2 through 40 years of age comparing postexposure efficacy of IGIM and HepA vaccine found that the efficacy of a single dose of HepA vaccine was similar to that of IGIM in preventing symptomatic infection when administered within 14 days after exposure.

People who have been exposed to HAV and previously have not received HepA vaccine should receive a single dose of single-antigen HepA vaccine or IGIM as soon as possible (see Table 3.17, p 395, for prophylaxis guidance and dosages). The efficacy of IGIM or vaccine for postexposure prophylaxis when administered more than 2 weeks after exposure has not been established. No data are available for people older than 40 years or people with underlying medical conditions.

- For **healthy people 12 months through 40 years of age,** HepA vaccine at the age-appropriate dose is preferred to IGIM because of vaccine advantages, including long-term protection and ease of administration.
- For **people older than 40 years,** IGIM is preferred because of the absence of data regarding vaccine performance in this age group and the increased risk of severe manifestations of hepatitis A with increasing age. However, HepA vaccine can be used if IGIM is unavailable.
- IGIM should be used for **children younger than 12 months,** immunocompromised people, people with chronic liver disease, and people for whom HepA vaccine is contraindicated.
- People who are receiving IGIM and for whom HepA vaccine also is recommended for other reasons should receive a dose of vaccine simultaneously with IGIM at a different site. For people who receive HepA vaccine, the second dose should be administered according to the licensed schedule to complete the series.
- **Household and sexual contacts.** All previously unimmunized people with close personal contact with a person with serologically confirmed HAV infection, such as household and sexual contacts, should receive HepA vaccine or IGIM within 2 weeks after the most recent exposure (Table 3.17, p 395). Serologic testing of contacts is not recommended, because testing adds unnecessary cost and may delay administration of postexposure prophylaxis.
- **Newborn infants of HAV-infected mothers.** Perinatal transmission of HAV is rare. Some experts advise giving IGIM (0.02 mL/kg) to an infant if the mother's symptoms began between 2 weeks before and 1 week after delivery. Efficacy in this circumstance has not been established. Severe disease in healthy infants is rare.
- **Child care center staff, employees, and children and their household contacts.** Outbreaks of HAV infection at child care centers have been recognized since the 1970s, but their frequency has decreased as HAV immunization rates in

---

[1]Centers for Disease Control and Prevention. Update: prevention of hepatitis A after exposure to hepatitis A virus and in international travelers. Updated recommendations of the Advisory Committee on Immunization Practices (ACIP). *MMWR Morb Mortal Wkly Rep.* 2007;56(41):1080–1084

children have increased and as hepatitis A incidence among children has declined. Because infections in children usually are mild or asymptomatic, outbreaks often are identified only when adult contacts (eg, parents) become ill. Serologic testing to confirm HAV infection in suspected cases is indicated.

Routine immunization of staff at child care centers is not recommended. HepA vaccine or IGIM (Table 3.17, p 395) should be administered to all previously unimmunized staff members and attendees of child care centers or homes if (1) one or more cases of hepatitis A are recognized in children or staff members; or (2) cases are recognized in 2 or more households of center attendees. In centers that provide care only to children who do not wear diapers, vaccine or IGIM needs to be administered only to classroom contacts of an index-case patient. When an outbreak occurs (ie, hepatitis A cases in 2 or more families), HepA vaccine or IGIM also should be considered for members of households that have children (center attendees) in diapers.

Children and adults with hepatitis A should be excluded from the center until 1 week after onset of illness, until the postexposure prophylaxis program has been completed in the center, or until directed by the health department (see Table 2.3, p 131). Although precise data concerning the onset of protection after postexposure prophylaxis are not available, allowing asymptomatic prophylaxis recipients to return to the child care center setting immediately after receipt of the vaccine or IGIM dose seems reasonable.

- **Schools.** Schoolroom exposure generally does not pose an appreciable risk of infection, and postexposure prophylaxis is not indicated when a single case occurs and the source of infection is outside the school. However, HepA vaccine or IGIM could be used for unimmunized people who have close contact with the index patient if transmission within the school setting is documented.

- **Hospitals.** Usually, health care-associated HAV in hospital personnel has occurred through spread from patients with acute HAV infection in whom the diagnosis was not recognized. Careful hygienic practices should be emphasized when a patient with jaundice or known or suspected hepatitis A is admitted to the hospital. When outbreaks occur, HepA vaccine or IGIM is recommended for people in close contact with infected patients (Table 3.17, p 395). Routine preexposure use of HepA vaccine for hospital personnel is not recommended.

- **Exposure to an infected food handler.** If a food handler is diagnosed with hepatitis A, HepA vaccine or IGIM should be provided to other food handlers at the same establishment (Table 3.17, p 395). Food handlers with acute HAV infection should be excluded for 1 week after onset of illness. Because common-source transmission to patrons is unlikely, postexposure prophylaxis with HepA vaccine or IGIM typically is not indicated but may be considered if the food handler directly handled food during the time when the food handler likely was infectious and had diarrhea or poor hygiene practices and if prophylaxis can be provided within 2 weeks of exposure. Routine HepA immunization of food handlers is not recommended.

- **Common-source exposure.** Postexposure prophylaxis (HepA vaccine or IGIM) can be considered if it can be administered to exposed people within 2 weeks of an exposure to the HAV-contaminated water or food. The efficacy of IGIM or vaccine when administered >2 weeks after exposure has not been established.

Hepatitis B

CLINICAL MANIFESTATIONS: People acutely infected with hepatitis B virus (HBV) may be asymptomatic or symptomatic. The likelihood of developing symptoms of acute hepatitis is age dependent: less than 1% of infants younger than 1 year, 5% to 15% of children 1 through 5 years of age, and 30% to 50% of people older than 5 years are symptomatic, although few data are available for adults older than 30 years. The spectrum of signs and symptoms is varied and includes subacute illness with nonspecific symptoms (eg, anorexia, nausea, or malaise), clinical hepatitis with jaundice, or fulminant hepatitis. Extrahepatic manifestations, such as arthralgia, arthritis, macular rashes, thrombocytopenia, polyarteritis nodosa, or glomerulonephritis, can occur early in the course of illness and may precede jaundice. Papular acrodermatitis (Gianotti-Crosti syndrome) is an extrahepatic manifestation of infection attributable to a number of viral infections, including hepatitis B. However, since the advent of universal HBV immunization in infants, papular acrodermatitis attributable to HBV is rare; it is more commonly caused by Epstein-Barr virus and less commonly by enteroviruses, cytomegalovirus, parvovirus B19, and others. Acute HBV infection cannot be distinguished from other forms of acute viral hepatitis on the basis of clinical signs and symptoms or nonspecific laboratory findings.

Chronic HBV infection is defined as persistence in serum for at least 6 months of any one of the following: hepatitis B surface antigen (HBsAg), HBV DNA, or hepatitis B e antigen (HBeAg). Chronic HBV infection is likely in the presence of HBsAg, HBV DNA, or HBeAg in serum from a person who tests negative for antibody of the immunoglobulin (Ig) M subclass to hepatitis B core antigen (IgM anti-HBc).

Age at the time of infection is the primary determinant of risk of progressing to chronic infection. Up to 90% of infants infected perinatally or in the first year of life will develop chronic HBV infection. Between 25% and 50% of children infected between 1 and 5 years of age become chronically infected, whereas 5% to 10% of infected older children and adults develop chronic HBV infection. Patients who become HBV infected while immunosuppressed or with an underlying chronic illness (eg, end-stage renal disease) have an increased risk of developing chronic infection. In the absence of treatment, up to 25% of infants and children who acquire chronic HBV infection will die prematurely from HBV-related hepatocellular carcinoma or cirrhosis.

The clinical course of untreated chronic HBV infection varies according to the population studied, reflecting differences in age at acquisition, rate of loss of HBeAg, and possibly HBV genotype. Most children have asymptomatic infection. Perinatally infected children usually have normal or minimally elevated alanine transaminase (ALT) concentrations and minimal or mild liver histologic abnormalities, with detectable HBeAg and high HBV DNA concentrations ($\geq$20 000 IU/mL) for years to decades after initial infection. Children with chronic HBV may exhibit growth impairment. Chronic HBV infection acquired during later childhood or adolescence usually is accompanied by more active liver disease and increased serum aminotransferase concentrations. Patients with detectable HBeAg *(HBeAg-positive chronic hepatitis B)* usually have high concentrations of HBV DNA and HBsAg in serum and are more likely to transmit infection. Because HBV-associated liver injury is thought to be immune mediated, in people coinfected with human immunodeficiency virus (HIV) and HBV, the return of immune competence with antiretroviral treatment of HIV infection may lead to a reactivation of HBV-related liver inflammation and damage. Over time (years to decades), HBeAg becomes undetectable in many chronically infected people. This transition often is accompanied by development of antibody to HBeAg (anti-HBe) and decreases in serum HBV DNA and serum aminotransferase concentrations and may be preceded by a temporary exacerbation of liver disease. These patients have *inactive chronic infection* but still may have exacerbations of hepatitis. Serologic reversion (reappearance of HBeAg) is more common if loss of HBeAg is not accompanied by development of anti-HBe; reversion with loss of anti-HBe also can occur.

Some patients who lose HBeAg may continue to have ongoing histologic evidence of liver damage and moderate to high concentrations of HBV DNA *(HBeAg-negative chronic hepatitis B)*. Patients with histologic evidence of chronic HBV infection, regardless of HBeAg status, remain at higher risk of death attributable to liver failure compared with HBV-infected people with no histologic evidence of liver inflammation and fibrosis.

Resolved hepatitis B is defined as clearance of HBsAg, normalization of serum aminotransferase concentrations, and development of antibody to HBsAg (anti-HBs). Chronically infected adults clear HBsAg and develop anti-HBs at the rate of 1% to 2% annually; during childhood, the annual clearance rate is less than 1%. Reactivation of resolved chronic infection is possible if these patients become immunosuppressed and also is well reported among HBsAg-positive patients receiving anti-tumor necrosis factor agents or disease-modifying antirheumatic drugs (12% of patients).

ETIOLOGY: HBV is a partially double-stranded DNA-containing 42-nm-diameter enveloped virus in the family *Hepadnaviridae*. Important components of the viral particle include an outer lipoprotein envelope containing HBsAg and an inner nucleocapsid consisting of hepatitis B core antigen (HBcAg).

EPIDEMIOLOGY: HBV is transmitted through infected blood or body fluids. Although HBsAg has been detected in multiple body fluids including human milk, saliva, and tears, the most potentially infectious include blood, serum, semen, vaginal secretions, and cerebrospinal, synovial, pleural, pericardial, peritoneal, and amniotic fluids. People with chronic HBV infection are the primary reservoirs for infection. Common modes of transmission include percutaneous and permucosal exposure to infectious body fluids; sharing or using nonsterilized needles, syringes, or glucose monitoring equipment or devices; sexual contact with an infected person; perinatal exposure to an infected mother; and household exposure to a person with chronic HBV infection. The risk of HBV acquisition when a susceptible child bites a child who has chronic HBV infection is unknown. A theoretical risk exists if HBsAg-positive blood enters the oral cavity of the biter, but transmission by this route has not been reported. Transmission by transfusion of contaminated blood or blood products is rare in the United States because of routine screening of blood donors and viral inactivation of certain blood products before administration.

Perinatal transmission of HBV is highly efficient and usually occurs from blood exposures during labor and delivery. In utero transmission accounts for less than 2% of all vertically transmitted HBV infections in most studies. Without postexposure prophylaxis, the risk of an infant acquiring HBV from an infected mother as a result of perinatal exposure is 70% to 90% for infants born to mothers who are HBsAg and HBeAg positive; the risk is 5% to 20% for infants born to HBsAg-positive but HBeAg-negative mothers.

Person-to-person spread of HBV can occur in settings involving interpersonal contact over extended periods, such as in a household with a person with chronic HBV infection. In regions of the world with a high prevalence of chronic HBV infection, transmission between children in household settings may account for a substantial amount of transmission. The precise mechanisms of transmission from child-to-child are unknown; however, frequent interpersonal contact of nonintact skin or mucous membranes with blood-containing secretions, open skin lesions, or blood-containing saliva are potential means of transmission. Transmission from sharing inanimate objects, such as razors or toothbrushes, also may occur. HBV can survive in the environment for 7 or more days but is inactivated by commonly used disinfectants, including household bleach diluted 1:10 with water. HBV is not transmitted by the fecal-oral route.

Transmission among children born in the United States is unusual because of high coverage with hepatitis B (HepB) vaccine administered at birth. Screening mothers during pregnancy for HBV infection allows for additional immunoprophylaxis with Hepatitis B Immune Globulin (HBIG), which, when administered with the hepatitis B vaccine in the immediate newborn period, enhances prevention of mother-to-infant HBV transmission. The risk of HBV transmission is higher in children who have not completed a vaccine series, children undergoing hemodialysis, institutionalized children with developmental disabilities, and children emigrating from regions and countries with endemic HBV (eg, Southeast Asia, China, Africa). Person-to-person transmission has been reported in child care settings, but risk of transmission in child care facilities in the United States has become negligible as a result of high infant hepatitis B immunization rates.

Acute HBV infection is reported most commonly among adults 30 through 49 years of age in the United States. Since 1990, the incidence of acute HBV infection has decreased in all age categories, with a 98% decline in children younger than 19 years and a 93% decline in young adults 20 through 29 years of age, with most of the decrease among people 20 through 24 years of age. Current statistics on hepatitis B case numbers and incidence rates can be found at **www.cdc.gov/hepatitis/statistics/2015surveillance/index.htm.** People at high risk for acute hepatitis B virus infection include people who inject drugs, people with multiple sexual partners, men who have sex with men, and those who reported surgery during the 6 weeks to 6 months before onset of symptoms. Others at increased risk include people with occupational exposure to blood or body fluids, staff of institutions and nonresidential child care programs for children with developmental disabilities, patients undergoing hemodialysis, and sexual or household contacts of people with an acute or chronic infection. Approximately 62% of case reports in 2014 with risk exposure or behavior information did not have a readily identifiable risk characteristic. HBV infection in adolescents and adults is associated with other sexually transmitted infections, including syphilis and HIV infection. Investigations have indicated an increased risk of HBV infection among adults with diabetes mellitus. Outbreaks in nonhospital health care settings, including assisted-living facilities and nursing homes, highlight the increased risk among people with diabetes mellitus undergoing assisted blood glucose monitoring.[1]

The prevalence of HBV infection and patterns of transmission vary markedly throughout the world (see Table 3.19). Approximately 45% of people worldwide live in regions of high HBV endemicity, where the prevalence of chronic HBV infection is 8% or greater. Historically in these regions, most new HBV infections occurred as a result of

---

[1]Centers for Disease Control and Prevention. Use of hepatitis B vaccination for adults with diabetes mellitus: recommendations of the Advisory Committee on Immunization Practices (ACIP). *MMWR Morb Mortal Wkly Rep.* 2011;60(50):1709–1711

perinatal or early childhood infections. In regions of intermediate HBV endemicity, where the prevalence of HBV infection is 2% to 7%, multiple modes of transmission (ie, perinatal, household, sexual, injection drug use, and health care associated) contribute to the burden of infection. In countries with low endemicity, where chronic HBV infection prevalence is less than 2% (including the United States) and where routine immunization has been adopted, new infections increasingly occur among unimmunized age groups. Many people born in countries with high endemicity live in the United States. Infant immunization programs in some of these countries have, in recent years, greatly reduced the seroprevalence of HBsAg, but many other countries with endemic HBV have yet to implement widespread routine childhood hepatitis B immunization programs.

The **incubation period** for acute HBV infection is 45 to 160 days, with an average of 90 days.

DIAGNOSTIC TESTS: Serologic protein antigen tests are available commercially to detect HBsAg and HBeAg. Serologic antibody assays also are available for detection of anti-HBs, total anti-HBc, IgM anti-HBc, and anti-HBe (see Table 3.20, p 405, Fig 3.2, p 406, and Fig 3.3, p 407). In addition, nucleic acid amplification testing (NAAT), polymerase chain reaction (PCR) assay, and branched DNA methods as well as hybridization assays are available to detect and quantify HBV DNA in plasma or serum. At least 2 PCR assays for quantitative detection of HBV DNA are cleared by the US Food and Drug Administration (FDA). These assays are used to monitor patients with chronic HBV infection and to evaluate their response to treatment regimens. The assays differ in their limits of detection, dynamic range, and target gene sequences detected. Because of variability in the different assays, it is best to use the same manufacturer's assay performed in the same laboratory to monitor an individual's patient's HBV load. Tests to quantify HBsAg and HBeAg currently are being developed but are not yet available commercially.

Table 3.19. Estimated International HBsAg Prevalence[a]

Region	Estimated HBsAg Prevalence[b]
North America	0.1%
Mexico and Central America	0.3%
South America	0.7%
Western Europe	0.7%
Australia and New Zealand	0.9%
Caribbean (except Haiti)	1.0%
Eastern Europe and North Asia	2.8%
South Asia	2.8%
Middle East	3.2%
Haiti	5.6%
East Asia	7.4%
Southeast Asia	9.1%
Africa	9.3%
Pacific Islands	12.0%

HBsAg indicates hepatitis B surface antigen.

[a]Centers for Disease Control and Prevention. A comprehensive immunization strategy to eliminate transmission of hepatitis B virus infection in the United States. Recommendations of the Advisory Committee on Immunization Practices (ACIP). Part II: immunization of adults. *MMWR Recomm Rep.* 2006;55(RR-16):1–33

[b]Level of HBV endemicity defined as high (≥8%), intermediate (2%–7%), and low (<2%).

Table 3.20. Diagnostic Tests for Hepatitis B Virus (HBV) Antigens and Antibodies

Factors To Be Tested	HBV Antigen or Antibody	Use
HBsAg	Hepatitis B surface antigen	Detection of acutely or chronically infected people; antigen used in hepatitis B vaccine; can be detected for up to 3 weeks after a dose of hepatitis B vaccine
Anti-HBs	Antibody to HBsAg	Identification of people who have resolved infections with HBV; determination of immunity after immunization
HBeAg	Hepatitis B e antigen	Identification of infected people at increased risk of transmitting HBV
Anti-HBe	Antibody to HBeAg	Identification of infected people with lower risk of transmitting HBV
Anti-HBc (total)	Antibody to HBcAg[a]	Identification of people with acute, resolved, or chronic HBV infection (not present after immunization); passively transferred maternal anti-HBc is detectable for as long as 24 months among infants born to HBsAg-positive women
IgM anti-HBc	IgM antibody to HBcAg	Identification of people with acute or recent HBV infections (including HBsAg-negative people during the "window" phase of infection; unreliable for detecting perinatal HBV infection)

HBcAg indicates hepatitis B core antigen; IgM, immunoglobulin M.
[a] No test is available commercially to measure HBcAg.

HBsAg is detectable during acute and chronic infection. If HBV infection is self-limited, HBsAg disappears in most patients within a few weeks to several months after infection, followed by appearance of anti-HBs. The time between disappearance of HBsAg and appearance of anti-HBs is termed the *window period* of infection. During the window period, the only marker of acute infection is IgM anti-HBc, which is highly specific for establishing the diagnosis of acute infection. However, IgM anti-HBc usually is not present in infants infected perinatally. People with chronic HBV infection have circulating HBsAg and circulating total anti-HBc (Fig 3.3, p 407); in a minority of chronically infected individuals, anti-HBs also is present. Both anti-HBs and total anti-HBc are present in people with resolved infection, whereas anti-HBs alone is present in people immunized with hepatitis B vaccine. The presence of HBeAg in serum correlates with higher concentrations of HBV DNA and greater infectivity. Tests for HBeAg and HBV DNA are useful in selection of candidates to receive antiviral therapy and to monitor response to therapy.

Transient HBsAg antigenemia can occur following receipt of HepB vaccine, with HBsAg being detected as early as 24 hours after and up to 3 weeks following administration of the vaccine.

TREATMENT: No specific therapy for uncomplicated *acute* HBV infection is available, and acute HBV infection usually does not warrant referral to a hepatitis specialist unless there is progression to acute liver failure. In that situation, treatment with a nucleoside or nucleotide analogue is indicated. Acute HBV infection may be difficult to distinguish from reactivation of HBV. If reactivation is a possibility, referral to a hepatitis specialist would be warranted. HBIG and corticosteroids are not effective treatment for acute or chronic disease.

Children and adolescents who have chronic HBV infection are at risk of developing serious liver disease, including primary hepatocellular carcinoma (HCC), with advancing age and, therefore, should receive hepatitis A vaccine. Although the peak incidence of primary HCC attributable to HBV infection is in the fifth decade of life, HCC occurs in children as young as 6 years who became infected perinatally or in early childhood. Several algorithms have been published describing the initial evaluation, monitoring, and criteria for treatment. Children with chronic HBV infection should be screened periodically for hepatic complications using serum aminotransferase tests, alpha-fetoprotein concentration, and abdominal ultrasonography. Definitive recommendations on the frequency and indications for specific tests are not yet available because of lack of data on their reliability in predicting sequelae. Patients with serum ALT concentrations persistently exceeding the upper limit of normal and patients with an increased serum alpha-fetoprotein concentration or abnormal findings on abdominal ultrasonography should be referred to a specialist in the management of chronic HBV infection.

The goal of treatment in chronic HBV infection is to prevent progression to cirrhosis, hepatic failure, and HCC. Current indications for treatment of chronic HBV infection include evidence of ongoing HBV viral replication, as indicated by the presence for longer

FIG 3.2. TYPICAL SEROLOGIC COURSE OF ACUTE HEPATITIS B VIRUS INFECTION WITH RECOVERY.

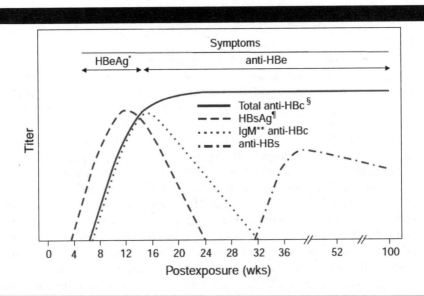

*Hepatitis B e antigen.
§Antibody to hepatitis B core antigen.
¶Hepatitis B surface antigen.
**Immunoglobulin M.
From Centers for Disease Control and Prevention. Recommendations for identification and public health management of persons with chronic hepatitis B virus infection. *MMWR Recomm Rep.* 2008;57(RR-8):1–20

FIG 3.3. TYPICAL SEROLOGIC COURSE OF ACUTE HEPATITIS B VIRUS (HBV) INFECTION WITH PROGRESSION TO CHRONIC HBV INFECTION

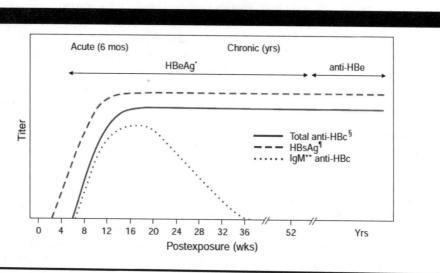

*Hepatitis B e antigen.
§Antibody to hepatitis B core antigen.
¶Hepatitis B surface antigen.
**Immunoglobulin M.
From Centers for Disease Control and Prevention. Recommendations for identification and public health management of persons with chronic hepatitis B virus infection. *MMWR Recomm Rep.* 2008;57(RR-8):1–20

than 6 months of serum HBV DNA greater than 20 000 IU/mL without HBeAg positivity, greater than 2000 IU/mL with HBeAg positivity, and elevated serum ALT concentrations for longer than 6 months or evidence of chronic hepatitis on liver biopsy. Children without necroinflammatory liver disease and children with immunotolerant chronic HBV infection (ie, normal ALT concentrations despite the presence of HBV DNA) usually do not warrant antiviral therapy. Treatment response is measured by biochemical, virologic, and histologic response. An important consideration in the choice of treatment is to avoid selection of antiviral-resistant mutations.

The FDA has approved 3 nucleoside analogues (entecavir, lamivudine, and telbivudine), 2 nucleotide analogues (tenofovir and adefovir), and 2 interferon-alfa drugs (interferon alfa-2b and pegylated interferon alfa-2a) for treatment of chronic HBV infection in adults. Tenofovir, entecavir, and pegylated interferon alfa-2a are preferred in adults as first-line therapy because of the lower likelihood of developing antiviral resistance mutations over long-term therapy. Of these, FDA licensure in the pediatric population is as follows: interferon alfa-2b, ≥1 year of age; lamivudine and entecavir, ≥2 years of age; adefovir and tenofovir disproxil fumarate, ≥12 years of age; and telbivudine, ≥16 years of age. Pediatric trials of telbivudine, tenofovir, and pegylated interferon currently are underway. Pegylated interferon alfa-2a is not approved for children with chronic HBV but is approved for children ≥5 years of age to treat chronic hepatitis C infection. Specific therapy guidelines for children coinfected with HIV and HBV can be accessed online (**https://aidsinfo.nih.gov/guidelines**). Developments in antiviral therapies of HBV may be found on the American Association for the Study of Liver Diseases Web site (**www.aasld.org**).

The optimal agent(s) and duration of therapy for chronic HBV infection in children remain unclear. There are few large randomized controlled trials of antiviral therapies for chronic hepatitis B in childhood. Studies indicate that approximately 17% to 58% of children with increased serum aminotransferase concentrations who are treated with interferon alfa-2b for 6 months lose HBeAg, compared with approximately 8% to 17% of untreated controls. Response to interferon-alfa is better for children from Western countries (20%–58%) as compared with Asian countries (17%). Children from Asian countries with HBV infection are more likely to: (1) have acquired infection perinatally; (2) have a prolonged immune-tolerant phase of infection; and (3) be infected with HBV genotype C. All 3 of these factors are associated with lower response rates to interferon-alfa, which is less effective for chronic infections acquired during early childhood, especially if serum aminotransferase concentrations are normal. Children with chronic HBV infection who were treated with lamivudine had higher rates of virologic response (loss of detectable HBV DNA and loss of HBeAg) after 1 year of treatment than did children who received placebo (23% versus 13%). Resistance to lamivudine can develop during treatment and may occur early. The high rates of lamivudine resistance (~70% after 3 years of therapy) have decreased enthusiasm for the use of this drug. Children coinfected with HIV and HBV should receive the lamivudine dose approved for treatment of HIV. Consultation with health care professionals with expertise in treating chronic hepatitis B in children is recommended.

ISOLATION OF THE HOSPITALIZED PATIENT: Standard precautions are indicated for patients with acute or chronic HBV infection. For infants born to HBsAg-positive mothers, no special care in addition to standard precautions, as described under Control Measures, is needed, other than removal of maternal blood by a gloved attendant.

CONTROL MEASURES:

Strategy for Prevention of HBV Infection. The primary goal of hepatitis B-prevention programs is to eliminate transmission of HBV, thereby decreasing rates of chronic HBV infection and HBV-related chronic liver disease. A secondary goal is prevention of acute HBV infection. In the United States over the past 2 decades, a comprehensive immunization strategy to eliminate HBV transmission has been implemented progressively and now includes the following 4 components[1-4]: (1) universal immunization of infants beginning at birth; (2) prevention of perinatal HBV infection through routine screening of all pregnant women and appropriate immunoprophylaxis of infants born to HBsAg-positive

---

[1]Centers for Disease Control and Prevention. A comprehensive immunization strategy to eliminate transmission of hepatitis B virus infection in the United States: recommendations of the Advisory Committee on Immunization Practices (ACIP). Part I: immunization of infants, children, and adolescents. *MMWR Recomm Rep.* 2005; 54(RR-16):1–31

[2]Centers for Disease Control and Prevention. A comprehensive immunization strategy to eliminate transmission of hepatitis B virus infection in the United States: recommendations of the Advisory Committee on Immunization Practices (ACIP). Part II: immunization of adults. *MMWR Recomm Rep.* 2006;55(RR-16):1–33

[3]Schillie S, Murphy TV, Fenlon N, et al. Update: shortened interval for postvaccination serologic testing of infants born to hepatitis B-infected mothers. *MMWR Morb Mortal Wkly Rep.* 2015;64(30):1118–1120

[4]American Academy of Pediatrics, Committee on Infectious Diseases. Elimination of perinatal hepatitis B: providing the first vaccine dose within 24 hours of birth. *Pediatrics.* 2017;140(3):e20171870

women and infants born to women with unknown HBsAg status; (3) routine immunization of children and adolescents who previously have not been immunized; and (4) immunization of previously unimmunized adults at increased risk of infection.

Hepatitis B Immunoprophylaxis. Two types of products are available for immunoprophylaxis. HBIG provides short-term protection (3–6 months) and is indicated only in specific postexposure circumstances (see Care of Exposed People, p 424). HepB vaccine is used for preexposure and postexposure protection and provides long-term protection. Preexposure immunization with HepB vaccine is the most effective means to prevent HBV transmission. Accordingly, HepB immunization is recommended for all infants, children, and adolescents through 18 years of age. Infants should receive HepB vaccine as part of the routine childhood immunization schedule. All children 11 through 12 years of age should have their immunization records reviewed and should complete the HepB vaccine series if they have not received the vaccine or did not complete the immunization series.

For infants born to women who are positive for both HBsAg and HBeAg, postexposure immunoprophylaxis either with HepB vaccine and HBIG or with HepB vaccine alone effectively prevents most infections after exposure to HBV. Use of both HepB vaccine and HBIG appears to provide greater protection than HepB vaccine alone. Effectiveness of postexposure immunoprophylaxis is related directly to the time elapsed between exposure and administration. Immunoprophylaxis of perinatal infection is most effective if administered within 12 hours of birth; data are limited on effectiveness when administered between 25 hours and 7 days of life. Serologic testing of all pregnant women for HBsAg early (eg, first trimester) during each pregnancy is essential for identifying women whose infants will require postexposure immunoprophylaxis beginning at birth (see Care of Exposed People, p 424).

Hepatitis B Immune Globulin.[1] HBIG is prepared from the plasma of donors with high concentrations of anti-HBs, with an anti-HBs titer of at least 1:100 000 by radioimmunoassay. Plasma donors are required to have negative serologic and nucleic acid test results for HIV and HCV. Additionally, the processes used to manufacture HBIG products are demonstrated to inactivate HBV, HIV, and HCV. Standard Immune Globulin is not effective for postexposure prophylaxis against HBV infection, because concentrations of anti-HBs are too low.

Hepatitis B Vaccine. Highly effective and safe HepB vaccines produced by recombinant DNA technology are licensed in the United States in single-antigen formulations and as components of combination vaccines. Plasma-derived HepB vaccines no longer are available in the United States but may be used successfully in a few countries. Recombinant vaccines contain 10 to 40 µg of HBsAg protein/mL, and a completed vaccine series results in production of anti-HBs of at least 10 mIU/mL in most people, which provides long-term protection for immunocompetent recipients. Single-dose formulations, including all pediatric formulations, contain no thimerosal as a preservative. Although the concentration of recombinant HBsAg protein differs among vaccine products, rates of seroprotection are equivalent when administered to immunocompetent infants, children, adolescents, or young adults in the doses recommended (see Table 3.21).

---

[1]Dosages recommended for postexposure prophylaxis are for products licensed in the United States. Because concentration of anti-HBs in other products may vary, different dosages may be recommended in other countries.

Table 3.21. Recommended Dosages of Hepatitis B Vaccines

Patients	Vaccine[a]		Combination Vaccines	
	Recombivax-HB[b] Dose, μg (mL)	Engerix-B[c] Dose, μg (mL)	Pediarix[d] Dose, μg/mL	Twinrix Dose, μg (mL)[e]
Infants of HBsAg-negative mothers and children and adolescents younger than 20 y	5 (0.5)	10 (0.5)	10 μg HBsAg (0.5)	Not applicable
Infants of HBsAg-positive mothers (HBIG [0.5 mL] also is recommended)	5 (0.5)	10 (0.5)	10 μg HBsAg (0.5)	Not applicable
Adolescents 11–15 y of age[b]	10 (1)	Not applicable	Not applicable	Not applicable
Adults 20 y or older	10 (1)	20 (1)	Not applicable	20 (1)
Adults undergoing dialysis and other immunosuppressed adults	40 (1)[f]	40 (2)[g]	Not applicable	Not applicable

HBsAg indicates hepatitis B surface antigen; HBIG, Hepatitis B Immune Globulin.

[a] Both vaccines are administered in a 3-dose schedule at 0, 1, and 6 months; 4 doses may be administered if a combination vaccine is used (at 2, 4, and 6 months) to complete the series. Only single-antigen hepatitis B vaccine can be used for the birth dose. Single-antigen or combination vaccine containing hepatitis B vaccine may be used to complete the series.

[b] Available from Merck & Co Inc (Whitehouse Station, NJ). A 2-dose schedule, administered at 0 months and then 4 to 6 months later, is licensed for adolescents 11 through 15 years of age using the adult formulation of Recombivax HB (10 μg [Merck & Co Inc]).

[c] Available from GlaxoSmithKline Biologicals (Research Triangle Park, NC). The US Food and Drug Administration also has licensed this vaccine for use in an optional 4-dose (0.5-mL dose) schedule at 0, 1, 2, and 12 months for all age groups. A 0-, 12-, and 24-month schedule is licensed for children 5 through 10 years of age at a 0.5-mL dose and for children 11 through 16 years of age at a 1.0-mL dose for whom an extended administration schedule is appropriate on the basis of risk of exposure.

[d] A combination of diphtheria and tetanus toxoids and acellular pertussis (DTaP), inactivated poliovirus (IPV), and hepatitis B (Engerix-B 10 μg) is approved for use at 2, 4, and 6 months of age (Pediarix [GlaxoSmithKline]). This vaccine should not be administered at birth, before 6 weeks of age, or at 7 years of age or older. For additional information, see Pertussis (p 620).

[e] A combination of hepatitis A (Havrix, 720 enzyme-linked immunosorbent assay units [ELU]) vaccine; Twinrix is licensed for use in people 18 years of age and older in a 3-dose schedule at 0, 1, and 6 months. Alternately, a 4-dose schedule at days 0, 7, and 21 to 30, followed by a booster dose at 12 months, may be used.

[f] Special formulation for adult dialysis patients administered at 0, 1, and 6 months.

[g] Two 1-mL doses administered in 1 or 2 injections in a 4-dose schedule at 0, 1, 2, and 6 months of age.

HepB vaccine can be administered concurrently with other vaccines (see Simultaneous Administration of Multiple Vaccines, p 35).

Vaccine Interchangeability. In general, the various brands of age-appropriate HepB vaccines are interchangeable within an immunization series. The immune response using 1 or 2 doses of a vaccine produced by one manufacturer followed by 1 or more subsequent doses from a different manufacturer is comparable to a full course of immunization with a single product. However, until additional data supporting interchangeability of acellular pertussis-containing HepB combination vaccines are available, vaccines from the same manufacturer should be used, whenever feasible, for at least the first 3 doses in the pertussis series (see Pertussis, p 620). In addition, a 2-dose schedule of the adult formulation of Recombivax HB (Merck & Co, Whitehouse Station, NJ) is licensed for adolescents 11 through 15 years of age (see Table 3.21).

Routes of Administration. Vaccine is administered intramuscularly in the anterolateral thigh for infants or deltoid area for children and adults (see Vaccine Administration, p 26). Administration in the buttocks or by the intradermal route is not recommended at any age.

Efficacy and Duration of Protection. HepB vaccines licensed in the United States have a 90% to 95% efficacy for preventing HBV infection and clinical HBV disease among susceptible children and adults. Immunocompetent people who achieve anti-HBs concentration $\geq$10 mIU/mL after preexposure vaccination have virtually complete protection against infection with HBV. Long-term studies of immunocompetent adults and children indicate that immune memory remains intact for 2 decades and protects against symptomatic acute and chronic HBV infection, even though anti-HBs concentrations may become low or undetectable over time. Breakthrough infections (detected by presence of anti-HBc or HBV DNA) have occurred in a limited number of immunized people, but these infections typically are transient and asymptomatic. Chronic HBV infection in immunized people has been documented in dialysis patients whose anti-HBs concentrations fell below 10 mIU/mL and rarely among people who did not respond to vaccination (eg, adults and infants born to HBsAg-positive mothers).

Booster Doses. For children and adults with normal immune status, routine booster doses of HepB vaccine are not recommended. For patients undergoing hemodialysis who are at continued risk of infection, the need for booster doses should be assessed by annual anti-HBs testing, and a booster dose should be administered when the anti-HBs concentration is <10 mIU/mL. For other immunocompromised people (eg, HIV-infected people, hematopoietic stem cell transplant recipients, and people receiving chemotherapy), the need for booster doses has not been determined. Annual anti-HBs testing and booster doses when anti-HBs concentrations decrease to <10 mIU/mL should be considered for immunocompromised people if they have an ongoing risk for HBV exposure. Similar consideration may be given to children with cystic fibrosis, liver disease, or celiac disease if there is an ongoing risk for HBV exposure. Children with celiac disease may not respond as well to HepB vaccine.

Adverse Events. Adverse effects most commonly reported in adults and children are pain at the injection site, reported by 3% to 29% of recipients, and a temperature greater than 37.7°C (99.8°F), reported by 1% to 6% of recipients. Anaphylaxis is uncommon, occurring in approximately 1 in 1.1 million recipients, according to vaccine adverse events passive reporting surveillance systems. Large, controlled epidemiologic studies and review by the Institute of Medicine,[1] now called the National Academy of Medicine (NAM [see Institute of Medicine Reviews of Adverse Events After Immunization, p 43]), found no evidence of an association between HepB vaccine and sudden infant death syndrome, type 1 diabetes mellitus, seizures, encephalitis, or autoimmune (eg, vasculitis) or demyelinating disease, including multiple sclerosis.

Immunization During Pregnancy or Lactation. No adverse effect on the developing fetus has been observed when pregnant women have been immunized. Because HBV infection may result in severe disease in the mother and chronic infection in the newborn infant, pregnancy is not a contraindication to immunization. Lactation is not a contraindication to immunization.

Serologic Testing. Susceptibility testing before immunization is not indicated routinely for children or adolescents. Testing for past or current infection may be considered for people in risk groups with high rates of HBV infection, including people born in countries with intermediate and high HBV endemicity (even if immunized, because the entire immunization series may not have been completed or the person may have failed to respond to the immunization), users of injection drugs, men who have sex with men, and household and sexual contacts of HBsAg-positive people, provided testing does not delay or impede immunization efforts. A substantial proportion of people with chronic HBV infection are unaware of their infection.

Routine postimmunization testing for anti-HBs is not necessary after routine vaccination of healthy people but is recommended 1 to 2 months after the final vaccine dose for the following specific groups: (1) hemodialysis patients; (2) people with HIV infection; (3) people at occupational risk of exposure from percutaneous injuries or mucosal or nonintact skin exposures (eg, certain health care and public safety workers); (4) other immunocompromised patients (eg, hematopoietic stem-cell transplant recipients or people receiving chemotherapy); and (5) sexual partners of HBsAg-positive people. If anti-HBs testing is performed on health care personnel at a time distant from immunization (ie, at the time of hire or matriculation for health care personnel vaccinated as an infant), further management is described in Fig 3.4. If immunized health care personnel are exposed to blood or body fluids from a person who is HBsAg-positive, management of the exposure is described in Table 3.22 (p 414).

Testing of infants born to HBsAg-positive mothers should occur at 1 to 2 months after the last vaccine dose; these infants should have postimmunization testing for HBsAg and anti-HBs performed at 9 to 12 months of age, generally at the next well-child visit after completion of the vaccine series (see Prevention of Perinatal HBV Infection, p 426).[2,3] Testing should not be performed before 9 months of age to maximize the likelihood of detecting late-onset HBV infections. HBsAg-negative infants with anti-HBs titers <10 mIU/mL after completing the 3-dose vaccine series should be revaccinated with a single dose of HepB vaccine and retested for anti-HBs antibody titers 1 to 2 months later. Infants who have anti-HBs titers ≥10 mIU/mL after this fourth dose of HepB vaccine do

[1]Institute of Medicine. *Adverse Effects of Vaccines: Evidence and Causality.* Washington, DC: National Academies Press; 2011

[2]Schillie S, Murphy TV, Fenlon N, et al. Update: shortened interval for postvaccination serologic testing of infants born to hepatitis B-infected mothers. *MMWR Morb Mortal Wkly Rep.* 2015;64(30):1118–1120

[3]American Academy of Pediatrics, Committee on Infectious Diseases. Elimination of perinatal hepatitis B: providing the first vaccine dose within 24 hours of birth. *Pediatrics.* 2017;140(3):e20171870

not need any additional doses of the HepB vaccine. Infants who fail to reach anti-HBs titers ≥10 mIU/mL after the fourth dose of HepB vaccine should receive 2 additional doses of the HepB vaccine followed by retesting for anti-HBs antibody titers 1 to 2 months later (see Fig 3.4). An alternate approach for children who have completed a 3-dose series of HepB vaccine but did not achieve anti-HBs titers ≥10 mIU/mL is to give

FIG 3.4. GUIDANCE FOR EVALUATING HEALTH CARE PERSONNEL FOR HEPATITIS B VIRUS PROTECTION AND FOR ADMINISTERING POSTEXPOSURE MANAGEMENT

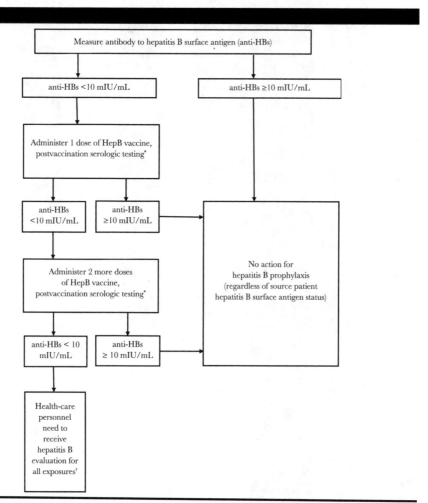

Reproduced from Schillie S, Murphy TV, Sawyer M, et al. CDC guidance for evaluating health-care personnel for hepatitis B virus protection and for administering post exposure management. *MMWR Recomm Rep*. 2013;62(RR-10):1–19.

*Should be performed 1–2 months after the last dose of vaccine using a quantitative method that allows detection of the protective concentration of anti-HBs (≥10 mIU/mL) (eg, enzyme-linked immunosorbent assay [ELISA]).

†A nonresponder is defined as a person with anti-HBs <10 mIU/mL after ≥6 doses of HepB vaccine. People who do not have a protective concentration of anti-HBs after revaccination should be tested for HBsAg. If positive, People should receive appropriate management or vaccination.

Table 3.22. Postexposure Management of Health-Care Personnel After Occupational Percutaneous or Mucosal Exposure to Blood and Body Fluids, by Health-Care Personnel HepB Vaccination and Response Status

Health Care Personnel Status	Postexposure Testing		Postexposure Prophylaxis		Postvaccination Serologic Testing[b]
	Source Patient (HBsAg)	HCP Testing (anti-HBs)	HBIG[a]	Vaccination	
Documented responder[c] after complete series (≥3 doses)	No action needed				
Documented nonresponder[d] after 6 doses	Positive/unknown	—[e]	HBIG x 2 separated by 1 month		No
	Negative	No action needed			
Response unknown after 3 doses	Positive/unknown	<10 mIU/mL[e]	HBIG x 1	Initiate revaccination	Yes
	Negative	<10 mIU/mL	None		
	Any result	≥10 mIU/mL	No action needed		

Table 3.22. Postexposure Management of Health-Care Personnel After Occupational Percutaneous or Mucosal Exposure to Blood and Body Fluids, by Health-Care Personnel HepB Vaccination and Response Status, continued

Health Care Personnel Status	Postexposure Testing Source Patient (HBsAg)	Postexposure Testing HCP Testing (anti-HBs)	Postexposure Prophylaxis HBIG[a]	Postexposure Prophylaxis Vaccination	Postvaccination Serologic Testing[b]
Unvaccinated/ incompletely vaccinated or vaccine refusers	Positive/ unknown	—[e]	HBIG x 1	Complete vaccination	Yes
	Negative	—	None	Complete vaccination	Yes

Reproduced from Centers for Disease Control and Prevention. CDC Guidance for Evaluating Health-Care Personnel for Hepatitis B Virus Protection and for Administering Post exposure Management. *MMWR Recomm Rep.* 2013;62(RR-10):1–19

HCP indicates health-care personnel; HBsAg, hepatitis B surface antigen; anti-HBs, antibody to hepatitis B surface antigen; HBIG, hepatitis B immune globulin.

[a] HBIG should be administered intramuscularly as soon as possible after exposure when indicated. The effectiveness of HBIG when administered >7 days after percutaneous, mucosal, or nonintact skin exposures is unknown. HBIG dosage is 0.06 mL/kg.

[b] Should be performed 1–2 months after the last dose of the HepB vaccine series (and 4–6 months after administration of HBIG to avoid detection of passively administered anti-HBs) using a quantitative method that allows detection of the protective concentration of anti-HBs (≥10 mIU/mL).

[c] A responder is defined as a person with anti-HBs ≥10 mIU/mL after ≥3 doses of HepB vaccine.

[d] A nonresponder is defined as a person with anti-HBs <10 mIU/mL after ≥6 doses of HepB vaccine.

[e] HCP who have anti-HBs <10 mIU/mL or who are unvaccinated or incompletely vaccinated and sustain an exposure to a source patient who is HBsAg-positive or has unknown HBsAg status should undergo baseline testing for HBV infection as soon as possible after exposure and follow-up testing approximately 6 months later. Initial baseline test consists of total anti-HBc; testing at approximately 6 months consists of HBsAg and total anti-HBc.

Table 3.23. Guidelines for Postexposure Prophylaxis[a] of People With Nonoccupational Exposures[b] to Blood or Body Fluids That Contain Blood, by Exposure Type and Vaccination Status

Exposure	Treatment	
	Unvaccinated Person[c]	Previously Vaccinated Person[d]
HBsAg-positive source		
Percutaneous (eg, bite or needlestick) or mucosal exposure to HBsAg-positive blood or body fluids	Administer hepatitis B vaccine series and hepatitis B immune globulin (HBIG)	Administer hepatitis B vaccine booster dose
Sexual or needle-sharing contact of an HBsAg-positive person	Administer hepatitis B vaccine series and HBIG	Administer hepatitis B vaccine booster dose
Victim of sexual assault/abuse by a perpetrator who is HBsAg positive	Administer hepatitis B vaccine series and HBIG	Administer hepatitis B vaccine booster dose
Source with unknown HBsAg status		
Victim of sexual assault/abuse by a perpetrator with unknown HBsAg status	Administer hepatitis B vaccine series	No treatment
Percutaneous (eg, bite or needlestick) or mucosal exposure to potentially infectious blood or body fluids from a source with unknown HBsAg status	Administer hepatitis B vaccine series	No treatment
Sex or needle-sharing contact of person with unknown HBsAg status	Administer hepatitis B vaccine series	No treatment

HBsAg indicates hepatitis B surface antigen.

[a]When indicated, immunoprophylaxis should be initiated as soon as possible, preferably within 24 hours. Studies are limited on the maximum interval after exposure during which postexposure prophylaxis is effective, but the interval is unlikely to exceed 7 days for percutaneous exposures or 14 days for sexual exposures. The hepatitis B vaccine series should be completed.

[b]These guidelines apply to nonoccupational exposures. Guidelines for occupational exposures can be found in Table 3.22.

[c]A person who is in the process of being vaccinated but who has not completed the vaccine series should complete the series and receive treatment as indicated.

[d]A person who has written documentation of a complete hepatitis B vaccine series and who did not receive postvaccination testing.

Source: Recommendations of the Advisory Committee on Immunization Practices (ACIP). Part II: immunization of adults. *MMWR Recomm Rep.* 2006;55(RR-16):30–31

3 additional doses of HepB vaccine and then retest for anti-HBs titers 1to 2 months after the third dose of this second series. Currently available data do not suggest any benefit from administration of additional HepB vaccine doses to infants who do not attain anti-HBs titers ≥10 mIU/mL following receipt of 2 complete 3-dose series (total of 6 doses) of HepB vaccine. For these infants, no additional HepB vaccine doses are recommended.

Management of Nonresponders. Vaccine recipients who do not develop a serum anti-HBs response (≥10 mIU/mL) after a primary vaccine series should be tested for HBsAg to rule out the possibility of a chronic infection as an explanation of failure to respond to the vaccine. If the HBsAg test result is negative, their management is detailed in Serologic

Testing (p 414), Fig 3.4 (p 413), and Table 3.22 (p 414) for health care personnel and Table 3.23 for nonoccupational exposures. Fewer than 5% of immunocompetent infants, children, and young adults receiving 6 doses of HepB vaccine administered appropriately fail to develop detectable antibody. People who remain anti-HBs negative 1 to 2 months after a reimmunization series are unlikely to respond to additional doses of vaccine and should be considered nonimmune if they are exposed to HBV in the future.

Altered Doses and Schedules. Larger vaccine doses are required to induce protective anti-HBs concentrations in adult hemodialysis patients and immunocompromised adults, including HIV-seropositive people (see Table 3.21, p 410). Humoral immune response to HepB vaccine also may be reduced in children and adolescents who are receiving hemodialysis or who are immunocompromised. However, few data exist concerning the response to higher doses of vaccine in children and adolescents, and no specific recommendations can be made for these age groups. For unvaccinated people with progressive chronic renal failure, and possibly cardiac or other transplant recipients, HepB vaccine should be administered as early as possible in the disease course to provide protection and potentially improve responses to vaccination.

Preexposure Universal Immunization of Infants, Children, and Adolescents. Immunization with HepB vaccine is recommended for all infants, children, and adolescents through 18 years of age, administered as a series of 3 doses (0.5 mL/dose) on a 0-, 1-, and 6-month schedule. Age-specific vaccine dosages are provided in Table 3.21 (p 410). Delivery hospitals should develop policies and procedures that ensure administration of a birth dose within 24 hours of age as part of the routine care of all medically stable infants weighing 2000 g or more at birth. For all medically stable infants weighing ≥2000 g at birth, regardless of mother's HBsAg status, the first dose of vaccine should be administered within 24 hours of birth.[1] Deferral to a time after birth or discharge from the hospital no longer is considered to be an acceptable option, because it might deprive an HBV-exposed infant of timely administration of HBV prophylaxis.

Determination of timing of the first dose of hepatitis B vaccine is predicated on the infant's birth weight and the mother's hepatitis B surface antigen status. Table 3.24 (p 420) details the appropriate timing of the first hepatitis B vaccine dose for infants weighing ≥2000 g and for infants <2000 g and infants born to mothers who are HBsAg-negative, HBsAg-positive, and HBsAg-unknown. Timing of administration of HBIG, if appropriate, also is detailed in the table. For preterm infants weighing <2000 g, the initial vaccine dose should not be counted in the required 3-dose schedule (a total of 4 doses of HepB vaccine should be administered), and the subsequent 3 doses should be administered in accordance with the schedule for immunization of infants weighing <2000 g. Only single-antigen HepB vaccine should be used for the birth dose. The HepB vaccine series (3 or 4 doses; see discussion about birth dose in next paragraph) for infants born to HBsAg-negative mothers should be completed by 6 to 18 months of age. All children and adolescents who have not been immunized against HBV should begin the series during any visit. See Special Considerations, p 421, for additional details on immunization at birth and prevention of perinatal HBV infection.

High seroconversion rates and protective concentrations of anti-HBs (10 mIU/mL or

---

[1] American Academy of Pediatrics, Committee on Infectious Diseases. Elimination of perinatal hepatitis B: providing the first vaccine dose within 24 hours of birth. *Pediatrics*. 2017;140(3):e20171870

greater) are achieved when HepB vaccine is administered in any of the various recommended schedules, including schedules begun soon after birth in term infants (see Table 3.21, p 410). Only single-antigen HepB vaccine can be used for doses administered between birth and 6 weeks of age. Single-antigen or combination vaccine may be used to complete the series; 4 doses of vaccine may be administered if a birth dose is administered and a combination vaccine containing a hepatitis B component is used to complete the series.[1] For guidelines for minimum scheduling time between vaccine doses for infants, see Table 1.11 (p 33). For immunizations of older children and adolescents, alternate administration schedules at 0, 1, and 4 months may be used (although shorter intervals between first and last doses result in lower immunogenicity). For younger children (birth through 10 years of age), an alternate administration schedule at 0, 1, 2, and 12 months is licensed for one single-antigen HepB vaccine. For older children and adolescents (5 through 16 years of age), an alternate administration schedule at 0, 12, and 24 months and for older children and adolescents (11 through 19 years of age), an alternate dosage (1.0 mL) and administration schedule at 0, 1, 2, and 12 months are licensed for one single-antigen HepB vaccine. A 2-dose alternate dosage (1.0 mL) and administration schedule at 0 and 4 to 6 months for another single-antigen HepB vaccine is licensed for children 11 through 15 years of age (see Table 3.21, p 410). These alternate dosage and administration schedules result in equivalent immunogenicity and can be used when acceptable on the basis of low risk of exposure and to facilitate adherence.

The recommended schedule for routine hepatitis B immunization of infants born to HBsAg-negative mothers is provided in the annual immunization schedule (**https://redbook.solutions.aap.org/SS/Immunization_Schedules.aspx**) (see Care of Exposed People, Postexposure Immunoprophylaxis, p 427, and Tables 3.24, p 420, and 3.25, p 422).

Combination products containing HepB vaccine may be administered in the United States, provided they are licensed by the FDA for the child's current age and administration of the other vaccine component(s) also is indicated. Children and adolescents who previously have not received HepB vaccine should be immunized routinely at any age with the age-appropriate doses and schedule. The vaccine schedule should be chosen with consideration of the need to achieve completion of the vaccine series. In all settings, immunization should be initiated, even though completion of the vaccine series might not be ensured.

Preexposure Immunization of Adults.[2]

- Hepatitis B immunization is recommended as a 3-dose series for all unimmunized adults at risk of HBV infection (see Table 3.26, p 423) and for all adults seeking protection from HBV infection. Acknowledgment of a specific risk factor is not a requirement for immunization.

- In settings in which a high proportion of adults are likely to have risk factors for HBV infection, all unimmunized adults should be assumed to be at risk and should receive hepatitis B immunization. These settings include: (1) sexually transmitted infection

---

[1]Centers for Disease Control and Prevention. General recommendations on immunization. Recommendations of the Advisory Committee on Immunization Practices (ACIP). *MMWR Recomm Rep.* 2011;60(RR-2):1–64

[2]Centers for Disease Control and Prevention. A comprehensive immunization strategy to eliminate transmission of hepatitis B virus infection in the United States: recommendations of the Advisory Committee on Immunization Practices (ACIP). Part II: immunization of adults. *MMWR Recomm Rep.* 2006;55(RR-16):1–33

treatment facilities; (2) HIV testing and treatment facilities; (3) facilities providing drug abuse treatment and prevention services; (4) health care settings targeting services to injection drug users; (5) correctional facilities; (6) health care settings serving men who have sex with men; (7) chronic hemodialysis facilities and end-stage renal disease programs; and (8) institutions and nonresidential care facilities for people with developmental disabilities.

- HepB vaccine should be administered to unimmunized adults with diabetes mellitus who are 19 through 59 years of age.[1] HepB vaccine may be administered at the discretion of the treating clinician to unimmunized adults with diabetes mellitus who are 60 years or older.
- Standing orders should be implemented to identify and immunize eligible adults in primary care and specialty medical settings. If ascertainment of risk for HBV infection is a barrier to immunization in these settings, health care professionals may use alternative immunization strategies, such as offering HepB vaccine to all unimmunized adults in age groups with highest risk of infection (eg, younger than 49 years).

Lapsed Immunizations. For infants, children, adolescents, and adults with lapsed immunizations (ie, the interval between doses is longer than that in one of the recommended schedules), the vaccine series should be completed without repeating doses, as long as minimum dosing intervals between the remaining doses necessary to complete the series are heeded (see Lapsed Immunizations, p 38).

SPECIAL CONSIDERATIONS:

Infants Weighing <2000 g at Birth. Studies demonstrate that decreased seroconversion rates might occur among preterm infants with a birth weight <2000 g after administration of HepB vaccine at birth. However, by the chronologic age of 1 month, all medically stable preterm infants, regardless of initial birth weight or gestational age, are as likely to respond to HepB immunization as are term and larger infants.

All infants weighing <2000 g who are born to an HBsAg-positive mother should receive immunoprophylaxis with HepB vaccine and HBIG within 12 hours after birth; the birth dose of HepB vaccine should not be counted toward completion of the HepB vaccine series, and 3 additional doses of HepB vaccine should be administered beginning when the infant is 1 month of age (see Table 3.24). Only monovalent HepB vaccines should be used from birth through 6 weeks of age.

If maternal HBsAg status is unknown at birth, the infant weighing <2000 g should receive HepB vaccine within 12 hours of birth. The mother's HBsAg status should be determined as quickly as possible. If the infant's birth weight is <2000 g and the maternal HBsAg status cannot be determined within 12 hours of life, HBIG also should be administered, because the less reliable immune response in preterm infants weighing <2000 g precludes the option of the 7-day waiting period for HBIG administration acceptable for term and larger preterm infants. Only monovalent HepB vaccine should be used from birth through 6 weeks of age.

All infants of HBsAg-negative mothers with a birth weight of less than 2000 g should receive the first dose of HepB vaccine series starting at 1 month of chronologic age or at hospital discharge if before 1 month of chronologic age. Infants born to HBsAg-negative

[1]Centers for Disease Control and Prevention. Use of hepatitis B vaccination for adults with diabetes mellitus: recommendations of the Advisory Committee on Immunization Practices (ACIP). *MMWR Morb Mortal Wkly Rep.* 2011;60(50):1709–1711

mothers do not need to have postimmunization serologic testing for anti-HBs. Table 3.24 provides a summary of the recommendations for immunization of infants on the basis of maternal hepatitis B status and infant birth weight. For information on use of combination vaccines containing HepB vaccine as a component to complete the series, see Table 3.25 (p 422).

Table 3.24. Hepatitis B Virus (HBV) Immunoprophylaxis Scheme by Infant Birth Weight[a]

Maternal Status	Infant Birth Weight 2000 g or More	Infant Birth Weight Less Than 2000 g
HBsAg positive	Hepatitis B vaccine + HBIG (within 12 h of birth). Continue vaccine series beginning at 1–2 mo of age according to recommended schedule for infants born to HBsAg-positive mothers (see Table 3.25).	Hepatitis B vaccine + HBIG (within 12 h of birth). Continue vaccine series beginning at 1–2 mo of age according to recommended schedule for infants born to HBsAg-positive mothers (ie, administer 3 additional hepatitis B vaccine doses with single-antigen vaccine at ages 1, 2–3, and 6 months, OR hepatitis B-containing combination vaccine at ages 2, 4, and 6 months (Pediarix) (see Table 3.25). Immunize with 4 vaccine doses; do not count birth dose as part of the 3-dose vaccine series.
	Check anti-HBs and HBsAg after completion of vaccine series (typically at 9–12 months of age).[b] HBsAg-negative infants with anti-HBs levels ≥10 mIU/mL are protected and need no further medical management. HBsAg-negative infants with anti-HBs levels <10 mIU/mL at 9 months of age should be reimmunized with a fourth-dose and retested. If the infant continues to have anti-HBs levels <10 mIU/mL, 2 additional doses should be administered and the infant retested. If after a sixth dose, the anti-HBs levels are <10 mIU/mL, no additional doses of hepatitis B vaccine are indicated. Infants who are HBsAg positive should receive appropriate follow-up, including medical evaluation for chronic liver disease.	Check anti-HBs and HBsAg after completion of vaccine series.[b] HBsAg-negative infants with anti-HBs levels ≥10 mIU/mL are protected and need no further medical management. HBsAg-negative infants with anti-HBs levels <10 mIU/mL at 9 months of age should be reimmunized with a fourth-dose and retested. If the infant continues to have anti-HBs levels <10 mIU/mL, 2 additional doses should be administered and the infant retested. If after a sixth dose, the anti-HBs levels are <10 mIU/mL, no additional doses of hepatitis B vaccine are indicated. Infants who are HBsAg positive should receive appropriate follow-up, including medical evaluation for chronic liver disease.

Table 3.24. Hepatitis B Virus (HBV) Immunoprophylaxis Scheme by Infant Birth Weight,ᵃ continued

Maternal Status	Infant Birth Weight 2000 g or More	Infant Birth Weight Less Than 2000 g
HBsAg status unknown	Test mother for HBsAg immediately after admission for delivery. Hepatitis B vaccine (within 12 h of birth). Administer HBIG (within 7 days) if mother tests HBsAg positive; if mother's HBsAg status remains unknown, some experts would administer HBIG (within 7 days). Continue the 3-dose vaccine series beginning at 1–2 mo of age according to recommended schedule based on mother's HBsAg result (see Table 3.25).	Test mother for HBsAg immediately after admission for delivery. Hepatitis B vaccine (within 12h of birth). Administer HBIG within 12 hours of birth if mother tests HBsAg positive or if mother's HBsAg result is not available/unknown within 12 h of birth. Continue vaccine series beginning at 1–2 mo of age according to recommended schedule based on mother's HBsAg result (ie, administer 3 additional hepatitis B vaccine doses with single-antigen vaccine at ages 1, 2–3, and 6 months, OR hepatitis B-containing combination vaccine at ages 2, 4, and 6 months (Pediarix) (see Table 3.25). Immunize with 4 vaccine doses; do not count birth dose as part of the 3-dose vaccine series
HBsAg negative	HBV vaccine at birth (within 24 h of birth). Continue vaccine series beginning at 1–2 mo of age (see Table 3.25). Follow-up anti-HBs and HBsAg testing not needed.	Delay first dose of hepatitis B vaccine until 1 mo of age or hospital discharge, whichever is first. Continue the 3-dose vaccine series beginning at 2 mo of age (see Table 3.25). Follow-up anti-HBs and HBsAg testing not needed.

HBsAg indicates hepatitis B surface antigen; HBIG, hepatitis B Immune Globulin; anti-HBs, antibody to HBsAg.

ᵃExtremes of gestational age and birth weight no longer are a consideration for timing of hepatitis B vaccine doses.

ᵇTest at 9 to 12 months of age, generally at the next well-child visit after completion of the primary series. Use testing method that allows determination of a protective concentration of anti-HBs (≥10 mIU/mL).

Considerations for High-Risk Groups:

Health Care Personnel and Others With Occupational Exposure to Blood. The risk of HBV exposure to a health care professional depends on the tasks the person performs and the HBsAg prevalence among the patient population served. Health care personnel who have the potential for contact with blood or other potentially infectious body fluids should be immunized. Because the risks of occupational HBV infection often are highest during the training period, immunization should be initiated as early as possible before or during training and before contact with blood, followed by postimmunization testing 1 to

2 months later for anti-HBs for health care personnel at risk of exposure. Health care personnel with anti-HBs <10 mIU/mL should be reimmunized with a single dose of vaccine and retested for anti-HBs within 1 to 2 months after that dose. Health care personnel whose anti-HBs remains <10 mIU/mL should receive 2 additional doses of vaccine (usually 6 doses total), followed by repeat anti-HBs testing 1 to 2 months after the last dose. Alternatively, it may be more practical for very recently vaccinated health care personnel with anti-HBs <10 mIU/mL to receive 3 consecutive additional doses of Hep B vaccine (usually 6 doses total), followed by anti-HBs testing 1 to 2 months after the last dose.

Patients Undergoing Hemodialysis. Immunization is recommended for susceptible patients undergoing hemodialysis. Immunization early in the course of renal disease is encouraged, because response is better than in advanced disease. Specific dosage recommendations have not been made for children undergoing hemodialysis. Some experts recommend increased doses of HepB vaccine for children receiving hemodialysis to increase immunogenicity.

Table 3.25. Hepatitis B Vaccine Schedules for Infants by Maternal Hepatitis B Surface Antigen (HBsAg) Status for Infants With Birth Weight ≥2000 g[a,b]

Maternal HBsAg Status	Single-Antigen Vaccine		Single-Antigen + Combination	
	Dose	Age	Dose	Age
Positive	1[c]	Birth (12 h or less)	1[c]	Birth (12 h or less) (Combination vaccine should not be used for birth dose)
	HBIG[d]	Birth (12 h or less)	HBIG[d]	Birth (12 h or less)
	2	1 through 2 mo	2	2 mo
	3[e]	6 mo	3	4 mo
			4[e]	6 mo (Pediarix)
Unknown[f]	1[c]	Birth (12 h or less)	1[c]	Birth (12 h or less) (Combination vaccine should not be used for birth dose)
	2	1 through 2 mo	2	2 mo
	3[e]	6 mo	3	4 mo
			4[e]	6 mo (Pediarix)
Negative	1[c]	Birth (24 h or less)	1[c]	Birth (24 h or less) (Combination vaccine should not be used for birth dose)
	2	1 through 2 mo	2	2 mo
	3[e]	6 through 18 mo	3	4 mo
			4[e]	6 mo (Pediarix)

HBIG indicates Hepatitis B Immune Globulin.

[a] Centers for Disease Control and Prevention. A comprehensive immunization strategy to eliminate transmission of hepatitis B virus infection in the United States: recommendations of the Advisory Committee on Immunization Practices (ACIP). Part 1: immunization of infants, children, and adolescents. *MMWR Recomm Rep.* 2005;54(RR-16):1–31.

[b] See Table 3.24 for vaccine schedules for preterm infants weighing less than 2000 g.

[c] Recombivax HB or Engerix-B should be used for the birth dose. Pediarix should not be administered at birth or before 6 weeks of age.

[d] HBIG (0.5 mL) administered intramuscularly in a separate site from vaccine.

[e] The final dose in the vaccine series should not be administered before 24 weeks (164 days) of age.

[f] Mothers should have blood drawn and tested for HBsAg as soon as possible after admission for delivery; if the mother is found to be HBsAg positive, the infant should receive HBIG as soon as possible but no later than 7 days of age.

Table 3.26. Adults Recommended to Receive Hepatitis B Virus (HBV) Vaccine

People at Risk of Infection by Sexual Exposure
- Sex partners of hepatitis B surface antigen (HBsAg)-positive people
- Sexually active people who are not in a long-term, mutually monogamous relationship (eg, people with more than 1 sex partner during the previous 6 months)
- People seeking evaluation or treatment for a sexually transmitted infection
- Men who have sex with men

People at Risk of Infection by Percutaneous or Mucosal Exposure to Blood
- Current or recent injection-drug users
- Household contacts of HBsAg-positive people
- Residents and staff of facilities for people with developmental disabilities
- Health care and public safety workers with reasonably anticipated risk of exposure to blood or blood-contaminated body fluids
- People with end-stage renal disease, including predialysis, hemodialysis, peritoneal dialysis, and home dialysis patients
- People with diabetes mellitus 19 through 59 years of age; people with diabetes mellitus 60 years of age and older may be immunized at the discretion of their physician

Others
- International travelers to regions with high or intermediate levels (HBsAg prevalence of 2% or greater) of endemic HBV infection (see Table 3.19, p 404)
- People with chronic liver disease
- People with human immunodeficiency (HIV) infection
- All other people seeking protection from HBV infection

Source: Centers for Disease Control and Prevention. A comprehensive immunization strategy to eliminate transmission of hepatitis B virus infection in the United States: recommendations of the Advisory Committee on Immunization Practices (ACIP). Part II: immunization of adults. *MMWR Recomm Rep.* 2006;55(RR-16):1–33

People Born in Countries Where the Prevalence of Chronic HBV Infection Is 2% or Greater. Foreign-born people (including immigrants, refugees, asylum seekers, and internationally adopted children) from countries where the prevalence of chronic HBV infection is 2% or greater (see Table 3.19, p 404) should be screened for HBsAg regardless of immunization status. Previously unimmunized family members and other household contacts should be immunized if a household member is found to be HBsAg positive. In addition, positive HBsAg test results are nationally notifiable (see Appendix IV, p 1069). People with positive HBsAg test results should be reported to the local or state health department and referred for medical management to reduce their risk of complications from chronic HBV infection and to reduce the risk of transmission.

Inmates in Juvenile Detention and Other Correctional Facilities. Unimmunized or underimmunized people in juvenile and adult correctional facilities should be immunized. If the length of stay is not sufficient to complete the immunization series, the series should be initiated, and follow-up mechanisms with a health care facility should be established to ensure completion of the series.

International Travelers. People traveling to areas where the prevalence of chronic HBV infection is 2% or greater (see Table 3.19, p 404) should be immunized. Ideally, HepB vaccination should be administered ≥6 months before travel so that a 3-dose regimen can

Table 3.27. Guide to Postexposure Immunoprophylaxis of Unimmunized People to Prevent Hepatitis B Virus (HBV) Infection

Type of Exposure	Immunoprophylaxis[a]
Household contact of HBsAg-positive person	Administer hepatitis B vaccine series
Discrete exposure to an HBsAg-positive source:	
• Percutaneous (eg, bite, needlestick, nonintact skin) or mucosal exposure to HBsAg-positive blood or body fluids	Administer hepatitis B vaccine + HBIG; complete vaccine series
• Sexual contact or needle sharing with an HBsAg-positive person	Administer hepatitis B vaccine + HBIG; complete vaccine series
• Victim of sexual assault/abuse by a perpetrator who is HBsAg positive	Administer hepatitis B vaccine + HBIG; complete vaccine series
Discrete exposure to a source with unknown HBsAg status:	
• Percutaneous (eg, bite, needlestick) or mucosal exposure to blood or body fluids with unknown HBsAg status	Administer hepatitis B vaccine series
• Victim of sexual assault/abuse by a perpetrator with unknown HBsAg status	Administer hepatitis B vaccine series
Susceptible child biting someone with chronic HBV infection	Initiate or complete the hepatitis B vaccine series Do not give HBIG (assumes no oral mucosal disease when the amount of blood transferred is small)

HBsAg indicates hepatitis B surface antigen; HBIG, Hepatitis B Immune Globulin.

[a]Immunoprophylaxis should be administered as soon as possible, and within 24 hours after exposure. Studies are limited on the maximum interval after exposure during which postexposure prophylaxis is effective, but the interval is unlikely to exceed 7 days for percutaneous exposures and 14 days for sexual exposures.

be completed (see Preexposure Universal Immunization, p 419). If immunization is initiated fewer than 4 months before departure, the alternative 4-dose schedule of 0, 1, 2, and 12 months, licensed for one vaccine (see Table 3.21, p 410), might provide protection if the first 3 doses can be administered before travel. Individual health care providers may choose to use an accelerated schedule (eg, doses at days 0, 7, and 21–30, with a booster at 12 months) for travelers who will depart before an approved immunization schedule can be completed. People who receive immunization on an accelerated schedule that is not licensed by the FDA also should receive a dose at 12 months after initiation of the series to promote long-term immunity.

Care of Exposed People (Postexposure Immunoprophylaxis) (Also See Table 3.27).

Prevention of Perinatal HBV Infection. Transmission of perinatal HBV infection can be prevented in approximately 95% of infants born to HBsAg-positive mothers by early active and passive immunoprophylaxis of the infant (ie, immunization and HBIG administration within 12 hours of birth). Immunization subsequently should be completed during the first 6 months of life. HepB vaccination alone, initiated at or shortly after birth, also is highly effective for preventing perinatal HBV infections. However, infants born to women with HBV DNA greater than 10^6 to 10^8 IU/mL or who are HBeAg positive have an increased risk of perinatal transmission even if appropriate active and passive vaccination is administered (~15%–30% risk of transmission versus less than 5% risk of transmission for women with lower HBV DNA or who are HBeAg negative). Tenofovir and telbivudine are the only nucleoside analogues that are not pregnancy category C drugs; these are category B drugs, and in small pilot studies, treatment of pregnant women in the third trimester with either of these drugs or lamivudine has been effective in preventing transmission to offspring of high-risk women. A recent small open-label study from China demonstrated that telbivudine (600 mg, orally, daily) given in the second and third trimester of pregnancy completely eliminated perinatal transmission of HBV in women who were both HBeAg and HBsAg positive, compared with a 9% transmission rate in a control group of women who did not receive the drug. All infants in both groups received HepB vaccine and HBIG within 6 hours of delivery.

Serologic Screening of Pregnant Women. Prenatal HBsAg testing of all pregnant women, regardless of HepB vaccination history, is recommended to identify newborn infants who require immediate postexposure prophylaxis. All pregnant women should be tested during an early prenatal visit with every pregnancy. Testing should be repeated at the time of admission to the hospital for delivery for HBsAg-negative women who are at high risk of HBV infection or who have had clinical hepatitis. Women who are HBsAg positive should be reported to local health departments for appropriate case management to ensure follow-up of their infants and immunization of sexual and household contacts. In populations where HBsAg testing of pregnant women is not feasible (eg, in remote areas without access to a laboratory), all infants should receive HepB vaccine within 12 hours of birth, should receive the second dose by 2 months of age, and should receive the third dose at 6 months of age. Pregnant women and their contacts who are HBsAg-positive should be referred for medical management to reduce their risk of chronic liver disease.

Management of Infants Born to HBsAg-Positive Women. Infants born to HBsAg-positive mothers, including infants weighing less than 2000 g, should receive the initial dose of HepB vaccine within 12 hours of birth (see Table 3.21, p 410, for appropriate dosages), and HBIG (0.5 mL) should be administered concurrently but at a different anatomic site. The effectiveness of HBIG diminishes the longer after exposure that it is initiated. The interval of effectiveness is unlikely to exceed 7 days. Subsequent doses of vaccine should be administered as recommended in Table 3.24 (p 420) and Table 3.25 (p 422). For infants who weigh <2000 g at birth, the initial vaccine dose should not be counted in the required 3-dose schedule (a total of 4 doses of HepB vaccine should be administered), and the subsequent 3 doses should be administered in accordance with the schedule for immunization of infants weighing <2000 g.

Infants born to HBsAg-positive women should be tested for anti-HBs and HBsAg at 9 to 12 months of age (generally at the next well-child visit after completion of the immunization series).[1,2] Testing should not be performed before 9 months of age to maximize

[1]Schillie S, Murphy TV, Fenlon N, et al. Update: shortened interval for postvaccination serologic testing of infants born to hepatitis B-infected mothers. *MMWR Morb Mortal Wkly Rep.* 2015;64(30):1118–1120

[2]American Academy of Pediatrics, Committee on Infectious Diseases. Elimination of perinatal hepatitis B: providing the first vaccine dose within 24 hours of birth. *Pediatrics.* 2017;140(3):e20171870

the likelihood of detecting late onset of HBV infections. Immunized infants with anti-HBs concentrations ≥10 mIU/mL and who are HBsAg negative are considered not to be infected and to have adequate vaccine-associated immune protection. Infants with anti-HBs concentrations <10 mIU/mL and who are HBsAg negative following a 3-dose hepatitis B vaccine series should receive 1 additional dose of hepatitis B vaccine (see Table 3.24, p 420) followed by testing for anti-HBs and HBsAg 1 to 2 months after the fourth dose. Infants with anti-HBs concentrations ≥10 mIU/mL and who are HBsAg negative after the fourth dose are considered not to be infected and to have adequate vaccine-associated immune protection. However, infants with anti-HBs concentrations <10 mIU/mL and who are HBsAg negative after the fourth dose should receive 2 additional doses of vaccine followed by testing for anti-HBs and HBsAg 1 to 2 months after the sixth dose. Subsequent doses of hepatitis B vaccine when anti-HBs concentrations are <10 mIU/mL after the sixth dose are not indicated.

Term Infants (Weighing ≥2000 g at Birth) Born to Mothers Not Tested During Pregnancy for HBsAg. Pregnant women whose HBsAg status is unknown at delivery should undergo blood testing as soon as possible to determine their HBsAg status. While awaiting results, the infant should receive the first HepB vaccine dose within 12 hours of birth, as recommended for infants born to HBsAg-positive mothers (see Table 3.21, p 410). Because HepB vaccine, when administered at birth, is highly effective for preventing perinatal infection in term infants, the possible added value and the cost of HBIG do not warrant its immediate use in term infants when the mother's HBsAg status is not known. If the woman is found to be HBsAg positive, term infants should receive HBIG (0.5 mL) as soon as possible, but within 7 days of birth, and should complete the HepB immunization series as recommended (see Tables 3.21, p 410, and 3.23, p 416). If the mother is found to be HBsAg negative, HepB immunization in the dose and schedule recommended for term infants born to HBsAg-negative mothers should be completed (see Table 3.21, p 410). If the mother's HBsAg status remains unknown, some experts would administer HBIG within 7 days of birth and complete the HepB immunization series as recommended for infants born to mothers who are HBsAg positive (Table 3.24, p 420).

Infants Weighing Less Than 2000 g Born to Mothers Not Tested During Pregnancy for HBsAg. Maternal HBsAg status should be determined as soon as possible. Infants weighing <2000 g born to mothers whose HBsAg status is unknown should receive HepB vaccine within the first 12 hours of life. Because of the potentially decreased immunogenicity of the HepB vaccine in infants weighing <2000 g at birth, these infants should receive HBIG (0.5 mL) if the mother's HBsAg status cannot be determined within the initial 12 hours of birth. In these infants, the initial vaccine dose should not be counted toward the 3 doses of HepB vaccine required to complete the immunization series. The subsequent 3 doses (for a total of 4 doses) are administered in accordance with recommendations for immunization of infants with a birth weight <2000 g, according to the HBsAg status of the mother (see Table 3.24, p 420). Follow-up HBsAg and anti-HBs testing on completion of the immunization series is recommended for all infants weighing <2000 g born to HBsAg-positive mothers (see Management of Infants Born to HBsAg-Positive Women, p 427).

Breastfeeding. Breastfeeding of the infant by an HBsAg-positive mother poses no additional risk of acquisition of HBV infection by the infant with appropriate administration of HepB vaccine and HBIG (see Human Milk, p 113).

Household Contacts and Sexual Partners of HBsAg-Positive People. Household and sexual contacts of HBsAg-positive people (with acute or chronic HBV infection) identified through prenatal screening, blood donor screening, or diagnostic or other serologic testing should be screened for HBV infection with anti-HBc or anti-HBs and HBsAg tests. Unvaccinated and uninfected people should be immunized. The first dose of vaccine should be administered after the blood for serologic tests is obtained while waiting on the results. People with chronic HBV should be referred for medical evaluation to prevent complications of the infection.

Prophylaxis with HBIG for other unimmunized household contacts of HBsAg-positive people is not indicated unless they have a discrete, identifiable exposure to the index patient (see next paragraph).

Postexposure Prophylaxis for People With Discrete Identifiable Exposures to Blood or Body Fluids. Management of people with a discrete, identifiable percutaneous (eg, needle stick, laceration, bite or nonintact skin), mucosal (eg, ocular or mucous membrane), or sexual exposure to blood or body fluids includes consideration of whether the HBsAg status of the person who was the source of exposure and the hepatitis B immunization and response status of the exposed person are known (also see Table 3.23, p 416). Immunization is recommended for any person who was exposed but not immunized previously. If possible, a blood specimen from the person who was the source of the exposure should be tested for HBsAg, and appropriate prophylaxis should be administered according to the hepatitis B immunization status and anti-HBs response status (if known) of the exposed person (see Table 3.23, p 416). Detailed guidelines for management of health care personnel and other people exposed to blood that is or might be HBsAg positive is provided in Table 3.22 and in the recommendations of the Advisory Committee on Immunization Practices of the Centers for Disease Control and Prevention.[1]

HBsAg-Positive Source. If the source is HBsAg positive, unimmunized people should receive both HBIG and HepB vaccine as soon as possible after exposure, preferably within 24 hours (see Table 3.23, p 416). The vaccine series should be completed using an age-appropriate dose and schedule. People who are in the process of being immunized but who have not completed the vaccine series should receive the appropriate dose of HBIG and should complete the vaccine series. Children and adolescents who have written documentation of a complete HepB vaccine series and who did not receive postimmunization testing should receive a single vaccine booster dose (Table 3.23, p 416).

Source With Unknown HBsAg Status. If the HBsAg status of the source is unknown, unimmunized people should begin the HepB vaccine series with the first dose initiated as soon as possible after exposure, preferably within 24 hours (see Table 3.23, p 416). The vaccine series should be completed using an age-appropriate dose and schedule. Children and adolescents with written documentation of a complete HepB vaccine series require no further treatment (Table 3.23, p 416).

Victims of Sexual Assault or Abuse. For unimmunized victims of sexual assault or abuse, active postexposure prophylaxis (ie, vaccine alone) should be initiated, with the first dose of HepB vaccine administered as part of the initial clinical evaluation. If the offender is known to be HBsAg positive, HBIG also should be administered. The vaccine series should be completed using an age-appropriate dose and schedule (see Table 3.23, p 416).

Child Care. All children, including children who attend child care, should receive HepB vaccine as part of their routine immunization. Immunization not only will decrease the

---

[1]Centers for Disease Control and Prevention. Immunization of health-care personnel: recommendations of the Advisory Committee on Immunization Practices (ACIP). *MMWR Recomm Rep.* 2011;60(RR-7):1–45

potential for HBV transmission after human bites but also will allay anxiety about transmission from attendees who may be HBsAg positive.

Children who are HBsAg positive and who have no behavioral or medical risk factors, such as unusually aggressive behavior (eg, frequent biting), generalized dermatitis, or a bleeding problem, should be admitted to child care without restrictions. Under these circumstances, the risk of HBV transmission in child care settings is negligible, and routine screening for HBsAg is not warranted. Admission of HBsAg-positive children with behavioral or medical risk factors should be assessed on an individual basis by the child's physician, in consultation with the child care staff.

Effectiveness of Hepatitis B Prevention Programs. Routine hepatitis B immunization programs have resulted in significant decreases in the prevalence of chronic HBV infection among children in populations with a high incidence of HBV infection. There is an association between higher coverage with HepB vaccine and larger decreases in HBsAg prevalence.

Although the long-term sequelae of chronic HBV infection usually are not recognized until adolescence and adulthood, cirrhosis and HCC occur in children. Worldwide, routine infant immunization programs and introduction of immunization schedules starting within the first 24 hours of life are expected to decrease significantly the incidence of death from cirrhosis and HCC attributable to HBV infection over the next 30 to 50 years.

The Centers for Disease Control and Prevention Division of Viral Hepatitis maintains a Web site (**www.cdc.gov/hepatitis**) with information on hepatitis for health care professionals and the public.

Hepatitis C

CLINICAL MANIFESTATIONS: Signs and symptoms of hepatitis C virus (HCV) infection are indistinguishable from those of hepatitis A or hepatitis B virus infections. Acute disease tends to be mild and insidious in onset, and most infections are asymptomatic. Jaundice occurs in less than 20% of patients with HCV infection, and abnormalities in serum alanine transaminase concentrations generally are less pronounced than in patients with hepatitis B virus infection. Persistent infection with HCV occurs in up to 80% of infected children, even in the absence of biochemical evidence of liver disease. Most children with chronic infection are asymptomatic. Although chronic HCV infection develops in approximately 75% to 85% of infected adults, limited data indicate that chronic HCV infection and cirrhosis occur less commonly in children, in part because of the usually indolent nature of infection in pediatric patients. Liver failure secondary to HCV infection is one of the leading indications for liver transplantation among adults in the United States.

ETIOLOGY: HCV is a small, single-stranded, positive-sense RNA virus and is a member of the family *Flaviviridae* in the genus *Hepacivirus*. At least 7 HCV genotypes exist with more than 50 subtypes. Distribution of genotypes and subtypes varies by geographic location, with genotype 1a being the most common in the United States.

EPIDEMIOLOGY: The incidence of acute symptomatic HCV infection in the United States was 0.8 per 100 000 in 2015 (**www.cdc.gov/hepatitis/statistics/2015surveillance/index.htm**). After asymptomatic infection and underreporting were considered, approximately 30 000 new cases were estimated to have occurred in 2014. For all age groups, the incidence of HCV infection decreased markedly in the United States since the 1990s and reached its lowest incidence in 2006–2010. However, after 2010, there was a 2.6-fold increase in reported cases of acute HCV in the United States by 2014. This increase was mostly seen in white, nonurban young people with a history of using injection drugs and opioid agonists such as oxycodone (**www.cdc.gov/ hepatitis/statistics/2011surveillance/commentary.htm**). A substantial burden of disease still exists in the United States because of the propensity of HCV to establish chronic infection and the high incidence of acute HCV infection through the 1980s. The prevalence of HCV infection in the general population of the United States is estimated at 1.3%, equating to an estimated 3.5 million people in the United States who have chronic HCV infection. Seroprevalence varies among populations according to risk factors. The pediatric prevalence of HCV corresponding to the National Health and Nutrition Examination Survey (NHANES) 1999–2002 was approximately 0.1%, although the numbers of HCV infections in the younger age groups were too small for reliable estimates. Worldwide, the prevalence of chronic HCV infection is highest in northern Africa, the Middle East, and parts of Asia.

HCV is transmitted primarily through percutaneous (parenteral) exposures to infectious blood that can result from injection drug use, needle stick injuries, and inadequate infection control in health-care settings. The most common risk factors for adults to acquire infection are injection drug use or receipt of blood products before 1992. The most common route of infection for children is maternal-fetal transmission. The current risk of HCV infection after blood transfusion in the United States is estimated to be less than 1 per 2 million units transfused because of exclusion of high-risk donors and of HCV-positive units after antibody testing as well as screening of pools of blood units by nucleic acid amplification test (NAAT). All intravenous and intramuscular Immune Globulin products available commercially in the United States undergo an inactivation procedure for HCV or are documented to be HCV RNA negative before release.

Approximately 60% of acute HCV cases reported to public health authorities are in acknowledged injection drug users who have shared needles or injection paraphernalia. For reported chronic HCV cases for which age is known, 63.5% were among people older than 40 years, and almost all infected people are outside the pediatric age range. Data from recent multicenter, population-based cohort studies indicate that approximately one third of young injection drug users 18 to 30 years of age are infected with HCV. People with sporadic percutaneous exposures, such as health care professionals (approximately 1% of cases), may be infected. Approximately half of the 18 000 people with hemophilia who received transfusions before adoption of heat treatment of clotting factors in 1987 are HCV-seropositive. Also, more recently appreciated has been the number of infections acquired in the health care setting, especially nonhospital clinics where infection control and needle and intravenous hygienic procedures have not been practiced strictly. Prevalence is high among people with frequent but smaller direct percutaneous exposures, such as patients receiving hemodialysis (10%–20%).

Sexual transmission of HCV between monogamous heterosexual partners is extremely rare. HCV virus has been identified in semen. However, studies show that the risk for HCV transmission is greater for parenteral transmission than sexual transmission. The risk for HCV acquisition by sexual transmission is increased with a high number of sexual partners, group sex, and coinfection with human immunodeficiency virus (HIV). Injection drug users may have a greater number of sex partners, so the role of sexual transmission is not fully understood. Sexual transmission of HCV among people coinfected with HIV has been described between HIV-infected men who have sex with men or HIV-infected heterosexual women.

Transmission among family contacts is uncommon but can occur from direct or inapparent percutaneous or mucosal exposure to blood.

Seroprevalence among pregnant women in the United States has been estimated at approximately 1% to 2%. The risk of perinatal transmission averages 5% to 6%, and transmission occurs only from women who are HCV RNA positive at the time of delivery. The exact timing of HCV transmission from mother to infant is not established. Factors that increase perinatal transmission include internal fetal monitoring, vaginal lacerations, and prolonged rupture of membranes (>6 hours). The method of delivery has no effect on perinatal infection risk. Serum antibody to HCV (anti-HCV) and HCV RNA have been detected in colostrum, but the risk of HCV transmission is similar in breastfed and formula-fed infants. Breastfeeding is safe as long as mother's nipples are not cracked or bleeding. When nipples are cracked or bleeding, mothers should stop breastfeeding and pump and discard their milk, and resume breastfeeding when the nipples have healed. Maternal coinfection with (untreated) HIV has been associated with increased risk of perinatal transmission of HCV, with transmission rates between 10% and 20%; transmission depends in part on the concentration of HCV RNA in the mother's blood.

All people with HCV RNA in their blood are considered to be infectious.

The **incubation period** for HCV infection averages 6 to 7 weeks, with a range of 2 weeks to 6 months. The time from exposure to development of viremia generally is 1 to 2 weeks.

DIAGNOSTIC TESTS[1]: The 2 types of tests available for laboratory diagnosis of HCV infections are immunoglobulin (Ig) G antibody enzyme immunoassays (EIA) or chemiluminescent immunoassays (CIA) for HCV and NAATs to detect HCV RNA. The diagnosis of HCV infection usually is made by serologic testing. Third-generation immunoassays cleared by the US Food and Drug Administration (FDA) are at least 97% sensitive and more than 99% specific. For some assays, a positive result is considered initially reactive, and repeat testing in duplicate is required. Final results are reported as reactive when at least 2 replicates are positive. Some of the newer assays with high performance allow for reporting of initial possible results without repeat testing. In June 2010, the FDA approved for use in people 15 years and older the OraQuick rapid blood test, which uses a test strip that produces a blue line within 20 minutes if anti-HCV antibodies are present. False-negative results early in the course of acute infection can result from any of the HCV serologic tests because of the prolonged interval between exposure and onset of illness and seroconversion. In a clinical setting where acute HCV infection is considered likely and the initial immunoassay result is negative, repeat testing with a third-generation immunoassay or NAAT should be performed. Within 15 weeks after exposure and within 5 to 6 weeks after onset of hepatitis, 80% of patients will have positive test results for serum anti-HCV antibody. Among infants born to anti-HCV–positive mothers, passively acquired maternal antibody may persist for up to 18 months.

FDA-licensed diagnostic NAATs for qualitative detection of HCV RNA are available commercially and recommended in the 2013 Centers for Disease Control and Prevention (CDC) HCV testing algorithm as follow-up for patients with a positive HCV serologic test result. HCV RNA can be detected in serum or plasma within 1 to 2 weeks after exposure

---

[1]Centers for Disease Control and Prevention. Testing for HCV Infection: an update of guidance for clinicians and laboratorians. *MMWR Morb Mortal Wkly Rep.* 2013;62(18):362–365

to the virus and weeks before onset of liver enzyme abnormalities or appearance of anti-HCV antibody. Assays for detection of HCV RNA are used commonly in clinical practice to: (1) detect HCV infection after needlestick or transfusion and before seroconversion; (2) identify anti-HCV–positive patients with active infection who are viremic; (3) identify infection in infants early in life (ie, perinatal transmission) when maternal antibody interferes with ability to detect antibody produced by the infant; and (4) monitor patients receiving antiviral therapy. However, false-positive and false-negative results of NAATs can occur from improper handling, storage, and contamination of test specimens. Viral RNA may be detected intermittently in acute infection (ie, in the first 6 or 12 months following infection); thus, a single negative assay result is not conclusive if performed during this acute infection period. Highly sensitive quantitative assays for measuring the concentration of HCV RNA have largely replaced qualitative assays. Quantitative RNA and genotyping assays of HCV are useful for determination of drug treatment regimens and duration of treatment. HCV genotyping has become extremely important in determining which direct-acting antiviral agents should be used in individual patients.

Because perinatally HCV-infected infants have a low risk of HCV acquisition, they usually do not exhibit symptoms for years, and there currently are no antiviral therapies available in the first 2 years of life, assessment of HCV infection may rely on serologic testing at 18 months of age. Prior to serologic testing, liver enzyme testing can be performed at approximately 6-month intervals to detect the rare perinatally HCV-infected infant who has significant liver injury prior to 18 months of age. In situations in which there may be concerns about the ability to maintain contact with perinatally HCV-exposed infant until 18 months of age, if the family is not willing to wait until 18 months of age to determine the child's HCV infection status, or if antiviral therapy becomes available to younger infants, quantitative RNA tests can be performed as early as 1 to 2 months of age. If the initial quantitative HCV RNA result is negative, serologic testing should be performed at 18 months of age.

TREATMENT: Patients with a diagnosis of HCV infection should be referred to a pediatric infectious disease specialist or gastroenterologist for clinical monitoring and consideration of enrollment into clinical trials of direct-acting oral hepatitis C antiviral therapy when available. Traditional interferon and ribavirin-based therapies are expensive, can have significant adverse reactions, and yield variable virologic response rates.

A number of highly effective interferon-free direct-acting antiviral drug regimens have been FDA approved for adults and are the current standard of care therapy for HCV in adults. These drugs are all oral, usually taken once daily, rarely associated with serious adverse effects, and most important, almost always curative (ie, sustained virologic response). Because this is a rapidly changing field, the American Association for the Study of Liver Disease and the Infectious Diseases Society of America are continually updating recommended antiviral drug treatment (**www.hcvguidelines.org**).

At present, the 3 direct-acting, all-oral combination drug therapy recommended for HCV genotypes 1a and 1b (>75% of all HCV in the United States) and genotype 4 (approximately 2%) include: ledipasvir and sofosubuvir (Harvoni [Gilead Sciences, Foster City, CA); ombitasvir, dasabuvir, and paritaprevir, with or without ribavirin (Viekira Pak [AbbVie, North Chicago, IL]); and grazoprevir and elbasvir (Zepatier [Merck & Co Inc, Whitehouse Station, NJ]). For people with (compensated) cirrhosis or who have failed previous antiviral therapy, treatment duration may vary from 12 to 24 weeks, depending on the treatment regimen used and the patient's previous receipt of HCV antiviral therapy. For adults with genotypes 2 (about 12% of all HCV patients) or 3 (7%), current therapy is sofosbuvir plus either ribavirin or daclatasvir for 12 to 24 weeks.

Together, these regimens offer hope for cure without significant adverse effects for a large population of adult and, ultimately, pediatric patients with HCV infection. At the current time, several of the all-oral anti-HCV regimens are being evaluated in clinical trials for use in children. A once-daily ledipasvir (90 mg)–sofosbuvir (400 mg) combination given for 12 weeks was well tolerated and resulted in 98% sustained viral response (cure) among 100 adolescent children 12 to 17 years of age with chronic hepatitis C caused by genotype 1. On April 7, 2017, sofosbuvir (Sovaldi) and ledipasvir and sofosbuvir (Harvoni) were approved by the FDA to treat hepatitis C virus in children 12 to 17 years of age.

Management of Chronic HCV Infection. Because of the very high rate of severe hepatitis in patients with HCV-associated chronic liver disease, all patients with chronic HCV infection should be immunized against hepatitis A and hepatitis B. With advancing age, chronic HCV infection increases the risk of liver-related morbidity and mortality, including cirrhosis and primary hepatocellular carcinoma. Among children, progression of liver disease appears to be accelerated when comorbid conditions, including HIV, childhood cancer, iron overload, or thalassemia, are present. Pediatricians should be alert to concomitant infections, alcohol abuse, and concomitant use of prescription and nonprescription drugs, such as acetaminophen, some antiretroviral agents (such as stavudine), and herbal medications, in patients with HCV infection that may worsen liver disease. Children with chronic infection should be followed closely, including sequential monitoring of serum alanine transaminase concentrations, because of the potential for chronic liver disease. The North American Society of Pediatric Gastroenterology, Hepatology and Nutrition published guidelines for children with HCV infection in 2012.[1] Evidence-based, consensus recommendations from the Infectious Diseases Society of America, the American Association for the Study of Liver Diseases, and the International Antiviral Society–USA for screening, treatment, and management of patients with HCV can be found online (**www.HCVguidelines.org**).

ISOLATION OF THE HOSPITALIZED PATIENT: Standard precautions are recommended.

CONTROL MEASURES:

Care of Exposed People.

Immunoprophylaxis. On the basis of lack of clinical efficacy in humans and data from animal studies, use of Immune Globulin for postexposure prophylaxis against HCV infection is not recommended. Furthermore, potential donors of immune globulin are screened for antibody to HCV and excluded from donation if positive, so Immune Globulin preparations are devoid of anti-HCV antibody.

Breastfeeding. Mothers infected with HCV should be advised that transmission of HCV by breastfeeding has not been documented. According to guidelines of the American Academy of Pediatrics and the CDC, maternal HCV infection is not a contraindication to breastfeeding. Mothers who are HCV infected and choose to breastfeed should interrupt

[1]Mack CL, Gonzalez-Peralta RP, Gupta N, et al; North American Society for Pediatric Gastroenterology, Hepatology, and Nutrition. NASPGHAN practice guidelines: diagnosis and management of hepatitis C infection in infants, children, and adolescents. *J Pediatr Gastroenterol Nutr.* 2012;54(6):838–855

breastfeeding temporarily if their nipples are bleeding or cracked and can consider expressing and discarding their milk until the nipples are healed. Once the nipples no longer are cracked or bleeding, HCV-infected mothers may fully resume breastfeeding.

Child Care. Exclusion of children with HCV infection from out-of-home child care is not indicated.

Serologic Testing for HCV Infection.

People Who Have Risk Factors for HCV Infection. HCV testing is recommended for anyone at increased risk for HCV infection and other populations, including[1-3]:

- People born from 1945 through 1965;
- People who have ever injected illegal drugs, including those who injected only once many years ago;
- Recipients of clotting factor concentrates made before 1987;
- Recipients of blood transfusions or solid organ transplants before July 1992;
- Patients who have ever received long-term hemodialysis treatment;
- People with known exposures to HCV, such as
  - ◆ Health care workers after needlesticks involving HCV-positive blood;
  - ◆ Recipients of blood or organs from a donor who later tested HCV-positive;
- All people with HIV infection;
- Patients with signs or symptoms of liver disease (eg, abnormal liver enzyme test results);
- Children born to HCV-positive mothers (to avoid detecting maternal antibody, these children should not be tested serologically before 18 months of age);
- Incarcerated people; and
- People who use intranasal illicit drugs or received tattoos from unregulated settings.

Pregnant Women. Routine serologic testing of pregnant women for HCV infection is not currently recommended.

Children Born to Women With HCV Infection. Children born to women previously identified to be HCV infected should be tested for HCV infection, because 5% to 6% of these children will acquire the infection. Transmission depends, in part, on the concentration of HCV RNA in the mother's blood, and if the mother does not have detectable HCV RNA at the time of delivery, then the likelihood of transmission to the infant is very low. The duration of passively acquired maternal antibody in infants can be as long as 18 months. Therefore, testing for anti-HCV antibodies should not be performed until after 18 months of age. If earlier diagnosis is desired, a NAAT to detect HCV RNA may be performed at or after the infant's first well-child visit at 1 to 2 months of age.

Adoptees. See Medical Evaluation for Infectious Diseases for Internationally Adopted, Refugee, and Immigrant Children (p 175) for specific situations when serologic testing is warranted.

---

[1]Centers for Disease Control and Prevention. Recommendations for the identification of chronic hepatitis C virus infection among persons born during 1945–1965. *MMWR Recomm Rep.* 2012;61(RR–4):1–32

[2]Centers for Disease Control and Prevention. Guidelines for prevention and treatment of opportunistic infections in HIV-infected adults and adolescents: recommendations from CDC, the National Institutes of Health, and the HIV Medicine Association of the Infectious Diseases Society of America. *MMWR Recomm Rep.* 2009;58(RR–4):1–207

[3]**https://aidsinfo.nih.gov/guidelines**

Counseling of Patients With HCV Infection. All people with HCV infection should be considered infectious, should be informed of the possibility of transmission to others, and should refrain from donating blood, organs, tissues, or semen and from sharing toothbrushes and razors.

Infected people should be counseled to avoid hepatotoxic agents, including medications, and should be informed of the risks of excessive alcohol ingestion. All patients with chronic HCV infection should be immunized against hepatitis A and hepatitis B.

Changes in sexual practices of infected people with a long-term, monogamous partner are not recommended; however, they should be informed of the possible risks and use of precautions to prevent transmission. People with multiple sexual partners should be advised to decrease the number of partners and to use condoms to prevent transmission. No data exist to support counseling a woman against pregnancy. Currently, HCV antiviral therapy is not recommended during pregnancy. Because HCV treatment regimens are becoming more convenient and better tolerated, HCV therapy, if shown to be safe in pregnancy and effective in reducing mother-to-infant HCV transmission, may eventually become available as a means of preventing perinatal HCV transmission.

The CDC Division of Viral Hepatitis maintains a Web site (**www.cdc.gov/hepatitis/HCV**) with information on hepatitis for health care professionals and the public, including specific information for people who have received blood transfusions before 1992. Information also can be obtained from the National Institutes of Health Web site (**www2.niddk.nih.gov/Research/ScientificAreas/DigestiveDiseases/Liver/VHID.htm**).

Evidence-based, consensus recommendations from the Infectious Diseases Society of America, the American Association for the Study of Liver Diseases, and the International Antiviral Society–USA for screening, treatment, and management of patients with HCV can be found online (**www.HCVguidelines.org**).

Hepatitis D

CLINICAL MANIFESTATIONS: Hepatitis D virus (HDV) causes infection only in people with acute or chronic hepatitis B virus (HBV) infection. HDV requires HBV surface antigen (HBsAg) for replication. The importance of HDV infection lies in its ability to convert an asymptomatic or mild chronic HBV infection into fulminant or more severe or rapidly progressive disease. Acute coinfection with HBV and HDV usually causes an acute illness indistinguishable from acute HBV infection alone, except that the likelihood of fulminant hepatitis can be as high as 5%.

ETIOLOGY: HDV measures 36 to 43 nm in diameter and consists of an RNA genome and a delta protein antigen, both of which are coated with HBsAg.

EPIDEMIOLOGY: HDV infection is present worldwide, in all age groups, and an estimated 15 to 20 million people are infected with the virus, according to surveys performed in the 1980s and 1990s. Over the past 20 years, HDV prevalence has decreased significantly in Western and Southern Europe because of long-standing hepatitis B vaccination programs, although HDV remains a significant health problem in resource-limited countries. At least 8 genotypes of HDV have been described, each with a typical geographic pattern, with genotype I being the predominant type in Europe and North America. HDV can cause an infection at the same time as the initial HBV infection (coinfection), or it can infect a person already chronically infected with HBV (superinfection). Acquisition of

HDV is by parenteral, percutaneous, or mucous membrane inoculation. HDV can be acquired from blood or blood products, through injection drug use, or by sexual contact, but only if HBV also is present. Transmission from mother to newborn infant is uncommon. Intrafamilial spread can occur among people with chronic HBV infection. High-prevalence areas include parts of Eastern Europe, South America, Africa, Central Asia, and the Middle East. In the United States, HDV infection is found most commonly in people who abuse injection drugs, people with hemophilia, and people who have emigrated from areas with endemic HDV infection.

The **incubation period** for HDV superinfection is approximately 2 to 8 weeks. When HBV and HDV viruses infect simultaneously, the incubation period is similar to that of HBV (45–160 days; average, 90 days).

DIAGNOSTIC TESTS: People with chronic HBV infection are at risk of HDV coinfection. Accordingly, their care should be supervised by an expert in hepatitis treatment. Consideration should be given to testing for anti-HDV immunoglobulin (Ig) G antibodies using a commercially available test if they have increased transaminase concentrations, particularly if they recently came from a country with high prevalence of HDV. Anti-HDV may not be present until several weeks after onset of illness, and acute and convalescent sera may be required to confirm the diagnosis. In a person with anti-HDV, the absence of IgM hepatitis B core antibody (anti-HBc), which is indicative of chronic HBV infection, suggests that the person has both chronic HBV infection and superinfection with HDV. Presence of anti-HDV IgG antibodies does not prove active infection, and thus, HDV RNA testing should be performed for diagnostic and therapeutic considerations. Patients with circulating HDV RNA should be staged for severity of liver disease, have surveillance for development of hepatocellular carcinoma, and be considered for treatment. Presence of anti-HDV IgM is of lesser utility, because it is present in both acute and chronic HDV infections.

TREATMENT: HDV has proven difficult to treat, and there are no approved therapies for use in children. Data suggest pegylated interferon-alfa may result in up to 40% of patients having a sustained response to treatment. Clinical trials suggest at least a year of therapy may be associated with sustained responses, and longer courses may be warranted if the patient is able to tolerate therapy. Further study of pegylated interferon monotherapy or as combination therapy with a direct-acting antiviral agent needs to be performed before treatment of HDV can be advised routinely. There are some preliminary data in adult volunteers suggesting that Myrcludex B (MYR GmbH [Burgwedel, Germany]), a lipomyristolated peptide containing 47 amino acids of the pre S1 domain of the HBV large surface protein, given either alone or in combination with pegylated interferon-alfa, significantly inhibits or clears HDV but has no effect on HBsAg. Ongoing studies may provide more insight into the long-term significance, if any, of this finding. Liver transplantation in individuals with liver failure attributable to coinfections of HBV and HDV has been reported.

ISOLATION OF THE HOSPITALIZED PATIENT: Standard precautions are recommended.

CONTROL MEASURES: The same control and preventive measures used for HBV infection are indicated. Because HDV cannot be transmitted in the absence of HBV infection, HBV immunization protects against HDV infection. People with chronic HBV infection should take extreme care to avoid exposure to HDV.

Hepatitis E

CLINICAL MANIFESTATIONS: Hepatitis E virus (HEV) infection causes an acute illness with symptoms including jaundice, malaise, anorexia, fever, abdominal pain, and arthralgia. Disease is more common among adults than among children and is more severe in pregnant women, in whom mortality rates can reach 10% to 25% during the third trimester. Chronic HEV infection mostly occurs in people with severe immunodeficiency. Approximately 60% of recipients of solid organ transplants fail to clear the virus and develop chronic hepatitis, and 10% will develop cirrhosis.

ETIOLOGY: HEV is a spherical, nonenveloped, positive-sense, single-stranded RNA virus. HEV is classified in the genus *Orthohepevirus* of the family *Hepeviridae*. *Orthohepevirus* A comprises 7 genotypes (based on phylogenetic analyses) that infect humans (HEV-1, -2, -3, -4, and -7), pigs (HEV-3 and -4), rabbits (HEV-3), wild boars (HEV-3, -4, -5, and -6), mongooses (HEV-3), deer (HEV-3), yaks (HEV-4), and camels (HEV-7).

EPIDEMIOLOGY: HEV is the most common cause of viral hepatitis in the world. Globally, an estimated 20 million HEV infections occur annually, resulting in 3.4 million cases of acute hepatitis, 70 000 deaths and 3000 stillbirths. In resource-limited countries, where almost all HEV infections occur, ingestion of fecally contaminated water is the most common route of HEV transmission, and large waterborne outbreaks occur frequently. Sporadic HEV infection has been reported throughout the world and is common in Africa and the Indian subcontinent. Person-to-person transmission appears to be much less efficient than with hepatitis A virus but occurs in sporadic and outbreak settings. Mother-to-infant transmission of HEV, mainly HEV-1, occurs frequently and accounts for a substantial number of fetal loss and perinatal mortality. HEV also is transmitted through blood and blood product transfusion. Transfusion-transmitted hepatitis E occurs primarily in countries with endemic disease and also is reported in areas without endemic infection. In the United States, serologic studies have demonstrated that approximately 6% of the population has immunoglobulin (Ig) G antibodies against HEV. However, symptomatic HEV infection in the United States is uncommon and generally occurs in people who acquire HEV-1 infection while traveling in countries with endemic HEV. Nonetheless, a number of people without a travel history have been diagnosed with acute hepatitis E, and evidence for the infection should be sought in cases of acute hepatitis with an unknown etiology. Hepatitis E may masquerade as drug-induced liver injury.

The **incubation period** is 2 to 6 weeks.

DIAGNOSTIC TESTS: HEV infection should be considered in any person with symptoms of viral hepatitis who has traveled to or from a region with endemic hepatitis E or from a region where an outbreak has been identified and who tests negative for serologic markers of hepatitis A, B, C, and other hepatotropic viruses. Testing for anti-HEV IgM and IgG is available through some research and commercial reference laboratories. Because anti-HEV assays are not approved by the US Food and Drug Administration and their performance characteristics are not well defined, results should be interpreted with caution, particularly in cases lacking a discrete onset of illness associated with jaundice or with no recent history of travel to a country with endemic HEV transmission. Definitive diagnosis may be made by demonstrating viral RNA in serum or stool samples by means of reverse transcriptase-polymerase chain reaction assay, which is available only in research settings (eg, with prior approval through the Centers for Disease Control and Prevention). Because virus circulates in the body for a relatively short period, the inability to detect HEV in serum or stool does not eliminate the possibility that the person was infected with HEV.

TREATMENT: Supportive. Some case reports and case series have indicated that modification of immunosuppressive medication and/or use of antiviral drugs, such as ribavirin, with or without interferon-alpha, may result in viral clearance in immunocompromised patients with chronic hepatitis E. However, no randomized controlled clinical trials have been performed.

ISOLATION OF THE HOSPITALIZED PATIENT: In addition to standard precautions, contact precautions are recommended for diapered and incontinent patients for the duration of illness.

CONTROL MEASURES: Provision of safe water is the most effective prevention measure. A safe and effective recombinant HEV vaccine has been approved for use by the Chinese Food and Drug Administration but is not approved for use in the United States. The World Health Organization recently published a position paper on hepatitis E vaccine development (**www.who.int/wer/2015/wer9018.pdf?ua=1**).

Herpes Simplex

CLINICAL MANIFESTATIONS:

Neonatal. In newborn infants, herpes simplex virus (HSV) infection can manifest as: (1) disseminated disease involving multiple organs, most prominently liver and lungs, and in 60% to 75% of cases also involving the central nervous system (CNS); (2) localized CNS disease, with or without skin, eye, or mouth involvement (CNS disease); or (3) disease localized to the skin, eyes, and/or mouth (SEM disease). Approximately 25% of cases of neonatal HSV manifest as disseminated disease, 30% manifest as CNS disease, and 45% manifest as SEM disease. In the absence of skin lesions, the diagnosis of neonatal HSV infection is challenging. More than 80% of neonates with SEM disease have skin vesicles; those without vesicles have infection limited to the eyes and/or oral mucosa. Approximately two thirds of neonates with disseminated or CNS disease have skin lesions, but these lesions may not be present at the time of onset of symptoms. Disseminated infection should be considered in neonates with sepsis syndrome with negative bacteriologic culture results, severe liver dysfunction, consumptive coagulopathy, or suspected viral pneumonia. HSV should be considered as a causative agent in neonates with fever (especially within the first 3 weeks of life), a vesicular rash, or abnormal cerebrospinal fluid (CSF) findings (especially in the presence of seizures or during a time of year when enteroviruses are not circulating in the community). Although asymptomatic HSV infection is common in older children, it rarely, if ever, occurs in neonates.

Neonatal herpetic infections often are severe, with attendant high mortality and morbidity rates, even when antiviral therapy is administered. Mortality rates from neonatal herpes increased between 2004 and 2013, compared with the 20 years prior to that. Recurrent skin lesions are common in surviving infants, occurring in approximately 50% of survivors, often within 1 to 2 weeks of completing the initial treatment course of parenteral acyclovir.

Initial signs of HSV infection can occur anytime between birth and approximately 6 weeks of age, although almost all infected infants develop clinical disease within the first month of life. Infants with disseminated disease and SEM disease have an earlier age of onset, typically presenting between the first and second weeks of life; infants with CNS disease usually present with illness between the second and third weeks of life.

Children Beyond the Neonatal Period and Adolescents. Most primary HSV childhood infections beyond the neonatal period are asymptomatic. Gingivostomatitis, which is the most common clinical manifestation of HSV during childhood, is caused by HSV type 1 (HSV-1) and is characterized by fever, irritability, tender submandibular adenopathy, and an ulcerative enanthem involving the gingiva and mucous membranes of the mouth, often with perioral vesicular lesions.

Genital herpes is characterized by vesicular or ulcerative lesions of the male or female genitalia, perineum, or both. Until recently, genital herpes most often was caused by HSV type 2 (HSV-2), but HSV-1 now accounts for more than half of all cases in the United States. Most cases of primary genital herpes infection in males and females are asymptomatic, so they are not recognized by the infected person or diagnosed by a health care professional.

Eczema herpeticum can develop in patients with atopic dermatitis who are infected with HSV, and can be difficult to distinguish from poorly controlled atopic dermatitis. Examination may reveal skin with punched-out erosions, hemorrhagic crusts, and/or vesicular lesions. Pustular lesions attributable to bacterial superinfection also may occur.

In immunocompromised patients, severe local lesions and, less commonly, disseminated HSV infection with generalized vesicular skin lesions and visceral involvement can occur.

After primary infection, HSV persists for life in a latent form. Reactivation of latent virus most commonly is asymptomatic. When symptomatic, recurrent HSV-1 herpes labialis manifests as single or grouped vesicles in the perioral region, usually on the vermilion border of the lips (typically called "cold sores" or "fever blisters"). Symptomatic recurrent genital herpes manifests as vesicular lesions on the penis, scrotum, vulva, cervix, buttocks, perianal areas, thighs, or back. Among immunocompromised patients, genital HSV-2 recurrences are more frequent and of longer duration. Recurrences may be heralded by a prodrome of burning or itching at the site of an incipient recurrence, identification of which can be useful in instituting early antiviral therapy.

Conjunctivitis and keratitis can result from primary or recurrent HSV infection. Herpetic whitlow consists of single or multiple vesicular lesions on the distal parts of fingers. Wrestlers can develop herpes gladiatorum if they become infected with HSV-1. HSV infection can be a precipitating factor in erythema multiforme, and recurrent erythema multiforme often is caused by symptomatic or asymptomatic HSV recurrences.

HSV encephalitis (HSE) occurs in children beyond the neonatal period, in adolescents, and in adults, and can result from primary or recurrent HSV-1 infection. One fifth of HSE cases occur in the pediatric age group. Symptoms and signs usually include fever, alterations in the state of consciousness, personality changes, seizures, and focal neurologic findings. Encephalitis commonly has an acute onset with a fulminant course, leading to coma and death in untreated patients. Patients who are comatose or semicomatose at initiation of therapy have a poorer outcome. HSE usually involves the temporal lobe, and magnetic resonance imaging is the most sensitive imaging modality to detect this. CSF pleocytosis with a predominance of lymphocytes is typical. Historically, erythrocytes in the CSF were considered suggestive of HSE, but with earlier diagnosis (prior to full manifestations of a hemorrhagic encephalitis), this finding is rare today.

HSV infection also can manifest as mild, self-limited aseptic meningitis, usually associated with genital HSV-2 infection. Unusual CNS manifestations of HSV include Bell's palsy, atypical pain syndromes, trigeminal neuralgia, ascending myelitis, transverse myelitis, postinfectious encephalomyelitis, and recurrent (Mollaret) meningitis.

ETIOLOGY: HSVs are large, enveloped, double-stranded DNA viruses. They are members of the family *Herpesviridae* and, along with varicella-zoster virus (human herpesvirus 3), are the subfamily *Alphaherpesviridae*. Two distinct HSV types exist: HSV-1 and HSV-2. Infections with HSV-1 traditionally involve the face and skin above the waist; however, an increasing number of genital herpes cases are attributable to HSV-1. Infections with HSV-2 usually involve the genitalia and skin below the waist in sexually active adolescents and adults. Both HSV-1 and HSV-2 cause herpetic disease in neonates. HSV-1 and HSV-2 establish latency following primary infection, with periodic reactivation to cause recurrent symptomatic disease or asymptomatic viral shedding. Genital HSV-2 infection is more likely to recur than is genital HSV-1 infection.

EPIDEMIOLOGY: HSV infections are ubiquitous and can be transmitted from people who are symptomatic or asymptomatic with primary or recurrent infections.

Neonatal. The incidence of neonatal HSV infection in the United States is estimated to range from 1 in 2000 to 1 in 3000 live births. HSV is transmitted to a neonate most often during birth through an infected maternal genital tract but can be caused by an ascending infection through ruptured or apparently intact amniotic membranes. Other less common sources of neonatal infection include postnatal transmission from a parent, sibling, or other caregiver, most often from a nongenital infection (eg, mouth or hands), and intrauterine infection causing congenital malformations.

The risk of transmission to a neonate born to a mother who acquires primary genital HSV infection near the time of delivery is estimated to be 25% to 60%. In contrast, the risk to a neonate born to a mother shedding HSV as a result of reactivation of infection acquired during the first half of pregnancy or earlier is less than 2%. Distinguishing between primary and recurrent HSV infections in women by history or physical examination alone may be impossible, because primary and recurrent genital infections may be asymptomatic or associated with nonspecific findings (eg, vaginal discharge, genital pain, or shallow ulcers). History of maternal genital HSV infection is not helpful in diagnosing neonatal HSV disease, because more than three quarters of infants who contract HSV infection are born to women with no history or clinical findings suggestive of genital HSV infection during or preceding pregnancy and who, therefore, are unaware of their infection.

Children Beyond the Neonatal Period and Adolescents. Patients with primary gingivostomatitis or genital herpes usually shed virus for at least 1 week and occasionally for several weeks. Patients with symptomatic recurrences shed virus for a shorter period, typically 3 to 4 days. Intermittent asymptomatic reactivation of oral and genital herpes is common and likely occurs throughout the remainder of a person's life. The greatest concentration of virus is shed during symptomatic primary infections and the lowest during asymptomatic reactivation.

Inoculation of abraded skin occurs from direct contact with HSV shed from oral, genital, or other skin sites. This contact can result in herpes gladiatorum among wrestlers, herpes rugbiorum among rugby players, or herpetic whitlow of the fingers in any exposed person.

The **incubation period** for HSV infection occurring beyond the neonatal period ranges from 2 days to 2 weeks.

DIAGNOSTIC TESTS: HSV grows readily in traditional cell culture. Special transport media are available that allow transport to local or regional laboratories for culture. Cytopathogenic effects typical of HSV infection usually are observed 1 to 3 days after inoculation. Methods of culture confirmation include fluorescent antibody staining, enzyme immunoassays (EIAs), and monolayer culture with typing. Cultures that remain negative by day 5 likely will remain negative. A spin amplification culture method involving centrifugation of the specimen onto glass coverslips in small vials (shell vial technique) followed by fluorescent antibody staining of the coverslips and fluorescent microscopy may be used to reduce time to detection to 24 to 48 hours. An alternative, commercially available rapid culture technique known as ELVIS (enzyme-linked, virus-inducible system) uses genetically engineered cells to allow for HSV gene expression and detection of infected cells by light microscopy. Sensitivity of culture is highly dependent on proper specimen collection, quality of reagents, and expertise of testing personnel, in addition to the stage of lesion development, with crusted lesions being less likely to be culture positive.

Polymerase chain reaction (PCR) assay usually can detect HSV DNA in CSF from neonates with CNS infection (neonatal HSV CNS disease) and from older children and adults with HSE and is the diagnostic method of choice for CNS HSV involvement. Most of these assays were developed by individual laboratories, and thus, performance varies depending on the individual test. PCR assay of CSF can yield negative results in cases of HSE, especially early in the disease course. In difficult cases in which repeated CSF PCR assay results are negative, histologic examination and viral culture of a brain tissue biopsy specimen is the most definitive method of confirming the diagnosis of HSE. There currently are 2 PCR assays cleared by the US Food and Drug Administration (FDA) for the detection of HSV in CSF; the first is a singleplex assay, and the second is a multiplex assay that is capable of detection HSV and a number of other bacterial and viral agents of meningitis and encephalitis in CSF. There are limited clinical data on the efficacy of these FDA-cleared assays, and results should be interpreted cautiously. Detection of intrathecal antibody against HSV also can assist in the diagnosis. Viral cultures of CSF from a patient with HSE usually are negative.

For diagnosis of neonatal HSV infection, all of the following specimens should be obtained for each patient: (1) swab specimens from the mouth, nasopharynx, conjunctivae, and anus ("surface specimens") for HSV culture (if available) or PCR assay; (2) specimens of skin vesicles for HSV culture (if available) or PCR assay; (3) CSF sample for HSV PCR assay; (4) whole blood sample for HSV PCR assay; and (5) whole blood sample for measuring alanine transaminase (ALT). The performance characteristics of PCR assay on skin and mucosal specimens from neonates has not been studied. Positive cultures obtained from any of the surface sites more than 12 to 24 hours after birth indicate viral replication and are, therefore, suggestive of infant infection rather than merely contamination after intrapartum exposure. As with any PCR assay, false-negative and false-positive results can occur. Any of the 3 manifestations of neonatal HSV disease (disseminated, CNS, SEM) can have associated viremia, so a positive whole blood PCR assay result does not define an infant as having disseminated HSV and, therefore, should not be used to determine extent of disease and duration of treatment; likewise, no data exist to support use of serial blood PCR assays to monitor response to therapy. Rapid diagnostic techniques are available, such as direct fluorescent antibody staining of vesicle scrapings or EIA detection of HSV antigens. These techniques are as specific but slightly less sensitive than culture. Radiographs and clinical manifestations can suggest HSV pneumonitis, and elevated transaminase values can suggest HSV hepatitis. Histologic examination of lesions for presence of multinucleated giant cells and eosinophilic intranuclear inclusions typical of HSV (eg, with Tzanck test) should not be performed because of low sensitivity.

HSV PCR assay and cell culture are the preferred tests for detecting HSV in genital lesions. The sensitivity of viral culture is low, especially for recurrent lesions, and declines rapidly as lesions begin to heal. PCR assays for HSV DNA are more sensitive and increasingly are used in many settings. There are currently several FDA-cleared PCR assays for the detection of HSV in skin, oral, and genital lesions in adults. Failure to detect HSV in genital lesions by culture or PCR assay does not rule out HSV infection, because viral shedding is intermittent.

Both type-specific and type-common antibodies to HSV develop during the first several weeks after infection and persist indefinitely. Approximately 20% of HSV-2 first episode patients seroconvert by 10 days, and the median time to seroconversion is 21 days with a type-specific enzyme-linked immunosorbent assay (ELISA); more than 95% of people seroconvert by 12 weeks following infection. Although type-specific HSV-2 antibody usually indicates previous anogenital infection, the presence of HSV-1 antibody does not distinguish anogenital from orolabial infection reliably, because a substantial proportion of initial genital infections and virtually all initial orolabial infections are caused by HSV-1. Type-specific serologic tests can be useful in confirming a clinical diagnosis of genital herpes caused by HSV-2. Additionally, these serologic tests can be used to evaluate individuals with recurrent or atypical genital tract symptoms with negative HSV culture or PCR evaluations and to manage sexual partners of people with genital herpes. Serologic testing is not useful in neonates.

Both laboratory-based assays and point-of-care tests that provide results for HSV-2 antibodies from capillary blood or serum are available. The sensitivities of these glycoprotein G type-specific tests for the detection of HSV-2 antibody vary from 80% to 98%. The most commonly used test, HerpeSelect 2 ELISA IgG (Focus Diagnostics, Cypress, CA), might be falsely positive at low index values (1.1–3.5). Such low values should be confirmed with another test, such as Biokit (Werfen, Barcelona, Spain) or the Western blot (University of Washington); the HerpeSelect 2 Immunoblot IgG should not be used for confirmation, because it uses the same antigen as the HerpeSelect 2 ELISA IgG. Repeat testing is indicated if recent acquisition of genital herpes is suspected. The HerpeSelect 1 ELISA IgG kit is insensitive. IgM testing for HSV-1 or HSV-2 is not useful, because IgM tests are not type-specific and might be positive during recurrent genital or oral episodes of herpes.

TREATMENT: For recommended antiviral dosages and duration of therapy with systemically administered acyclovir, valacyclovir, and famciclovir for different HSV infections, see Non-HIV Antiviral Drugs (p 966). Valacyclovir is an L-valyl ester of acyclovir that is metabolized to acyclovir after oral administration, resulting in higher serum concentrations than those achieved with oral acyclovir and similar serum concentrations as those achieved with intravenous administration of acyclovir. Famciclovir is converted rapidly to penciclovir after oral administration. Table 3.28 shows drugs for treatment of HSV by type of infection. Valacyclovir has been approved by the FDA for the treatment of cold sores (herpes labialis) in pediatric patients 12 years or older. In pediatric patients for whom a solid dosage form of valacyclovir is not appropriate, instructions for preparing a compounded liquid formulation of valacyclovir with a 28-day shelf-life are provided in the drug's package insert.

Neonatal. Parenteral acyclovir is the treatment for neonatal HSV infections. The dosage of acyclovir is 60 mg/kg per day in 3 divided doses (20 mg/kg/dose), administered intravenously for 14 days in SEM disease and for a minimum of 21 days in CNS disease or disseminated disease. All infants with neonatal HSV disease, regardless of disease classification, should have an ophthalmologic examination and neuroimaging to establish baseline brain anatomy; magnetic resonance imaging is the most sensitive imaging modality but may require sedation, so computed tomography or ultrasonography of the head are acceptable alternatives. All infants with CNS involvement should have a repeat lumbar puncture performed near the end of therapy to document that the CSF is negative for HSV DNA on PCR assay; in the unlikely event that the PCR result remains positive near the end of a 21-day treatment course, intravenous acyclovir should be administered for another week, with repeat CSF PCR assay performed near the end of the extended treatment period and another week of parenteral therapy if it remains positive. Parenteral antiviral therapy should not be stopped until the CSF PCR result for HSV DNA is negative. Consultation with a pediatric infectious diseases specialist is warranted in these cases.

Infants surviving neonatal HSV infections of any classification (disseminated, CNS, or SEM) should receive oral acyclovir suppression at 300 mg/m^2/dose, administered 3 times daily for 6 months after the completion of parenteral therapy for acute disease; the dose should be adjusted monthly to account for growth. Absolute neutrophil counts should be

Table 3.28. Recommended Therapy for Herpes Simplex Virus Infections[a]

Infection	Drug[b]
Neonatal	Parenteral acyclovir
Keratoconjunctivitis	Trifluridine[c] OR Topical ganciclovir
Genital	Acyclovir OR Famciclovir OR Valacyclovir
Mucocutaneous (immunocompromised or primary gingivostomatitis)	Acyclovir OR Famciclovir OR Valacyclovir
Acyclovir-resistant (severe infections, immunocompromised)	Parenteral foscarnet
Encephalitis	Parenteral acyclovir

[a] See text and Table 4.10 (p 966) for details.
[b] Famciclovir and valacyclovir are approved by the US Food and Drug Administration for treatment of adults.
[c] Treatment of herpes simplex virus ocular infection should involve an ophthalmologist.

assessed at 2 and 4 weeks after initiating suppressive acyclovir therapy and then monthly during the treatment period. Longer durations or higher doses of antiviral suppression do not further improve neurodevelopmental outcomes. Valacyclovir has not been studied for longer than 5 days in young infants, so it should not be used routinely for antiviral suppression in this age group.

Infants with ocular involvement attributable to HSV infection should receive a topical ophthalmic drug (1% trifluridine or 0.15% ganciclovir) as well as parenteral antiviral therapy. The older topical antiviral agents vidarabine and iododeoxyuridine no longer are available in the United States. An ophthalmologist should be involved in the management and treatment of acute neonatal ocular HSV disease.

Genital Infection.

Primary. Oral acyclovir therapy (400 mg, orally, 3 times/day for 7–10 days, or 200 mg, orally, 5 times/day for 7–10 days) shortens the duration of illness and viral shedding. Valacyclovir and famciclovir do not seem to be more effective than acyclovir but offer the advantage of less frequent dosing (famciclovir, 250 mg, orally, 3 times/day for 7–10 days; valacyclovir, 1 g, orally, 2 times/day for 7–10 days). Intravenous acyclovir is indicated for patients with a severe or complicated primary infection that requires hospitalization (5–10 mg/kg, intravenously, every 8 hours for 2–7 days or until clinical improvement is observed, followed by oral antiviral therapy to complete the treatment course). Treatment of primary herpetic lesions does not affect the subsequent frequency or severity of recurrences.

Recurrent. Antiviral therapy for recurrent genital herpes can be administered either episodically to ameliorate or shorten the duration of lesions or continuously as suppressive therapy to decrease the frequency of recurrences. Many patients benefit from antiviral therapy, and treatment options should be discussed with patients with recurrent disease. Suppressive therapy has the additional advantage of decreasing the risk of genital HSV-2 transmission to susceptible partners. Acyclovir and valacyclovir have been approved for suppression of genital herpes in immunocompetent adults. Either may be administered orally to pregnant women with first-episode genital herpes or severe recurrent herpes, and acyclovir should be administered intravenously to pregnant women with severe HSV infection.

Mucocutaneous.

Immunocompromised Hosts. Intravenous acyclovir is effective for treatment of mucocutaneous HSV infections. Acyclovir-resistant strains of HSV have been isolated from immunocompromised people receiving prolonged treatment with acyclovir. Foscarnet is the drug of choice for acyclovir-resistant HSV isolates.

Immunocompetent Hosts. Limited data are available on effects of acyclovir on the course of primary or recurrent nongenital mucocutaneous HSV infections in immunocompetent hosts. Therapeutic benefit has been noted in a limited number of children with primary gingivostomatitis treated with oral acyclovir. A small therapeutic benefit of oral acyclovir therapy has been demonstrated among adults with recurrent herpes labialis. When used as treatment for HSV orolabial disease, a dose of 80 mg/kg per day, in 4 divided doses, for 5 to 7 days, should be used, with a maximum of 3200 mg/day. Famciclovir or valacyclovir also can be considered. Topical acyclovir is ineffective. A topical formulation of penciclovir (Denavir [Prestium Pharma, Newtown, PA]) and a topical alcohol, docosanol (Abreva [GlaxoSmithKline, Research Triangle Park, NC]), have only limited activity for therapy of herpes labialis and are not recommended.

In a controlled study of a small number of adults with recurrent herpes labialis (6 or more episodes per year), suppressive acyclovir at a dosage of 400 mg, twice a day, was effective for decreasing the frequency of recurrent episodes. Although no studies of suppressive therapy have been performed in children, those with frequent recurrences may benefit from daily oral acyclovir therapy, with reevaluation being performed after 6 months to 1 year of continuous therapy; a dose of 30 mg/kg per day, in 3 divided doses, with a maximum 1000 mg/day, is reasonable to begin as suppressive therapy in children.

Other HSV Infections.

Central Nervous System. Patients with HSE should be treated for 21 days with intravenous acyclovir. For people with Bell palsy, the combination of acyclovir and prednisone may be considered.

Ocular. Treatment of eye lesions should be undertaken in consultation with an ophthalmologist. Several topical drugs, such as 1% trifluridine and 0.15% ganciclovir, have proven efficacy for superficial keratitis. The older topical antivirals vidarabine and iododeoxyuridine no longer are available in the United States. Topical corticosteroids administered without concomitant antiviral therapy are contraindicated in suspected HSV conjunctivitis; however, ophthalmologists may choose to use corticosteroids in conjunction with antiviral drugs to treat locally invasive infections. For children with recurrent ocular lesions, oral suppressive therapy with acyclovir may be of benefit and may be indicated for months or even years.

ISOLATION OF THE HOSPITALIZED PATIENT: In addition to standard precautions, the following recommendations should be followed.

Neonates With HSV Infection. Neonates with HSV infection should be hospitalized and managed with contact precautions if mucocutaneous lesions are present.

Neonates Exposed to HSV During Delivery. Infants born to women with active genital HSV lesions should be managed with contact precautions during the incubation period. Some experts believe that contact precautions are unnecessary if exposed infants were born by cesarean delivery, provided membranes were ruptured for less than 4 hours. The risk of HSV infection in infants born to mothers with a history of recurrent genital herpes who have no genital lesions at delivery is low, so special precautions are not necessary. Specific management options for neonates born to women with active genital HSV lesions are detailed in "Prevention of Neonatal Infection."

Women in Labor and Postpartum Women With HSV Infection. Women with active HSV lesions should be managed with contact precautions during labor, delivery, and the postpartum period. They should be instructed about the importance of careful hand hygiene before and after caring for their infants. The mother may wear a clean covering gown to help avoid contact of the infant with lesions or infectious secretions. A mother with herpes labialis or stomatitis should wear a disposable surgical mask when touching her newborn infant until the lesions have crusted. She should not kiss or nuzzle her newborn until lesions have cleared. Herpetic lesions on other skin sites should be covered.

Breastfeeding is acceptable if no lesions are present on the breasts and if active lesions elsewhere on the mother are covered (see Human Milk, p 113).

Children With Mucocutaneous HSV Infection. Contact precautions are recommended for patients with severe mucocutaneous HSV infection. Patients with localized recurrent lesions should be managed with standard precautions.

Patients With HSV Infection of the CNS. Standard precautions are recommended for patients with infection limited to the CNS.

CONTROL MEASURES:
Prevention of Neonatal Infection.

During Pregnancy. The absence of previous signs and symptoms of genital herpes infections has poor sensitivity in determining the risk of genital HSV infection in a pregnant woman. The American College of Obstetricians and Gynecologists recommends that women with active recurrent genital herpes be offered suppressive antiviral therapy at or beyond 36 weeks of gestation. However, cases of neonatal HSV disease have occurred among infants born to women who received such antiviral prophylaxis.

Care of Newborn Infants Whose Mothers Have Active Genital Lesions at Delivery. The risk of transmitting HSV to the newborn infant during delivery is influenced directly by the mother's classification of HSV infection (Table 3.29); women with primary genital HSV infections who are shedding HSV at delivery are 10 to 30 times more likely to transmit the virus to their newborn infants, compared with women with a recurrent infection. With the commercial availability of serologic tests that can reliably distinguish type-specific HSV antibodies, the means to further refine management of asymptomatic neonates delivered to women with active genital HSV lesions now is possible. The American Academy of Pediatrics developed algorithms (Fig 3.5 and 3.6) addressing evaluation and management of asymptomatic neonates following vaginal or cesarean delivery to women with active genital HSV lesions.[1] The algorithms are intended to outline one approach to the management of these neonates and may not be feasible in settings with limited access to PCR assays for HSV DNA or to the newer type-specific serologic tests. If, at any point during the evaluation outlined in the evaluation algorithm (Fig 3.5), an infant develops symptoms that could indicate neonatal HSV disease (eg, fever, hypothermia, lethargy, irritability, vesicular rash, seizures, etc), a full diagnostic evaluation should be undertaken and intravenous acyclovir therapy should be initiated. In applying this algorithm, obstetric and pediatric providers will need to work closely with their diagnostic laboratories to ensure that serologic and virologic testing is available and turnaround times are acceptable. In situations in which this is not possible, the approach detailed in the algorithm will have limited, and perhaps no, applicability.

Care of Newborn Infants Whose Mothers Have a History of Genital Herpes But No Active Genital Lesions at Delivery. An infant whose mother has known, recurrent genital infection but no genital lesions at delivery should be observed for signs of infection (eg, vesicular lesions of the skin, respiratory distress, seizures, or signs of sepsis) but should not have specimens for surface cultures for HSV obtained at 12 to 24 hours of life and should not receive empiric parenteral acyclovir. Education of parents and caregivers about the signs and symptoms of neonatal HSV infection during the first 6 weeks of life is prudent.

Infected Health Care Professionals.
Transmission of HSV in hospital nurseries from infected health care professionals to newborn infants rarely has been documented. The risk of transmission to infants by health care professionals who have herpes labialis or who are asymptomatic oral shedders of virus is low. Compromising patient care by excluding health care professionals with cold sores who are essential for the operation of the hospital nursery must be weighed against the potential risk of newborn infants becoming infected.

---

[1]Kimberlin DW, Baley J; American Academy of Pediatrics, Committee on Infectious Diseases. Guidance on management of asymptomatic neonates born to women with active genital herpes lesions. *Pediatrics.* 2013;131(2):e635–e646

Table 3.29. Maternal Infection Classification by Genital HSV Viral Type and Maternal Serologic Test Results[a]

Classification of Maternal Infection	PCR/Culture From Genital Lesion	Maternal HSV-1 and HSV-2 IgG Antibody Status
Documented first-episode primary infection	Positive, either virus	Both negative
Documented first-episode nonprimary infection	Positive for HSV-1	Positive for HSV-2 **AND** negative for HSV-1
	Positive for HSV-2	Positive for HSV-1 **AND** negative for HSV-2
Assumed first-episode (primary or nonprimary) infection	Positive for HSV-1 **OR** HSV-2	Not available
	Negative **OR** not available[b]	Negative for HSV-1 and/or HSV-2, **OR** not available
Recurrent infection	Positive for HSV-1	Positive for HSV-1
	Positive for HSV-2	Positive for HSV-2

HSV indicates herpes simplex virus; PCR, polymerase chain reaction (assay); IgG, immunoglobulin G.
[a]To be used for women without a clinical history of genital herpes.
[b]When a genital lesion is strongly suspicious for HSV, clinical judgment should supersede the virologic test results for the conservative purposes of this neonatal management algorithm. Conversely, if, in retrospect, the genital lesion was not likely to be caused by HSV and the PCR assay result/culture is negative, departure from the evaluation and management in this conservative algorithm may be warranted.

Health care professionals with cold sores who have contact with infants should cover and not touch their lesions and should comply with hand hygiene policies. Transmission of HSV infection from health care professionals with genital lesions is not likely as long as they comply with hand hygiene policies. Health care professionals with an active herpetic whitlow should not have responsibility for direct care of neonates or immunocompromised patients and should wear gloves and use hand hygiene during direct care of other patients.

Infected Household, Family, and Other Close Contacts of Newborn Infants. Household members with herpetic skin or mouth lesions (eg, stomatitis, herpes labialis, or herpetic whitlow) should be counseled about the risk of transmission and should avoid contact of their lesions with newborn infants by taking the same measures as recommended for infected health care professionals, as well as avoiding kissing and nuzzling the infant while they have active lip/mouth lesions or touching the infant while they have a herpetic whitlow. Cases of HSV transmission to the genitalia of male neonates have been reported following ritual circumcision (metzitzah b'peh) involving mouth suction of the site by the mohel performing the circumcision.

Care of People With Extensive Dermatitis. Patients with dermatitis are at risk of developing eczema herpeticum. If these patients are hospitalized, special care should be taken to avoid their exposure to HSV. These patients should not be kissed by people with cold sores or touched by people with herpetic whitlow.

FIG 3.5. ALGORITHM FOR THE <u>EVALUATION</u> OF ASYMPTOMATIC NEONATES FOLLOWING VAGINAL OR CESAREAN DELIVERY TO WOMEN WITH ACTIVE GENITAL HERPES LESIONS.

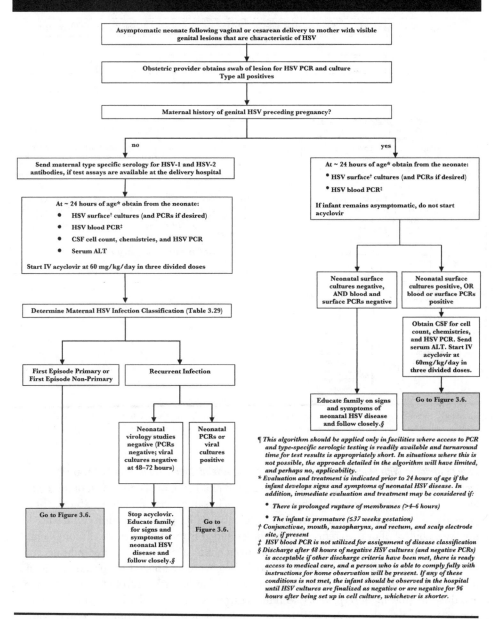

Reproduced from Kimberlin DW, Baley J; American Academy of Pediatrics, Committee on Infectious Diseases. Guidance on management of asymptomatic neonates born to women with active genital herpes lesions. *Pediatrics.* 2013;131(2):e635-e646

FIG 3.6. ALGORITHM FOR THE <u>TREATMENT</u> OF ASYMPTOMATIC NEONATES FOLLOWING VAGINAL OR CESAREAN DELIVERY TO WOMEN WITH ACTIVE GENITAL HERPES LESIONS.

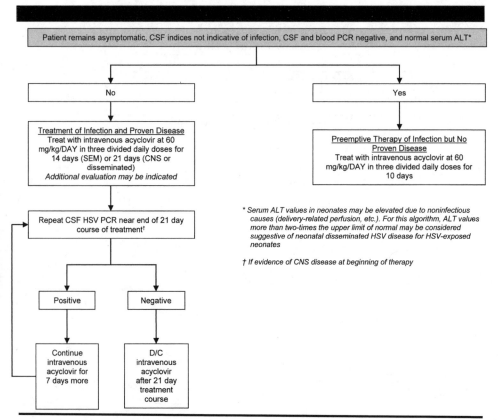

Reproduced from Kimberlin DW, Baley J; American Academy of Pediatrics, Committee on Infectious Diseases. Guidance on management of asymptomatic neonates born to women with active genital herpes lesions. *Pediatrics.* 2013;131(2):e635-e646

Care of Children With Mucocutaneous Infections Who Attend Child Care or School. Oral HSV infections are common among children who attend child care or school. Most of these infections are asymptomatic, with shedding of virus in saliva occurring in the absence of clinical disease. Only children with HSV gingivostomatitis (ie, primary infection) who do not have control of oral secretions should be excluded from child care. Exclusion of children with cold sores (ie, recurrent infection) from child care or school is not indicated. HSV lesions on other parts of the body should be covered with clothing or a bandage, if practical, for children attending school or day care. Additional control measures include avoiding the sharing of respiratory secretions through contact with objects and washing and sanitizing mouthed toys, bottle nipples, and utensils that have come in contact with saliva.

HSV Infections Among Wrestlers and Rugby Players.[1] HSV-1 has been identified as a cause of outbreak of skin infections among wrestlers (herpes gladiatorum) and rugby players (herpes rugbiorum) on numerous occasions, affecting up to 2.6% of high school and 7.6% of college wrestlers in the United States. During outbreaks, up to 34% of all high school wrestlers have been documented to be infected. The primary risk factor is direct skin-to-skin exposure to opponents with cutaneous lesions. Most outbreaks (96%) occur on the ventral surface of the body, with up to three quarters of the cases occurring on areas in direct contact when wrestlers are engaged in the lock-up position (head, face, and neck). Other body areas frequently involved are the extremities (42%) and trunk (28%). HSV conjunctivitis (5%) and blepharitis have also been reported. Between 25% and 40% of patients with herpes gladiatorum and herpes rugbiorum will develop constitutional symptoms including fever, chills, sore throat, and headaches.

Three to 8 days of exclusion from competition of infected athletes with primary outbreaks of herpes gladiatorum and herpes rugbiorum will contain more than 90% of outbreaks. Valacyclovir (500 mg, once daily for 7 days), when given within 24 hours of symptoms onset, has been shown to shorten the duration of time until HSV PCR clearance from lesions of adolescent and adult wrestlers with recurrent herpes gladiatorum. Wrestlers receiving valacyclovir should be advised about the importance of good hydration to minimize the likelihood of nephrotoxicity. Competitors often do not recognize or may deny possible infection. As a result, efforts to reduce transmission should include (1) examination of wrestlers and rugby players for vesicular or ulcerative lesions on exposed areas of their bodies and around their mouths or eyes before practice or competition by a person familiar with the appearance of mucocutaneous infections (including HSV, herpes zoster, and impetigo); (2) excluding athletes with these lesions from competition until all lesions are fully crusted or production of a physician's written statement indicating that their condition is noninfectious; and (3) cleaning of wrestling mats with a freshly prepared solution of household bleach (one quarter cup of bleach in 1 gallon of water), applied for a minimum contact time of 15 seconds at least daily, and preferably, between matches. Athletes with a history of *recurrent* herpes gladiatorum, herpes rugbiorum, or herpes labialis should be considered for suppressive antiviral therapy, again with cautionary guidance about the importance of maintaining good hydration to avoid the likelihood of nephrotoxicity.

Histoplasmosis

CLINICAL MANIFESTATIONS: *Histoplasma capsulatum* causes symptoms in fewer than 5% of infected people. Clinical manifestations are classified according to site (pulmonary or disseminated), duration (acute, subacute, or chronic), and pattern (primary or reactivation) of infection. Most symptomatic patients have acute pulmonary histoplasmosis, a brief, self-limited illness characterized by fever, chills, nonproductive cough, and malaise. Radiographic findings may consist of hilar or mediastinal adenopathy, or diffuse interstitial or reticulonodular pulmonary infiltrates. Most patients recover without treatment 2 to 3 weeks after onset of symptoms. Exposure to a large inoculum of conidia can cause severe pulmonary infection associated with high fevers, hypoxemia, diffuse reticulonodular

[1]Davies HD, Jackson MA; American Academy of Pediatrics, Committee on Infectious Diseases. Infectious Diseases Associated With Organized Sports and Outbreak Control. *Pediatrics*. 2017;140(4):e20172477

infiltrates, and acute respiratory distress syndrome (ARDS). Mediastinal involvement, a rare complication of pulmonary histoplasmosis, includes mediastinal lymphadenitis, which can cause airway encroachment in young children. Inflammatory syndromes (pericarditis and rheumatologic syndromes) can develop; erythema nodosum can occur in adolescents and adults. Primary cutaneous infections after trauma are rare. Chronic cavitary pulmonary histoplasmosis is extremely rare in children.

Progressive disseminated histoplasmosis (PDH) may occur in otherwise healthy infants and children younger than 2 years, or in older children with primary or acquired cellular immune dysfunction. It can be a rapidly progressive illness following acute infection, or can be a more chronic, slowly progressive disease. Early manifestations of PDH in children include prolonged fever, failure to thrive, and hepatosplenomegaly; if untreated, malnutrition, diffuse adenopathy, pneumonitis, mucosal ulceration, pancytopenia, disseminated intravascular coagulopathy, and gastrointestinal tract bleeding can ensue. PDH in adults occurs most often in people with underlying immune deficiency (eg, human immunodeficiency virus/acquired immunodeficiency syndrome, solid organ transplant, hematologic malignancy, and biologic response modifiers including tumor necrosis factor antagonists). Central nervous system involvement occurs in 5% to 25% of patients with chronic progressive disease. Chronic PDH generally occurs in adults with immune suppression and is characterized by prolonged fever, night sweats, weight loss, and fatigue; signs include hepatosplenomegaly, mucosal ulcerations, adrenal insufficiency, and pancytopenia. Clinicians should be alert to the risk of disseminated endemic mycoses in patients receiving tumor necrosis factor-alpha antagonists and disease-modifying antirheumatic drugs.

ETIOLOGY: *Histoplasma* strains, which may be classified into at least 7 distinct clades, are thermally dimorphic, endemic fungi that grow in the environment as a spore-bearing mold but convert to the yeast phase at 37°C.

EPIDEMIOLOGY: *H capsulatum* is encountered in most parts of the world (including Africa, the Americas, Asia, and Europe) and is highly endemic in the central and eastern United States, particularly the Mississippi, Ohio, and Missouri River valleys. *H capsulatum* var *duboisii* is found only in central and western Africa. Infection is acquired following inhalation of conidia that are aerosolized by disturbance of soil, especially when contaminated with bat guano or bird (especially chicken) droppings. The inoculum size, strain virulence, and immune status of the host affect the severity of the ensuing illness. Infections occur sporadically or rarely in point-source epidemics after exposure to activities that disturb contaminated sites. In regions with endemic disease, recreational and occupational activities, such as playing in hollow trees, caving, mud runs, construction, excavation, demolition, farming, and cleaning of contaminated buildings, have been associated with outbreaks. Person-to-person transmission does not occur except via transplantation of infected organs. Prior infection confers partial immunity; reinfection can occur but requires a larger inoculum.

The **incubation period** is variable but usually is 1 to 3 weeks.

DIAGNOSTIC TESTS: Detection of *H capsulatum* polysaccharide antigen in serum, urine, bronchoalveolar lavage fluid, or cerebrospinal fluid using a quantitative enzyme immunoassay is the preferred method of testing. Urine antigen detection is substantially more sensitive than serum antigen detection. Antigen detection is most sensitive for severe, acute pulmonary infections and for progressive disseminated infections. Results often are transiently positive early in the course of acute, self-limited pulmonary infections. A negative test result does not exclude infection. If the result initially is positive, the antigen test also is useful for monitoring treatment response and, thereafter, promptly identifying relapse or reinfection. Cross-reactions may occur in patients with blastomycosis, coccidioidomycosis, paracoccidioidomycosis, sporotrichosis, and penicilliosis; clinical and epidemiologic distinctions aid in differentiating these entities.

Serologic testing is available and is most useful in patients with subacute or chronic pulmonary disease. Complement fixation, immunodiffusion, and latex agglutination tests are available. The principal antigens used in these serologic tests are a soluble filtrate of mycelial grown broth culture known as histoplasmin and a killed yeast phase suspension of intact cells. A fourfold increase in either yeast-phase or mycelial-phase complement fixation titers or a single titer of ≥1:32 in either test is strong presumptive evidence of active or recent infection in patients exposed to or residing within regions of endemicity. Cross-reacting antibodies can result most commonly from *Blastomyces dermatitidis* and *Coccidioides* species but also rarely with *Aspergillus* and *Cryptococcus* infections. The immunodiffusion test is a qualitative method that is more specific, but slightly less sensitive, than the complement fixation test. It detects the H and M glycoproteins of *H capsulatum* found in histoplasmin. The M band develops with acute infection, generally by 6 weeks after infection, is often present in chronic forms of histoplasmosis, and persists for months to years after the infection has resolved. The H band is much less common, is rarely, if ever, found without an M band, and is indicative of chronic or severe acute forms of histoplasmosis. The immunodiffusion assay is approximately 80% sensitive but is more specific than the complement fixation assay. It commonly is used in conjunction with the complement fixation test. A latex agglutination test is commercially available for the detection of immunoglobulin (Ig) M antibodies to histoplasmin. It is used primarily for the diagnosis of acute histoplasmosis.

Culture is the definitive method of diagnosis. *H capsulatum* organisms from bone marrow, blood, sputum, and tissue specimens grow in the mycelia (mold) phase on standard mycologic media including Sabouraud dextrose or potato dextrose agar incubated at 25°C to 30°C in 1 to 6 weeks. The yeast phase of the organism can be recovered on primary culture using enriched media such as brain-heart infusion agar with blood (BHIB) incubated at 35°C to 37°C. Mycelial-phase organisms in culture can be confirmed as *H capsulatum* by conversion to yeast-phase organisms by repeated passage on BHIB at 35°C to 37°C. The lysis-centrifugation method is preferred for blood cultures. A DNA probe for *H capsulatum* permits rapid identification of mycelial-phase cultured isolates. Care should be taken in working with the organism in the laboratory, because mold-phase growth may release large numbers of infectious microconidia into the air.

Demonstration of typical intracellular yeast forms by examination with Wright or Giemsa stains of blood, bone marrow, or bronchoalveolar lavage specimens or with Gomori methenamine silver or other stains of tissue strongly supports the diagnosis of histoplasmosis when clinical, epidemiologic, and other laboratory studies are compatible.

TREATMENT: Immunocompetent children with uncomplicated or mild-to-moderate acute pulmonary histoplasmosis may not require antifungal therapy, because infection usually is self-limited. However, if the patient does not improve within 4 weeks, itraconazole should be given for 6 to 12 weeks.

In contrast, treatment is imperative for all forms of disseminated histoplasmosis, which can be either an acute (rapid onset and progression, usually in an immunocompromised patient) or chronic illness (slower evolution, usually in an immunocompetent patient). For severe acute pulmonary or disseminated infections, treatment with a lipid formulation of amphotericin B is recommended (see Table 4.7, p 942). Methylprednisolone during the first 1 to 2 weeks of therapy may be considered if severe respiratory complications develop but should be used only in conjunction with antifungals. After clinical improvement occurs in 1 to 2 weeks, itraconazole is recommended for an additional 12 weeks. Itraconazole is preferred over other mold-active azoles by most experts; when used in adults, itraconazole is more effective, has fewer adverse effects, and is less likely to induce resistance than is fluconazole. Serum trough concentrations of itraconazole should be 1 to 2 µg/mL. Concentrations should be checked after one to 2 weeks of therapy to ensure adequate drug exposure. When measured by high-pressure liquid chromatography, both itraconazole and its bioactive hydroxy-itraconazole metabolite are reported, the sum of which should be considered in assessing drug levels.

All patients with chronic pulmonary histoplasmosis (eg, progressive cavitation of the lungs) should be treated. Mild to moderate cases should be treated with itraconazole for 1 to 2 years. Severe cases should be treated initially with a lipid formulation amphotericin B followed by itraconazole for the same duration.

Mediastinal and inflammatory manifestations of infection generally do not need to be treated with antifungal agents. However, mediastinal adenitis that causes obstruction of a bronchus, the esophagus, or another mediastinal structure may improve with a brief course of corticosteroids. In these instances, itraconazole should be used concurrently and continued for 6 to 12 weeks thereafter. Dense fibrosis of mediastinal structures without an associated granulomatous inflammatory component does not respond to antifungal therapy, and surgical intervention may be necessary for severe cases. Pericarditis and rheumatologic syndromes may respond to treatment with nonsteroidal anti-inflammatory agents (indomethacin).

For treatment of moderately severe to severe progressive disseminated histoplasmosis (PDH) in an infant or child, a lipid formulation of amphotericin B is the drug of choice and usually is given for a minimum of 2 weeks. When the child has demonstrated substantial clinical improvement and a decline in the serum concentration of *Histoplasma* antigen, oral itraconazole is administered for 12 weeks. Prolonged therapy for up to 12 months may be required for patients with severe disease, primary immunodeficiency syndromes, acquired immunodeficiency that cannot be reversed, or patients who experience relapse despite appropriate therapy. For those with mild to moderate PDH, itraconazole for 12 months is recommended for treatment. After completion of treatment for PDH, urine antigen concentrations should be monitored for 6 months. Stable, low, and decreasing concentrations that are unaccompanied by signs of active infection may not necessarily require prolongation or resumption of treatment.

ISOLATION OF THE HOSPITALIZED PATIENT: Standard precautions are recommended.
CONTROL MEASURES: Histoplasmosis is a reportable disease in some states and countries. In outbreaks, investigation for a common source of infection is indicated. Exposure to soil and dust from areas with significant accumulations of bird and bat droppings should be avoided, especially by immunocompromised individuals, including those receiving tumor necrosis factor inhibitors or disease-modifying antirheumatic drugs. If exposure is unavoidable, it should be minimized through use of respiratory protection (eg, N95 respirator), gloves, and disposable clothing. Although N95 is adequate in most circumstances, in environments with extremely high inoculum, full-powered air purifying

respirators (PAPRs) with high efficiency particulate air (HEPA) filters are recommended. Areas suspected of being contaminated with *Histoplasma* species should be remediated. Old or abandoned structures likely to have been contaminated with bird or bat droppings should be saturated with water to reduce the aerosolization of spores during demolition. Guidelines for preventing histoplasmosis have been designed for health and safety professionals, environmental consultants, and people supervising workers involved in activities in which contaminated materials are disturbed. Additional information about the guidelines is available from the National Institute for Occupational Safety and Health (NIOSH; publication No. 2005-109, available from Publications Dissemination, 4676 Columbia Parkway, Cincinnati, OH 45226-1998; telephone 800-356-4674) and the NIOSH Web site (**www.cdc.gov/niosh/docs/2005-109/pdfs/2005-109.pdf**).

Hookworm Infections
(*Ancylostoma duodenale* and *Necator americanus*)

CLINICAL MANIFESTATIONS: Patients with hookworm infection often are asymptomatic; however, chronic hookworm infection is a common cause of moderate and severe hypochromic, microcytic anemia in people living in resource-limited tropical countries, and heavy infection can cause hypoproteinemia with edema. Chronic hookworm infection in children may lead to physical growth delay, deficits in cognition, and developmental delay. After contact with contaminated soil, initial skin penetration of larvae, often involving the feet, can cause a stinging or burning sensation followed by pruritus and a papulovesicular rash ("ground itch") that may persist for 1 to 2 weeks. Pneumonitis associated with migrating larvae (Löffler-like syndrome) is uncommon and usually mild, except in heavy infections. Colicky abdominal pain, nausea, diarrhea, and marked eosinophilia can develop 4 to 6 weeks after exposure. Blood loss secondary to hookworm infection develops 10 to 12 weeks after initial infection, and symptoms related to serious iron-deficiency anemia can develop in long-standing moderate or heavy hookworm infections. Pharyngeal itching, hoarseness, nausea, and vomiting can develop shortly after oral ingestion of infectious *Ancylostoma duodenale* larvae.

ETIOLOGY: *Necator americanus* is the major cause of hookworm infection worldwide, although *A duodenale* also is an important hookworm in some regions. Mixed infections can occur. Other species of hookworm also can infect humans (eg, *Ancylostoma ceylanicum)*. Each of these roundworms (nematodes) has a similar life cycle, with the exception of *A ceylanicum*, a zoonotic parasite. Other animal hookworm species cause cutaneous larva migrans when filariform larvae penetrate the skin and migrate in the upper dermis, causing an intensely pruritic track, although they do not develop further.

EPIDEMIOLOGY: Humans are the only reservoir for *A duodenale* and *N americanus*. Dogs, cats, and hamsters can harbor *A ceylanicum*. Hookworms are prominent in rural, tropical, and subtropical areas where soil contamination with human feces is common. *N americanus* is predominant in the Western hemisphere, sub-Saharan Africa, Southeast Asia, and a number of Pacific islands. *A duodenale* is the predominant species in the Mediterranean region, northern Asia, and selected foci of South America. *A ceylanicum* is found in Asia, Australia, some Pacific islands, South Africa, and Madagascar. Larvae and eggs survive in loose, sandy, moist, shady, well-aerated, warm soil (optimal temperature 23°C–33°C [73°F–91°F]). Hookworm eggs from stool hatch in soil in 1 to 2 days as rhabditiform larvae. These larvae develop into infective filariform larvae in soil within 5 to 7 days and can survive for 3 to 4 weeks. Percutaneous infection occurs after exposure to infectious larvae. *A duodenale* transmission can occur by oral ingestion and possibly through human milk. Untreated infected patients can harbor worms for 5 years or longer.

INCUBATION PERIOD: The time from exposure to development of noncutaneous symptoms is 4 to 12 weeks.

DIAGNOSTIC TESTS: Microscopic demonstration of hookworm eggs in feces is diagnostic. Adult worms or larvae rarely are seen. Approximately 5 to 8 weeks are required after infection for eggs to appear in feces. A direct stool smear with saline solution or potassium iodide saturated with iodine is adequate for diagnosis of heavy hookworm infection; light infections require concentration techniques. Quantification techniques (eg, Kato-Katz, Beaver direct smear, or Stoll egg-counting techniques) to determine the clinical significance of infection and the response to treatment may be available from state or reference laboratories. Cutaneous larva migrans is diagnosed clinically.

TREATMENT: Albendazole, mebendazole, and pyrantel pamoate all are effective treatments (see Drugs for Parasitic Infections, p 985). Mebendazole again is available in the United States. Albendazole must be taken with food; a fatty meal increases oral bioavailability. Pyrantel pamoate suspension can be mixed with milk or fruit juice. Although data suggest that these drugs are safe in children younger than 2 years, the risks and benefits of therapy should be considered before administration. In 1-year-old children, the World Health Organization recommends reducing the albendazole dose to half of that given to older children and adults. Reexamination of stool specimens 2 weeks after therapy to determine whether worms have been eliminated is helpful for assessing response to therapy. Retreatment is indicated for persistent infection. Nutritional supplementation, including iron, is important when moderate or severe anemia is present. Severely affected children may require blood transfusion.

ISOLATION OF THE HOSPITALIZED PATIENT: Standard precautions are recommended. Direct person-to-person transmission does not occur.

CONTROL MEASURES: Sanitary disposal of feces to prevent contamination of soil is necessary in areas with endemic infection. Treatment of all known infected people and screening of high-risk groups (ie, children and agricultural workers) in areas with endemic infection can help decrease environmental contamination. Wearing shoes protects against hookworm infection if no other parts of the body are in contact with contaminated soil; children playing in contaminated soil remain at risk if other body surfaces are in contact with the soil. Despite relatively rapid reinfection, periodic deworming treatments targeting preschool-aged and school-aged children have been advocated to prevent morbidity associated with heavy intestinal helminth infections. Certain populations immigrating to the United States (eg, refugees) receive presumptive treatment with albendazole prior to departure for the United States.

Human Herpesvirus 6 (Including Roseola) and 7

CLINICAL MANIFESTATIONS: Clinical manifestations of primary infection with human herpesvirus 6B (HHV-6B) include roseola (exanthem subitum) in approximately 20% of infected children, as well as a nonspecific febrile illness without rash or localizing signs. Acute HHV-6B infection may be accompanied by cervical and characteristic postoccipital lymphadenopathy, gastrointestinal tract or respiratory tract signs, and inflamed tympanic membranes. Fever often is high (temperature >39.5°C [103.0°F]) and persists for

3 to 7 days. Approximately 20% of all emergency department visits for febrile children 6 through 12 months of age are attributable to HHV-6B. Roseola is distinguished by an erythematous maculopapular rash that appears once fever resolves and can last hours to days. Febrile seizures, sometimes leading to status epilepticus, are the most common complication and reason for hospitalization among children with primary HHV-6B infection. Approximately 10% to 15% of children with primary HHV-6B infection develop febrile seizures, predominantly between the ages of 6 and 18 months. Other reported neurologic manifestations include a bulging fontanelle and encephalopathy or encephalitis, more commonly noted in Japanese infants than in the United States or Europe. Hepatitis has been reported as a rare manifestation of primary HHV-6B infection. Approximately 5% of mononucleosis syndrome cases are attributable to HHV-6B. Congenital infection with HHV-6B and HHV-6A, which occurs in approximately 1% of newborn infants, has not been linked to any clinical disease. Similarly, infection with HHV-6A has not been associated with any recognized disease.

The clinical manifestations occurring with human herpesvirus 7 (HHV-7) infection are less clear than with HHV-6B. Most primary infections with HHV-7 presumably are asymptomatic or mild and not distinctive. Some initial infections can present as typical roseola and may account for second or recurrent cases of roseola. Febrile illnesses associated with seizures also have been documented to occur during primary HHV-7 infection. Some investigators suggest that the association of HHV-7 with these clinical manifestations results from the ability of HHV-7 to reactivate latent HHV-6.

Following infection, HHV-6B, HHV-6A, and HHV-7 remain in a latent state and may reactivate. The clinical circumstances and manifestations of reactivation in healthy people are unclear. Illness associated with HHV-6B reactivation has been described primarily among recipients of solid organ and hematopoietic stem cell transplants. Clinical findings associated with HHV-6B reactivation in solid organ and hematopoietic stem cell transplants include fever, rash, hepatitis, bone marrow suppression, graft rejection, pneumonia, and encephalitis. The best characterized of these is post-transplantation acute limbic encephalitis, a specific syndrome associated with HHV-6B reactivation in the central nervous system characterized by anterograde amnesia, seizures, insomnia, confusion, and the syndrome of inappropriate antidiuretic hormone secretion. Patients undergoing cord blood transplantation are at an increased risk of developing post-transplantation acute limbic encephalitis, with significant morbidity and mortality attributed to this complication. Other clinical findings associated with HHV-6B reactivation in transplant patients are fever, rash, hepatitis, bone marrow suppression, graft rejection, pneumonia, and delirium. A few cases of central nervous system symptoms have been reported in association with HHV-7 reactivation in immunocompromised hosts, but clinical findings generally have been reported much less frequently with HHV-7 than with HHV-6B reactivation.

ETIOLOGY: HHV-6B, HHV-6A, and HHV-7 are lymphotropic viruses that are closely related members of the *Herpesviridae* family, subfamily *Betaherpesvirinae*. As betaherpesviruses, HHV-6B, HHV-6A, and HHV-7 are most closely related to cytomegalovirus. As with all human herpesviruses, they establish lifelong latency after initial acquisition. In 2012, HHV-6A and HHV-6B were recognized as distinct species rather than as variants of the same species. This increased the number of known human herpesviruses to 9. Essentially all postnatally acquired primary infections in children are caused by HHV-6B.

EPIDEMIOLOGY: HHV-6B and HHV-7 cause ubiquitous infections in children world-wide. Humans are the only known natural host. Nearly all children acquire HHV-6B in-fection within the first 2 years of life, probably resulting from asymptomatic shedding of infectious virus in secretions of a healthy family member or other close contact. During the acute phase of primary infection, HHV-6B and HHV-7 can be isolated from periph-eral blood mononuclear cells and HHV-7 from saliva of some children. Viral DNA subse-quently may be detected throughout life by polymerase chain reaction (PCR) assay in multiple body sites, including blood mononuclear cells, salivary glands, lung, skin, and the central nervous system. Virus-specific maternal antibody, which is present uniformly in the sera of infants at birth, provides transient partial protection. As maternal antibody concentration decreases during the first year of life, the infection rate increases rapidly, peaking between 6 and 24 months of age. Essentially all children are seropositive for HHV-6B before 4 years of age. Infections occur throughout the year without a seasonal pattern. Secondary cases rarely are identified. Occasional outbreaks of roseola have been reported.

Congenital infection occurs in approximately 1% of newborn infants, as determined by the presence of HHV-6A or HHV-6 B DNA in cord blood. The majority of HHV-6A infections in general appear to be attributable to chromosomal integration. Most congeni-tal infections appear to result from the germline passage of maternal or paternal chromo-somally integrated HHV-6 (ciHHV-6), a unique mechanism of transmission of human vi-ral congenital infection. Transplacental HHV-6 infection also may occur from reinfection or reactivation of maternal HHV-6 infection or from reactivated maternal ciHHV-6. HHV-6 has not been identified in human milk. Congenital infection typically is asympto-matic, and the implications of ciHHV-6 are not fully known.

HHV-7 infection usually occurs later in childhood than HHV-6B infection. By adult-hood, the seroprevalence of HHV-7 is approximately 85%. Infectious HHV-7 is present in more than 75% of saliva specimens obtained from healthy adults. Acquisition of virus via infected respiratory tract secretions of healthy contacts is the probable mode of trans-mission of HHV-7 to young children. HHV-7 has been detected in human milk, periph-eral blood mononuclear cells, cervical secretions, and other body sites. Congenital HHV-7 infection has not been demonstrated by the examination of large numbers of cord blood samples for HHV-7 DNA.

The mean **incubation period** for HHV-6B is 9 to 10 days. For HHV-7, the incu-bation period is not known.

DIAGNOSTIC TESTS: Multiple assays for detection of HHV-6 and HHV-7 have been de-veloped; some are available commercially, but because laboratory diagnosis of HHV-6 or HHV-7 usually does not influence clinical management (infections among the severely immunocompromised may be an exception), these tests have limited utility in clinical practice.

Reference laboratories offer diagnostic testing for HHV-6B, HHV-6A, and HHV-7 infections by detection of viral DNA in blood, cerebrospinal fluid (CSF), other body flu-ids, or tissue specimens. However, detection of HHV-6A, HHV-6B, or HHV-7 DNA by PCR assay might not differentiate between new infection, persistence of virus from past infection, or chromosomal integration of HHV-6. At least one multiplexed PCR diagnos-tic panel designed to detect agents of meningitis and encephalitis in CSF cleared by the US Food and Drug Administration contains HHV-6 as one of its target pathogens; how-ever, given the likelihood of ciHHV-6 (1%), which would give a positive CSF PCR result if cells are present, a positive test result should be interpreted with caution if there are no other findings to suggest encephalitis. DNA detection of HHV-6B or HHV-7 by PCR assay in conjunction with seroconversion or, in an infant with maternal antibodies, a fourfold titer increase confirms primary infection.

Chromosomal integration of HHV-6 is supported by consistently positive PCR test results for HHV-6 DNA in whole blood, tissue, or other fluids with high viral loads (eg, 1 x 10^6 copies in whole blood, which with a normal white blood cell count is approximately 1 copy of HHV-6 DNA per cell). ciHHV-6 can be confirmed by detection of HHV-6 DNA in hair follicles and can be suggested by testing whole blood from both parents to see if one of them has a high viral load. Quantitative PCR assay has been used for monitoring the effectiveness of antiviral treatment in immunocompromised patients.

Serologic tests include immunofluorescent antibody assay, neutralization, immunoblot, and enzyme immunoassay (EIA). A fourfold increase in serum antibody concentration alone does not necessarily indicate new infection, because an increase in titer may occur with reactivation and in association with other infections, especially other beta-herpesvirus infections. However, documented seroconversion is considered evidence of recent primary infection, and serologic tests may be useful for epidemiologic studies. Detection of specific immunoglobulin (Ig) M antibody is not reliable for diagnosing new infection, because IgM antibodies to HHV-6 and HHV-7 are not always detectable in children with primary infection, yet may be present in asymptomatic previously infected people. These antibody assays do not differentiate HHV-6A from HHV-6B infections. In addition, the diagnosis of primary HHV-7 infection in children with previous HHV-6B infection is confounded by concurrent increase in HHV-6 antibody titer from antigenic cross-reactivity or from reactivation of HHV-6B by a new HHV-7 infection. Detection of low-avidity HHV-6 or HHV-7 antibody with subsequent maturation to high-avidity antibody has been used in such situations to identify recent primary infection.

TREATMENT: Supportive. The use of ganciclovir (and, therefore, valganciclovir) or foscarnet may be beneficial for immunocompromised patients with HHV-6 disease and is recommended for treatment of encephalitis in hematopoietic stem cell transplant patients. Antiviral resistance may occur.

ISOLATION OF THE HOSPITALIZED PATIENT: Standard precautions are recommended.

CONTROL MEASURES: None.

Human Herpesvirus 8

CLINICAL MANIFESTATIONS: Human herpesvirus (HHV-8) is the etiologic agent associated with Kaposi sarcoma (KS), primary effusion lymphoma, multicentric Castleman disease (MCD), and "the Kaposi sarcoma herpesvirus-associated inflammatory cytokine syndrome (KICS)." MCD results in a proliferation of immune cells (both B and T lymphocytes) with multiorgan dysfunction that is associated with a hyperactive immune response resulting in excessive release of proinflammatory cytokines. HHV-8 also is one of the triggers of hemophagocytic lymphohistiocytosis (HLH). In regions with endemic HHV-8, a nonspecific primary infection syndrome in immunocompetent children consists of fever and a maculopapular rash, often accompanied by upper respiratory tract signs. Primary infection among immunocompromised people and men who have sex with men tends to have more severe manifestations, including pancytopenia, fever, rash, lymphadenopathy, splenomegaly, diarrhea, arthralgia, disseminated disease, and/or KS. In parts of

Africa, among children with and without human immunodeficiency virus (HIV) infection, KS is a frequent, aggressive malignancy. In the United States, KS is rare in children and occurs primarily in adults with poorly controlled HIV infection. Among organ transplant recipients and other immunosuppressed patients, KS is an important cause of cancer-related deaths. Primary effusion lymphoma is rare among children. MCD has been described in immunosuppressed and immunocompetent children, but the proportion of cases attributable to infection with HHV-8 is unknown.

ETIOLOGY: HHV-8 is a member of the family *Herpesviridae*, the *Gammaherpesvirinae* subfamily, and the *Rhadinovirus* genus, and is related closely to Epstein-Barr virus and to herpesvirus saimiri of monkeys.

EPIDEMIOLOGY: In areas of Africa, the Amazon basin, the Mediterranean, and the Middle East with endemic HHV-8, seroprevalence ranges from approximately 30% to 80%. Low rates of seroprevalence, generally less than 5%, have been reported in the United States, Northern and Central Europe, and most areas of Asia. Higher rates, however, occur in specific geographic regions, among adolescents and adults with or at high risk of acquiring HIV infection, injection drug users, and children adopted from some Eastern European countries.

Acquisition of HHV-8 in areas with endemic infection frequently occurs before puberty, likely by oral inoculation of saliva of close contacts, especially mothers and siblings. Virus is shed frequently in saliva of infected people and becomes latent for life in peripheral blood mononuclear cells, primarily CD19+ B lymphocytes, and lymphoid tissue. In areas where infection is not endemic, sexual transmission appears to be the major route of infection, especially among men who have sex with men. Studies from areas with endemic infection have suggested transmission may occur by blood transfusion, but in the United States, evidence for this is lacking. Transplantation of infected donor organs has been documented to result in HHV-8 infection in the recipient. HHV-8 DNA has been detected in blood drawn at birth from infants born to HHV-8 seropositive mothers, but vertical transmission seems to be rare. Viral DNA has been detected in human milk, but transmission via human milk is yet to be proven.

The **incubation period** of HHV-8 is unknown.

DIAGNOSTIC TESTS: Nucleic acid amplification testing and serologic assays for HHV-8 are available. Polymerase chain reaction (PCR) tests may be used on peripheral blood, fluid from body cavity effusions, and tissue biopsy specimens of patients with HHV-8–associated disease, such as KS. Detection of HHV-8 in peripheral blood specimens by PCR assay has been used to support the diagnosis of KS and to identify exacerbations of HHV-8-associated diseases, primarily MCD and KICS (especially at high copy number in these 2 diseases). However, HHV-8 DNA detection in the peripheral blood also occurs in asymptomatically infected people.

Currently available serologic assays measuring antibodies to HHV-8 include immunofluorescence antibody (IFA) assay, enzyme immunoassays (EIAs), and Western blot assays using recombinant HHV-8 proteins. These serologic assays detect both latent and lytic infection, but each has challenges with accuracy or convenience, with resulting limitations on their use in the diagnosis and management of acute clinical disease.

TREATMENT: No antiviral treatment is approved for HHV-8 disease. Several antiviral agents have in vitro activity against HHV-8. Ganciclovir has been shown to inhibit HHV-8 replication in the only randomized trial of an antiviral drug for this infection. Case reports document an effect of ganciclovir, ganciclovir combined with zidovudine, cidofovir, and foscarnet. Valacyclovir and famciclovir more modestly reduce HHV-8 replication. Retrospective cohort studies and in vitro assays suggest that antiretroviral therapy (particularly zidovudine and nelfinavir) may inhibit HHV-8 replication. Antiviral therapy may play a more significant role in the treatment of diseases associated with active HHV-8 replication, specifically MCD and KICS. HHV-8 associated malignancies can be treated with radiation and cancer chemotherapies.

ISOLATION OF THE HOSPITALIZED PATIENT: Standard precautions are recommended.

CONTROL MEASURES: Although there are no standard guidelines on preventing HHV-8 transmission, the extensive and consistent epidemiologic and virologic data implicating contact with saliva as the primary mode of HHV-8 acquisition have led some experts to recommend that persons at high-risk for the development of KS be counseled to avoid behavioral practices with exposure to saliva. Other experts, however, have questioned the feasibility or efficacy of such a strategy, which has never been evaluated. As such, no recommendations for measures to control transmission of HHV-8 infection can be recommended at this time.

Human Immunodeficiency Virus Infection[1]

CLINICAL MANIFESTATIONS: Human immunodeficiency virus (HIV) infection results in a wide array of clinical manifestations. HIV type 1 (HIV-1) is much more common in the United States than HIV type 2 (HIV-2). Unless otherwise specified, this chapter addresses HIV-1 infection. Acquired immunodeficiency syndrome (AIDS) is the name given to an advanced stage of HIV infection based on specific criteria for children, adolescents, and adults established by the Centers for Disease Control and Prevention (CDC).

Acute retroviral syndrome develops in 50% to 90% of adolescents and adults within the first few weeks after they become infected with HIV. Acute retroviral syndrome is characterized by nonspecific mononucleosis-like symptoms, including fever, malaise, lymphadenopathy, and skin rash.

With timely diagnosis of HIV infection in pregnant women, infants, and children and appropriate treatment, clinical manifestations of HIV infection, including the occurrence of AIDS-defining illnesses, now are rare among children in the United States and other industrialized countries. Early clinical manifestations of untreated pediatric HIV infection include unexplained fevers, generalized lymphadenopathy, hepatomegaly, splenomegaly, failure to thrive, persistent or recurrent oral and diaper candidiasis, recurrent diarrhea, parotitis, hepatitis, central nervous system (CNS) disease (eg, encephalopathy, hyperreflexia, hypertonia, floppiness, developmental delay), lymphoid interstitial pneumonia, recurrent invasive bacterial infections, and other opportunistic infections (OIs) (eg, viral, parasitic and fungal).[2]

In the era of combination antiretroviral therapy (cART), there has been a substantial

---

[1]For a complete listing of current policy statements from the American Academy of Pediatrics regarding human immunodeficiency virus and acquired immunodeficiency syndrome, see **http://pediatrics. aappublications.org/collection/committee-pediatric-aids.**

[2]Panel on Opportunistic Infections in HIV-Exposed and HIV-Infected Children. Guidelines for the Prevention and Treatment of Opportunistic Infections in HIV-Exposed and HIV-Infected Children. Department of Health and Human Services. Available at: **http://aidsinfo.nih.gov/contentfiles/lvguidelines/ oi_guidelines_pediatrics.pdf**

decrease in frequency of all OIs. The frequency of different OIs in the pre-cART era varied by age, pathogen, previous infection history, and immunologic status. In the pre-cART era, the most common OIs observed among children in the United States were infections caused by invasive encapsulated bacteria, *Pneumocystis jirovecii* (previously called *Pneumocystis carinii* pneumonia, hence the still-used acronym PCP), varicella-zoster virus, cytomegalovirus, herpes simplex virus, *Mycobacterium avium* complex, and *Candida* species. Less commonly observed opportunistic pathogens included Epstein-Barr virus (EBV), *Mycobacterium tuberculosis*, *Cryptosporidium* species, *Cystoisospora* (formerly *Isospora*) species, other enteric pathogens, *Aspergillus* species, and *Toxoplasma gondii*.

Immune reconstitution inflammatory syndrome (IRIS) is a paradoxical clinical deterioration often seen in severely immunosuppressed individuals that occurs shortly after the initiation of cART. Local and/or systemic symptoms develop secondary to an inflammatory response as cell-mediated immunity is restored. Underlying infection with mycobacteria (including *Mycobacterium tuberculosis),* herpesviruses, and fungi (including *Cryptococcal* species) predispose to IRIS.

Malignant neoplasms in children with HIV infection are relatively uncommon, but leiomyosarcomas and non-Hodgkin B-cell lymphomas of the Burkitt type (including some that occur in the CNS) occur more commonly in children with HIV infection than in immunocompetent children. Kaposi sarcoma, caused by human herpesvirus 8, is rare in children in the United States but has been documented in HIV-infected children who have emigrated from sub-Saharan African countries. The incidence of malignant neoplasms in HIV-infected children has decreased during the cART era.

The incidence of HIV encephalopathy is high among untreated HIV-infected infants and young children. In the United States, pediatric HIV encephalopathy has decreased substantially in the cART era, although other neurologic signs and symptoms have been appreciated, such as myelopathy or peripheral neuropathies, sometimes associated with antiretroviral therapy.

Without cART, the prognosis for survival is poor for untreated infants who acquired HIV infection through mother-to-child transmission (MTCT) and who have high viral loads (ie, >100 000 copies/mL) and severe suppression of CD4+ T-lymphocyte counts (see Table 3.30)[1]. In these children, AIDS-defining conditions developing during the first 6 months of life, including PCP, progressive neurologic disease, and severe wasting, are predictors of a poor outcome.

ETIOLOGY: HIV-1 and HIV-2 are cytopathic lentiviruses (genus *Lentivrus*) belonging to the family *Retroviridae* and are related closely to the simian immunodeficiency viruses, which infect a variety of nonhuman primate species in sub-Saharan Africa. Retroviruses are characterized by the presence of a viral reverse transcriptase (RT) enzyme that converts the single-stranded viral RNA genome into a double-stranded DNA copy. The double-stranded genome copy, termed the provirus, integrates into the host cell genome in a reaction catalyzed by the viral integrase enzyme.

Three distinct genetic groups of HIV exist worldwide: M (major), O (outlier), and N (new). Group M viruses are the most prevalent worldwide and comprise 8 genetic subtypes, or clades, known as A through K, each of which has a distinct geographic distribution.

---

[1]Centers for Disease Control and Prevention. Revised surveillance case definition for HIV infection—United States, 2014. *MMWR Recomm Rep.* 2014;63(RR-3):1–10

Table 3.30. HIV Infection Stage, Based on Age-Specific CD4+ T-Lymphocyte Count or CD4+ T-Lymphocyte Percentage of Total Lymphocytes[a,b]

| | Age on Date of CD4+ T-Lymphocyte Test | | | | | |
| | <1 y | | 1 Through 5 y | | 6 y Through Adult | |
Stage[a]	Cells/μL	%	Cells/μL	%	Cells/μL	%
1	≥1500	≥34	≥1000	≥30	≥500	≥26
2	750–1499	26–33	500–999	22–29	200–499	14–25
3	<750	<26	<500	<22	<200	<14

[a]The stage is based primarily on the CD4+ T-lymphocyte count; the CD4+ T-lymphocyte count takes precedence over the CD4+ T-lymphocyte percentage, and the percentage is considered only if the count is missing. If a Stage 3-defining opportunistic illness has been diagnosed, then the stage is 3 regardless of CD4+ T-lymphocyte test results.

[b]Source: Centers for Disease Control and Prevention. Revised surveillance case definition for HIV infection—United States, 2014. *MMWR Recomm Rep.* 2014;63(RR-3):1–10

HIV-2, the second AIDS-causing virus, is found predominantly in West Africa. The prevalence of HIV-2 in the United States is extremely low. HIV-2 is thought to have a milder disease course with a longer time to development of AIDS than HIV-1. Accurate diagnosis of HIV-2 is important clinically, because HIV-2 is resistant to nonnucleoside reverse transcriptase inhibitors (NNRTIs) and at least 1 fusion inhibitor (enfuvirtide). CDC guidelines state that HIV-2 serologic testing should be performed in patients who: (1) are from countries of high prevalence, mainly in Western Africa; (2) share needles or have sex partners known to be infected with HIV-2 or from areas with endemic infection; (3) received transfusions or nonsterile medical care in areas with endemic infection; or (4) are children of women with risk factors for HIV-2 infection.

EPIDEMIOLOGY: Humans are the only known reservoir for HIV-1 and HIV-2. Latent virus persists in peripheral blood mononuclear cells and in cells of the brain, bone marrow, and genital tract even when plasma viral load is undetectable. Only blood, semen, cervicovaginal secretions, and human milk have been implicated epidemiologically in transmission of infection.

Established modes of HIV transmission include: (1) sexual contact (vaginal, anal, or orogenital); (2) percutaneous blood exposure (from contaminated needles or other sharp instruments); (3) mucous membrane exposure to contaminated blood or other body fluids; (4) MTCT in utero, around the time of labor and delivery (perinatally), and postnatally through breastfeeding; and (5) transfusion with contaminated blood products. Cases of probable HIV transmission from HIV-infected caregivers to children through feeding blood-tinged premasticated food have been reported in the United States. As a result of highly effective screening assays and protocols, transfusion of blood, blood components, and clotting factors has virtually been eliminated as a cause of HIV transmission in the United States since 1985. In the United States, transmission of HIV has not been associated with normal activities in households, schools, or child care settings but has been documented after contact of nonintact skin with blood-containing body fluids.

Since the mid-1990s, the number of reported pediatric AIDS cases has decreased significantly, primarily because of prevention of MTCT of HIV. This decrease in rate of

MTCT of HIV in the United States was attributable to the development and implementation of antenatal HIV testing programs and other interventions to prevent transmission: antiretroviral (ARV) prophylaxis during the antepartum, intrapartum, and postnatal periods; cesarean delivery before labor and before rupture of membranes; and complete avoidance of breastfeeding. Currently in the United States, most HIV-infected pregnant women receive 3-drug cART regimens for treatment of their own HIV infection and for prevention of MTCT of HIV.

In the absence of breastfeeding, the risk of HIV infection for an infant born to an untreated HIV-infected mother in the United States is approximately 25%, with most transmission occurring around the intrapartum period. Maternal viral load is a critical determinant affecting the likelihood of MTCT of HIV, although transmission has been observed across the entire range of maternal viral loads. The risk of MTCT increases with each hour increase in the duration of ruptured membranes, which should be considered when evaluating the need for obstetric interventions. Cesarean delivery performed before onset of labor and before rupture of membranes has been shown to reduce MTCT. Current US guidelines recommend cesarean section before labor and before rupture of membranes at 38 completed weeks of gestation for HIV-infected women with a viral load >1000 copies/mL (irrespective of use of ARVs during pregnancy) and for women with unknown viral load near the time of delivery (**http://aidsinfo.nih.gov/ Guidelines**). Cesarean delivery before labor and before rupture of membranes is not routinely recommended for women with undetectable viral loads.

Postnatal transmission via breastfeeding is the most common mode of MTCT of HIV in resource-limited settings, where safe alternatives to human milk may not be readily available. HIV genomes have been detected in cell-associated and cell-free fractions of human milk, even in women receiving cART who have low HIV viral loads, and MTCT of HIV has been reported in a small percentage of these women. Therefore, replacement (formula) feeding continues to be recommended for US mothers receiving cART, because safe alternatives to human milk are readily available. In resource-limited settings, women whose HIV infection status is unknown are encouraged to breastfeed their infants exclusively for the first 6 months of life, because the morbidity associated with formula feeding is unacceptably high. In addition, these women should be offered HIV testing. The World Health Organization recommended in 2010 that HIV-infected mothers exclusively breastfeed their infants for the first 6 months of life if safe alternatives to human milk are not available. The introduction of complementary foods should occur after 6 months of life, and breastfeeding should continue through 12 months of life. Breastfeeding should be replaced only when a nutritionally adequate and safe diet can be maintained without human milk. In areas where ARVs are available, infants should receive daily nevirapine prophylaxis until 1 week after human milk consumption stops, and their mothers should receive ARV (consisting of an effective cART regimen) indefinitely. For infants known to be HIV infected, mothers are encouraged to breastfeed exclusively for the first 6 months of life, and after the introduction of complementary foods, breastfeeding should continue up to 2 years of age, as per recommendations for the general population.

Although the rate of acquisition of HIV infection among infants has decreased significantly in the United States, the rate of new HIV infections during adolescence and young adulthood continues to increase. HIV infection in adolescents occurs disproportionately among youth of minority race or ethnicity. Transmission of HIV to adolescents is attributable primarily to sexual exposure and secondarily to injection drug use. In 2014, it is estimated that for the 13- to 24-year age group, males accounted for the vast majority of those in whom HIV infection was diagnosed. Young men who have sex with men (MSM) are at particularly high risk of acquiring HIV infection, and the rates of HIV infection in this demographic group continue to increase. In the United States in 2014, for the 13- to 24-year age group, an estimated 95% of new HIV infection diagnoses among males were attributed to male-to-male sexual contact, accounting for 83% of all HIV diagnoses in this age group. In contrast, in the same year, 91% of diagnoses of HIV infection in women 13 to 24 years of age were attributed to heterosexual contact. In 2010, there were an estimated 40 144 adolescents and young adults 13 to 24 years of age living with a diagnosis of HIV infection in the United States and 6 dependent areas (American Samoa, Guam, the Northern Mariana Islands, Puerto Rico, the Republic of Palau, and the US Virgin Islands). Of these, 61% were black, 20% were Hispanic, and 14% were non-Hispanic white. Rates of HIV infection among adolescents are particularly high in the southeastern and northeastern United States. Most HIV-infected adolescents and young adults are asymptomatic and, without testing, remain unaware of their infection. In 2014, youth 13 to 24 years of age represented an estimated 22% of new HIV infections annually, and of these, almost half (44%) were unaware that they were infected.

INCUBATION PERIOD: The usual age of onset of symptoms is approximately 12 to 18 months of age[1] for untreated infants and children in the United States who acquire HIV infection through MTCT. However, some HIV-infected children become ill in the first few months of life, whereas others remain relatively asymptomatic for more than 5 years and, rarely, until early adolescence. Without therapy, a bimodal distribution of symptomatic infection has been described: 15% to 20% of untreated HIV-infected children die before 4 years of age, with a median age at death of 11 months (rapid progressors), and 80% to 85% of untreated HIV-infected children have delayed onset of milder symptoms and survive beyond 5 years of age (slower progressors).

Acute retroviral syndrome occurring in adolescents and adults following HIV acquisition occurs 7 to 14 days following viral acquisition and lasts for 5 to 7 days. Only a minority of patients are ill enough to seek medical care with acute retroviral syndrome, although more may recall a prior viral illness when queried later.

DIAGNOSTIC TESTS:

Serologic Assays. Immunoassays are used widely as the initial test for serum HIV antibody or for p24 antigen (see below) and HIV antibody. Serologic assays that are cleared by the FDA for the diagnosis of HIV include:

- Antigen/antibody combination immunoassays (fourth-generation tests) that detect HIV-1/HIV-2 antibodies as well as HIV-1 p24 antigen (see below): recommended for initial testing;
- HIV-1/HIV-2 immunoassays (third-generation antibody tests): alternative for initial testing;

---

[1]Centers for Disease Control and Prevention. HIV Surveillance Report, 2014; Vol 26. Atlanta, GA: Centers for Disease Control and Prevention; November 2015. Available at: **www.cdc.gov/hiv/library/reports/surveillance/**

- HIV-1/HIV-2 antibody differentiation immunoassay that differentiates HIV-1 antibodies from HIV-2 antibodies (Multispot HIV-1/HIV-2 test): recommended for supplemental confirmatory testing;
- HIV-1 Western blot and HIV-1 indirect immunofluorescent antibody assays (first-generation tests): alternative for supplemental confirmatory testing;
- HIV-1 and HIV-2 antibodies (separate results for each) as well as p24 antigen (fifth-generation test): FDA cleared for initial HIV screening, but not as a confirmatory test.

These tests are highly sensitive and specific. Repeated immunoassay testing in duplicate of initially reactive specimens is common practice and is followed by additional testing to establish the diagnosis of HIV. HIV antibody tests can be performed on samples of serum/plasma, whole blood, or oral fluid; antigen/antibody tests can be performed only on serum or plasma. Both laboratory and single-use device (point-of-care) rapid tests can deliver expedited test results. Rapid point-of-care tests have been approved for use in the United States; these tests are used widely throughout the world, particularly to screen mothers with unknown serostatus in maternity settings. As with laboratory immunoassays, additional testing is required after a reactive rapid test. Results from rapid tests are available from 1 to 20 minutes; in contrast, immunoassay results and follow-up testing might take 2 days or longer.

The 2014 CDC HIV laboratory testing algorithm recommends an initial HIV-1/HIV-2 antigen/antibody combination assay (fourth-generation assay) followed by an HIV-1/HIV-2 antibody differentiation assay. The fifth-generation immunoassay that provides separate results for HIV-1 and HIV-2 antibodies and p24 antigen is not yet reflected in the current CDC testing algorithm. If acute HIV infection or end-stage AIDS is suspected, virologic testing may be indicated because of false-negative antibody assay results in these populations.

Nucleic Acid Amplification Assays. Plasma HIV DNA or RNA assays have been used to diagnose HIV infection. Currently, there is one HIV-1 qualitative (not quantitative) RNA assay cleared by the FDA as a diagnostic test (APTIMA HIV-1 RNA Qualitative assay [Hologic Inc, Marlborough, MA]). The DNA polymerase chain reaction (PCR) assays can detect 1 to 10 DNA copies of proviral DNA in peripheral blood mononuclear cells, and are used qualitatively to diagnose HIV infection. In addition, RNA PCR quantitative (viral load) assays cleared by the FDA provide results that serve as a predictor of disease progression and are useful in monitoring changes in viral load during treatment with cART.

Antigen Detection. Detection of the p24 antigen (including immune complex-dissociated) is less sensitive than the HIV proviral DNA PCR assay or culture. False-positive test results occur in samples obtained from infants younger than 1 month. This test generally should not be used, although newer assays have been reported to have sensitivities similar to HIV proviral DNA PCR assays.

HIV-2 Detection. Most HIV immunoassays currently approved by FDA, including third-generation assays, detect but do not differentiate between HIV-1 and HIV-2 antibodies. It is important to notify the laboratory when ordering serologic tests for a patient in whom HIV-2 infection is a possibility. An HIV-1 Western blot performed as a supplemental confirmatory test following a positive immunoassay result might report a negative or indeterminate result or, in >60% of cases, misclassify the HIV-2 virus as HIV-1 (eg, detection of only p24 and gp160 bands). Therefore, FDA-approved HIV-1/HIV-2 antibody differentiation assays should be used in lieu of the Western blot to identify antibodies and distinguish HIV-1 from HIV-2. Nucleic acid amplification tests approved by the FDA for detection and quantitation of viral load are specific to HIV-1 and do not detect HIV-2. No nucleic acid amplification tests are approved by the FDA for HIV-2 viral load. Clinicians wishing to obtain assistance from the CDC laboratory to make an HIV-2 diagnosis should request a referral to the CDC laboratory from their local or state health department laboratory.

Diagnosis of Perinatally and Postnatally Acquired Infection. Because children born to HIV-infected mothers acquire passive maternal antibodies, antibody assays are not informative for the diagnosis of infection in children younger than 24 months unless assay results are negative. Therefore, laboratory diagnosis of HIV infection during the first 24 months of life is based on detection of the virus or viral nucleic acid (Table 3.31). In children 24 months and older, HIV antibody assays can be used for diagnosis. Historically, 18 months was considered the age at which a positive antibody assay could accurately distinguish between presence of maternal and infant antibodies. However, using medical record data for a cohort of HIV-uninfected infants born from 2000 to 2007, it was demonstrated that clearance of maternal HIV antibodies occurred later than previously reported. Despite a median age of seroreversion of 13.9 months, 14% of infants remained seropositive after 18 months, 4.3% remained seropositive after 21 months, and 1.2% remained seropositive after 24 months.

In the United States, the preferred test for diagnosis of HIV infection in children younger than 24 months is the HIV DNA PCR assay. The sensitivity of the test performed at birth is 55% but increases to more than 90% by 2 to 4 weeks of age and to 100% at 3 months of age. A positive result from a specimen obtained within 48 hours of life suggests in utero transmission. A single HIV DNA PCR assay has a sensitivity of 95%

Table 3.31. Laboratory Diagnosis of HIV Infection[a]

Test	Comment
HIV DNA PCR	Preferred test to diagnose HIV infection in infants and children younger than 18 months; highly sensitive and specific by 2 weeks of age and available; performed on peripheral blood mononuclear cells.
HIV p24 Ag	Less sensitive, false-positive results during first month of life, variable results; not recommended.
ICD p24 Ag	Negative test result does not rule out infection; not recommended.
HIV culture	Expensive, not readily available, requires up to 4 weeks for results; not recommended.
HIV RNA PCR	Preferred test to identify HIV-1 infections. Similar sensitivity and specificity to HIV DNA PCR in infants and children younger than 18 months, but DNA PCR is generally preferred because of greater clinical experience with that assay.

HIV indicates human immunodeficiency virus; PCR, polymerase chain reaction; Ag, antigen; ICD, immune complex dissociated.

[a]Read JS; American Academy of Pediatrics, Committee on Pediatric AIDS. Diagnosis of HIV-1 infection in children younger than 18 months in the United States, *Pediatrics*. 2007;120(6):e1547–e1562 (Reaffirmed April 2010). Available at: **http://pediatrics.aappublications.org/cgi/content/full/120/6/e1547**

and a specificity of 100% for samples collected from infected children 1 to 36 months of age. Results of DNA PCR assay, which detects cell-associated integrated HIV DNA, remain positive even among individuals with undetectable plasma viral loads.

Plasma HIV quantitative RNA assays also can be used to diagnose infection in HIV-exposed infants, with comparable sensitivity and specificity to DNA PCR regardless of the receipt of infant zidovudine prophylaxis. However, low levels of plasma viral load may result in false-negative RNA PCR assay results. In many cases, an HIV RNA assay is used as a supplemental test for an infant with positive DNA PCR assay results, providing both confirmation and an initial viral load measurement.

Plasma viral loads among untreated infants who acquire HIV infection through MTCT increase rapidly to very high levels (typically from several hundred thousand to more than 1 million copies/mL) after birth, decreasing only slowly to a "set point" by approximately 2 years of age. This contrasts with infection in adults, in whom the viral load generally does not reach the high levels that are seen in newly infected infants and for whom the "set point" occurs approximately 6 months after acquisition of infection. An HIV RNA assay result with only a low-level viral copy number in an HIV-exposed infant may indicate a false-positive result, reinforcing the importance of repeating any positive assay result to confirm the diagnosis of HIV infection in infancy. Like HIV DNA PCR assays, the sensitivity of HIV RNA assays for diagnosing infections in the first week of life is low (25%–40%), because transmission usually occurs around the time of delivery.

In HIV-exposed infants, diagnostic testing with HIV DNA or RNA assays is recommended at 14 to 21 days of age and, if results are negative, again at 1 to 2 months of age and at 4 to 6 months of age. An infant is considered infected if 2 samples from 2 different time points test positive by DNA or RNA PCR assay. In addition, viral diagnostic testing in the first 2 days of life is recommended by some experts to allow for early identification of infants with presumed in utero infection. If testing is performed shortly after birth, umbilical cord blood should not be used because of possible contamination with maternal blood. HIV-infected infants should be transitioned from neonatal ARV prophylaxis to cART treatment.

In nonbreastfed HIV-exposed children younger than 18 months with negative HIV virologic test results, *presumptive* exclusion of HIV infection is based on:

- Two negative HIV DNA or RNA virologic test results, from separate specimens, both of which were obtained at 2 weeks of age or older and one of which was obtained at 4 weeks of age or older; **OR**
- One negative HIV DNA or RNA virologic test result from a specimen obtained at 8 weeks of age or older; **OR**
- One negative HIV antibody test result obtained at 6 months of age or older; **AND**
- No other laboratory or clinical evidence of HIV infection (ie, no subsequent positive results from virologic tests if tests were performed and no AIDS-defining condition).

In nonbreastfed HIV-exposed children younger than 12 months with negative HIV virologic test results, *definitive* exclusion of HIV is based on:

- At least 2 negative HIV DNA or RNA virologic test results, from separate specimens, both of which were obtained at 1 month of age or older and one of which was obtained at 4 months of age or older; **OR**
- At least 2 negative HIV antibody test results from separate specimens obtained at 6 months of age or older;

AND

- No other laboratory or clinical evidence of HIV infection (ie, no subsequent positive results from virologic tests if tests were performed and no AIDS-defining condition).

In HIV-exposed children with 2 negative HIV DNA PCR test results, many clinicians will confirm the absence of antibody (ie, loss of passively acquired maternal antibody) to HIV on testing at 18 through 24 months of age ("seroreversion"). In addition, some clinicians have a slightly more stringent requirement that the 2 separate antibody-negative blood samples obtained after 6 months of age be drawn at least 1 month apart for a child to be considered HIV-uninfected.

Adolescents and HIV Testing. The American Academy of Pediatrics (AAP) recommends that routine screening be offered to all adolescents at least once by 16 through 18 years of age in health care settings. Use of any licensed HIV antibody test is appropriate. For any positive test result, referral to an HIV specialist is appropriate to confirm diagnosis and initiate management. Adolescents with behaviors that increase risk of HIV acquisition (eg, multiple sex partners, illicit drug use) should be tested at least annually. HIV testing is recommended and should be routine for all patients in sexually transmitted infection (STI) clinics and those seeking treatment for STIs in other clinical settings.

Suspicion of acute retroviral syndrome should prompt urgent assessment with an antigen/antibody immunoassay or HIV RNA in conjunction with an antibody test. If the immunoassay is negative or indeterminate, then testing for HIV RNA should follow. Clinicians should not assume that a laboratory report of a negative HIV antibody test result indicates that the necessary RNA screening for acute HIV infection has been conducted. HIV home-testing kits only detect HIV antibodies and therefore will not detect acute HIV infection.

Consent for Diagnostic Testing. The CDC recommends that diagnostic HIV testing and opt-out HIV screening be part of routine clinical care in all health care settings for patients 13 through 64 years of age. Patients or people responsible for the patient's care should be notified verbally that testing is planned, advised of the indication for testing and the implications of positive and negative test results, and offered an opportunity to ask questions and to decline testing. With such notification, the patient's general consent for medical care is considered sufficient for diagnostic HIV testing. Laws concerning consent and confidentiality for HIV care differ among states. Public health statutes and legal precedents allow for evaluation and treatment of minors for sexually transmitted infections without parental knowledge or consent, but not every state has explicitly defined HIV infection as a condition for which testing or treatment may proceed without parental consent.

TREATMENT:

Antiretroviral Therapy. Because HIV treatment options and recommendations change with time and vary with occurrence of ARV drug resistance and the adverse event profile, consultation with an expert in pediatric HIV infection is recommended in the care of HIV-infected infants, children, and adolescents. Current treatment recommendations for HIV-infected infants, children, and adolescents are available online (**http://aidsinfo. nih.gov**). Whenever possible, enrollment of HIV-infected infants, children, and adolescents in clinical trials should be encouraged. Information about trials for HIV-infected infants, children, and adolescents can be obtained by contacting the AIDS Clinical Trials Information Service (**https://aidsinfo.nih.gov/clinical-trials**).

cART is indicated for HIV-infected pediatric patients and should be provided as soon as possible after diagnosis of HIV infection is established. The principal objectives of therapy are to provide maximum suppression of viral replication, to restore and preserve immune function, to reduce HIV-associated morbidity and mortality, to minimize drug toxicity, to maintain normal growth and development, and to improve quality of life. Data from both observational studies and clinical trials indicate that very early initiation of therapy, regardless of presence or absence of HIV-related symptoms or immunosuppression, reduces morbidity and mortality compared with starting treatment when clinically symptomatic or immune suppressed. Effective administration of early therapy will maintain the viral load at low or undetectable concentrations and will reduce viral mutation and evolution.

Initiation of treatment of adolescents generally follows guidelines for adults, and initiation of treatment is recommended strongly for all HIV-infected adolescents or adults regardless of CD4+ T-lymphocyte count, as long as medication readiness is apparent. Dosages of ARVs can be prescribed according to age, weight, and body surface area or sexual maturity rating (previously Tanner stage). Adolescents in early puberty (sexual maturity ratings I and II) should be prescribed doses based on pediatric schedules, and adolescents in late puberty (sexual maturity rating III, IV, and V) should be prescribed doses based on adult schedules. In general, cART with at least 3 active drugs is recommended for all HIV-infected individuals requiring ARV therapy. ARV resistance testing (viral genotyping) is recommended before starting treatment. Suppression of virus to undetectable levels is the desired goal. A change in ARV therapy should be considered if there is evidence of disease progression (virologic, immunologic, or clinical), toxicity of or intolerance to drugs, development of drug resistance, or availability of data suggesting the possibility of a superior regimen.

Immunologic Classification for Opportunistic Infection and Vaccination Decision Making. For purposes of surveillance of pediatric HIV infection, the CDC uses a case definition that incorporates an immunologic classification system (Table 3.30, p 461),[1] which emphasizes the importance of the CD4+ T-lymphocyte count and percentage as critical determinants of prognosis. Data regarding plasma HIV-1 RNA concentration (viral load) are not included in this classification. The immune status of an HIV-infected child no longer is used to determine when to start antiretroviral therapy, because all children are started on ARV therapy at the time of diagnosis. Immune status still is used for initiation and discontinuation of prophylaxis for opportunistic infections and for determining whether it is safe to administer a live vaccine. Because the specific CD4+ T-lymphocyte count may vary for different opportunistic infections or live vaccines, recommendations for prophylaxis of opportunistic infections or safety of live vaccines can be found in the specific chapter for the opportunistic infection or live vaccine. More information can be obtained in "Guidelines for Prevention and Treatment of Opportunistic infections in HIV-Exposed and HIV-Infected Children" (**https://aidsinfo.nih.gov/guidelines/html/5/pediatric-oi-prevention-and-treatment-guidelines/0**).

Opportunistic Infections. Early diagnosis, prophylaxis, and aggressive treatment of OIs prolong survival. This is particularly true for PCP, which accounts for approximately one third of pediatric AIDS diagnoses overall and may occur early in the first year of life.

---

[1]Centers for Disease Control and Prevention. Revised surveillance case definition for HIV infection—United States, 2014. *MMWR Recomm Rep.* 2014;63(RR-3):1–10

Prophylaxis is not recommended for HIV-exposed infants who meet the criteria for presumptive or definitive absence of HIV infection. Thus, for infants with negative HIV diagnostic test results up through 4 weeks of age (eg, no positive test results or clinical symptoms), PCP prophylaxis would not need to be initiated. Because mortality rates are high, PCP chemoprophylaxis should be given to all HIV-exposed infants with indeterminate HIV infection status starting at 4 to 6 weeks of age but can be stopped if the child subsequently meets criteria for presumptive or definitive absence of HIV infection. All infants with HIV infection should receive PCP prophylaxis through 1 year of age regardless of immune status. The need for PCP prophylaxis for HIV-infected children 1 year and older is determined by the degree of immunosuppression from CD4+ T-lymphocyte percentage and count (see *Pneumocystis jirovecii* Infections, p 651).

Guidelines for prevention and treatment of OIs in children (**https://aidsinfo. nih.gov/guidelines/html/5/pediatric-oi-prevention-and-treatment-guidelines/0/**) and adolescents and adults (**https://aidsinfo.nih.gov/ guidelines/html/4/adult-and-adolescent-oi-prevention-and-treatment-guidelines/0**) provide indications for administration of drugs for infection with *Mycobacterium avium* complex, cytomegalovirus, *T gondii*, and other organisms.

Immunization Recommendations (also see Immunization in Special Clinical Circumstances, p 67, and Table 1.19, p 75).[1] All recommended childhood immunizations should be administered to HIV-exposed infants. If HIV infection is confirmed, guidelines for the HIV-infected child should be followed. Children and adolescents with HIV infection should be immunized as soon as is age appropriate with all inactivated vaccines. Inactivated influenza vaccine (IIV) should be administered annually according to the most current recommendations. The 3-dose series of human papillomavirus vaccine; tetanus toxoid, reduced diphtheria toxoid, and acellular pertussis (Tdap) vaccine; and meningococcal conjugate vaccine all are indicated in HIV-infected adolescents (**https://redbook.solutions. aap.org/SS/Immunization_Schedules.aspx**).

The live-virus measles-mumps-rubella (MMR) vaccine and monovalent varicella vaccine can be administered to asymptomatic HIV-infected children and adolescents without severe immunosuppression (that is, can be administered to children 1 through 13 years of age with a CD4+ T-lymphocyte percentage $\geq 15\%$ and to adolescents ≥ 14 years with a CD4+ T-lymphocyte count ≥ 200 lymphocytes/mm^3). Severely immunocompromised HIV-infected infants, children, adolescents, and young adults (eg, children 1 through 13 years of age with a CD4+ T-lymphocyte percentage $<15\%$ and adolescents ≥ 14 years with a CD4+ T-lymphocyte count <200 lymphocytes/mm^3) should not receive measles virus-containing vaccine, because vaccine-related pneumonia has been reported. The quadrivalent measles-mumps-rubella-varicella (MMRV) vaccine should not be administered to any HIV-infected infant, regardless of degree of immunosuppression, because of lack of safety data in this population.

Rotavirus vaccine should be administered to HIV-exposed and HIV-infected infants irrespective of CD4+ T-lymphocyte percentage or count.

All HIV-infected children should receive a dose of 23-valent polysaccharide pneumococcal vaccine after 24 months of age, with a minimal interval of 8 weeks since the last pneumococcal conjugate vaccine.

[1]Rubin LG, Levin MJ, Ljungman P, et al. 2013 IDSA clinical practice guideline for vaccination of the immunocompromised host. *Clin Infect Dis*. 2014;58(3):309–318

HIV-infected children who are 5 years and older and have not received Hib vaccine should receive 1 dose of Hib vaccine.

Infants and children with HIV infection 2 months of age or older should receive an age-appropriate series of the meningococcal ACWY conjugate vaccine (MenACWY) (see Meningococcal Infections, p 550).[1] The recommendations for children 2 months through 2 years of age and people 25 years or older are based on expert opinion, because the vaccine was not studied in HIV-infected people in these age groups. The same vaccine product should be used for all doses. However, if the product used for previous doses is unknown or unavailable, the vaccination series may be completed with any age- and formulation-appropriate meningococcal ACWY conjugate vaccine. Although no data on interchangeability of meningococcal conjugate vaccines in HIV-infected people are available, limited data from a postlicensure study in healthy adolescents suggests safety and immunogenicity of MenACWY-CRM are not adversely affected by prior immunization with MenACWY-D. For HIV-infected infants aged 2 through 23 months of age, only Men-ACWY-CRM (Menveo) can be used, because interference with immune response to pneumococcal conjugate vaccine occurs with MenACWY-D (Menactra).

Children Who Are HIV Uninfected Residing in the Household of an HIV-Infected Person. Members of households in which an adult or child has HIV infection can receive MMR vaccine, because these vaccine viruses are not transmitted person-to-person. To decrease the risk of transmission of influenza to patients with symptomatic HIV infection, all household members 6 months or older should receive yearly influenza immunization (see Influenza, p 476). Immunization with varicella vaccine of siblings and susceptible adult caregivers of patients with HIV infection is encouraged to prevent acquisition of wild-type varicella-zoster virus infection, which can cause severe disease in immunocompromised hosts. Transmission of varicella vaccine virus from an immunocompetent host to a household contact is very uncommon.

Postexposure Passive Immunization of HIV-Infected Children.

Measles (see Measles, p 537).[2] HIV-infected children who are exposed to measles require prophylaxis on the basis of immune status and measles vaccine history. HIV-infected children who have serologic evidence of immunity or who received 2 doses of measles vaccine after initiation of cART with no or moderate immunosuppression should be considered immune and will not require any additional measures to prevent measles. Asymptomatic mildly or moderately immunocompromised HIV-infected patients without evidence of immunity to measles should receive IGIM at a dose of 0.5 mL/kg (maximum 15 mL), regardless of immunization status. Severely immunocompromised patients (including HIV-infected people with CD4+ T-lymphocyte percentages <15% [all ages] or CD4+ T-lymphocyte counts <200/mm^3 [age >5 years] and those who have not received MMR vaccine since receiving cART) who are exposed to measles should receive IGIV prophylaxis, 400 mg/kg, after exposure to measles regardless of vaccination status, because they may not be protected by the vaccine. Some experts would include all

---

[1]Centers for Disease Control and Prevention. Recommendations for use of meningococcal conjugate vaccines in HIV-infected persons—Advisory Committee on Immunization Practices, 2016. *MMWR Morb Mortal Wkly Rep.* 2016;65(43):1189–1194

[2]Centers for Disease Control and Prevention. Prevention of measles, rubella, congenital rubella syndrome, and mumps, 2013 summary: recommendations of the Advisory Committee on Immunization Practices (ACIP). *MMWR Recomm Rep.* 2013;62(RR-4):1–34

HIV-infected people, regardless of immunologic status or MMR vaccine history, as needing IGIV prophylaxis. HIV-infected children who have received IGIV within 3 weeks of exposure do not require additional passive immunization.

Tetanus. HIV-infected children with severe immune suppression who sustain wounds classified as tetanus prone (see Tetanus, p 793, and Table 3.78, p 796) should receive Tetanus Immune Globulin regardless of immunization status.

Varicella. HIV-infected children without a history of previous varicella infection or who lack evidence of immunity to varicella should receive Varicella Zoster Immune Globulin (VariZIG), if available, ideally within 96 hours but potentially beneficial up to 10 days, after close contact with a person who has chickenpox or shingles (see Varicella-Zoster Infections, p 869). An alternative to VariZIG for passive immunization is IGIV, 400 mg/kg, administered once within 10 days after exposure. Children who have received IGIV for other reasons within 3 weeks of exposure do not require additional passive immunization.

ISOLATION OF THE HOSPITALIZED PATIENT: Standard precautions should be followed by all health care professionals regardless of suspected or confirmed HIV status of the patient. The risk to health care professionals of acquiring HIV infection from a patient is minimal, even after accidental exposure from a needlestick injury. Nevertheless, every effort should be made to avoid direct exposures to blood and other body fluids, especially those that could contain HIV. Guidelines for use of occupational and nonoccupational postexposure prophylaxis have been published by the CDC and should be started as soon as possible after the exposure but within 72 hours for maximal effectiveness (**www.cdc. gov/hiv/risk/pep/**). In addition, the University of California, San Francisco maintains a Clinician Consultation Center at 1-888-448-4911 seven days a week between 9 AM and 9 PM Eastern Time and can provide valuable support to providers.

CONTROL MEASURES: HIV is a nationally notifiable disease in the United States.

Interruption of MTCT of HIV. Development and implementation of efficacious interventions to prevent MTCT of HIV has resulted in a marked decrease in cases of MTCT of HIV infection in the United States. The following are the recommendations of the US Public Health Service, AAP, and American College of Obstetricians and Gynecologists for the prevention of MTCT of HIV.

The AAP and CDC recommend an opt-out approach for HIV testing of all pregnant women in all health care settings in the United States involving routine HIV screening for every pregnant woman after she is notified that testing will be performed, unless she declines. For women in labor with undocumented HIV infection status during the current pregnancy, immediate maternal HIV testing with opt-out consent, using a rapid HIV antibody test, is recommended. In many states, routinely offering HIV testing early and late during pregnancy is mandated by law. Education about HIV infection and testing should be part of a comprehensive program of health care for all women during their childbearing years.

Three efficacious interventions to prevent MTCT of HIV are utilized in the United States: antiretroviral prophylaxis; cesarean delivery at 38 completed weeks of gestation, before labor and before rupture of membranes; and complete avoidance of breastfeeding. It is important to diagnose HIV infection early in pregnancy to allow antenatal implementation of interventions to prevent transmission (cART as early in pregnancy as possible and cesarean delivery before labor and before rupture of membranes). In resource-limited countries where complete avoidance of breastfeeding (replacement feeding) may not always be safe or available, exclusive breastfeeding is associated with a lower risk of postnatal HIV transmission or infant morbidity/mortality compared with mixed breastfeeding and formula feeding. Both maternal cART and infant ARV prophylaxis during breastfeeding is effective in reducing MTCT of HIV.

Maternal ARV Therapy and MTCT Prophylaxis.

Management of Infected Mother. HIV-infected pregnant women should receive cART regimens, both for treatment of HIV infection and for prevention of MTCT of HIV. Virologic suppression is the goal both during pregnancy and following delivery for HIV-infected pregnant women. Detailed recommendations for use of ARVs in HIV-infected pregnant women can be found online (**http://aidsinfo.nih.gov**). Ideally, women initiating such a regimen during pregnancy should be tested for the presence of ARV resistance. However, initiation of cART should not be delayed pending results of resistance testing, especially if these decisions are being made late in pregnancy. Most women in industrialized nations are treated with potent cART started in the first trimester and continuing to delivery. HIV-infected women with HIV RNA ≥1000 copies/mL (or unknown HIV RNA) near delivery should receive intravenous (IV) zidovudine during labor, regardless of antepartum regimen or mode of delivery; in situations where IV administration is not possible, oral administration can be considered (Table 3.32, p 474). A pregnant woman already receiving treatment that does not include zidovudine need not have her ARV regimen changed if her viral load is suppressed.

The relative risk of first-trimester exposure and neural tube defects with efavirenz exposure is unclear. However, because this risk is restricted to the first 5 to 6 weeks of pregnancy and because unnecessary ARV drug changes occurring during pregnancy may lead to loss of viral control, efavirenz can be continued in pregnant women presenting after the first 6 weeks of pregnancy who conceive on an efavirenz-containing regimen with successful virologic suppression.

Intrapartum management of HIV-infected women and the immediate postnatal care of their newborn infants is multifaceted. Pediatric providers should collaborate with the regular HIV medical providers and the delivering physicians of pregnant women and establish protocols for management (including ARVs used) and communication. For women in labor with undocumented HIV infection status, a rapid HIV test should be performed as soon as possible. For an HIV-infected woman, routine oral ARVs should be continued on schedule. Any procedures that compromise the integrity of fetal skin during labor and delivery (eg, fetal scalp electrodes) or that increase the occurrence of maternal bleeding (eg, instrumented vaginal delivery, episiotomy) should be avoided when possible.

Management of Exposed Infant. The newborn infant should be bathed and cleaned of maternal secretions (especially bloody secretions) as soon as possible after birth. Newborn infants should begin ARV prophylaxis as soon as possible after birth, preferably within 12 hours. In the United States, neonatal prophylaxis generally consists of zidovudine for 6 weeks. Among infants whose mothers did not receive any ARVs before the onset of labor, neonatal postexposure prophylaxis with a 2- or 3-drug ARV regimen results in a lower rate of MTCT of HIV than zidovudine alone. A 2-drug regimen of zidovudine for 6 weeks with 3 doses of nevirapine during the first week of life (as soon as possible after birth, 48 hours after first dose, and 96 hours after second dose) is as effective but less toxic than a 3-drug regimen of zidovudine, lamivudine, and nelfinavir. Therefore, current recommendations for infants of HIV-infected women who did not receive any ARVs before the onset of labor are for administration of this 2-drug neonatal prophylaxis regimen

(Table 3.32, p 474). Likewise, in instances with maternal HIV RNA ≥1000 copies/mL (or unknown HIV RNA) near delivery, 3 doses of oral nevirapine are indicated for the infant within the first week of life, in addition to oral zidovudine. Detailed guidance is available regarding infant ARV prophylaxis regimens (**https://aidsinfo.nih.gov/ guidelines/html/3/perinatal-guidelines/0/#**). The mother should have the HIV drugs for both herself and her infant before leaving the hospital, and the infant should have an appointment for a postnatal visit at 2 to 4 weeks of age to monitor medication adherence and for HIV diagnostic testing.

For a newborn infant whose mother's HIV infection status is unknown, the mother or the newborn infant should be tested using a rapid HIV antibody test, with appropriate consent as required by state and local law. If the rapid HIV antibody test is positive, effective ARV prophylaxis should be administered to the infant as soon as possible, ideally within 12 hours. In some states, rapid testing of the neonate is required by law if the mother has refused to be tested.

The newborn infant's physician should be informed of the mother's HIV infection status so appropriate care and follow-up of the infant can be accomplished. Whenever possible, an HIV-infected mother and her infant should be referred to a facility that provides HIV-related services for both women and children.

Breastfeeding (also see Human Milk, p 113). Transmission of HIV by breastfeeding accounts for one third to one half of MTCT of HIV worldwide and is more likely among mothers who acquire HIV infection late in pregnancy or during the postpartum period. Late postnatal transmission is associated with reduced maternal CD4+ T-lymphocyte count, high plasma and human milk viral load, mastitis/breast abscess, and infant oral lesions (eg, oral thrush). Clinical trials in resource-limited settings have demonstrated the efficacy of ARV treatment of HIV-infected women while breastfeeding as well as ARV prophylaxis to breastfeeding children of HIV-infected women in prevention of MTCT. However, because such prophylaxis cannot be assumed to be completely protective against MTCT of HIV, in countries where safe alternative sources of infant feeding readily are available, affordable, and culturally accepted, such as the United States, HIV-infected women should be counseled not to breastfeed their infants or to donate to human milk banks. Similarly, women in industrialized countries who are receiving cART for their own health, even if they have undetectable HIV viral loads, also should be counseled not to breastfeed because of the continued possibility of HIV transmission. Because of social and cultural reasons, an HIV-infected pregnant woman may be pressured to or choose to breastfeed. It is, therefore, critical that providers keep open channels of communication with an HIV-infected pregnant mother. If, after counseling, a mother still chooses to breastfeed, it is important for the provider to be aware of this so that an appropriate plan of management can be developed, including encouraging prolonged use of ARVs in both the mother and infant while breastfeeding.

In general, women who are known to be HIV uninfected should be encouraged to breastfeed. However, women who are HIV uninfected but who are known to have HIV-infected sexual partners or bisexual partners or are active injection drug users should be counseled about the potential risk of acquiring HIV infection themselves and of then transmitting HIV through human milk. Such women should be counseled to use condoms and to undergo frequent HIV testing (eg, monthly to every 3 months) during the

Table 3.32. Zidovudine Regimen for Decreasing the Risk of Mother-to-Child Transmission (MTCT) of HIV[a,b]

Period of Time	Route	Dosage
For mother during pregnancy, initiate anytime and continue throughout pregnancy[c]	Oral	300 mg, 2 times per day
For mother during labor and delivery[d]	Intravenous	2 mg/kg during the first hour, then 1 mg/kg per hour until delivery
For the newborn infant ≥35 weeks' gestation, as soon as possible after birth[b,e]	Oral	4 mg/kg, twice daily, for the first 4–6 weeks of life[f]
For the newborn infant ≥30 to <35 weeks' gestation, as soon as possible after birth[b,e]	Oral	2 mg/kg, twice daily for 14 days, then increase to 3 mg/kg, twice daily, to complete a total of 6 weeks of treatment[f]
	Intravenous	1.5 mg/kg, twice daily (maximum of 6 weeks). When able to tolerate oral medications, the twice-daily dose is 2 mg/kg until 14 days of life and then 3 mg/kg to complete 6 weeks of treatment[f]
For the newborn infant <30 weeks' gestation, as soon as possible after birth[b,e]	Oral	2 mg/kg, twice daily for 28 days, then increase to 3 mg/kg, twice daily, to complete a total of 6 weeks of treatment[f]
	Intravenous	1.5 mg/kg, twice daily (maximum of 6 weeks). When able to tolerate oral medications, the twice-daily dose is 2 mg/kg until 28 days of life and then 3 mg/kg to complete a total of 6 weeks of treatment[f]

IV indicates intravenous; PO, oral.

[a]Modified from Panel on Treatment of HIV-Infected Pregnant Women and Prevention of Perinatal Transmission: Recommendations for Use of Antiretroviral Drugs in Pregnant HIV-1-Infected Women for Maternal Health and Interventions to Reduce Perinatal HIV Transmission in the United States. Washington, DC: US Department of Health and Human Services; 2015. Available at: **http://aidsinfo.nih.gov/contentfiles/PerinatalGL.pdf.** Information about other antiretroviral drugs for decreasing the rate of perinatal transmission of HIV can be found online (**http://aidsinfo.nih.gov).**

[b]For infants whose mothers received no antepartum antiretroviral prophylaxis, nevirapine in the following birth weight-based doses should be given as soon after delivery as possible, in addition to zidovudine. Weight-based dosing: birth weight 1.5–2 kg: 8 mg total for each dose; birth weight: >2 kg: 12 mg total for each dose. The first dose should be given as soon as possible after delivery up to 48 hours of life. The second dose should be given 48 hours after the first dose. The third dose should be given 96 hours after the second dose.

[c]Most women in industrialized nations are treated with potent combinations of 3 antiretroviral agents (cART) started at the first trimester and continuing to delivery. Oral zidovudine may be used as part of that therapy.

[d]IV zidovudine no longer is required for HIV-infected women receiving combination antiretroviral regimens who have HIV RNA <1000 copies/mL near delivery. HIV-infected women with HIV RNA ≥1000 copies/mL (or unknown HIV RNA) near delivery should be administered IV zidovudine during labor, regardless of antepartum regimen or mode of delivery. On the basis of pharmacokinetic data, in women with HIV RNA ≥1000 copies/mL near delivery for whom zidovudine is recommended, IV would be preferred to oral administration in the United States; in situations where IV administration is not possible, oral administration can be considered.

[e]The effectiveness of antiretroviral agents for prevention of MTCT of HIV decreases with delay in initiation after birth. Initiation of postexposure prophylaxis after the first 48 hours of life is not likely to be effective in preventing transmission.

[f]In the United Kingdom and many other European countries, a 4-week neonatal chemoprophylaxis regimen is recommended for infants born to mothers who have received antenatal combination ARV drug regimens. This approach also can be considered in cases in which adherence to or toxicity from the 6-week zidovudine prophylaxis regimen is a concern.

breastfeeding period to detect potential maternal HIV seroconversion. In addition, in the case of condom breakage during sexual intercourse with the HIV-infected discordant partner, women should be counseled to undergo immediate HIV testing and initiation of HIV postexposure prophylaxis within 72 hours of the condom breakage.

Premastication. Probable transmission of HIV by caregivers who premasticated food for infants has been described in 3 cases in the United States. In 2 of the cases, the caregivers had bleeding gums or sores in their mouths during the time they premasticated the food. The CDC recommends that in the United States, where safe alternative methods of feeding are available, HIV-infected caregivers be asked about whether they practice premastication and counseled not to premasticate food for infants.

HIV in the Athletic Setting. Athletes and staff of athletic programs can be exposed to blood during certain athletic activities. Recommendations have been developed by the AAP for prevention of transmission of HIV and other bloodborne pathogens in the athletic setting (see School Health, Infections Spread by Blood and Body Fluids, p 144).

Sexual Abuse. In cases of proven or suspected sexual abuse, the child should be tested serologically as soon as possible and then periodically for 6 months (eg, at 4 to 6 weeks, and at 3 months and 6 months after last known sexual contact) (see Evaluation of STIs in Adolescents, p 166). Serologic evaluation for HIV infection of the perpetrator should be attempted as soon after the incident as possible. Counseling of the child and family needs to be provided (see Prophylaxis of Children and Adolescents After Sexual Victimization, p 173).

Prevention of HIV Transmission Through Adult Behaviors (Sexual Activity). Abstinence from sexual activity is the only certain way to prevent sexual transmission of HIV. Safer sex practices, including use of condoms for all sexual encounters (vaginal, anal, and oral sex) can reduce HIV transmission significantly by reducing exposure to body fluids containing HIV. Suppressing HIV viral load to undetectable levels in the blood with cART regimens has resulted in decreases in transmission in discordant couples by as much as 96%. In MSM, continuous preexposure prophylaxis with ARV therapy (tenofovir and emtricitabine) was associated with reduction in HIV acquisition by 44% in the uninfected partner in a discordant couple. The efficacy of preexposure prophylaxis is higher with improved medication adherence. Preexposure prophylaxis also is effective in heterosexual couples and injection drug users. Because data on effectiveness and long-term safety of preexposure ARV prophylaxis in MSM are limited, preexposure prophylaxis should be performed using guidelines provided by the CDC (**www.cdc.gov/hiv/risk/prep/index.html**). ARV-based vaginal microbicides (1% tenofovir gel) have reduced HIV acquisition in uninfected women by 39%. Data from clinical trials conducted in African countries also provide evidence that medical male circumcision can reduce HIV acquisition in uninfected heterosexual males by 38% to 66% over 24 months.

Postexposure Prophylaxis for Possible Sexual or Other Nonoccupational Exposure to HIV. Decisions to provide ARVs after possible nonoccupational (ie, community) exposure to HIV must balance the potential benefits and risks. Decisions regarding the need for ARV prophylaxis in such instances are predicated on the probability that the source is infected or contaminated with HIV, the likelihood of transmission by the particular exposure, and the interval between exposure and initiation of therapy, balanced against expected adverse effects associated with the regimen.

The risk of transmission of HIV from a puncture wound attributable to a needle found in the community likely is lower than 0.3%, which is the estimated probability of

HIV transmission associated with a puncture wound involving a known HIV-contaminated needle in a health care setting. The actual risks of HIV infection in an infant or child after a needlestick injury or sexual abuse are unknown, but to date there are no confirmed transmissions of HIV from accidental nonoccupational needlestick injuries (needles found in the community). The estimated risk of HIV transmission per episode of receptive penile-anal sexual exposure is 138 per 10 000 exposures, whereas the estimated risk per episode of receptive vaginal exposure is 8 per 10 000 exposures.

Use of daily nevirapine for postexposure prophylaxis is not recommended because of the high incidence of severe (and rarely fatal) adverse effects in adults with normal CD4+ T-lymphocyte counts. Such adverse effects have not been reported with single-dose intrapartum/infant nevirapine used for prevention of MTCT of HIV.

ARVs generally should not be used if the risk of transmission is low (eg, trivial needlestick injury with a drug needle from an unknown nonoccupational source) or if care is sought more than 72 hours after the reported exposure. The benefits of postexposure prophylaxis are greatest when risk of infection is high, intervention is prompt, and adherence is likely. Consultation with an experienced pediatric HIV health care professional is essential. Detailed guidelines for postexposure prophylaxis for children can be found at **www.cdc.gov/hiv/pdf/programresources/cdc-hiv-npep-guidelines.pdf.**

Influenza

CLINICAL MANIFESTATIONS: Influenza typically begins with sudden onset of fever, often accompanied by chills or rigors, headache, malaise, diffuse myalgia, and nonproductive cough. Subsequently, respiratory tract signs and symptoms, including sore throat, nasal congestion, rhinitis, and cough, become more prominent. Conjunctival injection, abdominal pain, nausea, vomiting, and diarrhea less commonly are associated with influenza illness. In some children, influenza can appear as an upper respiratory tract illness or as a febrile illness with few respiratory tract symptoms. When influenza viruses are circulating in a community, the diagnosis of influenza should be considered in all children and adults (including health care personnel) with acute onset of respiratory symptoms, regardless of degree of symptoms, whether or not there is fever, and regardless of influenza vaccination status. Influenza is an important cause of otitis media. Acute myositis secondary to influenza can present with calf tenderness and refusal to walk. In infants, influenza can produce a nonspecific sepsis-like illness picture, and in infants and young children, influenza occasionally causes croup, pertussis like-illness, bronchiolitis, or pneumonia.

Although the large majority of children with influenza recover fully after 3 to 7 days, previously healthy children can have severe symptoms and complications. Neurologic complications associated with influenza range from febrile seizures to severe encephalopathy and encephalitis with status epilepticus, resulting in neurologic sequelae or death. Reye syndrome, which now is a very rare condition, has been associated with influenza infection and the use of aspirin therapy during the illness. Children with influenza or suspected influenza should not be given aspirin, and children with diseases that necessitate long-term aspirin therapy or salicylate-containing medication, including juvenile idiopathic arthritis or Kawasaki disease, should be recognized as being at increased risk for complications from influenza. Death from influenza-associated myocarditis has been reported. Invasive secondary infections or coinfections with group A streptococcus,

Staphylococcus aureus (including methicillin-resistant *S aureus* [MRSA]), *Streptococcus pneumoniae*, or other bacterial pathogens can result in severe disease and death.

ETIOLOGY: Influenza viruses are orthomyxoviruses of 3 genera or types (A, B, and C). Epidemic disease is caused by influenza virus types A and B, and both influenza A and B virus antigens are included in influenza vaccines. Type C influenza viruses cause sporadic mild influenza-like illness in children, and type C antigens are not included in influenza vaccines. Influenza A viruses are subclassified into subtypes by 2 surface antigens, hemagglutinin (HA) and neuraminidase (NA). Examples of these virus subtypes include H1N1 and H3N2 influenza A viruses. Specific antibodies to these various antigens, especially to hemagglutinin, are important determinants of immunity.

A minor antigenic variation within the same influenza A or B subtypes is termed *antigenic drift*. Antigenic drift occurs continuously and results in new strains of influenza A and B viruses, leading to seasonal epidemics. On the basis of ongoing global surveillance data, there have been only 5 times since 1986 that the vaccine strains in the influenza vaccine have not changed from the previous season.

Antigenic shifts, on the other hand, are major changes in influenza A viruses that result in new subtypes that contain a new HA alone or with a new NA. Antigenic shift occurs only with influenza A viruses and can lead to a pandemic if the new strain can infect humans and be transmitted efficiently from person to person in a sustained manner in the setting of little or no preexisting immunity. The virus type or subtype may have an effect on the number of hospitalizations and deaths that season. For example, seasons with influenza A (H3N2) as the predominant circulating strain have had 2.7 times higher average mortality rates than non–H3N2-predominant seasons. The 2009 influenza A (H1N1) pandemic combined both exceptional pediatric virulence and lack of immunity, which resulted in nearly 4 times as many pediatric deaths as usually recorded. Antigenic shift has produced 4 influenza pandemics in the 20th and 21st centuries. The 2009 pandemic was associated with 2 waves of substantial activity in the United States, which occurred in the spring and fall of 2009, extending well into winter 2010. During this time, more than 99% of virus isolates characterized were the 2009 pandemic influenza A (H1N1) virus. As with previous antigenic shifts, the 2009 pandemic influenza A (H1N1) viral strain subsequently has replaced the previously circulating seasonal influenza A (H1N1) strain in the ensuing influenza seasons.

Humans of all ages occasionally are infected with influenza A viruses of swine or avian origin. Human infections with swine influenza viruses have manifested as typical influenza-like illness, and confirmation of infection caused by an influenza virus of swine origin has been discovered retrospectively during routine surveillance typing of human influenza isolates. Human infections with avian influenza viruses are uncommon but may result in a spectrum of disease from mild respiratory symptoms and conjunctivitis to severe lower respiratory tract disease, acute respiratory distress syndrome (ARDS), and death. Most notable among avian influenza viruses are A (H5N1) and A (H7N9), both of which have been associated with severe disease and high case-fatality rates. Influenza A (H5N1) viruses emerged as human infections in 1997 and have since caused human disease in Asia, Africa, Europe, and the Middle East, areas where these viruses are present in domestic or wild birds. Influenza A (H7N9) infections were first detected in 2013 and have been associated with sporadic disease in China. As of 2017, Asian H7N9 is ranked as the influenza virus with the highest potential pandemic risk. No efficient or sustained human-to-human transmission has been detected, but when human infections occur, they are associated with severe illness and high mortality. Infection with a novel influenza A virus is a nationally notifiable disease and should be reported to the Centers for Disease Control and Prevention (CDC) through state health departments.

EPIDEMIOLOGY: Influenza is spread person to person, primarily through large-particle respiratory droplet transmission (eg, coughing or sneezing near a susceptible person), which requires close contact between the person who is the source and person who is the recipient, because droplets generally only travel short distances. Another indirect mode of transmission comes from hand transfer of influenza virus from droplet-contaminated surfaces to mucosal surfaces of the face (autoinoculation). Airborne transmission via small-particle aerosols in the vicinity of the infectious individual also may occur. Each year from 2010 through 2016, seasonal influenza epidemics were associated with an estimated 4.3 to 16.7 million medical visits, 140 000 to 710 000 hospitalizations, and 12 000 to 56 000 respiratory and circulatory deaths annually in the United States.

During community outbreaks of influenza, the highest incidence occurs among school-aged children. Secondary spread to adults and other children within a family is common. Incidence and disease severity depend in part on immunity developed as a result of previous experience (by natural disease) or recent influenza immunization with the circulating strain or a related strain. Influenza A and B viruses circulate worldwide, but the prevalence of each type and subtype can vary among communities and within a single community over the course of an influenza season. In temperate climates, seasonal epidemics usually occur during winter months. Peak influenza activity in the United States can occur anytime from November to May but most commonly occurs between January and March. Community outbreaks can last 4 to 8 weeks or longer. Circulation of 2 or 3 influenza virus strains in a community may be associated with a prolonged influenza season of 3 months or more and may produce bimodal peaks in activity. Influenza is highly contagious, especially among semienclosed institutionalized populations; other ongoing closed-group gatherings, such as schools and preschool/child care classrooms; or travelers who have returned from areas where influenza viruses may be circulating, including participants in organized tour groups, international mass gatherings, summer camps, or cruise or military ship passengers. Patients may be infectious 24 hours before onset of symptoms. Viral shedding in nasal secretions usually peaks during the first 3 days of illness and ceases within 7 days but can be prolonged in young children and immunodeficient patients for 10 days or even longer. Viral shedding is correlated directly with degree of fever.

Incidence of influenza in healthy children generally is 10% to 40% each year, but illness rates as low as 3% also have been reported, depending on the circulating strain. Tens of thousands of children visit medical clinics and emergency departments because of influenza illness each season. Influenza and its complications have been reported to result in a 10% to 30% increase in the number of courses of antimicrobial agents prescribed to children during the influenza season. Although bacterial coinfections with a variety of pathogens have been reported, medical care encounters for children with influenza are an important cause of inappropriate antimicrobial use.

Hospitalization rates among children younger than 2 years are similar to hospitalization rates among people 65 years and older. Rates vary among studies (190–480 per 100 000 population) because of differences in methodology and severity of influenza seasons. It is clear, however, that children younger than 24 months consistently are at a substantially higher risk of hospitalization than older children. Antecedent influenza infection sometimes is associated with development of pneumococcal or staphylococcal pneumonia in children. Methicillin-resistant staphylococcal community-acquired pneumonia, with a rapid clinical progression and a high fatality rate, has been reported in previously healthy children and adults with concomitant influenza infection. In the 2016–2017 influenza season, more than 40% of all children hospitalized with influenza had no known underlying conditions. Rates of hospitalization and morbidity attributable to complications, such as bronchitis and pneumonia, are greater in children with high-risk conditions, including pulmonary diseases such as asthma, metabolic diseases such as diabetes mellitus, hemoglobinopathies such as sickle cell disease, hemodynamically significant cardiac disease, immunosuppression, and neurologic and neurodevelopmental disorders.

Fatal outcomes, including sudden death, have been reported in both chronically ill and previously healthy children. Since 2004, the number of influenza-related deaths among children reported annually in nonpandemic seasons has ranged from 46 (2005–2006 season) to 171 (2012–2013 season); during the 2009–2010 season, the number of pediatric deaths recorded in the United States was 288. During the entire influenza A (H1N1) pandemic period lasting from April 2009 to August 2010, a total of 344 laboratory-confirmed, influenza-associated pediatric deaths were reported. Both influenza A and B viruses have been associated with deaths in children, most of which occurred in children younger than 5 years. Almost half of children who die do not have a high-risk condition as defined by the Advisory Committee on Immunization Practices (ACIP). All influenza-associated pediatric deaths are nationally notifiable and should be reported to the CDC through state health departments.

The **incubation period** usually is 1 to 4 days, with a mean of 2 days.

Influenza Pandemics. Influenza pandemics can lead to substantially increased morbidity and mortality rates compared with seasonal influenza. During the 20th century, there were 3 influenza pandemics, in 1918 (H1N1), 1957 (H2N2), and 1968 (H3N2). The pandemic in 1918 killed at least 20 million people in the United States and perhaps as many as 50 million people worldwide. The 2009 influenza A (H1N1) pandemic was the first in the 21st century, lasting from April 2009 to August 2010; there were 18 449 deaths among laboratory-confirmed influenza cases, although this is believed to represent only a fraction of the true number of deaths. On the basis of a modeling study from the CDC, it is estimated that the 2009 influenza A (H1N1) pandemic was associated with between 151 700 and 575 400 deaths worldwide. Public health authorities have developed plans for pandemic preparedness and response to a pandemic in the United States. Pediatric health care professionals should be familiar with national, state, and institutional pandemic plans, including recommendations for vaccine and antiviral drug use, health care surge capacity, and personal protective strategies that can be communicated to patients and families. Up-to-date information on pandemic influenza can be found at **www.pandemicflu.gov.**

DIAGNOSTIC TESTS: Influenza testing should be performed when the results are anticipated to influence clinical management (eg, to inform the decision to initiate antiviral therapy or pursue other diagnostic testing, to prescribe antibiotic agents, or to implement infection prevention and control measures). The decision to test is related to the level of suspicion for influenza, local influenza activity, and the sensitivity and specificity of commercially available influenza tests (Table 3.33, p 482), including rapid influenza molecular assays, reverse transcriptase-polymerase chain reaction (RT-PCR) assays, multiplex RT-PCR assays, immunofluorescence assays (direct fluorescent antibody [DFA] or indirect fluorescent antibody [IFA] staining), and rapid influenza diagnostic tests (RIDTs). Choice of influenza test depends on the clinical setting.

To diagnose influenza in the outpatient setting, upper respiratory tract (ie, nasopharyngeal or nasal) swab specimens should be collected as soon after illness onset as possible, preferably within 4 days of onset. The optimal respiratory tract swab specimen to collect depends on which influenza test is being used. Nasopharyngeal swab specimens have the highest yield of upper respiratory tract specimens for detection of influenza viruses. Midturbinate nasal swab specimens are acceptable. Testing with combined nasal and throat swab specimens may increase the detection of influenza viruses over single specimens from either site (particularly over throat swab specimens), depending on the test used, and is an option if nasopharyngeal swab specimens are not available. Using flocked swabs likely improves influenza virus detection over nonflocked swabs.

For inpatients without severe lower respiratory tract disease, nasopharyngeal, nasal, or combined nasal-throat swab specimens should be collected. For patients with respiratory failure receiving mechanical ventilation, including patients with negative influenza testing results on upper respiratory tract specimens, endotracheal aspirate or bronchoalveolar lavage (BAL) fluid specimens should be obtained. Nonrespiratory specimens such as blood, plasma, serum, cerebrospinal fluid, urine, and stool should not be collected or tested for seasonal influenza viruses. Specimens should be obtained, if possible, during the first 4 days of illness, because the quantity of virus shed decreases rapidly as illness progresses beyond that point.

Results of influenza testing should be properly interpreted in the context of clinical findings and local community influenza activity. Molecular tests have the best performance characteristics. RIDTs are significantly less sensitive than other methods and, therefore, produce more false-negative results. Some rapid diagnostic antigen tests cannot distinguish between influenza subtypes, a feature that can be critical during seasons with strains that differ in antiviral susceptibility and/or relative virulence (Table 3.33, p 482). Careful clinical judgment must be exercised, because the prevalence of circulating influenza viruses influences the positive and negative predictive values of these influenza screening tests. False-positive results are more likely to occur during periods of low influenza activity; false-negative results are more likely to occur during periods of peak influenza activity. Decisions regarding treatment and infection control can be made on the basis of positive rapid diagnostic test results. Positive results are helpful, because they may reduce additional testing to identify the cause of the child's influenza-like illness. Treatment should not be withheld in high-risk patients awaiting test results. Information about influenza surveillance is available through the CDC Voice Information System (influenza update, 888-232-3228) or through **www.cdc.gov/flu/**.

TREATMENT: In the United States, 2 classes of antiviral medications currently are approved for treatment or prophylaxis of influenza infections: neuraminidase inhibitors (oral oseltamivir, inhaled zanamivir, and intravenous peramivir) and adamantanes (amantadine and rimantadine). Guidance for use of these antiviral agents is summarized in Table 3.34. Oseltamivir remains the antiviral drug of choice. Zanamivir is an acceptable alternative but is more difficult to administer, especially in young children. Peramivir was approved in 2017 for use in children 2 years and older, although it has been approved for use in adults 18 years and older since 2014. Intravenous formulations are especially important for children who cannot absorb orally administered oseltamivir or cannot tolerate inhaled zanamivir. The US Food and Drug Administration (FDA) has approved oseltamivir for children as young as 2 weeks of age. Given preliminary pharmacokinetic data and limited safety data, oseltamivir can be used to treat influenza in both term and preterm infants from birth, because benefits of therapy are likely to outweigh possible risks of treatment.

Widespread resistance to adamantanes has been documented among H3N2 and H1N1 influenza viruses since 2005 (influenza B viruses intrinsically are not susceptible to adamantanes). Since January 2006, neuraminidase inhibitors have been the only influenza antiviral drugs recommended for use in influenza infections. Resistance to oseltamivir has been documented to be approximately 1% at most for any of the tested influenza viral samples during the past few years. These resistance patterns among circulating influenza A virus strains simplify antiviral treatment, as 2009 influenza A (H1N1), influenza A (H3N2), and influenza B all have been susceptible to neuraminidase inhibitors and resistant to adamantanes. Enhanced surveillance for influenza antiviral resistance is ongoing at the CDC in collaboration with local and state health departments. Each year, options for treatment or chemoprophylaxis of influenza in the United States will depend on influenza strain resistance patterns. Recommendations for influenza chemoprophylaxis and treatment can be found online (**www.cdc.gov/flu/professionals/antivirals/index.htm** or **www.aapredbook.org/flu**).

Treatment for influenza virus infection should be offered as early as possible, without waiting for confirmatory influenza testing, to any hospitalized child presumed clinically to have influenza disease or with serious, complicated, or progressive illness attributable to influenza, irrespective of influenza vaccination status or whether illness began greater than 48 hours before admission. Treatment also should be offered to influenza-infected children at high risk of complications from influenza, regardless of severity of illness. Treatment may be considered for any otherwise healthy child clinically presumed to have influenza disease. The greatest effect on outcome will occur if treatment can be initiated within 48 hours of illness onset, but treatment still should be considered if it is later in the course of progressive, symptomatic illness. Antiviral treatment also should be considered for children clinically presumed to have influenza disease and whose siblings or household contacts either are younger than 6 months or have underlying medical conditions that predispose them to complications of influenza. Children with severe influenza should be evaluated carefully for possible coinfection with bacterial pathogens (eg, *S aureus*) that might require antimicrobial therapy. Clinicians who want to have influenza isolates tested for susceptibility should contact their state health department.

If antiviral therapy is prescribed, treatment should be started as soon after illness on-. set as possible and should not be delayed while waiting for a definitive influenza test result, because early therapy provides the best outcomes.[1] The duration of treatment for the neuraminidase inhibitors oseltamivir and zanamivir is 5 days, and treatment with intravenous peramivir is 1 dose administered over 15 to 30 minutes. Recommended dosages for

---

[1]Centers for Disease Control and Prevention. Antiviral agents for the treatment and chemoprophylaxis of influenza: recommendations of the Advisory Committee on Immunization Practices (ACIP). *MMWR Recomm Rep.* 2011;60(RR-01):1–24

Table 3.33. Summary of Influenza Diagnostic Tests

Influenza Diagnostic Test	Method	Availability	Typical Processing Time	Sensitivity	Distinguishes Influenza A Virus Subtypes
Rapid influenza diagnostic tests[a]	Antigen detection	Wide	<15 min	10%–70%	No
Rapid influenza molecular assays[b]	RNA detection	Wide	<20 min	86%–100%	No
Nucleic acid amplification tests (including RT-PCR)	RNA detection	Limited	1–8 h	86%–100%	Yes
Direct and indirect Immunofluorescence assays	Antigen detection	Wide	1–4 h	70%–100%	No
Rapid cell culture (shell vials and cell mixtures)	Virus isolation	Limited	1–3 days	100%	Yes
Viral cell culture	Virus isolation	Limited	3–10 days	100%	Yes

RT-PCR indicates reverse transcriptase-polymerase chain reaction.

[a]Most rapid influenza diagnostic tests are Clinical Laboratory Improvement Amendments (CLIA) waived.

[b]Some rapid influenza molecular assays are CLIA waived, depending on the specimen.

Adapted from **www.cdc.gov/flu/professionals/diagnosis/rapidlab.htm.**

Table 3.34. Antiviral Drugs for Influenza[a]

Drug (Trade Name)	Virus	Administration	Treatment Indications	Chemoprophylaxis Indications	Adverse Effects
Oseltamivir (Tamiflu)	A and B	Oral	Birth or older[b]	3 mo or older	Nausea, vomiting
Zanamivir (Relenza)	A and B	Inhalation	7 y or older	5 y or older	Bronchospasm
Peramivir (Rapivab)	A and B[c]	Intravenous	2 y or older	N/A	Diarrhea; some reports of skin reactions
Amantadine[d] (Symmetrel)	A	Oral	1 y or older	1 y or older	Central nervous system, anxiety, gastrointestinal
Rimantadine[d] (Flumadine)	A	Oral	13 y or older	1 y or older	Central nervous system, anxiety, gastrointestinal

[a]For current recommendations about treatment and chemoprophylaxis of influenza, including specific dosing information, see **www.cdc.gov/flu/professionals/antivirals/index.htm** or **www.aapredbook.org/flu.**

[b]Approved by the FDA for children as young as 2 wk of age. Given preliminary pharmacokinetic data and limited safety data, the AAP believes that oseltamivir can be used to treat influenza in both term and preterm infants from birth because benefits of therapy are likely to outweigh possible risks of treatment.

[c]Peramivir efficacy is based on clinical trials in which the predominant influenza virus type was influenza A; a limited number of subjects infected with influenza B virus were enrolled.

[d]High levels of resistance to amantadine and rimantadine persist, and these drugs should not be used unless resistance patterns change significantly. Antiviral susceptibilities of viral strains are reported weekly at **www.cdc.gov/flu/weekly/fluactivitysurv.htm.**

drugs approved for treatment and prophylaxis of influenza are provided in Table 4.10 (p 966). Patients with any degree of renal insufficiency should be monitored for adverse events. Only zanamivir, which is administered by inhalation, does not require adjustment for people with severe renal insufficiency.

The most common adverse effects of oseltamivir are nausea and vomiting. Postmarketing reports, mostly from Japan, have noted self-injury and delirium with use of oseltamivir among pediatric patients, but other data suggest that these occurrences may have been related to influenza disease itself rather than antiviral therapy. An FDA review of controlled clinical trial data and ongoing surveillance has failed to establish a link between this drug (or any influenza antiviral medication) and neurologic or psychiatric events.[1] Zanamivir use has been associated with bronchospasm in some people and is not recommended for use in patients with underlying airway disease.

Control of fever with acetaminophen or another appropriate nonsalicylate-containing antipyretic agent may be important in some children, because fever and other symptoms of influenza could exacerbate underlying chronic conditions. Children and adolescents with influenza should not receive aspirin or any salicylate-containing products because of the potential risk of developing Reye syndrome.

ISOLATION OF THE HOSPITALIZED PATIENT: In addition to standard precautions, droplet precautions are recommended for children hospitalized with influenza or an influenza-like illness for the duration of illness.

CONTROL MEASURES:

Influenza Control in Peri- and Postpartum Settings. Strategies to decrease the likelihood of transmission from a mother to her newborn child during the birth hospitalization are provided at **www.cdc.gov/flu/professionals/infectioncontrol/peri-post-settings.htm.**

Influenza Vaccine. The influenza virus strains selected for inclusion in the seasonal vaccine may change yearly in anticipation of the predominant influenza strains expected to circulate in the United States in the upcoming influenza season.

The American Academy of Pediatrics (AAP) recommends annual use of inactivated influenza vaccines (IIVs) in all people 6 months and older. In the past, IIV contained the 3 virus strains (A [H3N2], A [H1N1], and B [1 of 2 lineages]), which were selected annually on the basis of influenza circulation in the southern hemisphere. In the 2013–2014 season, quadrivalent vaccines that contained both antigenically distinct lineages (ie, Victoria or Yamagata) of influenza B viruses, in addition to A (H3N2) and A (H1N1), were introduced. IIVs now are available in both trivalent (IIV3) and quadrivalent (IIV4) formulations. IIV4 is likely to offer broader protection than IIV3, especially if the circulating B strain is not included in the IIV3. Neither inactivated vaccine formation is preferred over the other.

IIVs contain no live virus. Those distributed in the United States are either subvirion vaccines, prepared by disrupting the lipid-containing membrane of the virus, or purified surface-antigen vaccines. The intramuscular (IM) IIV is licensed for administration to those 6 months and older and is available in both trivalent (IIV3) and quadrivalent (IIV4) formulations; the age indication varies among licensed IIVs for children. An intradermal

---

[1] Pediatric Advisory Committee Executive Summary for Tamiflu. Nutley, NJ: Hoffman-LaRoche Inc; November 2015. Available at: **www.fda.gov/ohrms/dockets/ac/05/briefing/2005-4180b_06_07_Tamiflu %20Executive%20Summary_Oct25.pdf**

(ID) formulation of IIV4 is licensed for use in people 18 through 64 years of age. This method of delivery involves a microinjection with a needle 90% shorter than needles used for IM administration. There is no preference for IM or ID immunization with IIV4 in people 18 years or older. A high-dose inactivated influenza vaccine is available for adults 65 years and older (**www.cdc.gov/flu/protect/vaccine/qa_fluzone.htm**).

An interim recommendation that intranasal quadrivalent live attenuated influenza vaccine (LAIV4) **not** be used in any setting in the United States was made in 2016 and continues through the 2017–2018 influenza season, although it is still licensed by the FDA for healthy people 2 through 49 years of age. In all pediatric age groups for the influenza seasons from 2013 through 2016, LAIV4 did not have any statistically significant benefit in preventing influenza, whereas IIV provided statistically significant protection, albeit to differing degrees by season. Children who received LAIV4 were almost 4 times more likely to become infected with an influenza virus than those who received IIV. No data have been published during the 2016–2017 season regarding laboratory-confirmed influenza to warrant rescinding this recommendation. The 4 vaccine strains in LAIV4 are attenuated, cold-adapted, temperature-sensitive viruses that replicate in the cooler temperature of the upper respiratory tract and stimulate both an immunoglobulin (Ig) A and IgG antibody response.

Two types of IIVs manufactured using egg-free technologies are available: cell culture-based inactivated influenza vaccine (ccIIV4) and recombinant influenza vaccine (RIV3 and RIV4). ccIIV4is indicated for people 4 years or older and is administered as an IM injection. ccIIV4 has comparable immunogenicity to US-licensed IIV4 comparator vaccines, and contraindications are similar to those for other IIVs. RIV3 and RIV4 are indicated for people 18 years or older and administered as an IM injection.

Immunogenicity in Children. Children 9 years and older require only 1 dose of influenza vaccine annually, regardless of their influenza immunization history. Children 6 months through 8 years of age who previously have **not** been immunized against influenza require 2 doses administered at least 4 weeks apart to produce a satisfactory antibody response (see Table 3.35). Significant protection against disease is achieved 1 to 2 weeks after the second dose. In subsequent years, children 6 months through 8 years of age may require 1 or 2 doses, depending on the child's age at the time of the first administered dose, his or her vaccine history, and the makeup of the current year's vaccine. A dosing algorithm for children 6 months through 8 years of age is prepared each year and can be found in the annual policy statement on influenza from the AAP published in September in *Pediatrics* and available at *Red Book* Online (**https://redbook.solutions.aap.org/redbook.aspx**).[1] Despite recent evidence for poor effectiveness of LAIV4, receipt of LAIV4 in the past is still expected to have primed a child's immune system and children who received 2 or more doses of LAIV4 in a previous season may receive only 1 dose of IIV for the current season. For children requiring 2 doses, vaccination should not be delayed to obtain a specific product for either dose. Any available, age-appropriate trivalent or quadrivalent vaccine can be used.

---

[1] American Academy of Pediatrics, Committee on Infectious Diseases. Recommendations for prevention and control of influenza in children, 2017–2018. *Pediatrics.* 2017;140(4):e20172550

Table 3.35. Schedule for Inactivated Influenza Vaccine (IIV) Dosage by Age[a]

Age	Dose, mL[b]	No. of Doses	Route[c]
6 through 35 mo	0.25	1–2[d]	Intramuscular (Fluzone)
	0.5	1–2[d]	Intramuscular (FluLaval, Fluarix)
3 through 8 y	0.5	1–2[d]	Intramuscular
9 y or older	0.5	1	Intramuscular
18 y or older (Intradermal)	0.1	1	Intradermal
18 y or older (Non–egg-based)	0.5	1	Intramuscular

[a]Manufacturers include Sanofi Pasteur (Fluzone Quadrivalent, split-virus vaccines licensed for people 6 months or older, Fluzone Intradermal Quadrivalent, split virus vaccine licensed for people 18 years and older, Fluzone High-Dose, split virus vaccine licensed for people 65 years and older), Sequirus (Afluria, split virus vaccine for people 5 years and older, Afluria Quadrivalent, split virus vaccine for people 18 years and older, Fluad, adjuvanted vaccine for people 65 years and older, Fluvirin, purified surface antigen, licensed for people 4 years or older, and Flucelvax, purified surface antigen, licensed for people 4 years and older), GlaxoSmithKline Biologicals (Fluarix Quadrivalent, split-virus vaccine licensed for people 6 months or older), ID Biomedical Corporation of Quebec (FluLaval Quadrivalent, split-virus vaccines licensed for people 6 months or older), and Protein Sciences (Flublok and Flublok Quadrivalent, recombinant vaccine licensed for people 18 years or older).

[b]From: Grohskopf LA, Sokolow LZ, Broder KR, et al. Prevention and control of seasonal influenza with vaccines: recommendations of the Advisory Committee on Immunization Practices—United States, 2017–18 influenza season. *MMWR Recomm Rep.* 2017;66(RR-2):1–20. Dosages are those recommended in recent years. Physicians should refer to the product circular each year to ensure that the appropriate dosage is given.

[c]For adults and older children, the recommended site of immunization is the deltoid muscle. For infants and young children, the preferred site is the anterolateral aspect of the thigh.

[d]Two doses administered at least 4 weeks apart are recommended for children younger than 9 years who are receiving IIV for the first time.

Vaccine Effectiveness. The effectiveness of influenza vaccines depends primarily on the age and immune competence of vaccine recipients, the degree of similarity between the viruses in the vaccine and those in circulation, and the outcome being measured. Protection against virologically confirmed influenza illness after immunization with IIV in healthy children older than 2 years ranges from 50% to 95%, depending on the closeness of vaccine strain match to the circulating wild strain. Effectiveness of IIV in children 6 through 23 months of age appears to be lower than in older children, although data are limited. The effectiveness of influenza immunization on acute respiratory tract illness is less evident in pediatric than in adult populations because of the frequency of upper respiratory tract infections and influenza-like illness caused by other viral agents in young children. Antibody titers for all seasonal influenza vaccines wane up to 50% of their original levels 6 to 12 months after immunization, necessitating annual influenza vaccination to maintain protection in all populations.

Coadministration With Other Vaccines. IIV can be administered simultaneously with other live and inactivated vaccines. During the 2 influenza seasons spanning 2010–2012, there were increased reports of febrile seizures in the United States in young children who received IIV and the 13-valent pneumococcal conjugate vaccine (PCV13) concomitantly, but this has not been observed in more recent seasons. Simultaneous administration of IIV and PCV13 continues to be recommended when both vaccines are indicated. Receipt of recommended childhood vaccines during a single visit has important benefits of protecting children against many infectious diseases; minimizing the number of visits that parents, caregivers, and children must make; and preventing febrile seizures by protecting children against influenza and pneumococcal infections, both of which can cause fever. Additional information can be found online (**www.cdc.gov/vaccinesafety/concerns/ FebrileSeizures.html**).

Recommendations for Influenza Immunization.[1,2] All people 6 months and older should receive influenza vaccine annually. Influenza vaccine should be administered as soon as available each year, preferably before the start of influenza season, at the time specified in the annual recommendations of the ACIP (**www.cdc.gov/flu/**). Providers should continue to offer vaccine until the vaccine expiration date (typically June 30, marking the end of the influenza season), because influenza is unpredictable. Protective immune responses persist throughout the influenza season, which can have more than 1 disease peak and may extend into March or later. Although the peak of influenza activity in the United States tends to occur in January through March, influenza activity can occur in early fall (ie, October and November) or late spring (eg, influenza circulated through the end of May during the 2013–2014 season). This approach also provides ample opportunity to administer a second dose of vaccine when indicated.

Particular focus should be on the administration of IIV for all children and adolescents with underlying medical conditions associated with an elevated risk of complications from influenza, including the following:

- Asthma or other chronic pulmonary diseases, such as cystic fibrosis.
- Hemodynamically significant cardiac disease.
- Immunosuppressive disorders or therapy (see Special Considerations, p 487).
- Human immunodeficiency virus (HIV) infection (see Human Immunodeficiency Virus Infection, p 459).
- Sickle cell anemia and other hemoglobinopathies.
- Diseases that necessitate long-term aspirin therapy or salicylate-containing medication, including juvenile idiopathic arthritis or Kawasaki disease, that may place a child at increased risk of Reye syndrome if infected with influenza.
- Chronic renal dysfunction.
- Chronic metabolic disease, including diabetes mellitus.
- Any condition that can compromise respiratory function or handling of secretions or can increase the risk of aspiration, such as neurodevelopmental disorders, spinal cord injuries, seizure disorders, or neuromuscular abnormalities.
- Pregnancy.

The AAP and CDC recommend vaccine administration at any visit to the medical home during influenza season when it is not contraindicated. Strategies to make seasonal influenza vaccine easily accessible for all children include alerts to families that vaccine is available (eg, e-mails, texts, and patient portals); creating walk-in influenza clinics; extending hours beyond routine times during peak vaccination periods; administering influenza vaccine during both well and sick visits; considering how to immunize parents, adult caregivers, and siblings at the same time in the same office setting as children; and working

---

[1]Centers for Disease Control and Prevention. Prevention and control of seasonal influenza with vaccines: recommendations of the Advisory Committee on Immunization Practices (ACIP)—United States, 2017–2018 influenza season. *MMWR Recomm Rep.* 2017;66(RR-2):1–20 (for updates, see **www.cdc.gov/flu**)

[2]American Academy of Pediatrics, Committee on Infectious Diseases. Recommendations for prevention and control of influenza in children, 2017–2018. *Pediatrics.* 2017;140(4):e20172550

with other institutions (eg, schools, child care programs, and religious organizations) or alternative care sites, such as emergency departments, to expand venues for administering vaccine. If a child or adult receives influenza vaccine outside of his or her medical home, such as at a pharmacy, retail-based clinic, or another practice, a system of patient record transfer is beneficial to ensuring maintenance of accurate immunization records.

Special Considerations. In children receiving immunosuppressive chemotherapy, influenza immunization may result in a less robust response than in immunocompetent children. The optimal time to immunize children with malignant neoplasms who must undergo chemotherapy is more than 3 weeks after chemotherapy has been discontinued, when the peripheral granulocyte and lymphocyte counts are greater than $1000/\mu L$ ($1.0 \times 10^9/L$). Children who no longer are receiving chemotherapy generally have high rates of seroconversion.

Children with hemodynamically unstable cardiac disease constitute a large group potentially at high risk of complications of influenza. The immune response to and safety of IIV in these children are comparable to immune response and safety in healthy children.

Corticosteroids administered daily for brief periods or every other day seem to have a minimal effect on antibody response to influenza vaccine. Prolonged administration of high doses of corticosteroids (ie, a dose of prednisone of either 2 mg/kg or greater or a total of 20 mg/day or greater or an equivalent) may impair antibody response. Influenza immunization can be deferred temporarily during the time of receipt of high-dose corticosteroids, provided deferral does not compromise the likelihood of immunization before the start of influenza season (see Vaccine Administration, p 26).

Pregnancy. Women, including adolescents, who will be pregnant or are considering pregnancy during influenza season should receive IIV, because pregnancy increases the risk of complications and hospitalization from influenza. Because intramuscular IIV is not a live-virus vaccine and rarely is associated with systemic reactions such as fever, influenza vaccine is considered safe during any stage of pregnancy. Studies have shown that infants born to women who received influenza vaccine have better influenza-related health outcomes. However, data suggest that only approximately half of pregnant women receive seasonal influenza vaccine, even though both pregnant women and their infants are at higher risk of complications, indicating that there remain opportunities to improve neonatal and infant health through vaccination of pregnant women. In addition, data from some studies suggest that influenza vaccination in pregnancy may decrease the risk of preterm birth as well as giving birth to infants who are small for gestational age. A 2017 case-control study found an association between spontaneous abortion in pregnant women and first trimester influenza vaccination when 2 consecutive annual influenza vaccinations were administered in the 2009–2019 and 2010–2011 influenza seasons, but not in the 2011–2012 season. Because of the small sample size and lack of biological plausibility, the ACIP and AAP have not recommended any changes to vaccination protocols as a result of this limited study. Further investigation is underway.

Close Contacts of High-Risk Patients. Immunization of people who are in close contact with children with high-risk conditions or with any child younger than 60 months (5 years) is an important means of protection for these children. In addition, immunization of pregnant women may benefit their unborn infants, because transplacentally acquired antibodies and human milk may protect infants from infection with influenza virus. Special outreach efforts for annual influenza immunization are recommended for the following people:

- Close contacts of infants younger than 6 months (see Recommendations for Influenza Immunization, p 486), because this high-risk group cannot be protected directly by immunization.
- Household contacts and out-of-home care providers of children younger than 5 years and at-risk children of all ages.
- Health care personnel (HCP) or health care volunteers.
- Any woman who is pregnant or considering pregnancy, is in the postpartum period, or is breastfeeding during the influenza season.
- Close contacts of immunosuppressed people.
- Children and adolescents of American Indian or Alaska Native heritage.
- Children who are members of households with high-risk adults (ie, adults with underlying medical conditions that predispose them to severe influenza infection or adults 50 years or older), any children 6 through 59 months of age, and children with HIV infection.

Health Care Personnel. The AAP recommends a mandatory annual immunization program for HCP, because they frequently come into contact with patients at high risk of influenza illness in their clinical settings.[1] Influenza vaccination of HCP has been shown to reduce both morbidity and mortality among patients. In the 2016–2017 influenza season, 42% of HCP reported having an influenza vaccination requirement at their institution. Since 2010, coverage among HCP who reported having such a requirement has exceeded 94% each year. Influenza vaccination coverage among HCP is not nearly as high in settings in which vaccination is promoted but not required (60%–84%), and is even lower in settings in which there is neither a requirement nor promotion (37%–57%). Higher coverage rates have been associated with offering vaccination on-site, over multiple days, and at no cost. A mandate is necessary to achieve herd immunity, reach *Healthy People 2020* objectives, and sufficiently protect people who come in contact with HCP. Influenza causes significant morbidity and mortality for both patients and HCP. A mandate is expected to cut costs and increase efficiency in health care settings. There has been widespread support and success by medical organizations and hospitals that have implemented mandatory influenza immunization for HCP.

Breastfeeding. Breastfeeding is not a contraindication for influenza immunization. Special effort should be made to vaccinate all women who are breastfeeding during the influenza season.

Reactions, Adverse Effects, and Contraindications. Although most IIV is produced in eggs and contains measurable amounts of egg protein, recent data have shown that IIV administered in a single, age-appropriate dose is well tolerated by recipients with egg allergy of any severity. Special precautions for egg-allergic recipients of IIV are not warranted, as the rate of anaphylaxis after IIV administration is no greater in egg-allergic than non–egg-allergic recipients or from other universally recommended vaccines. Standard immunization practice should include the ability to respond to rare acute hypersensitivity reactions. Patients who refuse to receive an egg-based vaccine may be vaccinated with age-appropriate recombinant or cell-cultured product.

Although a very slight increase in the number of cases of Guillain-Barré syndrome

---

[1]Bernstein HH; Starke JR; and the American Academy of Pediatrics, Committee on Infectious Diseases. Policy statement: influenza immunization for all health care personnel: keep it mandatory. *Pediatrics.* 2015;136(4):809–818

(GBS) was reported during the "swine flu" vaccine program of 1976, obtaining strong epidemiologic evidence for a possible limited increase in risk of a rare condition with multiple causes is difficult. GBS has an annual background incidence of 10 to 20 cases per 1 million adults, and during the 1976 swine influenza vaccine program, 1 case of GBS was reported per 100 000 people immunized. The risk of influenza vaccine-associated GBS was higher among people 25 years or older than among people younger than 25 years. If there is an association between seasonal influenza vaccine and GBS, the risk is rare, at no more than 1 to 2 cases per million doses. Whether influenza immunization specifically might increase the risk of recurrence of GBS is unknown. The decision not to immunize should be thoughtfully balanced against the potential morbidity and mortality associated with influenza for that individual.

Immunization of children who have asthma or cystic fibrosis with available IIV is not associated with a detectable increase in adverse events or exacerbations. IIV immunization for individuals with HIV infection is considered safe. HIV-infected children should receive annual influenza vaccination according to the HIV-specific recommended immunization schedule.

IIVs contain only inactivated subvirion or surface antigen particles and, therefore, cannot produce active influenza infection. The most common adverse events after IIV3 administration are local injection site pain and tenderness. Fever may occur within 24 hours after immunization in approximately 10% to 35% of children younger than 2 years but rarely in older children and adults. Mild systemic symptoms, such as nausea, lethargy, headache, muscle aches, and chills, may occur after administration of IIV3.

In children, the most common injection site adverse reactions associated with IIV4 administration are pain, redness, and swelling. The most common systemic adverse events are drowsiness, irritability, loss of appetite, fatigue, muscle aches, headache, arthralgia, and gastrointestinal tract symptoms. These events are reported with comparable frequency among participants receiving the licensed comparator trivalent vaccines.

The most common adverse events after administration of the ID formulation of IIV3 are redness, induration, swelling, pain, and itching, which occur at the site of administration; although all adverse events occur at a slightly higher rate with the IM formulation of IIV3, the rate of pain is similar between ID and IM. Headache, myalgia, and malaise may occur and tend to occur at the same rate as that with the IM formulation of IIV3. The most common solicited adverse reactions after ccIIV3 administration are injection site pain, erythema at the injection site, headache, fatigue, myalgia, and malaise. The most frequently reported adverse events for RIV3 are pain, headache, myalgia, and fatigue.

Chemoprophylaxis. Chemoprophylaxis should not be considered a substitute for immunization. If not contraindicated, influenza vaccine always should be offered, even after influenza virus has begun circulating in the community. Oseltamivir and zanamivir are important adjuncts to influenza immunization for control and prevention of influenza disease. However, recommendations for use of these drugs for chemoprophylaxis may vary by location and season, depending on susceptibility patterns. Pediatricians should inform recipients of antiviral chemoprophylaxis that the risk of influenza is lowered but still remains while taking medication, and susceptibility to influenza returns when medication is discontinued. Neither oseltamivir or zanamivir are a contraindication to immunization with IIV, and neither interferes with the immune response to IIV. For current recommendations about chemoprophylaxis against influenza, see

www.cdc.gov/flu/professionals/antivirals/index.htm or **www.aapredbook. org/flu/.**

Indications for Chemoprophylaxis. Although immunization is the preferred approach to prevention of infection, chemoprophylaxis during an influenza outbreak, as defined by the CDC, is recommended:

- For children at high risk of complications from influenza for whom influenza vaccine is contraindicated.
- For children at high risk during the 2 weeks after IIV immunization.
- For family members or HCP who are unimmunized and are likely to have ongoing, close exposure to:
  - unimmunized children at high risk; or
  - unimmunized infants and toddlers who are younger than 24 months.
- For control of influenza outbreaks for unimmunized staff and children in a closed institutional setting with children at high risk (eg, extended-care facilities).
- As a supplement to immunization among children at high risk, including children who are immunocompromised and may not respond to vaccine.
- As postexposure prophylaxis for family members and close contacts of an infected person if those people are at high risk of complications from influenza.
- For children at high risk and their family members and close contacts, as well as HCP, when circulating strains of influenza virus in the community are not matched with seasonal influenza vaccine strains, on the basis of current data from the CDC and local health departments.

These recommendations apply to routine circumstances, but it should be noted that guidance may change on the basis of updated recommendations from the CDC together with antiviral availability, local resources, clinical judgment, recommendations from local or public health authorities, risk of influenza complications, type and duration of exposure contact, and change in epidemiology or severity of influenza. Chemoprophylaxis is not recommended for infants younger than 3 months, unless the situation is judged critical, because of limited safety and efficacy data in this age group.

Kawasaki Disease

CLINICAL MANIFESTATIONS: Kawasaki disease is a self-limited vasculitis of medium-sized arteries, the diagnosis of which is made in patients with fever in addition to the presence of the following clinical criteria:

1. Bilateral injection of the bulbar conjunctivae with limbic sparing and without exudate;
2. Erythematous mouth and pharynx, strawberry tongue, and red, cracked lips;
3. A polymorphous, generalized, erythematous rash, often with accentuation in the groin, which can be morbilliform, maculopapular, scarlatiniform, or erythema multiform-like;
4. Changes in the peripheral extremities consisting of erythema of the palms and soles and firm, sometimes painful, induration of the hands and feet, often with periungual desquamation within 2 to 3 weeks after fever onset;
5. Acute, nonsuppurative, usually unilateral, anterior cervical lymphadenopathy with at least 1 node ≥1.5 cm in diameter.

The diagnosis of classic (or complete) Kawasaki disease is based on the presence of ≥5 days of fever and ≥4 of the 5 principal features described. In the presence of all 5 principal clinical criteria, particularly when erythema and swelling of the hands and feet are present and without an alternative explanation, the diagnosis may be made with only 4 days of fever. Individual clinical manifestations may appear and self-resolve rather than all being present simultaneously. It is important to question about previous presence of relevant manifestations when a patient seeks medical attention for persistent fever.

The correct diagnosis sometimes is delayed in patients who seek medical attention because of fever and unilateral neck swelling, which mistakenly is thought to be attributable to bacterial lymph node or para- or retropharyngeal infection. A distinguishing clinical and imaging feature in these cases is that suppuration is unlikely in Kawasaki disease. Concurrent viral upper respiratory infection sometimes is present in a patient with Kawasaki disease and, even if confirmed by virus detection, should not delay treatment of Kawasaki disease. (An exception is the patient with fever, exudative conjunctivitis, and exudative pharyngitis in whom adenovirus is detected. In such cases, Kawasaki disease is considered extremely unlikely.)

The following mucocutaneous or laboratory findings should prompt a search for an alternative diagnosis to Kawasaki disease: bullous, vesicular, or petechial rash; oral ulcers; pharyngeal or conjunctival exudates; generalized lymphadenopathy or splenomegaly; or leukopenia or relative lymphocyte predominance.

The diagnosis of incomplete Kawasaki disease should be considered in children with unexplained fever for ≥5 days plus fewer than 4 of the principal clinical criteria. Supportive laboratory data also are sought when considering the diagnosis of incomplete Kawasaki disease. In 2017, the American Heart Association (AHA) published updated guidelines for the diagnosis, treatment, and long-term management of Kawasaki disease.[1] The algorithm for diagnosis and treatment of suspected incomplete Kawasaki disease is reproduced in Fig 3.7. A high index of suspicion for Kawasaki disease should be maintained for infants, particularly those younger than 6 months, because compared with older children, infants have heightened risk of incomplete manifestations, delayed diagnosis, and development of coronary artery aneurysms. Kawasaki disease should be considered in infants younger than 6 months with prolonged unexplained fever, with or without aseptic meningitis, with evidence of systemic inflammation, even with fewer than 2 of the characteristic features of Kawasaki disease; in infants with a shock-like syndrome in whom an inciting infection is not confirmed; and in infants as well as older children when presumed cervical lymphadenitis or para- or retropharyngeal nonsuppurative infection fails to respond to appropriate antibiotic therapy.

If coronary artery aneurysm or ectasia is evident (z score ≥2.5) in any patient evaluated for fever, a presumptive diagnosis of Kawasaki disease should be made.

[1]McCrindle BW, Rowley AH, Newburger JW, et al; American Heart Association Rheumatic Fever, Endocarditis, and Kawasaki Disease Committee of the Council on Cardiovascular Disease in the Young; Council on Cardiovascular and Stroke Nursing; Council on Cardiovascular Surgery and Anesthesia; and Council on Epidemiology and Prevention. Diagnosis, treatment, and long-term management of Kawasaki disease: a scientific statement for health professionals from the American Heart Association. *Circulation*. Published online March 29, 2017; **http://circ.ahajournals.org/content/early/2017/03/29/CIR.0000000000000484**

FIG 3.7. EVALUATION OF SUSPECTED INCOMPLETE KAWASAKI DISEASE.[1,a]

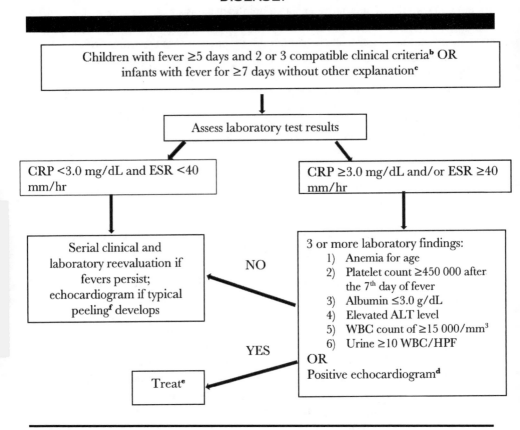

CRP indicates C-reactive protein; ESR, erythrocyte sedimentation rate; ALT, alanine transaminase; WBC, white blood cell; HPF, high-powered field.

[a]In the absence of a "gold standard" for diagnosis, this algorithm cannot be evidence based but rather represents the informed opinion of the expert committee. Consultation with an expert should be sought anytime assistance is needed.

[b]See text for clinical findings of Kawasaki disease.

[c]Infants ≤6 months of age are the most likely to develop prolonged fever without other clinical criteria for Kawasaki disease; these infants are at particularly high risk of developing coronary artery abnormalities.

[d]Echocardiography is considered positive for purposes of this algorithm if any of 3 conditions are met: z score of left anterior descending coronary artery or right coronary artery ≥2.5; coronary artery aneurysm is observed; or ≥3 other suggestive features exist, including decreased left ventricular function, mitral regurgitation, pericardial effusion, or z scores in left anterior descending coronary artery or right coronary artery of 2 to 2.5.

[e]Treatment should be given within 10 days of fever onset. See text for indications for treatment after the tenth day of fever.

[f]Typical peeling begins under the nail beds of fingers and toes.

[1]Source: McCrindle BW, Rowley AH, Newburger JW, et al; American Heart Association Rheumatic Fever, Endocarditis, and Kawasaki Disease Committee of the Council on Cardiovascular Disease in the Young; Council on Cardiovascular and Stroke Nursing; Council on Cardiovascular Surgery and Anesthesia; and Council on Epidemiology and Prevention. Diagnosis, treatment, and long-term management of Kawasaki disease: a scientific statement for health professionals from the American Heart Association. *Circulation.* Published online March 29, 2017; **http://circ.ahajournals.org/content/early/2017/03/29/CIR.0000000000000484**

A normal early echocardiographic study is typical and does not exclude the diagnosis but may be useful in evaluation of patients with suspected incomplete Kawasaki disease. In one study, 80% of patients with Kawasaki disease who ultimately developed coronary artery disease had abnormalities (z score $\geq$2.5) on an echocardiogram obtained during the first 10 days of illness.

Other clinical features of Kawasaki disease include irritability, abdominal pain, diarrhea, and vomiting. Other examination and laboratory findings include urethritis with sterile pyuria (70% of cases), mild anterior uveitis (80%), mild elevation of serum hepatic transaminase concentrations (50%), arthralgia or arthritis (10%–20%), meningismus with cerebrospinal fluid pleocytosis (40%), hydrops of the gallbladder (<10%), pericardial effusion of at least 1 mm (< 5%), myocarditis manifesting as congestive heart failure (< 5%), and cranial nerve palsy (< 1%). Persistent resting tachycardia and a hyperdynamic precordium are common findings, and an S3 gallop can be present. Fine desquamation in the groin area can occur in the acute phase of disease.[1] Inflammation or ulceration may be observed at the inoculation scar of previous bacille Calmette-Guérin immunization. Rarely, Kawasaki disease can present with acute shock; these children often have significant thrombocytopenia attributable to consumption coagulopathy, which also causes a low erythrocyte sedimentation rate (ESR). Group A streptococcal or *Staphylococcus aureus* toxic shock syndrome should be excluded in such cases.

The average duration of fever in untreated Kawasaki disease is 10 days; however, fever can last 2 weeks or longer. After fever resolves, patients can remain anorectic and/or irritable with decreased energy for 2 to 3 weeks. During this phase, branny desquamation of fingers, toes, hands, and feet and fine desquamation of other areas may occur. Transverse lines across the nails (Beau lines) sometimes are noted month(s) later. Recurrent disease develops in approximately 1% to 2% of patients in the United States a median of 1.5 years after the index episode. The recurrence rate is 3.5% in Asian and Pacific Islander people.

Coronary artery abnormalities are serious sequelae of Kawasaki disease, occurring in 20% to 25% of untreated children. Increased risk of developing coronary artery abnormalities is associated with male sex; age <12 months or >8 years; fever for more than 10 days; white blood cell count >15 000/mm^3; high relative neutrophil (>80%) and band count; low hemoglobin concentration (<10 g/dL); hypoalbuminemia, hyponatremia, or thrombocytopenia; and fever persisting or recurring >36 hours after completion of Immune Globulin Intravenous (IGIV) administration. Aneurysms of the coronary arteries most typically occur between 1 and 4 weeks after onset of illness; onset later than 6 weeks is extremely uncommon. Giant coronary artery aneurysms (internal diameter $\geq$8 mm) are highly predictive of long-term complications. Aneurysms occurring in other medium-sized arteries (eg, iliac, femoral, renal, and axillary vessels) are uncommon and generally do not occur in the absence of significant coronary abnormalities. In addition to coronary

---

[1] For further information on the diagnosis and management of Kawasaki disease, see McCrindle BW, Rowley AH, Newburger JW, et al; American Heart Association Rheumatic Fever, Endocarditis, and Kawasaki Disease Committee of the Council on Cardiovascular Disease in the Young; Council on Cardiovascular and Stroke Nursing; Council on Cardiovascular Surgery and Anesthesia; and Council on Epidemiology and Prevention. Diagnosis, treatment, and long-term management of Kawasaki disease: a scientific statement for health professionals from the American Heart Association. *Circulation.* Published online March 29, 2017; **http://circ.ahajournals.org/content/early/2017/03/29/CIR.0000000000000484**

artery disease, carditis can involve the pericardium, myocardium, or endocardium, and mitral or aortic regurgitation or both can develop. Carditis generally resolves when fever resolves.

In children with only mild coronary artery dilation, coronary artery dimensions often return to baseline within 6 to 8 weeks after onset of disease. Approximately 50% of coronary aneurysms (but only a small proportion of giant aneurysms) regress by echocardiography to normal luminal size within 1 to 2 years, although this process can result in luminal stenosis or a poorly compliant, fibrotic vessel wall or both.

The current case-fatality rate for Kawasaki disease in the United States and Japan is less than 0.2%. The principal cause of death is myocardial infarction resulting from coronary artery occlusion attributable to thrombosis or progressive stenosis. The relative risk of mortality is highest within 6 weeks of onset of acute symptoms, but myocardial infarction and sudden death can occur months to years after the acute episode. There is no current evidence that the vasculitis of Kawasaki disease predisposes to premature atherosclerotic coronary artery disease.

ETIOLOGY: The etiology is unknown. Epidemiologic and clinical features suggest an infectious and/or an environmental cause or trigger in genetically susceptible individuals.

EPIDEMIOLOGY: Peak age of occurrence in the United States is between 18 and 24 months. Fifty percent of patients are younger than 2 years, and 80% are younger than 5 years; cases are uncommon in children older than 8 years, but rare cases have occurred even in adults. The prevalence of coronary artery abnormalities is higher if treatment (IGIV) is delayed beyond the 10th day of illness. The male-to-female ratio is approximately 1.5:1. In the United States, 4000 to 5500 cases are estimated to occur each year; the incidence is highest in children of Asian ancestry. Kawasaki disease first was described in Japan, where a pattern of endemic occurrence with superimposed epidemic outbreaks was recognized. More cases, including clusters, occur during winter and spring. No evidence indicates person-to-person or common-source spread, although the incidence is tenfold higher in siblings of children with the disease than in the general population.

The **incubation period** is unknown.

DIAGNOSTIC TESTS: No specific diagnostic test is available. The diagnosis is established by fulfillment of the clinical criteria (see Clinical Manifestations, p 490) after consideration of other possible illnesses, such as staphylococcal or streptococcal toxin-mediated disease; drug reactions (eg, Stevens-Johnson syndrome); measles, adenovirus, Epstein-Barr virus, parvovirus B19, or enterovirus infections; rickettsial exanthems; leptospirosis; systemic-onset juvenile idiopathic arthritis; and reactive arthritis. The identification of a respiratory virus by molecular testing does not exclude the diagnosis of Kawasaki disease in infants and children who otherwise have met diagnostic criteria. A markedly increased ESR and/or serum C-reactive protein (CRP) concentration during the first 2 weeks of illness and an increased platelet count (>450 000/mm^3) on days 10 to 21 of illness are almost universal laboratory features. ESR and platelet count usually are normal within 6 to 8 weeks; CRP concentration returns to normal much sooner.

TREATMENT: Management during the acute phase is directed at decreasing inflammation of the myocardium and coronary artery wall and providing supportive care. Therapy should be initiated as soon as the diagnosis is established or strongly suspected. Once the acute phase has subsided, therapy is directed at prevention of coronary artery thrombosis.

Primary Treatment

Immune Globulin Intravenous (IGIV). A single dose of IGIV, 2 g/kg, administered over 10 to

12 hours, results in more rapid resolution of fever and other clinical and laboratory indicators of acute inflammation and has been proven to reduce the risk of coronary artery aneurysms from 17% to 4% in children with a normal first echocardiogram. IGIV plus aspirin (see below) is the treatment of choice and should be initiated as soon as possible in all patients when criteria of classic or incomplete Kawasaki disease are met and alternative diagnoses are unlikely, whether or not coronary artery abnormalities are detected. Despite prompt treatment with IGIV and aspirin, approximately 2% to 4% of patients develop coronary artery aneurysms even when treatment is initiated before the onset of coronary artery abnormalities.

Efficacy of therapy initiated later than the 10th day of illness or after detection of aneurysms has not been evaluated fully. However, therapy with IGIV and aspirin should be provided for patients in whom the diagnosis is made more than 10 days after the onset of fever (ie, the diagnosis was not made earlier) who have manifestations of continuing inflammation (ie, elevated ESR or CRP $\geq$3.0 mg/dL) plus either fever or coronary artery luminal dimension z score >2.5.

IGIV infusion reactions (fever, chills, hypotension) are not uncommon. A sometimes severe Coombs-positive hemolytic anemia can complicate IGIV therapy, especially in individuals with AB blood type, and usually occurs within 5 to 10 days of infusion. Aseptic meningitis can result from IGIV therapy and resolves quickly without neurologic sequelae. IGIV infusion results in elevation of the ESR; therefore, ESR is not a useful test to monitor disease activity after infusion; CRP is not affected by IGIV administration and can be used.

Aspirin. Aspirin is used for its anti-inflammatory (high-dose) and antithrombotic (low-dose) activity, although aspirin alone does not decrease the risk of coronary artery abnormalities. Aspirin is given in doses of 80 to 100 mg/kg per day in 4 divided doses when the diagnosis is made and concurrently with IGIV administration. Children with acute Kawasaki disease have decreased aspirin absorption and increased clearance and rarely achieve therapeutic serum concentrations. It generally is not necessary to monitor salicylate concentrations. High-dose aspirin therapy usually is given until the patient has been afebrile for 48 to 72 hours. Low-dose aspirin (3 to 5 mg/kg/day, in a single daily dose; maximum 81–325 mg/day) then is given until a follow-up echocardiogram at 6 to 8 weeks after onset of illness is normal or is continued indefinitely for children in whom coronary artery abnormalities are present. In general, ibuprofen should be avoided in children with coronary aneurysms taking aspirin, because ibuprofen and other nonsteroidal anti-inflammatory drugs with known or potential involvement of the cyclooxygenase pathway interfere with the antiplatelet effect of ASA to prevent thrombosis. Because of the theoretical risk of Reye syndrome in patients with influenza or varicella receiving salicylates, parents of children receiving aspirin should be instructed to contact their child's physician promptly if the child develops symptoms of or is exposed to either of these diseases. The child and all household contacts older than 6 months should receive influenza vaccine according to seasonal recommendations. The inactivated injectable influenza vaccine (not live attenuated vaccine) should be used in the child receiving aspirin. Family members can receive either inactivated or live attenuated (if recommended for that season; refer to the annual influenza policy statement from the American Academy of Pediatrics, usually published in September) influenza vaccine as appropriate for age and health status.

Adjunctive Therapies for Primary Treatment. The following are 2017 consensus recommendations of the AHA: (1) single-dose pulse methylprednisolone should not be administered with IGIV as routine primary therapy for patients with Kawasaki disease; and (2) administration of a longer course of corticosteroids (eg, prednisolone, 2 mg/kg/day, divided every 8 hours until afebrile, then an oral corticosteroid until CRP normalizes, with subsequent tapering over 2–3 weeks) together with IVIG and aspirin may be considered for treatment of high-risk patients with acute Kawasaki disease, when such risk can be identified before initiation of treatment.

Management of IGIV Resistance and Retreatment. Approximately 30% of patients who receive IGIV, 2 g/kg, plus aspirin have fever within the first 36 hours after completing the IGIV infusion, which is not an indication of therapeutic failure. However, 10% to 20% of treated patients have recrudescent or persistent fever beyond 36 hours after completion of their IGIV infusion and are termed IGIV-resistant. In these situations, the diagnosis of Kawasaki disease should be reevaluated. If Kawasaki disease still is considered to be most likely, retreatment with IGIV, 2 g/kg, usually is given and high-dose aspirin is continued. Several small series and observational studies have described children with IGIV-resistant Kawasaki disease in whom administration of a single dose of infliximab or a variety of regimens of corticosteroids was associated with an improvement of symptoms, without adverse events. Evidence of alteration of coronary artery outcomes associated with different therapies is limited.

Management of patients with Kawasaki disease refractory to a second dose of IGIV, infliximab, or a course of corticosteroids has included use of cyclosporine, another monoclonal drug (eg, anakinra), or plasma exchange.[1]

Cardiac Care.[1] Echocardiography should be performed at the time of suspected diagnosis and repeated at 2 weeks and 6 to 8 weeks after diagnosis. Children at higher risk—for example, children with persistent or recrudescent fever after initial IGIV or with baseline coronary artery abnormalities—may require more frequent echocardiograms to guide the need for additional therapies. Children should be assessed during this time for arrhythmias, congestive heart failure, and valvular regurgitation. The care of patients with significant cardiac abnormalities should involve a pediatric cardiologist experienced in management of patients with Kawasaki disease and in assessing echocardiographic studies of coronary arteries in children.

Long-term management of Kawasaki disease should be based on the extent of coronary artery involvement. In patients with persistent moderately large coronary artery aneurysms that are not large enough to warrant anticoagulation, clopidogrel (1 mg/kg, with consideration of lower dosing in infants) to antagonize ADP-mediated platelet activation in combination with prolonged low-dose aspirin are recommended.

Development of giant coronary artery aneurysms (luminal diameter ≥8 mm or larger in a child, but smaller diameter in an infant based on relative body surface area) usually

---

[1]For further information on the diagnosis and management of Kawasaki disease, see McCrindle BW, Rowley AH, Newburger JW, et al; American Heart Association Rheumatic Fever, Endocarditis, and Kawasaki Disease Committee of the Council on Cardiovascular Disease in the Young; Council on Cardiovascular and Stroke Nursing; Council on Cardiovascular Surgery and Anesthesia; and Council on Epidemiology and Prevention. Diagnosis, treatment, and long-term management of Kawasaki disease: a scientific statement for health professionals from the American Heart Association. *Circulation.* Published online March 29, 2017;
http://circ.ahajournals.org/content/early/2017/03/29/CIR.0000000000000484

requires addition of anticoagulant therapy, such as warfarin or low-molecular weight heparin, to prevent thrombosis. The AHA has provided recommendations regarding criteria for systemic anticoagulation and frequency of echocardiography in those with coronary aneurysms.[1]

Subsequent Immunization. Measles- and varicella-containing vaccines should be deferred until 11 months after receipt of IGIV, 2 g/kg, for treatment of Kawasaki disease because of possible interference with development of an adequate immune response. If the child's risk of exposure to measles or varicella within this period is high, the child should be immunized and then reimmunized at least 11 months after administration of IGIV (see Table 1.13, p 40). Live attenuated varicella-containing vaccines should be avoided during aspirin therapy because of a theoretical concern of Reye syndrome. If the child is receiving low-dose aspirin therapy and the risk of varicella exposure is high, or if aspirin therapy is prolonged beyond 11 months, benefits and theoretical risk of Reye syndrome should be discussed; usually, varicella vaccine is administered in this circumstance. The schedule for administration of inactivated childhood vaccines should not be interrupted.

ISOLATION OF THE HOSPITALIZED PATIENT: Standard precautions are indicated.

CONTROL MEASURES: None.

Kingella kingae Infections

CLINICAL MANIFESTATIONS: The most common infections attributable to *Kingella kingae* are pyogenic arthritis, osteomyelitis, and bacteremia. Other infections caused by *K kingae* include diskitis, endocarditis (*K kingae* belongs to the HACEK group of organisms), meningitis, and pneumonia. The vast majority of *K kingae* infections affect children between 6 and 48 months of age, with most cases occurring in children younger than 3 years.

K kingae is a primary cause of skeletal infections in the first 3 years of life. *K kingae* pyogenic arthritis generally is monoarticular and most commonly involves the knee, hip, or ankle. *K kingae* osteomyelitis most often involves the femur or tibia and has an unusual predilection for small bones, including the small bones of the foot. The clinical manifestations of *K kingae* pyogenic arthritis and osteomyelitis are similar to manifestations of skeletal infection attributable to other bacterial pathogens in immunocompetent children, although a subacute course may be more common. Brodie abscess of bone attributable to *K kingae* has been reported.

K kingae bacteremia can occur in previously healthy young children and in children with preexisting chronic medical problems. Children with *K kingae* bacteremia present with fever and frequently have concurrent symptoms of respiratory or gastrointestinal tract disease.

ETIOLOGY: *K kingae* is a gram-negative organism that belongs to the *Neisseriaceae* family. It is a fastidious, facultative anaerobic, β-hemolytic, small bacillus that appears as pairs or short chains with tapered ends and that often resists decolorization, sometimes resulting in misidentification as a gram-positive organism.

---

[1]Giglia TM, Massicotte MP, Tweddell JS, et al. Prevention and treatment of thrombosis in pediatric and congenital heart disease: a scientific statement from the American Heart Association. American Heart Association Congenital Heart Defects Committee of the Council on Cardiovascular Disease in the Young, Council on Cardiovascular and Stroke Nursing, Council on Epidemiology and Prevention, and Stroke Council. *Circulation.* 2013;128(24):2622–2703

EPIDEMIOLOGY: The usual habitat of *K kingae* is the human posterior pharynx. The organism colonizes young children more frequently than older children or adults and can be transmitted among children in child care centers, occasionally causing clusters of cases. Infection may be associated with preceding or concomitant stomatitis or upper respiratory tract infection.

The **incubation period** relative to acquisition of colonization is not well defined but presumably is variable.

DIAGNOSTIC TESTS: *K kingae* can be isolated from blood, synovial fluid, bone, cerebrospinal fluid, respiratory tract secretions, and other sites of infection. Organisms grow best in aerobic conditions with enhanced carbon dioxide. In patients with *K kingae* pyogenic arthritis or osteomyelitis, blood cultures often are negative. *K kingae* is difficult to isolate on routinely used solid media. Synovial fluid and bone aspirates from patients with suspected *K kingae* infection should be inoculated to both solid media and a blood culture system and held for 5 to 7 days to maximize recovery. Once recovered in culture, standard biochemical tests readily identify the organism; alternatively, mass spectrometry of bacterial cellular components may be used for rapid identification. When available, conventional and real-time polymerase chain reaction (PCR) methods markedly improve detection of *K kingae*, which should be suspected in young children with culture-negative skeletal infections. There currently are no PCR assays cleared by the US Food and Drug Administration for *K kingae*, and such tests are available only in specialty laboratories.

TREATMENT: Because some β-lactam antibiotic resistance is seen among isolates in the United States, ampicillin-sulbactam or a first-, second-, or third-generation cephalosporin is recommended for children with osteoarticular infections suspected to be attributable to *K kingae*. For more invasive or severe infections (eg, endocarditis), treatment with a third-generation cephalosporin or ampicillin plus an aminoglycoside should be considered.

K kingae usually is highly susceptible to penicillins and first-, second-, and third-generation cephalosporins. However, in vitro susceptibility to oxacillin is relatively reduced, and TEM-1 β-lactamase production has been reported in occasional isolates in parts of the United States and other countries, resulting in low-level resistance to penicillin and ampicillin. The TEM-1 β-lactamase is susceptible to β-lactamase inhibitors and lacks activity against second- and third-generation cephalosporins. Nearly all isolates are susceptible to aminoglycosides, macrolides, trimethoprim-sulfamethoxazole, tetracyclines, and fluoroquinolones. Between 40% and 100% of isolates are resistant to clindamycin, and virtually all isolates are resistant to vancomycin and trimethoprim (although most strains are susceptible to trimethoprim-sulfamethoxazole).

ISOLATION OF THE HOSPITALIZED PATIENT: Standard precautions are recommended.

CONTROL MEASURES: None. Although small clusters of cases have been reported in child care facilities in multiple countries, antimicrobial prophylaxis in contacts of a case is not standard practice. Prophylactic therapy has been used in the setting of an outbreak, and public health advice should be sought if more than a single case is identified in young children with close contact.

Legionella pneumophila Infections

CLINICAL MANIFESTATIONS: Legionellosis is associated primarily with 2 clinically and epidemiologically distinct illnesses: legionnaires' disease and Pontiac fever.

Legionnaires' disease varies in severity from mild to severe pneumonia characterized by fever, cough with or without chest pain, and progressive respiratory distress. Legionnaires' disease can be associated with chills and rigors, headache, myalgia, and gastrointestinal tract, central nervous system, and renal manifestations. Respiratory failure and death can occur. **Pontiac fever** is a milder febrile illness without pneumonia that is characterized by an abrupt onset of a self-limited, influenza-like illness (fever, myalgia, headache, weakness) resulting from host inflammation to the bacterium. Cervical lymphadenitis caused by *Legionella* species has been reported and may produce a syndrome clinically similar to nontuberculous mycobacterial infection.

ETIOLOGY: *Legionella* species are fastidious, small, aerobic bacilli that stain gram negative after recovery on buffered charcoal yeast extract (BCYE) media. They constitute a single genus in the family *Legionellaceae*. At least 20 of the more than 60 species have been implicated in human disease, but the most common species causing infections in the United States is *Legionella pneumophila*, with most isolates belonging to serogroup 1. Multiplication of *Legionella* organisms in water sources occurs optimally in temperatures between 25°C (77°F) and 42°C (108°F), although *Legionella* organisms have been recovered from water outside this temperature range.

EPIDEMIOLOGY: Legionnaires' disease is acquired through inhalation and microaspiration of aerosolized water contaminated with *Legionella* species. Only one case of possible person-to-person transmission has been reported. Most cases are sporadic and can be associated with travel or a stay in a health care facility; sporadic cases may be connected with unrecognized outbreaks or clusters. Outbreaks commonly are associated with buildings or structures that have complex water systems, like hotels and resorts, long-term care facilities, hospitals, and cruise ships. The most likely sources of infection include contaminated water aerosolized from showerheads, hot tubs, decorative fountains, and cooling towers (parts of centralized air-conditioning systems for large buildings). Health care-associated infections occur and often are related to contamination of the hot water supply. In patients who develop pneumonia during or after their hospitalization, legionnaires' disease should be considered in the differential diagnosis. Legionnaires' disease occurs most commonly in individuals who are elderly (≥50 years of age), are immunocompromised, have underlying lung or heart disease, are of male gender, are current or former cigarette smokers, exhibit end-stage renal failure, or have systemic malignancy. Infection in children is rare, with ≤1% cases of pneumonia caused by *Legionella*, and may be asymptomatic or mild and unrecognized. Severe disease has occurred in children with malignancy, severe combined immunodeficiency, chronic granulomatous disease, organ transplantation, end-stage renal disease, and underlying pulmonary disease and those treated with systemic corticosteroids or other immunosuppression. Health care-associated cases and outbreaks of infection in newborn infants have been associated with a contaminated water source and may result in severe illness.

The **incubation period** for legionnaires' disease (pneumonia) is 2 to 10 days, but may be up to 19 days; for Pontiac fever, the **incubation period** is 1 to 2 days but can be as short as 4 hours.

DIAGNOSTIC TESTS: When a patient is suspected of having legionnaires' disease, testing should include both culture of a lower respiratory tract swab specimen and urine antigen testing. Recovery of *Legionella* from respiratory tract secretions, lung tissue, pleural fluid, or other normally sterile fluid specimens by using supplemented BCYE media provides definitive evidence of infection, but the sensitivity of culture is laboratory dependent.

Specimens should be plated onto both supplemented, nonselective BCYE and selective BCYE containing appropriate antimicrobial agents and incubated at 35°C to 37°C for up to 14 days. Suspicious colonies commonly are identified by demonstrating growth dependence on L-cysteine followed by staining with specific fluorescein-labeled antibodies for *L pneumophila*.

Detection of *Legionella* lipopolysaccharide antigen in urine by commercially available immunoassays is highly specific. Such tests are sensitive for *L pneumophila* serogroup 1, but much less sensitive in patients infected with other *L pneumophila* serogroups or other *Legionella* species. Urinary antigen test sensitivity is also dependent on the assay method used and on the severity of disease.

Direct detection of the bacterium in respiratory tract swab specimens by direct immunofluorescent assay rarely is performed, because the specificity is technician dependent and the sensitivity is lower than that for culture or urine immunoassay.

Genus-specific polymerase chain reaction (PCR)-based assays have been developed that detect *Legionella* DNA in respiratory secretions as well as in blood and urine of some patients with pneumonia. There is a single PCR assay cleared by the US Food and Drug Administration available for detection of *Legionella* serotypes 1 through 14 in sputum.

Detection of serum immunoglobulin (Ig) M antibodies is not useful for diagnosis, and the positive predictive value of a single titer of ≥1:256 is low and does not provide definitive evidence of acute infection. A fourfold increase in antibody titer, as measured by indirect immunofluorescent antibody (IFA), confirms a recent infection. This serologic result is not useful for treatment decisions however, because convalescent titers take 3 to 4 weeks to increase (and the increase may be delayed for 8 to 12 weeks). Antibodies to several gram-negative organisms, including *Pseudomonas* species, *Bacteroides fragilis*, and *Campylobacter jejuni*, can cause false-positive IFA test results.

Because *Legionella* species are relatively inert biochemically, biochemical test systems are not helpful to identify *Legionella* organisms in culture. Mass spectrometry of cellular components shows promise as a rapid identification method.

TREATMENT: Patients with legionnaires' disease should receive antimicrobial agents. In immunocompetent patients, either intravenously administered azithromycin or levofloxacin (or another fluoroquinolone) is the drug of choice. Once the patient is improved clinically, oral therapy can be substituted. Levofloxacin (or another fluoroquinolone) is the drug of choice for immunocompromised children and adults and those with severe disease. Doxycycline and trimethoprim-sulfamethoxazole are alternative drugs. Duration of therapy is 5 to 10 days for azithromycin and 14 to 21 days for other drugs, with the longer courses of therapy for patients who are immunocompromised or who have severe disease. Doxycycline can be used for short durations (ie, 21 days or less) without regard to patient age (see Tetracyclines, p 905).

Antimicrobial treatment for patients with Pontiac fever is not recommended, because the disease results from host inflammation (not bacterial replication) and, thus, is self-limiting.

ISOLATION OF THE HOSPITALIZED PATIENT: Standard precautions are recommended.

CONTROL MEASURES: Adequate levels of disinfectant should be maintained in all building water systems. Hospitals should maintain hot water at the highest temperature allowable by state regulations or codes, preferably stored at 60°C (140°F) or greater with a minimum return temperature of 51°C (124°F); precaution should be taken to avoid scalding.

Cold water temperature should be maintained at less than 20°C (68°F) to minimize waterborne *Legionella* contamination. Occurrence of even a single laboratory-confirmed health care-associated case of legionellosis warrants consideration of an epidemiologic and environmental investigation. Hospitals with transplantation programs (solid organ or hematopoietic stem cell) should maintain a high index of suspicion of legionellosis, use sterile water for the filling and terminal rinsing of nebulization devices, and consider performing periodic culturing for *Legionella* species in the potable water supply of the transplant unit. Some hospitals may choose to perform periodic, routine culturing of water samples from the hospital's potable water system to detect *Legionella* species.

For emergency disinfection, superheating (to 71°C–77°C [160°F–170°F] or greater) and/or shock chlorination or targeted use of point-of-use water filters can be used. Measures for long-term decontamination of potable water supplies to prevent health care-associated cases are copper-silver ionization; addition of chlorine, monochloramine, or chlorine dioxide; and ultraviolet light. The most effective strategy for prevention of Legionnaires' disease in buildings with large or complex water systems is through the development and implementation of water management programs.[1]

Infection with *Legionella* species is a nationally notifiable disease in the United States.

Leishmaniasis

CLINICAL MANIFESTATIONS: The 3 main clinical syndromes are as follows:

- **Cutaneous leishmaniasis.** After inoculation by the bite of an infected female phlebotomine sand fly (approximately 2–3 mm long), parasites proliferate locally in mononuclear phagocytes, leading to an erythematous papule, which typically slowly enlarges to become a nodule and then an ulcerative lesion with raised, indurated borders. Ulcerative lesions may become dry and crusted or may develop a moist granulating base with an overlying exudate. Lesions can, however, persist as nodules, papules, or plaques and may be single or multiple. Lesions commonly appear on exposed areas of the body (eg, face and extremities) and may be accompanied by satellite lesions, sporotrichoid-like nodules, and regional adenopathy. Clinical manifestations of Old World and New World (American) cutaneous leishmaniasis generally are similar. Spontaneous resolution of lesions may take weeks to years—depending, in part, on the *Leishmania* species/strain—and usually results in a flat, atrophic scar.
- **Mucosal leishmaniasis (espundia)** traditionally refers to a metastatic sequela of New World cutaneous infection, which results from dissemination of the parasite from the skin to the naso-oropharyngeal/laryngeal mucosa; this form of leishmaniasis typically is caused by species in the *Viannia* subgenus. (Mucosal involvement attributable to local extension of cutaneous facial lesions has a different pathophysiology.) Mucosal disease usually becomes evident clinically months to years after the original cutaneous lesions have healed, although mucosal and cutaneous lesions may be noted simultaneously, and some affected people have had subclinical cutaneous infection. Untreated mucosal leishmaniasis can progress to cause ulcerative destruction of the mucosa (eg, perforation of the nasal septum) and facial disfigurement.

---

[1]Legionellosis: risk management for building water systems. ANSI/ASHRAE Standard 188–2015. Atlanta, GA: ASHRAE; 2015. Available at: **www.ashrae.org/resources--publications/bookstore/ansi-ashrae-standard-188-2015-legionellosis-risk-management-for-building-water-systems.**

- **Visceral leishmaniasis (kala-azar).** After cutaneous inoculation by an infected sand fly, the parasite spreads throughout the reticuloendothelial system (ie, within macrophages in spleen, liver, and bone marrow). The stereotypical clinical manifestations include fever, weight loss, hepatosplenomegaly, pancytopenia (anemia, leukopenia, and thrombocytopenia), hypoalbuminemia, and hypergammaglobulinemia. Peripheral lymphadenopathy is quite common in East Africa (eg, South Sudan). Some patients in South Asia (the Indian subcontinent) develop grayish discoloration of their skin; this manifestation gave rise to the Hindi term kala-azar ("black sickness"). Some patients develop post-kala-azar dermal leishmaniasis (referred to as PKDL) during or after treatment of visceral leishmaniasis. Untreated, advanced cases of visceral leishmaniasis almost always are fatal, either directly from the disease or from complications, such as secondary bacterial infections or hemorrhage. At the other end of the spectrum, visceral infection can be asymptomatic or oligosymptomatic. Latent visceral infection can reactivate years to decades after exposure in people who become immunocompromised (eg, because of coinfection with human immunodeficiency virus [HIV] or immunosuppressive/immunomodulatory therapy).

ETIOLOGY: In the human host, *Leishmania* species are obligate intracellular parasites of mononuclear phagocytes. Together with *Trypanosoma* species, they constitute the family *Trypanosomatidae*. Approximately 20 *Leishmania* species (in the *Leishmania* and *Viannia* subgenera) are known to infect humans. Cutaneous leishmaniasis typically is caused by Old World species *Leishmania tropica, Leishmania major,* and *Leishmania aethiopica* and by New World species *Leishmania mexicana, Leishmania amazonensis, Leishmania (Viannia) braziliensis, Leishmania (V) panamensis, Leishmania (V) guyanensis,* and *L (V) peruviana.* Mucosal leishmaniasis typically is caused by species in the *Viannia* subgenus (especially *L [V] braziliensis* but also *L [V] panamensis* and *L [V] guyanensis*). Most cases of visceral leishmaniasis are caused by *Leishmania donovani* or *Leishmania infantum (Leishmania chagasi* is synonymous). *L donovani* and *L infantum* also can cause cutaneous and mucosal leishmaniasis, although people with typical cutaneous leishmaniasis caused by these organisms rarely develop visceral leishmaniasis.

EPIDEMIOLOGY: In most settings, leishmaniasis is a zoonosis, with mammalian reservoir hosts, such as rodents or dogs. Some transmission cycles are anthroponotic: infected humans are the primary or only reservoir hosts of *L donovani* in South Asia (potentially also in East Africa) and of *L tropica.* Congenital and parenteral transmission also have been reported.

Overall, leishmaniasis is endemic in more than 90 countries in the tropics, subtropics, and southern Europe. Visceral leishmaniasis (0.2–0.4 million new cases annually) is found in focal areas of more than 60 countries: in the Old World, in parts of Asia (particularly South, Southwest, and Central Asia), Africa (particularly East Africa), the Middle East, and southern Europe, and in the New World, particularly in Brazil, with scattered foci elsewhere. Most (>90%) of the world's cases of visceral leishmaniasis occur in South Asia (India, Bangladesh, and Nepal), East Africa (Sudan, South Sudan, and Ethiopia), and Brazil.

Cutaneous leishmaniasis is more common (0.7 to 1.2 million new cases annually) and more widespread than visceral leishmaniasis. Cutaneous leishmaniasis is found in focal areas of more than 90 countries: in the Old World, in parts of the Middle East, Asia (particularly Southwest and Central Asia), Africa (particularly North and East Africa, with some cases elsewhere), and southern Europe, and, in the New World, in parts of Mexico, Central America, and South America (not in Chile or Uruguay). In addition, cases of cutaneous leishmaniasis have been acquired in Texas and occasionally in Oklahoma, and a cryptic case was diagnosed in a child in North Dakota. In general, the geographic distribution of leishmaniasis cases identified in the United States reflects immigration from and travel patterns to endemic regions.

The incubation periods for the various forms of leishmaniasis range from weeks to years. In cutaneous leishmaniasis, the primary skin lesions typically appear within several weeks of exposure. In visceral infection, the incubation period usually ranges from approximately 2 to 6 months.

DIAGNOSTIC TESTS: Definitive diagnosis is made by detecting the parasite (amastigote stages) in infected tissue (eg, of aspirates, touch preparations, or histologic sections) by light-microscopic examination of slides stained with Giemsa, hematoxylin, and eosin or other stains, by in vitro culture (not readily available), or increasingly by molecular methods (detection of parasite DNA by PCR testing). The latter are reported to be more sensitive than microscopy or culture, but none are currently cleared for use in the United States by the US Food and Drug Administration (FDA). In cutaneous and mucosal disease, tissue can be obtained by a 3-mm punch biopsy, lesion scrapings, or needle aspiration of the raised nonnecrotic edge of the lesion. In visceral leishmaniasis, although the sensitivity is highest (approximately 95%) for splenic aspiration, the procedure can be associated with life-threatening hemorrhage; bone marrow aspiration is safer and generally preferred. Other potential sources of specimens include liver, lymph node, and in some patients (eg, those coinfected with HIV), whole blood or buffy coat. Identification of the *Leishmania* species (eg, via isoenzyme analysis of cultured parasites or molecular approaches) may affect prognosis and influence treatment decisions. The Centers for Disease Control and Prevention (CDC) (**www.cdc.gov/parasites/leishmaniasis**) can assist in all aspects of diagnostic testing. Serologic testing usually is not helpful in the evaluation of potential cases of cutaneous leishmaniasis but can provide supportive evidence for the diagnosis of visceral or mucosal leishmaniasis, particularly if the patient is immunocompetent.

TREATMENT: Guidelines published in 2016 from the Infectious Diseases Society of America and the American Society of Tropical Medicine and Hygiene provide a detailed approach to diagnosis and treatment.[1] Systemic antileishmanial treatment always is indicated for patients with visceral or mucosal leishmaniasis, whereas not all patients with cutaneous leishmaniasis need to be treated or require systemic therapy (see Drugs for Parasitic Infections, p 985). Consultation with infectious disease or tropical medicine specialists and with staff of the CDC Division of Parasitic Diseases and Malaria is recommended (telephone: 404-718-4745; e-mail: **parasites@cdc.gov**; CDC Emergency Operations Center [after business hours and on weekends]: 770-488-7100). The relative merits of various treatment approaches/regimens for an individual patient should be considered, taking into account that the therapeutic response may vary, not only for different *Leishmania* species but also for the same species in different geographic regions. In addition, special considerations apply in the United States regarding the availability of particular

[1] Aronson N, Herwaldt BL, Libman M, et al. Diagnosis and treatment of leishmaniasis: clinical practice guidelines by the Infectious Diseases Society of America (IDSA) and the American Society of Tropical Medicine and Hygiene (ASTMH). *Clin Infect Dis.* 2016;63(12):e202-e264

medications. For example, the pentavalent antimonial compound, sodium stibogluconate, is not commercially available but can be obtained by US-licensed physicians through the CDC Drug Service (404-639-3670), under an investigational new drug (IND) protocol, for parenteral (intravenous or, less commonly, intramuscular) treatment of leishmaniasis. Liposomal amphotericin B is approved by the FDA for treatment of visceral leishmaniasis. The oral agent miltefosine is approved for treatment of cutaneous, mucosal, and visceral leishmaniasis; the FDA-approved indications are limited to infection caused by particular *Leishmania* species and to patients who are at least 12 years of age, weigh at least 30 kg (66 lb), and are not pregnant or breastfeeding during and for 5 months after the treatment course.

ISOLATION OF THE HOSPITALIZED PATIENT: Standard precautions are recommended.

CONTROL MEASURES: The best way for travelers to prevent leishmaniasis is by protecting themselves from sand fly bites. Vaccines and drugs for preventing infection are not available. To decrease the risk of being bitten, travelers should take the following measures:

- Stay in well-screened or air-conditioned areas when feasible. Avoid outdoor activities, especially from dusk to dawn, when sand flies generally are most active.
- When outside, wear long-sleeved shirts, long pants, and socks.
- Apply insect repellent on uncovered skin and under the ends of sleeves and pant legs. Follow instructions on the label of the repellent. The most effective repellents generally are those that contain the chemical N,N-diethyl-meta-toluamide (DEET) (see Prevention of Mosquitoborne and Tickborne Infections, p 195).
- Spray clothing items with a pyrethroid-containing insecticide several days before travel, and allow them to dry. The insecticide should be reapplied after every 5 washings. Permethrin should never be applied to skin.
- Spray living and sleeping areas with an insecticide.
- If not sleeping in an area that is well screened or air conditioned, a bed net tucked under the mattress is recommended. If at all possible, a bed net that has been soaked in or sprayed with a pyrethroid-containing insecticide should be used; the insecticide will be effective for several months if the bed net is not washed. Because sand flies are much smaller than mosquitoes and can penetrate through smaller holes, fine-mesh netting, which may be uncomfortable in hot weather, is needed for an effective physical barrier against sand flies (ie, if the bed net is not impregnated).
- Bed nets, repellents containing DEET, and permethrin should be purchased before traveling.

Leprosy

CLINICAL MANIFESTATIONS: Leprosy (Hansen disease) is a curable infection primarily involving skin, peripheral nerves, and mucosa of the upper respiratory tract. The clinical forms of leprosy reflect the cellular immune response to *Mycobacterium leprae* and, in turn, the number, size, structure, and bacillary content of the lesions. The organism has unique tropism for peripheral nerves, and all forms of leprosy exhibit nerve involvement. Leprosy lesions usually do not itch or hurt. They lack sensation to heat, touch, and pain but otherwise may be difficult to distinguish from other common maladies. There may be madarosis (loss of eyelashes or eyebrows). However, the stereotypical presentations of leonine facies with nasal deformity or clawed hands with loss of digits are manifestations of late-stage untreated disease that seldom are seen today. Although the nerve injury caused by leprosy is irreversible, early diagnosis and drug therapy can prevent sequelae.

Leprosy manifests over a broad clinical and histopathologic spectrum. In the United States, the Ridley-Jopling scale is used to classify patients according to the histopathologic features of their lesions and organization of the underlying granuloma. The scale includes: (1) tuberculoid, (2) borderline tuberculoid, (3) borderline, (4) borderline lepromatous, and (5) lepromatous. A simplified scheme introduced by the World Health Organization for circumstances in which pathologic examination and diagnosis is unavailable is based purely on clinical skin examination. Under this scheme, leprosy is classified by the number of skin patches seen on skin examination, classifying disease as either paucibacillary (1–5 lesions, usually tuberculoid or borderline tuberculoid) or multibacillary (>5 lesions, usually borderline, borderline lepromatous, or lepromatous). Patients in the tuberculoid spectrum have active cell-mediated immunity with low antibody responses to *M leprae* and few well-defined lesions containing few bacilli. Lepromatous spectrum cases have high antibody responses with little cell mediated immunity to *M leprae* and several somewhat-diffuse lesions usually containing numerous bacilli.

Serious consequences of leprosy occur from immune reactions and nerve involvement with resulting anesthesia, which can lead to repeated unrecognized trauma, ulcerations, fractures, and even bone resorption. Injuries can have a significant effect on life quality. Leprosy is a leading cause of permanent physical disability among communicable diseases worldwide. Eye involvement can occur, especially corneal scaring, and patients should be examined by an ophthalmologist. A diagnosis of leprosy should be considered in any patient with hypoesthetic or anesthetic skin rash or skin patches—especially those that do not respond to ordinary therapies—who have a history of residence in areas with endemic leprosy or where they may have had contact with armadillos.

Leprosy Reactions. Acute clinical exacerbations reflect abrupt changes in the immunologic balance. They are especially common during initial years of treatment but can occur in the absence of therapy. Two major types of leprosy reactions (LRs) are seen. Type 1 (reversal reaction, LR-1) is observed predominantly in borderline tuberculoid and borderline lepromatous leprosy and is the result of a sudden increase in effective cell-mediated immunity. Acute tenderness and swelling at the site of cutaneous and neural lesions with development of new lesions are major manifestations. Ulcerations can occur, but polymorphonuclear leukocytes are absent from the LR-1 lesion. Fever and systemic toxicity are uncommon. Type 2 (erythema nodosum leprosum, LR-2) occurs in borderline and lepromatous forms as a systemic inflammatory response. Tender, red dermal papules or nodules resembling erythema nodosum can occur along with high fever, migrating polyarthralgia, painful swelling of lymph nodes and spleen, iridocyclitis, and rarely, nephritis.

ETIOLOGY: Leprosy is caused by *M leprae*, an obligate intracellular rod-shaped bacterium that can have variable findings on Gram stain and is weakly acid-fast on standard Ziehl-Neelsen staining. It is best visualized using the Fite stain.[1] *M leprae* has not been cultured successfully in vitro. *M leprae* is the only bacterium known to infect Schwann cells of peripheral nerves, and demonstration of acid-fast bacilli in peripheral nerves is pathognomonic for leprosy. A newly described genomic variant, *Mycobacterium lepromatosis*, also has been implicated to cause leprosy, but the organism is not yet well characterized.

---

[1]Job CK, Chacko CJ. A modification of Fite's stain for demonstration of *M leprae* in tissue sections. *Indian J Lepr.* 1986;58(1):17–18

EPIDEMIOLOGY: Leprosy is considered a neglected tropical disease and is most prevalent in tropical and subtropical zones. It is not highly infectious. Several human genes have been identified that are associated with susceptibility to *M leprae,* and fewer than 5% of people appear to be genetically susceptible to the infection. Accordingly, spouses of leprosy patients are not likely to develop leprosy, but biological parents, children, and siblings who are household contacts of untreated patients with leprosy are at increased risk.

Transmission is thought to be most effective through long-term close contact with an infected individual and likely occurs through respiratory shedding of infectious droplets by untreated cases or individuals incubating subclinical infections. The 9-banded armadillo (*Dasypus novemcinctus*) is the only known nonhuman reservoir of *M leprae,* and zoonotic transmission is reported in the southern United States. There are unconfirmed reports of *M leprae* infection among 9-banded armadillos in Latin America as well as a 6-banded armadillo (*Euphractus sexcinctus*) in Brazil. People with human immunodeficiency virus (HIV) infection do not appear to be at increased risk of becoming infected with *M leprae.* However, concomitant HIV infection and leprosy can lead to worsening of leprosy symptoms during HIV treatment and result in immune reconstitution inflammatory syndrome. Like many other chronic infectious diseases, onset of leprosy is associated increasingly with use of anti-inflammatory autoimmune therapies and immunologic senescence among elderly patients.

There are approximately 6500 people with leprosy living in the United States, with 3500 under active medical management. During 1994–2011, there were 2323 new cases of leprosy, with an average annual incidence rate of 0.45 cases per 1 million people. Over this period, a decline in the rate of new diagnoses from 0.52 (1994–1996) to 0.43 (2009–2011) per million was observed. The annual incidence rate among foreign-born people in the United States decreased from 3.66 to 2.29, whereas the rate among people born in the United States was 0.16 in both 1994–1996 and 2009–2011.[1] Delayed diagnosis was more common among foreign-born people. The majority of leprosy cases reported in the United States occurred among residents of Texas, California, and Hawaii or among immigrants and other people who lived or worked in countries with endemic leprosy and likely acquired their disease while abroad. More than 65% of the world's leprosy patients reside in South and Southeast Asia, primarily India. Other areas of high endemicity include Angola, Brazil, the Central African Republic, Democratic Republic of Congo, Madagascar, Mozambique, the Republic of the Marshall Islands, South Sudan, the Federated States of Micronesia, and the United Republic of Tanzania.

The **incubation period** usually is 3 to 5 years but may range from 1 to 20 years. The average age at onset varies according to endemicity within the population. Younger patients (15 to 30 years of age) predominate in areas of high endemicity, and older average ages predominate in areas of low endemicity.

DIAGNOSTIC TESTS: There are no diagnostic tests or methods to detect subclinical leprosy. Histopathologic examination of a skin biopsy by an experienced pathologist is the best method of establishing the diagnosis and is the basis for classification of leprosy. These specimens can be sent to the National Hansen's Disease (Leprosy) Program (NHDP [800-642-2477; **www.hrsa.gov/hansensdisease**]) in formalin or embedded

---

[1]Centers for Disease Control and Prevention. Incidence of Hansen's disease—United States, 1994–2011. *MMWR Recomm Rep.* 2014;63(43):969–972

in paraffin. Acid-fast bacilli may be found in slit smears or biopsy specimens of skin lesions from patients with lepromatous forms of the disease but rarely are visualized from patients with tuberculoid and indeterminate forms of disease. A polymerase chain reaction test for *M leprae* is available to assist diagnosis after consultation with the NHDP and can be performed on the basis of clinical suspicion. Molecular tests for mutations causing drug resistance also are available, as is strain typing based on single nucleotide polymorphism and other genomic elements.

TREATMENT: Leprosy is curable. Therapy for patients with leprosy should be undertaken in consultation with an expert in leprosy. The National Hansen's Disease Program (NHDP; 800-642-2477) provides consultation on clinical and pathologic issues and information about local Hansen disease clinics and clinicians who have experience with the disease. Prevention of permanent nerve damage and disability is an important goal of treatment and care; a critical component of this is self-examination for any patient with loss of sensitivity in the foot. Combination antimicrobial multidrug therapy can be obtained free of charge from the NHDP in the United States and from the World Health Organization in other countries. Certain criteria must be met for physicians wishing to obtain the antimicrobial therapy from the NHDP (**www.hrsa.gov/hansensdisease/diagnosis/recommendedtreatment.html**).

It is important to treat *M leprae* infections with more than 1 antimicrobial agent to minimize development of antimicrobial-resistant organisms. Adults are treated with dapsone, rifampin, and clofazimine. Resistance to all 3 drugs has been documented but is extremely rare. The infectivity of leprosy patients ceases within a few days of initiating standard multidrug therapy.

Treatment Regimens Recommended by the NHDP.

Multibacillary Leprosy (6 Patches or More):

1. Dapsone, 1 mg/kg, orally, every 24 hours. Maximum dose: 100 mg/day for 24 months; **and**
2. Rifampin, 10 mg/kg per day for 24 months; 600 mg/day, orally, for 24 months; **and**
3. Clofazimine, which is available and may be obtained through the NHDP; clarithromycin for 24 months can be used in place of clofazimine for children.

Paucibacillary Leprosy (1–5 Patches):

1. Dapsone, 1 to 2 mg/kg, orally, every 24 hours (maximum dose: 100 mg/day for 12 months); **and**
2. Rifampin, 10 to 20 mg/kg per day, orally, for 12 months (maximum dose: 600 mg/day, orally, for 12 months).

Before beginning antimicrobial therapy, patients should be tested for glucose-6-phosphate dehydrogenase deficiency, have baseline complete blood cell counts and liver function test results (eg, transaminases) documented, and be evaluated for any evidence of tuberculosis infection, especially if infected with HIV. This consideration is important to avoid monotherapy of active tuberculosis with rifampin while treating active leprosy. Gastric upset and darkening of skin caused by daily clofazimine therapy are common adverse reactions to the therapy. Skin darkening typically resolves within several months of completing therapy.

Leprosy reactions should be treated aggressively to prevent peripheral nerve damage. Treatment with prednisone (1 mg/kg per day, orally) can be initiated. The severe type 2 reaction (erythema nodosum leprosum) occurs in patients with multibacillary leprosy. Treatment with thalidomide (100 mg/day for 4 days) is available for erythema nodosum leprosum under the Celgene S.T.E.P.S. Program (888-771-0141) and is used under strict supervision because of its teratogenicity. Thalidomide is not approved for use in children younger than 12 years. Most patients can be treated on an outpatient basis. Rehabilitative measures, including surgery and physical therapy, may be necessary for some patients.

All patients with leprosy should be educated about signs and symptoms of neuritis and cautioned to report signs and symptoms of neuritis immediately so that corticosteroid therapy can be instituted. Patients should receive counseling because of the social and psychological effects of this disease.

Relapse of disease after completing multidrug therapy is rare (0.01%–0.14%); the presentation of new skin patches usually is attributable to a late type 1 reaction (LR-1). When it does occur, relapse usually is attributable to reactivation of drug-susceptible organisms. People with relapses of disease require another course of multidrug therapy.

ISOLATION OF THE HOSPITALIZED PATIENT: Standard precautions are indicated; isolation is not required. Many patients suffer profound anxiety because of the stigma historically associated with leprosy.

CONTROL MEASURES: Leprosy is a reportable disease in the United States. Newly diagnosed cases should be reported to state public health authorities, the Centers for Disease Control and Prevention, and the NHDP. Normal hospital hygienic practices are advised. Hand hygiene is recommended for all people in contact with patients. Gloves are not required or recommended because of the associated stigma. Household contacts should be examined initially, but long-term follow-up of asymptomatic contacts is not warranted. Chemoprophylaxis is not recommended.

There are no vaccines approved for use in the United States. A single bacille Calmette-Guérin (BCG) immunization is reported to be from 28% to 60% protective against leprosy, and BCG is used as an adjunct to drug therapy in Brazil. However, BCG administration also may precipitate leprosy among subclinically infected individuals incubating the infection. The effectiveness of combined drug and immunotherapy is unknown.

Leptospirosis

CLINICAL MANIFESTATIONS: Leptospirosis is an acute febrile disease with varied manifestations. The severity of disease ranges from asymptomatic or subclinical to a self-limited febrile systemic illness (approximately 90% of patients) to a life-threatening illness that can include jaundice, renal failure (oliguric or nonoliguric), myocarditis, hemorrhage (particularly pulmonary), and refractory shock. Clinical presentation may be mono- or biphasic. Classically described biphasic leptospirosis has an acute septicemia phase usually lasting 1 week, during which time *Leptospira* organisms are present in blood, followed by a second immune-mediated phase that generally does not respond to antimicrobial therapy. Regardless of its severity, the acute phase is characterized by nonspecific symptoms, including fever, chills, headache, myalgia, nausea, vomiting, and conjunctival suffusion, occasionally accompanied by rash. Distinct clinical findings include notable conjunctival suffusion without purulent discharge (28%–99% of cases) and myalgia of the calf and lumbar regions (40%–97% of cases). Findings commonly associated with the immune-mediated phase include fever, aseptic meningitis, and uveitis; between 5% and 10% of

Leptospira-infected patients are estimated to experience severe illness; this phase usually requires supportive therapies. Severe manifestations include jaundice and renal dysfunction (Weil syndrome), pulmonary or other hemorrhage (which may involve gastrointestinal tract or brain), cardiac arrhythmias, and circulatory collapse. Abnormal potassium (high or low) and/or magnesium (low) levels may require aggressive management. The estimated case-fatality rate is 5% to 15% with severe illness, although it can increase to >50% in patients with pulmonary hemorrhage syndrome. Asymptomatic or subclinical infection with seroconversion is frequent, especially in settings of endemic infection.

ETIOLOGY: Leptospirosis is caused by pathogenic spirochetes of the genus *Leptospira*. Leptospires are classified by species and subdivided into more than 300 antigenically defined serovars and grouped into serogroups on the basis of antigenic relatedness. Currently, the molecular classification divides the genus into 23 named pathogenic (n=10), intermediate (n=5) and saprophytic (nonpathogenic; n=8) genomospecies as determined by DNA-DNA hybridization, 16S ribosomal gene phylogenetic clustering, and whole genome sequencing. This newer nomenclature supersedes the former division of these organisms into 2 species: *Leptospira interrogans*, comprising all pathogenic strains, and *Leptospira biflexa*, comprising all saprophytic stains found in the environment. All leptospires are tightly coiled spirochetes, obligate aerobic, with an optimum growth temperature of 28°C to 30°C.

EPIDEMIOLOGY: Leptospirosis is among the most globally important zoonoses, affecting people in resource-rich and resource-limited countries in both urban and rural contexts. It has been estimated that more than 1 million people annually worldwide are infected (95% confidence interval [CI], 434 000–1 750 000), with approximately 58 900 (95% CI, 23 800–95 900) deaths occurring each year. The reservoirs for *Leptospira* species include a wide range of wild and domestic animals, primarily rats, dogs, and livestock (cattle, pigs) that may shed organisms asymptomatically for years. *Leptospira* organisms excreted in animal urine may remain viable in moist soil or water for weeks to months in warm climates. Humans usually become infected via entry of leptospires through contact of mucosal surfaces (especially conjunctivae) or abraded skin with urine-contaminated environmental sources such as soil and water. Infection also may be acquired through direct contact with infected animals or their tissues, urine, or other body fluids. Epidemic exposure is associated with seasonal flooding and natural disasters, including hurricanes and monsoons. Populations in regions of high endemicity in the tropics likely encounter *Leptospira* organisms commonly during routine activities of daily living. People who are predisposed by occupation include abattoir and sewer workers, miners, veterinarians, farmers, and military personnel. Recreational exposures and clusters of disease have been associated with adventure travel, sporting events including triathlons, and wading, swimming, or boating in contaminated water, particularly during flooding or following heavy rainfall. Common history includes being submerged in or swallowing water during such activities. Person-to-person transmission is not convincingly described.

The **incubation period** usually is 5 to 14 days, range 2 to 30 days.

DIAGNOSTIC TESTS: Clinical features and routine laboratory findings of leptospirosis are not specific; a high index of suspicion must be maintained for the diagnosis. *Leptospira* organisms can be isolated from blood during the early septicemic phase (first week) of illness, from urine specimens 14 days or more after symptom onset, and from cerebrospinal fluid when clinical signs of aseptic meningitis are present. Specialized culture media are required but are not routinely available in most clinical laboratories. *Leptospira* organisms can be subcultured to specific *Leptospira* semi-solid medium (ie, EMJH) from blood culture bottles used in automated systems within 1 week of inoculation. However, isolation of the organism may be difficult, requiring incubation for up to 16 weeks, weekly darkfield microscopic examination, and avoidance of contamination. In addition, the sensitivity of culture for diagnosis is low. Isolated leptospires are identified by either serologic methods using agglutinating antisera or more recently by molecular methods.

For these reasons, serum specimens always should be obtained to facilitate diagnosis, and paired acute and convalescent sera are recommended. Antibodies can develop as early as 5 to 7 days after onset of illness; however, increases in antibody titer may not be detected until more than 10 days after onset, especially if antimicrobial therapy is initiated early. Antibodies can be measured by commercially available immunoassays, most of which are based on sonicates of the saprophyte *L biflexa*. These assays have variable sensitivity according to regional differences of the various *Leptospira* species. Further, in populations with high endemicity, background reactivity requires establishing regionally relevant diagnostic criteria and establishment of diagnostic versus background titers. Antibody increases can be transient, delayed, or absent in some patients, which may be related to antibiotic use, bacterial virulence, immunogenetics of the individual, or other unknown factors. Microscopic agglutination, the gold standard serologic test, is performed only in reference laboratories and seroconversion demonstrated between acute and convalescent specimens obtained at least 10 days apart is diagnostic.

Immunohistochemical and immunofluorescent techniques can detect leptospiral antigens in infected tissues. Polymerase chain reaction (PCR) assays for detection of *Leptospira* DNA in clinical specimens have been developed but are sensitive only in acute specimens and sometimes convalescent urine, are not approved by the FDA, and are available only in research laboratories. *Leptospira* DNA can be detected in whole blood during the first 7 days of illness, with highest sensitivity between days 1 and 4; *Leptospira* DNA can be found after 7 days of illness in urine and may be detectable for weeks to months in the absence of antimicrobial treatment.

TREATMENT: Antimicrobial therapy should be initiated as soon as possible after symptom onset. Intravenous penicillin is the drug of choice for patients with severe infection requiring hospitalization; penicillin has been shown to be effective in shortening duration of fever as late as 7 days into the course of illness. Penicillin G decreases the duration of systemic symptoms and persistence of associated laboratory abnormalities and may prevent development of leptospiruria. As with other spirochetal infections, a Jarisch-Herxheimer reaction (an acute febrile reaction accompanied by headache, myalgia, and an aggravated clinical picture lasting less than 24 hours) can develop after initiation of penicillin therapy. Parenteral cefotaxime, ceftriaxone, and doxycycline have been demonstrated in randomized clinical trials to be equal in efficacy to penicillin G for treatment of severe leptospirosis. For patients with mild disease, oral doxycycline has been shown to shorten the course of illness and decrease occurrence of leptospiruria; doxycycline can be used for short durations (ie, 21 days or less) without regard to patient age (see Tetracyclines, p 905). Ampicillin or amoxicillin also can be used to treat mild disease. Azithromycin has been demonstrated in a clinical trial to be as effective as doxycycline. Severe cases require appropriate supportive care, including fluid and electrolyte replacement. Patients with oliguric renal insufficiency require prompt dialysis, and those with pulmonary hemorrhagic syndrome may require mechanical ventilation to improve clinical outcome.

ISOLATION OF THE HOSPITALIZED PATIENT: In addition to standard precautions, contact precautions are recommended for contact with urine.

CONTROL MEASURES:

- Immunization of livestock and dogs can prevent clinical disease attributable to infecting serovars contained within the vaccine. However, immunization may not prevent the shedding of leptospires in urine of animals and, thus, contamination of environments with which humans may come in contact.
- In areas with known endemic infection, rodent-control programs may be useful in locations where they are an important contributor to human disease.
- Swimming, immersion, and swallowing water should be avoided in bodies of potentially contaminated fresh water.
- Protective clothing, boots, and gloves should be worn by people with potential occupational exposure to decrease their risk of infection.
- Doxycycline, 200 mg, administered orally once a week to adults, may provide effective prophylaxis against clinical disease and could be considered for high-risk groups (eg, triathletes) with short-term exposure, but infection may not be prevented, and adverse gastrointestinal tract events are common. Indications for prophylactic doxycycline use for children have not been established.

Listeria monocytogenes Infections
(Listeriosis)

CLINICAL MANIFESTATIONS: Listeriosis is a relatively uncommon but severe invasive infection caused by *Listeria monocytogenes*. Transmission predominantly is foodborne, and illness, especially with severe manifestations, occurs most frequently among pregnant women and their fetuses or newborn infants, older adults, and people with impaired cell-mediated immunity resulting from underlying illness or treatment (eg, organ transplant, hematologic malignancy, immunosuppression resulting from therapy with corticosteroid or anti-tumor necrosis factor agents, or acquired immunodeficiency syndrome). Pregnancy-associated infections can result in spontaneous abortion, fetal death, preterm delivery, and neonatal illness or death. In pregnant women, infections can be asymptomatic or associated with a nonspecific febrile illness with myalgia, back pain, and occasionally, gastrointestinal tract symptoms. Fetal infection results from transplacental transmission following maternal bacteremia. Approximately 65% of pregnant women with *Listeria* infection experience a prodromal illness before the diagnosis of listeriosis in their newborn infant. Amnionitis during labor, brown staining of amniotic fluid, or asymptomatic perinatal infection can occur.

Neonates can present with early-onset and late-onset syndromes similar to those of group B streptococcal infections. Preterm birth, pneumonia, and septicemia are common in early-onset disease (within the first week), with fatality rates of 14% to 56%. An erythematous rash with small, pale papules characterized histologically by granulomas, termed "granulomatosis infantisepticum," can occur in severe newborn infection. Late-onset infections occur at 8 to 30 days following term deliveries and usually result in meningitis with fatality rates of approximately 25%. Late-onset infection may result from acquisition of the organism during passage through the birth canal or, rarely, from environmental sources. Health care-associated nursery outbreaks have been reported.

Clinical features characteristic of invasive listeriosis outside the neonatal period or pregnancy are bacteremia and meningitis with or without parenchymal brain involvement, and less commonly brain abscess or endocarditis. *L monocytogenes* also can cause rhombencephalitis (brain stem encephalitis) in otherwise healthy adolescents and young adults. Outbreaks of febrile gastroenteritis caused by food contaminated with a very large inoculum of *L monocytogenes* have been reported. The prevalence of stool carriage of *L monocytogenes* among healthy, asymptomatic adults is estimated to be 1% to 5%.

ETIOLOGY: *L monocytogenes* is a facultatively anaerobic, nonspore-forming, nonbranching, motile, gram-positive rod that multiplies intracellularly. It has been assigned to the family *Listeriaceae* along with 5 other traditional and several newly named species. The organism grows readily on blood agar and produces incomplete hemolysis. *L monocytogenes* serotypes 1/2a, 4b, and 1/2b grow well at refrigerator temperatures (4°C–10°C).

EPIDEMIOLOGY: *L monocytogenes* causes approximately 1600 cases of invasive disease and 260 deaths annually in the United States. The saprophytic organism is distributed widely in the environment and is an important cause of illness in ruminants. Foodborne transmission causes outbreaks and sporadic infections in humans. Commonly incriminated foods include deli-style, ready-to-eat meats, particularly poultry; unpasteurized milk[1]; and soft cheeses, including Mexican-style cheese. Ice cream and fresh and frozen fruits and vegetables also have been implicated in recent outbreaks. Listeriosis is a relatively rare foodborne illness (approximately 1% of US cases) but is associated with a case-fatality rate of 16% to 20% (second only to *Vibrio vulnificus* at 35% to 39%) and causes 19% to 28% of all foodborne disease-related deaths. The US incidence of listeriosis decreased substantially during the 1990s, when US regulatory agencies began enforcing rigorous screening guidelines for *L monocytogenes* in processed foods and as better detection methods became available to identify contaminated foods.

The **incubation period** for invasive disease is longer for pregnancy-associated cases (2–4 weeks or occasionally longer) than for nonpregnancy-associated cases (1 to 14 days). The incubation period for self-limiting, febrile gastroenteritis following ingestion of a large inoculum is 24 hours; illness typically lasts 2 to 3 days.

DIAGNOSTIC TESTS: *L monocytogenes* can be recovered readily on blood agar from cultures of blood, cerebrospinal fluid (CSF), meconium, placental or fetal tissue specimens, amniotic fluid, and other infected tissue specimens, including joint, pleural, or peritoneal fluid. Attempts to recover the organism from clinical specimens from nonsterile body sites, including stool, should include the use of selective medium. Gram stain of meconium, placental tissue, biopsy specimens of the rash of early-onset infection, or CSF from an infected patient may demonstrate the organism. The organisms can be gram-variable and can resemble diphtheroids, cocci, or diplococci. Laboratory misidentification is not uncommon, and the isolation of a "diphtheroid" from blood or cerebrospinal fluid (CSF) should always alert one to the possibility that the organism is *L monocytogenes*.

A number of in-house developed polymerase chain reaction (PCR) assays have been described for detection of *L monocytogenes* in blood and CSF. At least one multiplexed PCR diagnostic panel designed to detect agents of meningitis and encephalitis in CSF cleared by the US Food and Drug Administration contains *L monocytogenes* as one of its target organisms; however, there are limited clinical data with the use of PCR for this purpose,

---

[1]American Academy of Pediatrics, Committee on Infectious Diseases and Committee on Nutrition. Consumption of raw or unpasteurized milk and milk products by pregnant women and children. *Pediatrics*. 2014;133(1): 175–179

and parallel culture of CSF also should be performed to allow for susceptibility testing and molecular characterization, especially for outbreak detection.

TREATMENT: No controlled trials have established the drug(s) of choice or duration of therapy for listeriosis. Combination therapy using ampicillin and a second agent is recommended for severe infections, including meningitis, encephalitis, endocarditis, and infections in neonates and immunocompromised patients. Therapy with intravenous ampicillin and an aminoglycoside, usually gentamicin, has been used traditionally. Use of an alternative second agent that is active intracellularly (eg, trimethoprim-sulfamethoxazole, fluoroquinolones, linezolid, or rifampin) is supported by case reports in adults. In the penicillin-allergic patient, options including either penicillin desensitization or use of either trimethoprim-sulfamethoxazole or a fluoroquinolone, both of which have been used successfully as monotherapy for *Listeria* meningitis and in the setting of brain abscess. If alternatives to gentamicin are used, susceptibility should be confirmed, because resistance to trimethoprim-sulfamethoxazole, fluoroquinolones, linezolid, or rifampin occasionally has been reported. Treatment failures with vancomycin have been reported. Cephalosporins are not active against *L monocytogenes*.

For bacteremia without associated central nervous system infection, 14 days of treatment is sufficient. For *L monocytogenes* meningitis, most experts recommend 21 days of treatment. Longer courses are necessary for patients with endocarditis or parenchymal brain infection (cerebritis, rhombencephalitis, brain abscess). Iron may enhance the pathogenicity of *L monocytogenes*; iron should be withheld from those with iron deficiency until treatment for listeriosis is complete. Diagnostic imaging of the brain near the end of the anticipated duration of therapy allows determination of parenchymal involvement of the brain and the need for prolonged therapy in neonates with complicated courses and immunocompromised patients.

ISOLATION OF THE HOSPITALIZED PATIENT: Standard precautions are recommended.

CONTROL MEASURES:

- Antimicrobial therapy for infection diagnosed during pregnancy may prevent fetal or perinatal infection and its consequences.
- Neonatal listeriosis complicating successive pregnancies is virtually unknown, and intrapartum antimicrobial therapy is not recommended for mothers with a history of perinatal listeriosis.
- General and specific guidelines for preventing listeriosis from foodborne sources are provided in Table 3.36.
- Trimethoprim-sulfamethoxazole, given as pneumocystis prophylaxis for those with acquired immunodeficiency syndrome, transplant recipients, or others on long-term, high-dose corticosteroids, effectively prevents listeriosis.
- Listeriosis is a nationally notifiable disease in the United States. Cases should be reported promptly to the state or local health department to facilitate early recognition and control of common-source outbreaks. Clinical isolates should be forwarded to a public health laboratory for molecular subtyping.

Table 3.36. Recommendations for Preventing Foodborne Listeriosis

General recommendations:
Washing and handling food
- **Rinse** raw produce, such as fruits and vegetables, thoroughly under running tap water before eating, cutting, or cooking. Even if the produce will be peeled, it should still be washed first.
- **Scrub** firm produce, such as melons and cucumbers, with a clean produce brush.
- **Dry** the produce with a clean cloth or paper towel.
- **Separate** uncooked meats and poultry from vegetables, cooked foods, and ready-to-eat foods.

Keep your kitchen and environment cleaner and safer
- Wash hands, knives, countertops, and cutting boards after handling and preparing uncooked foods.
- Be aware that *Listeria monocytogenes* can grow in foods in the refrigerator. Use an appliance thermometer, such as a refrigerator thermometer, to check the temperature inside your refrigerator. The refrigerator temperature should be 40°F or lower and the freezer temperature should be 0°F or lower.
- Clean up all spills in your refrigerator right away–especially juices from hot dog and lunch meat packages, raw meat, and raw poultry.
- Clean the inside walls and shelves of your refrigerator with hot water and liquid soap, then rinse.

Cook meat and poultry thoroughly
- Thoroughly cook raw food from animal sources, such as beef, pork, or poultry to a safe internal temperature. For a list of recommended temperatures for meat and poultry, visit the safe minimum cooking temperatures chart at **FoodSafety.gov (www.foodsafety.gov/keep/charts/mintemp.html)**.

Store foods safely
- Use precooked or ready-to-eat food as soon as you can. Do not store the product in the refrigerator beyond the use-by date; follow USDA refrigerator storage time guidelines:
  - ◆ Hot dogs – store opened package no longer than 1 week and unopened package no longer than 2 weeks in the refrigerator.
  - ◆ Luncheon and deli meat – store factory-sealed, unopened package no longer than 2 weeks. Store opened packages and meat sliced at a local deli no longer than 3 to 5 days in the refrigerator.
- Divide leftovers into shallow containers to promote rapid, even cooling. Cover with airtight lids or enclose in plastic wrap or aluminum foil. Use leftovers within 3 to 4 days.

Choose safer foods
- Do not drink raw (unpasteurized) milk[a] **(www.cdc.gov/foodsafety/rawmilk/raw-milk-index.html** and **http://pediatrics.aappublications.org/content/pediatrics/early/2013/12/10/peds.2013-3502.full.pdf)**, and do not eat foods that have unpasteurized milk in them.
- Find more specific information about this topic on the Listeriosis Prevention (**www.cdc.gov/foodsafety/specific-foods/listeria-and-food.html**) Web page.

Recommendations for people at higher risk, such as pregnant women, people with weakened immune systems, and older adults, in addition to the recommendations listed above:
Meats
- Do not eat hot dogs, luncheon meats, cold cuts, other deli meats (eg, bologna), or fermented or dry sausages unless they are heated to an internal temperature of 165°F or until steaming hot just before serving.
- Avoid getting fluid from hot dog and lunch meat packages on other foods, utensils, and food preparation surfaces, and wash hands after handling hot dogs, luncheon meats, and deli meats.

Table 3.36. Recommendations for Preventing Foodborne Listeriosis, continued

- Pay attention to labels. Do not eat refrigerated pâté or meat spreads from a deli or meat counter or from the refrigerated section of a store. Foods that do not need refrigeration, like canned or shelf-stable pâté and meat spreads, are safe to eat. Refrigerate after opening.

Soft cheeses

- Do not eat soft cheese, such as feta, queso blanco, queso fresco, brie, Camembert, blue-veined, or panela (queso panela) unless it is labeled as made with pasteurized milk. Make sure the label says, "MADE WITH PASTEURIZED MILK."
- Be aware that Mexican-style cheeses made from pasteurized milk, such as queso fresco, likely contaminated during cheese-making, have caused *Listeria* infections.

Seafood

- Do not eat refrigerated smoked seafood, unless it is contained in a cooked dish, such as a casserole, or unless it is a canned or shelf-stable product.
- Refrigerated smoked seafood, such as salmon, trout, whitefish, cod, tuna, and mackerel, is most often labeled as "nova-style," "lox," "kippered," "smoked," or "jerky." These fish typically are found in the refrigerator section or sold at seafood and deli counters of grocery stores and delicatessens. Canned and shelf-stable tuna, salmon, and other fish products are safe to eat.

Safety tips for eating melons

- Consumers and food preparers should wash their hands with warm water and soap for at least 20 seconds *before* and *after* handling any whole melon such as cantaloupe, watermelon, or honeydew.
- Scrub the surface of melons, such as cantaloupes, with a clean produce brush under running water and dry them with a clean cloth or paper towel before cutting. Be sure that your scrub brush is sanitized after each use to avoid transferring bacteria between melons.
- Promptly consume cut melon or refrigerate promptly. Keep your cut melon refrigerated at, or less than 40°F (32°F–34°F is best) for no more than 7 days.
- Discard cut melons left at room temperature for more than 4 hours.

[a]American Academy of Pediatrics, Committee on Infectious Diseases and Committee on Nutrition. Consumption of raw or unpasteurized milk and milk products by pregnant women and children. *Pediatrics*. 2014;133(1):175-179

Lyme Disease[1,2]

(Lyme Borreliosis, *Borrelia burgdorferi* sensu lato Infection)

CLINICAL MANIFESTATIONS: Clinical manifestations of Lyme disease are divided into 3 stages: early localized, early disseminated, and late manifestations. Early localized disease is characterized by a distinctive lesion, erythema migrans, at the site of a recent tick bite. Erythema migrans is by far the most common manifestation of Lyme disease in children. Erythema migrans begins as a red macule or papule that usually expands over days to weeks to form a large (≥5 cm in diameter) annular, erythematous lesion, sometimes with partial central clearing. The lesion usually but not always is painless, and it usually is not

[1]Wormser GP, Dattwyler RJ, Shapiro ED, et al. The clinical assessment, treatment, and prevention of Lyme disease, human granulocytic anaplasmosis, and babesiosis: clinical practice guidelines by the Infectious Diseases Society of America. *Clin Infect Dis*. 2006;43(9):1089–1134

[2]Lantos PM, Charini WA, Medoff G, et al. Final report of the Lyme Disease Review Panel of the Infectious Diseases Society of America. *Clin Infect Dis*. 2010;51(1):1–5

pruritic. Localized erythema migrans can vary greatly in size and shape and can be confused with cellulitis; lesions may have a purplish discoloration or central vesicular or necrotic areas. A classic "bulls-eye" appearance with concentric rings appears in a minority of cases. Factors that distinguish erythema migrans from local allergic reaction to a tick bite include larger size (≥ 5 cm), gradual expansion, less pruritus, and slower onset. Constitutional symptoms, such as malaise, headache, mild neck stiffness, myalgia, and arthralgia, often accompany erythema migrans. Fever may be present but is not universal and generally is mild.

In early disseminated disease, multiple erythema migrans lesions may appear several weeks after an infective tick bite and consist of secondary annular, erythematous lesions similar to but usually smaller than the primary lesion. Other manifestations of early disseminated illness (which may occur with or without a skin lesion) are palsies of the cranial nerves (most commonly cranial nerve VII), lymphocytic meningitis (often associated with cranial neuropathy or papilledema), and radiculitis. Carditis usually manifests as various degrees of atrioventricular block and can be life threatening. Although carditis occurs less commonly in children than in adults with Lyme disease, young adult males appear to be most prone. Systemic symptoms, such as low-grade fever, arthralgia, myalgia, headache, and fatigue may be present during the early disseminated stage.

Patients with early Lyme disease can be infected simultaneously with *Borrelia miyamotoi* and agents of babesiosis and anaplasmosis (see Babesiosis, p 235; *Ehrlichia, Anaplasma,* and Related Infections, p 323; and Borrelia Infections, p 252). These diagnoses should be suspected in patients who manifest high fever or hematologic abnormalities or who do not respond as expected to therapy prescribed for Lyme disease. Additionally, patients who contract Lyme disease may be coinfected with Powassan virus (deer tick virus) if bitten in the United States or with tickborne encephalitis virus if infection was acquired in Europe.

Late Lyme disease occurs in patients who are not treated at an earlier stage of illness and most commonly manifests as Lyme arthritis in children. Lyme arthritis is characterized by inflammatory arthritis that usually is mono- or pauciarticular and affects large joints, particularly the knees. Although arthralgia can be present at any stage of Lyme disease, Lyme arthritis has objective evidence of joint swelling as well as white blood cells in synovial fluid specimens. Arthritis can occur without a history of earlier stages of illness (including erythema migrans). Compared with pyogenic arthritis, Lyme arthritis tends to manifest with joint swelling/effusion out of proportion to pain or disability and with lower peripheral blood neutrophilia and erythrocyte sedimentation rate (ESR). Polyneuropathy, encephalopathy, and encephalitis are rare late manifestations. Children who are treated with antimicrobial agents in the early stage of disease almost never develop late manifestations.

Other clinical manifestations include ophthalmic conditions such as conjunctivitis, optic neuritis, keratitis, and uveitis.

Lyme disease is not thought to produce a congenital infection syndrome. No causal relationship between maternal Lyme disease and abnormalities of pregnancy or congenital disease caused by *Borrelia burgdorferi* sensu lato has been documented. No evidence exists that Lyme disease can be transmitted via human milk.

ETIOLOGY: In the United States, Lyme disease is caused by the spirochete *B burgdorferi* sensu stricto (hereafter referred to as *B burgdorferi*) and rarely by the recently discovered *Borrelia mayonii*. In Eurasia, *B burgdorferi, Borrelia afzelii,* and *Borrelia garinii* cause borreliosis. *Borrelia* species are members of the family *Spirochaetaceae,* which also includes *Treponema* species.

EPIDEMIOLOGY: In 2015, there were 28 453 confirmed cases of Lyme disease in the United States, although the actual number of cases may be up to 10-fold greater because of underreporting. Lyme disease occurs primarily in 2 distinct geographic regions of the United States, with more than 90% of cases occurring in New England and the eastern Mid-Atlantic States, as far south as Virginia. The disease also occurs, but with lower frequency, in the upper Midwest, especially Wisconsin and Minnesota. The geographic range is not static and has expanded considerably in the eastern and Midwestern states since 2000. Transmission also occurs at a low level on the west coast, especially northern California. The occurrence of cases in the United States correlates with the distribution and frequency of infected tick vectors—*Ixodes scapularis* in the east and Midwest and *Ixodes pacificus* in the west. In Southern states, *I scapularis* ticks are rarer than in the northeast; those ticks that are present do not commonly feed on competent reservoir mammals and are less likely to bite humans because of different questing habits. Reported cases from states without known endemic transmission may have been imported from endemic states or may be misdiagnoses resulting from false-positive serologic test results or results that are misinterpreted as positive.

The majority of cases of early localized and early disseminated Lyme disease occur between April and October; more than 50% of cases occur during June and July. People of all ages can be affected, but the incidence in the United States is highest among children 5 through 9 years of age and adults 55 through 59 years of age.

With lesion(s) similar to erythema migrans, "southern tick-associated rash illness" (STARI) has been reported in south central and southeastern states without endemic *B burgdorferi* infection.[1] The etiology is unknown. STARI results from the bite of the lone star tick, *Amblyomma americanum*, which is abundant in southern states and is biologically incapable of transmitting *B burgdorferi*. Patients with STARI may present with constitutional symptoms in addition to erythema migrans; however, STARI has not been associated with any of the disseminated complications of Lyme disease. Appropriate treatment of STARI is unknown.

B mayonii is a newly described species identified in a small number of patients from the upper Midwest with symptoms similar to those of Lyme disease. Patients with *B mayonii* infection can be expected to test positive for Lyme disease using the 2-tier serologic testing described below, and therapy used for Lyme disease is effective against *B mayonii*.

The **incubation period** from tick bite to appearance of single or multiple erythema migrans lesions ranges from 3 to 32 days, with a median time of 11 days. Late manifestations such as arthritis can occur months after the tick bite in people who do not receive antimicrobial therapy.

Lyme disease also is endemic in eastern Canada, Europe, states of the former Soviet Union, China, Mongolia, and Japan. The primary tick vector in Europe is *Ixodes ricinus*, and the primary tick vector in Asia is *Ixodes persulcatus*. Clinical manifestations of infection vary somewhat from manifestations seen in the United States. In particular, European Lyme disease can cause the skin lesions borrelial lymphocytoma and acrodermatitis chronica atrophicans and is more likely to produce neurologic disease, whereas arthritis is

---

[1]Lantos PM, Brinkerhoff RJ, Wormser GP, Clemen R. Empiric antibiotic treatment of erythema migrans-like skin lesions as a function of geography: a clinical and cost effectiveness modeling study. *Vector Borne Zoonotic Dis.* 2013;13(12):877–883

uncommon. These differences are attributable to the different genospecies of *Borrelia* responsible for European Lyme disease.

DIAGNOSTIC TESTS: The diagnosis of Lyme disease rests first and foremost on the recognition of a consistent clinical illness in people who have had plausible geographic exposure. Early Lyme disease in patients with erythema migrans is diagnosed clinically on the basis of recognition of the characteristic appearance of this skin lesion, and serologic testing is not recommended. Although erythema migrans is not strictly pathognomonic for Lyme disease, it is highly distinctive and characteristic. In areas with endemic Lyme disease, it is expected that the vast majority of erythema migrans occurring in the appropriate season is attributable to *B burgdorferi* infection, and presumptive treatment is appropriate. Current diagnostic testing is based on serology, but during early infection, the sensitivity is low. For children with solitary erythema migrans lesion, fewer than one-half will be seropositive, and diagnostic testing is not recommended. Patients who seek medical attention with one or more lesions of erythema migrans and without extracutaneous manifestations should be treated based on a clinical diagnosis of Lyme disease without serologic testing.

There is a broad differential diagnosis for extracutaneous manifestations of Lyme disease. The diagnosis of extracutaneous manifestations, including late-stage Lyme disease, requires a typical clinical illness, plausible geographic exposure, and a positive serologic test result.

The standard testing method for Lyme disease is a 2-tier serologic algorithm (**www. cdc.gov/lyme/healthcare/clinician_twotier.html**). The initial screening test identifies antibodies to a whole-cell sonicate, to peptide antigen, or to recombinant antigens of *B burgdorferi*. This test is performed using an enzyme-linked immunosorbent assay (ELISA or EIA) or immunofluorescent antibody (IFA) test. It should be noted that clinical laboratories vary somewhat in their description of this test. It may be described as "Lyme ELISA," "Lyme antibody screen," "total Lyme antibody," or "Lyme IgG/IgM." Many commercial laboratories offer EIA/IFA with reflex to Western immunoblot if the first-tier assay result is positive or equivocal.

Although the initial EIA or IFA test result may be reported quantitatively, its sole importance is to categorize the result as negative, equivocal, or positive. If the first-tier EIA result is negative, the patient is considered seronegative and no further testing is indicated. If the result is equivocal or positive, then a second-tier test is required to make the diagnosis of Lyme disease. Two-tier serologic testing increases test specificity. False-positive results are partly explained by antigenic components of *B burgdorferi* that are not specific to this species. Antibodies produced in response to other spirochetal infections, spirochetes in normal oral flora, other acute infections, and certain autoimmune diseases may be cross-reactive. In areas with endemic infection, previous subclinical infection with seroconversion may occur, and a seropositive patient's symptoms may be coincidental. Patients with active Lyme disease almost always have objective signs of infection (eg, erythema migrans, facial nerve palsy, arthritis). Nonspecific symptoms commonly accompany these specific signs but almost never are the only evidence of Lyme disease. Serologic testing for Lyme disease should not be performed for children without symptoms or signs suggestive of Lyme disease and plausible geographic exposure.

Serum specimens that yield positive or equivocal EIA or IFA results should be tested by the second-tier standardized Western immunoblot. Immunoblot testing should not be performed if the EIA or IFA test result is negative or without a prior EIA or IFA test, because specificity of immunoblot diminishes if the test is performed alone. The immunoblot assay tests for the presence of antibodies to specific *B burgdorferi* antigens, including immunoglobulin (Ig) M antibodies to 3 spirochetal antigens (the 23/24, 39, and 41 kDa polypeptides) and IgG antibodies to 10 spirochetal antigens (the 18, 23/24, 28, 30, 39, 41, 45, 60, 66, and 93 kDa polypeptides). Although some clinical laboratories report the presence of antibody to each of 13 bands, describing each band as positive or negative, a positive immunoblot result is defined as the presence of at least 2 IgM bands or 5 IgG bands. Physicians must be careful not to misinterpret a positive band as a positive test result or interpret a result as positive despite the presence of 4 or fewer IgG bands. It is noteworthy that IgG antibodies to flagella protein, the p41 band, is present in 30% to 50% of healthy people.

A positive IgM immunoblot can be falsely positive. The IgM assay is useful only for patients in the first 30 days after symptom onset. The IgM immunoblot result should be disregarded (or, if possible, not ordered) in patients who have had symptoms for longer than 4 to 6 weeks, or symptoms consistent with late Lyme disease, because false-positive IgM assay results are common, and because most untreated patients with disseminated Lyme disease will have a positive IgG result by week 4 to 6 after infection.

Lyme disease test results for *B burgdorferi* in patients treated for syphilis or other spirochete diseases are difficult to interpret. Consultation with an infectious diseases specialist is recommended. Although immunodeficiency theoretically could affect serologic testing results, reports have described infected patients who produced anti-*B burgdorferi* antibodies and had positive test results despite various immunocompromising conditions.

A licensed, commercially available serologic test (C6) that detects antibody to a peptide of the immunodominant conserved region of the variable surface antigen (VlsE) of *B burgdorferi* appears to have improved sensitivity for adults with early Lyme disease and Lyme disease acquired in Europe. However, when used alone, its specificity is slightly lower than that of standard 2-tier testing. Of interest, substitution of the C6 EIA for immunoblot testing in the 2-tier testing algorithm does not reduce the overall specificity.

No polymerase chain reaction (PCR) test for *B burgdorferi* currently is cleared by the US Food and Drug Administration (FDA). However, PCR testing of joint fluid from a patient with Lyme arthritis often has positive results and can be informative in establishing a diagnosis of Lyme arthritis. The role of a PCR assay on blood is not well established and is not routinely recommended. The yield of PCR testing on cerebrospinal fluid samples from patients with neuroborreliosis is too low to be useful in excluding this diagnosis.

Some patients who are treated with antimicrobial agents for early Lyme disease never develop detectable antibodies against *B burgdorferi;* they are cured and are not at risk of late disease. Development of antibodies in patients treated for early Lyme disease does not indicate lack of cure or presence of persistent infection. Ongoing infection without development of antibodies ("seronegative Lyme") has not been demonstrated. Most patients with early disseminated disease and virtually all patients with late disease have antibodies against *B burgdorferi*. Once such antibodies develop, they may persist for many years. Consequently, tests for antibodies should not be repeated or used to assess the success of treatment.

A number of tests for Lyme disease have been found to be invalid on the basis of independent testing or to be too nonspecific to exclude false-positive results. These include urine tests for *B burgdorferi*, CD57 assay, novel culture techniques, and antibody panels that differ from those recommended as part of standardized 2-tier testing. Although these tests are commercially available from some clinical laboratories, they are not FDA cleared and are not appropriate diagnostic tests for Lyme disease.

Current evidence indicates that patients with *B mayonii* infection develop a serologic response similar to that of patients infected with *B burgdorferi*. Two-tier testing can be expected to have positive results in patients with *B mayonii* infection.

TREATMENT: Consensus practice guidelines for assessment, treatment, and prevention of Lyme disease have been published by the Infectious Diseases Society of America.[1,2] Care of children should follow recommendations in Table 3.37. Antimicrobial therapy for non-specific symptoms or for asymptomatic seropositivity is not recommended. Antimicrobial agents administered for durations not specified in Table 3.37 are not recommended. Alternative diagnostic approaches or therapies without adequate validation studies and publication in peer-reviewed scientific literature are discouraged. Physicians have successfully treated patients with *B mayonii* infection with regimens used for Lyme disease.

Erythema Migrans (Single or Multiple). Doxycycline, amoxicillin, or cefuroxime can be used to treat children of any age who present with erythema migrans. Azithromycin generally is regarded as a second-line antimicrobial agent for erythema migrans in the United States, but further research on the efficacy of this agent is warranted. Selection of an oral antimicrobial agent for treatment of erythema migrans should be based on the following considerations: presence of neurologic disease (for which doxycycline is the drug of choice), drug allergy, adverse effects, frequency of administration (doxycycline and cefuroxime are administered twice a day, amoxicillin is administered 3 times a day), ability to minimize sun exposure (photosensitivity may be associated with doxycycline use), likelihood of coinfection with *Anaplasma phagocytophilum* or *Ehrlichia muris*-like agent (neither is sensitive to beta-lactam antimicrobial agents), and when *Staphylococcus aureus* cellulitis cannot be distinguished easily from erythema migrans (doxycycline is effective against most strains of methicillin-sensitive and methicillin-resistant *Staphylococcus aureus)*. Erythema migrans should be treated orally for 10 days if doxycycline is used and for 14 days if amoxicillin or cefuroxime is used. Because STARI may be indistinguishable from early Lyme disease and questions remain about appropriate treatment, some physicians treat STARI with the same antimicrobial agents orally as for Lyme disease.

Treatment of erythema migrans results in resolution of the skin lesion within several days of initiating therapy and almost always prevents development of later stages of Lyme disease.

Early Disseminated (Extracutaneous) Disease. Oral antimicrobial agents are appropriate and effective for most manifestations of disseminated Lyme disease, including multiple erythema migrans and for patients with Lyme carditis treated as outpatients. For patients requiring hospitalization for Lyme carditis (eg, high-grade atrioventricular block), initial therapy usually is parenteral but can be completed with oral therapy for a total course of 14 days (range: 14 to 21 days).

[1]Wormser GP, Dattwyler RJ, Shapiro ED, et al. The clinical assessment, treatment, and prevention of Lyme disease, human granulocytic anaplasmosis, and babesiosis: clinical practice guidelines by the Infectious Diseases Society of America. *Clin Infect Dis.* 2006;43(9):1089–1134

[2]Lantos PM, Charini WA, Medoff G, et al. Final report of the Lyme Disease Review Panel of the Infectious Diseases Society of America. *Clin Infect Dis.* 2010;51(1):1–5

Table 3.37. Recommended Treatment of Lyme Disease in Children

Disease Category	Drug(s) and Dose
Early localized disease	
Erythema migrans (single or multiple) (any age)	Doxycycline, 4.4 mg/kg per day, orally, divided into 2 doses (maximum 200 mg/day) for 10 days[a] **OR** Amoxicillin, 50 mg/kg per day, orally, divided into 3 doses (maximum 1.5 g/day) for 14 days[a] **OR** Cefuroxime, 30 mg/kg per day, orally, in 2 divided doses (maximum 1000 mg/day or 1 g/day) for 14 days[a] **OR**, for a patient unable to take a beta-lactam or doxycycline, Azithromycin, 10 mg/kg/day, orally, once daily for 7 days
Extracutaneous disease	
Isolated facial palsy	Doxycycline, 4.4 mg/kg per day, orally, divided into 2 doses (maximum 200 mg/day), for 14 days [a,b]
Arthritis	An oral agent as for early localized disease, for 28 days[c]
Persistent arthritis after first course of therapy	Retreat using an oral agent as for first-episode arthritis for 28 days[c] **OR** Ceftriaxone sodium, 50–75 mg/kg, IV, once a day (maximum 2 g/day) for 14–28 days
Atrioventricular heart block or carditis	An oral agent as for early localized disease, for 14 days (range 14–21 days) **OR** Ceftriaxone sodium, 50–75 mg/kg, IV, once a day (maximum 2 g/day) for 14 days (range 14–21 days for a hospitalized patient); oral therapy (using an agent as for early localized disease) can be substituted when the patient is stabilized or discharged, to complete the 14- to 21-day course
Meningitis	Doxycycline, 4.4 mg/kg per day, orally, divided into 1 or 2 doses (maximum 200 mg/day) for 14 days[a] **OR** Ceftriaxone sodium, 50–75 mg/kg, IV, once a day (maximum 2 g/day) for 14 days[a]

IV indicates intravenously.

[a]Represents a change from the 2006 Infectious Diseases Society of America (IDSA) guidelines by virtue of elimination of a longer range in duration of therapy of up to 21 days for erythema migrans, up to 21 days for facial palsy, and up to 28 days for meningitis or radiculopathy (Sanchez E, Vannier E, Wormser GP, Hu LT. Diagnosis, treatment, and prevention of Lyme disease, human granulocytic anaplasmosis, and babesiosis: a review. *JAMA*. 2016;315(16):1767-1777).

[b]Corticosteroids should not be given. Use of amoxicillin for facial palsy in children has not been studied. Treatment has no effect on the resolution of facial nerve palsy; its purpose is to prevent late disease.

[c]There are limited safety data on the use of doxycycline for >21 days in children <8 years of age.

Doxycycline is preferred therapy for facial nerve palsy caused by *B burgdorferi* in children of any age. The purpose of therapy for cranial nerve palsies is to reduce the risk of late disease. Amoxicillin has not been studied sufficiently for the treatment of facial nerve palsies in young children and is unlikely to reach therapeutic levels in the central nervous system.

A growing body of evidence suggests that oral doxycycline is effective for treatment of Lyme meningitis and may be used as an alternative to hospitalization and parenteral ceftriaxone therapy in children who are well enough to be treated as outpatients. In a child with a stiff neck and other symptoms of meningitis in whom the possibility of a bacterial (nonspirochetal) meningitis cannot be ruled out, a lumbar puncture is indicated. Neurologic disease is treated for 14 days.

Late Disseminated Disease. Children with Lyme arthritis are treated with oral antimicrobial agents for 28 days. Because of this duration, patients younger than 8 years should be treated with an oral agent other than doxycycline (eg, amoxicillin; see Table 3.37, footnote c). For patients 8 years and older, any of the oral options, including doxycycline, may be used (see Tetracyclines, p 905).

Patients who have responded incompletely or who respond and then relapse soon after stopping therapy can be given a second 28-day course of oral therapy. Patients who experience worsening of their arthritis can be treated with ceftriaxone parenterally for 14 to 28 days.

Approximately 10% to 15% of patients treated for Lyme arthritis will go on to have persistent synovitis that can last for months to years. Theories of pathophysiology include delayed resolution of inflammation because of slow clearance of nonviable bacteria following treatment versus an autoimmune mechanism. Misdiagnosis also should be considered (ie, Lyme antibodies in serum present from a previous infection or cross-reacting because of another disorder). Persisting synovitis following Lyme disease, termed "antibiotic-refractory Lyme arthritis," is a strongly HLA-associated phenomenon. Patients with persistent synovitis despite repeat treatment initially should be managed with nonsteroidal anti-inflammatory drugs. More severe cases should be referred to a rheumatologist. Methotrexate has been used successfully in some cases. Arthroscopic synovectomy is required rarely for more disabling or refractory cases.

Persistent Post-treatment Symptoms (Mistakenly Called "Chronic Lyme Disease"). Some patients have prolonged, persistent symptoms following standard treatment for Lyme disease. However, it is not clear whether this phenomenon is unique to Lyme disease or whether it is a more general occurrence during convalescence from other systemic illnesses. Persistent, treatment-refractory infection with *B burgdorferi* has not been substantiated scientifically. Patients with persistent symptoms following Lyme disease usually respond to symptomatic treatment and recover gradually.

Several double-blinded, randomized, placebo-controlled trials have found that retreatment with additional antimicrobial agents for patients with residual post-treatment Lyme disease subjective symptoms may be associated with harm and does not offer benefit.[1-4] Administration of additional antimicrobial agents to a patient with post-treatment

[1]Feder HM, Johnson BJ, O'Connell S, et al; Ad Hoc International Lyme Disease Group. A critical appraisal of "chronic Lyme disease." *N Engl J Med*. 2007;357(14):1422–1430

[2]Wormser GP, Dattwyler RJ, Shapiro ED, et al. The clinical assessment, treatment, and prevention of Lyme disease, human granulocytic anaplasmosis, and babesiosis: clinical practice guidelines by the Infectious Diseases Society of America. *Clin Infect Dis*. 2006;43(9):1089–1134

[3]Berende A, ter Hofstede HJ, Vos FJ, et al. Randomized trial of longer-term therapy for symptoms attributed to Lyme disease. *N Engl J Med*. 2016;374(13):1209–1220

[4]Marzec NS, Nelson C, Waldron PR, et al. Serious bacterial infections acquired during treatment of patients given a diagnosis of chronic Lyme disease—United States. *MMWR Morb Mortal Wkly Rep*. 2017;66(23):607–609

Lyme disease symptoms following standard treatment for Lyme disease is strongly discouraged.

Retreatment is appropriate for subsequent acute infections caused by *B burgdorferi*.

Pregnancy. Tetracyclines are contraindicated in pregnancy. Doxycycline has not been adequately studied during pregnancy to make a recommendation regarding its use. Otherwise, therapy is the same as recommended for nonpregnant people.

ISOLATION OF THE HOSPITALIZED PATIENT: Standard precautions are recommended.

CONTROL MEASURES: Lyme disease is a nationally notifiable disease in the United States.

Ticks. See Prevention of Mosquitoborne and Tickborne Infections (p 195).

Chemoprophylaxis. In areas of high endemicity (the coastal northeast), where 30% to 50% of *I scapularis* ticks harbor *B burgdorferi*, the overall risk of Lyme disease following a recognized tick bite is no higher than 3%. After a high-risk deer tick bite, defined as an engorged tick that has fed for >72 hours, the risk of infection may be 25% in an area with hyperendemic disease. The risk is extremely low after brief attachment, defined as <36 hours (eg, a flat, nonengorged deer tick is found). Testing of the tick for spirochete infection has a poor predictive value and is not recommended.

Studies of doxycycline prophylaxis have been conducted in adults and older children (≥12 years). In areas of high risk, a single prophylactic 200-mg dose (or 4.4 mg/kg for children weighing less than 45 kg) of doxycycline can be used in children of any age to reduce the risk of acquiring Lyme disease after the bite of an infected *I scapularis* tick. Benefits of prophylaxis may outweigh risks when the tick is engorged (ie, has been attached for at least 36 hours based on exposure history) and prophylaxis can be started within 72 hours of tick removal. Amoxicillin prophylaxis has been insufficiently studied, but it would likely require a longer course than doxycycline because of its shorter half-life and is not recommended. There are no clinical data to support antibiotic prophylaxis specifically for anaplasmosis, ehrlichiosis, babesiosis or Rocky Mountain spotted fever.

Blood Donation. To date, no documented cases of *B burgdorferi* transmission have occurred as a result of spirochete transmission via blood transfusion. Nevertheless, because spirochetemia occurs in early Lyme disease, patients with active disease should not donate blood. Patients who have been treated for Lyme disease can be considered for blood donation.

Vaccines. A Lyme disease vaccine was licensed by the US Food and Drug Administration 1998 for people 15 to 70 years of age but was withdrawn in 2002, principally because of poor sales and unsubstantiated public concerns about adverse effects. A phase I/II trial of a new vaccine performed in Europe found the vaccine to be immunogenic and without safety concerns.

Lymphatic Filariasis
(Bancroftian, Malayan, and Timorian)

CLINICAL MANIFESTATIONS: Lymphatic filariasis (LF) is caused by infection with the filarial parasites *Wuchereria bancrofti*, *Brugia malayi*, or *Brugia timori*. Adult worms cause lymphatic dilatation and dysfunction, which result in abnormal lymph flow and eventually may lead to lymphedema in the legs, scrotal area (for *W bancrofti* only), and arms. Recurrent secondary bacterial infections hasten progression of lymphedema to the more severe form known as elephantiasis. Although the infection occurs commonly in young children living in areas with endemic LF, chronic manifestations of infection, such as hydrocele and lymphedema, occur infrequently in people younger than 20 years. Most filarial infections remain clinically asymptomatic, but even then they commonly cause subclinical lymphatic dilatation and dysfunction. Lymphadenopathy, most frequently of the inguinal, crural, and axillary lymph nodes, is the most common clinical sign of lymphatic filariasis in children. There can be an acute inflammatory response that progresses from the lymph node distally (retrograde) along the affected lymphatic vessel, usually in the limbs. Accompanying systemic symptoms, such as headache or fever, generally are mild. In postpubertal males, adult *W bancrofti* organisms are found most commonly in the intrascrotal lymphatic vessels; thus, inflammation around dead or dying adult worms may present as funiculitis (inflammation of the spermatic cord), epididymitis, or orchitis. A tender granulomatous nodule may be palpable at the site of dying or dead adult worms. Chyluria can occur as a manifestation of bancroftian filariasis. Tropical pulmonary eosinophilia, characterized by cough, fever, wheezing, marked eosinophilia, and high serum immunoglobulin (Ig) E concentrations, is a rare manifestation of lymphatic filariasis.

ETIOLOGY: Filariasis is caused by 3 filarial nematodes in the family *Filaridae*: *W bancrofti*, *B malayi*, and *B timori*.

EPIDEMIOLOGY: The parasite is transmitted by the bite of infected mosquitoes of various genera, including *Culex*, *Aedes*, *Anopheles*, and *Mansonia*. *W bancrofti*, the most prevalent cause of lymphatic filariasis, is found in Haiti, the Dominican Republic, Guyana, northeast Brazil, sub-Saharan and North Africa, and Asia, extending from India through the Indonesian archipelago to the western Pacific islands. Humans are the only definitive host for the parasite. *B malayi* is found mostly in Southeast Asia and parts of India. *B timori* is restricted to certain islands at the eastern end of the Indonesian archipelago. Live adult worms release microfilariae into the bloodstream. Adult worms live for an average of 5 to 8 years, and reinfection is common. Microfilariae that can infect mosquitoes may be present in a patient's blood for decades, although individual microfilariae have a lifespan between 3 and 12 months. The adult worm is not transmissible from person to person or by blood transfusion, but microfilariae may be transmitted by transfusion.

The **incubation period** is not well established; the period from acquisition to the appearance of microfilariae in blood can be 3 to 12 months, depending on the species of parasite.

DIAGNOSTIC TESTS: Diagnosis requires epidemiologic risk and consistent laboratory findings (identification of microfilariae or antibody). Microfilariae generally can be detected microscopically on blood smears obtained at night (10 PM–4 AM), although variations in the periodicity of microfilaremia have been described depending on the parasite strain and the geographic location. Adult worms or microfilariae can be identified based on general morphology, size, and the presence or absence of a sheath in Giemsa-stained fluid or tissue specimens obtained at biopsy. Serologic enzyme immunoassays are available, but interpretation of results is affected by cross-reactions of filarial antibodies with antibodies against other helminths. Determination of serum antifilarial IgG is available through the Parasitic Diseases Laboratory at the National Institutes of Health (301-496-5398) or through the Centers for Disease Control and Prevention (CDC [**www.dpd. cdc.gov/dpdx;** 404-718-4745; **parasites@cdc.gov**]). Assays for circulating parasite antigen of *W bancrofti* are available commercially but are not cleared for use by the US Food and Drug Administration (FDA), nor are they available in the United States. Polymerase chain reaction assays can detect parasite-specific DNA in fluids and tissues with high sensitivity and specificity, but none are FDA cleared. Ultrasonography can be used to visualize adult worms. Patients with lymphedema may no longer have microfilariae or antifilarial antibody present.

TREATMENT: The main goal of treatment of an infected person is to kill the adult worm. Diethylcarbamazine citrate (DEC), which is both microfilaricidal and active against the adult worm, is the drug of choice for lymphatic filariasis (see Drugs for Parasitic Infections, p 985). DEC is no longer sold in the United States but can be obtained from the CDC (404-718-4745; **parasites@cdc.gov;** or **www.cdc.gov/parasites/ lymphaticfilariasis**). DEC is contraindicated in patients who may also have onchocerciasis or loiasis because of the possibility of exacerbation of skin or eye involvement or severe adverse effects. Treatment with DEC should be undertaken by a tropical medicine specialist with experience in treating lymphatic filariasis, because DEC therapy has been associated with life-threatening adverse events, including encephalopathy and renal failure, particularly in people with circulating *Loa loa* microfilaria concentrations >2500/mm^3. Ivermectin is effective against the microfilariae of *W bancrofti* and the 2 *Brugia* species but has no effect on the adult parasite. Albendazole has demonstrated macrofilaricidal activity. Combination therapy with single-dose DEC-albendazole or ivermectin-albendazole has been shown to be more effective than any one drug alone in suppressing microfilaremia and is the basis for the Global Programme for Elimination of Lymphatic Filariasis. Doxycycline, a drug that targets the *Wolbachia* (intracellular rickettsial-like bacteria) endosymbiont in adult worms, has been shown to be macrofilaricidal as well and has been used in combination with DEC.

Antifilarial chemotherapy has been shown to have limited efficacy for reversing or stabilizing the lymphedema in its early forms. Doxycycline, in limited studies, has been shown to decrease the severity of lymphedema. Complex decongestive physiotherapy can be effective for treating lymphedema and requires strict attention to hygiene in the affected anatomical areas. Chyluria originating in the bladder responds to fulguration; chyluria originating in the kidney is difficult to correct. Prompt identification and treatment of bacterial superinfections, particularly streptococcal and staphylococcal infections, and careful treatment of intertriginous and ungual fungal infections are important aspects of therapy for lymphedema. For management of hydrocele, surgery may be indicated.

ISOLATION OF THE HOSPITALIZED PATIENT: Standard precautions are recommended.

CONTROL MEASURES: Control measures have been instituted on the basis of annual mass drug administration of DEC and albendazole (worldwide in areas with endemic infection except Africa) or albendazole and ivermectin (in Africa) to decrease or possibly eliminate transmission. The use of insecticide-treated bed nets also has been shown to decrease transmission. No vaccine is available for lymphatic filariasis.

Lymphocytic Choriomeningitis

CLINICAL MANIFESTATIONS: Child and adult infections with lymphocytic choriomeningitis virus (LCMV) are asymptomatic in approximately one third of cases. Symptomatic infection may result in a mild to severe illness, which can include fever, malaise, myalgia, retro-orbital headache, photophobia, anorexia, and nausea and vomiting. Sore throat, cough, arthralgia or arthritis, and orchitis also may occur. Initial symptoms may last from a few days to 3 weeks. Leukopenia, lymphopenia, thrombocytopenia, and elevation of lactate dehydrogenase and aspartate transaminase occur frequently. A biphasic febrile course is common; after a few days without symptoms, the second phase may occur in up to half of symptomatic patients, consisting of neurologic manifestations that vary from aseptic meningitis to severe encephalitis. Transverse myelitis, eighth nerve deafness, Guillain-Barré syndrome, and hydrocephalus also have been reported, but a causal link remains to be established. Extraneural disease has included reports of myocarditis and dermatitis. Rarely, LCMV has caused a disease resembling viral hemorrhagic syndrome. Transmission of LCMV through organ transplantation and infection in other immunocompromised populations can result in fatal disseminated infection with multiple organ failure.

Current prevalence is not known, because diagnostic testing is not often performed. Seasonality is not certain. However, because other etiologic agents responsible for aseptic meningitis are more prevalent in summer months, LCMV may result in a higher proportion of aseptic meningitis in winter months. Convalescence may take several weeks, with asthenia, poor cognitive function, headaches, and arthralgia. Recovery without sequelae is the usual outcome. LCMV infection should be suspected in presence of: (1) aseptic meningitis or encephalitis during the fall-winter season; (2) febrile illness, followed by brief remission, followed by onset of neurologic illness; and (3) cerebrospinal fluid (CSF) findings of lymphocytosis and hypoglycorrhachia.

Infection during pregnancy has been associated with spontaneous abortion. Congenital infection may cause severe abnormalities, including hydrocephalus, chorioretinitis, intracranial calcifications, microcephaly, and mental retardation. Congenital LCMV should be included in the differential diagnosis whenever intrauterine infections with toxoplasma, rubella, cytomegalovirus, herpes simplex, enterovirus, parechovirus, Zika virus, dengue, syphilis, and parvovirus B19 are also being considered.

ETIOLOGY: LCMV is a single-stranded RNA virus that belongs to the family *Arenaviridae* (so named because of its appearance on electron microscopy, which resembles grains of sand). Other members of this family include Lassa virus and the Tacaribe group.

EPIDEMIOLOGY: LCMV is a chronic infection of common house mice, which often are infected asymptomatically and chronically shed virus in urine and other excretions. Congenital murine infection is common and results in a normal-appearing litter with chronic viremia and particularly high virus excretion. In addition, pet hamsters, laboratory mice, guinea pigs, and colonized golden hamsters can have chronic infection and can be sources of human infection. Humans are infected mostly by inhalation of aerosol generated by rodents shedding virus from the urine, feces, blood, or nasopharyngeal secretions. Other less likely routes of entry of infected secretions include conjunctival and other mucous membranes, ingestion, and occult cuts. The disease is observed more frequently in young adults. Human-to-human transmission has occurred during pregnancy from infected mothers to their fetus and through solid organ transplantation from an undiagnosed, acutely LCMV-infected organ donor. Several such clusters of cases have been described following transplantation, and one case was traced to a pet hamster purchased by the donor. A number of laboratory-acquired LCMV infections have occurred, both through infected laboratory animals and contaminated tissue-culture stocks.

The **incubation period** usually is 6 to 13 days and occasionally is as long as 3 weeks.

DIAGNOSTIC TESTS: Patients with central nervous system disease have a mononuclear pleocytosis with 30 to 8000 cells in CSF. Hypoglycorrhachia, as well as mild increase in protein, may occur. LCMV usually can be isolated from CSF obtained during the acute phase of illness and, in severe disseminated infections, also from blood, urine, and naso-pharyngeal secretion specimens. Reverse transcriptase-polymerase chain reaction assays available through reference or commercial laboratories can be used on serum during the acute stage and on CSF during the neurologic phase; however, none of these assays are cleared by the US Food and Drug Administration (FDA). Serum specimens from the acute and convalescent phases of illness can be tested for increases in antibody titers by enzyme immunoassays and neutralization tests. Demonstration of virus-specific immuno-globulin M antibodies in serum or CSF specimens is useful. In congenital infections, diagnosis usually is suspected at the sequela phase, and diagnosis usually is made by serologic testing. In immunosuppressed patients, seroconversion can take several weeks. Diagnosis can be made retrospectively by immunohistochemical assay of fixed tissues obtained from necropsy.

TREATMENT: Supportive. Limited data suggest a possible role for ribavirin in immuno-suppressed patients infected with LCMV. However, ribavirin is not FDA approved for treatment of LCMV.

ISOLATION OF THE HOSPITALIZED PATIENT: Standard precautions are recommended.

CONTROL MEASURES: Infection can be controlled by preventing rodent infestation in animal and food storage areas. Because the virus is excreted for long periods of time by rodent hosts, attempts should be made to monitor laboratory and wholesale colonies of mice and hamsters for infection. Pet rodents or wild mice in a patient's home should be considered likely sources of infection. Guidelines for minimizing risk of human LCMV infection associated with rodents are available[1] (also see Diseases Transmitted by Animals [Zoonoses], p 1093). Although the risk of LCMV infection from pet rodents is low, pregnant women should avoid exposure to wild or pet rodents and their aerosolized excreta. Pregnant women also should avoid working in the laboratory with LCMV.

Malaria

CLINICAL MANIFESTATIONS: The classic symptoms of malaria are high fever with chills, rigor, sweats, and headache, which may be paroxysmal. If appropriate treatment is not administered, fever and paroxysms may occur in a cyclic pattern. Depending on the infecting species, fever classically appears every day (*Plasmodium knowlesi*), every other day (*Plasmodium falciparum*, *Plasmodium vivax*, and *Plasmodium ovale*), or every third day (*Plasmodium malariae*), although in general practice this pattern is infrequently observed, especially in children. Other manifestations, particularly as the clinical disease progresses, can include nausea, vomiting, diarrhea, cough, tachypnea, arthralgia, myalgia, and abdominal and back pain. Anemia and thrombocytopenia, along with pallor and jaundice caused by hemolysis, are common in severe illness. Hepatosplenomegaly is frequently present in infected children in areas with endemic malaria and may be present in adults and in people not previously infected with malaria. More severe disease frequently occurs in people without immunity acquired as a result of previous infection, in young children and in primigravid women, or in those who are immunocompromised.

---

[1]Centers for Disease Control and Prevention. Update: interim guidance for minimizing risk for human lympho-cytic choriomeningitis virus infection associated with pet rodents. *MMWR Morb Mortal Wkly Rep.* 2005;54(32): 799–801

Infection with *P falciparum*, one of the 5 *Plasmodium* species that infect humans, potentially is fatal and most commonly manifests as a febrile nonspecific illness without localizing signs. Severe disease (most commonly caused by *P falciparum*) may manifest as one of the following clinical syndromes, all of which are medical emergencies and may be fatal unless treated:

- **Cerebral malaria,** characterized by unarousable coma and manifesting with a range of neurologic signs and symptoms, including generalized seizures, signs of increased intracranial pressure (confusion and progression to stupor, coma), and death;
- **Hypoglycemia,** which can present with metabolic acidosis and hypotension associated with hyperparasitemia; it also can be a consequence of quinine or quinidine-induced hyperinsulinemia;
- **Renal failure** caused by acute tubular necrosis (rare in children younger than 8 years);
- **Respiratory failure,** without pulmonary edema;
- **Metabolic acidosis,** usually attributed to lactic acidosis, hypovolemia, liver dysfunction, and impaired renal function;
- **Severe anemia** attributable to high parasitemia and hemolysis, sequestration of infected erythrocytes to capillaries, and hemolysis of infected erythrocytes associated with hypersplenism; or
- **Vascular collapse and shock** associated with hypothermia and adrenal insufficiency; people with asplenia who become infected may be at increased risk of more severe illness and death.

Syndromes primarily associated with *P vivax* and *P ovale* infection are as follows:

- **Anemia** attributable to acute parasitemia;
- **Hypersplenism** with danger of splenic rupture; and
- **Relapse of infection,** for as long as 3 to 5 years after the primary infection, attributable to latent hepatic stages (hypnozoites).

Syndromes associated with *P malariae* infection include:

- **Chronic asymptomatic parasitemia** for as long as decades after the primary infection; and
- **Nephrotic syndrome** resulting from deposition of immune complexes in the kidney.

Plasmodium knowlesi is a nonhuman primate malaria parasite that also can infect humans. *P knowlesi* malaria has been misdiagnosed commonly as the more benign *P malariae* malaria. Disease can be characterized by very rapid replication of the parasite and hyperparasitemia resulting in severe disease. Severe disease in patients with *P knowlesi* infection should be treated aggressively, because hepatorenal failure and subsequent death have been well documented.

Congenital malaria resulting from perinatal transmission occurs infrequently, with increased risk among primigravidae. Most congenital cases have been caused by *P vivax* and *P falciparum; P malariae* and *P ovale* account for fewer than 20% of such cases. Manifestations can resemble those of neonatal sepsis, including fever and nonspecific symptoms of poor appetite, irritability, and lethargy.

ETIOLOGY: The genus *Plasmodium* includes species of intraerythrocytic parasites that infect a wide range of mammals, birds, and reptiles. The 5 species that infect humans are

P falciparum, P vivax, P ovale, P malariae, and *P knowlesi.* Coinfection with multiple species increasingly is documented among residents of areas with endemic disease as polymerase chain reaction technology is applied to the diagnosis of malaria infection.

EPIDEMIOLOGY: Malaria is endemic throughout the tropical areas of the world and is acquired from the bite of the female nocturnal-feeding *Anopheles* genus of mosquito. Half of the world's population lives in areas where transmission occurs. Worldwide, 212 million cases and 429 000 deaths were reported in 2015. Approximately 10% of these are cases of severe malaria, which have a significantly higher chance of death. Most deaths occur in young children. Infection by the malaria parasite poses substantial risks to pregnant women, especially primigravida women in areas with endemic infection, and their fetuses and may result in spontaneous abortion and stillbirth. Malaria also contributes to low birth weight in countries where *P falciparum* is endemic.

The risk of malaria is highest, but variable, for travelers to sub-Saharan Africa, Papua New Guinea, the Solomon Islands, and Vanuatu; the risk is intermediate on the Indian subcontinent and is low in most of Southeast Asia and Latin America. The potential for malaria reintroduction can occur in areas where malaria previously was eliminated if infected people return and the mosquito vector is still present. These conditions have resulted in recent cases in travelers to areas such as Jamaica, Greece, and the Bahamas.

Health care professionals should check the CDC Web site for the most current information (**www.cdc.gov/malaria**) to determine malaria endemicity when providing pretravel malaria advice or evaluating a febrile returned traveler. Transmission is possible in more temperate climates, including areas of the United States where *Anopheles* mosquitoes are present.

Nearly all of the approximately 1500 annual reported cases in the United States result from infection acquired abroad.[1] Uncommon modes of malaria transmission are congenital, through transfusions, or through the use of contaminated needles or syringes.

P vivax and *P falciparum* are the most prevalent species worldwide. *P vivax* malaria is prevalent on the Indian subcontinent and in Central America. *P falciparum* malaria is prevalent in Africa, Papua New Guinea, and on the island of Hispaniola (Haiti and the Dominican Republic). *P vivax* and *P falciparum* species are the most common malaria species in southern and Southeast Asia, Oceania, and South America. *P malariae,* although much less common, has a wide distribution. *P ovale* malaria occurs most frequently in West Africa but has been reported in other areas. Reported cases of human infections with *P knowlesi* have been from certain countries of Southeast Asia, specifically Borneo, Malaysia, Philippines, Thailand, the Thai-Burmese border, Singapore, and Cambodia.

Relapses may occur in *P vivax* and *P ovale* infections because of a persistent hepatic (hypnozoite) stage of infection. Recrudescence of *P falciparum* and *P malariae* infection occurs when a persistent low-concentration parasitemia produces recurrence of blood parasite replication and symptoms of the disease or when drug resistance prevents elimination of the parasite. In areas of Africa and Asia with hyperendemic transmission, repeated infection in people with partial immunity results in a high prevalence of asymptomatic parasitemia.

Drug resistance in both *P falciparum* and *P vivax* has been evolving throughout areas

[1]Centers for Disease Control and Prevention. Malaria surveillance—United States, 2014. *MMWR Surveill Summ.* 2017;66(SS-12):1–24

with endemic malaria, generally proportional to the use of particular drugs in a population. The spread of chloroquine-resistant *P falciparum* strains throughout the world dates back to the 1960s. *P falciparum* resistance to sulfadoxine-pyrimethamine is distributed throughout Africa. Mefloquine resistance has been documented in Myanmar (Burma), Lao People's Democratic Republic (Laos), Thailand, Cambodia, China, and Vietnam. Resistance to artemisinins has been reported from the 5 countries of Greater Mekong Subregions (GMS), which consist of Cambodia, Laos, Myanmar, Thailand, and Vietnam. Chloroquine-resistant *P vivax* has been reported in Indonesia, Papua New Guinea, the Solomon Islands, Myanmar, India, and Guyana.

The **incubation period** (time to onset of malaria symptoms) is as soon as 7 days after exposure in an area with endemic malaria to as late as several months after departure. More than 80% of cases in the United States occur in people who have onset of symptoms after their return to the United States.

DIAGNOSTIC TESTS: Definitive parasitological diagnosis has historically been based on identification of *Plasmodium* parasites microscopically on stained blood films. Both thick and thin blood films should be examined. The thick film allows for concentration of the blood to find parasites that may be present at low density, whereas the thin film is most useful for species identification and determination of the density of red blood cells infected with parasites. If initial blood smears test negative for *Plasmodium* species but malaria remains a possibility, the smear should be repeated every 12 to 24 hours during a 72-hour period.

Confirmation and identification of the species of malaria parasites on the blood smear is essential in guiding therapy. Serologic testing generally is not helpful, except in epidemiologic surveys. Polymerase chain reaction (PCR) assay is available in reference laboratories and many state health departments. Additionally, there is an increasing range of rapid diagnostic test methods available. Species confirmation and antimalarial drug resistance testing are available free of charge at the Centers for Disease Control and Prevention (CDC) for all cases of malaria diagnosed in the United States. A US Food and Drug Administration (FDA)-approved test for rapid antigen detection is available in the United States. It is the only antigen-detection kit available and is approved for use by hospitals and commercial laboratories. Rapid diagnostic testing is recommended to be conducted in parallel with routine microscopy to provide further information needed for patient treatment, such as the percentage of erythrocytes harboring parasites. Both positive and negative rapid diagnostic test results should be confirmed by microscopic examination, because low-level parasitemia may not be detected (ie, false-negative result), false-positive results occur, and mixed infections may not be detected accurately. Information about the sensitivity of rapid diagnostic tests for the 2 less common species of malaria, *P ovale* and *P malariae*, is limited. Additional information about rapid diagnostic testing for malaria is available on the CDC Web site (**www.cdc.gov/malaria/diagnosis_ treatment/index.html**).

TREATMENT: The choice of malaria chemotherapy is based on the infecting species, possible drug resistance, and severity of disease (see Drugs for Parasitic Infections, p 985). Severe malaria (largely a consideration for *P falciparum* infections) is defined as any one or more of the following: parasitemia greater than 5% of red blood cells infected, signs of central nervous system or other end-organ involvement, shock, acidosis, thrombocytopenia, and/or hypoglycemia. Patients with severe malaria require intensive care and parenteral treatment with intravenous quinidine until the parasite density decreases to less than 1% and they are able to tolerate oral therapy. Important safety precautions when using quinidine are available at **www.cdc.gov/malaria/diagnosis_treatment/clinicians3.html.** The manufacturer of intravenous quinidine is ceasing production, and it will no longer be available after March 2019. Please consult the CDC malaria Web site for therapeutic options thereafter, including intravenous artesunate (see next paragraph). Concurrent treatment with tetracycline, doxycycline, or clindamycin should begin orally or intravenously if oral treatment is not tolerated (see Drugs for Parasitic Infections, p 985). A recent review of available literature suggests exchange transfusion for severe disease is not efficacious in patients with end-organ involvement.

For patients with severe malaria in the United States who do not tolerate or cannot easily access quinidine, intravenous artesunate is available through a CDC investigational new drug (IND) protocol. Clinicians may contact the physician on call through the CDC malaria hotline (770-488-7788, Monday–Friday, 9:00 AM–5:00 PM Eastern Time; or 770-488-7100 at all other times) for additional information and release of the drug.[1] For patients with *P falciparum* malaria, sequential blood smears to determine percentage of erythrocytes infected with parasites are monitored to assess therapeutic efficacy. Assistance with management of malaria is available 24 hours a day through the CDC Malaria Hotline (770-488-7788). Guidelines for the treatment of malaria are available on the CDC Web site (**www.cdc.gov/malaria/resources/pdf/treatmenttable.pdf**).

ISOLATION OF THE HOSPITALIZED PATIENT: Standard precautions are recommended.

CONTROL MEASURES: Malaria is a nationally notifiable disease in the United States. There is no licensed vaccine against malaria. Effective measures to reduce the risk of acquiring malaria include control of *Anopheles* mosquito populations, protection against mosquito bites, treatment of infected people, and chemoprophylaxis of travelers to areas with endemic infection (see Table 3.38). Measures to prevent contact with mosquitoes, especially from dusk to dawn (because of the nocturnal biting habits of most female *Anopheles* mosquitoes), through use of bed nets impregnated with insecticide, mosquito repellents (see Prevention of Mosquitoborne and Tickborne Infections, p 195), and protective clothing also are beneficial and should be optimized. The most current information on country-specific malaria transmission, drug resistance, and resulting recommendations for travelers can be obtained by contacting the CDC (**www.cdc.gov/malaria** or the Malaria Hotline at 770-488-7788).

***Chemoprophylaxis for Travelers to Areas With Endemic Malaria.*[2]** Drugs for the prevention of malaria currently available in the United States include chloroquine, mefloquine, doxycycline, atovaquone-proguanil, and primaquine. Table 3.38 details use of these drugs for prophylaxis against malaria.

More than 80% of malaria-infected patients reported in the United States did not follow a CDC-recommended prophylaxis regimen. The appropriate chemoprophylactic regimen is determined by the traveler's risk of acquiring malaria in the area(s) to be

---

[1]Centers for Disease Control and Prevention. Notice to readers: new medication for severe malaria available under an investigational new drug protocol. *MMWR Morb Mortal Wkly Rep.* 2007;56(30):769–770

[2]For further information on prevention of malaria in travelers, see the biennial publication of the US Public Health Service, *Health Information for International Travel*, 2014. Atlanta, GA: US Department of Health and Human Services, Public Health Service, Centers for Disease Control and Prevention, National Center for Infectious Diseases, Division of Global Migration and Quarantine; 2014. Oxford University Press. Available at: **wwwnc.cdc.gov/travel/page/yellowbook-home**

Table 3.38. Drugs to Consider for Use in Children for Malaria Prophylaxis[a]

Locale	Drug	Dosing	Timing	Adverse Effects and Contraindications	Other Considerations
Only chloroquine-sensitive areas	Chloroquine or hydroxychloroquine	Chloroquine dose: 5 mg/kg base (8.3 mg/kg salt), orally, once weekly, up to maximum adult dose 300 mg base Hydroxychloroquine dose: 5 mg/kg base (6.5 mg/kg salt), orally, once weekly, up to maximum 310 mg base	Begin 1–2 weeks before travel and take weekly throughout and for 4 weeks after leaving area	Most common adverse effects: gastrointestinal tract disturbance, headache, dizziness, blurred vision, pruritus, insomnia Can exacerbate psoriasis	Take with meals Hydroxychloroquine considered better tolerated than chloroquine

Table 3.38. Drugs to Consider for Use in Children for Malaria Prophylaxis,[a] continued

Locale	Drug	Dosing	Timing	Adverse Effects and Contraindications	Other Considerations
Only mefloquine-sensitive areas	Mefloquine	≤9 kg: 4.6 mg/kg base (5 mg/kg salt), once weekly >9–19 kg: ¼ tablet, once weekly >19–30 kg: ½ tablet, once weekly >30–45 kg: ¾ tablet, once weekly >45 kg: 1 tablet, once weekly Each tablet contains 228 mg base (250 mg salt)	Begin ≥2 wk before travel, then weekly on same day each wk throughout and for 4 wk after leaving area Initiating 2–3 wk before travel can help assess tolerability	Most common adverse effects: gastrointestinal tract disturbance, headache, insomnia, vivid dreams, visual disturbance, anxiety, dizziness CONTRAINDICATED in travelers with a known hypersensitivity to the drug, and in those with active or recent history depression, anxiety disorder, psychosis, schizophrenia, other major psychiatric disorder or seizures Do not use in those with cardiac conduction defects	Black box warning: persistent dizziness Patients must be given copy of FDA medication guide May be given in all trimesters of pregnancy Alternatives if not tolerated: doxycycline or atovaquone-proguanil

Table 3.38. Drugs to Consider for Use in Children for Malaria Prophylaxis,[a] continued

Locale	Drug	Dosing	Timing	Adverse Effects and Contraindications	Other Considerations
All areas	Atovaquone-proguanil	Pediatric tablets, 62.5 mg atovaquone and 25 mg proguanil hydrochloride 5–8 kg: ½ tab >8–10 kg: ¾ tab >10–20 kg: 1 tab >20–30 kg: 2 tabs >30–40 kg: 3 tabs >40 kg: 1 adult tab (250 mg atovaquone/100 mg proguanil)	Start 1–2 days before travel, take daily throughout travel and for 7 days after leaving area	Most common adverse effects: abdominal pain, nausea, vomiting, headache Do not use in those with creatinine clearance <30 mL/min; not recommended infants <5 kg, pregnant women, or women breastfeeding infants <5 kg	Generally well tolerated Proguanil can increase warfarin effect; dosage adjustment may be needed
All areas	Doxycycline	2.2 mg/kg, up to maximum adult dose 100 mg/day	Start 1–2 days before travel, take daily throughout travel and for 4 weeks after leaving area	Most common adverse effects: photosensitivity, gastrointestinal disturbance Not recommended for pregnant women, or for children <8 years since duration of prophylaxis exceeds 21 days	Take with meals Also active against rickettsiae and leptospirae (hikers, campers, fresh water swimmers) Complete oral typhoid vaccine before starting doxycycline

Licensed for 4 months' use but may be safely given up to 2 years

Table 3.38. Drugs to Consider for Use in Children for Malaria Prophylaxis,[a] continued

Locale	Drug	Dosing	Timing	Adverse Effects and Contraindications	Other Considerations
Short-duration travel to areas with *P vivax*	Primaquine	0.5 mg/kg base (0.8 mg/kg salt) up to adult dose of 30 mg base (52.6 mg salt) daily	Start 1–2 days before travel, take daily throughout travel and for 7 days after leaving area	CONTRAINDICATED in those with G6PD deficiency and pregnant women Should not be given to lactating woman unless infant has normal G6PD level	Also used for presumptive therapy (ie, terminal prophylaxis) to decrease risk of *P vivax* or *P ovale* relapse

G6PD indicates glucose-6-phosphate dehydrogenase.

[a]No drug is 100% effective; always combine chemoprophylaxis with personal protection measures.

visited and by local prevalence of drug resistance. The travel itinerary should be reviewed in detail and compared with information on where malaria transmission occurs within a given country to determine whether the traveler will be traveling in a part of the country where malaria occurs and if antimalarial drug resistance has been reported in that location (see the chapter "Yellow Fever and Malaria Information, by Country" in the CDC *Yellow Book* **[wwwnc.cdc.gov/travel/yellowbook/2018/infectious-diseases-related-to-travel/yellow-fever-malaria-information-by-country]**). Additional factors to consider are the patient's other medical conditions, medications being taken (to assess potential drug interactions), the cost of the medicines, and the potential adverse effects. Indications for prophylaxis for children are identical to those for adults. Pediatric dosages should be calculated on the basis of the child's current weight, and children's dosages should never exceed adult dosages. Drugs used for malaria chemoprophylaxis generally are well tolerated, although adverse reactions can occur. Minor adverse reactions do not require stopping or adjusting drug dosage. Travelers with serious adverse reactions should be advised to contact their physician.

Medications for chemoprophylaxis of malaria should not be obtained at overseas locations, as the quality of these products is unknown. Travelers also should avoid additional medications and combinations that are commonly prescribed abroad but not recommended in the United States. Chemoprophylaxis should begin before arrival in the area with endemic malaria (starting at least 2 weeks before arrival for mefloquine, 1 week before arrival for chloroquine, and 1–2 days before arrival for doxycycline and atovaquone-proguanil), allowing time to develop efficacious blood concentrations of the drug(s). If there is a desire to ensure tolerance of the antimalarial drug to be used for prophylaxis, then the drug should be started earlier so that there is time to assess any adverse events before departure and to change to alternative effective drug(s). For example, if there is concern about individual tolerance with mefloquine, then prophylaxis can be started 3 weeks before travel. Most adverse events will occur during the first 3 doses, and if the person does not tolerate mefloquine, then there still is time to prescribe alternative therapy before travel.

Prophylaxis During Pregnancy and Lactation. Malaria during pregnancy carries significant risks of morbidity and mortality for both the mother and fetus. Malaria may increase the risk of adverse outcomes in pregnancy, including abortion, preterm birth, and stillbirth. For these reasons and because no chemoprophylactic regimen is absolutely effective, women who are pregnant or likely to become pregnant should try to avoid travel to areas where they could contract malaria.

Women traveling to areas where drug-resistant *P falciparum* has not been reported may take chloroquine prophylaxis. Harmful effects on the fetus have not been demonstrated when chloroquine is given in the recommended doses for malaria prophylaxis. Pregnancy and lactation, therefore, are not contraindications for malaria prophylaxis with chloroquine.

For pregnant women who travel to areas where chloroquine-resistant *P falciparum* exists, the CDC recommends mefloquine chemoprophylaxis in all trimesters of pregnancy when exposure to chloroquine-resistant *P falciparum* is unavoidable. Lactating mothers of infants weighing more than 5 kg also may use atovaquone-proguanil or mefloquine for prophylaxis when exposure to chloroquine-resistant *P falciparum* is unavoidable.

Reliable Antimalarial Supply While Traveling. Travelers to areas with endemic malaria should seek medical attention immediately if they develop fever. Malaria treatment can be effective if begun early in the course of disease, and delay of appropriate treatment can have serious or even fatal consequences. Travelers who do not take an antimalarial drug for prophylaxis, who are on a less-than-effective regimen, or who may be in very remote areas can be given an adequate supply of atovaquone-proguanil or artemether-lumefantrine. If they contract malaria while traveling, they will have a medicine that will not interact with their other medications, is of good quality, and is not depleting local resources.

Travelers taking atovaquone-proguanil as their chemoprophylactic drug regimen should not take atovaquone-proguanil for treatment and should use an alternative anti-malarial regimen recommended by a travel medicine expert.

Travelers should be advised that any fever or influenza-like illness that develops within 3 months of departure from an area with endemic malaria requires immediate medical evaluation, including blood smears to rule out malaria.

Prevention of Relapses. There is no test to determine the potential for relapses of *P vivax* or *P ovale* infection, but to prevent relapses after departure from areas where these species are endemic, travelers with prolonged exposure and normal G6PD concentrations should receive presumptive antirelapse therapy (terminal prophylaxis) with primaquine for 14 days. Rarely, travelers exposed to primaquine-resistant or -tolerant parasites may require high-dose primaquine. Primaquine can cause hemolysis in patients with G6PD deficiency; thus, all patients should be screened for this condition before primaquine therapy is initiated.

Personal Protective Measures. All travelers to areas where malaria is endemic should be advised to use personal protective measures, including the following: (1) using insecticide-impregnated mosquito nets while sleeping; (2) remaining in well-screened areas at dusk and at night; (3) wearing protective clothing, preferably permethrin treated; and (4) using mosquito repellents. To be effective, most repellents require frequent reapplications (see Prevention of Mosquitoborne and Tickborne Infections, p 195).

Measles

CLINICAL MANIFESTATIONS: Measles is an acute viral disease characterized by fever, cough, coryza, and conjunctivitis, followed by a maculopapular rash beginning on the face and spreading cephalocaudally and centrifugally. During the prodromal period, a pathognomonic enanthema (Koplik spots) may be present. Complications of measles, including otitis media, bronchopneumonia, laryngotracheobronchitis (croup), and diarrhea, occur commonly in young children and immunocompromised hosts. Acute encephalitis, which often results in permanent brain damage, occurs in approximately 1 of every 1000 cases. In the postelimination era, death, predominantly resulting from respiratory and neurologic complications, has occurred in 1 to 3 of every 1000 cases reported in the United States. Case-fatality rates are increased in children younger than 5 years, pregnant women, and immunocompromised children, including children with leukemia, human immunodeficiency virus (HIV) infection, and severe malnutrition (including vitamin A deficiency). Sometimes the characteristic rash does not develop in immunocompromised patients. Individuals with incomplete immunity from immunization with inactivated measles vaccine may have an atypical presentation with some but not all symptoms following exposure to wild-type measles.

Subacute sclerosing panencephalitis (SSPE) is a rare degenerative central nervous system disease characterized by behavioral and intellectual deterioration and seizures that occurs 7 to 11 years after wild-type measles virus infection, occurring at a rate of 4 to 11 per 100 000 measles cases, with higher rates if measles occurs before 2 years of age. Widespread measles immunization has led to the virtual disappearance of SSPE in the United States.

ETIOLOGY: Measles virus is an enveloped RNA virus with 1 serotype, classified as a member of the genus *Morbillivirus* in the *Paramyxoviridae* family.

EPIDEMIOLOGY: The only natural host of measles virus is humans. Measles is transmitted by direct contact with infectious droplets or, less commonly, by airborne spread. Measles is one of the most highly communicable of all infectious diseases; the attack rate in a susceptible individual exposed to measles is 90%. Population immunity of greater than 95% is needed to stop ongoing transmission. In temperate areas, the peak incidence of infection usually occurs during late winter and spring. In the prevaccine era, most cases of measles in the United States occurred in preschool- and young school-aged children, and few people remained susceptible by 20 years of age. Following implementation of routine childhood vaccination in the United States at age 12 to 15 months, the age of peak measles incidence during epidemics in the United States shifted to 6 to 12 months. This susceptibility approximates the time at which transplacentally acquired maternal antibodies no longer are present if the mother has vaccine-induced immunity. The childhood and adolescent immunization program in the United States began with licensure of the measles vaccine in 1963 and has resulted in a greater than 99% decrease in the reported incidence of measles, with interruption of endemic disease transmission being declared in 2000.

From 1989 to 1991, the incidence of measles in the United States increased because of low immunization rates in preschool-aged children, especially in urban areas, and because of primary vaccine failures after one measles vaccine dose. Following improved coverage in preschool-aged children and implementation of a routine second dose of measles-mumps-rubella (MMR) vaccine for children, the incidence of measles declined to extremely low levels (<1 case per 1 million population). In 2000, an independent panel of internationally recognized experts reviewed available data and unanimously agreed that measles no longer was endemic (defined as continuous, year-round transmission) in the United States. Compared with earlier postelimination years (2001–2008), when the annual median number of cases reported was 56 cases/year (range, 37–140), a median of 130 measles cases were reported annually (range, 55–667) during 2009–2014. In 2011, 2013, and 2014, the numbers of reported cases were 220, 187, and 667, respectively; these larger numbers of cases were attributable to an increase in the number of importations and/or spread from importations. The median number of measles outbreaks (defined as 3 or more cases linked in time and space) that occurred during 2009–2014 was 10 per year (range, 4–23) and was higher than the annual median number of outbreaks that occurred in earlier postelimination years (median, 4 outbreaks per year; range, 2–10 outbreaks). Of the 1264 cases reported during 2009–2014, 1204 (95%) were import associated (including 275 [22%] directly imported cases), and 60 (5%) cases were of an unknown source; among 1173 cases in US residents, 74% were in unvaccinated people, 16% were in people with unknown vaccination status (83% of those were adults), and 10% were in vaccinated people (with ≥1 dose of a measles-containing vaccine). During the same period, among 917 cases in vaccine-eligible US residents, 65% were in people reported as having a philosophical or religious objection to vaccination. In 2015, 188 people from 24 states and the District of Columbia were reported to have measles. This large, multistate measles outbreak was linked to an amusement park in California. The outbreak likely started from a traveler who became infected overseas with measles, then visited the amusement park while infectious; however, no source was identified. In 2016, 86 people from 16 states were reported to have measles, and in 2017, 120 people from 15 states and the District of Columbia were reported to have measles.

Progress continues toward global control and regional measles elimination. In 2016, there were 89 780 measles deaths globally, marking the first year measles deaths have fallen below 100 000 per year. Measles vaccination resulted in an 84% drop in measles deaths between 2000 and 2016 worldwide. In 2016, approximately 85% of the world's children received one dose of measles vaccine by their first birthday through routine health services, up from 72% in 2000. During 2000–2016, measles vaccination prevented an estimated 20.4 million deaths. All World Health Organization (WHO) regions have established goals to eliminate measles by 2020. Resuming progress toward 2020 milestones and elimination goals will require countries and their partners to raise the visibility of measles elimination, address barriers to measles vaccination, and make substantial and sustained additional investments in strengthening health systems.

Inadequate response to vaccine (ie, primary vaccine failure) occurs in as many as 7% of people who have received a single dose of vaccine at 12 months or older. Most cases of measles in previously immunized children seem to be attributable to primary vaccine failures, but waning immunity after immunization (ie, secondary vaccine failure) may be a factor in some cases. Primary vaccine failure was the main reason a 2-dose vaccine schedule was recommended routinely for children and high-risk adults.

Patients infected with wild-type measles virus are contagious from 4 days before the rash through 4 days after appearance of the rash. Immunocompromised patients who may have prolonged excretion of the virus in respiratory tract secretions can be contagious for the duration of the illness. Patients with SSPE are not contagious.

The **incubation period** generally is 8 to 12 days from exposure to onset of symptoms. In family studies, the average interval between appearance of rash in the index case and subsequent cases is 14 days, with a range of 7 to 21 days. In SSPE, the mean incubation period of 84 cases reported between 1976 and 1983 was 10.8 years.

DIAGNOSTIC TESTS: Measles virus infection can be confirmed by: (1) detection of measles viral RNA by reverse transcriptase-polymerase chain reaction (RT-PCR); (2) detection of measles-specific immunoglobulin (Ig) M; (3) a fourfold increase in measles IgG antibody concentration in paired acute and convalescent serum specimens (collected at least 10 days apart); or (4) isolation of measles virus in cell culture. Detection of IgM in serum samples by enzyme immunoassay has been the preferred method for case confirmation; however, as the incidence of disease decreases, the positive predictive value of IgM detection also decreases. For this reason, detection of viral RNA in blood; throat, nasal, and posterior nasopharyngeal swab specimens; bronchial lavage samples; or urine samples (respiratory samples are preferred specimens, and sampling more than 1 site may increase sensitivity) is playing an increasing role in case confirmation, especially in countries that have achieved measles elimination. A serum sample as well as a throat swab specimen should be obtained from any patient in whom measles infection is suspected. Additionally, it is ideal to obtain a urine sample, because sampling from all 3 sites will increase the likelihood of establishing a diagnosis. State public health laboratories and the Measles Laboratory at the Centers for Disease Control and Prevention (CDC) can perform RT-PCR assays to detect measles RNA. Isolation of measles virus in cell culture is not recommended for routine case confirmation (ie, clinical diagnosis), because isolation can take up to 2 weeks to complete. However, viral isolates are important for monitoring the genetic characteristics of circulating measles viruses.

Ideally, both a serum sample for IgM detection and serum and throat swab samples for RNA detection should be taken at first contact with a suspected case. The sensitivity of measles IgM assays varies by timing of specimen collection, immunization status of the patient, and the assay method itself. Up to 20% of assays for IgM may have a false-negative result in the first 72 hours after rash onset. If the measles IgM result is negative and the patient has a generalized rash lasting more than 72 hours, a second serum specimen should be obtained, and the measles IgM test should be repeated. Measles IgM is detectable for at least 1 month after rash onset in unimmunized people but might be absent or present only transiently in people immunized with 1 or 2 vaccine doses. Therefore, a negative IgM test result should not be used to rule out the diagnosis in immunized people.

Detection of viral RNA by RT-PCR provides a relatively rapid and sensitive method for case confirmation. It is important to collect samples for RNA detection as soon as possible after rash onset, because viral shedding declines with time after rash. Specimen timing and quality greatly influence the results of RT-PCR testing, so a negative result should not be the only criterion used to rule out a case of measles. Another advantage of collecting samples for molecular detection of the virus is that these samples can also be used to genotype the virus. Genotype information is used to help identify patterns of importation and transmission. For example, analysis by CDC scientists showed that the measles virus type in the 2015 outbreak (B3) was identical to the virus type that caused the large measles outbreak in the Philippines in 2014. Genome sequencing can be used to differentiate between wild-type and vaccine virus infection in suspected cases with a history of recent vaccination.

In populations with high vaccine coverage, such as those in the United States, comprehensive serologic and virologic testing generally is not available locally and requires submitting specimens to state public health laboratories or the CDC. Individuals with a febrile rash illness who are seronegative for measles IgM and have negative RT-PCR assay results for measles should be tested for rubella using the same specimens. All cases of suspected measles should be reported immediately to the local or state health department without waiting for results of diagnostic tests. Measles is on the list of nationally notifiable diseases that should be reported to the CDC within 24 hours.

TREATMENT: No specific antiviral therapy is available. Measles virus is susceptible in vitro to ribavirin, which has been given by the intravenous and aerosol routes to treat severely affected and immunocompromised children with measles. However, no controlled trials have been conducted, and ribavirin is not licensed by the US Food and Drug Administration for treatment of measles.

Vitamin A. Vitamin A treatment of children with measles in resource-limited countries has been associated with decreased morbidity and mortality rates. Low serum concentrations of vitamin A also have been found in children in the United States, and children with more severe measles illness have lower vitamin A concentrations. The WHO currently recommends vitamin A for all children with acute measles, regardless of their country of residence. Vitamin A for treatment of measles is administered once daily for 2 days, at the following doses:

- 200 000 IU for children 12 months or older;
- 100 000 IU for infants 6 through 11 months of age; and
- 50 000 IU for infants younger than 6 months.
- An additional (ie, a third) age-specific dose should be given 2 through 4 weeks later to children with clinical signs and symptoms of vitamin A deficiency.

Even in countries where measles is not usually severe, vitamin A should be given to all children with severe measles (eg, requiring hospitalization). Parenteral and oral formulations of vitamin A are available in the United States.

ISOLATION OF THE HOSPITALIZED PATIENT: In addition to standard precautions, airborne transmission precautions are indicated for 4 days after the onset of rash in otherwise healthy children and for the duration of illness in immunocompromised patients. Exposed susceptible patients should be placed on airborne precautions from day 5 after first exposure until day 21 after last exposure.[1]

CONTROL MEASURES:

Evidence of Immunity to Measles.[2] Evidence of immunity to measles includes any of the following:

1. Documentation of age-appropriate vaccination with a live measles virus-containing vaccine:
   - preschool-aged children: 1 dose administered after the first birthday;
   - school-aged children (grades K-12): 2 doses; the first dose administered after the first birthday and the second dose administered at least 28 days after the first dose;
2. Laboratory evidence of immunity;
3. Laboratory confirmation of disease; or
4. Born before 1957.

Care of Exposed People.

Use of Vaccine. Available data suggest that measles vaccine, if administered within 72 hours of measles exposure to susceptible individuals, will provide protection or disease modification in some cases. Measles vaccine should be considered in all exposed individuals who are vaccine eligible and who have not been vaccinated or have received only 1 dose of vaccine (the second measles vaccine dose can be administered ≥28 days after the first measles vaccine dose). If the exposure does not result in infection, the vaccine should induce protection against subsequent measles exposures. Immunization is the intervention of choice for control of measles outbreaks in schools and child care centers and for vaccine-eligible people 12 months and older and has been used starting at 6 months of age with good efficacy in previous measles epidemics in the United States.

Use of Immune Globulin. Immune Globulin (IG) can be administered either intramuscularly (IGIM) or intravenously (IGIV) within 6 days of exposure to prevent or modify measles in people who do not have evidence of measles immunity. The recommended dose of IGIM is 0.50 mL/kg (the maximum dose by volume is 15 mL). IGIV is the recommended IG preparation for pregnant women without evidence of measles immunity and

---

[1]Centers for Disease Control and Prevention. Immunization of health-care personnel: recommendations of the Advisory Committee on Immunization Practices (ACIP). *MMWR Recomm Rep.* 2011;60(RR-7):1–45

[2]Centers for Disease Control and Prevention. Prevention of measles, rubella, congenital rubella syndrome, and mumps, 2013 summary: recommendations of the Advisory Committee on Immunization Practices (ACIP). *MMWR Recomm Rep.* 2013;62(RR-4):1–34

for severely immunocompromised hosts,[1] regardless of immunologic or vaccination status, including patients with severe primary immunodeficiency; patients who have received a bone marrow transplant, until at least 12 months after finishing all immunosuppressive treatment, or longer in patients who have developed graft-versus-host disease; patients on treatment for acute lymphoblastic leukemia, within and until at least 6 months after completion of immunosuppressive chemotherapy; individuals who have received a solid organ transplant; people with human immunodeficiency virus (HIV) infection or acquired immunodeficiency syndrome (AIDS) who have severe immunosuppression; and patients younger than 12 months whose mothers received biologic response modifiers during pregnancy. IGIV is recommended for these groups because they may be at higher risk of severe measles and complications, and people who weigh >30 kg will receive less than the recommended dose with IGIM preparations. IGIV is administered at a dose of 400 mg/kg. For patients who already are receiving IGIV at regularly scheduled intervals, the usual dose of 400 mg/kg should be adequate for measles prophylaxis after exposures occurring within 3 weeks of receiving IGIV. For people routinely receiving Immune Globulin Subcutaneous (IGSC) therapy, administration of at least 200 mg/kg for 2 consecutive weeks before measles exposure should be sufficient. IG is not indicated for household or other close contacts who have received 1 dose of vaccine at 12 months or older unless they are severely immunocompromised (as defined previously).

For children who receive IGIM for modification or prevention of measles after exposure, measles vaccine (if not contraindicated) should be administered 6 months after IGIM administration, provided the child is at least 12 months of age. Intervals vary between administration of IGIV or other biologic products and measles-containing vaccines (see Table 1.13, p 40).

HIV Infection.[1] HIV-infected children who are exposed to measles require prophylaxis on the basis of immune status and measles vaccine history. HIV-infected children who have serologic evidence of immunity or who received 2 doses of measles vaccine after initiation of combination antiretroviral therapy (cART) with no or moderate immunosuppression (see Human Immunodeficiency Virus Infection, p 459) should be considered immune and will not require any additional measures to prevent measles. Asymptomatic mildly or moderately immunocompromised HIV-infected patients without evidence of immunity to measles should receive IGIM at a dose of 0.5 mL/kg (maximum 15 mL), regardless of immunization status. Severely immunocompromised patients (including HIV-infected people with CD4+ T-lymphocyte percentages <15% [all ages] or CD4+ T-lymphocyte counts <200/mm^3 [age >5 years] and those who have not received MMR vaccine since receiving cART) who are exposed to measles should receive IGIV prophylaxis, 400 mg/kg, after exposure to measles regardless of vaccination status, because they may not be protected by the vaccine. Some experts would include all HIV-infected people, regardless of immunologic status or MMR vaccine history, as needing IGIV prophylaxis. HIV-infected children who have received IGIV within 3 weeks of exposure do not require additional passive immunization.

Health Care Personnel. To decrease health care-associated infection, immunization programs should be established to ensure that all people who work or volunteer in health

[1]Centers for Disease Control and Prevention. Prevention of measles, rubella, congenital rubella syndrome, and mumps, 2013 summary: recommendations of the Advisory Committee on Immunization Practices (ACIP). *MMWR Recomm Rep.* 2013;62(RR-4):1–34

Table 3.39. Recommendations for Measles Immunization[a]

Category	Recommendations
Unimmunized, no history of measles (12 through 15 mo of age)	MMR or MMRV vaccine is recommended at 12 through 15 mo of age; a second dose is recommended at least 28 days after the first dose (or 90 days for MMRV) and usually is administered at 4 through 6 y of age
Children 6 through 11 mo of age in epidemic situations[b] or before international travel	Immunize with MMR vaccine, but this dose is not considered valid, and 2 valid doses administered on or after the first birthday are required. The first valid dose should be administered at 12 through 15 mo of age; the second valid dose is recommended at least 28 days later and usually is administered at 4 through 6 y of age. MMRV should not be administered to children <12 mo of age.
Students in kindergarten, elementary, middle, and high school who have received 1 dose of measles vaccine at 12 mo of age or older	Administer the second dose
Students in college and other postsecondary institutions who have received 1 dose of measles vaccine at 12 mo of age or older	Administer the second dose
History of immunization before the first birthday	Dose not considered valid; immunize (2 doses)
History of receipt of inactivated measles vaccine or unknown type of vaccine, 1963–1967	Dose not considered valid; immunize (2 doses)
Further attenuated or unknown vaccine administered with IG	Dose not considered valid; immunize (2 doses)
Allergy to eggs	Immunize; no reactions likely (see text for details)
Neomycin allergy, nonanaphylactic	Immunize; no reactions likely (see text for details)
Severe hypersensitivity (anaphylaxis) to neomycin or gelatin	Avoid immunization
Tuberculosis	Immunize (see Tuberculosis, p 829); if patient has untreated tuberculosis disease, start antituberculosis therapy before immunizing
Measles exposure	Immunize or give IG, depending on circumstances (see Care of Exposed People, p 541)
HIV infected	Immunize (2 doses) unless severely immunocompromised (see text, p 542); administration of IG if exposed to measles is based on degree of immunosuppression and measles vaccine history (see text, p 542)
Personal or family history of seizures	Immunize; advise parents of slightly increased risk of seizures
Immunoglobulin or blood recipient	Immunize at the appropriate interval (see Table 1.13, p 40)

MMR indicates measles-mumps-rubella vaccine; MMRV, measles-mumps-rubella-varicella vaccine; IG, Immune Globulin; HIV, human immunodeficiency virus.

[a]See text for details and recommendations for use of MMRV vaccine.

[b]See Outbreak Control (p 550).

care facilities (including students) have presumptive evidence of immunity to measles (see Immunization in Health Care Personnel, p 97).

Measles Vaccine Recommendations (see Table 3.39 for summary).

Use of MMR Vaccine. The only measles vaccine licensed in the United States is a live fur-ther-attenuated strain prepared in chicken embryo cell culture. Measles vaccines provided through the Expanded Programme on Immunization in resource-limited countries meet the WHO standards and usually are comparable with the vaccine available in the United States. Measles vaccine is available in combination formulations, which include measles-mumps-rubella (MMR) and measles-mumps-rubella-varicella (MMRV) vaccines. Single-antigen measles vaccine no longer is available in the United States. Measles-containing vaccine in a dose of 0.5 mL is administered subcutaneously. Measles-containing vaccines can be administered simultaneously with other immunizations in a separate syringe at a separate site (see Simultaneous Administration of Multiple Vaccines, p 35).

Serum measles antibodies develop in approximately 95% of children immunized at 12 months of age and 98% of children immunized at 15 months of age. Protection con-ferred by a single dose is durable in most people. A small proportion (5% or less) of im-munized people may lose protection after several years. For measles control and elimina-tion, 2 doses of vaccine are required. More than 99% of people who receive 2 doses (sepa-rated by at least 28 days, and the first dose administered on or after the first birthday) de-velop serologic evidence of measles immunity. The second dose provides protection to those failing to respond to their primary measles immunization and, therefore, is not a booster dose. Immunization is not deleterious for people who already are immune. Im-munized people do not shed or transmit measles vaccine virus.

Improperly stored vaccine may fail to protect against measles. Since 1979, an im-proved stabilizer has been added to the vaccine that makes it more resistant to heat inac-tivation. For recommended storage of MMR and MMRV vaccines, see the manufactur-ers' package labels. MMRV vaccine must be stored frozen between −58°F and +5°F.

Age of Routine Immunization. The first dose of MMR vaccine should be administered at 12 through 15 months of age. Delays in administering the first dose contributed to large outbreaks in the United States from 1989 to 1991. The second dose is recommended rou-tinely at school entry (ie, 4 through 6 years of age) but can be administered at any earlier age (eg, during an outbreak or before international travel), provided the interval between the first and second MMR doses is at least 28 days. Catch-up second dose immunization should occur for all school children (elementary, middle, high school) who have received only 1 dose, including at the adolescent visit at 11 through 12 years of age and beyond. If a child receives a dose of measles vaccine before 12 months of age, this dose is not counted toward the required number of doses; the universally recommended 2 doses are still required in the US beginning at 12 through 15 months of age and separated by at least 28 days.

Use of MMRV Vaccine.[1,2]

---

[1]Centers for Disease Control and Prevention. Use of combination measles, mumps, rubella, and varicella vac-cine: recommendations of the Advisory Committee on Immunization Practices (ACIP). *MMWR Recomm Rep.* 2010;59(RR–3):1–12

[2]American Academy of Pediatrics, Committee on Infectious Diseases. Prevention of varicella: update of recom-mendations for use of quadrivalent and monovalent varicella vaccines in children. *Pediatrics.* 2011;128(3):630–632

- MMRV vaccine is indicated for simultaneous immunization against measles, mumps, rubella, and varicella among children 12 months through 12 years of age; MMRV vaccine is not indicated for people outside this age group. See Varicella-Zoster Infections, p 869, for recommendations for use of MMRV vaccine for the first dose.
- Children with HIV infection also should not receive MMRV vaccine because of lack of safety data of the quadrivalent vaccine in children infected with HIV.
- MMRV vaccine may be administered with other vaccines recommended at 12 through 15 months of age and before or at 4 through 6 years of age (**https:// redbook.solutions.aap.org/SS/Immunization_Schedules.aspx**).
- At least 28 days should elapse between a dose of measles-containing vaccine, such as MMR vaccine, and a dose of MMRV vaccine. However, the recommended minimal interval between MMRV vaccine doses is 90 days.
- Febrile seizures occur in 7 to 9 per 10 000 children receiving the first dose of MMRV vaccine at 12 through 23 months of age and in 3 to 4 per 10 000 children receiving the first dose of MMR and varicella vaccines administered separately at the same visit at 12 through 23 months of age. Thus, 1 additional febrile seizure is expected to occur per approximately 2300 to 2600 children 12 through 23 months of age immunized with a first-dose MMRV vaccine, compared with separate MMR and monovalent varicella vaccines. The period of risk for febrile seizures is from 5 to 12 days following receipt of the vaccine. Febrile seizures do not predispose to epilepsy or neurodevelopmental delays later in life and have no lasting medical consequence. The benefit of using MMRV instead of MMR and monovalent varicella vaccines separately is that the quadrivalent product results in 1 fewer injection. The American Academy of Pediatrics recommends that for the first dose of measles, mumps, rubella, and varicella vaccines at ages 12 through 47 months, either MMR and varicella vaccines or MMRV vaccine be used. Pediatricians should discuss risks and benefits of the vaccine choices with the parents or caregivers. For the first dose of measles, mumps, rubella, and varicella vaccines at ages 48 months and older and for dose 2 at any age (15 months through 12 years), use of MMRV vaccine generally is preferred over separate injections of MMR and varicella vaccines to minimize the number of injections. Children 4 through 6 years of age who received MMRV did not have an increased risk of febrile seizures when compared with children of the same age who received separate injections of MMR and varicella vaccine. However, it might be prudent to administer separate MMR and varicella vaccines to children with a personal of family history of febrile seizures or epilepsy, because the risk of febrile seizures is higher in this group.

Colleges and Other Institutions for Education Beyond High School. Colleges and other educational institutions should require that all entering students have documentation of evidence of measles immunity (see Evidence of Immunity to Measles, p 541). Students without documentation of measles immunity should receive MMR vaccine on entry, followed by a second dose 28 days later, if not contraindicated.

Immunization During an Outbreak. During an outbreak, MMR vaccine should be offered to all people exposed or in the outbreak setting who lack evidence of measles immunity. During a community-wide outbreak that affects infants, MMR vaccine has been shown to be efficacious and may be recommended for infants 6 through 11 months of age (see Outbreak Control, p 550). However, because of the presence of maternal antibody in some children, seroconversion rates after MMR immunization are lower in children immunized before the first birthday than in children immunized on or after the first birthday.

For this reason, doses received prior to the first birthday should not count toward the recommended 2-dose series. Children immunized before their first birthday should be reimmunized with MMR or MMRV vaccine at 12 through 15 months of age (at least 28 days after the initial measles immunization) and again at school entry (4 through 6 years of age).

International Travel. People traveling internationally (any country outside of the United States) should be immune to measles prior to travel. Infants 6 through 11 months of age should receive 1 dose of MMR vaccine before departure, and then they should receive a second dose of measles-containing vaccine at 12 through 15 months of age (at least 28 days after the initial measles immunization) and a third dose at 4 through 6 years of age. Children 12 through 15 months of age should receive their first dose of MMR vaccine before departure and again by 4 through 6 years of age. Children 12 months or older who have received 1 dose and are traveling to areas where measles is endemic or epidemic should receive their second dose before departure, provided the interval between doses is 28 days or more.

International Adoptees. The US Department of State requires that internationally adopted children 10 years and older receive several vaccines, including MMR, before entry into the United States. Internationally adopted children who are younger than 10 years are exempt from Immigration and Nationality Act regulations pertaining to immunization of immigrants before arrival in the United States (see Children Who Received Immunizations Outside the United States or Whose Immunization Status is Unknown or Uncertain, p 100); adoptive parents are required to sign a waiver indicating their intention to comply with US immunization recommendations after their child's arrival in the United States.

Health Care Personnel.[1] Adequate presumptive evidence of immunity to measles for people who work in health care facilities is: (1) documented administration of 2 doses of live-virus measles vaccine with the first dose administered at ≥12 months of age and the second dose at least 28 days after the first; (2) laboratory evidence of immunity or laboratory confirmation of disease; or (3) birth before 1957. Birth before 1957 is not a guarantee of measles immunity, and therefore, facilities should consider vaccinating unimmunized personnel born before 1957 who lack laboratory evidence of immunity with 2 doses of MMR vaccine at the appropriate interval (see Immunization in Health Care Personnel, p 97). For recommendations during an outbreak, see Outbreak Control (p 550).

Adverse Events. A body temperature of 39.4°C (103°F) or higher develops in approximately 5% to 15% of vaccine recipients, usually between 6 and 12 days after receipt of MMR vaccine; fever generally lasts 1 to 2 days but may last as long as 5 days. Most people with fever otherwise are asymptomatic. Transient rashes have been reported in approximately 5% of vaccine recipients. Recipients who develop fever and/or rash are not considered contagious. Febrile seizures 5 to 12 days after immunization occur in 1 in 3000 to 4000 people immunized with MMR vaccine. Transient thrombocytopenia occurs in 1 in 22 000 to 40 000 people after administration of measles-containing vaccines, specifically MMR (see Thrombocytopenia, p 548). There is no evidence that reimmunization increases the risk of adverse events in people already immune to these diseases. Data indicate that only people who are not immune to the viruses in MMR tend to have adverse

[1]Centers for Disease Control and Prevention. Immunization of health-care personnel: recommendations of the Advisory Committee on Immunization Practices (ACIP). *MMWR Recomm Rep.* 2011;60(RR–07):1–45

effects. Thus, events following a second dose of MMR vaccine would be expected to be substantially lower than after a first dose, because most people who received a first dose would be immune.

Rates of most local and systemic adverse events for children immunized with MMRV vaccine are comparable with rates for children immunized with MMR and varicella vaccines administered concomitantly. However, recipients of a first dose of MMRV vaccine have a greater rate of fever 102°F (38.9°C) or higher than do recipients of MMR and varicella administered concomitantly (22% vs 15%, respectively), and measles-like rash is observed in 3% of recipients of MMRV vaccine and 2% of recipients of MMR and varicella vaccines administered concomitantly.

The reported frequency of central nervous system conditions, such as encephalitis and encephalopathy, after measles immunization is less than 1 per million doses administered in the United States. Because the incidence of encephalitis or encephalopathy after measles immunization in the United States is lower than the observed incidence of encephalitis of unknown cause, some or most of the rare reported severe neurologic disorders may be related temporally, rather than causally, to measles immunization. Multiple studies, as well as an Institute of Medicine (now called the National Academy of Medicine) Vaccine Safety Review, refute a causal relationship between autism and MMR vaccine or between inflammatory bowel disease and MMR vaccine. The original 1998 study claiming such a relationship was retracted by the publishing journal in 2010, and the lead author has had his medical license revoked in Great Britain.

Seizures. Risk of febrile seizures following receipt of MMR and MMRV vaccines at 12 through 23 months of age is discussed earlier in the chapter (see Use of MMRV Vaccine, p 544). Children with histories of seizures or children whose first-degree relatives have histories of seizures may be at a slightly increased risk of a seizure and should nevertheless be immunized with separate MMR and varicella vaccines, because the benefits of immunization greatly outweigh the risks of a febrile seizure.

Subacute Sclerosing Panencephalitis. Measles vaccine, by protecting against measles, decreases significantly the possibility of developing SSPE. Vaccine-strain measles virus has never been confirmed in a case of SSPE.

Precautions and Contraindications.

Febrile Illnesses. Children with minor illnesses, such as upper respiratory tract infections, may be immunized. Fever is not a contraindication to immunization. However, if other manifestations suggest a more serious illness, immunization should be deferred until the illness has resolved.

Allergic Reactions. Hypersensitivity reactions occur rarely and usually are minor, consisting of wheal-and-flare reactions or urticaria at the injection site. Reactions have been attributed to trace amounts of neomycin or gelatin or some other component in the vaccine formulation. Anaphylaxis is rare. Measles vaccine is produced in chicken embryo cell culture and does not contain significant amounts of egg white (ovalbumin) cross-reacting proteins. Children with egg allergy are at low risk of anaphylactic reactions to measles-containing vaccines (including MMR and MMRV). Skin testing of children for egg allergy is not predictive of reactions to MMR vaccine and is not recommended before administering MMR or other measles-containing vaccines. People with allergies to chickens or feathers are not at increased risk of reaction to the vaccine.

People who have had a significant hypersensitivity reaction after the first dose of measles vaccine should: (1) be tested for measles immunity, and if immune, should not receive a second dose; or (2) receive evaluation and possible skin testing before receiving a second dose. People who have had an immediate anaphylactic reaction to previous measles immunization should not be reimmunized but should be tested to determine whether they are immune.

People who have experienced anaphylactic reactions to gelatin or topically or systemically administered neomycin should receive measles vaccine only in settings where such reactions can be managed and after consultation with an allergist or immunologist. Most often, however, neomycin allergy manifests as contact dermatitis, which is not a contraindication to receiving measles vaccine.

Thrombocytopenia. Rarely, MMR vaccine can be associated with thrombocytopenia within 2 months of immunization, with a temporal clustering 2 to 3 weeks after immunization. On the basis of case reports, the risk of vaccine-associated thrombocytopenia may be higher for people who previously experienced thrombocytopenia, especially if it occurred in temporal association with earlier MMR immunization. The decision to immunize these children should be based on assessment of immunity after the first dose and the benefits of protection against measles, mumps, and rubella in comparison with the risks of recurrence of thrombocytopenia after immunization. The risk of thrombocytopenia is higher after the first dose of vaccine than after the second dose. There have been no reported cases of thrombocytopenia associated with receipt of MMR vaccine that have resulted in hemorrhagic complications or death in otherwise healthy people.

Recent Administration of IG. IG preparations interfere with the serologic response to measles vaccine for variable periods, depending on the dose of IG administered. Suggested intervals between IG or blood-product administration and measles immunization are provided in Table 1.13 (p 40). If vaccine is administered at intervals shorter than those indicated, as may be warranted if the risk of exposure to measles is imminent, the child should be reimmunized at or after the appropriate interval for immunization (and at least 28 days after the earlier immunization) unless serologic testing indicates that measles-specific antibodies were produced.

MMR vaccine should be administered at least 2 weeks before planned administration of IG, blood transfusion, or other blood products because of the theoretical possibility that antibody will neutralize vaccine virus and interfere with successful immunization; if IG must be administered within 14 days after administration of MMR or MMRV, these vaccines should be administered again after the interval specified in Table 1.13 (p 40).

Tuberculosis. Tuberculin skin testing is not a prerequisite for measles immunization. Antituberculosis therapy should be initiated before administering MMR vaccine to people with untreated tuberculosis infection or disease. Tuberculin skin testing, if otherwise indicated, can be performed any time before or on the day of immunization. Otherwise, testing should be postponed for 4 to 6 weeks, because measles immunization temporarily may suppress tuberculin skin test reactivity. The effects of measles vaccination on interferon gamma release assay (IGRA) characteristics have not been determined; the same precautions as for tuberculin skin testing should be followed.

Altered Immunity. Immunocompromised patients with disorders associated with increased severity of viral infections should not receive live-virus measles vaccine (the exception is people with HIV infection, unless they have evidence of severe immunosuppression; see Immunization and Other Considerations in Immunocompromised Children, p 72, and HIV Infection, below). The risk of exposure to measles for immunocompromised patients can be decreased by immunizing their close susceptible contacts.

Immunized people do not shed or transmit infectious measles vaccine virus. Management of immunodeficient and immunosuppressed patients exposed to measles can be facilitated by previous knowledge of their immune status. If possible, children should receive measles vaccine before initiating treatment with biological response modifiers, such as tumor necrosis factor antagonists, and before transplantation, ideally with 2 doses. Susceptible patients who are immunocompromised should receive IG after measles exposure (see Care of Exposed People, p 541).

Corticosteroids. For patients who have received high doses of corticosteroids (≥ 2 mg/kg of body weight or ≥ 20 mg/day of prednisone or its equivalent for people who weigh ≥ 10 kg) for 14 days or more and who otherwise are not immunocompromised, the recommended interval between stopping the corticosteroids and immunization is at least 4 weeks (see Immunization and Other Considerations in Immunocompromised Children, p 72). In general, inhaled steroids do not cause immunosuppression and are not a contraindication to measles immunization.

HIV Infection.[1] Measles immunization (administered as MMR vaccine) is recommended for all people ≥ 12 months of age with HIV infection who do not have evidence of measles immunity and who do not have evidence of severe immunosuppression, because measles can be severe and often is fatal in patients with HIV infection (see Human Immunodeficiency Virus Infection, p 459). For vaccination purposes, severe immunosuppression is defined in children 1 through 13 years of age as a CD4+ T-lymphocyte percentage <15% and in adolescents ≥ 14 years as a CD4+ T-lymphocyte count <200 lymphocytes/mm^3. Severely immunocompromised HIV-infected infants, children, adolescents, and young adults should not receive measles virus-containing vaccine, because vaccine-related pneumonia has been reported (see Human Immunodeficiency Virus Infection, p 459). The quadrivalent measles-mumps-rubella-varicella (MMRV) vaccine should not be administered to any HIV-infected infant, regardless of degree of immunosuppression, because of lack of safety data in this population. The first dose of MMR vaccine should be administered at age 12 through 15 months and the second dose at age 4 through 6 years, or as early as 28 days after the first dose. Children, adolescents, and adults with newly diagnosed HIV infections and without evidence of measles immunity should complete a 2-dose schedule with MMR vaccine as soon as possible after diagnosis, unless they have evidence of severe immunosuppression. People with perinatally acquired HIV infection who were vaccinated against measles before initiation of cART should be considered unvaccinated and should be revaccinated with 2 doses of MMR vaccine once effective cART has been administered, unless they have other acceptable current evidence of measles immunity. All members of the household of an HIV-infected person should receive 2 doses of MMR unless they are HIV infected and severely immunosuppressed, were born before 1957, have laboratory evidence of measles immunity, have had age-appropriate immunizations, or have a contraindication to measles vaccine. Because measles vaccine virus is not shed after immunization, HIV-infected people are not at risk of measles vaccine virus infection if household members are immunized.

Personal or Family History of Seizures. Children with a personal or family history of seizures should be immunized after parents or guardians are advised that the risk of seizures after measles immunization is increased slightly. Risk of febrile seizures following receipt of

---

[1]Rubin LG, Levin MJ, Ljungman P, et al. 2013 IDSA clinical practice guideline for vaccination of the immunocompromised host. *Clin Infect Dis.* 2014;58(3):309–318

MMR and MMRV vaccine at 12 through 23 months of age is discussed earlier in the chapter (see Use of MMRV Vaccine, p 544). Children receiving anticonvulsants should continue such therapy after measles immunization.

Pregnancy. A measles-containing vaccine should not be administered to women known to be pregnant. Women who receive MMR vaccine should not become pregnant for at least 28 days. This precaution is based on the theoretical risk of fetal infection, which applies to administration of any live-virus vaccine to women who might be pregnant or who might become pregnant shortly after immunization. No data from women who were inadvertently vaccinated while pregnant substantiate this theoretical risk. When immunizing adolescents and young adults against measles, recommended precautions include asking women if they are pregnant, excluding women who are, and explaining the theoretical risks to others.

Outbreak Control. Every suspected measles case should be reported immediately to the local health department, and every effort must be made to obtain laboratory evidence that would confirm that the illness is measles (including obtaining specimens for virus detection), especially if the illness may be the first case in the community. Subsequent prevention of spread of measles depends on prompt immunization of people at risk of exposure or people already exposed who cannot readily provide documentation of measles immunity, including the date of immunization. People who have not been immunized, including those who have been exempted from measles immunization for medical reasons, should be excluded from school, child care, and health care settings until at least 21 days after the onset of rash in the last case of measles. Extra doses of measles vaccine administered to previously immunized people are not associated with an increased risk of reactions.

Schools and Child Care Facilities. During measles outbreaks in child care facilities, schools, and colleges and other institutions of higher education, all students, their siblings, and personnel born in 1957 or after who cannot provide documentation that they received 2 doses of measles-containing vaccine on or after their first birthday or other evidence of measles immunity should be immunized. People receiving their second dose, as well as unimmunized people receiving their first dose as part of the outbreak-control program, may be readmitted immediately to the school or child care facility.

Health Care Facilities. If an outbreak occurs in an area served by a hospital or within a hospital, all employees and volunteers who cannot provide documentation that they have received 2 doses of measles vaccine, with the first dose administered on or after their first birthday, or laboratory evidence of immunity to measles should receive 2 doses of MMR vaccine. Because some health care personnel born before 1957 have acquired measles in health care facilities, immunization with 2 doses of MMR vaccine is recommended for health care personnel without serologic evidence of immunity in this age category during outbreaks. Serologic testing before immunization is not recommended during an outbreak, because rapid immunization is required to halt disease transmission. Health care personnel without evidence of immunity who have been exposed should be relieved of direct patient contact from the fifth to the 21st day after exposure, regardless of whether they received vaccine or IG after the exposure. Health care personnel who become ill should be relieved of patient contact until 4 days after rash develops.

Meningococcal Infections

CLINICAL MANIFESTATIONS: Invasive infection usually results in septicemia (~35%–

40% of cases), meningitis (~50% of cases), or both. Bacteremic pneumonia is less common (~9% of cases). Rarely, young children have occult bacteremia. Onset of invasive infections can be insidious and nonspecific, but onset of septicemia (meningococcemia) typically is abrupt, with fever, chills, malaise, myalgia, limb pain, prostration, and a rash that initially can be macular or maculopapular but typically becomes petechial or purpuric within hours. A similar rash can occur with viral infections or with severe sepsis attributable to other bacterial pathogens. In fulminant cases, purpura, limb ischemia, coagulopathy, pulmonary edema, shock, coma, and death can ensue within hours despite appropriate management. Signs and symptoms of meningococcal meningitis are indistinguishable from those associated with pneumococcal meningitis. In severe and fatal cases of meningococcal meningitis, raised intracranial pressure is a predominant presenting feature. Less common manifestations of meningococcal infection include conjunctivitis, septic arthritis, and chronic meningococcemia. Invasive infections can be complicated by arthritis, myocarditis, pericarditis, and endophthalmitis. The overall case-fatality rate for meningococcal disease is ~15% and is somewhat higher in late adolescence and in adults. Mortality is higher with infection caused by serogroup C and Y strains than serogroup B strains. Risk factors for mortality include coma, hypotension, leukopenia, thrombocytopenia, and absence of meningitis. A self-limiting postinfectious inflammatory syndrome occurs in fewer than 10% of cases, begins a minimum 4 days after onset of meningococcal infection, and most commonly presents as fever and arthritis or vasculitis with less common manifestations including iritis, scleritis, conjunctivitis, pericarditis, and polyserositis.

Sequelae associated with meningococcal disease occur in up to 19% of survivors and include hearing loss, neurologic disability, digit or limb amputations, and skin scarring. In addition, patients may experience subtle long-term neurologic deficits, such as impaired school performance, behavioral problems, and attention deficit disorder.

ETIOLOGY: *Neisseria meningitidis* is a gram-negative diplococcus with 13 serogroups based on capsular type.

EPIDEMIOLOGY: In the United States, *N meningitidis* is the leading cause of bacterial meningitis in children 11 through 17 years of age and remains an important cause of septicemia. *N meningitidis* disease rates are highest in infants, adolescents, young adults 16 through 21 years of age, and adults older than 65 years. Household contacts of cases have 500 to 800 times the rate of disease for the general population. A predominance of US cases is observed in the winter, often noted 2 to 3 weeks following onset of influenza outbreaks, with peak of cases in January, February, and March. Patients with persistent complement-component deficiencies (eg, C3, C5–C9, properdin, or factor D or factor H deficiencies), with anatomic or functional asplenia, or treated with eculizumab are at increased risk of invasive and recurrent meningococcal disease. Asymptomatic colonization of the upper respiratory tract is most common in older adolescents and young adults and is the reservoir from which the organism is spread. Transmission occurs from person to person through droplets from the respiratory tract and requires close contact. Patients should be considered capable of transmitting the organism for up to 24 hours after initiation of effective antimicrobial treatment.

Distribution of meningococcal serogroups in the United States has shifted in the past 2 decades. Serogroups B, C, and Y each account for approximately 30% of reported cases, but serogroup distribution varies by age, location, and time. Approximately 90% of cases among adolescents and young adults are caused by serogroups B, C, Y, or W and, therefore, potentially are preventable with available vaccines. In infants and children younger than 60 months, approximately two thirds of cases are caused by serogroup B.

During the past 60 years, the annual incidence of meningococcal disease in the United States has varied from ≤0.3 to 1.5 cases per 100 000 population. Since the early 2000s, annual incidence rates have decreased, and during 2012 to 2014, rates were at a historic low, with fewer than 600 cases annually in the United States; 375 cases were reported in 2015. The decrease in cases in the United States started before the 2005 introduction of meningococcal vaccine into the routine immunization schedule and the 2011 recommendation for a booster vaccine for age 16 years. Reasons for this decrease are postulated to be related to the increased use of influenza vaccine, reduction in the carriage rates, the use of meningococcal conjugate vaccines in preadolescents and adolescents, immunity of the population to circulating meningococcal strains unrelated to vaccination, and changes in behavioral risk factors (eg, decreases in smoking and exposure to secondhand smoke among adolescents and young adults).

Strains belonging to groups A, B, C, Y, and W are implicated most commonly in invasive disease worldwide. Serogroup A has been associated frequently with epidemics outside the United States, primarily in sub-Saharan Africa. A serogroup A meningococcal conjugate vaccine was introduced in the "meningitis belt" of sub-Saharan Africa in December 2010, and its widespread use has been associated with a marked reduction in serogroup A disease rates; recent outbreaks in the meningitis belt have been associated with serogroups C, W, and most recently, the rarely reported serogroup X. In Europe, Australia, and South America, the incidence of meningococcal disease ranged from 0.3 to 3 cases per 100 000 population in recent years. Serogroups B and C are the most commonly reported in these regions, although increased rates of serogroups W and Y have been observed in some countries.

Most cases of meningococcal disease are sporadic, with fewer than 5% associated with outbreaks. Outbreaks occur in communities and institutions, including child care centers, schools, colleges, and military recruit camps. More recently, several outbreaks of serogroup B meningococcal disease have occurred on college campuses, and clusters/outbreaks of serogroup C meningococcal disease have been reported among men who have sex with men.

The **incubation period** is 1 to 10 days, usually less than 4 days.

DIAGNOSTIC TESTS: Cultures of blood and cerebrospinal fluid (CSF) are indicated for patients with suspected invasive meningococcal disease. Cultures of a petechial or purpuric lesion scraping, synovial fluid, and other usually sterile body fluid specimens sometimes are positive. Specimens for culture should be plated onto both sheep blood and chocolate agar and incubated at 35°C to 37°C with 5% carbon dioxide in a moist atmosphere. The organism is readily identified with standard biochemical tests as well as by the newer method of mass spectrometry of bacterial cell components. Isolates should be submitted to a reference laboratory for serogrouping for epidemiologic purposes. A Gram stain of a petechial or purpuric scraping, CSF, and buffy coat smear of blood can be positive. Because *N meningitidis* can be a component of the nasopharyngeal flora, isolation of *N meningitidis* from this site is not helpful diagnostically. Antigen detection tests, primarily by latex agglutination, to detect select meningococcal polysaccharide types in CSF were developed more than 2 decades ago. These assays no longer are commonly used because of concerns about test sensitivity and specificity. A serogroup-specific polymerase chain reaction (PCR) test to detect *N meningitidis* from clinical specimens is used routinely in the United Kingdom and some European countries, where up to 56% of cases are confirmed by PCR testing alone. PCR testing is useful particularly in patients who receive antimicrobial therapy before cultures are obtained. In the United States, PCR-based assays are available in some research and public health laboratories. A multiplex PCR assay has been developed that appears to have a sensitivity and specificity approaching 100% for detection of serogroups A, B, C, W, and Y.

Surveillance case definitions for invasive meningococcal disease are provided in Table 3.40. Serologic typing, multilocus sequence typing, multilocus enzyme electrophoresis, pulsed-field gel electrophoresis of enzyme-restricted DNA fragments, and whole genome sequencing can be useful epidemiologic tools during a suspected outbreak to detect concordance among invasive strains.

TREATMENT: The priority in management of meningococcal disease is treatment of shock in meningococcemia and of raised intracranial pressure in severe meningitis. Empirical therapy for suspected meningococcal disease should include cefotaxime or ceftriaxone. Once the microbiologic diagnosis is established, definitive treatment with penicillin G (300 000 U/kg/day; maximum, 12 million U/day, divided every 4–6 hours), ampicillin, cefotaxime, or ceftriaxone is recommended. Five to 7 days of antimicrobial therapy is adequate. Some experts recommend susceptibility testing before switching to penicillin, although resistance of *N meningitidis* to penicillin is rare in the United States. Additionally, susceptibility testing is not standardized, and the clinical significance of intermediate susceptibility to penicillin is unknown. Ceftriaxone clears nasopharyngeal carriage effectively after 1 dose. For patients with a life-threatening penicillin allergy characterized by anaphylaxis, meropenem or ceftriaxone can be used with caution as the rate of cross-reactivity in penicillin-allergic adults is very low. In meningococcemia, early and rapid fluid resuscitation and early use of inotropic and ventilatory support may reduce mortality.

Table 3.40. Surveillance Case Definitions for Invasive Meningococcal Disease

Confirmed case

A clinically compatible case and isolation of *Neisseria meningitidis* from a usually sterile site, for example:
- Blood
- Cerebrospinal fluid (CSF)
- Synovial fluid
- Pleural fluid
- Pericardial fluid
- Isolation from skin scraping of petechial or purpuric lesions

OR

Detection of *N meningitidis*-specific nucleic acid in a specimen obtained from a normally sterile body site (eg, blood or CSF), using a validated polymerase chain reaction (PCR) assay

Probable case

A clinically compatible case with EITHER a positive result of antigen test OR immunohistochemistry of formalin-fixed tissue

Suspect

- A clinically compatible case and gram-negative diplococci in any sterile fluid, such as CSF, synovial fluid, or scraping from a petechial or purpuric lesion
- Clinical purpura fulminans without a positive culture

The postinfectious inflammatory syndromes associated with meningococcal disease often respond to nonsteroidal anti-inflammatory drugs. Treating physicians should consider evaluating for conditions that increase risk of disease, such as underlying complement component deficiencies.

ISOLATION OF THE HOSPITALIZED PATIENT: In addition to standard precautions, droplet precautions are recommended until 24 hours after initiation of effective antimicrobial therapy.

CONTROL MEASURES:

Care of Exposed People.

Postexposure Chemoprophylaxis. Regardless of immunization status, close contacts including household contacts of all people with invasive meningococcal disease (see Table 3.41), whether endemic or in an outbreak situation, are at high risk of infection and should promptly receive chemoprophylaxis. Chemoprophylaxis should be provided even if the close contact has received meningococcal vaccine, because currently licensed vaccines are not 100% effective. Ceftriaxone clears nasopharyngeal carriage effectively after 1 dose. The decision to give chemoprophylaxis to other contacts is based on risk of contracting invasive disease related to specific exposure to the secretions from infected patient. Throat and nasopharyngeal cultures are not recommended, because these cultures are of no value in deciding who should receive chemoprophylaxis.

Chemoprophylaxis is warranted for people who have been exposed directly to a patient's oral secretions through close social contact, such as kissing or sharing of toothbrushes or eating utensils, as well as for child care and preschool contacts during the 2 to 3 days before onset of disease in the index case. People who frequently slept in the same

Table 3.41. Disease Risk for Contacts of People With Invasive Meningococcal Disease

High risk: chemoprophylaxis recommended (close contacts)
- Household contact, especially children younger than 2 years
- Child care or preschool contact at any time during 7 days before onset of illness
- Direct exposure to index patient's secretions through kissing or through sharing toothbrushes or eating utensils, markers of close social contact, at any time during 7 days before onset of illness
- Mouth-to-mouth resuscitation, unprotected contact during endotracheal intubation at any time 7 days before onset of illness or within 24 h of initiation of effective antimicrobial therapy
- Frequently slept in same dwelling as index patient during 7 days before onset of illness
- Passengers seated directly next to the index case during airline flights lasting more than 8 hours (gate to gate)

Low risk: chemoprophylaxis not recommended
- Casual contact: no history of direct exposure to index patient's oral secretions (eg, school or work)
- Indirect contact: only contact is with a high-risk contact, no direct contact with the index patient
- Health care personnel without direct exposure to patient's oral secretions

In outbreak or cluster
- Chemoprophylaxis for people other than people at high risk should be administered only after consultation with local public health authorities

Table 3.42. Recommended Chemoprophylaxis Regimens for High-Risk Contacts and People With Invasive Meningococcal Disease

Age of Infants, Children, and Adults	Dose	Duration	Efficacy, %	Cautions
Rifampin[a]				
<1 mo	5 mg/kg, orally, every 12 h	2 days		Discussion with an expert for infants <1 mo
≥1 mo	15–20 mg/kg (maximum 600 mg), orally, every 12 h	2 days	90–95	Can interfere with efficacy of oral contraceptives and some seizure and anticoagulant medications; can stain soft contact lenses
Ceftriaxone				
<15 y	125 mg, intramuscularly	Single dose	90–95	To decrease pain at injection site, dilute with 1% lidocaine
≥15 y	250 mg, intramuscularly	Single dose	90–95	To decrease pain at injection site, dilute with 1% lidocaine
Ciprofloxacin[a,b]				
≥1 mo	20 mg/kg (maximum 500 mg), orally	Single dose	90–95	
Azithromycin	10 mg/kg (maximum 500 mg)	Single dose	90	Not recommended routinely; equivalent to rifampin for eradication of *Neisseria meningitidis* from nasopharynx in one study of young adults

[a]Not recommended for use in pregnant women.

[b]Use only if fluoroquinolone-resistant strains of *N meningitidis* have not been identified in the community.

dwelling as the infected person within this period also should receive chemoprophylaxis. Routine prophylaxis is not recommended for health care personnel unless they have had intimate exposure to respiratory tract secretions, such as occurs with unprotected mouth-to-mouth resuscitation, intubation, or suctioning before or less than 24 hours after antimicrobial therapy was initiated. Chemoprophylaxis ideally should be initiated within 24 hours after the index patient is identified; prophylaxis is not indicated more than 2 weeks after exposure.

Antimicrobial Regimens for Prophylaxis (see Table 3.42). Rifampin, ceftriaxone, or ciprofloxacin are appropriate drugs for chemoprophylaxis in adults; neither rifampin nor ciprofloxacin are recommended for pregnant women. The drug of choice for most children is rifampin or ciprofloxacin; ceftriaxone also may be used (Table 3.42). Rifampin alters the pharmacokinetics of a number of medications. Rifampin requires 4 doses over 2 days to eradicate nasopharyngeal carriage, but ceftriaxone and ciprofloxacin require only a single dose. If antimicrobial agents other than ceftriaxone or cefotaxime (each of which will eradicate nasopharyngeal carriage) are used for treatment of invasive meningococcal disease, the child should receive chemoprophylaxis before hospital discharge to eradicate nasopharyngeal carriage of *N meningitidis*.

Ciprofloxacin-resistant strains of *N meningitidis* were detected in 2 states several years ago[1]; if ciprofloxacin resistance is found, this drug should not be used for chemoprophylaxis. Use of azithromycin as a single oral dose has been shown to be effective for eradication of nasopharyngeal carriage in one study and can be used where ciprofloxacin resistance has been detected.

Postexposure Immunoprophylaxis. Because secondary cases can occur several weeks or more after onset of disease in the index case, meningococcal vaccine is recommended when an outbreak is caused by a serogroup prevented by a meningococcal vaccine. For control of meningococcal outbreaks caused by serogroups A, C, Y, and W, the preferred vaccine in adults and children 2 months and older is a meningococcal conjugate vaccine (see Tables 3.43 and 3.44). The Centers for Disease Control and Prevention (CDC) Advisory Committee on Immunization Practices has recommended that either of the 2 licensed serogroup B vaccines be used in people 10 years and older during a serogroup B meningococcal disease outbreak; the same vaccine product should be used for all doses.

Immunoprophylaxis During Eculizumab Therapy.[2] Sixteen cases of meningococcal disease were identified in eculizumab recipients in the United States during 2008–2016; among these, 11 were caused by nongroupable *N meningitidis*. Fourteen patients had documentation of receipt of at least 1 dose of meningococcal vaccine before disease onset. Providers should continue to follow recommendations for eculizumab recipients to receive both MenACWY and MenB vaccines. Providers could also consider antimicrobial prophylaxis (usually penicillin prophylaxis) for the duration of eculizumab treatment, and until immunocompetence is restored once eculizumab is stopped, to potentially reduce the risk for meningococcal disease.

Meningococcal Vaccines. In the United States, 2 meningococcal vaccines are licensed and available for use in children and adults against serogroups A, C, W, and Y (MenACWY), and 2 vaccines are licensed for people 10 through 25 years of age against serogroup B (MenB). Both MenACWY vaccines are protein conjugate vaccines, while the 2 MenB vaccines utilize 2 different technologies. An additional MenACWY polysaccharide vaccine (Menomune) was discontinued in the United States in 2017.

Serogroup A, C, W, and Y Vaccines. MenACWY-D (Menactra, Sanofi Pasteur) is licensed for use in people 9 months through 55 years of age, while MenACWY-CRM (Menveo, Novartis Vaccines) is licensed for use in people 2 months through 55 years of age. Each is administered intramuscularly as a 0.5-mL dose. MenACWY-D is administered as a 2-dose primary series, 3 months apart, among children 9 through 23 months of age. When MenACWY-D and Daptacel (DTaP, Sanofi Pasteur) are being administered to children 4 through 6 years of age, preference should be given to simultaneous administration of the 2 vaccines or administration of MenACWY-D before administration of Daptacel, because administration of MenACWY-D 1 month after Daptacel has been shown to reduce meningococcal antibody response to MenACWY-D.

MenACWY-CRM is licensed for infants as a 4-dose series at 2, 4, 6, and 12 months of age. Dosing during the primary series varies by product, age, and underlying risk for

[1]Centers for Disease Control and Prevention. Emergence of fluoroquinolone-resistant *Neisseria meningitidis*—Minnesota and North Dakota, 2007–2008. *MMWR Morb Mortal Wkly Rep.* 2008;57(7):173–175

[2]McNamara LA, Topaz N, Wang X, Hariri S, Fox L, MacNeil JR. High risk for invasive meningococcal disease among patients receiving eculizumab (Soliris) despite receipt of meningococcal vaccine. *MMWR Morb Mortal Wkly Rep.* 2017;66(27):734–737

disease (see Tables 3.43 and 3.44).

Recommendations for use of a meningococcal conjugate vaccine are as follows[1-4] (Tables 3.43 and 3.44):

- Adolescents should be immunized routinely at the 11- through 12-year health care visit (see **https://redbook.solutions.aap.org/SS/Immunization_ Schedules.aspx**), when immunization status and other preventive health services can be addressed (Table 3.43). A booster dose at 16 years of age is recommended for adolescents immunized at 11 through 12 years of age.

- Adolescents 13 through 18 years of age should be immunized routinely with a meningococcal conjugate vaccine if not previously immunized. Adolescents who receive the first dose at 13 through 15 years of age should receive a 1-time booster dose at 16 through 18 years of age.

- Adolescents who receive their first dose of meningococcal conjugate vaccine at or after 16 years of age do not need a booster dose unless they have risk factors (Table 3.44).

- Routine childhood immunization with meningococcal conjugate vaccines is not recommended for children 2 months through 10 years of age because of the low proportion of infections that are preventable with vaccination; approximately two thirds of disease among children 59 months and younger is caused by serogroup B, which is not prevented with licensed vaccines approved for use in those ages in the United States.

- People at increased risk of invasive meningococcal disease (defined, by age, in the subgroup column of Table 3.44) should be immunized with a meningococcal conjugate vaccine beginning at 2 months of age.

- For high-risk individuals younger than 2 years, only MenACWY-CRM (Menveo) should be used, because interference with immune response to pneumococcal conjugate vaccine occurs with MenACWY-D (Menactra).

Serogroup B Meningococcal Vaccines. MenBFHbp (Trumenba, Pfizer, Philadelphia, PA) is based on a surface-exposed lipoprotein named factor H binding protein (FHbp) that is expressed in more than 97% of invasive meningococcal B strains and functions as an important meningococcal virulence factor. It can be administered as either a 2- or 3-dose series (0 and 6 months or 0, 1–2, and 6 months), depending on risk factors for disease and on outbreak conditions (see Tables 3.43 and 3.44). FHbp sequences segregate into 2 genetically and immunologically distinct subfamilies, A and B. MenB-FHbp contains 2 lipidated FHbp variants (A05 and B01), 1 from each subfamily. It has been used in several outbreaks on US college campuses.

MenB-4C (Bexsero, Novartis Vaccines and Diagnostics, Siena, Italy) contains 4 antigenic components: 1 FHbp fusion protein, NadA, NHBA fusion protein, and the outer

[1]Centers for Disease Control and Prevention. Infant meningococcal vaccination: Advisory Committee on Immunization Practices (ACIP) recommendations and rationale. *MMWR Morb Mortal Wkly Rep.* 2013;62(3):52–54

[2]Centers for Disease Control and Prevention. Prevention and control of meningococcal disease: recommendations of the Advisory Committee on Immunization Practices (ACIP). *MMWR Recomm Rep.* 2013;62(RR-02):1–28

[3]Centers for Disease Control and Prevention. Use of MenACWY-CRM vaccine in children aged 2 through 23 months at increased risk for meningococcal disease: recommendations of the Advisory Committee on Immunization Practices, 2013. *MMWR Morb Mortal Wkly Rep.* 2014;63(24):527–530

[4]American Academy of Pediatrics, Committee on Infectious Diseases. Updated recommendations on the use of meningococcal vaccines. *Pediatrics.* 2014;134(2):400–403

Table 3.43. Recommended Meningococcal Vaccines for Immunocompetent Children and Adults

Age	Vaccine	Status
2 mo through 10 y	MenACWY-D[a] (Menactra, Sanofi Pasteur, Swiftwater, PA) or MenACWY-CRM[b] (Menveo, Novartis, Cambridge, MA)	**Not routinely recommended;** see Table 3.44 (p 559) for recommendations for people at increased risk
11 through 21 y	MenACWY-D or MenACWY-CRM	Primary: 11 through 12 y of age, 1 dose 13 through 18 y of age, 1 dose, if not previously immunized 19 through 21 y of age, not routinely recommended but may be administered as catch-up immunization for those who have not received a dose after their 16th birthday Booster: 1 dose recommended for adolescents if first dose administered prior to 16th birthday
16 through 23 y	MenB-FHbp (Trumenba, Pfizer Inc, Philadelphia, PA) or MenB-4C (Bexsero, Novartis Vaccines and Diagnostics, Siena, Italy)	Category B recommendation; optional; if administered, preferred age 16 through 18 y and 2-dose series recommended For MenB-4C (Bexsero, Novartis Vaccines and Diagnostics, Siena, Italy), dose 1 administered initially, then followed by dose 2 administered ≥1 month later For MenB-FHbp (Trumenba, Pfizer Inc, Philadelphia, PA), dose 1 administered initially, then followed by dose 2 administered 6 months later; in setting of serogroup B meningococcal outbreak, a 3-dose vaccine series administered at 0, 1–2, and 6 months See Table 3.44 (p 559) for recommendations for people at increased risk
22 through 55 y	MenACWY-D or MenACWY-CRM	Not recommended routinely; see Table 3.44 (p 559) for people at increased risk
≥56 y	MenACWY-D or MenACWY-CRM	Not recommended routinely; see Table 3.44 for people at increased risk

[a]Licensed only for people 9 months through 55 years of age, but should not be used before 2 y of age to avoid interference with the immune response to the pneumococcal conjugate vaccine (PCV) series.
[b]Licensed only for people 2 months through 55 years of age.

Table 3.44. Recommended Immunization Schedule and Intervals for People at Increased Risk of Invasive Meningococcal Disease[a]

Age	Subgroup	Primary Immunization	Booster Dose[b]
2 through 23 mo of age, with high-risk conditions	Children who: • have persistent complement deficiencies • have functional or anatomic asplenia • have human immunodeficiency virus (HIV) infection • travel to or are residents of countries where meningococcal disease is hyperendemic or epidemic • are at risk during a community outbreak attributable to a vaccine serogroup	4 doses of MenACWY-CRM (Menveo) at 2, 4, 6, and 12 mo In children initiating vaccination at 7 through 23 mo of age, MenACWY-CRM is to be administered as a 2-dose series, with the second dose administered in the second year of life and at least 3 mo after the first dose MenACWY-D (Menactra) should not be used before 2 y of age to avoid interference with the immune response to the pneumococcal conjugate vaccine (PCV) series	Person remains at increased risk and first dose received at age: • **2 mo through 6 y of age:** Should receive additional dose of MenACWY 3 y after primary immunization. Boosters should be repeated every 5 y thereafter. • **≥7 y of age:** Should receive additional dose of MenACWY 5 y after primary immunization. Boosters should be repeated every 5 y thereafter.
2 through 55 y with high-risk conditions and not immunized previously	People who: • have persistent complement deficiencies • have functional or anatomic asplenia • have HIV infection	2 doses of either MenACWY-CRM or MenACWY-D, 8–12 wk apart MenACWY-D (Menactra) may be used if at least 4 wk after completion of PCV doses	
10 y or older with high-risk conditions and not immunized previously	People who: • have persistent complement deficiencies • have functional or anatomic asplenia • are at increased risk because of a serogroup B meningococcal disease outbreak • are laboratory workers routinely exposed to isolates of *Neisseria meningitidis*	2-dose series of MenB-4C, 1 mo apart OR 3-dose series of MenB-FHbp, with 2nd and 3rd doses administered 1–2 and 6 mo after initial doses	

[a]Includes children who have persistent complement deficiencies (eg, C3, C5-C9, properdin, or factor D or factor H or receiving eculizumab) or anatomic or functional asplenia; travelers to or residents of countries in which meningococcal disease is hyperendemic or epidemic; and children who are part of a community outbreak of a vaccine-preventable serogroup.
[b]If child remains at increased risk of meningococcal disease.

membrane vesicle that was part of the New Zealand vaccine. It is administered as a 2-dose series (0, 1 month [see Tables 3.43 and 3.44]).

Effectiveness against clinical disease endpoints and duration of protection for either vaccine in the age groups for which they are licensed in the United States are limited. Potential differences in immunogenicity and breadth of coverage between these 2 serogroup B meningococcal vaccines are not completely known. Recommendations for use of a serogroup B meningococcal vaccine are as follows[1-3] (Tables 3.43 and 3.44):

- People 10 years and older at increased risk for meningococcal disease should receive a meningococcal serogroup B vaccine, using the same vaccine for all doses in the vaccination series (Table 3.44). Vaccination may further activate complement, and as a result, patients with complement-mediated diseases may experience increased symptoms of their underlying disease, such as hemolysis, following vaccination. A temporary increase in hemolysis has been reported in some patients who received serogroup B meningococcal vaccine while on eculizumab therapy.

- A MenB vaccine series may be considered for people 16 through 23 years (category B recommendation), with a preferred age at vaccination of 16 through 18 years (Table 3.43).

    Immunization During outbreaks. For control of meningococcal outbreaks caused by vaccine-preventable serogroups (A, C, Y, or W), a meningococcal conjugate vaccine containing the outbreak serogroup should be used for people 2 months through 55 years of age. For outbreaks of meningococcal disease caused by serogroup B in people 10 years and older, a MenB series using either licensed MenB vaccine can be administered.

    Reimmunization/Booster Doses. Children previously immunized with a meningococcal conjugate vaccine who are at ongoing increased risk for meningococcal disease should receive booster immunizations. Children who remain at increased risk should receive a first booster dose of MenACWY-D or Men-ACWY-CRM 3 years after the primary series if they received their primary series before their 7th birthday, then every 5 years thereafter. If the primary series was administered after the 7th birthday, then the first booster dose should be 5 years later and then every 5 years thereafter. If a child was vaccinated for an outbreak or travel at <10 years of age, he or she would still need the adolescent doses.

    Adverse Events. Common adverse events after quadrivalent meningococcal conjugate vaccines include pain, erythema, and swelling at the injection site; headache; fatigue; and irritability. Similar adverse effects are observed after MenB vaccines but are more common and may be more severe. Syncope can occur after any vaccination and is most common among adolescents and young adults. Adolescents should be seated or lying down during vaccination, and having vaccine recipients sit or lie down for at least 15 minutes after immunization could avert many syncopal episodes and secondary injuries. If

[1]Folaranmi T, Rubin L, Martin SW, Patel M, MacNeil JR. Use of serogroup B meningococcal vaccines in persons aged ≥10 years at increased risk for serogroup B meningococcal disease: recommendations of the Advisory Committee on Immunization Practices, 2015. *MMWR Morb Mortal Wkly Rep.* 2015;64(22):608–612

[2]MacNeil JR, Rubin L, Folaranmi T, Ortega-Sanchez IR, Patel M, Martin SW. Use of serogroup B meningococcal vaccines in adolescents and young adults: recommendations of the Advisory Committee on Immunization Practices, 2015. *MMWR Morb Mortal Wkly Rep.* 2015;64(41):1171–1176

[3]Patton ME, Stephens D, Moore K, MacNeil JR. Updated recommendations for use of MenB-FHbp serogroup B meningococcal vaccine—Advisory Committee on Immunization Practices, 2016. *MMWR Morb Mortal Wkly Rep.* 2017;66(19):509–513

syncope develops, patients should be observed until symptoms resolve.[1] Syncope following receipt of a vaccine is not a contraindication to subsequent doses.

Precautions. No randomized controlled clinical trials have been conducted to evaluate use of MenB vaccines in pregnant or lactating women. Vaccination should be deferred in pregnant women unless the woman is at increased risk and, after consultation with her health care provider, the benefits of vaccination are considered to outweigh the potential risks.

Reporting. All confirmed, presumptive, and probable cases of invasive meningococcal disease (see Table 3.40, p 553) must be reported to the appropriate health department. Timely reporting can facilitate early administration of chemoprophylaxis to close contacts, recognition and containment of outbreaks, and serogrouping of isolates so that appropriate prevention recommendations can be implemented rapidly.

Counseling and Public Education. When a case of invasive meningococcal disease is detected, the physician should provide accurate and timely information about meningococcal disease and the risk of transmission to families and contacts of the infected person, provide or arrange for chemoprophylaxis, and contact the local public health department, which will advise about immunization. Some experts recommend that patients with invasive meningococcal disease be evaluated for a complement component deficiency; screening can be accomplished with inexpensive CH50 and AH50 testing. If a specific complement component deficiency is detected, patients should receive a meningococcal conjugate vaccine series if 2 months or older and a MenB series if 10 years or older. Patients and parents should be counseled about the risk of recurrent invasive meningococcal disease and the need for immediate medical evaluation when fever develops. Public health questions, such as whether a mass immunization program or an expanded chemoprophylaxis program is needed, should be referred to the local health department. In appropriate situations, early provision of information in collaboration with the local health department to schools or affected groups and to the media may help minimize public anxiety and unrealistic or inappropriate demands for intervention.

Human Metapneumovirus

CLINICAL MANIFESTATIONS: Human metapneumovirus (hMPV) causes acute respiratory tract illness in people of all ages and is one of the leading causes of bronchiolitis in infants. hMPV also causes pneumonia, asthma exacerbations, croup, and upper respiratory tract infections (URIs) with concomitant acute otitis media in children. Similar to influenza, infection with hMPV has been associated with invasive secondary bacterial infections, including *Streptococcus pneumoniae*, that can result in severe disease. hMPV is associated with acute exacerbations of chronic obstructive pulmonary disease (COPD) and pneumonia in adults. Otherwise healthy young children infected with hMPV usually have mild or moderate respiratory symptoms, but some young children have severe disease requiring hospitalization. hMPV infection in immunosuppressed people may result in severe disease, and fatalities have been reported in hematopoietic stem cell or lung transplant recipients. Preterm birth and underlying cardiopulmonary disease are risk factors for more severe disease. Children with a history of gestational age <32 weeks are at

---

[1] Centers for Disease Control and Prevention. Syncope after vaccination—United States, January 2005–July 2007. *MMWR Morb Mortal Wkly Rep.* 2008;57(17):457–460

higher risk for hospitalization, suffer more severe disease, and require longer stays and more supplementary oxygen. Preterm birth is associated with more severe disease not only in infancy but also in later years of life. Recurrent infection occurs throughout life and, in previously healthy people, usually is mild or asymptomatic.

ETIOLOGY: hMPV is an enveloped single-stranded negative-sense RNA virus in the genus *Metapneumovirus* of the family *Paramyxoviridae*. hMPV comprises at least 4 genetic lineages in 2 major antigenic subgroups (designated A1, A2, B1, and B2) based on sequence differences in the fusion (F) and attachment (G) surface glycoproteins. Viruses from these different lineages cocirculate each year in varying proportions.

EPIDEMIOLOGY: Humans are the only source of infection. Spread occurs by direct or close contact with contaminated secretions. Health care-associated infections have been reported.

hMPV infections usually occur annually during late winter and early spring in temperate climates, overlapping with parts of the respiratory syncytial virus (RSV) season, but typically 1 to 2 months later than RSV. Sporadic infection may occur throughout the year. In otherwise healthy infants, the duration of viral shedding is 1 to 2 weeks. Prolonged shedding (weeks to months) has been reported in severely immunocompromised hosts.

Serologic studies suggest that most children are infected at least once by 5 years of age. The population incidence of hospitalizations attributable to hMPV is lower than that attributable to RSV, but comparable to that of influenza and parainfluenza 3 in children younger than 5 years. Large studies have shown that hMPV is detected in 6% to 12% of children with lower respiratory tract illnesses who are hospitalized or seen in outpatient settings and emergency departments. Overall annual rates of hospitalization associated with hMPV infection are about 1 per 1000 children 1 to 5 years of age, 2 per 1000 children 6 to 11 months of age, and 3 per 1000 infants younger than 6 months. Coinfection with RSV and other respiratory viruses occurs.

The **incubation period** is estimated to be 3 to 5 days in most cases.

DIAGNOSTIC TESTS: Reverse transcriptase-polymerase chain reaction (RT-PCR) assays are the diagnostic method of choice for hMPV. Several RT-PCR assays for hMPV are available commercially and have been cleared for use by the US Food and Drug Administration. These include a test for hMPV alone and multiplexed tests for hMPV and other diverse respiratory pathogens. hMPV can be difficult to isolate in cell culture. Immunofluorescence assays using monoclonal antibodies for hMPV antigen for direct detection in respiratory tract specimens are available, with reported sensitivities varying from 65% to 95%. Some of these assays also may be used for confirmation of hMPV recovered in cell culture. Testing of acute and convalescent serum specimens for titer increases is only used in research settings to confirm hMPV infections.

TREATMENT: Treatment is supportive. In vitro studies and animal models have shown that ribavirin and some preparations of Immune Globulin Intravenous have activity against hMPV, but no controlled clinical data are available to assess whether these have any therapeutic benefit, and their use is not recommended. Antimicrobial agents are not indicated in the treatment of infants hospitalized with uncomplicated hMPV bronchiolitis or pneumonia unless evidence exists for the presence of a concurrent bacterial infection.[1]

---

[1]American Academy of Pediatrics, Subcommittee on Diagnosis and Management of Bronchiolitis. Clinical practice guideline: the diagnosis, management, and prevention of bronchiolitis. *Pediatrics*. 2014;134(5):e1474–e1502

Isolation of the Hospitalized Patient. In addition to standard precautions, contact precautions are recommended for the duration of hMPV-associated illness. Prolonged shedding of virus in respiratory tract secretions may occur, particularly in immunocompromised people, and the duration of contact precautions should be extended in these situations.

CONTROL MEASURES: Appropriate respiratory hygiene and cough etiquette should be followed. Control of health care-associated hMPV infection depends on adherence to contact precautions. Exposure to hMPV-infected people, including other patients, staff, and family members, may not be recognized, because illness may be mild.

Preventive measures include limiting exposure to settings where contact with hMPV may occur (eg, child care centers) and emphasizing hand hygiene in all settings, including the home, especially when contacts of high-risk children have respiratory tract infections.

Microsporidia Infections
(Microsporidiosis)

CLINICAL MANIFESTATIONS: Microsporidia infections can be asymptomatic and may be more common than previously believed. Patients with symptomatic intestinal infection have watery, nonbloody diarrhea, generally without fever. Abdominal cramping can occur. Symptomatic intestinal infection, often protracted diarrhea, is most common in immunocompromised people, especially in organ transplant recipients and people who are infected with human immunodeficiency virus (HIV) with low CD4+ lymphocyte counts (<100 cells/μL). Complications include malnutrition, progressive weight loss, and failure to thrive. Different infecting microsporidia species may result in different clinical manifestations, including ocular, muscle, and genitourinary involvement (see Table 3.45). Chronic infection in immunocompetent people is rare.

ETIOLOGY: Microsporidia are obligate intracellular, spore-forming organisms classified as fungi. *Enterocytozoon bieneusi* and *Encephalitozoon intestinalis* are the most commonly reported pathogens in humans and are most often associated with chronic diarrhea in HIV-infected people. Multiple genera, including *Encephalitozoon, Enterocytozoon, Nosema, Pleistophora, Trachipleistophora, Anncaliia, Vittaforma,* and *Microsporidium,* have been implicated in human infection, as have unclassified species.

EPIDEMIOLOGY: Most microsporidia infections are transmitted by oral ingestion of spores. *Microsporidium* spores commonly are found in surface water, and strains responsible for human infection have been identified in municipal water supplies and ground water. Several studies indicate that waterborne transmission occurs. Donor-derived infections in organ transplant recipients have been documented. Person-to-person spread by the fecal-oral route also occurs. Spores also have been detected in other body fluids, but their role in transmission is unknown. Data suggest the possibility of zoonotic transmission.

The **incubation period** is unknown.

DIAGNOSTIC TESTS: Infection with gastrointestinal tract microsporidia can be documented by identification of organisms in biopsy specimens from the small intestine. Microsporidia spores can be detected in formalin-fixed stool specimens or duodenal aspirates stained with a chromotrope-based stain (a modification of the trichrome stain) and examined by an experienced microscopist. Several histologic stains, including calcofluor, hematoxylin-eosin, Gram, acid-fast, periodic acid-Schiff, Warthin-Starry silver, and Giemsa

Table 3.45. Clinical Manifestations of Microsporidia Infections

Microsporidia species	Clinical Manifestation
Anncaliia algerae	Keratoconjunctivitis, skin and deep muscle infection
Enterocytozoon bieneusi	Diarrhea, acalculous cholecystitis
Encephalitozoon cuniculi and *Encephalitozoon hellem*	Keratoconjunctivitis, infection of respiratory and genitourinary tract, disseminated infection
Encephalitozoon intestinalis (synonym *Septata intestinalis*)	Infection of the gastrointestinal tract causing diarrhea, and dissemination to ocular, genitourinary, and respiratory tracts
Microsporidium (M ceylonensis and *M africanum)*	Infection of the cornea
Nosema species *(N ocularum)*, *Anncaliia connori*	Ocular infection
Pleistophora species	Muscular infection
Trachipleistophora anthropophthera	Disseminated infection
Trachipleistophora hominis	Muscular infection, stromal keratitis, (probably disseminated infection)
Tubulinosema acridophagus	Disseminated infection
Vittaforma corneae (synonym *Nosema corneum*)	Ocular infection, urinary tract infection

Source: **www.cdc.gov/dpdx/microsporidiosis/**

stains, can be used to detect organisms in tissue sections. Organisms often are not noticed because they are small (0.8–4 µm), stain poorly, and evoke minimal inflammatory response. Use of stool concentration techniques does not seem to improve the ability to detect *E bieneusi* spores. Polymerase chain reaction assay can be used for diagnosis, but none is cleared by the US Food and Drug Administration. Identification and diagnostic confirmation of species requires transmission electron microscopy or molecular techniques. The isolation of select microsporidia species has been accomplished using cell culture. Similarly, the value of serologic testing, when available, has not been substantiated.

TREATMENT: Restoration of immune function is critical for control of any microsporidia infection. Effective antiretroviral therapy is the primary initial treatment for these infections in people infected with HIV. Albendazole is the drug of choice for infections caused by microsporidia other than *E bieneusi* and *Vittaforma corneae* infections, which may respond to fumagillin. However, fumagillin is associated with bone marrow toxicity, recurrence of diarrhea is common after therapy is discontinued, and the drug for systemic use is not available in the United States. None of these therapies have been studied in children with microsporidia infection. Topical fumagillin eye drops (available on an investigational basis in the United States) can be considered for local treatment of keratoconjunctivitis. The addition of oral albendazole to topical fumagillin can be considered for keratoconjunctivitis caused by microsporidia other than *E bieneusi* or *V corneae*, because microsporidia may persist systemically despite clearance from the eye with topical therapy alone. Supportive care for malnutrition and dehydration may be necessary. Antimotility agents may be useful to control chronic diarrhea.

ISOLATION OF THE HOSPITALIZED PATIENT: In addition to standard precautions, contact precautions are recommended for diapered and incontinent children for the duration of illness.

CONTROL MEASURES: None have been documented. In HIV-infected and other immunocompromised people, decreased exposure may result from attention to hand hygiene, drinking bottled or boiled water, and avoiding unpeeled fruits and vegetables. No chemoprophylactic regimens are known to be effective in preventing microsporidiosis, although continuation of treatment regimens is recommended as secondary prophylaxis in HIV-infected individuals until immune reconstitution.

Molluscum Contagiosum

CLINICAL MANIFESTATIONS: Molluscum contagiosum is a benign viral infection of the skin with no systemic manifestations. It usually is characterized by 1 to 20 discrete, 2- to 5-mm-diameter, flesh-colored to translucent, dome-shaped papules, some with central umbilication. Lesions commonly occur on the trunk, face, and extremities but rarely are generalized. Molluscum contagiosum is a self-limited epidermal infection that usually resolves spontaneously in 6 to 12 months but may take as long as 4 years to disappear completely. The average duration for a single lesion is approximately 2 months. An eczematous reaction encircles lesions in approximately 10% of patients. People with atopic dermatitis and immunocompromising conditions, including human immunodeficiency virus infection and patients with congenital DOCK8 deficiency, tend to have more widespread and prolonged eruptions, which often are recalcitrant to therapy.

ETIOLOGY: Molluscum contagiosum virus (MCV) is the sole member of the genus *Molluscipoxvirus*, family *Poxviridae*. DNA subtypes of MCV can be differentiated, but the specific subtype probably is insignificant in pathogenesis. Other poxviruses include the agents of smallpox, monkeypox, vaccinia, and cowpox.

EPIDEMIOLOGY: Humans are the only known source of the virus, which is spread by direct contact, scratching, shaving, sexual contact, or fomites. Vertical transmission has been linked with neonatal molluscum contagiosum infection. Lesions can be disseminated by autoinoculation. Infectivity generally is low, but occasional outbreaks may occur in facilities such as child care centers. The period of communicability is unknown.

The **incubation period** varies between 2 and 7 weeks, but may be as long as 6 months.

DIAGNOSTIC TESTS: The diagnosis usually can be made clinically from the characteristic appearance of umbilicated papules. Wright or Giemsa staining of cells expressed from the central core of a lesion reveals characteristic intracytoplasmic inclusions. Electron microscopic examination of these cells identifies typical poxvirus particles. The virus does not grow readily in culture. Serologic testing is not available routinely for clinical practice. If questions persist, nucleic acid testing by polymerase chain reaction is available at certain reference centers. Adolescents and young adults with genital molluscum contagiosum should have screening tests for other sexually transmitted infections.

TREATMENT: There is no consensus on management of molluscum contagiosum in children and adolescents. Genital lesions should be treated to prevent spread to sexual contacts. Treatment of nongenital lesions is sometimes provided for cosmetic reasons. Lesions in healthy people typically are self-limited, so treatment may be unnecessary. However, therapy may be warranted to: (1) alleviate discomfort, including itching; (2) reduce auto-inoculation; (3) limit transmission of the virus to close contacts; (4) reduce cosmetic concerns; and (5) prevent secondary infection.

Physical destruction of the lesions is the most rapid and effective means of curing molluscum contagiosum. Modalities available include curettage, cryodestruction with liquid nitrogen, electrodesiccation, and chemical agents designed to initiate a local inflammatory response (podophyllin, tretinoin, cantharidin, 25%–50% trichloroacetic acid, liquefied phenol, silver nitrate, tincture of iodine, or potassium hydroxide). Most data available for any of these modalities are anecdotal. Randomized trials generally are limited because of small sample sizes. These treatments require an experienced provider; they can result in postprocedural pain, irritation, hyperpigmentation, and scarring. Because physical destruction of the lesions is painful, appropriate local anesthesia may be required, particularly in young children. Open-label and observational studies indicate that cantharidin can be an effective treatment for molluscum contagiosum; however, in 1 small randomized controlled trial of 29 patients, the improvement seen with cantharidin, although greater than with placebo, was not found to be statistically significant. Data from large randomized, vehicle-controlled, double-blind trials have failed to demonstrate efficacy of imiquimod cream, a local immune modulator, for molluscum contagiosum in children 2 to 12 years of age. Cidofovir is a cytosine nucleotide analogue with in vitro activity against molluscum contagiosum; successful intravenous treatment of immunocompromised adults with severe involvement has been reported. However, use of cidofovir should be reserved for extreme cases because of potential carcinogenicity and known toxicities (neutropenia and potentially permanent nephrotoxicity) associated with systemic administration of cidofovir. Successful treatment using topical cidofovir, in a combination vehicle, has been reported in both adult and pediatric cases, most of whom were immunocompromised. Solitary genital lesions in children usually are not acquired by sexual transmission and do not necessarily denote sexual abuse, as other modes of direct contact with the virus, including autoinoculation, may result in genital infection.

ISOLATION OF THE HOSPITALIZED PATIENT: Standard precautions are recommended.

CONTROL MEASURES: No control measures are known for isolated cases. For outbreaks, which are common in the tropics, restricting direct person-to-person contact and sharing of potentially contaminated fomites, such as towels and bedding, may decrease spread. Molluscum contagiosum should not prevent a child from attending child care or school or from swimming in public pools. Covering lesions is not necessary for child care, but when possible, localized lesions not covered by clothing may be covered with a gas-permeable dressing followed by underwrap and tape when participating in sports activities.[1] The bandage should be changed daily or when soiled.

Moraxella catarrhalis Infections

CLINICAL MANIFESTATIONS: *Moraxella catarrhalis* commonly is implicated in acute otitis media (AOM), otitis media with effusion, and sinusitis. AOM caused by *M catarrhalis* occurs predominantly in younger infants and frequently is recovered in mixed infections.

[1]Davies HH, Jackson MA, Rice SG; American Academy of Pediatrics, Committee on Infectious Diseases. Infectious diseases associated with organized sports and outbreak control. *Pediatrics*. 2017;140(4):e20172477

Since introduction of 13-valent pneumococcal conjugate vaccine (PCV13), it appears to be recovered in a greater proportion of children undergoing tympanocentesis; however, it is unclear whether this represents an increase in cases attributable to *M catarrhalis* or a decrease in pneumococcal disease. *M catarrhalis* can cause pneumonia and bacteremia in healthy children, but is more commonly reported in children with chronic lung disease or impaired host defenses, such as leukemia with neutropenia or congenital immunodeficiency. In immunocompetent patients, bacteremia usually is associated with a respiratory tract focus; in immunocompromised children, most often no focus of infection is identified. Other clinical manifestations include hypotension with or without a rash indistinguishable from that observed in meningococcemia, neonatal meningitis, and focal infections, such as preseptal cellulitis, bacterial tracheitis, urethritis, osteomyelitis, or septic arthritis. Rare manifestations include endocarditis, peritonitis, shunt-associated ventriculitis, meningitis, and mastoiditis.

ETIOLOGY: *M catarrhalis* is a gram-negative aerobic diplococcus. Nearly 100% of strains produce beta-lactamase that mediates resistance to the penicillins, including amoxicillin.

EPIDEMIOLOGY: *M catarrhalis* is part of the normal microbiota of the upper respiratory tract of humans. Two thirds of children are colonized within the first year of life. The mode of transmission is presumed to be direct contact with contaminated respiratory tract secretions or droplet spread. Infection is most common in infants and young children but also occurs in immunocompromised people at all ages. The duration of carriage by children with infection or colonization and the period of communicability are unknown. Recent studies suggest early colonization with *M catarrhalis* is associated with a stable microbiome and low risk for recurrent respiratory tract infection.

DIAGNOSTIC TESTS: The organism can be isolated on blood or chocolate agar culture media after incubation in air or with increased carbon dioxide. On Gram stain, *Moraxella* species are short and plump gram-negative rods, usually occurring in pairs or short chains, and are mostly catalase and cytochrome oxidase positive. Culture of middle ear or sinus aspirates is indicated for patients with unusually severe infection, for patients with infection that fails to respond to treatment, and for immunocompromised children. *M catarrhalis* often is recovered as part of mixed infections. Polymerase chain reaction tests for *M catarrhalis* have been developed but currently are used for research purposes only.

TREATMENT: Almost all strains of *Moraxella* species produce beta-lactamase and are resistant to amoxicillin. When beta-lactamase–producing *M catarrhalis* is isolated from appropriately obtained specimens (middle ear fluid, sinus aspirates, or lower respiratory tract secretions), in vitro data indicate that cefotaxime and ceftriaxone are likely to be effective if parenteral antimicrobial therapy is needed. Pharmacokinetic and pharmacodynamic studies support the use of amoxicillin-clavulanate, cefixime, azithromycin, cefdinir, cefpodoxime, trimethoprim-sulfamethoxazole, or a fluoroquinolone. These studies also suggest that cefuroxime axetil, high-dose amoxicillin, and cefaclor are likely to be ineffective. The organism is resistant to clindamycin, vancomycin, and oxacillin.

ISOLATION OF THE HOSPITALIZED PATIENT: Standard precautions are recommended.

CONTROL MEASURES: None.

Mumps

CLINICAL MANIFESTATIONS: Mumps is a systemic disease characterized by swelling of one or more of the salivary glands, usually the parotid glands. Approximately one third of infections do not cause clinically apparent salivary gland swelling and may be asymptomatic (subclinical) or manifest primarily as respiratory tract infection. More than 50% of people with mumps have cerebrospinal fluid pleocytosis, but fewer than 10% have symptoms of viral meningitis. Orchitis is a commonly reported complication after puberty, although sterility rarely results. Rare complications include arthritis, thyroiditis, mastitis, glomerulonephritis, myocarditis, endocardial fibroelastosis, thrombocytopenia, cerebellar ataxia, transverse myelitis, encephalitis, pancreatitis, oophoritis, and permanent hearing impairment. In the absence of an immunization program, mumps typically occurs during childhood. Infection in adults is more likely to result in complications. Although mumps virus can cross the placenta, no evidence exists that this transmission results in congenital malformation.

ETIOLOGY: Mumps is an RNA virus in the genus *Rubulavirus* in the family *Paramyxoviridae*. The genus also includes human parainfluenza virus types 2 and 4. Other infectious causes of parotitis include Epstein-Barr virus, cytomegalovirus, parainfluenza virus types 1 and 3, influenza A virus, enteroviruses, lymphocytic choriomeningitis virus, human immunodeficiency virus (HIV), nontuberculous mycobacterium, gram-positive bacteria, and less often, gram-negative bacteria.

EPIDEMIOLOGY: Mumps occurs worldwide, and humans are the only known natural hosts. The virus is spread by contact with infectious respiratory tract secretions and saliva. Mumps virus is the only known cause of epidemic parotitis. Historically, the peak incidence of mumps was between January and May and among children younger than 10 years. Mumps vaccine was licensed in the United States in 1967 and recommended for routine childhood immunization in 1977. After implementation of the 2-dose measles-mumps-rubella (MMR) vaccine recommendation in 1989 for measles control in the United States, mumps further declined to extremely low levels, with an incidence of 0.1/100 000 by 1999. From 2000 to 2005, seasonality no longer was evident, and there were fewer than 300 reported cases per year (incidence, 0.1/100 000), representing a greater than 99% reduction in disease incidence compared with the prevaccine era. In early 2006, a large-scale mumps outbreak occurred in the Midwestern United States, with 6584 reported cases (incidence of 2.2/100 000). Most of the cases occurred among people 18 through 24 years of age, many of whom were college students who had received 2 doses of mumps vaccine. Another outbreak in 2009–2010 affected more than 3500 people, mainly students in grades 6 through 12 who were members of traditional observant religious communities in New York and New Jersey and who also had received 2 doses of vaccine. Beginning in 2016, even larger outbreaks of mumps have occurred in the United States. In 2016, there were 6353 cases, and between January 1 and December 2, 2017, the preliminary number of cases is 4980. There were 67 mumps outbreaks reported in 2016, including 35 university outbreaks, 7 outbreaks in close-knit communities, 21 outbreaks in other close-contact settings (eg, churches, workplaces, fitness centers, etc), and 4 community-wide outbreaks. Available data from 1 outbreak indicate that cases occurred primarily in young adults with high 2-dose MMR vaccination coverage. Two doses of vaccine are approximately 88% effective in preventing disease. In settings of high immunization coverage, such as the United States, it is predictable that most mumps cases will occur in people who have received 2 doses of vaccine.

The **incubation period** usually is 16 to 18 days, but cases may occur from 12 to 25 days after exposure. The period of maximum communicability begins several days before parotitis onset. The recommended isolation period is 5 days after onset of parotid swelling. However, virus has been isolated from saliva from 7 days before through 8 days after onset of swelling.

DIAGNOSTIC TESTS: Despite localized outbreaks, mumps remains an uncommon infection in the United States, and most parotitis has other etiologies, including other infectious agents. People with parotitis without other apparent cause should undergo diagnostic testing to confirm mumps virus as the cause or to diagnose other etiologies. Successful detection of mumps virus depends primarily on the timing of collection and quality of the clinical sample. Mumps can be confirmed by detection of mumps virus nucleic acid by reverse transcriptase-polymerase chain reaction (RT-PCR) assay in specimens from buccal swabs (Stenson duct exudates), throat washings, saliva, or cerebrospinal fluid. The mumps RT-PCR test, as developed and available at the Centers for Disease Control and Prevention (CDC), is sensitive and specific. Other RT-PCR assays for mumps may be available at local clinical and reference laboratories, but none are currently cleared by the US Food and Drug Administration (FDA). Failure to detect mumps virus RNA by RT-PCR in samples from a person with clinically compatible mumps symptoms does not rule out mumps as a diagnosis. Mumps virus may be isolated in cell culture using a variety of cell types, using either standard or rapid isolation and identification techniques. However, clinical laboratories in the United States generally do not have experience with mumps virus cell culture methods, and RT-PCR is more sensitive than culture.

Mumps can be diagnosed by testing for mumps-specific immunoglobulin (Ig) M antibody or by a significant increase between acute and convalescent serum mumps IgG antibody titer determined by standard quantitative or semiquantitative serologic assay. In highly immunized populations, confirming the diagnosis of mumps by serologic testing can be challenging, because the IgM response may be absent or short lived; acute IgG titers already might be high, so no significant increase can be detected between acute and convalescent specimens. In immunized people or previously infected individuals presenting with clinically compatible mumps, a negative IgM result does not rule out acute mumps.

TREATMENT: Supportive.

ISOLATION OF THE HOSPITALIZED PATIENT: In addition to standard precautions, droplet precautions are recommended until 5 days after onset of parotid swelling.

CONTROL MEASURES: Mumps is a nationally notifiable disease in the United States.

Evidence of Immunity to Mumps.[1] Presumptive evidence of immunity to mumps includes any of the following:

1. Documentation of age-appropriate vaccination with a live mumps virus-containing vaccine:
   - preschool-aged children: 1 dose after their first birthday;
   - school-aged children (grades K–12) and adults at high risk (ie, health care personnel, international travelers, and students at postsecondary educational institutions): 2 doses after their first birthday, with the second dose administered at least 28 days after the first dose;
   - adults not at high risk: 1 dose;

---

[1] Centers for Disease Control and Prevention. Prevention of measles, rubella, congenital rubella syndrome, and mumps, 2013 summary: recommendations of the Advisory Committee on Immunization Practices (ACIP). *MMWR Recomm Rep.* 2013;62(RR-4):1–34

2. Laboratory evidence of immunity;

3. Laboratory confirmation of disease; or

4. Born before 1957.

School and Child Care. Children and young adults should be excluded for 5 days from onset of parotid gland swelling.

Exclusion. When determining means to control outbreaks, exclusion of unimmunized students without evidence of immunity from affected schools and schools judged by local public health authorities to be at risk of transmission should be considered. Excluded students can be readmitted immediately after immunization. Students who remain unimmunized should be excluded until at least 26 days after onset of parotitis in the last person with mumps in the affected school.

Care of Exposed People. Mumps vaccine has not been demonstrated to be effective in preventing infection or decreasing the severity of infection if administered after exposure. However, susceptible people still should receive MMR vaccine (or measles-mumps-rubella-varicella [MMRV] vaccine, if thought to be susceptive to varicella and 12 months through 12 years of age) even after exposure, because immunization will provide protection against subsequent exposures. Immunization during the incubation period presents no increased risk of adverse events.

During an outbreak, the first dose of MMR vaccine (or MMRV, if age appropriate) should be offered to all unimmunized people 12 months and older, and a second dose of MMR vaccine (or MMRV, if age appropriate) should be offered to all students (including those in postsecondary school) and to all health care personnel born in or after 1957 who have only received 1 dose of MMR vaccine. Health care personnel born before 1957 without a history of 2 doses of MMR and who lack laboratory evidence of mumps immunity or laboratory confirmation of disease should receive 2 appropriately spaced doses of MMR vaccine. A second dose of MMR also may be considered during outbreaks for preschool aged children who have received 1 MMR dose. People previously vaccinated with 2 doses of a mumps-containing vaccine who are identified by public health as at increased risk for mumps because of an outbreak should receive a third dose of a mumps-containing vaccine to improve protection against mumps disease and related complications.

Immune Globulin (IG) preparations are not effective as postexposure prophylaxis for mumps.

Mumps Vaccine. Live attenuated mumps vaccine containing the Jeryl-Lynn strain has been licensed in the United States since 1967. Vaccine is administered by subcutaneous injection of 0.5 mL of MMR vaccine (licensed for people 12 months or older) or MMRV vaccine (licensed for children 12 months through 12 years of age). Monovalent mumps vaccine no longer is available in the United States. Postlicensure data indicate that the effectiveness of 1 dose of mumps vaccine has been approximately 78% (range, 49%–92%), and 2-dose vaccine effectiveness is 88% (range, 66%–95%). Some studies and investigations conducted during the recent mumps outbreaks indicate that vaccine-induced immunity might wane, possibly explaining the recent occurrence of mumps in the 15- through 24-year age group.

Vaccine Recommendations.

- The first dose of MMR or MMRV vaccine (see MMRV vaccine recommendations in Varicella-Zoster Infections, p 869) should be administered routinely to children at 12

through 15 months of age, with a second dose of MMR or MMRV vaccine administered at 4 through 6 years of age. The second dose of MMR or MMRV vaccine may
be administered before 4 years of age, provided at least 28 days have elapsed since the
first dose. MMR or MMRV vaccine is not harmful if administered to a person already
immune to one or more of the viruses from previous infection or immunization.

- People should be immunized unless they have evidence of mumps immunity (p 569).
  Adequate immunization is 2 doses of mumps-containing vaccine (≥28 days apart) for
  school-aged children and adults at high risk (ie, health care personnel, students at postsecondary educational institutions, and international travelers). Because mumps is endemic throughout most of the world, unless they have evidence of immunity, people
  12 months or older should be offered 2 doses of MMR vaccine before beginning
  travel. Children younger than 12 months need not receive mumps vaccine before
  travel, but they may receive it as MMR vaccine starting at 6 months of age if measles
  immunization is indicated. If a child receives a dose of mumps vaccine before 12
  months of age, this dose is not counted toward the required number of doses, and 2
  additional doses are required beginning at 12 through 15 months of age and separated
  by at least 28 days.
- Health care personnel born before 1957 should receive 2 doses of MMR vaccine unless they have laboratory evidence of immunity or disease.
- A mumps-containing vaccine may be administered with other vaccines at different injection sites and with separate syringes (see Simultaneous Administration of Multiple
  Vaccines, p 35).

Adverse Reactions. Adverse reactions associated with the mumps component of US-licensed MMR or MMRV vaccines are rare. Orchitis, parotitis, and low-grade fever may
occur. Causality has not been established for temporally related reactions, including febrile seizures, nerve deafness, aseptic meningitis, encephalitis, rash, pruritus, and purpura.
Allergic reactions also are rare (see Measles, Precautions and Contraindications [p 547],
and Rubella, Precautions and Contraindications [p 710]). Other reactions that occur after immunization with MMR or MMRV vaccine may be attributable to other components of the vaccines (see Measles, p 537, Adverse Events, p 546, Rubella, p 705, and
Varicella-Zoster Infections, p 869).

A second dose of MMR or MMRV vaccine is not associated with an increased incidence of reactions relative to the first dose.

Precautions and Contraindications. See Measles, p 537, Rubella, p 705, and, if MMRV is
used, Varicella-Zoster Infections, p 869.

Febrile Illness. Children with minor illnesses with or without fever, such as upper respiratory tract infections, should be immunized. Fever is not a contraindication to immunization. However, if other manifestations suggest a more serious illness, the child should not
be immunized until recovered.

Allergies. Hypersensitivity reactions occur rarely and usually are minor, consisting of
wheal-and-flare reactions or urticaria at the injection site. Reactions have been attributed
to trace amounts of neomycin or gelatin or some other component in the vaccine formulation. Anaphylaxis is rare; MMR and MMRV vaccines are produced in chicken embryo
cell culture and do not contain significant amounts of egg white (ovalbumin) cross-reacting proteins, so children with egg allergy are at low risk of anaphylactic reactions. Skin
testing of children for egg allergy is not predictive of reactions to MMR or MMRV vaccine and, therefore, is not required before administering vaccine. People with allergies to

chickens or feathers are not at increased risk of reaction to the vaccine. People who have experienced anaphylactic reactions to gelatin or topically or systemically administered neomycin should receive mumps vaccine only in settings where such reactions could be managed and after consultation with an allergist or immunologist. Most often, however, neomycin allergy manifests as contact dermatitis, which is not a contraindication to receiving mumps vaccine (see Measles, p 537).

Recent Administration of IG. Administration of MMR or MMRV vaccine should be delayed from 3 to 11 months following receipt of specific blood products or IG (see Table 1.13, p 40). MMR vaccine should be administered at least 2 weeks before planned administration of IG, blood transfusion, or other blood products because of the theoretical possibility that antibody will neutralize vaccine virus and interfere with successful immunization; if IG must be administered within 14 days after administration of MMR or MMRV, these vaccines should be readministered after the interval specified in Table 1.13 (p 40).

Altered Immunity. Patients with immunodeficiency diseases and those receiving immunosuppressive therapy or expected to receive such therapy within 4 weeks, including high doses of systemically administered corticosteroids, alkylating agents, antimetabolites, or radiation, or people who otherwise are immunocompromised should not receive live attenuated vaccines including MMR or MMRV (see Immunization and Other Considerations in Immunocompromised Children, p 72).

Exceptions are patients with human immunodeficiency virus (HIV) infection who are not severely immunocompromised. The live-virus measles-mumps-rubella (MMR) vaccine can be administered to asymptomatic HIV-infected children and adolescents without severe immunosuppression (that is, can be administered to children 1 through 13 years of age with a CD4+ T-lymphocyte percentage $\geq$15% and to adolescents $\geq$14 years with a CD4+ T-lymphocyte count $\geq$200 lymphocytes/mm^3). Severely immunocompromised HIV-infected infants, children, adolescents, and young adults (eg, children 1 through 13 years of age with a CD4+ T-lymphocyte percentage <15% and adolescents $\geq$14 years with a CD4+ T-lymphocyte count <200 lymphocytes/mm^3) should not receive measles virus-containing vaccine, because vaccine-related pneumonia has been reported. The quadrivalent measles-mumps-rubella-varicella (MMRV) vaccine should not be administered to any HIV-infected infant, regardless of degree of immunosuppression, because of lack of safety data in this population (see Human Immunodeficiency Virus Infection, p 459).

The risk of mumps exposure for patients with altered immunity can be decreased by immunizing their close susceptible (ie, household) contacts. Vaccine recipients cannot transmit mumps vaccine virus.

After cessation of immunosuppressive therapy, MMR immunization should be deferred for at least 3 months (with the exception of corticosteroid recipients [see next paragraph]). This interval is based on the assumptions that immunologic responsiveness will have been restored in 3 months and the underlying disease for which immunosuppressive therapy was given is in remission or under control. However, because the interval can vary with the intensity and type of immunosuppressive therapy, radiation therapy, underlying disease, and other factors, a definitive recommendation for an interval after cessation of immunosuppressive therapy when mumps vaccine (as MMR) can be administered safely and effectively often is not possible.

Corticosteroids. Children receiving $\geq$2 mg/kg per day of prednisone or its equivalent, or $\geq$20 mg/day if they weigh 10 kg or more, for 14 days or more and who otherwise are not immunocompromised should not receive live-virus vaccines until 4 weeks after discontinuation (see Immunization and Other Considerations in Immunocompromised Children, p 72).

Pregnancy. Conception should be avoided for 4 weeks after mumps immunization because of the theoretical risk associated with live-virus vaccine. Susceptible postpubertal females should not be immunized if they are known to be pregnant. However, mumps immunization during pregnancy has not been associated with congenital malformations (see Immunization in Pregnancy, p 69).

Mycoplasma pneumoniae and Other *Mycoplasma* Species Infections

CLINICAL MANIFESTATIONS: *Mycoplasma pneumoniae* is a frequent cause of upper and lower respiratory tract infections in children, including pharyngitis, acute bronchitis, and pneumonia. Acute otitis media is uncommon. Bullous myringitis, once considered pathognomonic for mycoplasma, now is known to occur with other pathogens as well. Sinusitis and croup are rare. Symptoms are variable and include cough, malaise, fever, and occasionally headache. Acute bronchitis and upper respiratory tract illness caused by *M pneumoniae* generally are mild and self-limited. Approximately 10% of infected school-aged children will develop pneumonia with cough and rales on physical examination within days after onset of constitutional symptoms. Cough, initially nonproductive, can become productive, persist for 3 to 4 weeks, and be accompanied by wheezing. Approximately 10% of children with *M pneumoniae* infection will exhibit a rash, which most often is maculopapular. Radiographic abnormalities are variable; bilateral diffuse infiltrates or focal abnormalities, such as consolidation, effusion, or hilar adenopathy, can occur.

Unusual manifestations include nervous system disease (eg, aseptic meningitis, encephalitis, acute disseminated encephalomyelitis, cerebellar ataxia, transverse myelitis, and peripheral neuropathy) as well as myocarditis, pericarditis, arthritis, erythema nodosum, polymorphous mucocutaneous eruptions (including classic and atypical Stevens-Johnson syndrome), hemolytic anemia, thrombocytopenic purpura, and hemophagocytic syndromes. Severe pneumonia with pleural effusion can occur, particularly in patients with sickle cell disease, Down syndrome, immunodeficiencies, and chronic cardiorespiratory disease. Acute chest syndrome and pneumonia have been associated with *M pneumoniae* in patients with sickle cell disease. Infection also has been associated with exacerbations of asthma.

Several other *Mycoplasma* species colonize mucosal surfaces of humans and can produce disease in children. *Mycoplasma hominis* infection has been reported in neonates (especially at scalp electrode monitor site) and children (both immunocompetent and immunocompromised). Intra-abdominal abscess, septic arthritis, endocarditis, pneumonia, meningoencephalitis, brain abscess, and surgical wound infection have been reported to be attributable to *M hominis*.

ETIOLOGY: Mycoplasmas, including *M pneumoniae,* are pleomorphic bacteria that lack a cell wall. They are classified in the family *Mycoplasmataceae,* which includes the *Mycoplasma* and *Ureaplasma* genera.

EPIDEMIOLOGY: Mycoplasmas are ubiquitous in animals and plants, but *M pneumoniae* causes disease only in humans. *M pneumoniae* is transmissible by respiratory droplets during close contact with a symptomatic person. Outbreaks have been described in hospitals, military bases, colleges, and summer camps. Occasionally, *M pneumoniae* causes ventilator-associated pneumonia. *M pneumoniae* is a leading cause of pneumonia in school-aged children and young adults but is an infrequent cause of community-acquired pneumonia in children younger than 5 years. In the United States, an estimated 2 million infections are caused by *M pneumoniae* each year. Overall, approximately 20% of hospitalized community-acquired pneumonia is thought to be caused by *M pneumoniae*. Infections occur throughout the world, in any season, and in all geographic settings. In family studies, approximately 30% of household contacts develop pneumonia. Asymptomatic carriage after infection may occur for weeks to months. Immunity after infection is not long lasting.

The **incubation period** usually is 2 to 3 weeks (range, 1–4 weeks), which can contribute to lengthy outbreaks.

DIAGNOSTIC TESTS: Nucleic acid amplification tests (NAATs), including polymerase chain reaction (PCR) tests for *M pneumoniae*, are available commercially and increasingly are replacing other tests, because PCR tests performed on respiratory tract specimens (nasal wash, nasopharyngeal swab, pharyngeal swab) are rapid, have sensitivity and specificity between 80% and 100%, and yield positive results earlier in the course of illness. Several assays are cleared by the US Food and Drug Administration (FDA) for diagnostic use, including an assay targeting *M pneumoniae* alone and multiplex assays that simultaneously target other respiratory pathogens. Identification of *M pneumoniae* by NAAT or culture in a patient with compatible clinical manifestations suggests causation. However, attributing a nonclassic clinical disorder to *M pneumoniae* is problematic, because the organism can colonize the respiratory tract for several weeks after acute infection (even after appropriate antimicrobial therapy) and has been detected by PCR in 17% to 25% of asymptomatic children 3 months to 16 years of age. Performance characteristics of PCR assays that have not been cleared by the FDA are not generalizable. PCR assays to detect point mutations associated with macrolide resistance have been developed, but none have been cleared by the FDA. PCR assay of body fluids for *M hominis* is available at reference laboratories and may be helpful diagnostically.

Serologic tests using immunofluorescence and enzyme immunoassays that detect *M pneumoniae*-specific immunoglobulin (Ig) M and IgG antibodies are available commercially. IgM antibodies generally are not detectable within the first 7 days after onset of symptoms. Although the presence of IgM antibodies may indicate recent *M pneumoniae* infection, false-positive test results occur, and antibodies persist in serum for several months and may not indicate current infection. IgM antibodies may not be elevated in older children and adults who have had recurrent *M pneumoniae* infection. Serologic diagnosis is best accomplished by demonstrating a fourfold or greater increase in antibody titer between acute and convalescent serum specimens. Complement-fixation assay results should be interpreted cautiously, because the assay is both less sensitive and less specific than is immunofluorescent assay or enzyme immunoassay. IgM antibody titer peaks at approximately 3 to 6 weeks and persists for 2 to 3 months after infection but should be interpreted cautiously because of frequent false-positive results. Measurement of serum cold hemagglutinin titer has limited value, because titers of ≥1:64 are present in only 50% to 75% of patients with pneumonia caused by *M pneumoniae,* and lower titers are nonspecifically present during respiratory viral infections.

Mycoplasma organisms are not visible by cell-wall specific stains (eg, Gram stain) using light microscopy. *M pneumoniae* and *M hominis* can be grown in special enriched broth and agar media such as SP4 or on commercially available mixed liquid broth/agar slant media. However, most clinical laboratories lack the capacity to perform culture isolation; culture and identification may take longer than 21 days.

The diagnosis of mycoplasma-associated central nervous system disease is challenging, both because disease may not be the result of direct invasion and because there is no reliable single test for cerebrospinal fluid to establish a diagnosis.

TREATMENT: *Mycoplasma* infection is an infrequent cause of community-acquired pneumonia (CAP) in preschool-aged children. Evidence of benefit of antimicrobial therapy for nonhospitalized children with lower respiratory tract disease attributable to *M pneumoniae* is limited. Some data suggest benefit of appropriate antimicrobial therapy in hospitalized children. Antimicrobial therapy is not recommended for preschool-aged children with CAP, because viral pathogens are responsible for the great majority of cases.[1] There is no evidence that treatment of other possible manifestations of *M pneumoniae* infection (eg, upper respiratory tract infection, extrapulmonary infection) with antimicrobial agents alters the course of illness.

Because *Mycoplasma* organisms lack a cell wall, they inherently are resistant to beta-lactam agents. Macrolides, including azithromycin, clarithromycin, and erythromycin, are the preferred antimicrobial agents for treatment of *Mycoplasma* pneumonia in school-aged children who have moderate to severe infection and those with underlying conditions, such as sickle cell disease.[1] Fluoroquinolones and doxycycline are effective in vitro. Macrolide-resistant strains are increasingly common although the effect of resistance on treatment outcome is not known. The usual course of antimicrobial therapy for pneumonia is 7 to 10 days, except for azithromycin, for which it usually is 5 days.

M hominis usually is resistant to erythromycin and azithromycin but is variably susceptible to clindamycin, tetracyclines, and fluoroquinolones.

ISOLATION OF THE HOSPITALIZED PATIENT: In addition to standard precautions, droplet precautions are recommended for the duration of symptomatic illness.

CONTROL MEASURES: Hand hygiene decreases household transmission of respiratory pathogens and should be encouraged.

Tetracycline or azithromycin prophylaxis for close contacts has been shown to limit transmission in family and institutional outbreaks. However, antimicrobial prophylaxis for asymptomatic exposed contacts is not recommended routinely, because most secondary illnesses will be mild and self-limited. Prophylaxis with a macrolide or tetracycline can be considered for people at increased risk of severe illness with *M pneumoniae*, such as children with sickle cell disease who are close contacts of a person who is acutely ill with *M pneumoniae* infection.

Nocardiosis

CLINICAL MANIFESTATIONS: Immunocompetent children typically develop cutaneous or lymphocutaneous disease with pustular or ulcerative lesions following soil contamination of a skin injury. Deep-seated tissue infection may follow traumatic soil-contaminated wounds. Immunocompromised people may develop invasive disease (pulmonary disease,

---

[1]Bradley JS, Byington CL, Shah SS, et al. The management of community-acquired pneumonia in infants and children older than 3 months of age: clinical practice guidelines by the Pediatric Infectious Diseases Society and the Infectious Diseases Society of America. *Clin Infect Dis.* 2011;53(1):e25-e76

which may disseminate); at-risk people include those with chronic granulomatous disease, human immunodeficiency virus infection, or disease requiring long-term systemic cortico-steroid therapy or organ transplantation, or people having received tumor necrosis factor inhibitors, especially infliximab. Pulmonary disease commonly manifests as rounded nod-ular infiltrates that can undergo cavitation; the infection may be acute, subacute, or chronic. Hematogenous spread may occur from the lungs to the brain (single or multiple abscesses), to the skin (pustules, pyoderma, abscesses, mycetoma), or occasionally to other organs. Some experts recommend cerebrospinal fluid examination and/or neuroimaging in patients with pulmonary disease, even with a nonfocal neurologic examination, given the propensity of these organisms to infect the central nervous system. *Nocardia* organisms can be recovered from respiratory specimens of patients with cystic fibrosis, but the clini-cal significance of this pathogen in these patients is unclear.

ETIOLOGY: *Nocardia* are gram-positive, filamentous bacteria that belong to a group infor-mally known as the aerobic actinomycetes. The cell walls of *Nocardia* organisms contain mycolic acid and thus may be described as "acid fast" or "partially acid fast" using special staining techniques and light microscopy.

EPIDEMIOLOGY: *Nocardia* species are ubiquitous environmental saprophytes, living in soil, organic matter, and water. Infections caused by *Nocardia* species typically are the result of environmental exposure through inhalation of soil or dust particles or through traumatic inoculation with a soil-contaminated object. The most prevalent species reported from human clinical sources in the United States are the *Nocardia asteroides* complex, which in-cludes *Nocardia nova, Nocardia farcinica, Nocardia cyriacigeorgica,* and *Nocardia abscessus.* Primary cutaneous infection most often is associated with *Nocardia brasiliensis.* Other less common pathogenic species include *Nocardia brevicatena, Nocardia otitidiscaviarum, Nocardia pseudobrasili-ensis, Nocardia transvalensis* complex, and *Nocardia veterana.*

Person-to-person and animal-to-human transmission is not known to occur.

The **incubation period** is unknown.

DIAGNOSTIC TESTS: Isolation of *Nocardia* species from clinical specimens can require ex-tended incubation periods because of their slow growth. Specimens from sterile sites can be inoculated directly onto solid media such as sheep blood, chocolate, brain-heart infu-sion, Sabouraud dextrose agars, and buffered charcoal yeast extract (BCYE) agar. Speci-mens from nonsterile or contaminated sites, such as tissue or sputum, should be inocu-lated onto selective media, such as Thayer Martin or BCYE with vancomycin, with a minimum incubation of 3 weeks. Recovery of *Nocardia* species from tissue can be im-proved if the laboratory is requested to observe cultures for up to 4 weeks in an appropri-ate liquid medium at optimal growth temperature (between 25°C and 35°C for most spe-cies). Stained smears of sputum, body fluids, or pus demonstrating beaded, branching rods that stain weakly gram-positive and partially acid-fast by the modified Kinyoun method suggest the diagnosis. Because of the difficulty in interpretation of the acid-fast stain, positive and negative staining controls are suggested. The Brown-Brenn tissue gram-stain method and Grocott-Gomori methenamine silver stains are recommended to demonstrate microorganisms in tissue specimens.

Accurate identification of *Nocardia* isolates paired with antimicrobial susceptibility test-ing greatly enhances the selection of appropriate antimicrobial therapy, thereby increas-ing the likelihood of favorable patient care outcomes. Because of the variability of pheno-typic traits and the difficulty growing the organisms on commercial biochemical testing media, accurate identification is accomplished through molecular methods. For *Nocardia* species, 16S rRNA gene sequence analysis of a nearly full-length (~1440 bp) sequence can identify the isolate to the species level. Mass spectrometry of cellular components for the identification of *Nocardia* species has not been well-studied. Serologic tests for *Nocardia* species are not useful.

TREATMENT: Rapid and accurate identification of *Nocardia* isolates along with antimicrobial susceptibility testing are essential tools for successful treatment of nocardiosis. *Nocardia* species possess intrinsic resistance to multiple drugs. Antimicrobial susceptibility testing recommended by the Clinical and Laboratory Standards Institute is complex and generally requires a specialty or reference laboratory. Such testing should guide therapy and is recommended for all non-*asteroides Nocardia* strains, all strains from patients with invasive disease, when patients are unable to tolerate a sulfonamide, or for patients in whom sulfonamide therapy fails.

Trimethoprim-sulfamethoxazole (TMP/SMX) or a sulfonamide alone (eg, sulfisoxazole or sulfamethoxazole) is the drug of choice for mild infections. Sulfonamides that are less urine soluble, such as sulfadiazine, should be avoided. Certain *Nocardia* species including *N farcinica, N nova,* and *N otitidiscaviarum* may demonstrate resistance to TMP/SMX. If infection does not respond to TMP/SMX, imipenem, meropenem, and fluoroquinolones may be considered. Other agents with specific *Nocardia* coverage include clarithromycin *(N nova)* and amoxicillin-clavulanate *(N brasiliensis* and *N abscessus).* Linezolid has excellent activity against all *Nocardia* species. Pediatric data are lacking for many of these agents in treatment of nocardiosis. Immunocompetent patients with lymphocutaneous disease usually respond after 6 to 12 weeks of monotherapy.

Combination drug therapy is recommended for patients with serious disease (pulmonary infection, disseminated disease, central nervous system involvement). Combination therapy also is recommended for infection in immunocompromised hosts. Initial combination treatment should include imipenem (resistance noted for some strains of *N brasiliensis*), amikacin, and TMP/SMX. Linezolid, ceftriaxone or cefotaxime (resistance noted for some strains of *N farcinica, N transvalensis,* and *N otitidiscaviarum*), meropenem, or minocycline are alternative agents. Immunocompromised patients and patients with serious disease should be treated for 6 to 12 months and for at least 3 months after apparent cure because of the propensity for relapse. Patients with human immunodeficiency virus infection may need even longer therapy, and suppressive therapy should be considered for life. Patients with central nervous system disease should be monitored with serial neuroimaging studies.

Drainage of abscesses is beneficial, and removal of infected foreign bodies (eg, central venous catheters) is recommended.

ISOLATION OF THE HOSPITALIZED PATIENT: Standard precautions are recommended.

CONTROL MEASURES: People with weakened immune systems should be advised to cover their skin when working with soil.

Norovirus and Sapovirus Infections

CLINICAL MANIFESTATIONS: Abrupt onset of vomiting accompanied by watery diarrhea, abdominal cramps, and nausea are characteristic of norovirus gastroenteritis. Acute diarrhea without vomiting may also occur, most notably in children. Symptoms can last from 24 to 60 hours, but usually no more than 48 hours. However, more prolonged courses of illness can occur, particularly among elderly people, young children, and hospitalized patients. Norovirus illness also is recognized as an important cause of chronic gastroenteritis in immunocompromised patients. Systemic manifestations, including fever, myalgia, malaise, anorexia, and headache, may accompany gastrointestinal tract symptoms. Since the introduction of rotavirus vaccines, noroviruses have become the leading cause of gastroenteritis in the United States.[1,2]

ETIOLOGY: Noroviruses are 27- to 40-nm, nonenveloped, single-stranded RNA viruses of the family *Caliciviridae*. This family is classified into 5 known genera (*Lagovirus, Nebovirus, Vesivirus, Sapovirus,* and *Norovirus*) and 5 additional proposed genera (*Valovirus, Secalivirus, Recovirus, Nacovirus,* and *Bavovirus*). *Norovirus* and *Sapovirus* are the genera known to cause human infection. Noroviruses are genetically diverse, with 6 known (I–VI) and 3 proposed genogroups (VII–IX). Viruses from 4 genogroups (I, II, IV, and VIII) can cause human illness. Sapoviruses are divided into 5 major genogroups (I–V), of which viruses from 4 (GI, GII, GIV, and GV) cause disease in humans. At least 17 different sapovirus genotypes have been recognized.

EPIDEMIOLOGY: Norovirus causes an estimated 1 in 15 US residents to become ill each year as well as 56 000 to 71 000 hospitalizations and 570 to 800 deaths, predominantly among young children and the elderly.[3] As a result of the success of rotavirus vaccines, noroviruses have become the predominant agent of pediatric viral gastroenteritis in the United States, causing both sporadic cases and outbreaks.[4] Norovirus genogroup II, genotype 4 (GII.4) has been predominant worldwide during the past decade. Sapovirus infections also cause outbreaks, albeit significantly fewer than norovirus, and are a contributor to sporadic acute diarrhea in children. Asymptomatic norovirus excretion is common across all age groups, with the highest prevalence in children. Outbreaks with high attack rates tend to occur in semiclosed populations, such as long-term care facilities, schools, and cruise ships. Transmission is by person-to-person spread via the fecal-oral or vomitus-oral routes, through contaminated food or water, or by touching surfaces contaminated with norovirus and then touching the mouth. Norovirus is recognized as the most common cause of foodborne illness and foodborne disease outbreaks in the United States.[5] Common-source outbreaks have been described after ingestion of ice, shellfish, and a variety of ready-to-eat foods, including salads, berries, and bakery products, usually contaminated by infected food handlers. Transmission via vomitus has been documented, and exposure to contaminated surfaces and aerosolized vomitus has been implicated in some outbreaks.

Norovirus recognizes and binds to histo-blood group antigens, which are expressed

[1]Lopman B. Global Burden of Norovirus and Prospects for Vaccine Development. Available at: **www.cdc.gov/norovirus/downloads/global-burden-report.pdf**

[2]Shah MP, Wikswo ME, Barclay L, et al. Near real-time surveillance of U.S. norovirus outbreaks by the Norovirus Sentinel Testing and Tracking Network—United States, August 2009–July 2015. *MMWR Morb Mortal Wkly Rep.* 2017;66(7):185–189

[3]Centers for Disease Control and Prevention. Vital Signs: foodborne norovirus outbreaks—United States, 2009–2012. *MMWR Morb Mortal Wkly Rep.* 2014;63(22):491–495

[4]Payne DC, Vinje J, Szilagyi PG, et al. Norovirus and medically attended gastroenteritis in U.S. children. *N Engl J Med.* 2013;368(12):1121–1130

[5]Centers for Disease Control and Prevention. Surveillance for foodborne disease outbreaks—United States, 2009–2010. *MMWR Morb Mortal Wkly Rep.* 2013;62(3):41–47

by the fucosyltransferase 2 (FUT2) gene, and individuals with a functional FUT2 gene are referred to as "secretors." FUT2 polymorphisms have been associated with increased host susceptibility to certain norovirus strains.

The **incubation period** is 12 to 48 hours. Viral shedding may start before onset of symptoms, peaks several days after exposure, and may persist for 4 weeks or more. Prolonged shedding (>6 months) has been reported in immunocompromised hosts. Infection occurs year-round but is more common during the colder months of the year.

DIAGNOSTIC TESTS: Molecular diagnostic methods are the most sensitive way to detect norovirus or sapovirus. In children, interpretation of test results may be complicated by the frequent detection of viruses in fecal samples from asymptomatic children and the detection of multiple viruses in a single sample. Multiple multiplex nucleic acid-based assays for the detection of gastrointestinal pathogens are cleared by the US Food and Drug Administration (FDA), with the majority including norovirus testing and a select few including sapovirus.

State and local public health laboratories use real-time reverse transcriptase-polymerase chain reaction (RT-PCR) for detection of norovirus and sapovirus RNA in stool. Viral genotypes are identified by Sanger sequencing of relatively small regions of the capsid gene. Laboratory and epidemiologic support for investigation of suspected viral gastroenteritis outbreaks is available at the Centers for Disease Control and Prevention (CDC) by request.

Norovirus was recently able to be cultured using human B cells and commensal bacteria; however, this diagnostic approach is not commercially available. Only select human strains of sapovirus have been cultured.

TREATMENT: Supportive therapy includes oral or intravenous rehydration solutions to replace and maintain fluid and electrolyte balance.

ISOLATION OF THE HOSPITALIZED PATIENT: In addition to standard precautions, contact precautions are recommended for suspected cases of acute gastroenteritis attributable to norovirus infection until 48 hours after symptom resolution.

CONTROL MEASURES: Appropriate hand hygiene is the most important method to prevent norovirus infection and control transmission. Reducing any norovirus present on hands is best accomplished by thorough handwashing with running water and plain or antiseptic soap. Washing hands with soap and water after contact with a patient with norovirus infection is more effective than using alcohol-based hand sanitizers for reducing transmission.

Several factors favor transmission of noroviruses, including low infectious dose, large numbers of virus particles excreted, and prolonged shedding. The spread of infection can be decreased by standard measures for control of diarrhea, such as educating child care providers and food handlers about infection control, maintaining cleanliness of surfaces and food preparation areas, using appropriate disinfectants (principally sodium hypochlorite [chlorine bleach]), excluding caregivers or food handlers who are ill and for a period after recovery (eg, 48 hours), and exercising appropriate hand hygiene, as discussed previously. If a source of transmission can be identified (eg, contaminated food or water) during an outbreak, then specific interventions to interrupt transmission can be effective.

Infants and children should be excluded from child care centers until stools are contained in the diaper or when toilet-trained children no longer have accidents using the toilet and when stool frequency becomes no more than 2 stools above that child's normal frequency for the time the child is in the program, even if the stools remain loose.

Candidate norovirus virus-like-particle vaccines are in clinical development. Sporadic cases are not nationally notifiable, but outbreaks should be reported to local and state public health authorities as required and to the CDC via the National Outbreak Reporting System (NORS), and virus genotyping data should be submitted to CaliciNet (**www.cdc.gov/norovirus/reporting/calicinet/index.html**). Guidance on norovirus is available on the CDC Web site (**www.cdc.gov/mmwr/pdf/rr/rr6003. pdf**).[1] A toolkit designed to help health care professionals control and prevent norovirus gastroenteritis in health care settings is available (**www.cdc.gov/hai/pdfs/ norovirus/229110-ANorovirusIntroLetter508.pdf**).

Onchocerciasis
(River Blindness, Filariasis)

CLINICAL MANIFESTATIONS: The disease involves skin, subcutaneous tissues, lymphatic vessels, and eyes. Subcutaneous, nontender nodules that can be up to several centimeters in diameter containing male and female worms develop 6 to 12 months after initial infection. In patients in Africa, nodules tend to be found on the lower torso, pelvis, and lower extremities, whereas in patients in Central and South America, the nodules more often are located on the upper body (the head and trunk) but also may occur on the extremities. After the worms mature, fertilized females produce embryos called microfilariae that migrate to the dermis and may cause a papular dermatitis. Pruritus often is highly intense, resulting in patient-inflicted excoriations over the affected areas. After a period of years, skin can become lichenified and hypo- or hyperpigmented. Microfilariae may invade ocular structures, leading to inflammation of the cornea, iris, ciliary body, retina, choroid, and optic nerve. Loss of visual acuity and blindness can result over time if the disease is left untreated.

ETIOLOGY: *Onchocerca volvulus* is a filarial nematode and 1 of 8 species of filarial worms that commonly infect humans.

EPIDEMIOLOGY: *O volvulus* has no significant animal reservoir. Microfilariae in human skin infect *Simulium* species flies (black flies) when they take a blood meal; microfilariae then, in 10 to 14 days, develop in the vector into infectious larvae that are transmitted with subsequent bites. Black flies breed in fast-flowing streams and rivers (hence, the colloquial name for the disease, "river blindness"). The disease occurs primarily in equatorial Africa, but small foci are found in Venezuela, Brazil, and Yemen. Prevalence is greatest among people who live near vector breeding sites. The infection is not transmissible by person-to-person contact or blood transfusion.

The **incubation period** from larval inoculation to microfilariae in the skin usually is 12 to 18 months but can be as long as 3 years.

DIAGNOSTIC TESTS: Direct examination of a 1- to 2-mg shaving or biopsy specimen of the epidermis and upper dermis (usually taken from the posterior iliac crest area) can reveal microfilariae. Microfilariae are not found in blood. Adult worms may be demonstrated in excised nodules that have been sectioned and stained. A slit-lamp examination of an involved eye may reveal motile microfilariae in the anterior chamber or "snowflake" corneal lesions. Eosinophilia is common. Specific serologic tests and polymerase

---

[1]Centers for Disease Control and Prevention. Updated norovirus outbreak management and disease prevention guidelines. *MMWR Recomm Rep.* 2011;60(3):1–15

chain reaction techniques for detection of microfilariae in skin are available in the United States only in research and public health laboratories, including those of the National Institutes of Health and Centers for Disease Control and Prevention.

TREATMENT: Ivermectin, a microfilaricidal agent, is the drug of choice for treatment of onchocerciasis. Treatment decreases dermatitis and the risk of developing severe ocular disease but does not kill the adult worms (which can live for more than a decade) and, thus, is not curative. One single oral dose of ivermectin (150 μg/kg) should be given every 6 to 12 months until asymptomatic. Adverse reactions to treatment are caused by death of microfilariae and can include rash, edema, fever, myalgia, and rarely, asthma exacerbation and hypotension. Such reactions are more common in people with higher skin loads of microfilaria and decrease with repeated treatment in the absence of reexposure. Precautions to ivermectin treatment include pregnancy (class C drug), central nervous system disorders, and high levels of circulating *Loa* microfilaremia (determined by examining a Giemsa-stained thick blood smear between 10 AM and 2 PM; see Drugs for Parasitic Infections, p 985). Treatment of patients with high levels of circulating *L loa* microfilaremia with ivermectin rarely can result in fatal encephalopathy. Referral to a tropical medicine specialist would be indicated for people coinfected with *Onchocerca volvulus* and *Loa loa*. The American Academy of Pediatrics notes that ivermectin usually is compatible with breastfeeding. Because low levels of drug are found in human milk after maternal treatment, some experts recommend delaying maternal treatment until the infant is 7 days of age, but risk versus benefit should be considered. Safety and effectiveness of ivermectin in pediatric patients weighing less than 15 kg have not been established.

A 6-week course of doxycycline (100–200 mg/day) can be used to kill adult worms through depletion of the endosymbiotic rickettsia-like bacteria *Wolbachia*, which appear to be required for survival of *O volvulus*. Doxycycline can be used for short durations (ie, 21 days or less) without regard to patient age, but for the longer treatment durations required in for treatment of *O volvulus*, for whom the alternative treatment of ivermectin exists, doxycycline is not recommended for children younger than 8 years (see Tetracyclines, p 905). Doxycycline may be used for children 8 years or older and nonpregnant adults to obviate the need for years of ivermectin treatment. Doxycycline treatment may be initiated 1 week after treatment with ivermectin; for patients without symptoms, a 6-week course of doxycycline may be given, followed by a dose of ivermectin. There are no studies of the safety of simultaneous treatment.

Diethylcarbamazine is contraindicated, because it may cause adverse ocular reactions. Nodules can be removed surgically, but not all nodules may be clinically detectable or surgically accessible.

ISOLATION OF THE HOSPITALIZED PATIENT: Standard precautions are recommended.

CONTROL MEASURES: Repellents and protective clothing (long sleeves and pants) can decrease exposure to bites from black flies, which bite by day. Treatment of vector breeding sites with larvicides is effective for controlling black fly populations. Vector control, however, largely has been supplanted by community-wide mass ivermectin administration programs. A highly successful global initiative being led by the World Health Organization has distributed hundreds of millions of ivermectin treatments (donated by the drug manufacturer for this purpose) safely to communities with onchocerciasis. As a result of these programs, transmission largely has been eliminated from the Americas (where most mass treatment programs now have halted) and markedly curtailed throughout Africa.

Human Papillomaviruses

CLINICAL MANIFESTATIONS: Most human papillomavirus (HPV) infections are subclinical, and 90% resolve spontaneously within 2 years. However, persistent HPV infection can cause benign epithelial proliferation (warts) of the skin and mucous membranes as well as cancers of the lower anogenital tract and the head and neck. HPVs can be grouped into cutaneous and mucosal types. The cutaneous types cause common skin warts, plantar warts, flat warts, and thread-like (filiform) warts. These cutaneous warts are benign. Certain mucosal types (low risk) are associated with warts or papillomas of mucous membranes, including the upper respiratory tract and anogenital, oral, nasal, and conjunctival areas. Other mucosal types (high risk) are associated with precancers and cancers, including cervical, anogenital, and oropharyngeal cancers.

Common **skin warts** are dome-shaped with conical projections that give the surface a rough appearance. Skin warts usually are painless and multiple, occurring commonly on the hands and around or under the nails. When small dermal vessels become thrombosed, black dots appear in the warts.

Plantar warts on the foot often are larger than warts at other sites and may not project through much of the skin surface. They can be painful when walking and are characterized by marked hyperkeratosis, sometimes with black dots.

Flat warts ("juvenile warts") commonly are found on the face and extremities of children and adolescents. Flat warts usually are small, multiple, and flat topped, seldom exhibit papillomatosis, and rarely cause pain. **Filiform warts** occur on the face and neck.

Anogenital warts, also called **condylomata acuminata,** are skin-colored warts with a papular, flat or cauliflower-like surface that range in size from a few millimeters to several centimeters; these warts often occur in groups. In males, these warts may be found on the penis, scrotum, or anal or perianal area. In females, these lesions may occur on the vulvar, anal, or perianal areas and less commonly in the vagina or on the cervix. Warts usually are painless, although they may cause itching, burning, local pain, or bleeding.

Invasive cancers attributable to HPV include those of cervix, vagina, vulva, penis, anus, and oropharynx (back of throat, base of tongue, and tonsils). Cervical cancer is the most common HPV-attributable cancer among women, and oropharyngeal cancer is the most common HPV-attributable cancer among men. Anogenital **low-grade squamous intraepithelial lesions (LSILs)** can result from persistent infection with low-risk or high-risk HPV types, whereas **high-grade squamous intraepithelial lesions (HSILs)** can result from persistent infection with high-risk HPV types. In the cervix, HSILs typically indicate the presence of **cervical intraepithelial neoplasia (CIN)** grades 2 or 3, which are precancerous lesions. These lesions are detected through routine screening with cytologic testing (Papanicolaou [Pap] test) and/or clinical HPV tests; tissue biopsy is required to make the diagnosis. Endocervical glandular precancer, **adenocarcinoma in situ (AIS)**, also can result from persistent infection with high-risk HPV types.

Recurrent respiratory papillomatosis is a rare condition characterized by recurring papillomas in the larynx or other areas of the upper respiratory tract. Recurrent respiratory papillomatosis is called juvenile onset when it occurs before 18 years of age, versus adult onset. Juvenile onset recurrent respiratory papillomatosis is believed to result from vertical transmission of HPV types 6 or 11 from a mother to her infant at the time of delivery and is diagnosed most commonly in children between 2 and 5 years of age, with manifestations of voice change (eg, hoarseness), stridor, or abnormal cry. Respiratory papillomas can cause respiratory tract obstruction in young children, and repeated surgeries often are needed.

Epidermodysplasia verruciformis is a rare, inherited disorder believed to be a consequence of a deficiency of cell-mediated immunity resulting in an abnormal susceptibility to certain HPV types and manifesting as chronic cutaneous lesions and skin cancers. Lesions may resemble flat warts or pigmented plaques covering the torso and upper extremities. Most appear during the first decade of life, but malignant transformation, which occurs in 30% to 60% of affected people, usually is delayed until adulthood.

ETIOLOGY: HPVs are small, nonenveloped, double-stranded DNA viruses of the *Papillomaviridae* family, which can be grouped into a number of types based on DNA sequence variation. Different types display different specific tissue tropism. Types 6 and 11 cause condylomata acuminata, recurrent respiratory papillomatosis, and conjunctival papillomas but rarely are found in cancer; they are referred to as low-risk types. High-risk types (types 16, 18, 31, 33, 35, 39, 45, 51, 52, 56, 58, 59, 66, and 68, which are included in clinical HPV tests), can cause low-grade cervical cell abnormalities, high-grade cervical cell abnormalities that are precursors to cancer, and anogenital cancers. High-risk HPV types are detected in 99% of cervical precancers and 90% of invasive cervical cancer. Approximately 50% of cervical cancers worldwide are attributable to HPV type 16, and 70% are attributable to types 16 and 18. The majority of other HPV-related cancers—anogenital cancers (vulvar, vaginal, penile, anal) and oropharyngeal cancers—are attributable to HPV type 16. Infection with a high-risk HPV type is considered necessary but not sufficient to cause cancer, because the vast majority of people with an HPV infection will not develop cancer. Risk of developing cancer precursors or cancers is greater in people with certain immunocompromising conditions, such as human immunodeficiency virus (HIV) infection or cellular immune deficiencies.

EPIDEMIOLOGY: Virtually all adults will be infected with some type of HPV during their lives. In the United States, HPV infection prevalence is 79 million, and annual incidence is 14 million infections. HPV types involved in common hand and foot warts are quite different from mucosal types.

Nongenital hand and foot warts occur commonly among school-aged children, in whom prevalence is as high as 50%. Acquisition can occur through casual contact and is facilitated by minor skin trauma. Autoinoculation can result in spread of lesions. The intense and often widespread appearance of cutaneous warts in people with compromised cellular immunity (particularly those who have undergone transplantation or who have HIV infection) suggests that alterations in T-lymphocyte immunity may impair clearance of infection.

Genital HPV infections are transmitted primarily by skin-to-skin contact, usually through sexual intercourse and other close genital contact. In US females, the highest prevalence of infection is in 20- to 24-year-olds. Most infections are subclinical and clear spontaneously within 2 years. Cancer is an uncommon outcome of infection that generally requires decades of persistent infection with high-risk HPV types. There are nearly 31 000 cases of HPV-attributable cancers annually in the United States. Cervical cancer accounts for approximately 12 000 new cases and 4000 deaths annually in the United States. HPV also is the cause of most vulvar, vaginal, penile, and anal cancers as well as 70% of oropharyngeal cancers.

Rarely, HPV infection is transmitted to a child through the birth canal during delivery or transmitted from nongenital sites. When anogenital warts are identified in a child, sexual abuse must be considered while noting the possibility of vertical transmission to neonates (see Social Implications of STIs in Children, p 56).

The **incubation period** for symptoms of HPV infection is estimated to range from 3 months to several years.

DIAGNOSTIC TESTS: Most cutaneous and anogenital warts can be diagnosed through clinical inspection. Serologic testing for HPV does not inform clinical decisions and is not commercially available. Routine cervical cancer screening guidelines have been established by multiple professional societies. These guidelines direct the interval at which cytologic screening (Pap testing) should be performed, when HPV clinical tests ("cotesting") should be added, and when colposcopic evaluation with biopsy should be performed. Vulvar, vaginal, penile, and anal lesions may be identified using visual inspection, sometimes using magnification; in some cases, cytologic screening is used and suspicious lesions are biopsied, but there is no routine screening recommended for cancers at these sites. For all anogenital lesions, diagnosis is made on the basis of histologic findings. Respiratory papillomatosis is diagnosed using endoscopy and biopsy.

Although cytologic and histologic changes can be suggestive of HPV, these findings are not diagnostic of HPV. Detection of HPV infection is based on detection of viral nucleic acid (DNA or RNA). Clinical tests for high-risk HPV types may be used in combination with Pap testing for cervical cancer screening in women 30 years or older and for triage of equivocal Pap test abnormalities (atypical squamous cells of undetermined significance [ASCUS]) in women 21 years or older.[1] The benefit of adding HPV testing to the Pap test is that the rate of false-negative results with the Pap test is reduced with a negative test result for high-risk HPV types, allowing longer intervals (eg, 5 years) between routine Pap test screenings. Previously, without HPV testing, the relatively high false-negative rate directed that frequent consecutive Pap testing be performed to ensure that no lesion was missed.

A number of HPV DNA or mRNA detection and genotyping assays have been cleared for use in the United States by the US Food and Drug Administration (FDA). Liquid-based cytology collection and transport kits permit performance of Pap smear cytology and HPV detection and genotyping on the same specimen. There are differences in the appropriate clinical applications for each of these assays, including whether they can be used as an initial standalone test (ie, without cervical cytology) or in a primary screening algorithm; none is recommended for use in women younger than 21 years or for men.

TREATMENT[2]**:** There is no treatment for HPV infection. Treatment may be directed toward lesions caused by HPV.

Regression of **nongenital and genital warts** occurs in approximately 30% of

---

[1]Massad LS, Einstein MH, Huh WK, et al; 2012 American Society for Colposcopy and Cervical Pathology (ASCCP) Consensus Guidelines Conference. 2012 updated consensus guidelines for the management of abnormal cervical cancer screening tests and cancer precursors. *J Low Genit Tract Dis.* 2013;17(5):S1-S27. Available at: **www.asccp.org/asccp-guidelines**

[2]Centers for Disease Control and Prevention. Sexually Transmitted Diseases Treatment Guidelines, 2015. *MMWR Recomm Rep.* 2015; 2015;64:1–137. Available at: **www.cdc.gov/mmwr/preview/mmwrhtml/rr6403a1.htm**

cases within 6 months. Most methods of treatment of cutaneous warts use chemical or physical destruction of the infected epithelium, including cryotherapy with liquid nitrogen, laser or surgical removal of warts, application of salicylic acid products, or application of topical immune-modulating agents. Daily treatment with tretinoin has been useful for widespread flat warts in children. Care should be taken to avoid deleterious cosmetic results with therapy. Systemic treatments for refractory warts, including cimetidine, have been used with varying success.

Treatments for genital warts are characterized as patient-applied or provider administered. Interventions include ablational/excisional treatments or topical antiproliferative or immune-modulating medications. Oral warts can be removed through cryotherapy, electrocautery, or surgical excision.

Many agents used for treatment of warts have not been tested for safety and efficacy in children, and some are contraindicated in pregnancy.

Although most forms of therapy are successful for initial removal of warts, treatment may not eradicate HPV infection from the surrounding tissue. Recurrences are common and may be attributable to reactivation rather than reinfection. Follow-up visits during and after treatment for genital warts may be advantageous, because treatments can result in local symptoms or adverse effects.

Cancer precursor lesions that are identified in the cervix (HSILs, AIS) or elsewhere in the genital tract may require excision or destruction. Treatment of cervical lesions can cause substantial economic, emotional, and reproductive adverse effects, including higher risk of preterm birth. Management of invasive cervical and other anogenital and orpharyngeal cancers requires a specialist and should be conducted according to current guidance.

Respiratory papillomatosis is difficult to treat and is best managed by an experienced otolaryngologist. Local recurrence is common, and repeated surgical debulking procedures are necessary to relieve airway obstruction. Extension or dissemination of respiratory papillomas from the larynx into the trachea, bronchi, or lung parenchyma is rare but can result in increased morbidity and mortality; malignant transformation occurs rarely. Intralesional interferon, oral indole-3-carbinole, photodynamic therapy, and intralesional cidofovir have been used as investigational treatments, but the lack of adequately powered controlled trials with any of these interventions makes conclusions regarding efficacy difficult.

ISOLATION OF THE HOSPITALIZED PATIENT: Standard precautions are recommended.

CONTROL MEASURES AND CARE OF EXPOSED PEOPLE: Sexual abuse should be considered if anogenital warts are found in a child. Suspected child sexual abuse should be reported to the appropriate local agency if anogenital warts are found in a child who is prepubertal (see Social Implications of STIs in Children, p 56).

Certain HPV infections can be prevented by vaccination (see below). Abstaining from sex, delaying sexual debut, and minimizing the lifetime number of sex partners are other modes of reducing risk of disease caused by anogenital HPV infections. Consistent and correct use of latex condoms may reduce the risk of anogenital HPV infection when infected areas are covered or protected by the condom. Use of latex condoms has been associated with a decrease in the risk of genital warts and cervical cancer. The degree and duration of contagiousness in patients with a history of genital HPV infection is unknown. People with genital warts should refrain from sex with new partners while warts are present, and inform their current sex partners, who also may benefit from a clinical evaluation for anogenital warts or other sexually transmitted infections.

Although respiratory papillomatosis is believed to be caused by transmission of HPV types 6 and 11 during passage through the birth canal, this condition has occurred in infants born by cesarean delivery. Because the preventive value of cesarean delivery is unknown, it should not be performed solely to prevent transmission of HPV to the newborn infant.

Cervical Cancer Screening. Women who have received HPV vaccine should continue to have regular cervical cancer screening. HPV vaccines do not necessarily provide protection against all HPV types associated with development of cervical cancer nor alter the course of infections existing before vaccination. Several professional organizations offer guidance on cervical cancer screening, including the American College of Obstetricians and Gynecologists (**www.acog.org**), the American Cancer Society (**www.cancer. org**), and the US Preventive Services Task Force (**www.uspreventiveservicestask-force.org**). These organizations recommend that Pap testing begin at 21 years of age for all healthy women, regardless of sexual history. Female adolescents with a recent diagnosis of HIV infection should undergo cervical Pap test screening at the time of diagnosis and again in the next 6 to 12 months (**http://aidsinfo.nih.gov/guidelines**). Sexually active female adolescents who have had an organ transplant or are receiving long-term corticosteroid therapy also should undergo similar cervical Pap test screening. If cytologic screening has been initiated before 21 years of age, patients with abnormal Pap test results should be cared for by a physician who is knowledgeable in the management of cervical dysplasia.

HPV Vaccines. Three HPV vaccines are licensed by the FDA for use in the United States. A quadrivalent vaccine (4vHPV [types 6, 11, 16, and 18], Gardasil [Merck & Co Inc, Whitehouse Station, NJ]) was licensed by the FDA in 2006 for use in females 9 through 26 years of age and in 2009 for use in males 9 through 26 years of age. A bivalent vaccine (2vHPV [types 16 and 18], Cervarix [GlaxoSmithKline Biologicals, Rixensart, Belgium]) was licensed in 2009 for use in females 10 through 25 years of age. A 9-valent HPV vaccine (9vHPV [types 6, 11, 16, 18, 31, 33, 45, 52, and 58], Gardasil 9 [Merck & Co Inc, Whitehouse Station, NJ]) was licensed by the FDA in 2014 for use in females and males and is indicated for females and males ages 9 through 26 years. Although 4vHPV and 2vHPV still are licensed for use, they are no longer being sold in the United States, leaving 9vHPV as the only available product.

Immunogenicity. More than 97% of healthy vaccine recipients develop antibodies to HPV vaccine types after vaccination. Antibody titers are higher in adolescent females and males aged 9 through 15 years compared with females and males aged 16 through 26 years.

Antibody titers for all HPV vaccines decrease over time but plateau by 18 to 24 months. Follow-up studies through 8 and 10 years after 4vHPV and 2vHPV vaccination, respectively, have shown no waning of protection. However reassuring, the clinical significance of antibody titers is not clear, because a serologic correlate of protection has not been established. Studies of all 3 HPV vaccines have found that antibody titers after 2 doses administered 6 to 12 months apart to 9- through 14-year-olds are similar to 3 doses administered to women 16 through 26 years of age, the age group in which efficacy was demonstrated in clinical trials.

Efficacy. 4vHPV and 2vHPV have been shown to be highly effective in preventing cervical precancers related to HPV types 16 and 18 in clinical trials among females 15 or 16 through 25 or 26 years of age. 4vHPV has been shown to be highly effective in preventing genital warts related to HPV types 6 and 11 in clinical trials among females and males 16 through 26 years of age. 4vHPV also has been shown to be highly effective in preventing anal precancers in males 16 through 26 years of age. 9vHPV has been shown in a clinical trial to provide 97% protection against the additional 5 HPV types in the 9-valent product (31, 33, 45, 52, and 58) and has noninferior immunogenicity for the 4 HPV types in the quadrivalent product (6, 11, 16, and 18). HPV vaccines have not been proven to have therapeutic effect on existing HPV infection or disease and do not offer protection against progression of infection to disease from HPV acquired before immunization. Therefore, HPV vaccines are most effective when administered well before most people are exposed to HPV through sexual contact.

In countries with early adoption and high uptake of HPV vaccines, rates of precancers have declined markedly in vaccinated cohorts. Incidence of genital warts in 4vHPV-immunized cohorts has been reduced by 90%. Assessment of the full impact of HPV vaccination on anogenital and oropharyngeal cancers may take decades, given the natural history of HPV oncogenesis. In the United States, prevalence of vaccine-type HPV decreased by approximately 60% in 14- to 19-year-old girls within the first 6 years after the vaccination program began in 2006; decreases also have been observed in genital warts and cervical precancers.

Long-term follow-up studies are being conducted to determine the duration of efficacy for all HPV vaccines.

Vaccine Recommendations.[1-3] The American Academy of Pediatrics and the Advisory Committee on Immunization Practices (ACIP) of the Centers for Disease Control and Prevention recommend routine HPV vaccination for females and males. The AAP recommends starting the series between 9 and 12 years, at an age that the provider deems optimal for acceptance and completion of the vaccination series. The ACIP recommends starting the series at age 11 or 12 years of age and states that vaccination can be administered starting at age 9 years. When HPV vaccine is begun at 9 or 10 years of age, other adolescent vaccines (eg, MenACWY and Tdap) still are recommended to be administered only at 11 to 12 years of age.

Providers are encouraged to recommend use of HPV vaccine as they do all other routine childhood and adolescent vaccines. Research has demonstrated that parents are influenced by the strong recommendations and personal testimonials of their child's pediatrician. Opportunities to prevent cancers and deaths are being missed by clinicians who focus on HPV vaccine as a sexually transmitted infection vaccine rather than a cancer prevention vaccine, or who solicit parents' opinion about HPV vaccine rather than announce vaccination as routinely indicated.

---

[1]American Academy of Pediatrics, Committee on Infectious Diseases. HPV vaccine recommendations. *Pediatrics.* 2012;129(3):602–605

[2]Centers for Disease Control and Prevention. Human papillomavirus vaccination: recommendations of the Advisory Committee on Immunization Practices (ACIP). *MMWR Recomm Rep.* 2014;63(RR-5):1–30

[3]Meites E, Kempe A, Markowitz LE. Use of a 2-dose schedule for human papillomavirus vaccination—updated recommendations of the Advisory Committee on Immunization Practices. *MMWR Morb Mortal Wkly Rep.* 2016;65(49):1405–1408

HPV vaccination is also recommended for females through age 26 years and for males through age 21 years of age who were not previously immunized. Males 22 through 26 years of age may be immunized.

HPV vaccination is recommended for men who have sex with men (including men who identify as gay or bisexual, or who intend to have sex with men) and transgender people and people who are immunocompromised through 26 years of age.

In the United States, no HPV vaccines are licensed for use in people older than 26 years.

Dosage and Administration. HPV vaccine is administered in either 2 or 3 doses of 0.5 mL, intramuscularly, preferably in a deltoid muscle.

- For people initiating vaccination before their 15th birthday, the recommended schedule is 2 doses of HPV vaccine, with the second dose administered 6 to 12 months after the first dose (minimum interval 5 months).
- For people initiating vaccination on or after their 15th birthday, the recommended schedule is 3 doses of HPV vaccine. In a 3-dose schedule, the second dose should be administered at least 1 to 2 months after the first dose (minimum interval 4 weeks), and the third dose should be administered 6 months after the first dose (minimum interval 5 months after first dose, and 12 weeks after second dose).
- Dose(s) of vaccine administered after a shorter-than-recommended minimum interval should be repeated after another minimum interval elapses.
- People considered adequately vaccinated:
    - People who initiated vaccination before their 15th birthday and received 2 doses of any HPV vaccine (9vHPV, 4vHPV, or 2vHPV) at the recommended dosing schedule (0, 6–12 months), or 3 doses of any HPV vaccine at the recommended dosing schedule (0, 1–2, 6 months).
    - People who initiated vaccination on or after their 15th birthday and received 3 doses of any HPV vaccine (9vHPV, 4vHPV, or 2vHPV) at the recommended dosing schedule (0, 1–2, 6 months).
- If the vaccine schedule is interrupted, the vaccine series does not need to be restarted.
- 9vHPV may be used to complete a series started with 4vHPV or 2vHPV.
- There is no recommendation regarding additional vaccination with 9vHPV for people who previously completed a 4vHPV tor 2vHPV vaccination series.
- Evidence of past HPV exposure or current HPV infection or disease, such as abnormal Pap test results, cervical lesions, anogenital warts, or a positive HPV DNA test result, are not contraindications to HPV immunization. Men and women in the recommended age ranges still should receive HPV vaccine to protect against any HPV types not already acquired.
- HPV vaccines are available in single-dose vials and prefilled syringes and contain no antimicrobial agents or preservative.
- HPV vaccines should be stored at 2°C to 8°C (36°F–46°F) and not frozen.
- HPV vaccines can be coadministered with any live or inactivated vaccine indicated at the same visit.

Recommendations for Special Populations. HPV vaccines are not live vaccines. HPV vaccines are recommended for people in the recommended age groups who are immunocompromised as a result of infection (including HIV), disease, or medications. Immune response and vaccine efficacy in immunocompromised people might be less than that in immunocompetent people. For immunocompromised people ages 9 through 26 years (including people with primary or secondary immunocompromising conditions that might reduce cell-mediated or humoral immunity, such as B-lymphocyte antibody deficiencies, T-lymphocyte complete or partial defects, HIV infection, malignant neoplasms, transplantation, autoimmune disease, or immunosuppressive therapy), a 3-dose schedule of HPV vaccine is recommended. There are ongoing evaluations on duration of efficacy and immunogenicity in immunocompromised populations, including those with HIV infection.

Children younger than 15 years with asplenia, asthma, chronic granulomatous disease, chronic liver disease, chronic lung disease, chronic renal disease, central nervous system anatomic barrier defects (eg, cochlear implant), complement deficiency, diabetes, heart disease, or sickle cell disease should receive a 2-dose schedule of HPV vaccine, rather than a 3-dose schedule.[1]

Children who are victims of sexual abuse or assault are recognized to be at greater risk for subsequent unsafe and unprotected intercourse and to have these behaviors at an earlier age than nonabused children. For children with a history of sexual abuse or assault, the HPV vaccination series should be started at 9 years of age.

Vaccine Adverse Events, Precautions, and Contraindications. Studies of more than 15 000 people in clinical trials for each of the HPV vaccines have shown no serious safety concerns. More than 90 million doses of HPV vaccines have been distributed in the United States. Injection site discomfort or pain, redness, and swelling are the most commonly reported local adverse events. Systemic symptoms after HPV vaccine can include headache, fever, nausea, dizziness, and fatigue/malaise. Syncope (fainting) has been reported in adolescents after receipt of recommended vaccines, including HPV vaccine. HPV vaccines can be administered to people with minor acute illnesses.

- Immunization of people with moderate or severe acute illnesses should be deferred until after their condition improves.
- HPV vaccines are contraindicated in people with a history of immediate hypersensitivity to any vaccine component; 9vHPV is produced in yeast and should not be administered to anyone with a severe yeast allergy.
- HPV vaccines are not recommended for use during pregnancy. The health care professional should inquire about pregnancy in sexually active patients, but a pregnancy test is not required before starting the immunization series. If a vaccine recipient becomes pregnant, subsequent doses should be postponed until she is no longer pregnant. If a dose has been administered inadvertently during pregnancy, no intervention is needed. Data to date show no evidence of adverse effect of any HPV vaccine on outcomes of pregnancy. Health care professionals can report pregnant women who received 9vHPV by calling the manufacturer at 1-800-986-8999. The CDC will continue to monitor pregnancy outcomes through reports to VAERS and through studies in the Vaccine Safety Datalink (see Vaccine Adverse Event Reporting System, p 45, and Vaccine Safety Datalink Project, p 46).
- Vaccine providers, particularly when vaccinating adolescents, should observe patients (with patients seated or lying down) for 15 minutes after vaccination to decrease the

[1]Centers for Disease Control and Prevention. Use of a 2-dose schedule for human papillomavirus vaccination—updated recommendations of the Advisory Committee on Immunization Practices. *MMWR Morb Mortal Wkly Rep.* 2016;65(49):1405–1408

risk for injury should they faint. If syncope develops, patients should be observed until symptoms resolve.

- 9vHPV can be administered to lactating women.

Paracoccidioidomycosis
(Formerly Known as South American Blastomycosis)

CLINICAL MANIFESTATIONS: Disease occurs primarily in adults, in whom the site of initial infection is the lungs. Disease is infrequent in children, in whom approximately 5% to 10% of all cases occur. Clinical patterns can include subclinical infection or progressive disease that can be either acute-subacute (juvenile type) or chronic (adult type). In both adult and juvenile forms, constitutional symptoms, such as fever, malaise, anorexia, and weight loss, are common. In the juvenile form, the initial pulmonary infection usually is asymptomatic, and manifestations are related to dissemination of infection to the reticuloendothelial system, resulting in enlarged lymph nodes and involvement of liver, spleen, and bone marrow. Skin lesions are observed regularly and are located typically on the face, neck, and trunk. Involvement of bones, joints, and mucous membranes is less common. Enlarged lymph nodes occasionally coalesce and form abscesses or fistulas. The chronic form of the illness can be localized to the lungs or can disseminate. Oral mucosal lesions are observed in half of the cases. Skin involvement is common but occurs in a smaller proportion than in patients with the acute-subacute form. Infection can be latent for years before causing illness.

ETIOLOGY: *Paracoccidioides brasiliensis* is a thermally dimorphic fungus with yeast and mycelia (mold) phases. A new species, *Paracoccidioides lutzii*, also causes paracoccidioidomycosis.

EPIDEMIOLOGY: The infection occurs in Latin America, from Mexico to Argentina, with 80% of cases in Brazil. The natural reservoir is unknown, although soil is suspected. The mode of transmission is unknown, but most likely occurs via inhalation of contaminated soil or dust; person-to-person transmission does not occur.

The **incubation period** is highly variable, ranging from 1 month to decades, so prior residence in Latin America is important to determine.

DIAGNOSTIC TESTS: A number of serologic tests are available; quantitative immunodiffusion is the preferred test. The antibody titer by immunodiffusion usually is ≥1:32 in acute infection. Round, multiple-budding yeast cells with a distinguishing pilot's wheel appearance can be seen in preparations of sputum, bronchoalveolar lavage specimens, scrapings from ulcers, and material from lesions or in tissue biopsy specimens. Several procedures, including wet or KOH wet preparations, or histologic staining with hematoxylin and eosin, silver, or periodic-acid Schiff, are adequate for visualization of fungal elements. The mycelia form of *P brasiliensis* can be cultured on most enriched media, including blood agar at 37°C and Mycosel or Sabouraud dextrose agar at 25°C to 30°C. Cultures should be held at least 4 weeks. Its appearance is not distinctive, and confirmation requires conversion to the yeast phase or DNA sequence determination.

TREATMENT: Amphotericin B is preferred by many experts for initial treatment of severe paracoccidioidomycosis (see Antifungal Drugs for Systemic Fungal Infections, p 938). An alternative is intravenous trimethoprim-sulfamethoxazole (8–10 mg/kg/day of the trimethoprim component, divided into 3 daily doses). Children treated initially by the intravenous route can transition to orally administered therapy after clinical improvement has been observed, usually after 3 to 6 weeks, and the duration of total acute treatment usually lasts for 6 to 12 months.

Oral therapy with itraconazole (5–10 mg/kg, twice daily; maximum dose, 200 mg) is the treatment of choice for less severe or localized infection and to complete treatment when amphotericin B is used initially. Itraconazole oral solution is preferred to capsules. Serum trough concentrations of itraconazole should be 1 to 2 μg/mL. Concentrations should be checked after 1 to 2 weeks of therapy to ensure adequate drug exposure. When measured by high-pressure liquid chromatography, both itraconazole and its bioactive hydroxy-itraconazole metabolite are reported, the sum of which should be considered in assessing drug concentrations.

Prolonged therapy for 6 to 12 months is necessary to minimize the relapse rate. Children with severe disease can require a longer course. Voriconazole is as well tolerated and as effective as itraconazole in adults, but data for its use in children with paracoccidioidomycosis are not available. Similarly, isavuconazole has been efficacious in adults, but there are no pediatric data for paracoccidioidomycosis. Trimethoprim-sulfamethoxazole orally (10 mg/kg/day of the trimethoprim component divided into 2 doses daily, maximum dose 160 mg trimethoprim and 800 mg sulfamethoxazole) is an alternative, but treatment must be continued for 2 years or longer to lessen the risk of relapse, which occurs in 10% to 15% of optimally treated patients. Ketoconazole and fluconazole generally are not recommended.

Serial serologic testing by quantitative immunodiffusion is useful for monitoring the response to therapy. The expected response is a progressive decline in titers after 1 to 3 months of treatment with stabilization at a low titer for years or even lifelong.

ISOLATION OF THE HOSPITALIZED PATIENT: Standard precautions are recommended.
CONTROL MEASURES: None.

Paragonimiasis

CLINICAL MANIFESTATIONS: There are 2 major forms of paragonimiasis: (1) disease principally attributable to *Paragonimus westermani, Paragonimus heterotremus, Paragonimus africanus, Paragonimus uterobilateralis,* and *Paragonimus kellicotti,* causing primary pulmonary disease with or without extrapulmonary manifestations; and (2) disease attributable to other species of *Paragonimus,* most notably *Paragonimus skrjabini,* for which humans are accidental hosts and manifestations generally are extrapulmonary, resulting in a larva migrans syndrome similar to that caused by *Toxocara canis.* The former disease is especially likely to have an insidious onset and a chronic course. Pulmonary disease is associated with chronic cough and dyspnea, but most infections probably are inapparent or result in mild symptoms. During worm migration in the lungs, migratory infiltrates may be noted on serial imaging. Heavy infestations cause paroxysms of coughing, which often produce blood-tinged sputum that is brown because of the presence of the pigmented *Paragonimus* eggs and hemosiderin. Hemoptysis can be severe. Eosinophilic pleural effusion, pneumothorax, bronchiectasis, and pulmonary fibrosis with clubbing can develop.

Extrapulmonary manifestations may involve the liver, spleen, abdominal cavity, intestinal wall, intra-abdominal lymph nodes, skin, and central nervous system, with meningoencephalitis, seizures, and space-occupying tumors attributable to invasion of the brain by adult flukes, usually occurring within a year of pulmonary infection. Symptoms tend to subside after approximately 5 years but can persist for as many as 20 years. Extrapulmonary paragonimiasis also is associated with migratory allergic subcutaneous nodules, which contain juvenile worms.

ETIOLOGY: Paragonimiasis is caused by the lung fluke (trematode, flat worm) *Paragonimus*. In Asia, classical paragonimiasis is caused by adult flukes and eggs of *P westermani* and *P heterotremus*. In Africa, the adult flukes and eggs of *P africanus* and *P uterobilateralis* produce the disease, whereas in North America the endemic species is *P kellicotti*. In North America, disease also has been caused by *P westermani*, present in imported crab. The adult flukes of *P westermani* are up to 12 mm long and 7 mm wide and occur throughout Asia. A triploid parthenogenetic form of *P westermani*, which is larger, produces more eggs, and elicits greater disease, has been described in Japan, Korea, Taiwan, and parts of eastern China. *P heterotremus* occurs in Southeast Asia and adjacent parts of China.

Extrapulmonary paragonimiasis (ie, visceral larva migrans) is caused by larval stages of *P skrjabini* and *Paragonimus miyazakii*. The worms rarely mature in infected human tissues. *P skrjabini* occurs in China, whereas *P miyazakii* occurs in Japan. *Paragonimus mexicanus* and *Paragonimus ecuadoriensis* occur in Mexico, Costa Rica, Ecuador, and Peru. *P kellicotti*, a lung fluke of mink, opossums, and other animals in the United States, can cause infection in humans.

EPIDEMIOLOGY: Transmission occurs when raw or undercooked freshwater crabs or crayfish containing larvae (metacercariae) are ingested. Numerous cases have been associated with ingestion of uncooked or undercooked crawfish and during exposure to river water during canoeing or camping trips in the Midwestern United States. The metacercariae excyst in the small intestine and penetrate the abdominal cavity, where they remain for a few days before migrating through the diaphragm to the lungs. *P westermani* and *P heterotremus* mature within the lungs over 6 to 10 weeks, when they then begin egg production. Eggs escape from pulmonary capsules into the bronchi and exit from the human host in sputum or feces. Eggs hatch in freshwater within 3 weeks, giving rise to miracidia. Miracidia penetrate freshwater snails and emerge several weeks later as cercariae, which encyst within the muscles and viscera of freshwater crustaceans before maturing into infective metacercariae. A less common mode of transmission that also may occur is human infection through ingestion of raw pork, usually from wild pigs, containing the juvenile stages of *Paragonimus* species (described as occurring in Japan).

Humans are accidental ("dead-end") hosts for *P skrjabini* and *P miyazakii* in visceral larva migrans. These flukes cannot mature in humans and, hence, do not produce eggs.

Paragonimus species infect a variety of other mammals, such as canids, mustelids, felids, and rodents, which serve as animal reservoir hosts.

The **incubation period** is variable. Egg production begins by approximately 8 weeks after ingestion of *P westermani* metacercariae.

DIAGNOSIS: Paragonimiasis should be considered in patients with unexplained fever, cough, eosinophilia, and pleural effusion or other chest radiographic abnormalities who have eaten raw or undercooked crayfish. Microscopic examination of stool, sputum, pleural fluid, cerebrospinal fluid, and other tissue specimens may reveal eggs. A Western blot serologic antibody test based on *P westermani* antigen, available at the Centers for Disease Control and Prevention (CDC), is sensitive and specific; antibody concentrations detected by immunoblot decrease slowly after the infection is cured by treatment. Charcot-Leyden crystals and eosinophils in sputum are useful diagnostic elements. Peripheral blood eosinophilia also is characteristic. Chest radiographs may appear normal or may resemble radiographs from patients with tuberculosis or malignancy.

TREATMENT: Praziquantel in a 2- to 3-day course is the treatment of choice (see Drugs for Parasitic Infections, p 985) and is associated with high cure rates, as demonstrated by disappearance of egg production and radiographic lesions in the lungs. The drug also is effective for some extrapulmonary manifestations. An alternative drug for patients unable to take praziquantel (eg, because of previous allergic reaction) is triclabendazole, given in 1 or 2 doses. Triclabendazole is not available commercially in the United States; however, it is available to US-licensed physicians through the CDC Drug Service, under a special protocol that requires both the CDC and US Food and Drug Administration to agree that the drug is indicated for treatment of a particular patient. For patients with central nervous system paragonimiasis, a short course of steroids may be beneficial in addition to the praziquantel, to reduce the inflammatory response associated with the dying flukes.

ISOLATION OF THE HOSPITALIZED PATIENT: Standard precautions are recommended.

CONTROL MEASURES: Cooking of crabs and crayfish for several minutes until the meat has congealed and turned opaque kills metacercariae. Meat from wild pigs should be well cooked before eating (internal temperature of at least 160°F [71°C]). Control of animal reservoirs is not possible.

Parainfluenza Viral Infections

CLINICAL MANIFESTATIONS: Parainfluenza viruses (PIVs) are the major cause of laryngotracheobronchitis (croup) and may cause bronchiolitis and pneumonia as well as upper respiratory tract infection.[1] PIV type 1 (PIV1) and, to a lesser extent, PIV type 2 (PIV2) are the most common pathogens associated with croup. PIV type 3 (PIV3) most commonly is associated with bronchiolitis and pneumonia in infants and young children. Infections with PIV type 4 (PIV4) are less well characterized but have been associated with mild upper respiratory tract infections as well as lower respiratory tract infections. Longitudinal studies have demonstrated that upper respiratory infections caused by viruses, including PIVs, can be associated with acute otitis media, which is frequently a mixed viral-bacterial infection. Rarely, PIVs have been isolated from patients with parotitis, myopericarditis, aseptic meningitis, encephalitis, or Guillain-Barré syndrome. PIV infections can exacerbate symptoms of chronic lung disease and asthma in children and adults. In children with immunodeficiency and recipients of hematopoietic stem cell transplants, PIVs can cause refractory infections with persistent shedding, severe pneumonia with viral dissemination, and even fatal disease, most commonly caused by PIV3. PIV infections do not confer complete protective immunity; therefore, reinfections can occur with all serotypes and at any age, but reinfections usually are mild and limited to the upper respiratory tract.

ETIOLOGY: PIVs are enveloped single-stranded negative-sense RNA viruses classified in the family *Paramyxoviridae*. Four antigenically distinct types—1, 2, 3, and 4 (with 2 subtypes, 4A and 4B)—that infect humans have been identified. PIV-1 and PIV-3 are in the genus *Respirovirus* and PIV-2 and PIV-4 are placed in the genus *Rubulavirus*.

---

[1]American Academy of Pediatrics, Subcommittee on Diagnosis and Management of Bronchiolitis. Clinical practice guideline: the diagnosis, management, and prevention of bronchiolitis. *Pediatrics.* 2014;134(5):e1474-e1502

EPIDEMIOLOGY: PIVs are transmitted from person to person by direct contact and exposure to contaminated nasopharyngeal secretions through respiratory tract droplets and fomites. PIV infections can be sporadic or associated with outbreaks of acute respiratory tract disease. Seasonal patterns of infection are distinct, predictable, and cyclic in temperate regions. Different serotypes have distinct epidemiologic patterns. PIV1 tends to produce outbreaks of respiratory tract illness, usually croup, in the autumn of every other year. A major increase in the number of cases of croup in the autumn usually indicates a PIV1 outbreak. PIV2 also can cause outbreaks of respiratory tract illness in the autumn, often in conjunction with PIV1 outbreaks, but PIV2 outbreaks tend to be less severe, irregular, and less common. PIV3 is endemic and usually is prominent during spring and summer in temperate climates but often continues into autumn, especially in years when autumn outbreaks of PIV1 or PIV2 are absent. PIV4 seasonal patterns are not as well characterized, but a recent study has shown that infections with PIV4 had year-round prevalence with peaks during the fall of odd-numbered years.

The age of primary infection varies with serotype. Primary infection with all types usually occurs by 5 years of age. Infection with PIV3 more often occurs in infants and is a frequent cause of bronchiolitis and pneumonia in this age group. By 12 months of age, 50% of infants have acquired PIV3 infection. Infections between 1 and 5 years of age more commonly are associated with PIV1 and, to a lesser extent, PIV2. Acquisition of PIV4 also occurs during preschool years following the pattern observed with PIV1 and PIV2. Rates of PIV-associated hospitalizations for children vary depending on clinical syndrome, PIV type, and patient age.

Immunocompetent children with primary PIV infection may shed virus for up to 1 week before onset of clinical symptoms and for 1 to 3 weeks after symptoms have disappeared, depending on serotype. Severe lower respiratory tract disease with prolonged shedding of the virus can develop in immunodeficient people. In these patients, infection may spread beyond the respiratory tract to the liver and lymph nodes.

The **incubation period** ranges from 2 to 6 days.

DIAGNOSTIC TESTS: Reverse transcriptase-polymerase chain reaction (RT-PCR) assays are the preferred diagnostic method for detection and differentiation of PIVs. PIVs may be isolated from nasopharyngeal secretions in cell culture, usually within 4 to 7 days of culture inoculation. Time to detection in cell culture may be decreased with fluorescein-labeled antibodies or use of centrifugation of the specimen onto a monolayer of susceptible cells with subsequent staining for viral antigen (rapid shell vial assay). In general, such antigen-based culture identification methods detect PIV1, -2, and -3, but not PIV4. Similarly, rapid direct antigen detection techniques, including immunofluorescence assays, can be used to detect the virus directly in nasopharyngeal secretions, but sensitivities of the tests vary compared with cell culture, and PIV4 generally is not detected. PIVs are included in many respiratory pathogen panels. Serologic diagnosis, made retrospectively by a significant increase in antibody titer between serum specimens obtained during acute infection and convalescence, is less useful, because results are delayed and infection may not always be accompanied by a significant homotypic antibody response.

TREATMENT: Specific antiviral therapy is not available, although several antiviral agents with activity against PIVs currently are in development. Most infections are self-limited and require no treatment. Monitoring for hypoxia and hypercapnia in more severely affected children with lower respiratory tract disease may be helpful.

Racemic epinephrine aerosol commonly is given to severely affected hospitalized patients with laryngotracheobronchitis to decrease airway obstruction. Parenteral, oral, and nebulized corticosteroids have been demonstrated to lessen the severity and duration of symptoms and hospitalization in patients with moderate to severe laryngotracheobronchitis. Oral steroids also are effective for outpatients with less severe croup. Management otherwise is supportive.

Antimicrobial agents should be reserved for documented secondary bacterial infections. Use of ribavirin (usually inhaled), with or without concomitant administration of Immune Globulin Intravenous (IGIV), has been reported anecdotally in immunocompromised patients with severe pneumonia; however, controlled studies are lacking.

ISOLATION OF THE HOSPITALIZED PATIENT: In addition to standard precautions, contact precautions are recommended for hospitalized infants and young children diagnosed with PIV for the duration of illness. Before a specific pathogen has been identified, contact and droplet precautions are required if influenza virus or adenovirus infections are considered. In immunocompromised patients, the duration of contact precautions should be extended because of possible prolonged shedding. Hospitalized immunocompromised patients with PIV infection should be isolated to prevent spread to other patients.

CONTROL MEASURES: Appropriate respiratory hygiene and cough etiquette should be followed. Exposure to PIV-infected people, including other patients, staff, and family members, may not be recognized, because illness may be mild. Additional infection control measures should be considered in certain settings (eg, child care centers, nursing homes) when respiratory infections have been identified to limit spread. Several vaccine candidates targeting PIV1, -2, and -3 are being evaluated in clinical studies.

Parasitic Diseases

Parasites are among the most common causes of morbidity and mortality in various and diverse geographic locations worldwide. Outside the tropics and subtropics, parasitic diseases are common among travelers, immigrants, and immunocompromised people. Toxocariasis may be quite common in the southern United States and can affect impoverished populations in this region. Malaria infections in the United States occur among people who have traveled to regions with ongoing malaria transmission, and the diagnosis should be considered when evaluating fever in a returned traveler. Certain infections such as Chagas disease, neurocysticercosis, schistosomiasis, and *Strongyloides stercoralis*, have long latency periods and are commonly encountered in immigrants from regions with endemic infection. Physicians and clinical laboratory personnel need to be aware of where these infections may be acquired, their clinical presentations, and methods of diagnosis and should advise people on how to prevent infection. Table 3.46 provides details on some infrequently encountered parasitic diseases.

Consultation and assistance in diagnosis and management of parasitic diseases are available from the Centers for Disease Control and Prevention (CDC), state health departments, and university departments or hospitals that have divisions of geographic medicine, tropical medicine, pediatric infectious diseases, international health, and public health.

Table 3.46. Selected Parasitic Diseases Not Covered Elsewhere[a]

Disease and/or Agent	Where Infection May Be Acquired	Definitive Host	Intermediate Host	Modes of Human Infection	Directly Communicable (Person to Person)	Diagnostic Laboratory Tests in Humans	Causative Form of Parasite	Manifestations in Humans
Angiostrongylus cantonensis (neurotropic disease)	Widespread in the tropics, particularly Pacific Islands, Southeast Asia, Central and South America, the Caribbean, and the United States	Rodents	Snails and slugs	Eating improperly cooked infected mollusks or food contaminated by mollusk secretions containing larvae; prawns, fish, and land crabs that have ingested infected mollusks also may be infectious	No	Eosinophils in CSF; rarely, identification of larvae in CSF or at autopsy; RT-PCR of CSF, serologic testing – ELISA	Larval worms	Eosinophilia, eosinophilic meningoencephalitis

Table 3.46. Selected Parasitic Diseases Not Covered Elsewhere,[a] continued

Disease and/or Agent	Where Infection May Be Acquired	Definitive Host	Intermediate Host	Modes of Human Infection	Directly Communicable (Person to Person)	Diagnostic Laboratory Tests in Humans	Causative Form of Parasite	Manifestations in Humans
Angiostrongylus costaricensis (gastrointestinal tract disease)	Central and South America	Rodents	Snails and slugs	Eating improperly cooked infected mollusks or food contaminated by mollusk secretions containing larvae	No	Gel diffusion; identification of larvae and eggs in tissue	Larval worms	Abdominal pain, eosinophilia
Anisakiasis	Cosmopolitan, most common where eating raw fish is practiced	Marine mammal	Certain saltwater fish, squid, and octopus	Eating uncooked or inadequately treated infected marine fish	No	Identification of recovered larvae on endoscopy or identified in granulomas	Larval worms	Acute gastrointestinal tract disease

Table 3.46. Selected Parasitic Diseases Not Covered Elsewhere,[a] continued

Disease and/or Agent	Where Infection May Be Acquired	Definitive Host	Intermediate Host	Modes of Human Infection	Directly Communicable (Person to Person)	Diagnostic Laboratory Tests in Humans	Causative Form of Parasite	Manifestations in Humans
Clonorchis sinensis, Opisthorchis viverrini, Opisthorchis felineus (flukes)	East Asia, Eastern Europe, Russian Federation	Humans, cats, dogs, other mammals	Certain freshwater snails	Eating uncooked infected freshwater fish	No	Eggs in stool or duodenal fluid Serologic testing – ELISA	Larvae and mature flukes	Abdominal pain; hepatobiliary disease; cholangiocarcinoma
Dracunculiasis (*Dracunculus medinensis*) (guinea worm)	Foci in Africa; global eradication nearly achieved	Humans	Crustacea (copepods)	Drinking water infested with infected copepods	No	Identification of emerging or adult worm in subcutaneous tissues	Adult female worm	Emerging roundworm; inflammatory response; systemic and local blister or ulcer in skin

Table 3.46. Selected Parasitic Diseases Not Covered Elsewhere,ᵃ continued

Disease and/or Agent	Where Infection May Be Acquired	Definitive Host	Intermediate Host	Modes of Human Infection	Directly Communicable (Person to Person)	Diagnostic Laboratory Tests in Humans	Causative Form of Parasite	Manifestations in Humans
Fascioliasis (liver fluke; *Fasciola hepatica*)	Worldwide; predominantly in the tropics	Sheep and cattle most important; other mammals	Snails	Freshwater plants; watercress; drinking contaminated water	No	Identifying eggs in stool, duodenal fluid, or bile; serologic testing; examination of surgical specimens	Migrating metacercariae cause liver parenchymal destruction; adult worms can obstruct bile ducts	Acute: fever, right upper quadrant pain, hepatosplenomegaly; anorexia, nausea, vomiting, myalgia, cough, urticaria; eosinophilia Chronic: bile duct obstruction; gastrointestinal tract symptoms
Fasciolopsiasis (*Fasciolopsis buski*)	East Asia	Humans, pigs, dogs	Certain freshwater snails, plants	Eating uncooked infected plants	No	Eggs or worm in feces or duodenal fluid; serologic testing – ELISA	Larvae and mature worms	Diarrhea, constipation, vomiting, anorexia, edema of face and legs, ascites

Table 3.46. Selected Parasitic Diseases Not Covered Elsewhere,[a] continued

Disease and/or Agent	Where Infection May Be Acquired	Definitive Host	Intermediate Host	Modes of Human Infection	Directly Communicable (Person to Person)	Diagnostic Laboratory Tests in Humans	Causative Form of Parasite	Manifestations in Humans
Intestinal capillariasis (*Capillaria philippinensis*)	Philippines, Thailand	Humans, fish-eating birds	Fish	Ingestion of uncooked infected fish	Uncertain	Eggs and parasite in feces	Larvae and mature worms	Protein-losing enteropathy, diarrhea, malabsorption, ascites, emaciation

CSF indicates cerebrospinal fluid; RT-PCR, reverse-transcriptase polymerase chain reaction; ELISA, enzyme-linked immunosorbent assay.

[a]For recommended drug treatment, see Drugs for Parasitic Infections (p 985).

Through authorized investigational new drug mechanisms, the CDC distributes several drugs that are not available commercially in the United States for treatment of parasitic diseases. To request these drugs, a physician must contact the CDC Parasitic Diseases Inquiries office (see Appendix I, Directory of Resources, p 1051; 404-718-4745; e-mail: **parasites@cdc.gov**). Consultation with a medical officer from the CDC is required before a drug is released for a patient.

Important human parasitic infections are discussed in individual chapters in Section 3; the diseases are arranged alphabetically, and the discussions include recommendations for drug treatment. Drugs for Parasitic Infections can be found beginning on p 985 and are compiled from recommendations on the CDC Web site and other sources. Recommendations for treatment of parasitic infections may differ between sources because of differences of opinion among experts and because a number of drugs used commonly for treatment of parasitic infections may not be approved for that specific organism or for the age group under consideration. Specific expertise or multiple sources should be consulted especially when there is a lack of familiarity with the parasite or the drugs recommended for treatment.

Human Parechovirus Infections

CLINICAL MANIFESTATIONS: Human parechoviruses (HPeVs) primarily cause disease in young infants and present in a similar manner to enterovirus or disseminated herpes simplex virus infection, with a febrile illness, exanthem, sepsis-like syndrome, and/or central nervous system manifestations such as meningitis (typically with little or no pleocytosis), encephalitis, intractable seizures, and paralytic disease, often with brain imaging abnormalities. Infections (particularly with HPeV type 3) may be severe and include sepsis, hepatitis and coagulopathy, myocarditis, pneumonia, and/or meningoencephalitis, with long-term sequelae. HPeV infections have been associated with respiratory and gastrointestinal tract disease and a variety of other less severe manifestations, although causation has not been established consistently.

ETIOLOGY: HPeVs are a group of small, nonenveloped, single-stranded, positive-sense RNA viruses in the family *Picornaviridae*. The *Parechovirus* genus includes at least 16 HPeV types (designated 1–16). HPeV types 1 and 2 previously were classified as echoviruses 22 and 23, respectively. HPeV types 1 and 3 have been implicated in disease most frequently with available surveillance.

EPIDEMIOLOGY: Humans are the primary reservoir for HPeV, although infection in primates has been demonstrated. HPeV infections have been reported worldwide. Seroepidemiologic studies suggest that HPeV infections occur commonly during early childhood. In some studies, most school-aged children have serologic evidence of prior infection, but seroprevalence appears to vary by geographic region and specific HPeV type. Infections frequently are asymptomatic. Clinical reports suggest that most severe disease occurs in infants and young children. Transmission appears to occur via the fecal-oral and respiratory routes, and on the basis of reports of very early onset neonatal disease, in utero transmission also may occur. HPeVs may circulate throughout the year, but infections by certain types occur more commonly during summer and fall months. Multiple HPeV types may circulate in a community during the same time period. Community outbreaks and health care-associated transmission in neonatal and pediatric hospital units have been described. Virus is shed from the upper respiratory tract for 1 to 3 weeks and in stool for less than 2 weeks to 5 months. Shedding may occur in the absence of illness.

The **incubation period** for HPeV infections has not been defined.

DIAGNOSTIC TESTS: Reverse-transcriptase polymerase chain reaction (RT-PCR) assays that detect HPeVs, available at the Centers for Disease Control and Prevention and select reference and hospital-based laboratories, represent the best diagnostic modality currently available. Some of the assays may not detect all 16 serotypes. Enterovirus PCR assays will not detect HPeV. There is at least one RT-PCR assay cleared by the US Food and Drug Administration available in the United States for detecting HPeVs. This assay is a multiplexed, multiple-pathogen assay designed to detect a number of bacterial and viral agents of meningitis and encephalitis in cerebrospinal fluid. Clinical data on the use of this assay are limited. HPeVs can be detected by RT-PCR in stool, throat swab specimens, nasopharyngeal aspirates, tracheal secretions, cerebrospinal fluid, and blood. As with the enteroviruses, the HPeVs can be shed in throat and particularly from the gastrointestinal tract for prolonged periods, so detection does not necessarily represent a current invasive disease attributable to HPeVs. The HPeV type can be identified by partial genomic sequencing or by neutralization assay of a viral isolate, although neutralizing antisera are not available for all serotypes. Viral culture can be used, but recovery in culture is less sensitive than PCR assay, requires multiple cell lines, and may take several days. Furthermore, most HPeV types were identified by molecular methods and have never been propagated in culture. Serologic assays have been developed for research but are not available commercially for diagnostic purposes.

TREATMENT: No specific therapy is available for HPeV infections. Immune Globulin Intravenous (IGIV) has been used in some published case reports of neonates with severe HPeV infections, often complicated by myocarditis.

ISOLATION OF THE HOSPITALIZED PATIENT: In addition to standard precautions, contact precautions are appropriate for infants and young children for the duration of HPeV illness. Cohorting of infected neonates may be effective in controlling hospital nursery outbreaks.

CONTROL MEASURES: Hand hygiene is important in decreasing spread of HPeVs within families and institutions. No vaccine for HPeVs is available.

Parvovirus B19

(Erythema Infectiosum, Fifth Disease)

CLINICAL MANIFESTATIONS: Infection with human parvovirus B19 is recognized most often as erythema infectiosum (EI), or fifth disease, which is characterized by a distinctive rash that may be preceded by mild systemic symptoms, including fever in 15% to 30% of patients. The facial rash can be intensely red with a "slapped cheek" appearance that often is accompanied by circumoral pallor. A symmetric, macular, lace-like, and often pruritic rash occurs on the trunk, moving peripherally to involve the arms, buttocks, and thighs. The rash can fluctuate in intensity and recur with environmental changes, such as temperature and exposure to sunlight, for weeks to months. A brief, mild, nonspecific illness consisting of fever, malaise, myalgia, and headache often precedes the characteristic exanthem by approximately 7 to 10 days. Arthralgia and arthritis occur in fewer than 10% of infected children but commonly occur among adults, especially women. Knees are involved most commonly in children, but a symmetric polyarthropathy of knees, fingers, and other joints is common in adults.

Human parvovirus B19 can cause asymptomatic or subclinical infections. Other manifestations (Table 3.47) include a mild respiratory tract illness with no rash, a rash atypical for EI that may be rubelliform or petechial, popular-purpuric gloves-and-socks syndrome (PPGSS; painful and pruritic papules, petechiae, and purpura of hands and feet, often with fever and an enanthem), polyarthropathy syndrome (arthralgia and arthritis in adults in the absence of other manifestations of EI), chronic erythroid hypoplasia with severe anemia in immunodeficient patients (eg, patients with human immunodeficiency virus [HIV] infection, patients receiving immune suppressive therapy), and transient aplastic crisis lasting 7 to 10 days in patients with hemolytic anemias (eg, sickle cell disease and autoimmune hemolytic anemia). For children with other conditions associated with low hemoglobin concentrations, including hemorrhage and severe anemia, parvovirus B19 infection usually will not result in aplastic crisis but might result in prolongation of recovery from the anemia. Patients with transient aplastic crisis may have a prodromal illness with fever, malaise, and myalgia, but rash usually is absent. In addition, human parvovirus B19 infection sometimes has been associated with decreases in numbers of platelets, lymphocytes, and neutrophils. In rare cases, parvovirus B19 infection has been associated with acute hepatitis and myocarditis in children. Human parvovirus B19 infection occurring during pregnancy can cause fetal hydrops, intrauterine growth restriction, isolated pleural and pericardial effusions, and death, but the virus is not a proven cause of congenital anomalies. The risk of fetal death is between 2% and 6% when infection occurs during pregnancy. The greatest risk appears to occur during the first half of pregnancy.

ETIOLOGY: Human parvovirus B19 is a small, nonenveloped, single-stranded DNA virus in the family *Parvoviridae*, genus *Erythroparvovirus*. Three distinct genotypes of the virus have been described, but there is no evidence of differences of virologic or disease characteristics among the genotypes. Parvovirus B19 replicates in human erythrocyte precursors, which accounts for some of the clinical manifestations following infection. Human parvovirus B19-associated red blood cell aplasia is related to caspase-mediated apoptosis of erythrocyte precursors.

Table 3.47. Clinical Manifestations of Human Parvovirus B19 Infection

Conditions	Usual Hosts
Erythema infectiosum (fifth disease, EI)	Immunocompetent children
Polyarthropathy syndrome	Immunocompetent adults (more common in women)
Chronic anemia/pure red cell aplasia	Immunocompromised hosts
Transient aplastic crisis	People with hemolytic anemia (ie, sickle cell anemia)
Hydrops fetalis/congenital anemia	Fetus (first 20 weeks of pregnancy)
Petechial, papular-purpuric gloves-and-socks syndrome (PPGSS)	Immunocompetent children and young adults

EPIDEMIOLOGY: Parvovirus B19 is distributed worldwide and is a common cause of infection in humans, who are the only known hosts. Modes of transmission include contact with respiratory tract secretions, percutaneous exposure to blood or blood products, and vertical transmission from mother to fetus. Human parvovirus B19 infections are ubiquitous, and cases of EI can occur sporadically or in outbreaks in elementary or junior high schools during late winter and early spring. Secondary spread among susceptible household members is common, with infection occurring in approximately 50% of susceptible contacts in some studies. The transmission rate in schools is lower, but infection can be an occupational risk for school and child care personnel, with approximately 20% of susceptible contacts becoming infected. In young children, antibody seroprevalence generally is 5% to 10%. In most communities, approximately 50% of young adults and often more than 90% of elderly people are seropositive.

The **incubation period** from acquisition of parvovirus B19 to onset of initial symptoms (rash or symptoms of aplastic crisis) is between 4 and 14 days but can be as long as 21 days. Timing of the presence of high-titer parvovirus B19 DNA in serum and respiratory tract secretions indicates that people with EI are infectious before rash onset and are unlikely to be infectious after onset of the rash and/or joint symptoms. In contrast, patients with aplastic crises are contagious from before the onset of symptoms through at least the week after onset. Symptoms of PPGSS can occur in association with viremia and before development of antibody response, and affected patients should be considered infectious.

DIAGNOSTIC TESTS: In the immunocompetent host, detection of serum parvovirus B19-specific immunoglobulin (Ig) M antibodies is the preferred diagnostic test for an acute or recent parvovirus B19-associated rash illness. A positive IgM test result indicates that infection probably occurred within the previous 2 to 3 months. On the basis of immunoassay results, IgM antibodies may be detected in 90% or more of patients at the time of the EI rash and by the third day of illness in patients with transient aplastic crisis. Serum IgG antibodies appear by approximately day 2 of EI and persist for life; therefore, presence of parvovirus B19 IgG is not necessarily indicative of acute infection. These assays are available through commercial laboratories and through some state public health department and research laboratories. However, their sensitivity and specificity may vary, particularly for IgM.

Serum IgM and IgG assays are not reliable in immunocompromised patients. The optimal method for detecting transient aplastic crisis or chronic infection in the immunocompromised patient is demonstration of high titer of viral DNA by polymerase chain reaction (PCR) assays. Such patients generally have $>10^6$ parvovirus B19 DNA copies/mL of plasma. Currently, there are no PCR assays cleared by the US Food and Drug Administration for the qualitative or quantitative detection of parvovirus B19 DNA, but such assays are available through select commercial and reference laboratories and sometimes in larger hospital-based laboratories. With the availability of a World Health Organization (WHO) nucleic acid standard for parvovirus B19 DNA, assay results can be reported in international units per mL (IU/mL) to allow for straightforward comparison across assays. The WHO also offers an International Reference Panel for parvovirus B19 nucleic acid amplification assays to allow laboratories to ensure that all 3 genotypes are detected in their assays. Because parvovirus B19 DNA can be detected at low levels by PCR assay in serum for months and even years after the acute viremic phase, detection does not necessarily indicate acute infection. Low levels of parvovirus B19 DNA also can be detected by PCR in tissues (skin, heart, liver, bone marrow), independent of active disease. Qualitative PCR may be used on amniotic fluid as an aid to diagnosis of hydrops fetalis. Parvovirus B19 cannot be propagated in standard cell culture.

TREATMENT: For most patients, only supportive care is indicated. Patients with aplastic crisis may require transfusions of blood products. For treatment of chronic infection in immunodeficient patients, Immune Globulin Intravenous (IGIV) therapy often is effective and should be considered. Some cases of parvovirus B19 infection concurrent with hydrops fetalis have been treated successfully with intrauterine blood transfusions of the fetus.

ISOLATION OF THE HOSPITALIZED PATIENT: In addition to standard precautions, droplet precautions are recommended for hospitalized children with aplastic crises, children with PPGSS, or immunosuppressed patients with chronic infection and anemia for the duration of hospitalization. For patients with transient aplastic or erythrocyte crisis, these precautions should be maintained for 7 days or until the reticulocyte count has recovered from suppression to at least 2%. Neonates who had hydrops attributable to parvovirus B19 in utero do not require isolation if the hydrops is resolved at the time of birth.

Pregnant health care workers should be informed of the potential risks to their fetus from human parvovirus B19 infections and about preventive measures that may decrease these risks (eg, attention to strict infection control procedures and not caring for immunocompromised patients with chronic parvovirus B19 infection or patients with parvovirus B19-associated aplastic crises, because patients in both groups are likely to be contagious).

CONTROL MEASURES:

- Women who are exposed to children at home or at work (eg, teachers or child care providers) are at increased risk of infection with parvovirus B19. However, because school or child care center outbreaks often indicate wider spread in the community, including inapparent infection, women are at some degree of risk of exposure from other sources at home or in the community. In view of the high prevalence of parvovirus B19 infection, the low incidence of adverse effects on the fetus, and the fact that avoidance of child care or classroom teaching can decrease but not eliminate the risk of exposure, routine exclusion of pregnant women from the workplace where EI is occurring is not recommended. Women of childbearing age who are concerned can undergo serologic testing for IgG antibody to parvovirus B19 to determine their susceptibility to infection.

- Pregnant women who discover that they have been in contact with children who were in the incubation period of EI or with children who were in aplastic crisis should have the relatively low potential risk of infection explained to them. The American College of Obstetricians and Gynecologists recommends that pregnant women exposed to parvovirus B19 should have serologic testing performed to determine susceptibility and possible evidence of acute parvovirus B19 infection.[1] Pregnant women with evidence of acute parvovirus B19 infection should be monitored closely (eg, serial ultrasonographic examinations) by their obstetric provider. In pregnant women with suspected or proven intrauterine parvovirus B19 infection, amniotic fluid and fetal tissues should be considered infectious, and contact precautions should be used in addition to standard precautions if exposure is likely.

---

[1]American College of Obstetricians and Gynecologists. Cytomegalovirus, parvovirus B19, varicella zoster, and toxoplasmosis in pregnancy. Practice Bulletin No. 151. *Obstet Gynecol.* 2015;125(6):1510–1525

- Children with EI may attend child care or school, because they no longer are contagious once the rash appears.
- Transmission of parvovirus B19 is likely to be decreased through use of routine infection-control practices, including hand hygiene and proper disposal of used facial tissues.
- The FDA has issued guidance for nucleic acid amplification testing to reduce the possible risk of parvovirus B19 transmission by plasma-derived products (**www.fda. gov/ucm/groups/fdagov-public/@fdagov-bio-gen/documents/ document/ucm078510.pdf**). The goal is to identify and prevent the use of plasma-derived products containing high levels of virus. Human parvovirus B19 viral loads in manufacturing pools should not exceed 10^4 IU/mL.

Pasteurella Infections

CLINICAL MANIFESTATIONS: The most common manifestation is cellulitis at the site of a bite or scratch of a cat, dog, or other domestic or wild animal. Cellulitis typically develops within 24 hours of the injury and includes swelling, erythema, tenderness, and serosanguinous to purulent drainage at the wound site. Regional lymphadenopathy, chills, and fever can occur. The most frequent local complications are abscesses and tenosynovitis, but septic arthritis and osteomyelitis also are reported. Other less common manifestations of infection include septicemia, central nervous system infections (meningitis is the most common; however, brain abscess and subdural empyema have been observed), ocular infections (eg, conjunctivitis, corneal ulcer, endophthalmitis), endocarditis, respiratory tract infections (eg, pneumonia, pulmonary abscesses, pleural empyema, epiglottitis), appendicitis, hepatic abscess, peritonitis, and urinary tract infection. People with liver disease, solid organ transplant, or underlying host defense abnormalities are predisposed to bacteremia with *Pasteurella multocida*.

ETIOLOGY: The genus *Pasteurella* is one of 4 genera of human pathogens classified in the family *Pasteurellaceae*; the other genera are *Actinobacillus*, *Aggregatibacter*, and *Haemophilus*. Members of the genus *Pasteurella* are nonmotile, facultatively anaerobic, mostly catalase and oxidase positive, gram-negative coccobacilli that are primarily respiratory tract colonizers and pathogens in animals. The most common human pathogen is *Pasteurella multocida*. Most human infections are caused by the following species or subspecies: *P multocida* subspecies *multocida* (causing more than 50% of infections), *P multocida* subspecies *septica*, *Pasteurella canis*, *Pasteurella stomatis*, and *Pasteurella dagmatis*.

EPIDEMIOLOGY: *Pasteurella* species have a worldwide distribution. They colonize the upper respiratory tract of 70% to 90% of cats, 25% to 50% of dogs, and many other wild and domestic animals. Transmission most frequently occurs from the bite or scratch or licking of a previous wound by a cat or dog. Infected cat bite wounds contain *Pasteurella* species more often than do dog bite wounds. Rarely, respiratory tract spread occurs from animals to humans, and in a significant proportion of cases, no animal exposure can be identified. Human-to-human transmission has been documented vertically from mother to neonate, horizontally from colonized humans, and by contaminated blood products.

The **incubation period** usually is less than 24 hours.

DIAGNOSTIC TESTS: The isolation of *Pasteurella* species from a normally sterile body site (eg, blood, joint fluid, cerebrospinal fluid, pleural fluid, or suppurative lymph nodes) establishes the diagnosis of systemic infection. Recovery of the organism from a superficial site, such as drainage from a skin lesion subsequent to an animal bite, must be interpreted in the context of other potential pathogens isolated; however, mixed infection may occur. *Pasteurella* species are somewhat fastidious but may be cultured on several media generally used in clinical laboratories, including tryptic soybean digest agar with 5% sheep blood and chocolate agars, at 35°C to 37°C without increased carbon dioxide concentration. Although they resemble several other organisms morphologically, laboratory identification to the genus level generally is not difficult; however, species and subspecies differentiation is more challenging with standard biochemical testing alone. Newer laboratory methods, including PCR amplification of the 16S rRNA gene followed by sequencing, and identification of cellular components by matrix-assisted laser desorption/ionization time of flight (MALDI-TOF) mass spectroscopy, have significantly improved specific identification.

TREATMENT: The drug of choice is penicillin. Penicillin resistance is rare, but beta-lactamase–producing strains have been recovered, especially from adults with pulmonary disease. Other oral agents that usually are effective include ampicillin, amoxicillin, amoxicillin/clavulanate, cefuroxime, cefixime, cefpodoxime, doxycycline, and fluoroquinolones. Parenteral third-generation cephalosporins, including ceftriaxone and cefotaxime, demonstrate excellent in vitro activity. Oral and parenteral antistaphylococcal penicillins and first-generation cephalosporins including cephalexin are not as active and are not recommended for treatment. *Pasteurella* species are usually resistant to vancomycin, clindamycin, and erythromycin. For patients who are allergic to beta-lactam agents, azithromycin, trimethoprim-sulfamethoxazole, and the fluoroquinolones are alternative choices, but clinical experience with these agents is limited. For suspected polymicrobial infected bite wounds, oral amoxicillin-clavulanate or, for severe infection, intravenous ampicillin-sulbactam or piperacillin-tazobactam can be given. The duration of therapy usually is 7 to 10 days for local infections and 10 to 14 days for more severe infections. Antimicrobial therapy should be continued for 4 to 6 weeks for bone and joint infections. Wound drainage or débridement may be necessary.

ISOLATION OF THE HOSPITALIZED PATIENT: Standard precautions are recommended.

CONTROL MEASURES: Limiting contact with wild animals and education about appropriate contact with domestic animals can help to prevent *Pasteurella* infections (see Bite Wounds, p 189). Wounds from animal bites and scratches should be irrigated, cleansed, and débrided promptly. Antimicrobial prophylaxis for selected children, depending on the type of animal bite wound, should be initiated according to the recommendations in Table 2.11, p 189.

Pediculosis Capitis[1]

(Head Lice)

CLINICAL MANIFESTATIONS: Itching is the most common symptom of head lice infestation, but many children are asymptomatic. Adult lice (2–3 mm long, tan to grayish-white) or eggs (match hair color) and nits (empty egg shells, white) are found on the hair and are most readily apparent behind the ears and near the nape of the neck. Excoriations and crusting caused by secondary bacterial infection may occur and often are associated with

[1]Devore CD, Schutze GE; American Academy of Pediatrics, Committee on School Health and Committee on Infectious Diseases. Clinical report: head lice. *Pediatrics*. 2015;135(5):e1355-e1365

regional lymphadenopathy. Head lice usually deposit their eggs on a hair shaft 4 mm or less from the scalp. Because hair grows at a rate of approximately 1 cm per month, the duration of infestation can be estimated by the distance of the nit from the scalp.

ETIOLOGY: *Pediculus humanus capitis* is the head louse. Both nymphs and adult lice feed on human blood.

EPIDEMIOLOGY: In the United States, head lice infestation is most common in children attending child care and elementary school. Head lice infestation is not a sign of poor hygiene. All socioeconomic groups are affected. Head lice infestation is not influenced by hair length or frequency of shampooing or brushing. Head lice are not a health hazard and are not responsible for spread of any disease. Head lice are only able to crawl; therefore, transmission occurs mainly by direct head-to-head contact with hair of infested people. Transmission by contact with personal belongings, such as combs, hair brushes, sporting gear, and hats, is uncommon. Away from the scalp, head lice survive <1 day at room temperature, and their eggs generally become nonviable within a week and cannot hatch at a lower ambient temperature than that near the scalp.

The **incubation period** from the laying of eggs to hatching of the first nymph usually is about 1 week (6 to 9 days). Lice mature to the adult stage approximately 7 days later. Adult females then may lay eggs (nits), but these will develop only if the female has mated.

DIAGNOSTIC TESTS: Identification of eggs, nymphs, and adult lice with the naked eye is possible; diagnosis can be confirmed by using a hand lens, dermatoscope (epiluminescence microscope), or traditional microscope. Nymphal and adult lice shun light and move rapidly to conceal themselves. Wetting the hair with water, oil, or a conditioner may "slow down" the movement of the lice. In combination with using a fine-tooth comb, examiners may improve their ability to diagnose infestation and shorten inspection time. It is important to differentiate nits from dandruff, hair casts (a layer of follicular cells that slide easily off the hair shaft), plugs of desquamated cells, external hair debris, and fungal infections of the scalp. Because nits remain firmly affixed to hair, their mere presence is not a sign of an active infestation.

TREATMENT: A number of effective pediculicidal agents are available to treat head lice infestation (see Drugs for Parasitic Infections, p 985). Costs vary by product (see Table 3.48). Safety is a major concern with pediculicides, because the lice infestation itself presents minimal risk to the host. Pediculicides should be used only as directed and with care. Instructions on proper use of any product should be explained carefully. Therapy can be initiated with over-the-counter 1% permethrin lotion or with pyrethrin combined with piperonyl butoxide, both of which have good safety profiles. Resistance to these compounds has been documented in the United States; health care providers should be aware of regional patterns of clinical resistance. For treatment failures not attributable to improper use of an over-the-counter pediculicide, malathion, benzyl alcohol lotion, spinosad suspension, or ivermectin lotion should be used. When lice are resistant to all topical agents, oral ivermectin may be used in children weighing more than 15 kg. Drugs that have residual activity may kill nymphs as they emerge from eggs. No treatment is 100% ovicidal. Retreatment (with benzyl alcohol lotion, spinosad suspension, or malathion lotion) is performed commonly 7 to 10 days after treatment—that is, after eggs present at the time of initial treatment have hatched but before new eggs are produced. Rinsing of hair after topical pediculicide application should always be done over a sink rather

Table 3.48. Pediculicides for the Treatment of Head Lice

Product	Brand Name	Recommended Age Range	Retreatment Interval (If Needed)	Availability	Cost Estimate[a]
Permethrin 1% lotion	Nix (Prestige Brands, Greenburgh, NY)	≥2 mo	9–10 days	Over the counter	$
Pyrethrins + piperonyl butoxide	Rid (Bayer Group, Leverkusen, Germany)	≥24 mo	9–10 days	Over the counter	$
Malathion 0.5%	Ovide (Taro Pharmaceutical Industries Ltd, Haifa Bay, Israel)	≥2 y	7–9 days if live lice are seen after initial dose	Prescription	$$$$
Benzyl alcohol 5%	Ulesfia (Contract Pharmaceuticals Ltd, Mississauga, Ontario, Canada)	≥6 mo	9–10 days	Prescription	$$ – $$$$[b]
Spinosad 0.9% suspension	Natroba (ParaPRO, Carmel, IN)	≥6 mo	7 days if live lice are seen after initial dose	Prescription	$$$$
Ivermectin 0.5% lotion	Sklice (Arbor Pharmaceuticals, Atlanta, GA)	≥6 mo	Single use	Prescription	$$$$
Ivermectin (oral)	Stromectol (Merck & Co Inc, Whitehouse Station, NJ)	Any age, if weight >15 kg	9–10 days	Prescription	$$$$

[a]$ = ≤$25; $$ = $26–$99; $$$ = $100–$199; $$$$ = $200–$299.
[b]Cost varies by length of hair, which impacts number of units of product required.

than during a shower or bath to limit skin exposure and with warm water rather than hot water to minimize skin absorption attributable to vasodilatation.

- **Permethrin (1%).** Permethrin is available without a prescription in a 1% lotion. The infested hair and scalp is first washed with a nonconditioning shampoo and towel-dried. Permethrin is then applied to the scalp and entire length of wet hair, left for 10 minutes, and then rinsed off with water. Permethrin has a low potential for toxic effects and can be highly effective. Resistance has been reported in the United States, but prevalence is unknown. Although residual permethrin is designed to kill emerging nymphs, many experts advise a second treatment 9 to 10 days after the first treatment, especially if hair is washed within a week after the first treatment or if live lice are seen. Permethrin 1% is approved by the FDA for use on children 2 months or older.
- **Pyrethrin-based products.** Pyrethrins are natural extracts from the chrysanthemum flower, formulated with piperonyl butoxide, and are available without a

prescription as shampoos or mousse preparations. The product is applied to dry hair in sufficient amounts to saturate the scalp and entire length of the hair, left for 10 minutes, and then rinsed off with water. Pyrethrins have no residual activity; repeat application 9 to 10 days after the first application is necessary to kill newly hatched lice. Pyrethrins are contraindicated in people who are allergic to chrysanthemums or ragweed and should only be used on children 24 months of age or older.

- **Malathion (0.5%).** This organophosphate pesticide, which is both pediculicidal and partially ovicidal, is available only by prescription as a lotion and is highly effective as formulated in the United States. Malathion lotion is applied to dry hair in sufficient amounts to saturate the scalp and entire length of the hair, left to dry naturally, and then removed 8 to 12 hours later by washing and rinsing the hair. The product can be reapplied 7 to 9 days later only if live lice are still seen. The high alcohol content of the lotion makes it highly flammable; therefore, the lotion or lotion-coated hair during treatment should not be exposed to lighted cigarettes (no smoking around the individual during hair treatment), open flames, or electric heat sources such as hair dryers or curling irons. The safety and effectiveness of malathion lotion have not been assessed by the FDA in children younger than 6 years; experts have recommended its use in children as young as 24 months of age. Malathion is contraindicated in children younger than 24 months because of the possibility of increased scalp permeability and absorption.
- **Benzyl alcohol lotion (5%).** Benzyl alcohol is available by prescription in a lotion formulated with mineral oil and is highly effective as a pediculicide. The lotion is applied to dry hair in sufficient amounts to saturate the scalp and entire length of the hair, left for 10 minutes, and then rinsed off with water. Retreatment at 9 to 10 days is recommended to kill any newly hatched lice. This agent has been approved by the FDA for use in children 6 months or older. Benzyl alcohol should not be used in infants younger than 6 months, because it has been associated with neonatal gasping syndrome.
- **Spinosad suspension (0.9%).** Spinosad is a novel neurotoxin derived from *Saccharopolyspora spinosa*. Spinosad suspension contains benzyl alcohol and is both pediculicidal and ovicidal. The suspension is applied to dry hair in sufficient amounts to saturate the scalp and entire length of the hair, left for 10 minutes, and then rinsed off with water. A second treatment is applied at 7 days if live lice still are seen. Spinosad suspension is FDA approved for topical treatment of head lice in people 6 months and older. Because of the association of benzyl alcohol with neonatal gasping syndrome, this product should not be used in infants younger than 6 months.
- **Ivermectin lotion (0.5%).** Ivermectin interferes with the function of invertebrate nerve and muscle cells. It is used widely as an anthelmintic agent. The 0.5% lotion is FDA approved as a single-application, topical treatment of head lice in people 6 months and older. The lotion is applied to dry hair in sufficient amounts to saturate the scalp and entire length of the hair, left for 10 minutes, and then rinsed off with water.
- **Oral ivermectin.** Ivermectin may be effective against head lice if sufficient concentration is present in the blood at the time a louse feeds, although it has not been evaluated by the FDA as a pediculicide. It has been given as a single oral dose of 200 µg/kg or 400 µg/kg, with a second dose given after 9 to 10 days. Fewer failures occur at the 400 µg/kg-dose compared with the lower dose. Because it blocks essential neural

transmission if it crosses the blood-brain barrier and young children may be at higher risk of this adverse drug reaction, ivermectin should not be used in children weighing less than 15 kg.

- Lindane no longer is recommended by the American Academy of Pediatrics for use as treatment of head lice.
- Data are lacking to determine whether suffocation of lice by application of occlusive agents, such as petroleum jelly, olive oil, butter, or fat-containing mayonnaise, is effective as a method of treatment.

Because pediculicides kill lice shortly after application, detection of living lice on scalp inspection 24 hours or more after treatment suggests either incorrect use of pediculicide, hatching of lice after treatment, reinfestation, or resistance to therapy. In such situations, after excluding incorrect use, immediate retreatment with a different pediculicide followed by a second application 7 to 10 days later (with the exception of single-use ivermectin) is recommended.

Itching or mild burning of the scalp caused by inflammation of the skin in response to topical therapeutic agents can persist for many days after lice are killed; this is not a reason for retreatment. Topical corticosteroid and oral antihistamine agents may be beneficial for relieving these signs and symptoms.

Manual removal of nits after successful treatment with a pediculicide is helpful to decrease diagnostic confusion and to decrease the small risk of self-reinfestation and social stigmatization. Fine-toothed nit combs designed for this purpose are available. Other products, such as vinegar, should not be used to help remove nits, because these may interfere with effectiveness of the pediculicide.

ISOLATION OF THE HOSPITALIZED PATIENT: In addition to standard precautions, contact precautions are recommended until the patient has been treated with an appropriate pediculicide.

CONTROL MEASURES: Household and other close contacts should be examined and treated if infested. Bedmates of infested people should be treated prophylactically at the same time as the infested household members and contact, even if bedmates do not have identifiable live lice. Prophylactic treatment of other noninfested people is not recommended. Children should not be excluded or sent home early from school because of head lice, because head lice have a low contagion within classrooms. Parents of children with infestation (ie, at least 1 live, crawling louse) should be notified and informed that their child should be treated. The presence of nits alone does not justify treatment.

"No-nit" policies requiring that children be free of nits before they return to a child care facility or school should be discouraged. Egg cases (nits) farther from the scalp are easier to discover but are of no consequence. Routine classroom or schoolwide screening for lice is discouraged, because it is not an accurate or cost-effective way of lowering the incidence of head lice in the school setting. However, parents who are educated on the diagnosis of lice infestation may screen their own children's heads for lice on a regular basis and if the child is symptomatic.

Supplemental measures generally are not required to eliminate an infestation. Head lice rarely are transferred via fomites from shared headgear, clothing, combs, or bedding. Special handling of such items, therefore, is not likely to be useful; protective headgear should not be refused because of fear of head lice. If desired, hats, bedding, clothing, and towels worn or used by the infested person in the 2-day period just before treatment is started can be machine-washed and dried using the hot water and hot air cycles, respectively, because lice and eggs are killed by exposure for 5 minutes to temperatures greater than 130°F. Vacuuming furniture and floors can remove an infested person's hairs that might have viable eggs attached. Pediculicide spray is not necessary and should not be used. Treatment of dogs, cats, or other pets is not indicated, because they do not play a role in transmission of human head lice.

Pediculosis Corporis
(Body Lice)

CLINICAL MANIFESTATIONS: Patients affected with pediculosis corporis characteristically come to medical attention because of intense itching, particularly at night. Bites manifest as small erythematous macules, papules, and excoriations, primarily on the trunk. In heavily bitten areas, typically around the mid-section of the body (waist, groin, upper thighs), the skin can become thickened and discolored. Secondary bacterial infection of the skin (pyoderma) caused by scratching is common.

ETIOLOGY: *Pediculus humanus corporis* (or *humanus*) is the body louse. Both nymphs and adult lice feed on human blood.

EPIDEMIOLOGY: Body lice generally are restricted to people living in crowded conditions without access to regular bathing or changes of clothing (refugees, victims of war or natural disasters, homeless people). Under these conditions, body lice can spread rapidly through direct contact or contact with contaminated clothing or bedding. Body lice live in clothes or bedding, lay their eggs on or near the seams of clothing, and only move to the skin to feed. Body lice cannot survive away from a blood source for longer than approximately 5 to 7 days at room temperature. In contrast with head and pubic lice, body lice are well-recognized vectors of disease (eg, epidemic typhus, trench fever, epidemic relapsing fever, and bacillary angiomatosis).

The **incubation period** from laying eggs to hatching of the first nymph is approximately 1 to 2 weeks, depending on ambient temperature. Lice mature and are capable of reproducing 9 to 19 days after hatching, depending on whether infested clothing is removed for sleeping.

DIAGNOSTIC TESTS: Seams of clothing should be examined for eggs (nits), nymphs, and adult lice (2–4 mm) if body louse infestation is suspected. Nits and lice may be seen with the naked eye; diagnosis can be confirmed by using a hand lens, dermatoscope (epiluminescence microscope), or a traditional microscope. Adult and nymphal body lice seldom are seen on the body, because they generally are sequestered in clothing.

TREATMENT: Treatment consists of improving hygiene, including bathing and regular changes of clean clothes and bedding. Infested materials can be discarded or decontaminated by washing in hot water (at least 128°F–130°F), by machine drying at hot temperatures, by dry cleaning, or by pressing with a hot iron. Temperatures exceeding 128°F for 5 minutes are lethal to lice and eggs. Pediculicides usually are not necessary if materials are laundered at least weekly (see Drugs for Parasitic Infections, p 985). People with abundant body hair may require full-body treatment with a pediculicide, because lice and eggs may occasionally adhere to body hair. The only such treatment approved by the US Food and Drug Administration is pyrethrin with piperonyl butoxide.

ISOLATION OF THE HOSPITALIZED PATIENT: In addition to standard precautions, contact precautions are recommended and should continue until the patient's clothing and bedding has been reliably cleaned.

CONTROL MEASURES: The most important factor in the control of body lice infestation is the ability to change and wash clothing. Close contacts should be examined and treated appropriately; clothing and bedding should be laundered using hot water and dried using the hot cycle. Clothing and items that are not washable can be dry cleaned. Fumigation or dusting with chemical insecticides sometimes is necessary to control and prevent certain diseases (epidemic typhus) that are spread by body lice.

Pediculosis Pubis
(Pubic Lice, Crab Lice)

CLINICAL MANIFESTATIONS: Pruritus of the anogenital area is a common symptom in pubic lice infestations ("crabs" or "phthiriasis"). Adult lice (1–2 mm long and flattened, tan to grayish-white) or eggs (match hair color) and nits (empty egg shells, white) are found on hair. The parasite most frequently is found in the pubic region, but infestation can involve the eyelashes, eyebrows, beard, axilla, perianal area, and rarely, the scalp. A characteristic sign of heavy pubic lice infestation is the presence of bluish or slate-colored macules (maculae ceruleae) on the chest, abdomen, or thighs.

ETIOLOGY: *Pthirus pubis* is the pubic or crab louse. Both nymphs and adult lice feed on human blood. Pubic lice are not a health hazard and are not responsible for the spread of any disease.

EPIDEMIOLOGY: Pubic lice infestations are more prevalent in adults and usually are transmitted through sexual contact. Transmission by contact with contaminated items, such as towels, is uncommon. Pubic lice on the eyelashes or eyebrows of children may be evidence of sexual abuse, although other modes of transmission are possible. Adult pubic lice can survive away from a host for up to 48 hours, and their eggs can remain viable for up to 10 days under suitable environmental conditions.

The **incubation period** from the laying of eggs to the hatching of the first nymph is approximately 6 to 10 days. Adult lice become capable of reproducing approximately 2 to 3 weeks after hatching.

DIAGNOSTIC TESTS: Identification of eggs (nits), nymphs, and lice with the naked eye is possible; the diagnosis can be confirmed by using a hand lens, traditional microscope, or dermatoscope (epiluminescence microscope). Pubic lice may be difficult to find because of low numbers, and they do not crawl as quickly as head and body lice. If crawling lice are not seen, finding nits in the pubic area strongly suggests infestation and should lead to treatment.

TREATMENT: All areas of the body with coarse hair should be examined for evidence of pubic lice infestation. Lice and their eggs can be removed manually, or the hairs can be shaved to eliminate infestation immediately. Caution should be used when inspecting, removing or treating lice on or near the eyelashes. Pediculicides used to treat other kinds of louse infestations are effective for treatment of pubic lice (see Pediculosis Capitis, p 607; and Drugs for Parasitic Infections, p 985) although treatment is off-label for all products except pyrethrin with piperonyl butoxide. After treatment, patients should put on clean underwear and clothing (as per "Control Measures" below). Retreatment is recommended as for head lice.

Topical pediculicides should not be used for treatment of pubic lice infestation of eyelashes; an ophthalmic-grade petrolatum ointment (only available by prescription) applied to the eyelashes 2 to 4 times daily for 10 days is effective.

Infested people should be examined for other sexually transmitted infections (see Sexually Transmitted Infections in Adolescents and Children, p 165). Pubic lice on the eyelashes or eyebrows of children should prompt evaluation for sexual abuse (see Evaluation of STIs in Adolescents, p 54).

ISOLATION OF THE HOSPITALIZED PATIENT: In addition to standard precautions, contact precautions are recommended until the patient has been treated with an appropriate pediculicide.

CONTROL MEASURES: All sexual contacts should be examined and treated, as needed. Patients should be advised to avoid sexual contact until they and their sex partners have been treated successfully. Bedding, towels, and clothing can be decontaminated by machine washing and drying using the hot water and hot air cycles, respectively, because lice and eggs are killed by exposure for 5 minutes at temperatures greater than 130°F. Clothing and items that are not washable can be dry cleaned.

Pelvic Inflammatory Disease

CLINICAL MANIFESTATIONS: Pelvic inflammatory disease (PID) comprises a spectrum of inflammatory disorders of the female upper genital tract, including any combination of endometritis, parametritis, salpingitis, oophoritis, tubo-ovarian abscess, and pelvic peritonitis. Acute PID is difficult to diagnose because of the wide variation in symptoms and signs. Symptoms of acute PID include unilateral or bilateral lower abdominal or pelvic pain, fever, vomiting, abnormal vaginal discharge, irregular vaginal bleeding, and pain with intercourse. The severity of symptoms varies widely and may range from indolent to severe. Patients occasionally present with right upper quadrant abdominal pain resulting from perihepatitis (Fitz-Hugh-Curtis syndrome). Many episodes of PID go undiagnosed and untreated because the patient and/or health care professional fails to recognize the implications of mild or nonspecific symptoms and signs. Subclinical PID is a term that can be applied to females with very minimal or no symptoms, and there is a growing body of evidence that this represents a large proportion of all PID cases. In both clinically apparent and subclinical PID, inflammation occurs within the reproductive tract that scars or damages the fallopian tubes or surrounding structures. Clinicians need to recognize the implication of mild or nonspecific findings, particularly in a young female who might provide an incomplete or inaccurate sexual history.

Examination findings vary but may include oral temperature >101°F (>38.3°C), lower abdominal tenderness with or without peritoneal signs, abnormal cervical or vaginal discharge, tenderness with lateral motion of the cervix, uterine tenderness, unilateral or bilateral adnexal tenderness, and adnexal fullness. Pyuria (presence of white blood cells [WBCs] on urine microscopy), abundant WBCs on saline microscopy of vaginal fluid, an elevated erythrocyte sedimentation rate, elevated C-reactive protein, and/or an adnexal mass demonstrated by abdominal or transvaginal ultrasonography are findings that support a diagnosis of PID.

Complications of PID include perihepatitis (Fitz-Hugh-Curtis syndrome) and tubo-ovarian abscess/complex formation. Long-term sequelae include tubal scarring that can cause infertility in an estimated 20% of females, ectopic pregnancy in an estimated 9%, and chronic pelvic pain in an estimated 18%. Factors that may increase the likelihood of infertility are delay in diagnosis or delay in initiation of antimicrobial therapy, younger age at time of infection, chlamydial infection, recurrent PID, and PID determined to be severe by laparoscopic examination.

Any prepubertal girl with PID needs to be assessed for sexual abuse. Mandatory reporters should follow their state's regulations for reporting.

ETIOLOGY: *Neisseria gonorrhoeae* and *Chlamydia trachomatis* are the pathogens most commonly associated with PID, although the proportion of PID cases attributable to these pathogens is declining. Numerous other organisms have been isolated from upper genital tract cultures of females with PID, including anaerobes, *Gardnerella vaginalis*, *Haemophilus influenzae*, *Streptococcus agalactiae*, enteric gram-negative rods, cytomegalovirus, *Mycoplasma genitalium*, *Mycoplasma hominis*, and *Ureaplasma urealyticum*. Polymicrobial infection is common. However, in more than half of cases, no organism is identified in lower genital tract swab specimens (ie, endocervical or vaginal specimens). More recent data suggest that *M genitalium* may play a role in the pathogenesis of PID, although there currently is no direct detection assay such as antigen or nucleic acid detection cleared by the US Food and Drug Administration for *M genitalium*.

EPIDEMIOLOGY: Although many of the issues pertaining to high-risk sexual behavior and acquisition of sexually transmitted infections (STIs) are common to both adolescents and adults, they often are intensified among adolescents because of both behavioral and biological predispositions. Adolescents and young women can be at higher risk of STIs and PID because of behavioral factors such as inconsistent barrier contraceptive use, douching, greater number of current and lifetime sexual partners, and use of alcohol and other substances that may impair judgment while engaging in sexual activity. Latex condoms may reduce the risk of PID. Adolescent and young adult females also have an increased biologic susceptibility to STIs. Cervical ectopy increases risk of chlamydia and gonorrhea infection by exposing columnar epithelium to a potential infectious inoculum. Although the risk of developing PID is minimally elevated during the initial 20 days following intrauterine device (IUD) insertion, the Centers for Disease Control and Prevention (CDC) advises that the benefits of IUDs in adolescents generally outweigh the risks.

An **incubation period** for PID is undefined.

DIAGNOSTIC TESTS[1]**:** Diagnostic criteria recommended by the CDC are presented in Table 3.49. No single symptom, sign, or laboratory or imaging finding is sensitive and specific for the diagnosis of acute PID. The diagnosis of PID typically is accomplished by using a combination of clinical symptoms and signs, physical examination, and laboratory tests. A clinical diagnosis of symptomatic PID has a positive predictive value (PPV) for salpingitis of 65% to 90% but generally is higher among populations at risk, such as sexually active females 25 years and younger, females attending STD clinics, and females who live in communities with high gonorrhea or chlamydia rates.

The minimum clinical criteria on pelvic examination to make the diagnosis of PID include cervical motion tenderness, or uterine or adnexal tenderness. Additional criteria can be used to make the diagnosis of PID more specific (Table 3.49). Most females with PID have either mucopurulent cervical discharge or evidence of WBCs on a microscopic evaluation of a saline preparation of vaginal fluid (ie, wet prep). If a patient's cervical discharge appears normal and no WBCs are observed on the wet prep of vaginal fluid, the

---

[1]Centers for Disease Control and Prevention. Sexually transmitted diseases treatment guidelines, 2015. *MMWR Morb Mortal Wkly Rep.* 2015;64(RR-3):1–137

Table 3.49. Criteria for Clinical Diagnosis of Pelvic Inflammatory Disease (PID)[a]

Minimum Criteria

Empiric treatment of PID should be initiated in sexually active young women if they are experiencing pelvic or lower abdominal pain, if one or more of the following **minimum criteria** are present, and no other cause(s) for the illness can be identified:

- Uterine tenderness

  or

- Adnexal tenderness

  or

- Cervical motion tenderness

Additional Criteria

These criteria may be used to enhance the specificity of the minimum criteria. Additional criteria that support a diagnosis of PID include the following:

- Oral temperature greater than 38.3°C (101°F)
- Mucopurulent cervical or vaginal discharge
- Presence of white blood cells (WBCs) on saline microscopy of vaginal secretions
- Elevated erythrocyte sedimentation rate
- Elevated C-reactive protein
- Laboratory documentation of cervical infection with *Neisseria gonorrhoeae* or *Chlamydia trachomatis*

Most females with PID have mucopurulent cervical discharge or evidence of WBCs on a microscopic evaluation of a saline preparation of vaginal fluid. If the cervical discharge appears normal **and** no WBCs are found on the wet preparation, the diagnosis of PID is unlikely, and alternative causes of pain should be sought.

The **most specific criteria** for diagnosing PID include the following:

- Endometrial biopsy with histopathologic evidence of endometritis
- Transvaginal ultrasonography or magnetic resonance imaging techniques showing thickened, fluid-filled tubes with or without free pelvic fluid or tubo-ovarian complex, or Doppler ultrasonography suggests increased fallopian tube blood flow suggestive of infection (eg, tubal hyperemia)
- Laparoscopic findings consistent with PID

A diagnostic evaluation that includes some of these more extensive studies may be warranted in some cases.

[a]Adapted from Centers for Disease Control and Prevention. Sexually transmitted diseases treatment guidelines, 2015. *MMWR Recomm Rep.* 2015;64(RR-3):1-137

diagnosis of PID is unlikely, and alternative causes of pain should be considered. A cervical or vaginal swab specimen should be obtained from all patients with suspected PID to perform a nucleic acid amplification test (NAAT) for *C trachomatis* and *N gonorrhoeae*. A swab specimen for culture *of N gonorrhoeae* may be collected from the cervix or vagina to allow susceptibility testing to be performed. When the diagnosis of PID is in doubt, there is concern for a tubo-ovarian abscess, or the patient is not responding to conventional therapy, further diagnostic evaluation using transvaginal ultrasonography or magnetic resonance imaging (MRI) may be helpful to evaluate for thickened, fluid-filled tubes with or without free pelvic fluid or tubo-ovarian complex or using Doppler ultrasonography to evaluate for evidence of increased fallopian tube blood flow suggestive of infection (eg, tubal hyperemia). Laparoscopy is the gold standard for diagnosis, allowing direct visualization of the adnexal structures as well as allowing bacteriologic specimens to be obtained directly from tubal exudate or the cul-de-sac. Endometrial biopsy may demonstrate histopathologic evidence of endometritis and may be the only sign of PID in some females. Because of their high cost and invasive nature, however, these procedures are not indicated for diagnosis of most PID cases. Pregnancy must be ruled out in all patients evaluated for PID. In addition to determining whether WBCs are present in cervico- vaginal secretion, wet mount will assist in the diagnosis or exclusion of the commonly associated trichomonas or bacterial vaginosis. Serologic testing for human immunodeficiency virus (HIV) and syphilis also should be performed.

TREATMENT[1]**:** A sexually active adolescent or young adult female with lower abdominal pain who exhibits uterine, adnexal, or cervical motion tenderness on bimanual examination should be treated for PID if no other cause is identified. To minimize risks of progressive infection and subsequent infertility, treatment should be initiated at the time of clinical diagnosis, and therapy should be completed, regardless of the STI test results.

Among females with mild to moderate PID, there is no difference in clinical course, recurrent PID, chronic pelvic pain, or infertility rates between females hospitalized and those treated as outpatients for PID. No evidence is available to suggest that adolescents benefit from hospitalization for PID management. The decision to hospitalize adolescents with acute PID should be made on the basis of the same criteria used for older women and should be based on the provider's judgment and whether the patient meets any of the following suggested criteria:

- The patient is experiencing a surgical emergency, such as ectopic pregnancy or appendicitis, or another serious condition cannot be excluded;
- The patient's illness is severe (eg, vomiting, severe pain, overt peritonitis, or high fever);
- The patient has a tubo-ovarian abscess;
- The patient is pregnant;
- The patient is unable to follow or tolerate an outpatient regimen; or
- The patient has failed to respond clinically to outpatient therapy.

The antimicrobial regimen chosen should provide empiric, broad-spectrum coverage directed against the most common causative agents, including *N gonorrhoeae* and *C trachomatis*, even if these pathogens are not identified in lower genital tract specimens (Table 3.50, and Table 3.51). As a result of the emergence of quinolone-resistant *N gonorrhoeae*, fluoroquinolones no longer are recommended as first-line treatment of PID.

For patients with severe cephalosporin allergy, the use of a fluoroquinolone (levofloxacin, 500 mg, orally, once daily; ofloxacin, 400 mg, twice daily; or moxifloxacin, 400 mg, orally, once daily) with metronidazole (500 mg, orally, twice daily) for 14 days can be considered, provided the community prevalence as well as individual risk for gonococcal infection are low and patient follow up is likely. If the *N gonorrhoeae* culture is positive, antimicrobial susceptibility testing should guide therapy. If the isolate is determined to be a quinolone-resistant strain of *N gonorrhoeae* or if antimicrobial susceptibility cannot be assessed (eg, if only NAAT testing is available), consultation with an infectious disease specialist and the local or state health department is recommended. Clinicians should follow public health reporting guidelines for positive *N gonorrhoeae* results.

---

[1]Centers for Disease Control and Prevention. Sexually transmitted diseases treatment guidelines, 2015. *MMWR Morb Mortal Wkly Rep.* 2015;64(RR-3):1–137

Table 3.50. Recommended Parenteral Treatment of Pelvic Inflammatory Disease (PID)[a,b]

Cefotetan, 2 g, IV, every 12 h **OR Cefoxitin**, 2 g, IV, every 6 h

PLUS

Doxycycline, 100 mg, orally or IV, every 12 h to complete 14 days

OR

Clindamycin, 900 mg, IV, every 8 h
PLUS
Gentamicin: loading dose, IV or IM (2 mg/kg), followed by maintenance dose (1.5 mg/kg) every 8 h. Single daily dosing (3–5 mg/kg) can be substituted.

NOTE

Parenteral therapy may be discontinued 24 h after clinical improvement; continuing oral therapy should consist of doxycycline (100 mg, orally, twice a day) or clindamycin (450 mg, orally, 4 times a day) to complete a total of 14 days of therapy. If tubo-ovarian abscess is present, clindamycin (450 mg, orally 4 times daily) or metronidazole (500 mg, twice daily) should be used to complete at least 14 days of therapy with doxycycline to provide more effective anaerobic coverage than doxycycline alone.

IV indicates intravenous; IM, intramuscular.

[a]Additional regimens may be found in: Centers for Disease Control and Prevention. Sexually transmitted diseases treatment guidelines, 2015. *MMWR Recomm Rep.* 2015;64(RR-3):1-137 (see **www.cdc.gov/std/treatment**).

[b]Hospitalization and parenteral treatment is recommended if patient has severe illness such as tubo-ovarian abscess, is pregnant, or is unable to tolerate or follow ambulatory regimens.

Adapted from Centers for Disease Control and Prevention. Sexually transmitted diseases treatment guidelines, 2015. *MMWR Morb Mortal Wkly Rep.* 2015;64(RR-3):1-137.

Table 3.51. Recommended Intramuscular/Oral Regimens for Treatment of Pelvic Inflammatory Disease (PID)[a,b]

Ceftriaxone, 250 mg, IM, once **OR Cefoxitin**, 2 g, IM, and **probenecid**, 1 g, orally, in a single dose concurrently **OR** Other parenteral third-generation **cephalosporin** (eg, **ceftizoxime** or **cefotaxime**)

PLUS

Doxycycline, 100 mg, orally, twice a day for 14 days

WITH or WITHOUT

Metronidazole, 500 mg, orally, twice a day for 14 days[c]

IV indicates intravenous; IM, intramuscular.

[a]Additional regimens may be found in: Centers for Disease Control and Prevention. Sexually transmitted diseases treatment guidelines, 2015. *MMWR Recomm Rep.* 2015;64(RR-3):1-137 (see **www.cdc.gov/std/treatment**).

[b]Patients with inadequate response to outpatient therapy after 72 hours should be reevaluated for possible misdiagnosis and may require parenteral therapy.

[c]The recommended third-generation cephalosporins are limited in the coverage of anaerobes. Therefore, the addition of metronidazole to treatment regimens with third-generation cephalosporins should be considered.

Adapted from Centers for Disease Control and Prevention. Sexually transmitted diseases treatment guidelines, 2015. *MMWR Morb Mortal Wkly Rep.* 2015;64(RR-3):1-137.

Parenteral Treatment. The CDC recommends several regimens for parenteral therapy (Table 3.50). Because of pain associated with intravenous doxycycline infusion, doxycycline should be administered orally when possible. Transition to oral therapy usually can be initiated within 24 to 48 hours of clinical improvement. When using the parenteral cefotetan or cefoxitin regimens, oral therapy with doxycycline (100 mg, twice daily) can be used to complete the 14 days of therapy. For the clindamycin/gentamicin regimen, oral clindamycin (450 mg, orally, 4 times daily) or doxycycline (100 mg, twice daily) can be used to complete the 14 days of therapy. However, when tubo-ovarian abscess is present, clindamycin (450 mg, orally, 4 times daily) or metronidazole (500 mg, twice daily) should be used to complete at least 14 days of therapy with doxycycline to provide more effective anaerobic coverage.

Intramuscular/Oral Treatment. The CDC recommends several regimens for intramuscular/oral treatment (Table 3.51). Evidence is limited for alternative outpatient regimens. Limited data demonstrate that azithromycin (1 g, orally, once a week for 2 weeks) in combination with ceftriaxone (250 mg, intramuscularly, in a single dose) is effective for the outpatient treatment of PID.[1] This regimen can be considered if compliance with a 2-week daily oral regimen is unlikely. However, the CDC recommends considering the addition of metronidazole to this regimen to provide anaerobic coverage.

A critical component to the outpatient management is short-term follow-up, especially in the adolescent population. Outpatients should be reevaluated after 72 hours of therapy, including repeating the bimanual examination of the pelvis; hospitalization and/or further diagnostics should be considered in females without clinical improvement.

Pregnant women with PID are at high risk for preterm delivery and severe infection. They should be hospitalized to receive intravenous antibiotic therapy. Doxycycline should not be used during pregnancy unless it is essential for the mother's welfare.

A diagnosis of Fitz-Hugh-Curtis syndrome does not alter the treatment regimen. Patients with tubo-ovarian abscesses should be treated with inpatient parenteral treatment that includes anaerobic coverage, and antimicrobial therapy can be switched to the oral route after 24 hours of clinical improvement; at the time of discharge, patients should complete a 14-day course of doxycycline (100 mg, twice a day) or clindamycin (450 mg, orally, 4 times a day). If an IUD user receives a diagnosis of PID, the IUD does not need to be removed. However, the woman should receive treatment according to these recommendations and should have close clinical follow-up. If no clinical improvement occurs within 48 to 72 hours of initiating treatment, providers should consider removing the IUD.

ISOLATION OF THE HOSPITALIZED PATIENT: Standard precautions are recommended.

CONTROL MEASURES[2]:

- Male sexual partners of patients with PID should receive diagnostic evaluation for gonococcal and chlamydial urethritis and should be treated presumptively for both infections if they had sexual contact with the patient during the 60 days preceding onset of symptoms in the patient. If a woman's last sexual intercourse was >60 days before onset of symptoms or diagnosis, the most recent sex partner should be treated. A large

[1]Savaris RF, Teixeira LM, Torres TG, et al. Comparing ceftriaxone plus azithromycin or doxycycline for pelvic inflammatory disease: a randomized controlled trial. *Obstet Gynecol* 2007;110(1):53–60

[2]Centers for Disease Control and Prevention. Recommendations for partner services programs for HIV infection, syphilis, gonorrhea, and chlamydial infection. *MMWR Recomm Rep.* 2008;57(RR-9):1–63

proportion of male contacts will be asymptomatic.
- The patient should abstain from sexual intercourse until she and her partner(s) have completed treatment.
- The patient and her partner(s) should be encouraged to use condoms consistently and correctly.
- The patient should be screened for other STIs, including HIV.
- Unimmunized or incompletely immunized patients should complete the immunization series for human papillomavirus and hepatitis B (see **https://redbook.solutions. aap.org/SS/Immunization_Schedules.aspx**).
- Because of the high risk of reinfection, patients who have positive test results for *N gonorrhoeae* or *C trachomatis* should be retested 3 months after completing treatment or at their next clinical encounter within 12 months of treatment.
- The diagnosis of PID provides an opportunity to educate the adolescent about prevention of STIs, including abstinence, consistent use of barrier methods of protection, immunization, and the importance of receiving periodic screening for STIs.

Pertussis (Whooping Cough)

CLINICAL MANIFESTATIONS: Pertussis begins with mild upper respiratory tract symptoms similar to the common cold (catarrhal stage) and progresses to cough, usually paroxysms of cough (paroxysmal stage), characterized by inspiratory whoop (gasping) after repeated cough on the same breath, which commonly is followed by vomiting. Fever is absent or minimal. Symptoms wane gradually over weeks to months (convalescent stage). Cough illness in immunized children and adults can range from typical to mild and unrecognized. The duration of classic pertussis is 6 to 10 weeks. Approximately half of adolescents with pertussis cough for 10 weeks or longer. Complications among adolescents and adults include syncope, weight loss, sleep disturbance, incontinence, rib fractures, and pneumonia; among adults, complications increase with age. Pertussis is most severe when it occurs during the first 6 months of life, particularly in preterm and unimmunized infants. Disease in infants younger than 6 months can be atypical with a short catarrhal stage, followed by gagging, gasping, bradycardia, or apnea (67%) as prominent early manifestations; absence of whoop; and prolonged convalescence. Sudden unexpected death can be caused by pertussis. Complications among infants include pneumonia (23%) and pulmonary hypertension as well as complications related to severe coughing spells, such as conjunctival bleeding, hernia, and severe coughing spells leading to hypoxia and complications such as seizures (2%), encephalopathy (less than 0.5%), apnea, and death. More than two thirds of infants with pertussis are hospitalized. Case-fatality rates are approximately 1% in infants younger than 2 months and less than 0.5% in infants 2 through 11 months of age. Maternal immunization during pregnancy and an infant's previous immunization reduce morbidity and mortality in young infants.

ETIOLOGY: Pertussis is caused by a fastidious, gram-negative, pleomorphic bacillus, *Bordetella pertussis*. Other causes of sporadic prolonged cough illness include *Bordetella parapertussis*, *Mycoplasma pneumoniae*, *Chlamydia trachomatis*, *Chlamydia pneumoniae*, *Bordetella bronchiseptica* (the cause of kennel cough), *Bordetella holmesii*, and certain respiratory tract viruses, particularly adenoviruses and respiratory syncytial viruses.

EPIDEMIOLOGY: Humans are the only known hosts of *B pertussis*. Transmission occurs by close contact with cases via large respiratory droplets generated by coughing or sneezing.

Cases occur year-round, typically with a late summer-autumn peak. Neither infection nor immunization provides lifelong immunity. Waning immunity, particularly when acellular pertussis vaccine is used for the entire immunization series, is predominantly responsible for increased cases reported in school-aged children, adolescents, and adults. Additionally, waning maternal immunity of mothers who have not received Tdap vaccine during that pregnancy results in low concentrations of transplacentally transmitted antibody and an increase in pertussis in very young infants. Reports of pertussis increased in the United States in recent years with notable epidemic peaks in disease; more than 48 000 cases of pertussis were reported in 2012, the highest number in over 50 years. Pertussis is highly contagious. As many as 80% of previously immunized household contacts of symptomatic infant cases are infected with *B pertussis,* with symptoms in these contacts varying from mild to classic pertussis. Siblings and adults with cough illness are important sources of pertussis infection for young infants. Infected people are most contagious during the catarrhal stage through the third week after onset of paroxysms. Factors affecting the length of communicability include age, immunization status or previous infection, and receipt of appropriate antimicrobial therapy.

The **incubation period** is 7 to 10 days, with a range of 5 to 21 days.

DIAGNOSTIC TESTS: Culture was considered the "gold standard" for laboratory diagnosis of pertussis but is not optimally sensitive, because *B pertussis* is a fastidious organism. Culture requires collection of an appropriate nasopharyngeal specimen, obtained either by aspiration or with polyester or flocked rayon swabs or calcium alginate swabs. Specimens must be placed into special transport media (such as Regan-Lowe) immediately and not allowed to dry during prompt transport to the laboratory. Culture results can be negative if taken from a previously immunized person, if antimicrobial therapy has been started, if more than 2 weeks has elapsed since cough onset, or if the specimen is not collected or handled appropriately.

Nucleic acid amplification tests (NAATs), including polymerase chain reaction (PCR) assay, now are commercially available and cleared by the FDA as standalone tests or as multiplex assays, and are the most commonly used laboratory method for detection of *B pertussis* because of greater sensitivity and more rapid turnaround time. The PCR test requires collection of an adequate nasopharyngeal specimen using a Dacron swab or nasopharyngeal wash or aspirate. Calcium alginate swabs can be inhibitory to PCR and should not be used for PCR tests. The PCR test has optimal sensitivity during the first 3 weeks of cough, is unlikely to be useful if antimicrobial therapy has been given for more than 5 days, and has lower sensitivity in previously immunized people, but still is more sensitive than culture. The Centers for Disease Control and Prevention (CDC) has released a "best practices" document to guide pertussis PCR assays (**www.cdc.gov/ pertussis/clinical/diagnostic-testing/diagnosis-pcr-bestpractices.html**) as well as a video demonstrating optimal specimen collection. Some PCR assays target only a multicopy insertion gene sequence (IS 481) found in *B pertussis* as well as the less commonly encountered *B holmesii* and some strains of *B bronchiseptica*. Multiple DNA target sequences are required to distinguish among *Bordetella* species. Direct fluorescent antibody (DFA) testing no longer is recommended.

Commercial serologic tests for pertussis infection can be helpful for diagnosis, especially late in illness and in adolescents and adults in whom antibody concentrations from prior immunization have waned. Most assays are formulated as enzyme immunoassays.

However, no commercial kit is cleared by the FDA for diagnostic use, and little is understood about the clinical accuracy of these kits. In the absence of recent immunization, an elevated serum immunoglobulin (Ig) G antibody to pertussis toxin (PT) present 2 to 8 weeks after onset of cough is suggestive of recent *B pertussis* infection. For single serum specimens, an IgG anti-PT value of approximately 100 IU/mL or greater (using standard reference sera as a comparator) has been recommended. Positive paired serologic results based on the World Health Organization pertussis case definition may also be considered diagnostic. IgA and IgM assays lack adequate sensitivity and specificity and should not be used for the diagnosis of pertussis.

An increased white blood cell count attributable to absolute lymphocytosis is suggestive of pertussis in infants and young children but often is absent in older people with pertussis and can be only mildly abnormal in some young infants at the time of presentation. A markedly elevated white blood cell count is associated with a poor prognosis in young infants.

TREATMENT: Antimicrobial therapy administered during the catarrhal stage may ameliorate the disease. Antimicrobial therapy is indicated before test results are received if the clinical history is strongly suggestive of pertussis or the patient is at high risk of severe or complicated disease (eg, is an infant). A 5-day course of azithromycin is the appropriate first-line choice for treatment and for postexposure prophylaxis (PEP [see Table 3.52, p 625]).[1] After the paroxysmal cough is established, antimicrobial agents have no discernible effect on the course of illness but are recommended to limit spread of organisms to others. Resistance of *B pertussis* to macrolide antimicrobial agents has been reported, but rarely. Penicillins and first- and second-generation cephalosporins are not effective against *B pertussis*.

Azithromycin should be used with caution in people with prolonged QT interval and proarrhythmic conditions. An association between orally administered erythromycin and azithromycin with infantile hypertrophic pyloric stenosis (IHPS) has been reported,[2] but azithromycin remains the drug of choice for treatment or prophylaxis of pertussis in very young infants because the risk of developing severe pertussis and life-threatening complications outweighs the potential risk of pyloric stenosis (odds ratio, 2.9–8.3), and azithromycin has a lower odds ratio than erythromycin for pyloric stenosis. Health care providers should be alert to the possible development of pyloric stenosis in infants from birth up to 6 weeks of age who have received azithromycin or erythromycin. Cases of IHPS should be reported to MedWatch (see MedWatch, p 1026).

Trimethoprim-sulfamethoxazole is an alternative for patients older than 2 months who cannot tolerate macrolides or who are infected with a macrolide-resistant strain, but studies evaluating trimethoprim-sulfamethoxazole as treatment for pertussis are limited.

Young infants are at increased risk of respiratory failure attributable to apnea or secondary bacterial pneumonia and are at risk of cardiopulmonary failure and death from severe pulmonary hypertension. Hospitalized young infants with pertussis should be managed in a setting/facility where these complications can be recognized and managed ur-

---

[1]Centers for Disease Control and Prevention. Recommended antimicrobial agents for the treatment and postexposure prophylaxis of pertussis: 2005 CDC guidelines. *MMWR Recomm Rep.* 2005;54(RR–14):1–16

[2]Eberly MD, Eide MB, Thompson JL, Nylund CM. Azithromycin in early infancy and pyloric stenosis. *Pediatrics.* 2015;135(3):483–486

gently. Exchange transfusions or leukopheresis have been reported to be life-saving in infants with progressive pulmonary hypertension and markedly elevated lymphocyte counts.

Because data on the clinical effectiveness of antibiotic treatment on *B parapertussis* are limited, treatment decisions should be based on clinical judgment, with particular attention toward special populations that may be at increased risk for severe *B parapertussis* disease, including infants, elderly, and immunocompromised people. Treatment may be warranted to prevent severe outcomes and decrease duration of illness in these patients. Limited available data suggest that *B parapertussis* is less susceptible to antimicrobial agents than *B pertussis*, although some studies indicate that macrolides, trimethoprim-sulfamethoxazole, and ciprofloxacin generally have activity against *B parapertussis*.

ISOLATION OF THE HOSPITALIZED PATIENT: In addition to standard precautions, droplet precautions are recommended for 21 days from onset of cough if appropriate antimicrobial therapy is not administered or for 5 days after initiation of effective therapy.

CONTROL MEASURES: Pertussis is a nationally notifiable disease in the United States.

Care of Exposed People

Household and Other Close Contacts. Close contacts who are unimmunized or underimmunized should have pertussis immunization initiated or continued using age-appropriate products according to the recommended schedule as soon as possible; this includes off-label use of tetanus toxoid, reduced-content diphtheria toxoid, and acellular pertussis vaccine (Tdap) in children 7 through 9 years of age who did not complete the diphtheria and tetanus toxoids and acellular pertussis vaccine (DTaP) series (see Table 3.53, p 626).

PEP is recommended for all household contacts of the index case and other close contacts, including children in child care, regardless of immunization status. (**www.cdc.gov/pertussis/outbreaks/pep.html**). When considering borderline degree of exposure for a nonhousehold contact, PEP should be administered if the contact personally is at high risk or lives in a household with a person at high risk of severe pertussis (eg, young infant, pregnant woman, person who has contact with infants). If 21 days have elapsed since onset of cough in the index case, PEP has limited value but should be considered for households with high-risk contacts. The agents, doses, and duration of PEP are the same as for treatment of pertussis (see Table 3.52). Prophylaxis for people exposed to *B parapertussis* is not recommended currently.

People who have been in contact with an infected person should be monitored closely for respiratory tract symptoms for 21 days after last contact with the infected person. Close contacts with cough should be evaluated.

Child Care. Pertussis vaccine and chemoprophylaxis should be administered as recommended for household and other close contacts. Child care providers and exposed children, especially incompletely immunized children, should be observed for respiratory tract symptoms for 21 days after last contact with the index case while infectious. Children and child care providers who are symptomatic or who have confirmed pertussis should be excluded from child care pending physician evaluation and completion of 5 days of the recommended course of antimicrobial therapy. Untreated children and providers should be excluded until 21 days have elapsed from cough onset.

Schools. Students and staff members with pertussis should be excluded from school until they have completed 5 days of the recommended course of antimicrobial therapy. People who do not receive appropriate antimicrobial therapy should be excluded from school for 21 days after onset of symptoms. Use of PEP for large groups of students usually is not recommended, especially in the setting of widespread community transmission, but exceptions for individuals can be considered. This occurs when close contact simulates a household exposure or when pertussis in the exposed person would have severe medical consequences. Public health officials should be consulted for recommendations to control pertussis transmission in schools; their additional recommendations could include use of Tdap in children after their 4- to 6-year DTaP booster but before they are 10 years of age (off label), Tdap administration at 10 years of age, and institution of the DTaP series in siblings who are 6 weeks of age. The immunization status of close contacts should be reviewed, and appropriate vaccines administered when indicated. Parents and teachers should be notified about possible exposures to pertussis. Exclusion of exposed people with cough illness should be considered pending evaluation by a physician.

Health Care Settings.[1] Health care facilities should maximize efforts to immunize all health care personnel (HCP) with Tdap. All HCP should observe respiratory precautions when examining a patient with a cough illness. People exposed to a patient with pertussis should be evaluated by infection-control personnel for postexposure management and follow-up. Data on the need for PEP in Tdap-immunized HCP are inconclusive. Some immunized HCP still are at risk of *B pertussis* infection. Receipt of Tdap may not preclude the need to administer PEP.

Recommendations of the CDC are as follows:

- PEP is recommended for all HCP (even if immunized with Tdap) who have been exposed to pertussis and are likely to expose other patients at risk of severe pertussis (eg, hospitalized neonates and pregnant women). Other exposed HCP either should receive PEP or should be monitored daily for 21 days after exposure and treated at the onset of signs and symptoms of pertussis.
- Other people (patients, caregivers) defined as close contacts or high-risk contacts of a patient or HCP with pertussis should receive chemoprophylaxis (and immunization when indicated), as recommended for household contacts (see Table 3.52, p 625).
- HCP with symptoms of pertussis (or HCP with any respiratory illness within 21 days of exposure to pertussis who did not receive PEP) should be excluded from work for at least the first 5 days of the recommended antimicrobial therapy. HCP with symptoms of pertussis who do not accept antimicrobial therapy should be excluded from work for 21 days from onset of cough. Use of a respiratory mask is not sufficient protection during this time.

Immunization

Vaccine Products. Purified acellular-component pertussis vaccines (DTaP) replaced previously used diphtheria, tetanus, and whole-cell pertussis vaccine (DTwP or DTP) exclusively in 1997 and contain 3 or more immunogens derived from *B pertussis* organisms: inactivated pertussis toxin (toxoid), filamentous hemagglutinin, fimbrial proteins (agglutinogens), and pertactin (an outer membrane 69-kd protein); see Table 3.53 (p 627) for products. Acellular pertussis vaccines are adsorbed onto aluminum salts and must be administered intramuscularly. All pertussis vaccines in the United States are combined with diphtheria and tetanus toxoids; none contains thimerosal as a preservative. DTaP products may be formulated as combination vaccines containing one or more of inactivated

---

[1]Centers for Disease Control and Prevention. Immunization of health-care personnel. Recommendations of the Advisory Committee on Immunization Practices (ACIP). *MMWR Recomm Rep*. 2011;60(RR-07):1–45

Table 3.52. Recommended Antimicrobial Therapy and Postexposure Prophylaxis for Pertussis in Infants, Children, Adolescents, and Adults[a]

Age	Azithromycin	Recommended Drugs Erythromycin	Clarithromycin	Alternative TMP-SMX
Younger than 1 mo	10 mg/kg/day as a single dose daily for 5 days[b,c]	40 mg/kg/day in 4 divided doses for 14 days	Not recommended	Contraindicated at younger than 2 mo
1 through 5 mo	10 mg/kg/day as a single dose daily for 5 days[b]	40 mg/kg/day in 4 divided doses for 14 days	15 mg/kg/day in 2 divided doses for 7 days	2 mo or older: TMP, 8 mg/kg/day; SMX, 40 mg/kg/day in 2 doses for 14 days
6 mo or older and children	10 mg/kg as a single dose on day 1 (maximum 500 mg), then 5 mg/kg/day as a single dose on days 2 through 5 (maximum 250 mg/day)[b,d]	40 mg/kg/day in 4 divided doses for 7–14 days (maximum 1–2 g/day)	15 mg/kg/day in 2 divided doses for 7 days (maximum 1 g/day)	2 mo or older: TMP, 8 mg/kg/day; SMX, 40 mg/kg/day in 2 doses for 14 days
Adolescents and adults	500 mg as a single dose on day 1, then 250 mg as a single dose on days 2 through 5[b,d]	2 g/day in 4 divided doses for 7–14 days	1 g/day in 2 divided doses for 7 days	TMP, 320 mg/day; SMX, 1600 mg/day in 2 divided doses for 14 days

TMP indicates trimethoprim; SMX, sulfamethoxazole.

[a]Centers for Disease Control and Prevention. Recommended antimicrobial agents for the treatment and postexposure prophylaxis of pertussis: 2005 CDC guidelines. *MMWR Recomm Rep.* 2005;54(RR-14):1–16

[b]Azithromycin should be used with caution in people with prolonged QT interval and certain proarrhythmic conditions.

[c]Preferred macrolide for this age because of risk of idiopathic hypertrophic pyloric stenosis associated with erythromycin.

[d]A 3-day course of azithromycin for PEP or treatment has not been validated and is not recommended.

Table 3.53. Composition and Recommended Use of Vaccines With Tetanus Toxoid, Diphtheria Toxoid, and Acellular Pertussis Components Licensed and Available in the United States[a,b]

Pharmaceutical	Manufacturer	Pertussis Antigens	Recommended Use
DTaP Vaccine for Children Younger Than 7 Years			
DTaP (Infanrix)	GlaxoSmithKline Biologicals	PT, FHA, pertactin	**All 5 doses**, children 6 wk through 6 y of age
DTaP (Daptacel)	Sanofi Pasteur	PT, FHA, pertactin, fimbriae types 2 and 3	**All 5 doses**, children 6 wk through 6 y of age
DTaP-hepatitis B-IPV (Pediarix)	GlaxoSmithKline Biologicals	PT, FHA, pertactin	**First 3 doses, children 6 wk through 6 y of age; usual use** at 6- to 8-wk intervals beginning at 2 mo of age; then 2 doses of DTaP are needed to complete the 5-dose series before 7 y of age
DTaP-IPV/Hib (Pentacel)	Sanofi Pasteur	PT, FHA, pertactin, fimbriae types 2 and 3	**First 4 doses, children 6 wk through 4 y of age; usual use** at 2, 4, 6, and 15 through 18 mo of age; then 1 dose of DTaP is needed to complete the 5-dose series before 7 y of age
DTaP-IPV (Kinrix)	GlaxoSmithKline Biologicals	PT, FHA, pertactin	**Booster dose** for **fifth dose** of DTaP and **fourth dose** of IPV at 4 through 6 y of age
DTaP-IPV (Quadracel)	Sanofi Pasteur	PT, FHA, pertactin, fimbriae types 2 and 3	**Booster dose** for **fifth dose** of DTaP and **fourth dose** of IPV at 4 through 6 y of age
Tdap Vaccines for Adolescents			
Tdap (Boostrix)	GlaxoSmithKline Biologicals	PT, FHA, pertactin	**Single dose** at 11 through 12 y of age
Tdap (Adacel)	Sanofi Pasteur	PT, FHA, pertactin, fimbriae types 2 and 3	**Single dose** at 11 through 12 y of age

DTaP indicates pediatric formulation of diphtheria and tetanus toxoids and acellular pertussis vaccines; PT, pertussis toxoid; FHA, filamentous hemagglutinin; Hib, *Haemophilus influenzae* type b vaccine; IPV, inactivated poliovirus; Tdap, adolescent/adult formulation of tetanus toxoid, reduced diphtheria toxoid, and acellular pertussis vaccine; Td, tetanus and reduced diphtheria toxoids (for children 7 years of age or older and adults).

ª DTaP recommended schedule is 2, 4, 6, and 15 through 18 months and 4 through 6 years of age. The fourth dose can be administered as early as 12 months of age, provided 6 months have elapsed since the third dose was administered. The fifth dose is not necessary if the fourth dose was administered on or after the fourth birthday. Refer to manufacturers' product information for comprehensive product information regarding indications and use of the vaccines listed.

ᵇ Tripedia and TriHibit are licensed but no longer are available in the United States.

poliovirus vaccine, hepatitis B vaccine, and *Haemophilus influenzae* type b vaccine. Recommendations for the series of DTaP for children younger than 7 years are provided in the annual immunization schedule for children and adolescents **(https://redbook. solutions.aap.org/SS/Immunization_Schedules.aspx).** Adolescent and adult formulations, known as Tdap vaccines, contain reduced quantities of diphtheria toxoid and some pertussis antigens compared with DTaP. A single dose is recommended universally for people 11 years and older, including adults of any age, in place of a decennial tetanus and diphtheria vaccine (Td). The preferred schedule is to administer Tdap at the 11- or 12- year-old preventive visit, with catch-up of older adolescents. Booster doses of Tdap are not recommended for any group of people except pregnant women (see subsequent sections).

Dose and Route. Each 0.5-mL dose of DTaP or Tdap is administered intramuscularly. Use of a decreased volume of individual doses of pertussis vaccines or multiple doses of decreased-volume (fractional) doses is not recommended.

Interchangeability of Acellular Pertussis Vaccines. Insufficient data exist on the safety, immunogenicity, and efficacy of DTaP vaccines from different manufacturers when administered interchangeably for the primary series in infants. In circumstances in which the type of DTaP product(s) received previously is unknown or the previously administered product(s) is not readily available, any DTaP vaccine licensed for use in the primary series may be used. There is no need to match Tdap vaccine manufacturer with DTaP vaccine manufacturer used for earlier doses.

Recommendations for Routine Childhood Immunization With DTaP. Five doses of pertussis-containing vaccine are recommended prior to entering school: 4 doses of DTaP before 2 years of age and 1 dose of DTaP before school entry. The first dose of DTaP may be administered as early as 6 weeks of age, followed by 2 additional doses at intervals of approximately 2 months. The fourth dose of DTaP is recommended at 15 through 18 months of age, and the fifth dose of DTaP is administered before school entry (kindergarten or elementary school) at 4 through 6 years of age. The fourth dose can be administered as early as 12 months of age, provided 6 months have elapsed since the third dose was administered. If the fourth dose of pertussis vaccine is delayed until after the fourth birthday, the fifth dose is not recommended.

Other recommendations are as follows:

- Simultaneous administration of DTaP and all other recommended vaccines is acceptable. Vaccines should not be mixed in the same syringe unless the specific combination is licensed by the FDA (see Simultaneous Administration of Multiple Vaccines, p 35, and *Haemophilus influenzae* Infections, p 367).
- Inadvertent administration of Tdap instead of DTaP to a child younger than 7 years as either dose 1, 2, or 3 of DTaP does not count as a valid dose; DTaP should be administered as soon as is feasible.
- Inadvertent administration of Tdap instead of DTaP to a child younger than 7 years of age as either dose 4 or 5 can be counted as valid for DTaP dose 4 or 5.
- During a pertussis outbreak in the community, public health authorities may recommend starting DTaP immunization as early as 6 weeks of age, with doses 2 and 3 in the primary series administered at intervals as short as 4 weeks.
- Children younger than 7 years who have begun but not completed their primary immunization schedule with DTwP outside the United States should receive DTaP to complete the pertussis immunization schedule.

- DTaP is not licensed or recommended for people 7 years or older.
- Children between 7 and 10 years of age who have not completed their primary immunization schedule or have an unknown vaccine history should receive a single dose of Tdap. If they require additional tetanus and diphtheria toxoid doses, Td should be used.

Combined Vaccines. Several pertussis-containing combination vaccines are licensed for use (see Table 3.53, p 626) and may be used when feasible and when any components are indicated and none is contraindicated.

Recommendations for Scheduling Pertussis Immunization for Children Younger Than 7 Years in Special Circumstances

- For children whose pertussis immunization schedule is resumed after deferral or interruption of the recommended schedule, the next dose in the sequence should be administered, regardless of the interval since the last dose—that is, the schedule is not restarted (see Lapsed Immunizations, p 38).
- For children who have received fewer than the recommended number of doses of pertussis vaccine but who have received the recommended number of diphtheria and tetanus toxoid (DT) vaccine doses for their age, DTaP should be administered to complete the recommended pertussis immunization schedule.
- The total number of doses of diphtheria and tetanus toxoids (as DT, DTaP, or DTwP) should not exceed 6 before the seventh birthday.
- Although *B pertussis* infection confers protection against recurrent infection, the duration of protection is unknown. Age-appropriate DTaP dose(s) or a Tdap dose should be administered to complete the standard or catch-up immunization series on schedule in people who have had pertussis infection. No interval between disease and immunization is needed.

Medical Records. Charts of children for whom pertussis immunization has been deferred should be flagged, and the immunization status of these children should be assessed periodically to ensure that they are immunized appropriately.

Adverse Events After DTaP Immunization in Children Younger Than 7 Years

- **Local and febrile reactions.** Reactions to DTaP can occur within several hours of immunization and subside spontaneously within 48 hours without sequelae. Most commonly, these include redness, swelling, induration, and tenderness at the injection site as well as drowsiness. Less common reactions include fretfulness, anorexia, vomiting, crying, and slight to moderate fever.

   Swelling involving the entire thigh or upper arm has been reported in 2% to 3% of vaccine recipients after administration of the fourth and fifth doses of DTaP. Limb swelling can be accompanied by erythema, pain, and fever; it is not an infection. Although thigh swelling may interfere with walking, most children have no limitation of activity; the condition resolves spontaneously and has no sequelae. Entire limb swelling after a fourth dose of DTaP is associated with a modestly increased risk of a similar reaction or an injection-site reaction >5 cm after the fifth dose. Entire limb swelling is not a contraindication to further DTaP, Tdap, or Td immunization.

   A review by the Institute of Medicine (IOM) based on case-series reports found evidence of a rare yet likely causal relationship between receipt of tetanus toxoid-containing vaccines and brachial neuritis. However, the frequency of this event has not been determined. Brachial neuritis is listed in the Vaccine Injury Table.

- **Other reactions.** The rate of anaphylaxis following DTwP was estimated to be approximately 2 cases per 100 000 injections; the incidence of anaphylaxis after immunization with DTaP or Tdap is unknown. The Institute of Medicine report titled "Adverse Effects of Vaccines: Evidence and Causality" links tetanus-containing vaccines to anaphylaxis.[1] Severe anaphylactic reactions and resulting deaths, if any, are rare after pertussis immunization. Transient urticarial rashes that occur occasionally after pertussis immunization, unless appearing immediately (ie, within minutes), are unlikely to be anaphylactic (IgE mediated) in origin.

- **Seizures.** The incidence of seizures occurring within 48 hours of administration of DTwP was estimated to be 1 case per 1750 doses administered. These usually are simple febrile seizures and have not been demonstrated to result in recurrent afebrile seizures (ie, epilepsy) or other neurologic sequelae.

    Seizures have been reported substantially less often after DTaP, and a postlicensure study of children 6 to 23 months of age who received DTaP during 1997–2001 did not show an increased risk for seizures. A small increased risk for febrile seizures after DTaP when administered simultaneously with inactivated influenza vaccine was observed in a study in the Vaccine Safety Datalink. However, neither the CDC Advisory Committee on Immunization Practices (ACIP) nor the American Academy of Pediatrics recommends administering vaccines on separate days.

- **Hypotonic-hyporesponsive episode.** A hypotonic-hyporesponsive episode (HHE) (also termed "collapse" or "shock-like state") was reported to occur at a frequency of 1 per 1750 doses of DTwP administered, although reported rates varied widely. A follow-up study of a group of children who experienced an HHE following DTwP immunization demonstrated no evidence of subsequent serious neurologic sequelae or intellectual impairment. HHEs occur significantly less often after immunization with DTaP than with DTwP and are not a contraindication to subsequent dose(s).

- **Temperature 40.5°C (104.8°F) or higher.** The rate of temperature to 40.5°C (104.8°F) or higher after administration of DTaP is less than 0.1%.

- **Prolonged crying.** The frequency of inconsolable crying for 3 or more hours within 48 hours of receipt of DTaP is 0.2% or less. The significance of persistent crying is unknown, has been noted after receipt of vaccinations other than pertussis vaccine, is not known to be associated with sequelae, and is not a contraindication to subsequent dose(s).

    Evaluation of Adverse Events Temporally Associated With Pertussis Immunization. Appropriate diagnostic studies should be performed to establish the cause of serious adverse events occurring temporally after immunization, rather than assuming that they are caused by the vaccine.[2] The CDC has established independent Clinical Immunization Safety Assessment (CISA) centers to assess people with selected adverse events and offer recommendations for management. Genetic testing of several cases of encephalopathy temporally associated with DTwP revealed a genetic defect in neuronal sodium channels (Dravet syndrome); fever associated with DTwP likely unmasked the genetic condition and was not the cause of encephalopathy. The cause of events temporally related to immunization,

---

[1]Institute of Medicine. *Adverse Effects of Vaccines: Evidence and Causality.* Washington, DC: The National Academies Press; 2011

[2]Williams SE, Edwards KM, Baxter RP, et.al. Comprehensive assessment of serious adverse events following immunization by health care providers. *J Pediatr.* 2013;162(6):1276–1281

even when unrelated to the immunization received, cannot always be established, even after extensive diagnostic and investigative studies.

The preponderance of evidence does not support a causal relationship between immunization with DTwP and sudden infant death syndrome, infantile spasms, or serious acute neurologic illness resulting in permanent neurologic injury. Active surveillance performed by the IMPACT network of Canadian pediatric centers screening more than 12 000 admissions for neurologic disorders between 1993 and 2002 found no case of encephalopathy attributable to DTaP after administration of more than 6.5 million doses.

Contraindications and Precautions to DTaP Immunization.

Contraindications to DTaP and Tdap:

- **Severe allergic reaction (eg, anaphylaxis)** to a dose of DTaP or to a vaccine component. (DT or Td) is a contraindication to DTaP, DT, or Td. Because of the importance of tetanus vaccination, people who experience anaphylactic reactions should be referred to an allergist to determine whether they have a specific allergy to tetanus toxoid and can be desensitized to tetanus toxoid.
- Encephalopathy (eg, coma, decreased level of consciousness, or prolonged seizures) not attributable to another identifiable cause within 7 days after administration of a previous dose of diphtheria and tetanus toxoids and pertussis vaccine (DTwP, DTaP, or Tdap) is a contraindication to the pertussis component.

Precautions:

- **Guillain-Barré syndrome** within 6 weeks after a previous dose of tetanus toxoid-containing vaccine is a **precaution** to further doses of DTaP, Tdap, DT, or Td.
- Moderate or severe acute illness with or without a fever is a reason to defer administration of any vaccine until the person has recovered.
- **Evolving neurologic disorder** generally is a reason to defer DTaP or Tdap immunization temporarily to reduce confusion about reason(s) for a change in the clinical course. If deferred in the first year of life, DT should not be administered, because in the United States, the risk of acquiring diphtheria or tetanus by children younger than 1 year is remote. The decision to administer DTaP should be revisited, and if deferral is chosen after 1 year of age, DT immunization should be completed according to the recommended schedule (see Diphtheria, p 319, and/or Tetanus, p 793).

Recommendations for Routine Adolescent Immunization With Tdap.[1] Adolescents 10 years and older should receive a single dose of Tdap instead of Td for booster immunization against tetanus, diphtheria, and pertussis. The preferred age for Tdap immunizations is 11 through 12 years of age.

- Adolescents who received Td but not Tdap should receive a single dose of Tdap to provide protection against pertussis regardless of time since receipt of Td.
- Simultaneous administration of Tdap and all other recommended vaccines is recommended when feasible. Vaccines should not be mixed in the same syringe. Other indicated vaccine(s) that are not available and, therefore, cannot be administered at the time of administration of Tdap, can be administered anytime thereafter.
- Inadvertent administration of DTaP instead of Tdap in people 7 years and older is counted as a valid dose of Tdap

---

[1]Centers for Disease Control and Prevention. Updated recommendations for the use of tetanus toxoid, reduced diphtheria toxoid and acellular pertussis (Tdap) vaccine from the Advisory Committee on Immunization Practices, 2010. *MMWR Morb Mortal Wkly Rep.* 2011;60(1):13–15

- Outside of pregnancy, a second dose of Tdap is not recommended. See the following sections for special situations.

Recommendations for Scheduling Tdap in Children 7 Years and Older Who Did Not Complete Recommended DTaP Doses Before 7 Years of Age. Children 7 through 10 years of age who have not completed their immunization schedule with DTaP before 7 years of age (see previous section) or who have an unknown vaccine history should receive a single dose of Tdap. If further dose(s) of tetanus and diphtheria toxoids are needed in a catch-up schedule, Td is used. The preferred schedule is Tdap followed by Td (if needed) at 2 months and 6 to 12 months, but a single dose of Tdap could be substituted for any dose in the series. Children who receive Tdap at 7 through 10 years of age may receive the standard Tdap booster at 11 or 12 years of age.

Recommendations for Adolescent and Adult Immunization With Tdap in Special Situations. Currently, Tdap vaccines are licensed for only a single dose. Special situations for use of Tdap, or repeated use of Tdap off label, are provided in the following sections.

Use of Tdap in Pregnancy.[1] Providers of prenatal care should implement a Tdap immunization program for all pregnant women. The ACIP recommends that a dose of Tdap be administered during **each** pregnancy, irrespective of the mother's prior history of receiving Tdap. Tdap should be administered preferably early in the interval between 27 and 36 weeks' gestation, although Tdap may be administered at any time during pregnancy. Current evidence suggests that immunization early in the interval between 27 and 36 weeks' gestation will maximize passive antibody transfer to the infant. For women not previously vaccinated with Tdap and in whom Tdap was not administered during pregnancy, Tdap should be administered immediately postpartum. Postpartum Tdap is not recommended for women who previously received Tdap at any time.

Protection of Young Infants: The Cocoon Strategy. Tdap vaccination during each pregnancy is the preferred strategy for protecting young infants from pertussis in the early months of life. In addition, the AAP, CDC, American College of Obstetricians and Gynecologists, and American Academy of Family Physicians recommend the "cocoon" strategy to help protect infants from pertussis. This strategy may offer indirect protection through immunization of their family members to decrease their likelihood of acquisition and subsequent transmission of *B pertussis* to young infants, who have high risk of severe or fatal pertussis. Immunizing parents or other adult family contacts in the pediatric office setting could increase immunization coverage for this population.[2]

- Underimmunized children younger than 7 years should receive DTaP, and underimmunized children 7 years and older should receive Tdap (see previous discussion).
- All adolescents and adults should have received a single dose of Tdap. To ensure receipt, all adolescents and adults who have or anticipate having close contact with an infant younger than 12 months (eg, parents, siblings, grandparents, child care providers, and HCP) and who previously have not received Tdap should receive a single dose of Tdap, ideally at least 2 weeks before beginning close contact with the infant.

---

[1]Centers for Disease Control and Prevention. Updated recommendations for use of tetanus toxoid, reduced diphtheria toxoid, and acellular pertussis vaccine (Tdap) in pregnant women--Advisory Committee on Immunization Practices (ACIP), 2012. *MMWR*. 2013;62(7):131–135

[2]Lessin HR; Edwards KM; American Academy of Pediatrics, Committee on Practice and Ambulatory Medicine, Committee on Infectious Diseases. Immunizing parents and other close family contacts in the pediatric office setting. *Pediatrics*. 2012;129(2):e247-e253

There is no minimum interval required between Tdap and prior Td.
- Cough illness in contacts of neonates should be investigated and managed aggressively, with consideration given for azithromycin prophylaxis for the neonate if pertussis contact is likely (see Control Measures).

Special Situations.
- **Wound management in people who previously received Tdap.** In the setting when tetanus prophylaxis is required following a wound in a person who previously received Tdap ≥5 years earlier or in whom Tdap history is uncertain, Tdap can be used if Td is not readily available.
- **Wound management for pregnant women.** As part of standard wound management care to prevent tetanus, if a tetanus toxoid-containing vaccine is indicated in a pregnant woman who has not received at Td-containing vaccine within 5 years, Tdap should be administered.
- **Pregnant women for whom tetanus booster is due.** If Td booster immunization is indicated during pregnancy (ie, more than 10 years since previous Td), Tdap should be administered, preferably between weeks 27 and 36 of gestation.
- **Pregnant women with unknown or incomplete tetanus vaccination.** To ensure protection against maternal and neonatal tetanus, pregnant women who never have been immunized against tetanus should receive 3 doses of Td-containing vaccines during pregnancy. The recommended schedule is 0, 4 weeks, and 6 to 12 months. Tdap should replace 1 dose of Td, preferably between weeks 27 and 36 of gestation.

Health Care Professionals. The CDC recommends a single dose of Tdap as soon as is feasible for HCP of any age who previously have not received Tdap. There is no minimum interval suggested or required between Tdap and prior Td. After receipt of Tdap, HCP should receive routine decennial Td booster immunization. The decision not to recommend decennial Tdap for HCP is not related to safety concerns but rather to poor cost effectiveness.

In certain cases (eg, documented transmission in the health care setting), revaccination of HCP with Tdap may be considered (**www.cdc.gov/vaccines/vpd/pertussis/tdap-revac-hcp.html**). In such a case, Tdap is not a substitute for infection prevention and control measures, including postexposure antimicrobial prophylaxis for exposed HCP. If implemented, HCP who work with infants or pregnant women should be prioritized for revaccination.

Hospitals and ambulatory care facilities should provide Tdap for HCP and maximize immunization rates (eg, education about the benefits of immunization or mandatory requirement, convenient access, and provision of Tdap at no charge).

Recommendations for Adult Immunization With Tdap. The CDC recommends administration of a single dose of Tdap universally for adults of any age who previously have not received Tdap, with no minimum interval required between Tdap and prior dose of Td.

When available, Boostrix (GlaxoSmithKline, Research Triangle Park, NC) is the preferred Tdap vaccine for adults 65 years and older, because Boostrix is FDA approved for this indication; however, providers should not miss an opportunity to vaccinate and can use any available Tdap product. A dose of either vaccine is considered valid.

Adverse Events After Administration of Tdap. Local adverse events after administration of Tdap in adolescents and adults are common but usually are mild. Systemic adverse events also are common but usually are mild (eg, any fever, 3%–14%; any headache, 40%–44%;

tiredness, 27%–37%). Postmarketing data suggest that these events occur at approximately the same rate and severity as following receipt of Td.

Syncope can occur after immunization, is more common among adolescents and young adults, and can result in serious injury. Vaccine recipients should be seated and observed for 15 minutes after immunization. If syncope occurs, patients should be observed until symptoms resolve.

Contraindications, Precautions, and Deferral of Use of Tdap in Adolescents and Adults. Anaphylaxis that occurred after any component of the vaccine is a **contraindication** to Tdap (see Tetanus, p 793, for additional recommendations regarding tetanus immunization). In **latex-allergic** individuals, package inserts should be consulted regarding latex content.

History of **Guillain-Barré** syndrome within 6 weeks of a dose of a tetanus toxoid vaccine is a **precaution** to Tdap immunization. If the decision is made to continue tetanus toxoid immunization, Tdap is preferred if indicated. A history of severe **Arthus hypersensitivity reaction** after a previous dose of a tetanus or diphtheria toxoid-containing vaccine administered less than 10 years previously should lead to **deferral** of Tdap or Td immunization for 10 years after administration of the tetanus or diphtheria toxoid-containing vaccine.

Pinworm Infection

(*Enterobius vermicularis*)

CLINICAL MANIFESTATIONS: Although some people are asymptomatic, pinworm infection (enterobiasis) may cause pruritus ani and, rarely, pruritus vulvae. Bacterial superinfections can result from scratching and excoriation of the area. Pinworms have been found in the lumen of the appendix, and in some cases, these intraluminal parasites have been associated with signs of acute appendicitis, but they have also been observed in histologically normal appendices removed for incidental reasons. Many clinical findings, such as grinding of teeth at night, weight loss, and enuresis, have been attributed to pinworm infections, but proof of a causal relationship has not been established. Urethritis, vaginitis, salpingitis, or pelvic peritonitis may occur from aberrant migration of an adult worm from the perineum. Eosinophilic enterocolitis has been reported, although peripheral eosinophilia generally is not seen.

ETIOLOGY: *Enterobius vermicularis* is a nematode or roundworm.

EPIDEMIOLOGY: Enterobiasis occurs worldwide and commonly clusters within families. Prevalence rates are higher in preschool- and school-aged children, in primary caregivers of infected children, and in institutionalized people; up to 50% of these populations may be infected.

The adult female and egg induce intense perianal pruritus, leading to transmission by the fecal-oral route via contaminated hands. Alternative modes of transmission include person-to-person or sexual transmission. Female pinworms usually die after depositing up to 10 000 fertilized eggs within 24 hours on the perianal skin. Eggs adhere to the anal region and embryonate within 6 hours, becoming infective, leading to person-to-person spread or reinfection by autoinfection. A person remains infectious as long as female nematodes are discharging eggs on perianal skin. Eggs remain infective in an indoor environment usually for 2 to 3 weeks. Humans are the only known natural hosts.

The **incubation period** from ingestion of an egg until an adult gravid female migrates to the perianal region is 1 to 2 months or longer.

DIAGNOSTIC TESTS: Diagnosis is established via the classic cellulose tape (clear adhesive cellophane tape) test or with a commercially available pinworm paddle test, which is a clear plastic paddle coated with an adhesive surface on one side that is pressed in the perianal region during the night or at the time of waking, prior to bathing. The paddle is then pressed on a slide and eggs can be visualized by microscopy. Eggs are 50 x 25 microns and flattened on one side, giving them a "bean-shaped" appearance. Testing on 3 different days will increase the yield. The adult females, which are white and measure 8 to 13 mm, also can be seen in the perineal region. Stool examinations are of limited value, because worms or eggs are infrequently found in the stool. Peripheral eosinophilia is unusual and should not be attributed to pinworm infection.

TREATMENT: Several drugs of choice are available for treatment (see Drugs for Parasitic Infections, p 985) of pinworms, including pyrantel pamoate (11 mg/kg; maximum 1 g), which is available over the counter, albendazole (400 mg), and mebendazole (100 mg). Albendazole and mebendazole currently are significantly more costly than pyrantel pamoate. Each medication is recommended to be given in a single dose and repeated in 2 weeks, because these drugs are not completely effective against the egg or developing larvae stages. For children younger than 2 years, in whom experience with these drugs is limited, risks and benefits should be considered before drug administration. Ivermectin has been evaluated and is effective. Despite effective therapy, reinfection is common; therefore, treatment of the entire household should be considered, given the high transmission rate in families. Hygienic prevention, such as bathing in the morning to remove eggs, frequent hand hygiene, and clipping of fingernails all are helpful for decreasing the risk of autoinfection and continued transmission. Repeated infections should be treated by the same method as the first infection. All household members should be treated as a group in situations in which multiple or repeated symptomatic infections occur. Vaginitis is self-limited and does not require separate treatment.

ISOLATION OF THE HOSPITALIZED PATIENT: Standard precautions are indicated.

CONTROL MEASURES: Control is difficult in child care centers and schools, because the rate of reinfection is high. In institutions, mass and simultaneous treatment, repeated in 2 weeks, can be effective. Hand hygiene is the most effective method of prevention. Bed linens and underclothing of infected children should be handled carefully, should not be shaken (to avoid spreading ova into the air), and should be laundered promptly.

Pityriasis Versicolor
(Formerly Tinea Versicolor)

CLINICAL MANIFESTATIONS: Pityriasis versicolor (formerly tinea versicolor) is a common and benign superficial infection of the skin, classically manifesting on the upper trunk and neck. In infants and children, the infection is likely to involve the face, particularly the bilateral temples. Infection can include other areas, including the scalp, genital area, and thighs. Symmetrical involvement with ovoid discrete or coalescent lesions of varying size is typical; these macules or patches vary in color, even in the same person. White, pink, tan, or brown coloration is often surmounted by faint dusty scales. Lesions fail to tan during the summer and are relatively darker than the surrounding skin during the winter, hence the term versicolor. The differential diagnosis includes pityriasis alba, vitiligo, seborrheic dermatitis, pityriasis rosea, progressive macular hypopigmentation, and pityriasis lichenoides. Folliculitis also can occur, particularly in immunocompromised patients. Systemic infections can occur in neonates, particularly those receiving total parenteral nutrition with lipids.

ETIOLOGY: The cause of pityriasis versicolor is a number of species of the *Malassezia furfur* complex, a group of lipid-dependent yeasts that exist on healthy skin in yeast phase and cause clinical lesions only when substantial growth of hyphae occurs. Moisture, heat, and the presence of lipid-containing sebaceous secretions encourage rapid overgrowth of hyphae.

EPIDEMIOLOGY: Pityriasis versicolor can occur in any climate or age group but tends to favor adolescents and young adults, particularly in tropical climates. The **incubation period** is unknown.

DIAGNOSTIC TESTS: The presence of symmetrically distributed faintly scaling macules and patches of varying color concentrated on the upper back and chest is close to diagnostic. The "evoked scale" sign consists of stretching or scraping the involved skin, which readily elicits a visible layer of thin scale. Involved areas fluoresce yellow-green under Wood lamp evaluation. Potassium hydroxide wet mount prep of scraped scales reveals the classic "spaghetti and meatballs" short hyphae and clusters of yeast forms. Because this yeast is a common inhabitant of the skin, culture from the skin surface is nondiagnostic. Samples from pustules or sterile sites should be placed in media enriched with olive oil or another long-chain fatty acid.

TREATMENT: Multiple topical and systemic agents are efficacious, and recommendations vary substantially. For uncomplicated cases, most experts recommend initiating therapy with topical agents. The most cost-effective treatments are selenium sulfide shampoo/lotion and clotrimazole cream. Selenium sulfide shampoo is used for 3 to 7 days; application is once daily for 5 to 10 minutes, followed by rinsing. Topical azole therapy (eg, clotrimazole cream) is applied twice daily for 2 to 3 weeks. Adherence with these agents may be low because of unpleasant adverse effects (the shampoo has a sulfur-like odor) or duration and anatomic extent of required therapy. Other effective topical agents include ketoconazole, bifonazole, miconazole, econazole, oxiconazole, clotrimazole, terbinafine, and ciclopirox, as well as zinc pyrithione shampoo. Shampoos are easier to disperse, particularly on wet skin, than topical creams and may increase compliance.

Recurrence following discontinuation of therapy may approach 60% to 80%, and preventive treatments sometimes are used to decrease recurrences. Off-label regimens to decrease recurrence include use of the aforementioned shampoos/lotions on a weekly or monthly basis. The family must be counseled that return of pigment to the previously affected sites can take months.

Systemic therapy is reserved for resistant infection or extensive involvement. Medications, including fluconazole, ketoconazole, itraconazole, and pramiconazole, are not approved by the US Food and Drug Administration for pityriasis versicolor. Single oral doses do not appear to be as efficacious as multiple doses over several days or weeks. Fluconazole can be administered at 300 mg weekly for 2 to 4 weeks, and ketoconazole can be administered at 200 mg daily for 10 days. Although oral agents may be easier to use than topical agents, they are not necessarily more effective and have possible serious adverse effects. In several studies, topical therapy has appeared to be equivalent or superior to systemic therapy. Drug interactions can occur when using oral drugs, and monitoring for liver toxicity must be considered in patients receiving systemic therapy, particularly if they receive multiple courses.

ISOLATION OF THE HOSPITALIZED PATIENT: Standard precautions are recommended.
CONTROL MEASURES: The organism that causes pityriasis versicolor is commensal and resides on normal skin.

Plague

CLINICAL MANIFESTATIONS: Naturally acquired plague most commonly manifests in the **bubonic form,** with acute onset of high fever and a painful swollen regional lymph node (bubo). Buboes develop most commonly in the inguinal region but also occur in axillary or cervical areas. Less commonly, plague manifests in the **septicemic form** (hypotension, acute respiratory distress, purpuric skin lesions, intravascular coagulopathy, organ failure) or as **pneumonic plague** (cough, fever, dyspnea, and hemoptysis) and rarely as **meningeal**, **pharyngeal**, **cutaneous, ocular**, or **gastrointestinal plague.** Abrupt onset of fever, chills, headache, and malaise are characteristic in all cases. Occasionally, patients have symptoms of mild lymphadenitis or prominent gastrointestinal tract symptoms, which may obscure the correct diagnosis. Untreated, plague often progresses to overwhelming sepsis and death. Plague has been referred to as the Black Death.

ETIOLOGY: Plague is caused by *Yersinia pestis,* a pleomorphic, bipolar-staining (with Giemsa, Wright, and Watson stains), gram-negative coccobacillus. *Y pestis* is a member of the *Enterobacteriaceae* family, along with more common *Yersinia* species and other enteric bacteria.

EPIDEMIOLOGY: Plague is a zoonotic infection primarily maintained in rodents and their fleas. Humans are incidental hosts who develop bubonic or primary septicemic manifestations typically through the bite of infected rodent fleas or through direct contact with tissues of infected animals. Secondary pneumonic plague arises from hematogenous seeding of the lungs with *Y pestis* in patients with untreated bubonic or septicemic plague. Primary pneumonic plague is acquired by inhalation of respiratory tract droplets from a human or animal with pneumonic plague. Only the pneumonic form has been shown to be transmitted from person to person. Plague occurs worldwide with enzootic foci in parts of Asia, Africa, and the Americas. Most human plague cases are reported from rural, underdeveloped areas and mainly occur as isolated cases or in small, focal clusters. In the United States, plague is endemic in western states, with most cases reported from New Mexico, Colorado, Arizona, and California.[1] Cases of plague have been identified in travelers returning to states without endemic plague.

The **incubation period** is 2 to 8 days for bubonic plague and 1 to 6 days for primary pneumonic plague.

DIAGNOSTIC TESTS: Diagnosis of plague usually is confirmed by culture of *Y pestis* from blood, bubo aspirate, sputum, or another clinical specimen. The organism is slow growing but not fastidious and can be isolated on sheep blood and chocolate agars with typical "fried-egg" colonies appearing after 48 to 72 hours of incubation. *Y pestis* has a bipolar (safety-pin) appearance when stained with Wright-Giemsa or Wayson stains. A positive direct fluorescent antibody test result for the presence of *Y pestis* in direct smears or cultures of blood, bubo aspirate, sputum, or another clinical specimen provides presumptive

[1]Kwit N, Nelson C, Kugeler K, et al. Human plague—United States, 2015. *MMWR Morb Mortal Wkly Rep.* 2015;64(33):918–919

evidence of *Y pestis* infection. Automated, commercially available biochemical identification systems are not recommended, because they can misidentify *Y pestis*. Identification of suspected isolates of *Y pestis* should be based on guidelines recommended for "sentinel level" clinical microbiology laboratories using preliminary characterization tests, followed by definitive identification performed at the state or federal public health laboratory. Polymerase chain reaction assay and immunohistochemical staining for rapid diagnosis of *Y pestis* are available in some reference or public health laboratories.

A single positive serologic test result from a passive hemagglutination assay or enzyme immunoassay also provides presumptive evidence of infection. Seroconversion, defined as a fourfold increase in antibody titer between serum specimens obtained at least 2 weeks apart, also confirms the diagnosis of plague.

In the United States, *Y pestis* is classified as a select agent, and the possession and transport of the organism requires adherence to strict federal guidelines. Laboratory-acquired cases, including fatal cases, have been reported. Clinical laboratories must handle a suspected or confirmed isolate using at least biosafety level 2 guidelines with particular attention to preventing aerosolization of the organism. Isolates suspected as *Y pestis* should be reported immediately to the state health department and submitted to the Division of Vector-Borne Infectious Diseases of the Centers for Disease Control and Prevention (CDC) following procedures for transfer of select agents.

TREATMENT: For children, gentamicin and streptomycin, administered intramuscularly or intravenously, appear to be equally effective. Alternative drugs approved by the US Food and Drug Administration (FDA) include ciprofloxacin, levofloxacin, moxifloxacin, tetracycline, doxycycline, chloramphenicol, and trimethoprim-sulfamethoxazole. Fluoroquinolones have been shown to be highly effective in animal and in vitro studies. Trimethoprim-sulfamethoxazole should not be considered a first-line treatment option when treating bubonic plague and should not be used as monotherapy to treat pneumonic or septicemic plague because of higher treatment failure rates than with other antimicrobial agents. The usual duration of antimicrobial treatment is 10 to 14 days or until several days after resolution of fever. Chloramphenicol is considered the treatment of choice for plague meningitis, but when chloramphenicol is unavailable, fluoroquinolones, particularly a drug such as levofloxacin, which attains higher cerebrospinal fluid concentrations, should be considered as alternative therapy.

Drainage of abscessed buboes may be necessary; drainage material is infectious until effective antimicrobial therapy has been administered.

ISOLATION OF THE HOSPITALIZED PATIENT: For patients with bubonic plague, standard precautions are recommended. For patients with suspected pneumonic plague, respiratory droplet precautions should be initiated immediately and continued for 48 hours after initiation of effective antimicrobial treatment.

CONTROL MEASURES:

Care of Exposed People. All people with exposure to a known or suspected plague source, such as *Y pestis*-infected fleas or infectious tissues, in the previous 6 days, should be offered antimicrobial prophylaxis or be cautioned to report fever greater than 38.3°C (101.0°F) or other illness to their physician. People with close exposure (less than 2 meters) to a patient with pneumonic plague and who are within the incubation period should receive antimicrobial prophylaxis, but isolation of asymptomatic people is not recommended. Pneumonic transmission typically occurs in the end stage of disease in patients with hemoptysis, thereby placing caregivers and health care professionals at high risk. For adults and children, including those younger than 8 years, doxycycline or ciprofloxacin is recommended (see Tetracyclines, p 905, and Fluoroquinolones, p 904). The benefits of prophylactic therapy should be weighed against the risks. Prophylaxis is administered for 7 days and in the usual therapeutic doses.

Other Measures. State public health authorities should be notified immediately of any suspected cases of human plague. People living in areas with endemic plague should be informed about the importance of eliminating sources of rodent food and harborage near residences, the role of dogs and cats in bringing plague-infected rodent fleas into peridomestic environments, the need for flea control and confinement of pets, and the importance of avoiding contact with sick and dead animals. Other preventive measures include surveillance of rodent populations and use of rodent control measures and insecticides by health authorities when surveillance indicates the occurrence of plague epizootics.

Vaccine. There is no vaccine currently licensed for use in the United States. New vaccines based on recombinant capsular subunit protein F1 and the low-calcium response V antigen (LcrV) are under evaluation.

Pneumococcal Infections[1,2]

CLINICAL MANIFESTATIONS: *Streptococcus pneumoniae* is a common bacterial cause of acute otitis media, sinusitis, community-acquired pneumonia, and pediatric conjunctivitis; pleural empyema, mastoiditis, and periorbital cellulitis occur. It is the most common cause of bacterial meningitis in infants and children ages 2 months to 11 years in the United States.[3] *S pneumoniae* also may cause endocarditis, pericarditis, peritonitis, pyogenic arthritis, osteomyelitis, soft tissue infection, and neonatal septicemia. Overwhelming septicemia in patients with splenic dysfunction is noted, and hemolytic-uremic syndrome can accompany pneumococcal pneumonia with or without pleural empyema or meningitis.

ETIOLOGY: *S pneumoniae* organisms (pneumococci) are lancet-shaped, gram-positive, catalase-negative diplococci. More than 90 pneumococcal serotypes have been identified on the basis of unique polysaccharide capsules.

EPIDEMIOLOGY: Nasopharyngeal carriage rates in children range from 21% in industrialized countries to more than 90% in resource-limited countries. Transmission is from person to person by respiratory droplet contact. Viral upper respiratory tract infections, including influenza, can predispose to pneumococcal infection and transmission. Pneumococcal infections are most prevalent during winter months. The period of communicability is unknown and may be as long as the organism is present in respiratory tract secretions but probably is less than 24 hours after effective antimicrobial therapy is begun. During the prepneumococcal conjugate vaccine era, among young children who acquired a new pneumococcal serotype in the nasopharynx, otitis media or other pneumococcal

---

[1]American Academy of Pediatrics, Committee on Infectious Diseases. Policy statement: recommendations for the prevention *Streptococcus pneumoniae* infections in infants and children: use of 13-valent pneumococcal conjugate vaccine (PCV13) and pneumococcal polysaccharide vaccine (PPSV23). *Pediatrics.* 2010;126(1):186–190

[2]Centers for Disease Control and Prevention. Prevention of pneumococcal disease among infants and children—use of 13-valent pneumococcal conjugate vaccine and 23-valent pneumococcal polysaccharide vaccine. *MMWR Recomm Rep.* 2010;59(RR-11):1–18

[3]Thigpen MC, Whitney CG, Messonnier NE, et al; Emerging Infections Programs Network. Bacterial meningitis in the United States, 1998–2007. *N Engl J Med.* 2011;364(21):2016–2025

infection occurred in approximately 15%, usually within a few days of acquisition.

The incidence and severity of infections are increased in people with congenital or acquired humoral immunodeficiency, human immunodeficiency virus (HIV) infection, absent or deficient splenic function (eg, sickle cell disease, congenital or surgical asplenia), certain complement deficiencies, diabetes mellitus, chronic liver disease, chronic renal failure or nephrotic syndrome, or abnormal innate immune responses. Children with cochlear implants, particularly those who had placement of an older model that involved a cochlear electrode, have high rates of pneumococcal meningitis, as do children with congenital or acquired cerebrospinal fluid (CSF) leaks.[1] Other categories of children at presumed high risk or at moderate risk of developing invasive pneumococcal disease are outlined in Table 3.54. Infection rates are highest in infants, young children, elderly people, and black, Alaska Native, and some American Indian populations. Since introduction of the heptavalent pneumococcal conjugate vaccine (PCV7), which included the most common serotypes associated with invasive infection (4, 6B, 9V, 14, 18C, 19F, and 23F), in 2000 and 13-valent pneumococcal conjugate vaccine (PCV13), which includes the additional serotypes 1, 3, 5, 6A, 7F, and 19A, in 2010, racial disparities have diminished; however, rates of invasive pneumococcal disease (IPD) among some American Indian (Alaska Native, Navajo, and White Mountain Apache) populations remain more than fivefold higher than the rate among children in the general US population, especially for serotypes not included in the vaccine. Factors associated with this increased risk include household crowding, poverty, and lack of in-home piped water.

By 7 years after the introduction of PCV7 in 2000, the incidence of vaccine-type invasive pneumococcal infections decreased by 99%, and the incidence of all IPD decreased by 76% in children younger than 5 years. In adults 65 years and older, IPD caused by PCV7 serotypes decreased 92% compared with baseline and all IPD decreased by 37%. The reduction in cases in these latter groups indicates the significant indirect benefits of PCV7 immunization by interruption of transmission of pneumococci from children to adults. After introduction of PCV13, further reductions in IPD disease in children younger than 5 years occurred, in large part because of reductions in IPD caused by serotype 19A. There have also been reductions in IPD in unvaccinated older children and adults indicative of herd protection.

The **incubation period** varies by type of infection but can be as short as 1 to 3 days.

DIAGNOSTIC TESTS: Recovery of *S pneumoniae* from a normally sterile site (eg, blood, CSF, peritoneal fluid, middle ear fluid, joint fluid) or from a suppurative focus confirms the diagnosis. The finding of lancet-shaped gram-positive organisms and white blood cells in expectorated sputum (older children and adults) or pleural exudate suggests pneumococcal pneumonia. Recovery of pneumococci by culture of an upper respiratory tract swab specimen is not sufficient to assign an etiologic diagnosis of pneumococcal disease involving the middle ear, upper or lower respiratory tract, or sinus. The organism is isolated readily on sheep blood agar, where it produces a zone of "alpha" hemolysis (greening of the agar); however, it cannot be differentiated from other species of viridans-group

---

[1]American Academy of Pediatrics, Committee on Infectious Diseases. Policy statement: cochlear implants in children: surgical site infections and prevention and treatment of acute otitis media and meningitis. *Pediatrics*. 2010;126(2):381–391

Table 3.54. Underlying Medical Conditions That Are Indications for Immunization with 23-Valent Pneumococcal Polysaccharide Vaccine (PPSV23)[a] Among Children, by Risk Group[b]

Risk group	Condition
Immunocompetent children	Chronic heart disease[c]
	Chronic lung disease[d]
	Diabetes mellitus
	Cerebrospinal fluid leaks
	Cochlear implant
Children with functional or anatomic asplenia	Sickle cell disease and other hemoglobinopathies
	Chronic or acquired asplenia, or splenic dysfunction
Children with immunocompromising conditions	HIV infection
	Chronic renal failure and nephrotic syndrome
	Diseases associated with treatment with immunosuppressive drugs or radiation therapy, including malignant neoplasms, leukemias, lymphomas, and Hodgkin disease; or solid organ transplantation
	Congenital immunodeficiency[e]

[a]PPSV23 is indicated starting at 24 months of age.
[b]Centers for Disease Control and Prevention. Licensure of a 13-valent pneumococcal conjugate vaccine (PCV13) and recommendations for use among children. Advisory Committee on Immunization Practices (ACIP). *MMWR Morb Mortal Wkly Rep.* 2010;59(9):258-261
[c]Particularly cyanotic congenital heart disease and cardiac failure.
[d]Including asthma if treated with prolonged high-dose oral corticosteroids.
[e]Includes B- (humoral) or T-lymphocyte deficiency; complement deficiencies, particularly C_1, C_2, C_3, and C_4 deficiency; and phagocytic disorders (excluding chronic granulomatous disease).

streptococci on the basis of colonial morphologic characteristics (see Table 3.72, p 758). Definitive identification requires determination of optochin susceptibility (optochin disk test) or bile solubility (sodium deoxycholate lysis); the latter method demonstrates better sensitivity and specificity and is recommended. Commercial biochemical test systems and mass spectrometry of cellular components have also been applied to identification of *S pneumoniae*, but there are reports of misidentification with these methods.

There are at least 2 US Food and Drug Administration (FDA)-cleared multiplexed nucleic acid amplification tests designed to identify *S pneumoniae* and other bacterial and fungal pathogens directly from positive blood culture bottles. At least one real-time polymerase chain reaction (PCR) assay is cleared by the FDA for detection of *S pneumoniae* in CSF. The assay is a multiplexed PCR designed to detect a number of agents of bacterial and viral meningitis or encephalitis. There is limited clinical experience with this assay, and there were several falsely positive results for *S pneumoniae* during the clinical trials leading to FDA clearance. Therefore, this assay should be used cautiously and be accompanied by culture of CSF to obtain an isolate, which is needed for antimicrobial susceptibility testing. Other PCR tests designed to detect *lyt*A or other gene targets are investigational but may be specific and significantly more sensitive than culture of pleural fluid,

CSF, blood, or other normally sterile body fluid particularly in patients who have received recent antimicrobial therapy.

Detection of C-polysaccharide (common to all pneumococci) in urine for diagnosis of pneumococcal pneumonia may have some utility in adults but is not useful in children, because asymptomatically colonized children may have positive test results. Similarly, commercially available antigen detection tests performed on CSF or blood are not recommended for routine use because of low sensitivity.

Susceptibility Testing. All *S pneumoniae* isolates from normally sterile body fluids (eg, CSF, blood, middle ear fluid, mastoid, pleural, joint fluid, pericardial fluid) should be tested for antimicrobial susceptibility to determine the minimum inhibitory concentration (MIC) of penicillin, cefotaxime or ceftriaxone, and clindamycin. CSF isolates also should be tested for susceptibility to vancomycin, meropenem, and rifampin. *Nonsusceptibility* includes both *intermediate* and *resistant* isolates. Breakpoints vary depending on whether an isolate is from a nonmeningeal or meningeal site; in children with meningitis presentations, the breakpoints for meningeal isolates should be used (eg, a blood isolate in a patient with meningitis). Accordingly, current definitions by the Clinical and Laboratory Standards Institute (CLSI) for susceptibility and nonsusceptibility are provided in Table 3.55 for nonmeningeal and meningitis presentations. *S pneumoniae* strains that are nonsusceptible to penicillin G, cefotaxime, ceftriaxone, and other antimicrobial agents using meningitis breakpoints have been identified throughout the United States and worldwide.

For patients with meningitis caused by an organism that is nonsusceptible to penicillin, susceptibility testing of rifampin also should be performed. If the patient has a nonmeningeal infection caused by an isolate that is nonsusceptible to penicillin, cefotaxime, and ceftriaxone, susceptibility testing to other agents such as clindamycin, erythromycin, trimethoprim-sulfamethoxazole, linezolid, meropenem, and vancomycin should be performed.

Table 3.55. Clinical and Laboratory Standards Institute Definitions of in Vitro Susceptibility and Nonsusceptibility of Pneumococcal Isolates in Nonmeningeal and Meningeal Cases[a,b]

Drug and Isolate Location	Susceptible, µg/mL	Nonsusceptible, µg/mL	
		Intermediate	Resistant
Penicillin (oral)[c]	≤0.06	0.12–1.0	≥2.0
Penicillin (intravenous)[d]			
Nonmeningeal cases	≤2.0	4.0	≥8.0
Meningitis cases	≤0.06	None	≥0.12
Cefotaxime **OR** ceftriaxone			
Nonmeningeal cases	≤1.0	2.0	≥4.0
Meningitis cases	≤0.5	1.0	≥2.0

[a]Clinical and Laboratory Standards Institute. *Performance Standards for Antimicrobial Susceptibility Testing: 27th Informational Supplement.* CLSI Publication No. M100-S27. Wayne, PA: Clinical and Laboratory Standards Institute; 2016
[b]Centers for Disease Control and Prevention. Effects of new penicillin susceptibility breakpoints for *Streptococcus pneumoniae*— United States, 2006–2007. *MMWR Morb Mortal Wkly Rep.* 2008;57(50):1353–1355
[c]Without meningitis.
[d]Treated with intravenous penicillin.

Quantitative MIC testing using reliable methods, such as broth microdilution or antimicrobial gradient strips, should be performed on isolates from children with invasive infections. For isolates from noninvasive infections, quantitative MIC testing or a qualitative screening testing can be used; the latter uses a 1-μg oxacillin disk on an agar plate to reliably identify all penicillin-*susceptible* pneumococci using meningitis breakpoints (ie, diskzone diameter of 20 mm or greater). Organisms with an oxacillin disk-zone size of less than 20 mm potentially are nonsusceptible to penicillins and cephalosporins for treatment of meningitis and require quantitative susceptibility testing.

TREATMENT:

Bacterial Meningitis Possibly or Proven to Be Caused by S pneumoniae. For all children with bacterial meningitis presumed to be caused by *S pneumoniae*, vancomycin should be administered in addition to cefotaxime (or ceftriaxone for those >1 month) because of the possibility of *S pneumoniae* resistant to penicillin, cefotaxime, and ceftriaxone.

For children with serious hypersensitivity reactions to beta-lactam antimicrobial agents (ie, penicillins and cephalosporins), the combination of vancomycin and rifampin should be considered. Vancomycin should not be given alone, because bactericidal concentrations in CSF are difficult to sustain, and clinical experience to support use of vancomycin as monotherapy is minimal. Rifampin also should not be given as monotherapy, because resistance can develop during therapy. Meropenem is an alternative drug in a patient with hypersensitivity to other beta-lactam antimicrobial agents. Penicillin desensitization can be considered.

A repeat lumbar puncture should be considered after 48 hours of therapy in the following circumstances:

- The organism is penicillin nonsusceptible by oxacillin disk or quantitative (MIC) testing, and results from cefotaxime and ceftriaxone quantitative susceptibility testing are not yet available or the isolate is cefotaxime and ceftriaxone nonsusceptible; or
- The patient's condition has not improved or has worsened; or
- The child has received dexamethasone, which can interfere with the ability to interpret the clinical response, such as resolution of fever.

Once results of susceptibility testing are available, therapy should be modified according to the guidance in Table 3.56. If the organism is susceptible to penicillin, vancomycin should be discontinued and either penicillin or cefotaxime or ceftriaxone should be continued; if the isolate is penicillin nonsusceptible, cefotaxime or ceftriaxone should be continued.

If the organism is nonsusceptible to penicillin and cefotaxime or ceftriaxone, vancomycin should be continued. Addition of rifampin to the combination of vancomycin and cefotaxime or ceftriaxone after 24 to 48 hours of therapy should be considered if the organism is susceptible to rifampin and: (1) after 24 to 48 hours, despite therapy with vancomycin and cefotaxime or ceftriaxone, the clinical condition has worsened; (2) the subsequent culture of CSF indicates failure to eradicate or to decrease substantially the number of organisms; or (3) the organism has a high cefotaxime or ceftriaxone MIC (≥ 2 μg/mL or ≥ 4 μg/mL) indicating resistance. Consultation with an infectious disease specialist should be considered for all children with bacterial meningitis.

Dexamethasone. For infants and children 6 weeks and older, adjunctive therapy with dexamethasone may be considered after weighing the potential benefits and risks. Some experts recommend use of corticosteroids in pneumococcal meningitis, but this issue is

Table 3.56. Antimicrobial Therapy for Infants and Children With Meningitis Caused by *Streptococcus pneumoniae* on the Basis of Susceptibility Test Results

Susceptibility Test Results	Antimicrobial Management[a]
Susceptible to penicillin	**Discontinue vancomycin** **AND** Begin penicillin (and discontinue cephalosporin) **OR** Continue cefotaxime or ceftriaxone alone[b]
Nonsusceptible to penicillin (*intermediate* or *resistant*) **AND** *Susceptible* to cefotaxime and ceftriaxone	**Discontinue vancomycin** **AND** Continue cefotaxime or ceftriaxone
Nonsusceptible to penicillin (*intermediate* or *resistant*) **AND** *Nonsusceptible* to cefotaxime and ceftriaxone (*intermediate* or *resistant*) **AND** *Susceptible* to rifampin	Continue vancomycin and high-dose cefotaxime or ceftriaxone **AND** Rifampin may be added in selected circumstances (see text)

[a]Initial empiric therapy of nonallergic children older than 1 month of age with presumed bacterial meningitis should be vancomycin and cefotaxime or ceftriaxone. See Table 3.57, for dosages. Some experts recommend the maximum dosages (see Bacterial Meningitis Possibly or Proven to Be Caused by *S pneumoniae*, p 643).

[b]Some physicians may choose this alternative for convenience and cost savings but only in treatment of meningitis.

controversial and data are not sufficient to make a routine recommendation for children. The Infectious Diseases Society of America recommends use of dexamethasone in adults with suspected or proven pneumococcal meningitis. If used, dexamethasone should be administered before or concurrently with the first dose of antimicrobial agents.

Nonmeningeal Invasive Pneumococcal Infections Requiring Hospitalization. For nonmeningeal invasive infections in previously healthy children who are not critically ill, antimicrobial agents currently used to treat infections with *S pneumoniae* and other potential pathogens should be initiated at the usually recommended dosages (see Table 3.57).

For critically ill infants and children with invasive infections potentially attributable to *S pneumoniae*, vancomycin, in addition to empiric antimicrobial therapy (eg, cefotaxime or ceftriaxone or others), can be considered. Such patients include those with presumed septic shock, severe pneumonia with empyema, or significant hypoxia or myopericardial involvement. If vancomycin is administered, it should be discontinued as soon as antimicrobial susceptibility test results demonstrate effective alternative agents.

If the organism has in vitro resistance to penicillin, cefotaxime, and ceftriaxone according to guidelines of the CLSI, therapy should be modified on the basis of clinical response, susceptibility to other antimicrobial agents, and results of follow-up cultures of blood and other infected body fluids. Consultation with an infectious disease specialist should be considered.

Table 3.57. Dosages of Intravenous Antimicrobial Agents for Invasive Pneumococcal Infections in Infants and Children[a]

Antimicrobial Agent	Meningitis		Nonmeningeal Infections	
	Dose/kg per day	Dose Interval	Dose/kg per day	Dose Interval
Penicillin G	250 000–400 000 U[b] (max 24 million U/day)	4–6 h	250 000–400 000 U[b] (max 24 million U/day)	4–6 h
Ampicillin	300 mg (max 12 g/day)	6 h	200 mg (max 12 g/day)	6 h
Cefotaxime	225–300 mg (max 2 g/dose)	8 h	75–225 mg (max 2 g/dose)	8 h
Ceftriaxone	100 mg (max 2 g/dose, 4 g/day)	12–24h	50–75 mg (max 2 g/dose, 4 g/day)	12–24 h
Vancomycin	60 mg	6 h	40–45 mg	6–8 h
Rifampin[c]	20 mg	12 h	Not indicated	...
Chloramphenicol[d]	75–100 mg	6 h	75–100 mg	6 h
Clindamycin	Not indicated	...	30–40 mg (max 1800 mg/day, orally)	6–8 h
Meropenem[e]	120 mg (max 2 g/dose)	8 h	60 mg (max 2 g/dose)	8 h

[a]Doses are for children 1 month or older.
[b]Because 1 U = 0.6 µg, this range is equal to 150 to 240 mg/kg per day.
[c]Indications for use are not defined completely.
[d]Drug should be considered only for patients with life-threatening allergic response after administration of beta-lactam antimicrobial agents.
[e]Drug is approved for pediatric patients 3 months and older.

For children with severe hypersensitivity to beta-lactam antimicrobial agents (ie, penicillins and cephalosporins), initial management should include vancomycin or clindamycin, in addition to antimicrobial agents for other potential pathogens, as indicated. Vancomycin should not be continued if the organism is susceptible to other appropriate non–beta-lactam antimicrobial agents. Consultation with an infectious disease specialist should be considered.

Dosages for Invasive Pneumococcal Disease. The recommended dosages of intravenous antimicrobial agents for treatment of invasive pneumococcal infections are provided in Table 3.57.

Acute Otitis Media.[1] According to clinical practice guidelines of the American Academy of Pediatrics (AAP) and the American Academy of Family Physicians (AAFP) on acute suppurative otitis media (AOM), amoxicillin (80–90 mg/kg/day) is recommended for infants

---

[1]Lieberthal AS, Carroll AE, Chonmaitree T, et al. Clinical practice guideline: diagnosis and management of acute otitis media. *Pediatrics.* 2013;131(3):e964-e999

<6 months of age and for those 6 through 23 months of age with bilateral disease. A watch-and-wait option can be considered for older children and those with nonsevere disease. Optimal duration of therapy is uncertain. For younger children and children with severe disease at any age, a 10-day course is recommended; for children 6 years and older with mild or moderate disease, a duration of 5 to 7 days is appropriate. Otalgia should be treated in all cases.

Patients who fail to respond to initial management should be reassessed at 48 to 72 hours to confirm the diagnosis of AOM and exclude other causes of illness. If AOM is confirmed in the patient managed initially with observation, amoxicillin should be administered. If the patient has failed initial antibacterial therapy, a change in antibacterial agent is indicated. Suitable alternative agents should be active against penicillin-nonsusceptible pneumococci as well as beta-lactamase–producing *Haemophilus influenzae* and *Moraxella catarrhalis*. Such agents include high-dose oral amoxicillin-clavulanate; oral cefdinir, cefpodoxime, or cefuroxime; or intramuscular ceftriaxone in a 3-day course. Amoxicillin-clavulanate should be administered at 80 to 90 mg/kg per day of the amoxicillin component in the 14:1 formulation to decrease the incidence of diarrhea. The maximum amount of clavulinate per dose is 125 mg. Patients who continue to fail to respond to therapy with one of the aforementioned oral agents should be treated with a 3-day course of parenteral ceftriaxone. Macrolide resistance among *S pneumoniae* is high, so clarithromycin and azithromycin are not considered appropriate alternatives for initial therapy even in patients with a type I (immediate, anaphylactic) reaction to a beta-lactam agent. In such cases, treatment with clindamycin (if susceptibility is known) or levofloxacin is preferred. For patients with a history of non-type I allergic reaction to penicillin, agents such as cefdinir, cefuroxime, or cefpodoxime can be used orally.

Myringotomy or tympanocentesis should be considered for children failing to respond to second-line therapy, for severe cases to obtain cultures to guide therapy, and for patients with invasive pneumococcal infection. For multidrug-resistant strains of *S pneumoniae*, use of levofloxacin or other agents should be considered in consultation with an infectious diseases expert and based on the specific susceptibility profile.

Sinusitis. Antimicrobial agents effective for treatment of AOM also are likely to be effective for acute sinusitis and are recommended when a child meets clinical criteria for diagnosis.

Pneumonia.[1] Oral amoxicillin at a dose of 45 mg/kg/day or 90 mg/kg/day in 3 equally divided portions is likely to be effective in ambulatory children with pneumonia caused by susceptible and relatively resistant pneumococci (MICs of 2.0 µg/mL), respectively. Ampicillin is used for intravenous therapy of community acquired pneumonia. Cefotaxime or ceftriaxone is used for treatment of inpatients infected with pneumococci suspected or proven to be penicillin-resistant strains, for serious infections including empyema, or in those not fully immunized with PCV13. Vancomycin should be included in those with life-threatening infection. For patients with isolates resistant to penicillin (MICs of 4.0 µg/mL or higher) or significant allergy to beta lactam antimicrobials, treatment with clindamycin (if susceptible) or levofloxacin should be considered, assuming that concurrent meningitis has been excluded.

---

[1]Bradley JS, Byington CL, Shah SS, et al. The management of community-acquired pneumonia in infants and children older than 3 months of age: clinical practice guidelines by the Pediatric Infectious Diseases Society and the Infectious Diseases Society of America. *Clin Infect Dis.* 2011;53(7):e25–e76

ISOLATION OF THE HOSPITALIZED PATIENT: Standard precautions are recommended, including for patients with infections caused by drug-resistant *S pneumoniae*.

CONTROL MEASURES:

Active Immunization. Two pneumococcal vaccines are available for use in children in the United States: the 13-valent pneumococcal conjugate vaccine (PCV13) and 23-valent pneumococcal polysaccharide vaccine (PPSV23). PCV13 is licensed for use in infants and children 6 weeks and older as well as in adults 50 years and older. PCV13 is composed of the 7 purified capsular polysaccharide serotypes that were in PCV7 (4, 6B, 9V, 14, 18C, 19F, and 23F) plus another 6 (1, 3, 5, 6A, 7F, and 19A), all individually conjugated to a nontoxic variant of diphtheria toxin carrier protein, CRM_{197} (~34 µg). PCV13 is available in single-dose, prefilled syringes that do not contain latex or preservative but contain 100 µg polysorbate 80, 0.125 mg of aluminum (as aluminum phosphate adjuvant), and 295 µg succinate buffer. PPSV23 is licensed for use in children 2 years and older and adults. PPSV23 is composed of 23 capsular polysaccharides in isotonic saline solution containing 0.25% phenol as preservative. Each available vaccine is recommended in a dose of 0.5 mL to be administered intramuscularly. Immunization with PPSV23 does not induce immunologic memory or boosting with subsequent doses, and no effects on nasopharyngeal carriage or indirect protection of unimmunized groups have been documented.

Routine Immunization With Pneumococcal Conjugate Vaccine. PCV13 is recommended for all infants and children 2 through 59 months of age. For infants, the vaccine should be administered at 2, 4, 6, and 12 through 15 months of age; catch-up immunization is recommended for all children 59 months of age or younger (Table 3.58). Infants should begin the PCV13 immunization series in conjunction with other recommended vaccines at the time of the first regularly scheduled health maintenance visit after 6 weeks of age. Infants of very low birth weight (1500 g or less) should be immunized when they attain a chronologic age of 6 to 8 weeks, regardless of their gestational age at birth. PCV13 can be administered concurrently with all other age-appropriate childhood immunizations using a separate syringe and a separate injection site.

Immunization of Children Unimmunized or Incompletely Immunized With PCV13. For toddlers 2 through 59 months of age who have not received PCV13, the dose schedule is outlined in Table 3.58. PCV13 is recommended for all children younger than 18 years who are at high risk or presumed high risk of acquiring invasive pneumococcal infection (Table 3.59), as defined in Table 3.54 (p 642).

Immunization of Children 6 Through 18 Years of Age With High-Risk Conditions[1]

PPSV23-Naïve Children. For children 6 through 18 years of age who previously have not received PCV13 or PPSV23 and who are at increased risk of IPD because of anatomic or functional asplenia (including sickle cell disease [SCD]), HIV infection, cochlear implant, CSF leak, or other immunocompromising conditions (Table 3.54, p 641), administration of a single PCV13 dose followed by a dose of PPSV23 at least 8 weeks after the PCV13 dose is recommended. A second PPSV23 dose is recommended 5 years after the first PPSV23 dose for children with anatomic or functional asplenia (including SCD), HIV infection, or other immunocompromising conditions. No more than a total of 2 PPSV23

---

[1]Centers for Disease Control and Prevention. Use of 13-valent pneumococcal conjugate vaccine and 23-valent pneumococcal polysaccharide vaccine among children aged 6–18 years with immunocompromising conditions: recommendations of the Advisory Committee on Immunization Practices (ACIP). *MMWR Morb Mortal Wkly Rep*. 2013;62(25):521–524

doses should be administered before 65 years of age.

Previous Vaccination With PPSV23. Children 6 through 18 years of age who previously received ≥1 dose of PPSV23 and no prior PCV13 immunizations and who are at increased risk for IPD because of anatomic or functional asplenia, including SCD, HIV infection, CSF leaks, cochlear implants, or other immuncompromising conditions, should receive a single dose of PCV13 at least 8 weeks after the last PPSV23 dose, even if they have received PCV7 previously. If a second PPSV23 dose is indicated, it should be administered at least 5 years after the first PPSV23 dose; no more than a total of 2 PPSV23 doses should be administered before 65 years of age.

Immunization of Children 2 Through 18 Years of Age Who Are at Increased Risk of IPD With PPSV23 After PCV7 or PCV13.[1] Children 2 years or older with an underlying medical condition increasing the risk of IPD should receive PPSV23 after completing all recommended doses of PCV13. These children should receive a single dose of PPSV23 at least 8 weeks after

Table 3.58. Recommended Schedule for Doses of PCV13, Including Catch-up Immunizations in Previously Unimmunized and Partially Immunized Children 2 Through 59 Months of Age

Age at Examination	Immunization History	Recommended Regimen[a,b]
2 through 6 mo	0 doses	3 doses, 8 wk apart; fourth dose at 12 through 15 mo of age
	1 dose	2 doses, 8 wk apart; fourth dose at 12 through 15 mo of age
	2 doses	1 dose, 8 wk after the most recent dose; fourth dose at 12 through 15 mo of age
7 through 11 mo	0 doses	2 doses, 4 wk apart; third dose at 12 mo of age
	1 or 2 doses before age 7 mo	1 dose at age 7 through 11 mo, with another dose at 12 through 15 mo of age (≥2 mo later)
12 through 23 mo	0 doses	2 doses, ≥8 wk apart
	1 dose at <12 mo	2 doses, ≥8 wk apart
	1 dose at ≥12 mo	1 dose, ≥8 wk after the most recent dose
	2 or 3 doses at <12 mo	1 dose, ≥8 wk after the most recent dose
24 through 59 mo[c]		
Healthy children	Any incomplete schedule	1 dose, ≥8 wk after the most recent dose[c]

PCV13 indicates 13-valent pneumococcal conjugate vaccine.

[a] For children immunized at younger than 12 months, the minimum interval between doses is 4 weeks. Doses administered at 12 months or older should be at least 8 weeks apart.

[b] Centers for Disease Control and Prevention. Licensure of a 13-valent pneumococcal conjugate vaccine (PCV13) and recommendations for use among children. Advisory Committee on Immunization Practices (ACIP). *MMWR Morb Mortal Wkly Rep.* 2010;59(RR-11):1-18

[c] A single dose should be administered to all healthy children 24 through 59 months of age with any incomplete schedule.

[1] American Academy of Pediatrics, Committee on Infectious Diseases. Immunization for *Streptococcus pneumoniae* infections in high-risk children. *Pediatrics.* 2014;134(6):1230–1233

Table 3.59. Recommendations for Pneumococcal Immunization with PCV13 and/or PPSV23 Vaccine for Children at High Risk or Presumed High Risk of Pneumococcal Disease, as Defined in Table 3.54 (p 641)

Age	Previous Dose(s) of Any Pneumococcal Vaccine	Recommendations
23 mo or younger	None	PCV13, as in Table 3.58 (p 648)
24 through 71 mo	4 doses of PCV13	1 dose of PPSV23 vaccine at 24 mo of age, ≥8 wk after last dose of PCV13
24 through 71 mo	3 previous doses of PCV13 before 24 mo of age	1 dose of PCV13 1 dose of PPSV23, ≥8 wk after the last dose of PCV13
24 through 71 mo	<3 doses of PCV13 before 24 mo of age	2 doses of PCV13, ≥8 wk after last dose of PCV13 (if applicable) 1 dose of PPSV23 vaccine, ≥8 wk after the last dose of PCV13
24 through 71 mo	1 dose of PPSV23	2 doses of PCV13, 8 wk apart, beginning at 8 wk after last dose of PPSV23
6 years through 18 years with immunocompromising conditions[a,b]	No previous doses of PCV13 or PPSV23	1 dose of PCV13 followed by 1 dose of PPSV23 at least 8 weeks later and a second dose of PPSV23 5 years after the first[c]
	1 dose of PCV13	1 dose of PPSV23 and a second dose of PPSV23 5 years after the first
	≥1 dose of PPSV23 and no previous dose of PCV13	1 dose of PCV13 (even if PCV7 previously administered) ≥8 weeks after the last PPSV23 dose; if a second PPSV23 dose is indicated, it should be administered ≥5 years after the first PPSV23 dose

PCV13 indicates 13-valent pneumococcal conjugate vaccine; PPSV23, 23-valent pneumococcal polysaccharide vaccine.

[a]Includes anatomic or functional asplenia, HIV infection, cochlear implant, CSF leak, nephrotic syndrome, chronic renal failure, or other immunocompromising conditions.

[b]AAP Committee on Infectious Diseases. Policy Statement—Immunization for *Streptococcus pneumoniae* Infections in High-Risk Children. *Pediatrics*. 2014;134(6):1230–1233

[c]A second dose of PPSV23 5 years after the first dose is recommended only for children who have functional or anatomic asplenia, HIV infection, or other immunocompromising conditions (Table 3.54, p 641). No more than 2 doses of PPSV23 are recommended. All other children with underlying medical conditions should receive 1 dose of PPSV23.

the most recent dose of PCV13. In children who are candidates for solid organ transplantation and in cases when a splenectomy is planned for a patient older than 2 years, PPSV23 should be administered at least 2 weeks before transplant or splenectomy. In candidates for solid organ transplantation not previously vaccinated with PCV13, a dose of PCV13 should be administered, even for those older than 6 years.

If a child previously has received PPSV23, the child also should receive the recommended doses of PCV13. A second dose of PPSV23 is recommended 5 years after the first dose in children with sickle cell disease or functional or anatomic asplenia, HIV infection, or other immunocompromising conditions, but no more than a total of 2 PPSV23 doses should be administered before 65 years of age.

Control of Transmission of Pneumococcal Infection and Invasive Disease Among Children Attending Out-of-Home Child Care. Antimicrobial chemoprophylaxis is not recommended for contacts of children with IPD, regardless of their immunization status.

General Recommendations for Use of Pneumococcal Vaccines.

- Either PPSV23 or PCV13 can be administered concurrently with other childhood vaccines, with one exception. For children for whom quadrivalent meningococcal conjugate vaccine is indicated, MenACWY-D (Menactra [Sanofi Pasteur, Swiftwater, PA]) should not be administered concomitantly OR within 4 weeks of administration of PCV13 immunization, to avoid potential interference with the immune response to PCV13. Concomitant administration of PCV7 and MenACWY-D (Menactra) was shown to interfere with the immune response to some PCV7 serotypes. Because of their high risk for invasive pneumococcal disease, children with functional or anatomic asplenia should not be immunized with MenACWY-D (Menactra) before 2 years of age so that they can complete their PCV13 series; MenACWY-CRM (Menveo [Novartis Vaccines and Diagnostics, Cambridge, MA]) can be used before 2 years of age, however, because it has not been shown to interfere with the immune response to PCV13.

- When elective splenectomy is performed for any reason, immunization with PCV13 should be completed at least 2 weeks before splenectomy. Immunization also should precede initiation of immune-compromising therapy or placement of a cochlear implant by at least 2 weeks. PPSV23 can be administered 8 or more weeks after PCV13 (see Immunization and Other Considerations in Immunocompromised Children, p 72).

- Generally, pneumococcal vaccines should be deferred during pregnancy. Other inactivated or killed vaccines, including licensed polysaccharide vaccines, have been administered safely during pregnancy. However, a pregnant woman who has an underlying medical condition that predisposes to IPD is at risk for severe disease and should receive PPSV23 if it has been >5 years since prior PPSV23 and she has not previously received 2 doses.

Case Reporting. Cases of IPD in children younger than 5 years and drug-resistant infection in all ages should be reported according to state standards. The vast majority of cases of invasive disease cases are caused by non-PCV13 serotypes. Therefore, the overwhelming majority of invasive pneumococcal disease cases occurring among immunized children do not represent vaccine failures. To differentiate PCV13 failure in an immunized child from disease caused by a serotype not included in PCV13, the isolate should be serotyped. A protocol for serotyping pneumococci using PCR is available for state public health laboratories on the CDC Web site (**www.cdc.gov/streplab/downloads/triplex-pcr-us.pdf**). If the invasive isolate is a serotype included in the vaccine, an evaluation of the patient's HIV status and immunologic function should be considered, if the child had received an age-appropriate regimen of PCV13 at least 2 weeks before the onset of the invasive infection.

Adverse Reactions to Pneumococcal Vaccines. Adverse reactions after administration of polysaccharide or conjugate vaccines generally are mild to moderate. The most commonly reported adverse reactions are local reactions of injection site, pain, redness, or swelling in addition to irritability, decreased appetite, or impaired sleep. Fever may occur within the first 1 to 2 days after injections, particularly after use of conjugate vaccine. Other systemic reactions include fatigue, headache, generalized muscle pain, decreased appetite, and chills.

Passive Immunization. Intravenous administration of Immune Globulin is recommended for preventing pneumococcal infection in patients with certain congenital or acquired immunodeficiency diseases, including children with HIV infection who have recurrent pneumococcal infections (**https://aidsinfo.nih.gov/guidelines/html/5/pediatric-oi-prevention-and-treatment-guidelines/397/bacterial-infections**).

Chemoprophylaxis. Daily antimicrobial prophylaxis is recommended for children with functional or anatomic asplenia, regardless of their immunization status, for prevention of pneumococcal disease on the basis of results of a large, multicenter study (see Asplenia and Functional Asplenia, p 88). Oral penicillin V (125 mg, twice a day, for children younger than 3 years; 250 mg, twice a day, for children 3 years and older) is recommended. The study, performed before routine use of PCV7 or PCV13 in the United States, demonstrated that oral penicillin V given to infants and young children with sickle cell disease decreased the incidence of pneumococcal bacteremia by 84% compared with the placebo control group. Although overall incidence of IPD is decreased after penicillin prophylaxis, cases of penicillin-resistant IPD and nasopharyngeal carriage of penicillin-resistant strains in patients with sickle cell disease have increased since these studies were conducted. Parents should be informed that penicillin prophylaxis may not be effective in preventing all cases of IPD. In children with suspected or proven penicillin allergy, erythromycin is an alternative agent for prophylaxis.[1]

The age at which prophylaxis is discontinued is an empiric decision. Most children with sickle cell disease who have received all recommended pneumococcal vaccines for age and who had received penicillin prophylaxis for prolonged periods, who are receiving regular medical attention, and who have not had a previous severe pneumococcal infection or a surgical splenectomy may discontinue prophylactic penicillin safely at 5 years of age. However, they must be counseled to seek medical attention promptly for all febrile events. The duration of prophylaxis for children with asplenia attributable to other causes is unknown. Some experts continue prophylaxis throughout childhood or longer.

Pneumocystis jirovecii Infections

CLINICAL MANIFESTATIONS: Symptomatic infection is extremely rare in healthy people. Disease in immunocompromised infants and children is a respiratory illness characterized by dyspnea, tachypnea, significant hypoxemia, nonproductive cough, and fever. The intensity of these signs and symptoms may vary, and in some immunocompromised children and adults, the onset may be acute and fulminant. Most children with *Pneumocystis* pneumonia are significantly hypoxic. Chest radiographs often show bilateral diffuse interstitial or alveolar disease but may appear normal in early disease. Atypical radiographic findings may include lobar, miliary, cavitary, and nodular lesions. The mortality rate in immunocompromised patients ranges from 5% to 40% in treated patients and approaches 100% without therapy.

ETIOLOGY: Nomenclature for *Pneumocystis* species has evolved. Human *Pneumocystis* is called *Pneumocystis jirovecii*, although the familiar acronym PCP (originally *Pneumocystis carinii* pneumonia) still is used commonly among clinicians. *P jirovecii* is an atypical fungus

---

[1] American Academy of Pediatrics, Committee on Genetics. Health supervision for children with sickle cell disease. *Pediatrics.* 2002;109(3):526–535 (Reaffirmed January 2011, February 2016)

(based on DNA sequence analysis) with several morphologic and biologic similarities to protozoa, including susceptibility to a number of antiprotozoal agents but resistance to most antifungal agents. In addition, the organism exists as 2 distinct morphologic forms: the 5- to 7-μm-diameter cysts, which contain up to 8 intracystic bodies or sporozoites, and the smaller, 1- to 5-μm-diameter trophozoite or trophic form.

EPIDEMIOLOGY: *Pneumocystis* species are ubiquitous in mammals worldwide and have a tropism for respiratory tract epithelium. *Pneumocystis* isolates recovered from mice, rats, and ferrets differ genetically from each other and from human *P jirovecii*. Asymptomatic or mild human infection occurs early in life, with more than 85% of healthy children showing seropositivity by 20 months of age. Animal models and studies of patients with acquired immunodeficiency syndrome (AIDS) do not support the existence of latency, and suggest that disease after the second year of life is likely re-infection.

The single most important factor in susceptibility to PCP is the status of cell-mediated immunity of the host, reflected by a marked decrease in percentage and numbers CD4+ T-lymphocytes, or a decrease in CD4+ T-lymphocyte function. In resource-limited countries and in times of famine, *Pneumocystis* pneumonia (also referred to as PCP, maintaining the same acronym as previously was used for the organism) can occur in epidemics, primarily affecting malnourished infants and children. In industrialized countries, PCP occurs almost entirely in immunocompromised people with deficient cell-mediated immunity, particularly people with human immunodeficiency virus (HIV) infection, recipients of immunosuppressive therapy after solid organ transplantation or during treatment for malignancy, and children with primary immunodeficiency syndromes. Although decreasing in frequency because of effective prophylaxis and antiretroviral therapy, PCP remains one of the most common serious opportunistic infections in infants and children with perinatally acquired HIV infection and adolescents with advanced immunosuppression. Although onset of disease can occur at any age, PCP most commonly occurs in HIV-infected children in the first year of life, with peak incidence at 3 through 6 months of age. In patients with cancer, the disease can occur during remission or relapse of the malignancy.

Animal studies have demonstrated animal-to-animal transmission by the airborne route; human-to-human transmission has been suggested by molecular epidemiology and global clustering of PCP cases in several studies. Outbreaks in hospitals have been reported. Vertical transmission has been postulated but never proven. The period of communicability is unknown.

The **incubation period** is unknown, but outbreaks of PCP in transplant recipients have demonstrated a median of 53 days from exposure to clinically apparent infection.

DIAGNOSTIC TESTS: A definitive diagnosis of PCP is made by visualization of organisms (*Pneumocystis* cysts) in lung tissue or respiratory tract secretion specimens. The most sensitive and specific diagnostic procedures involve specimen collection from open lung biopsy and, in older children, transbronchial biopsy. However, bronchoscopy with bronchoalveolar lavage, induction of sputum in older children and adolescents, and intubation with deep endotracheal aspiration are less invasive, can be diagnostic, and are sensitive in patients with HIV infection, who tend to have heavier organism burdens. Methenamine silver stain, toluidine blue stain, and fluorescently conjugated monoclonal antibody are useful tools for identifying the thick-walled cysts of *P jirovecii*. Sporozoites (within cysts) and trophozoites are identified with Giemsa or modified Wright-Giemsa stain. The sensitivity of all microscopy-based methods depends on the skill of the laboratory technician.

Pneumocystis species cannot be cultivated continuously outside the mammalian lung.

Polymerase chain reaction (PCR) assays have been shown to be highly sensitive and cost-effective with a variety of specimen types from the respiratory tract. However, there are currently no US Food and Drug Administration (FDA)-cleared PCR tests for *P jirovecii*. Because highly sensitive PCR assays may detect colonization with these organisms, results from such assays must be interpreted in the context of clinical presentation.

Limited data suggest that serum 1,3-β-D-glucan (BG) assay, which is available as an FDA-cleared test in the United States for invasive fungal infections, may be a potential marker for *Pneumocystis* infection. This compound is a component of the cell wall of the cyst stage of the organism and may be found in high concentrations in serum of patients infected with *P jirovecii*; however, most other fungi also secrete the compound during infection, so correlation with clinical presentation is imperative.

TREATMENT[1]: The drug of choice is trimethoprim-sulfamethoxazole (TMP-SMX), usually administered intravenously. Oral therapy should be reserved for patients with mild disease who do not have malabsorption or diarrhea, and for patients with a favorable clinical response to initial intravenous therapy. Duration of therapy is 21 days. The rate of adverse reactions to TMP-SMX (eg, rash, neutropenia, anemia, thrombocytopenia, renal toxicity, hepatitis, nausea, vomiting, and diarrhea) is higher in HIV-infected children than in non–HIV-infected patients. It is not necessary to discontinue therapy for mild adverse reactions (eg, vomiting). At least half of patients with more severe reactions that include rash require interruption of therapy. Desensitization to TMP-SMX may be considered after the acute reaction has abated.

Pentamidine, administered intravenously, is an alternative drug for children and adults who cannot tolerate TMP-SMX or who have severe disease and have not responded to TMP-SMX after 4 to 8 days of therapy. The therapeutic efficacy of intravenous pentamidine in adults with PCP is similar to that of TMP-SMX. Pentamidine is associated with a high incidence of adverse reactions, including pancreatitis, diabetes mellitus, renal toxicity, electrolyte abnormalities, hypoglycemia, hyperglycemia, hypotension, cardiac arrhythmias, fever, and neutropenia. Aerosolized pentamidine should not be used for treatment, because its efficacy is limited.

Atovaquone is approved for oral treatment of mild to moderate PCP in adults who are intolerant of TMP-SMX. Experience with use of atovaquone in children is limited, although a study comparing the efficacy of bacterial prophylaxis of atovaquone-azithromycin versus TMP-SMX noted that prevention of PCP was equivalent between the 2 drug regimens. Adverse reactions to atovaquone are limited to rash, nausea, and diarrhea.

Other potentially useful drugs in adults include clindamycin with primaquine (adverse reactions are rash, nausea, and diarrhea), dapsone with trimethoprim (associated with neutropenia, anemia, thrombocytopenia, methemoglobinemia, rash, and transaminase elevation), and trimetrexate with leucovorin. Experience with the use of these combinations in children is limited.

On the basis of studies in both adults and children, a course of corticosteroids is recommended in patients with moderate to severe PCP (as defined by an arterial oxygen

---

[1]Panel on Opportunistic Infections in HIV-Exposed and HIV-Infected Children. Guidelines for the Prevention and Treatment of Opportunistic Infections (OIs) in HIV-Exposed and HIV-Infected Children. 2013. Available at: **https://aidsinfo.nih.gov/guidelines/html/5/pediatric-opportunistic-infection/415/ pneumocystis-jirovecii-pneumonia**

pressure [PaO$_2$] of less than 70 mm Hg in room air or an arterial-alveolar gradient ≥35 mm Hg). The recommended scheduled dosing of oral prednisone during treatment is presented in Table 3.60.

Coinfection with other organisms, such as cytomegalovirus or pneumococcus, has been reported in HIV-infected children. Children with dual infections may have more severe disease.

Chemoprophylaxis. Chemoprophylaxis is highly effective in preventing PCP among high-risk groups. Prophylaxis against a first episode of PCP is indicated for many patients with significant immunosuppression, including people with HIV infection (see Human Immunodeficiency Virus Infection, p 459) and people with primary or acquired cell-mediated immunodeficiency.

In HIV-infected children, risk of PCP is associated with age-specific CD4+ T-lymphocyte cell counts and percentages that define severe immunosuppression (Immune Category 3 [see Table 3.30, p 461]). Because CD4+ T-lymphocyte cell counts and percentages can decline rapidly in HIV-infected infants, prophylaxis for PCP is recommended for all infants born to HIV-infected women beginning at 4 to 6 weeks of age and continuing until 12 months of age unless a diagnosis of HIV has been excluded presumptively or definitively, in which case prophylaxis should be discontinued (see Table 3.61). Children who are HIV infected or whose HIV status is indeterminate should continue prophylaxis throughout the first year of life.

For HIV-infected children aged 12 months or older, PCP prophylaxis should be continued or initiated in the following circumstances:

- Children 1 through 5 years of age with CD4+ T-lymphocyte counts <500 cells/mm^3 or CD4+ T-lymphocyte percentage <15%
- Children 6 years or older with CD4+ T-lymphocyte counts <200 cells/mm^3 or CD4+ T-lymphocyte percentage <15% (see Human Immunodeficiency Virus Infection, Table 3.30, p 461, and Table 3.61).

For HIV-infected children aged 12 months or older, discontinuation of PCP prophylaxis should be considered when, after receiving combination antiretroviral therapy for >6 months, the following parameters have been sustained for >3 consecutive months:

- Children 1 through 5 years of age with CD4+ T-lymphocyte counts ≥500 cells/mm^3 or CD4+ T-lymphocyte percentage ≥15%
- Children aged 6 years or older with CD4+ T-lymphocyte counts ≥200 cells/mm^3 or CD4+ T-lymphocyte percentage ≥15%

HIV-infected children older than 1 year who are not receiving PCP prophylaxis (eg, children not previously identified as infected or children whose PCP prophylaxis was discontinued) should begin or resume prophylaxis if their CD4+ T-lymphocyte cell counts and percentages reach the targeted values for PCP prophylaxis initiation (see Table 3.61).

Table 3.60. Dosing of Oral Prednisone in the Treatment of *Pneumocystis* pneumonia[a]

Age	Days 1–5	Days 6–10	Days 11–21
<13 y	1 mg/kg/dose, twice daily	0.5 mg/kg/dose, twice daily	0.5 mg/kg/dose daily
≥13 y	40 mg, twice daily	40 mg daily	20 mg daily

[a]The maximum doses should not exceed the dose for children older than 13 years.

Table 3.61. Recommendations for *Pneumocystis jirovecii* Pneumonia (PCP) Prophylaxis for Human Immunodeficiency Virus (HIV)-Exposed Infants and Children, by Age and HIV Infection Status[a]

Age and HIV Infection Status	PCP prophylaxis[b]
Birth through 4 to 6 wk of age, HIV exposed or HIV infected	No prophylaxis
4 to 6 wk through 12 mo of age	
HIV infected or indeterminate	Prophylaxis
HIV infection presumptively or definitively excluded[c]	No prophylaxis
1 through 5 y of age, HIV infected	Prophylaxis if: CD4+ T-lymphocyte count is less than 500 cells/μL or percentage is less than 15%[d]
6 y of age or older, HIV infected	Prophylaxis if: CD4+ T-lymphocyte count is less than 200 cells/μL or percentage is less than 15%[d]

[a]Guidelines for prevention and treatment of opportunistic infections in HIV-exposed and HIV-infected children. Recommendations from the National Institutes of Health, Centers for Disease Control and Prevention, the HIV Medicine Association of the Infectious Diseases Society of America, the Pediatric Infectious Diseases Society, and the American Academy of Pediatrics. *Pediatr Infect Dis J.* 2013;32(Suppl 2):i-KK4. Available at: **https://aidsinfo.nih.gov/guidelines/html/5/pediatric-opportunistic-infection/415/pneumocystis-jirovecii-pneumonia**

[b]Children who have had PCP should receive lifelong ("secondary") PCP prophylaxis unless/until their CD4+ T-lymphocyte cell counts and percentages achieve and maintain designated age-specific values greater than those indicative of severe immunosuppression (Immune Category 3) for at least 6 months (see Human Immunodeficiency Virus Infection, Table 3.30, p 461).

[c]In nonbreastfeeding HIV-exposed infants with no positive virologic test results or other laboratory or clinical evidence of HIV infection, HIV presumptively can be excluded on the basis of 2 negative virologic test results, 1 performed at 2 weeks of age or older and 1 performed at 4 weeks of age or older, on 1 negative virologic test result performed at 8 weeks of age or older, or on 1 negative HIV antibody test performed at 6 months of age or older. HIV definitively can be excluded on the basis of 2 negative virologic test results, 1 performed at 4 weeks of age or older and 1 performed at 4 months of age or older, or on 2 negative HIV antibody test results from 2 separate specimens obtained at 6 months of age or older (see Human Immunodeficiency Virus Infection, p 459).

[d]Prophylaxis should be considered on a case-by-case basis for children who might otherwise be at risk of PCP, such as children with rapidly declining CD4+ T-lymphocyte cell counts or percentages or children with Clinical Category C status of HIV infection.

In patients with AIDS, prophylaxis should be initiated at the end of therapy for acute infection and should be continued until 6 months after CD4+ T-lymphocyte cell count and percentage exceed the values designated as requiring prophylaxis (see Table 3.61) or lifelong if CD4+ T-lymphocyte cells do not exceed these thresholds in response to antiretroviral therapy.

Prophylaxis for PCP is recommended for children who have received hematopoietic stem cell transplants (HSCTs)[1] or solid organ transplants; children with hematologic

---

[1]Center for International Blood and Marrow Research; National Marrow Donor program; European Blood and Marrow Transplant Group; American Society of Blood and Marrow Transplantation; Canadian Blood and Marrow Transplant Group; Infectious Diseases Society of America; Society for Healthcare Epidemiology of America; Association of Medical Microbiology and Infectious Disease Canada; Centers for Disease Control and Prevention. Guidelines for preventing infectious complications among hematopoietic cell transplant recipients: a global perspective. *Biol Blood Marrow Transplant.* 2009;15(10):1143–1238

malignancies (eg, leukemia or lymphoma) and some nonhematologic malignancies; children with severe cell-mediated immunodeficiency, including children who received adrenocorticotropic hormone for treatment of infantile spasm; and children who otherwise are immunocompromised and who have had a previous episode of PCP. For this diverse group of immunocompromised hosts, the risk of PCP varies with duration and intensity of chemotherapy, with other immunosuppressive therapies, with coinfection with immunosuppressive viruses (eg, cytomegalovirus), and local epidemiologic rates of PCP. Guidelines for allogeneic HSCT recipients recommend that PCP prophylaxis be initiated at engraftment (or before engraftment, if engraftment is delayed) and administered for at least 6 months. It should be continued in all children receiving ongoing or intensified immunosuppressive therapy (eg, prednisone or cyclosporine) or in children with chronic graft-versus-host disease. Guidelines for PCP prophylaxis for solid organ transplant recipients are less definitive, but some authorities suggest durations ranging from 6 months to 1 year following renal transplantation, and from 1 year to lifelong following heart, lung, liver, and intestinal transplantation.

The recommended drug regimen for PCP prophylaxis for all immunocompromised patients is TMP-SMX. Acceptable dosing intervals and schedules are presented in Table 3.62. For patients who cannot tolerate TMP-SMX, alternative oral choices include atovaquone or dapsone. Atovaquone is effective and safe but expensive. Dapsone is effective and inexpensive but associated with more serious adverse effects than atovaquone. Aerosolized pentamidine is recommended for children who cannot tolerate TMP-SMX, atovaquone, or dapsone and are old enough to use a Respirgard II nebulizer. Intravenous pentamidine has been used but generally is not recommended for prophylaxis. Other drug combinations with potential for prophylaxis include pyrimethamine plus dapsone plus leucovorin or pyrimethamine-sulfadoxine. Experience with these drugs in adults and children for this indication is limited. These agents should be considered only in situations in which recommended regimens are not tolerated or cannot be used for other reasons.

ISOLATION OF THE HOSPITALIZED PATIENT: Standard precautions are recommended. Some experts recommend that because of the theoretical risk for transmission, patients with PCP should not share a room with other immunocompromised patients, especially patients who are not receiving PCP prophylaxis. Data are insufficient to support this recommendation as standard practice.

CONTROL MEASURES: Appropriate therapy for infected patients and prophylaxis in immunocompromised patients are the only available means of control. Detailed guidelines for children, adolescents, and adults infected with HIV have been issued by the Centers for Disease Control and Prevention and the Infectious Diseases Society of America.[1,2]

---

[1] Panel on Opportunistic Infections in HIV-Exposed and HIV-Infected Children. Guidelines for the Prevention and Treatment of Opportunistic Infections (OIs) in HIV-Exposed and HIV-Infected Children. 2013. Available at: **https://aidsinfo.nih.gov/guidelines/html/5/pediatric-opportunistic-infection/415/pneumocystis-jirovecii-pneumonia**

[2] Panel on Opportunistic Infections in HIV-Infected Adults and Adolescents. Guidelines for the prevention and treatment of opportunistic infections in HIV-infected adults and adolescents: recommendations from the Centers for Disease Control and Prevention, the National Institutes. Available at: **https://aidsinfo.nih.gov/guidelines/html/4/adult-and-adolescent-opportunistic-infection/321/pcp**

Table 3.62. Drug Regimens for *Pneumocystis jirovecii* Pneumonia Prophylaxis for Children 4 Weeks and Older[a]

Recommended daily dose:

Trimethoprim-sulfamethoxazole (trimethoprim, 5–10 mg/kg per day; and sulfamethoxazole, 25–50 mg/kg per day, orally). The total daily dose should not exceed 320 mg TMP and 1600 mg SMX.

Acceptable dosing intervals and schedules:

- In divided doses twice daily, given 3 days per week on consecutive days or on alternate days
- In divided doses twice daily, given 2 days per week on consecutive days or on alternate days
- Total dose once daily, given 7 days per week

Alternative regimens if trimethoprim-sulfamethoxazole is not tolerated:

- **Dapsone (children 1 mo or older)**

  2 mg/kg (maximum 100 mg), orally, once a day or 4 mg/kg (maximum 200 mg), orally, every week

- **Aerosolized pentamidine (children 5 y or older)**

  300 mg, inhaled monthly via Respirgard II nebulizer

- **Atovaquone**

  ♦ **children 1 through 3 mo of age and older than 24 mo through 12 y of age:** 30–40 mg/kg (maximum 1500 mg), orally, once a day

  ♦ **children 4 through 24 mo of age:** 45 mg/kg (maximum 1500 mg), orally, once a day

  ♦ **children older than 12 y:** 1500 mg, orally, once a day

[a]Panel on Opportunistic Infections in HIV-Exposed and HIV-Infected Children. Guidelines for the Prevention and Treatment of Opportunistic Infections (OIs) in HIV-Exposed and HIV-Infected Children. 2013. Available at: **https://aidsinfo.nih.gov/guidelines/html/5/pediatric-opportunistic-infection/415/pneumocystis-jirovecii-pneumonia.**

Poliovirus Infections

CLINICAL MANIFESTATIONS: Approximately 70% of poliovirus infections in susceptible children are asymptomatic. Nonspecific illness with low-grade fever and sore throat (minor illness) occurs in approximately 25% of infected people, and viral meningitis (nonparalytic polio), sometimes accompanied by paresthesias, occurs in 1% to 5% of patients a few days after the minor illness has resolved. Rapid onset of asymmetric acute flaccid paralysis with areflexia of the involved limb (paralytic poliomyelitis) occurs in fewer than 1% of infections, with residual paresis in approximately two thirds of patients. Classical paralytic polio begins with a minor illness characterized by fever, sore throat, headache, nausea, constipation, and/or malaise for several days, followed by a symptom-free period of 1 to 3 days. Rapid onset of paralysis then follows. Typically, paralysis is asymmetric and affects the proximal muscles more than the distal muscles. Cranial nerve involvement (bulbar poliomyelitis) and paralysis of the diaphragm and intercostal muscles may lead to impaired respiration requiring assisted ventilation. Sensation usually is intact. The cerebrospinal fluid (CSF) profile is characteristic of viral meningitis, with mild pleocytosis and lymphocytic predominance.

Adults who contracted paralytic poliomyelitis during childhood may develop the noninfectious postpolio syndrome 15 to 40 years later, characterized by slow and irreversible exacerbation of weakness in the muscle groups affected during the original infection. Muscle and joint pain also are common manifestations. The estimated incidence of post-polio syndrome in poliomyelitis survivors is 25% to 40%.

ETIOLOGY: Polioviruses are classified as members of the family *Picornaviridae*, genus *Enterovirus*, in the species enterovirus C, and include 3 serotypes. They are nonenveloped, positive-sense, single-stranded RNA viruses that are highly stable in a liquid environment. Acute paralytic disease may be caused by naturally occurring (wild) polioviruses, by oral poliovirus (OPV) vaccine viruses that cause rare cases of vaccine-associated paralytic poliomyelitis (VAPP) in vaccine recipients or their close contacts, or by circulating vaccine-derived polioviruses (cVDPVs) that have acquired virulence properties (neurovirulence and transmissibility) that are indistinguishable from naturally occurring polioviruses as a result of sustained person-to-person circulation in the absence of adequate population immunity. People with primary B-lymphocyte immunodeficiencies are at increased risk both of VAPP and of chronic infection (immunodeficiency-associated vaccine-derived polioviruses, or iVDPVs) from vaccine virus. With ongoing progress in the World Health Organization (WHO) Global Polio Eradication Initiative, more cases of paralytic disease are caused by vaccine-related viruses (VAPP and cVDPV) than by wild polioviruses.

EPIDEMIOLOGY: Humans are the only natural reservoir for poliovirus. Spread is by contact with feces and/or respiratory secretions. Infection is more common in infants and young children and occurs at an earlier age among children living in poor hygienic conditions. In temperate climates, poliovirus infections are most common during summer and autumn; in the tropics, the seasonal pattern is less pronounced.

The last reported case of poliomyelitis attributable to indigenously acquired, naturally occurring wild poliovirus in the United States occurred in 1979 during an outbreak among unimmunized people that resulted in 10 paralytic cases. With the exception of very rare imported cases, all poliomyelitis cases acquired in the United States have been attributable to VAPP, which, until 1998, occurred in an average of 6 to 8 people annually. Fewer VAPP cases were reported in 1998 and 1999, after a shift in US immunization policy in 1997 from use of OPV to a sequential inactivated poliovirus (IPV) vaccine/OPV schedule. Implementation of an all-IPV vaccine schedule in 2000 halted the occurrence of VAPP cases in the United States.

Circulation of indigenous wild poliovirus strains ceased in the United States several decades ago, and the risk of contact with imported wild polioviruses and cVDPV viruses has decreased in parallel with the success of the global eradication program. Of the 3 poliovirus serotypes, type 2 wild poliovirus has been declared eradicated globally by the Global Certification Commission, with the last naturally occurring case detected in 1999 in India. No cases of type 3 wild poliovirus have been detected since 2012, suggesting this type may also be eradicated. Type 1 poliovirus now accounts for all polio cases attributable to wild poliovirus. Because the only source of disease from type 2 poliovirus is related to vaccine use, the world switched from trivalent OPV (tOPV) to bivalent OPV (bOPV) on April 1, 2016, thus ending all routine immunization with live type 2 poliovirus-containing oral vaccines. Similarly, following this vaccine change, the only remaining risk of type 2 infection would come from vaccine manufacturers and laboratories. For this reason, containment of all type 2 poliovirus infectious and potentially infectious materials into accredited essential facilities has been initiated globally.

Communicability of poliovirus is greatest shortly before and after onset of clinical illness, when the virus is present in the throat and excreted in high concentrations in feces.

Virus persists in the throat for approximately 1 to 2 weeks after onset of illness and is excreted in feces for 3 to 6 weeks. Patients potentially are contagious as long as fecal excretion persists. In recipients of OPV, virus also persists in the throat for 1 to 2 weeks and is excreted in feces for several weeks, although in rare cases, excretion for more than 2 months can occur. Immunocompromised patients with significant primary B-lymphocyte immune deficiencies have excreted iVDPV for periods of more than 25 years.

The **incubation period of nonparalytic poliomyelitis** is 3 to 6 days. For the onset of poliomyelitis, the **incubation period to paralysis** usually is 7 to 21 days (range, 3–35 days).

DIAGNOSTIC TESTS: Poliovirus can be detected in specimens from the pharynx and feces, less commonly from urine, and rarely from CSF by isolation in cell culture. The relatively low sensitivity of isolation in cell culture from cerebrospinal fluid is likely attributable to low viral load, presence of neutralizing antibodies, and an inadequate volume of cerebrospinal fluid for optimal recovery on cell culture. Fecal material and pharyngeal swab specimens are most likely to yield virus in cell culture.

The diagnostic test of choice for confirming poliovirus disease is viral culture of stool specimens and throat swab specimens obtained early in the course of illness as possible. There currently are FDA-cleared nucleic acid amplification tests (NAATs) for enteroviruses from cerebrospinal fluid and at least one multiplexed assay that detects enteroviruses, in addition to a number of other bacterial and viral agents causing meningitis or encephalitis. Such commonly used molecular tests for enteroviruses will detect poliovirus but will not differentiate poliovirus from other enteroviruses and, therefore, are insufficient to demonstrate that poliovirus is the etiology of disease. In these situations, additional virus testing will be necessary to confirm the diagnosis of poliovirus-related disease. Interpretation of acute and convalescent serologic test results can be difficult because of high levels of population immunity.

Real-time reverse transcriptase-polymerase chain reaction (RT-PCR) assays generally have sensitivity that is nearly comparable to or better than cell culture and may be more likely to identify polioviruses in CSF. Two or more stool and throat swab specimens for enterovirus isolation or detection by RT-PCR should be obtained at least 24 hours apart from patients with suspected paralytic poliomyelitis as early in the course of illness as possible, ideally within 14 days of onset of symptoms. Poliovirus may be excreted intermittently, and a single negative test result does not rule out infection.

Identification and typing of poliovirus isolated in cell culture historically was performed by neutralization assay. Molecular methods have largely replaced neutralization for identification and typing to differentiate wild-type from vaccine-like virus strains.

Because OPV no longer is available in the United States, the chance of exposure to vaccine-type polioviruses has become remote. Therefore, if a poliovirus is isolated in the United States, the isolate should be reported immediately to the state health department and sent to the Centers for Disease Control and Prevention (CDC) through the state health department for further testing. Paralytic poliomyelitis and detection of polioviruses are nationally reportable conditions in the United States.

TREATMENT: Supportive.

ISOLATION OF THE HOSPITALIZED PATIENT: In addition to standard precautions, contact precautions are indicated for infants and young children for the duration of hospitalization.

CONTROL MEASURES:
Immunization of Infants and Children.

Vaccines. Of the 2 poliovirus vaccine types, only IPV is available in the United States. IPV contains the 3 serotypes, which are grown in Vero cells or human diploid cells and inactivated with formaldehyde. IPV also is available in combination with other childhood vaccines (see Table 1.12, p 37). As of May 16, 2016, bivalent live attenuated oral poliovirus vaccine (bOPV), which contains types 1 and 3 poliovirus serotypes, is now the primary vaccine used in low- and middle-income countries. bOPV is produced in monkey kidney cells or human diploid cells.

Immunogenicity and Efficacy. Both IPV and OPV, in their recommended schedules, are highly immunogenic and effective in preventing poliomyelitis. Administration of IPV results in seroconversion in 95% or more of vaccine recipients to each of the 3 serotypes after 2 doses and results in seroconversion in 99% to 100% of recipients after 3 doses. Immunity probably is lifelong. Following exposure to live polioviruses, most IPV-immunized children will excrete virus from stool but not from the oropharynx. Stool excretion quantities and duration are somewhat reduced compared with shedding from unimmunized people. Immunization with 3 or more doses of OPV induces excellent serum antibody responses and a variable degree of intestinal immunity against poliovirus reinfection. A 3-dose series of OPV, as formerly used in the United States, results in sustained, probably lifelong immunity. After 3 doses of OPV in tropical countries, seroconversion rates are lower than in the United States, likely because of interference by other enteric pathogens with the replication of vaccine strains at the level of the gastrointestinal tract or other enteropathies.

Administration With Other Vaccines. Either IPV or OPV may be administered concurrently with other routinely recommended childhood vaccines (see Simultaneous Administration of Multiple Vaccines, p 35). For administration of combination vaccines containing IPV (see Table 1.12, p 37) with other vaccines and interchangeability of the combined vaccine with other vaccine products, see Pertussis (p 620), Hepatitis B (p 401), *Haemophilus influenzae* Infections (p 367), and Pneumococcal Infections (p 639).

Adverse Reactions. Serious adverse events associated with use of IPV are extremely rare. Because IPV may contain trace amounts of streptomycin, neomycin, and polymyxin B, allergic reactions are possible in recipients with hypersensitivity to one or more of these antimicrobial agents.

OPV can cause VAPP. Before exclusive use of IPV in the United States beginning in 2000, the overall risk of VAPP associated with OPV was approximately 1 case per 2.4 million doses of OPV distributed. The rate of VAPP following the first dose, including vaccine recipient and contact cases, was approximately 1 case per 750 000 doses.

Schedule.[1] Four doses of IPV are recommended for routine immunization of all infants and children in the United States.

Refugee and Immigrant Children. Refugee and immigrant children should meet recommendations of the Advisory Committee on Immunization Practices of the CDC for poliovirus vaccination, which include protection against all 3 poliovirus types by age-appropriate

---

[1]Centers for Disease Control and Prevention. Updated recommendations of the Advisory Committee on Immunization Practices (ACIP) regarding routine poliovirus vaccination. *MMWR Morb Mortal Wkly Rep.* 2009;58(30):829–830

vaccination with IPV or tOPV (trivalent oral polio vaccine). Some countries have provided mOPV (monovalent polio vaccine) or bOPV (bivalent oral polio vaccine) during polio vaccination campaigns after April 1, 2016. Only written documentation of receipt of IPV or tOPV constitutes proof of vaccination according to the US polio vaccination recommendations. If OPV was administered prior to April 1, 2016, OPV can be counted as tOPV. If OPV was administered after April 1, 2016, it may not be counted as tOPV unless the written documentation denotes that it is tOPV. For children incompletely immunized with tOPV, the series should be completed with IPV according to the catch-up schedule outlined below. In the absence of adequate written vaccination records, vaccination or revaccination in accordance with the age-appropriate IPV schedule for the United States is recommended. Serologic testing to assess immunity no longer is available and, therefore, no longer is recommended by the CDC.[1]

- The first 2 doses of the 4-dose IPV series should be administered at 2-month intervals beginning at 2 months of age (minimum age, 6 weeks), and a third dose is recommended at 6 through 18 months of age. Doses may be administered at 4-week intervals when accelerated protection is indicated.
- Administration of the third dose at 6 months of age has the potential advantage of enhancing the likelihood of completion of the primary series and does not compromise seroconversion.
- A fourth and final dose in the series should be administered at 4 years or older and at a minimum interval of 6 months from the third dose.
- The final dose in the IPV series at 4 years or older should be administered regardless of the number of previous doses; a fourth dose is not necessary if the third dose was administered at 4 years or older and a minimum of 6 months after the second dose.
- When IPV is administered in combination with other vaccines at 2, 4, 6, and 12 through 15 months of age, it is necessary to administer a fifth and final dose of IPV at 4 years or older. The minimum interval from dose 4 to dose 5 should be at least 6 months.
- If a child misses an IPV dose at 4 through 6 years of age, the child should receive a booster dose as soon as feasible.

OPV remains the vaccine of choice for global eradication, although the Strategic Advisory Group of Experts (SAGE) on Immunization of the WHO has recommended that all countries currently using OPV introduce at least 1 dose of IPV into their routine immunization schedules in preparation for stopping all use of OPV after global certification that all wild polioviruses have been eradicated.[2]

Children Incompletely Immunized. Children who have not received the recommended doses of poliovirus vaccines on schedule should receive sufficient doses of IPV to complete the immunization series for their age (see **http://aapredbook.aappublications.org/site/resources/izschedules.xhtml**).

Vaccine Recommendations for Adults. Most adults residing in the United States are presumed

[1]Marin M, Patel M, Oberste S, Pallansch MA. Guidance for assessment of poliovirus vaccination status and vaccination of children who have received poliovirus vaccine outside the United States. *MMWR Morb Mortal Wkly Rep.* 2017;66(1):23–25

[2]Orenstein WA, Seib KG; American Academy of Pediatrics, Committee on Infectious Diseases. Eradicating polio: how the world's pediatricians can help stop this crippling illness forever. *Pediatrics.* 2015;135(1):196–202

to be immune to poliovirus from previous immunization and have only a small risk of exposure to wild poliovirus in the United States. However, immunization is recommended for adults who may be traveling to areas where polio infection occurs. Travelers to polio-affected areas should receive polio vaccination or a booster polio vaccination before travel according to CDC guidance (**wwwnc.cdc.gov/travel/yellowbook/2014/chapter-3-infectious-diseases-related-to-travel/poliomyelitis**). Countries are considered to have active wild poliovirus circulation if they have ongoing endemic circulation, active polio outbreaks, or environmental evidence of active wild poliovirus circulation. Travelers working in health care settings, refugee camps, or other humanitarian aid settings in these countries may be at particular risk.

For unimmunized adults, primary immunization with IPV is recommended. Adults without documentation of vaccination history should be considered unimmunized. Two doses of IPV should be administered at intervals of 1 to 2 months (4–8 weeks); a third dose is administered 6 to 12 months after the second dose. If time does not allow 3 doses of IPV to be administered according to the recommended schedule before protection is required, the following alternatives are recommended:

- If protection is not needed until 8 weeks or more, 3 doses of IPV should be administered at least 4 weeks apart (eg, at weeks 0, 4, and 8).
- If protection is not needed for 4 to 8 weeks, 2 doses of IPV should be administered at least 4 weeks apart (eg, at weeks 0 and 4).
- If protection is needed in fewer than 4 weeks, a single dose of IPV should be administered.

The remaining doses of IPV to complete the primary immunization schedule should be administered subsequently at the recommended intervals if the person remains at an increased risk.

Recommendations in other circumstances are as follows:

- **Incompletely immunized adults.** Adults who previously received less than a full primary series of OPV or IPV should receive the remaining required doses of IPV regardless of the interval since the last dose and the type of vaccine that was received previously.
- **Adults who are at an increased risk of exposure to wild or vaccine-derived polioviruses and who previously completed primary immunization with OPV or IPV.** These adults can receive a single dose of IPV. Available data do not indicate the need for more than a single lifetime booster dose with IPV.

Travelers also may be affected by new WHO and CDC polio vaccination recommendations for people residing for 4 or more consecutive weeks in countries with ongoing poliovirus transmission and who are leaving those countries to go to polio-free countries.[1]

- All residents and long-term visitors (defined as a duration of more than 4 weeks) should receive an additional dose of IPV between 4 weeks and 12 months before international travel and have the dose documented.
- Residents and long-term visitors who currently are in those countries who must travel with fewer than 4 weeks' notice and have not been vaccinated with OPV or IPV within the previous 4 week to 12 months should receive a dose at least by the time of departure.

---

[1]Centers for Disease Control and Prevention. Interim CDC guidance for polio vaccination for travel to and from countries affected by wild poliovirus. *MMWR Morb Mortal Wkly Rep*. 2014;63(27):591–594

The list of countries affected by this new recommendation can be found online (**www. polioeradication.org/infectedcountres/PolioEmergency.aspx**).

Precautions and Contraindications to Immunization.

Immunocompromised People. Immunocompromised patients, including people with human immunodeficiency virus (HIV) infection; combined immunodeficiency; abnormalities of immunoglobulin synthesis (ie, antibody deficiency syndromes); leukemia, lymphoma, or generalized malignant neoplasm; or people receiving immunosuppressive therapy with pharmacologic agents (see Immunization and Other Considerations in Immunocompromised Children, p 72) or radiation therapy should receive IPV. OPV should not be used. The immune response to IPV in an immunocompromised patient may vary based on their level of immunosuppression.

Household Contacts of Immunocompromised People or People With Altered Immune States, Immunosuppression Attributable to Therapy for Other Disease, or Known HIV Infection. IPV is recommended for these people, and OPV should not be used. If OPV inadvertently is introduced into a household of an immunocompromised or HIV-infected person, close contact between the patient and the OPV recipient should be minimized for approximately 4 to 6 weeks after immunization. Household members should be counseled on practices that will minimize exposure of the immunocompromised or HIV-infected person to excreted poliovirus vaccine. These practices include exercising hand hygiene after contact with the child by all and avoiding diaper changing by the immunosuppressed person.

Pregnancy. Immunization during pregnancy generally should be avoided. However, there is no evidence that IPV is unsafe in pregnant women or their developing fetuses. If immediate protection against poliomyelitis is needed, IPV is recommended.

Hypersensitivity or Anaphylactic Reactions to IPV Vaccine or Antimicrobial Agents Contained in IPV. IPV is contraindicated for people who have experienced an anaphylactic reaction after a previous dose of IPV attributable to any component of the vaccine.

Breastfeeding. Breastfeeding and mild diarrhea are not contraindications to IPV or OPV administration.

Reporting of Adverse Events After Immunization. All cases of VAPP and other serious adverse events associated temporally with poliovirus vaccine should be reported (see Vaccine Adverse Event Reporting System [VAERS], p 45).

Case Reporting and Investigation. A suspected case of poliomyelitis or a nonparalytic poliovirus infection, regardless of whether the virus is suspected to be wild poliovirus or VDPV, should be considered a **public health emergency** and reported immediately to the state health department, which then results in an immediate epidemiologic investigation. Poliomyelitis should be considered in the differential diagnosis of all cases of acute flaccid paralysis, including Guillain-Barré syndrome, transverse myelitis, and acute flaccid myelitis (acute neurologic illness of unknown etiology associated with limb weakness in children; see Enterovirus [Nonpoliovirus], p 331).[1] If the course is compatible clinically with poliomyelitis, specimens should be obtained for virologic studies (see Diagnostic Tests, p 659). If evidence implicates wild poliovirus or a VDPV infection, an intensive investigation will be conducted, and a public health decision will be made about the need for supplementary immunizations, choice of vaccine, and other actions. Because the vast majority of people who transmit poliovirus either are clinically asymptomatic or have a

---

[1] Centers for Disease Control and Prevention. Acute neurologic illness of unknown etiology in children—Colorado, August–September 2014. *MMWR Morb Mortal Wkly.* 2014;63(40):901–902

minor illness, the source person who transmitted virus to the patient with paralytic polio may be very difficult to identify (eg, there may be no known contact with someone who traveled to an area with endemic or epidemic polio). Therefore, pediatricians should be guided by the clinical presentation in deciding whether a child with acute paralysis might have polio and might warrant reporting the suspected case to public health authorities. It is important to collect 2 stool specimens 24 hours apart for detection of polio. The Centers for Disease Control and Prevention has developed a comprehensive Web site for assessing and managing patients with acute flaccid myelitis as part of its emerging infection surveillance efforts (eg, West Nile virus, enterovirus D68) and in preparation for the final efforts to eradicate polioviruses worldwide (**www.cdc.gov/acute-flaccid-myelitis/hcp/index.html**).

Polyomaviruses (BK, JC, and Other Polyomaviruses)

CLINICAL MANIFESTATIONS: BK virus (BKV) infection and JC virus (JCV) infection in humans usually occur in childhood and seemingly result in lifelong persistence. Primary infection with BKV in immunocompetent children generally is asymptomatic. However, because of the tropism of BKV for the genitourinary tract epithelium, it may occasionally cause asymptomatic hematuria or cystitis in healthy children. More than 90% of adults are seropositive for BKV. BKV is more likely to cause disease in immunocompromised people, including hemorrhagic cystitis in hematopoietic stem cell transplant recipients and interstitial nephritis and ureteral stenosis in renal transplant recipients. The primary symptom of BKV-associated hemorrhagic cystitis among immunocompromised children is painful hematuria. Passage of blood clots in the urine and secondary obstructive nephropathy can occur in patients with BKV-associated hemorrhagic cystitis. BKV-associated nephropathy occurs in 3% to 8% of renal transplant recipients and less frequently in other solid organ transplant recipients. BKV-associated nephropathy should be suspected in any renal transplant recipient with allograft dysfunction. More than half of renal allograft patients with BKV-associated nephropathy may experience allograft loss.

JCV is the cause of progressive multifocal leukoencephalopathy (PML), a demyelinating disease of the central nervous system that occurs in severely immunocompromised patients, including patients with acquired immunodeficiency syndrome (AIDS), patients receiving intensive chemotherapy, bone marrow or solid organ transplant recipients, and patients receiving various monoclonal antibody therapies for treatment of autoimmune, oncologic, and neurologic diseases. PML, the only known disease caused by JCV, occurs in approximately 3% to 5% of untreated adults with AIDS but is rare in children with AIDS. Symptoms include cognitive disturbance, hemiparesis, ataxia, cranial nerve dysfunction, and aphasia. Lytic infection of oligodendrocytes by JCV is the primary mechanism of pathogenesis for PML. In the absence of restored T-lymphocyte function, PML almost always is fatal. PML is an AIDS-defining illness in human immunodeficiency virus (HIV)-infected people.[1] Most adults are infected by JCV, with infections being acquired

[1] Guidelines for prevention and treatment of opportunistic infections in HIV-exposed and HIV-infected children. Recommendations from the National Institutes of Health, Centers for Disease Control and Prevention, the HIV Medicine Association of the Infectious Diseases Society of America, the Pediatric Infectious Diseases Society, and the American Academy of Pediatrics. *Pediatr Infect Dis J.* 2013;32(Suppl 2):i-KK4. Available at: **https://aidsinfo.nih.gov/guidelines/html/5/pediatric-opportunistic-infection/416/progressive-multifocal-leukoencephalopathy**

during adolescence and early adulthood.

To date, 13 polyomaviruses have been detected in humans, but only a few have been associated with disease, including BK and JC viruses. The Merkel cell polyomavirus (MCPyV) has been detected in >80% of Merkel cell carcinomas, which are rare neuroendocrine tumors of the skin. The trichodysplasia spinulosa-associated polyomavirus (TSPyV) has been identified in tissue from patients with trichodysplasia spinulosa, a rare follicular disease of immunocompromised patients that primarily affects the face. The KI polyomavirus (KIPyV) and WU polyomavirus (WUPyV) have been identified in respiratory tract secretions, primarily in association with known pathogenic viruses of the respiratory tract. Human polyomaviruses 6 and 7 (HPyV6 and HPyV7) have been detected as asymptomatic inhabitants of human skin. Human polyomavirus 9 (HPyV9) has been detected in the serum of some renal transplant recipients. The natural history, prevalence, and pathogenic potential of these recently discovered human polyomaviruses have not yet been established.

ETIOLOGY: Polyomaviruses are members of the family *Polyomaviridae*, which has a single genus, *Polyomavirus*. They are nonenveloped viruses with a circular double-stranded DNA genome with icosahedral symmetry of the capsid ranging 40 to 50 nm in diameter. The genome of the polyomaviruses is approximately 5 kilobase pairs in length and encodes 5 major proteins: 3 for capsid proteins VP1, VP2, and VP3, and 2 for large T and small t antigens that facilitate viral genome replication and transformation. One of the biological characteristics of the polyomaviruses is the maintenance of a chronic viral infection in their host with little or no symptoms. Symptomatic disease caused by human polyomavirus infections almost exclusively occurs in immunosuppressed people.

EPIDEMIOLOGY: Humans are the only known natural hosts for BKV and JCV. The mode of transmission of BKV and JCV is uncertain, but the respiratory route and the oral route by water or food have been postulated for their transmission. BKV and JCV are ubiquitous in the human population, with BKV infection occurring in early childhood and JCV infection occurring primarily in adolescence and adulthood. BKV persists in the kidney and gastrointestinal tract of healthy subjects, with urinary excretion occurring in 3% to 5% of healthy adults. JCV persists in the kidney and brain of healthy people. The prevalence of urinary excretion of JCV increases with age.

DIAGNOSTIC TESTS: Detection of BKV T-antigen by immunohistochemical analysis of renal biopsy material is the gold standard for diagnosis of BKV-associated nephropathy, but nucleic acid-based polymerase chain reaction (PCR) assays are the most sensitive tools for rapid viral screening for polyomaviruses and quantification of viral load. Prospective monitoring of BK viral load in plasma using PCR commonly is used after renal transplantation to monitor for BKV-associated nephropathy. Detection of BKV nucleic acid in plasma by PCR assay is associated with an increased risk of BKV-associated nephropathy, especially when BKV viral loads exceed 10 000 genomes/mL. However, detection of BKV in urine of renal transplant recipients is common and does not predict BKV disease after renal transplantation. Both BKV and JCV can be propagated in cell culture. However, culture plays no role in the laboratory diagnosis of infection attributable to these agents. Antibody assays commonly are used to detect the presence of specific antibodies against individual viruses.

The diagnosis of BKV-associated hemorrhagic cystitis is made clinically when other causes of urinary tract bleeding are excluded. Among hematopoietic stem cell transplant recipients, detection of BKV by PCR in urine is common (more than 50%), but BKV-associated hemorrhagic cystitis is much less common (10%–15%). Prolonged urinary shedding of BKV and detection of BKV in plasma after hematopoietic stem cell transplantation has been associated with increased risk of developing BKV-associated hemorrhagic cystitis. Urine cytologic testing may suggest urinary shedding of BKV on the basis of presence of decoy cells, which resemble renal carcinoma cells. However, decoy cells do not have high sensitivity or specificity for BKV disease.

A confirmed diagnosis of PML attributable to JCV requires a compatible clinical syndrome and magnetic resonance imaging or computed tomographic findings showing lesions in the brain white matter coupled with brain biopsy findings. JCV can be demonstrated by in situ hybridization, electron microscopy, or immunohistochemistry of brain biopsy or autopsy material. However, there are no FDA-cleared NAATs for detection of JCV. Diagnosis of PML can be facilitated when JCV DNA is detected in cerebrospinal fluid by a nucleic acid amplification test, which may obviate the need for a brain biopsy. Early in the course of PML, false-negative PCR assay results have been reported, so repeat testing is warranted when clinical suspicion of PML is high. Measurement of JCV DNA concentrations in cerebrospinal fluid samples may be a useful marker for managing PML in patients with AIDS who are receiving combination antiretroviral therapy.

TREATMENT: Multiple studies evaluating treatment options (eg, cidofovir, leflunomide, adoptive cellular immunotherapy) are ongoing **(www.clinicaltrials.gov).** In patients with biopsy-confirmed BKV-associated nephropathy, reduction of immune suppression may prevent allograft loss. The use of fluoroquinolones or Immune Globulin Intravenous (IGIV) in the treatment of BKV-associated nephropathy provide little to no benefit. In renal transplant patients with BKV plasma viral loads greater than 10 000 genomes/mL, judicious reduction of immune suppression has been shown to prevent development of BKV-associated nephropathy without increasing the risk of rejection.

Most patients with BKV-hemorrhagic cystitis after hematopoietic stem cell transplantation require only supportive care, because restoration of immune function by stem cell engraftment ultimately will control BKV replication. In severe cases, surgical intervention may be required to stop bladder hemorrhage. Cidofovir has been used for treatment; however, definitive data on its efficacy and safety are lacking.

Restoration of immune function (eg, combination antiretroviral therapy for patients with AIDS) is necessary for survival of patients with PML. Cidofovir sometimes is used for the treatment of PML but has not been shown to be effective in producing clinical improvement. For patients with monoclonal antibody-associated PML, plasmapheresis and/or immune stimulatory agents (eg, granulocyte colony-stimulating factor) may be useful to improve outcomes.

ISOLATION OF THE HOSPITALIZED PATIENT: Standard precautions are recommended.
CONTROL MEASURES: None.

Prion Diseases: Transmissible Spongiform Encephalopathies

CLINICAL MANIFESTATIONS: Transmissible spongiform encephalopathies (TSEs or prion diseases) constitute a group of rare, rapidly progressive, universally fatal neurodegenerative diseases of humans and animals that are characterized by neuronal degeneration, spongiform vacuolation in the cerebral gray matter, reactive proliferation of astrocytes and microglia, and accumulation of abnormal misfolded protease-resistant prion protein (protease-resistant prion protein [PrP^{res}]. This protease-resistant prion protein, variably called prion, scrapie prion protein [PrP^{sc}], or as suggested by the World Health Organization, TSE-associated PrP [PrP^{TSE}]), distributes diffusely throughout the brain or forms plaques of various morphology.

Human prion diseases include several diseases: Creutzfeldt-Jakob disease (CJD), Gerstmann-Sträussler-Scheinker disease, fatal familial and sporadic fatal insomnia, kuru, and variant CJD (vCJD, presumably caused by the agent of bovine spongiform encephalopathy [BSE], commonly called "mad cow" disease). Classic CJD can be sporadic (approximately 85% of cases), familial (approximately 15% of cases), or iatrogenic (fewer than 1% of cases). Sporadic CJD most commonly is a disease of older adults (median age of death in the United States, 68 years) but also rarely has been described in adolescents older than 13 years and young adults. Iatrogenic CJD has been acquired through intramuscular injection of contaminated cadaveric pituitary hormones (growth hormone and human gonadotropin), dura mater allografts, corneal transplantation, and use of contaminated instrumentation at neurosurgery or during depth-electrode electroencephalographic recording. In 1996, an outbreak of vCJD linked to exposure to tissues from BSE-infected cattle was reported in the United Kingdom. Since the end of 2003, 4 presumptive cases of transfusion-transmitted vCJD have been reported: 3 clinical cases as well as 1 asymptomatic case in which PrP^{TSE} was detected in the spleen and lymph nodes but not brain tissues. A fifth possible iatrogenic vCJD infection in a hemophiliac patient in the United Kingdom, also asymptomatic, with a finding of PrP^{TSE} in spleen, was attributed to treatment with potentially vCJD-contaminated, United Kingdom-sourced fractionated plasma products. The best-known prion diseases affecting animals include scrapie of sheep and goats BSE and a chronic wasting disease (CWD) of North American deer, elk, and moose (**www.cdc.gov/prions/index.html**). CWD recently was detected in reindeer and a European elk (moose) in Norway. Except for vCJD, no other human prion disease has been attributed to infection with an agent of animal origin.

CJD manifests as a rapidly progressive neurologic disease with escalating defects in memory, personality, and other higher cortical functions. At presentation, approximately one third of patients have cerebellar dysfunction, including ataxia and dysarthria. Iatrogenic CJD also may manifest as dementia with cerebellar signs. Myoclonus develops in at least 80% of affected patients at some point in the course of disease. Death usually occurs in weeks to months (median, 4–5 months); approximately 10% to 15% of patients with sporadic CJD survive for more than 1 year.

vCJD is distinguished from classic CJD by younger age of onset (median age at death around 28 years), early "psychiatric" manifestations, and other features, such as painful sensory symptoms, delayed onset of overt neurologic signs, relative absence of diagnostic electroencephalographic changes, and a more prolonged duration of illness (median, 13–14 months). In vCJD, but not in classic CJD, a high proportion of people exhibit high signal abnormalities on T2-weighted brain magnetic resonance imaging in the pulvinar region of the posterior thalamus (known as the "pulvinar sign"). In vCJD, the neuropathologic examination reveals highly reproducible pathology with spongiform vacuolation and numerous "florid" plaques (compact amyloid plaque surrounded by vacuoles) and exceptionally striking punctate deposition of PrP^{TSE} in the basal ganglia. In addition, PrP^{TSE} is detectable in the tonsils, appendix, spleen, and lymph nodes of patients with vCJD.

ETIOLOGY: The infectious particle or prion responsible for human and animal prion diseases is believed to consist of a misfolded form (PrP^{TSE}) of a normal ubiquitous cellular prion protein (PrP^C) found in high quantities on the surfaces of cells of the central nervous system and in spermatogenetic cells in both humans and animals. The precise protein structure and mechanism of propagation is unknown. It has been postulated that sporadic CJD arises from a spontaneous structural change of a host-encoded sialoglycoprotein, PrP^C, into the pathogenic PrP^{TSE} form. Prion propagation is proposed to occur by a "recruitment" reaction (the nature of which is under investigation), in which abnormal PrP^{TSE} serves as a template or lattice for the conversion of neighboring PrP^C molecules into misfolded protein with high potential to aggregate.

EPIDEMIOLOGY: Classic CJD is rare, occurring in the United States at a rate of approximately 1 to 1.5 cases per million people annually. The onset of disease peaks in the 60- through 74-year age group. Case-control studies of sporadic CJD have not identified any consistent environmental risk factor. No statistically significant increase in cases of sporadic CJD has been observed in people previously treated with blood, blood components, or plasma derivatives. The incidence of sporadic CJD is not increased in patients with several diseases associated with frequent exposure to blood or blood products, specifically hemophilia A and B, thalassemia, and sickle cell disease, suggesting that the risk of transfusion transmission of classic CJD, if any, must be very low and appropriately regarded as theoretical. CJD has not been reported in infants born to infected mothers. Familial forms of prion diseases are expressed as autosomal-dominant disorder with variable penetrance associated with a variety of mutations of the PrP-encoding gene (PRNP) located on chromosome 20. Onset of familial CJD occurs approximately 10 years earlier than sporadic CJD.

As of June 2016 (**www.cjd.ed.ac.uk/surveillance**), the total number of vCJD cases reported was in 178 patients in the United Kingdom, 27 in France, 5 in Spain, 4 in Ireland, 4 in the United States, 3 in the Netherlands, 3 in Italy, 2 in Portugal, 2 in Canada, and 1 each in Taiwan, Japan, and Saudi Arabia. Two of the 4 patients in the United States, 2 of the 4 in Ireland, and 1 each of the patients in France, Canada, and Taiwan are believed to have acquired vCJD during residence in the United Kingdom. The Centers for Disease Control and Prevention (CDC) and Health Canada have concluded that one of the vCJD patients in the United States and another in Canada probably were infected during their childhood residencies in Saudi Arabia. Another US patient might have been infected while a student in Kuwait. Authorities suspect that the Japanese patient was infected during a short visit of 24 days to the United Kingdom in 1990, 12 years before the onset of vCJD. Most patients with vCJD were younger than 30 years, and several were adolescents. All but 3 of the primary 174 United Kingdom patients with noniatrogenic vCJD died before 60 years of age. All but 14 patients died before 50 years of age, and 151 patients (87%) died before the age of 40. The median age at death of the 174 primary vCJD cases was 27 years. The ages at death of the 3 iatrogenic vCJD transfusion transmission cases were 32, 69, and 75 years. On the basis of animal inoculation studies, comparative PrP immunoblotting, and epidemiologic investigations, almost all cases of vCJD are believed to have resulted from exposure to tissues from cattle infected with BSE. As noted, 3 clinically symptomatic patients and 1 patient with no clinical signs of neurologic disease are believed to have been infected with vCJD through transfusion of nonleukoreduced red blood cells, and 1 hemophiliac patient, also with no clinical signs of prion disease, was probably infected through injections of human plasma-derived clotting factors.

The **incubation period** for iatrogenic CJD varies by route of exposure and ranges from about 14 months to up to at least 42 years.

DIAGNOSTIC TESTS: The diagnosis of human prion diseases can be made with certainty only by neuropathologic examination of affected brain tissue, usually obtained at autopsy. Immunodetection methods such as immunohistochemistry and Western blot can be used to test brain tissues. Electroencephalography (EEG), magnetic resonance imaging (MRI), and cerebrospinal fluid (CSF) testing can be used to diagnose prion disease in live patients. In most patients with classic CJD, a characteristic 1-cycle to 2-cycles per second triphasic sharp-wave discharge on EEG tracing is regarded as indicative of CJD. The likelihood of finding this abnormality is enhanced when serial EEG recordings are obtained. Validated assays that detect 2 protein markers, 14-3-3 and Tau, in CSF showed 83% to 90% sensitivity and 78% diagnostic accuracy. These proteins are surrogate and nonspecific markers found in CSF as a result of the death of neurons. Specific disease marker PrP^{TSE} was demonstrated in CSF of 80% CJD cases. Testing for this marker now is performed in a few laboratories using sophisticated techniques that detect minute amounts of the protein. No validated blood test is available, but a prototype test for vCJD that captures, enriches, and detects disease-associated prion protein from whole blood using stainless steel powder is being developed.[1] Recent promising developments exploit the in vivo prion replication process to amplify and detect even minute amounts of prions in biological samples. One such technique, real-time quaking-induced conversion (RT-QuIC), has been successfully applied in the clinical diagnosis of CJD in CSF samples with high specificity and sensitivity. RT-QuIC also has been applied to diagnose CJD in olfactory epithelium brushings and, with additional validation, may be used in clinical settings.[2] A progressive neurologic syndrome in a person bearing a pathogenic mutation of the PRNP gene (not a normal polymorphism) is presumed to be prion disease. Because no unique nucleic acid has been detected in prions (the infectious particles) causing TSEs, nucleic acid amplification studies such as polymerase chain reaction tests are not possible. Consideration of brain biopsies for patients with possible CJD should be given when other potentially treatable diseases remain in the differential diagnosis. Complete postmortem examination of the brain is encouraged to confirm the clinical diagnosis and to detect emerging forms of CJD, such as vCJD. State-of-the-art diagnostic testing, including assays of 14-3-3, tau and PrP^{TSE} proteins in CSF, PRNP gene sequencing, Western blot analysis to identify and characterize PrP^{TSE} from the brain, and histologic processing of brain tissues with expert neuropathologic consultation, are offered by the National Prion Disease Pathology Surveillance Center (telephone, 216-368-0587; **www.cjdsurveillance.com**). Clinical specimens that may contain prions, particularly specimens with significant amounts of infectious prions, including brain, spinal cord, and possibly CSF, should be handled with extreme caution. Prions can be significantly but not completely inactivated by physical or chemical means commonly used in the laboratory. Potentially contaminated laboratory waste should be both autoclaved and then incinerated.

TREATMENT: No treatment has been shown in humans to slow or stop the progressive neurodegeneration in prion diseases. Experimental treatments are being studied. Sup-

[1] Jackson GS, Burk-Rafel J, Edgeworth JA, et al. Population screening for variant Creutzfeldt-Jakob disease using a novel blood test: diagnostic accuracy and feasibility study. *JAMA Neurol.* 2014;71(4):421–428

[2] Orrú CD, Bongianni M, Tonoli G, et al. A test for Creutzfeldt-Jakob disease using nasal brushings [erratum in: *N Engl J Med.* 2014;371(19):1852]. *N Engl J Med.* 2014;371(6):519–295

portive therapy is necessary to manage dementia, spasticity, rigidity, and seizures occurring during the course of the illness. Psychological support may be offered to families of affected people. Genetic counseling is indicated in familial disease, taking into account that penetrance has been variable in some families in which people with a PRNP mutation survived to an advanced age without developing neurodegenerative disease. A family support and patient advocacy group, the CJD Foundation (telephone 800-659-1991; **www.cjdfoundation.org**), offers helpful information and advice together with information for professionals.

ISOLATION OF THE HOSPITALIZED PATIENT: Standard precautions are recommended. Available evidence indicates that even prolonged intimate contact with CJD-infected people has not resulted in transmission of disease. Tissues associated with high levels of infectivity (eg, brain, eyes, and spinal cord of affected people) and instruments in contact with those tissues are considered biohazards; incineration, prolonged autoclaving at high temperature and pressure after thorough cleaning, and especially exposure to a solution of 1 N or greater sodium hydroxide or a solution of 5.25% or greater sodium hypochlorite (undiluted household chlorine bleach) for 1 hour has been reported to decrease markedly or eliminate infectivity of contaminated surgical instruments (**www.cdc.gov/prions/index.html**). Detailed recommendations for CJD infection-control, distribution of infectivity in various tissues, and specific decontamination protocols are available online (**www.cdc.gov/prions/cjd/infection-control.html** and **www.who.int/csr/resources/publications/bse/WHO_CDS_CSR_APH_2000_3/en/**). Person-to-person transmission of classic sporadic CJD by blood, milk, saliva, urine, or feces has not been reported. These body fluids should be handled using standard infection control procedures; universal blood precautions should be sufficient to prevent bloodborne transmission.

CONTROL MEASURES: Immunization against prion diseases is not available, and no protective immune response to infection has been demonstrated. Iatrogenic transmission of CJD through cadaveric pituitary hormones has been obviated by use of recombinant products. Recognition that CJD can be spread by transplantation of infected dura and corneas and that vCJD can be spread by blood transfusion has led to more stringent donor selection criteria and improved collection protocols. Health care professionals should follow their state's prion disease reporting requirements and indicate CJD or other prion disease diagnoses appropriately on death certificates; US mortality data are used to help monitor occurrences of prion diseases. In addition, any suspected or confirmed diagnosis of a prion disease of special public health concern (eg, suspected iatrogenic disease or vCJD) should be reported promptly to the appropriate state or local health departments and to the CDC (telephone, 404-639-3091 or 404-639-4435; **www.cdc.gov/prions/cjd/index.html**). Current precautionary policies of the US Food and Drug Administration to reduce the risk of transmitting CJD by human blood or blood products are available online (**www.fda.gov/downloads/biologicsbloodvaccines/guidancecomplianceregulatoryinformation/guidances/blood/ucm307137.pdf**). General information about BSE is available from the Food and Drug Administration (**www.fda.gov/AnimalVeterinary/ResourcesforYou/AnimalHealthLiteracy/ucm136222.htm**), from the USDA (**www.fsis.usda.gov/wps/portal/fsis/topics/food-safety-education/get-answers/food-safety-fact-sheets/production-and-inspection/bovine-spongiform-encephalopathy-bse/bse-resources**), from the CDC (**www.cdc.gov/**

prions/bse/index.html), and from the World Organization for Animal Health (www.oie.int/en/animal-health-in-the-world/bse-portal/).

Q Fever (*Coxiella burnetii* Infection)

CLINICAL MANIFESTATIONS: Approximately half of acute Q fever infections result in symptoms. Acute and persistent (chronic) forms of the disease exist and both can present as fever of unknown origin. Q fever in children typically is characterized by abrupt onset of fever, often accompanied by chills, headache, weakness, cough, and other nonspecific systemic symptoms. Illness typically is self-limited, although a relapsing febrile illness lasting for several months has been documented in children. Gastrointestinal tract symptoms, such as diarrhea, vomiting, abdominal pain, and anorexia, are reported in 50% to 80% of children. Rash has been observed in some patients with Q fever. Q fever pneumonia usually manifests with a mild cough and shortness of breath but can progress to respiratory distress. Chest radiographic patterns are variable; chest computed tomography may show multilobar airspace consolidation. In immunocompromised patients, a nodular pattern accompanied by a halo of ground-glass opacification and vessel connection, or findings suggestive of a necrotizing process, may be seen. More severe manifestations of acute Q fever are rare but include hepatitis, hemolytic-uremic syndrome, myocarditis, pericarditis, cerebellitis, encephalitis, meningitis, hemophagocytosis, lymphadenitis, acalculous cholecystitis, and rhabdomyolysis. Persistent, localized (chronic) Q fever is rare in children but can present as blood culture-negative endocarditis, chronic relapsing or multifocal osteomyelitis, or chronic hepatitis. Children who are immunocompromised or have underlying valvular heart disease may be at higher risk of persistent, localized Q fever.

ETIOLOGY: *Coxiella burnetii*, the cause of Q fever, previously was considered to be a rickettsial organism but is a gram-negative intracellular bacterium that belongs to the order *Legionellales*, family *Coxiellaceae*. It shares many features, including relatedness of several virulence genes, with *Legionella pneumophila*. The infectious form of *C burnetii* is highly resistant to heat, desiccation, and disinfectant chemicals and can persist for long periods of time in the environment. *C burnetii* is classified as a category B bioterrorism agent by the Centers for Disease Control and Prevention (CDC).

EPIDEMIOLOGY: Q fever is a zoonotic infection that has been reported worldwide, including in every state in the United States. The "Q" comes from "query" fever, the name of the disease until its etiologic agent was identified in the 1930s. *C burnetii* infection usually is asymptomatic in animals. Many different species can be infected, although cattle, sheep, and goats are the primary reservoirs for human infection. Tick vectors may be important for maintaining animal and bird reservoirs but are not thought to be important in transmission to humans. Humans most often acquire infection by inhalation of fine-particle aerosols of *C burnetii* generated from birthing fluids or other excreta of infected animals or through inhalation of dust contaminated by these materials. Infection can occur by exposure to contaminated materials, such as wool, straw, bedding, or laundry. Windborne particles containing infectious organisms can travel prolonged distances, contributing to sporadic cases for which no apparent animal contact can be demonstrated. Unpasteurized dairy products can contain the organism. Seasonal trends occur in farming areas with predictable frequency, and the disease often coincides with the livestock birthing season in spring.

The **incubation period** is 14 to 22 days, with a range from 9 to 39 days, depending on the inoculum size. Persistent, localized (chronic) Q fever can develop months to years after initial infection.

DIAGNOSTIC TESTS: Serologic evidence of a fourfold increase in phase II immunoglobulin (Ig) G via immunofluorescent assay (IFA) tests between paired sera taken 3 to 6 weeks apart is the diagnostic gold standard to confirm diagnosis of acute Q fever. A single high serum phase II IgG titer ($\geq$1:128) by IFA in the convalescent stage may be considered as evidence of probable infection. Confirmation of persistent (chronic) Q fever is based on an increasing phase I IgG titer (typically $\geq$1:1024) that often is higher than the phase II IgG titer *and* an identifiable nidus of infection (eg, endocarditis, vascular infection, osteomyelitis, chronic hepatitis). Polymerase chain reaction (PCR) testing on whole blood (because the organism is an intracellular pathogen) or serum may be useful in the first 2 weeks of symptom onset and before antimicrobial administration. Although a positive PCR assay result can confirm the diagnosis, a negative PCR test result will not rule out Q fever. Currently, there are no PCR assays cleared by the US Food and Drug Administration for *C burnetii*, and PCR testing generally is available only in select reference or public health laboratories. Detection of *C burnetii* in tissues (eg, heart valve) by immunohistochemistry or PCR assay can also confirm a diagnosis of chronic Q fever. However, PCR test results may be negative in up to 66% of patients with endocarditis attributable to Q fever. Isolation of *C burnetii* from blood can be performed only in special laboratories with biological safety level 3 facilities using specialized culture methods, embryonated eggs, or animal inoculation because of the potential hazard to laboratory workers.

TREATMENT: Acute Q fever generally is a self-limited illness, and many patients recover without antimicrobial therapy. However, early treatment is effective in shortening illness duration and symptom severity and should be initiated in all symptomatic patients. For patients with suspected disease, immediate empiric therapy should be given, because laboratory results are often negative early in illness onset pending production of quantifiable antibody. Doxycycline (100 mg, orally, 2 times/day for children $\geq$8 years; or 4.4 mg/kg per day, orally, divided 2 times/day for children <8 years, with a maximum dose of 100 mg) administered for 14 days is the drug of choice for severe infections in patients and can be used for acute Q fever regardless of patient age (see Tetracyclines, p 905). Children younger than 8 years with mild illness, pregnant women, and patients allergic to doxycycline can be treated with trimethoprim-sulfamethoxazole.

Persistent (chronic) Q fever is much more difficult to treat, and relapses can occur despite appropriate therapy, necessitating repeated courses of therapy. The recommended therapy for Q fever endocarditis is a combination of doxycycline and hydroxychloroquine for a minimum of 18 months. Surgical replacement of the infected valve may be necessary in some patients.

ISOLATION OF THE HOSPITALIZED PATIENT: Standard precautions are recommended.

CONTROL MEASURES: Strict adherence to proper hygiene when handling infected parturient animals or their excreta can help decrease the risk of infection in the farm setting, as can ensuring that people do not consume unpasteurized milk and milk products. Improved prescreening of animal herds used by research facilities may decrease the risk of infection. Special safety practices are recommended for nonpropagative laboratory procedures involving *C burnetii* and for all propagative procedures, during aerosol-generating procedures performed on infected patients, and during high-risk worker exposures in biomedical facilities that house sheep and goats. Vaccines for domestic animals and people working in high-risk occupations have been developed but are not licensed in the United

States. Q fever is a nationally reportable disease, and all human cases should be reported to the state health department. Additional information about Q fever is available on the CDC Web site (**www.cdc.gov/qfever/index.html**).

Rabies[1]

CLINICAL MANIFESTATIONS: Infection with rabies virus and other lyssaviruses characteristically produces an acute illness with rapidly progressive central nervous system manifestations, including anxiety, radicular pain, dysesthesia or pruritus, hydrophobia, and dysautonomia. Some patients may have paralysis. Illness almost invariably progresses to death. The differential diagnosis of acute encephalitic illnesses of unknown cause or with features of Guillain-Barré syndrome should include rabies.

ETIOLOGY: Rabies virus is a single-stranded RNA virus classified in the *Rhabdoviridae* family, *Lyssavirus* genus. The genus *Lyssavirus* currently contains 14 species divided into 3 phylogroups.

EPIDEMIOLOGY: Understanding the epidemiology of rabies has been aided by viral variant identification using monoclonal antibodies and nucleotide sequencing. In the United States, human cases have decreased steadily since the 1950s, reflecting widespread immunization of dogs and the availability of effective prophylaxis after exposure to a rabid animal. From 2000 through 2014, 31 of 44 cases of human rabies reported in the United States were acquired indigenously. Among the 31 indigenously acquired cases, all but 4 were associated with bats. Despite the large focus of rabies in raccoons in the eastern United States, only 3 human deaths have been attributed to the raccoon rabies virus variant. Historically, 2 cases of human rabies were attributable to probable aerosol exposure in laboratories, and 2 unusual cases have been attributed to possible airborne exposures in caves inhabited by millions of bats, although alternative infection routes cannot be discounted. Transmission also has occurred by transplantation of organs, corneas, and other tissues from patients dying of undiagnosed rabies. Person-to-person transmission by bite has not been documented in the United States, although the virus has been isolated from saliva of infected patients.

Wildlife rabies perpetuates throughout all of the 50 United States except Hawaii, which remains "rabies free." Wildlife, including bats, raccoons, skunks, foxes, coyotes, bobcats, and mongoose, are the most important potential sources of infection for humans and domestic animals in the United States and its territories. Rabies in small rodents (squirrels, hamsters, guinea pigs, gerbils, chipmunks, rats, and mice) and lagomorphs (rabbits, pikas, and hares) is rare. Rabies may occur in woodchucks or other large rodents in areas where raccoon rabies is common. The virus is present in saliva and is transmitted by bites or, rarely, by contamination of mucosa or skin lesions by saliva or other potentially infectious material (eg, neural tissue). Worldwide, most rabies cases in humans result from dog bites in areas where canine rabies is enzootic (**www.who.int/rabies/ Presence_dog_transmitted_human_Rabies_2014.png?ua=1**). Most rabid dogs, cats, and ferrets shed virus for a few days before there are obvious signs of illness. No case of human rabies in the United States has been attributed to a dog, cat, or ferret that

---

[1]For further information, see Centers for Disease Control and Prevention. Human rabies prevention: United States, 2008. Recommendations of the Advisory Committee on Immunization Practices. *MMWR Recomm Rep.* 2008;57(RR-3):1–28

has remained healthy throughout the standard 10-day period of confinement after an exposure.

The **incubation period** in humans averages 1 to 3 months but ranges from days to years.

DIAGNOSTIC TESTS: Infection in animals can be diagnosed by demonstration of the presence of rabies virus antigen in brain tissue using a direct fluorescent antibody (DFA) test. Suspected rabid animals should be euthanized in a manner that preserves brain tissue for appropriate laboratory diagnosis. Virus can be isolated in suckling mice or in tissue culture from saliva, brain, and other specimens and can be detected by identification of viral antigens by immunofluorescence or immunoperoxidase staining or nucleotide sequences by reverse transcriptase-polymerase chain reaction (RT-PCR) in affected tissues. Diagnosis in suspected human cases can be made postmortem by either immunofluorescent or immunohistochemical examination of brain tissue or by detection of viral nucleotide sequences. The latter generally is performed by RT-PCR, but only after DFA testing has failed to confirm the diagnosis of a suspected case. Antemortem diagnosis can be made by DFA testing on skin biopsy specimens from the nape of the neck, by isolation of the virus from saliva, by detection of antibody in serum (neutralization or IFA methods generally are used) in unvaccinated people and in cerebrospinal fluid (CSF) in all infected people, and by detection of viral nucleotide sequences in saliva, skin, or other tissues. RT-PCR plays a greater role in the diagnosis of rabies in such antemortem specimens in the absence of a brain biopsy specimen. No single test is sufficiently sensitive because of the unique nature of rabies pathobiology. Laboratory personnel and state health or local health departments should be consulted before submission of specimens to the Centers for Disease Control and Prevention (CDC) so appropriate collection and transport of materials can be arranged.

TREATMENT: There is no specific treatment. Once symptoms have developed, neither rabies vaccine nor Rabies Immune Globulin (RIG) improves the prognosis. A combination of sedation and intensive medical intervention may be valuable adjunctive therapy.[1] Details of one management protocol used can be found at **www.mcw.edu/rabies.** Eleven people have survived rabies in association with incomplete rabies vaccine schedules. Eight people who had not received rabies postexposure prophylaxis have survived rabies. Approximately half of survivors have normal cognition.

ISOLATION OF THE HOSPITALIZED PATIENT: Standard precautions (ie, gowns, gloves, goggles, and masks) are recommended for the duration of illness. If the patient has bitten another person or potentially infectious material from the patient has contaminated an open wound or mucous membrane, the involved area should be washed thoroughly with soap and water, and risk assessment should be completed to determine whether postexposure prophylaxis should be administered (see Care of Exposed People, p 677).

CONTROL MEASURES: In the United States, animal rabies is common. Education of children to avoid contact with stray or wild animals is of primary importance. Inadvertent contact of family members and pets with potentially rabid animals, such as raccoons, foxes, coyotes, and skunks, may be decreased by securing garbage and pet food outdoors to decrease attraction of domestic and wild animals. Similarly, chimneys and other potential entrances for wildlife, including bats, should be identified and covered. Bats should be

[1]Centers for Disease Control and Prevention. Recovery of a patient from clinical rabies—California, 2011. *MMWR Morb Mortal Wkly Rep.* 2012;61(4):61–65

excluded from human living quarters. International travelers to areas with enzootic canine rabies should be warned to avoid exposure to stray dogs, and if traveling to an area with enzootic infection where immediate access to medical care and biologic agents is limited, preexposure prophylaxis is indicated.

Exposure Risk and Decisions to Administer Prophylaxis. Exposure to rabies results from a break in the skin caused by the teeth of a rabid animal or by contamination of scratches, abrasions, or mucous membranes with saliva or other potentially infectious material, such as neural tissue, from a rabid animal. The decision to immunize a potentially exposed person should be made in consultation with the local health department, which can provide information on risk of rabies in a particular area for each species of animal and in accordance with the guidance in Table 3.63. Consultation with experts at the CDC may be helpful to guide decisions on prophylaxis (**www.cdc.gov/rabies/resources/contacts.html**).

In the United States and Puerto Rico, all mammals are believed to be susceptible, but bats, raccoons, skunks, foxes, coyotes, and mongooses are more likely to be infected than are other animals.[1] According to the CDC, all bites by such wildlife must be considered a possible exposure to the rabies virus. Postexposure prophylaxis should be initiated as soon as possible following exposure to these animals unless the animal has already been tested and determined not to be rabid. If postexposure prophylaxis has been initiated and

Table 3.63. Rabies Postexposure Prophylaxis Guide

Animal Type	Evaluation and Disposition of Animal	Postexposure Prophylaxis Recommendations
Dogs, cats, and ferrets	Healthy and available for 10 days of observation	Prophylaxis only if animal develops signs of rabies[a]
	Rabid or suspected of being rabid[b]	Immediate immunization and RIG[c]
	Unknown (escaped)	Consult public health officials for advice
Bats, skunks, raccoons, coyotes, foxes, mongooses, and most other carnivores; woodchucks	Regarded as rabid unless geographic area is known to be free of rabies or until animal proven negative by laboratory tests[b]	Immediate immunization and RIG[c]
Livestock, rodents, and lagomorphs (rabbits, hares, and pikas)	Consider individually	Consult public health officials; bites of squirrels, hamsters, guinea pigs, gerbils, chipmunks, rats, mice and other rodents, rabbits, hares, and pikas almost never require rabies postexposure prophylaxis

RIG indicates Rabies Immune Globulin.

[a]During the 10-day observation period, at the first sign of rabies in the biting dog, cat, or ferret, prophylaxis of the exposed person with RIG (human) and vaccine should be initiated. The animal should be euthanized immediately and tested.

[b]The animal should be euthanized and tested as soon as possible. Holding for observation is not recommended. Immunization is discontinued if immunofluorescent test result for the animal is negative.

[c]See text.

[1]Centers for Disease Control and Prevention. Human rabies—Puerto Rico, 2015. *MMWR Morb Mortal Wkly Rep.* 2017;65(52):1474–1476

subsequent testing shows that the exposing animal was not rabid, postexposure prophylaxis can be discontinued. Cattle, dogs, cats, ferrets, and other animals occasionally are infected. Bites of small rodents (such as squirrels, hamsters, guinea pigs, gerbils, chipmunks, mice, and rats) and lagomorphs (rabbits, hares, and pikas) rarely require prophylaxis, because these animals almost never are found to be infected with rabies and have not been known to transmit rabies to humans. Additional factors must be considered when deciding whether immunoprophylaxis is indicated. An unprovoked attack may be more suggestive of a rabid animal than a bite that occurs during attempts to feed or handle an animal. Properly immunized dogs, cats, and ferrets have only a minimal chance of developing rabies. However, in rare instances, rabies has developed in properly immunized animals.

Postexposure prophylaxis for rabies is recommended for all people bitten by wild mammalian carnivores or bats or by domestic animals that are suspected to be rabid unless laboratory tests prove that the animal does not have rabies. Postexposure prophylaxis also is recommended for people who report an open wound, scratch, or mucous membrane that has been contaminated with saliva or other potentially infectious material (eg, brain tissue) from a rabid animal. The injury inflicted by a bat bite or scratch may be small and not readily evident, or the circumstances of contact with a bat may preclude accurate recall (eg, a bat in a room of a deeply sleeping or medicated person or a previously unattended child, especially an infant or toddler who cannot reliably communicate about a potential bite). Hence, postexposure prophylaxis may be indicated, following proper risk assessment, for situations in which a bat physically is present in the same room if a bite or mucous membrane exposure cannot reliably be excluded, unless prompt testing of the bat has excluded rabies virus infection. Prophylaxis should be initiated as soon as possible after bites by known or suspected rabid animals.

Risk assessment for the administration of postexposure prophylaxis is recommended for people who report a possibly infectious exposure (eg, bite, scratch, or open wound or mucous membrane contaminated with saliva or other infectious material, such as tears, CSF, or brain tissue) to a human with rabies. Rabies virus transmission after exposure to a human with rabies has not been documented convincingly in the United States, except after tissue or organ transplantation from donors who died of unsuspected rabies encephalitis. Casual contact with an infected person (eg, by touching a patient) or contact with noninfectious fluids or tissues (eg, blood or feces) alone does not constitute an exposure and is not an indication for prophylaxis.

Handling of Animals Suspected of Having Rabies. A dog, cat, bat, or ferret that is suspected of having rabies and has bitten a human should be captured, confined, euthanized, and tested or should be observed by a veterinarian for 10 days by order of public health authorities. If signs of rabies develop, the animal should be euthanized in a manner to allow its head to be removed and shipped under refrigeration (not frozen, which would delay testing) to a qualified laboratory for examination.

Other biting animals that may have exposed a person to rabies virus should be reported immediately to the local health department. Management of animals depends on the species, the circumstances of the bite, and the epidemiology of rabies in the area. Previous immunization of an animal may not preclude the necessity for euthanasia and testing. Because clinical manifestations of rabies in a wild animal cannot be interpreted reliably, a wild mammal suspected of having rabies should be euthanized at once, and its brain should be examined for evidence of rabies virus infection. The exposed person need not receive prophylaxis if the result of rapid examination of the brain by DFA testing is negative for rabies virus infection.

Risk Assessments for Contacts of Humans With Rabies. Administration of postexposure prophylaxis to hospital contacts of patients with rabies is required only in situations in which potentially infectious material (such as saliva, CSF, or brain tissue) comes into direct contact with broken skin or mucous membranes. It is expected that in cases in which people are using appropriate protective equipment, there will likely be no risk of exposure (see Care of Exposed People).

Care of Exposed People.

Local Wound Care. The immediate objective of postexposure prophylaxis is to prevent virus from entering neural tissue. Prompt and thorough local treatment of all lesions is essential, because virus may remain localized to the area of the bite for a variable time. All wounds should be flushed thoroughly and cleaned with soap and water. Quaternary ammonium compounds (such as benzalkonium chloride) no longer are considered superior to soap. The need for tetanus prophylaxis and measures to control bacterial infection should be considered. The wound, if possible, should not be sutured. For severe facial wounds, which often also are infected with bacteria, better cosmesis results from single sutures, widely placed, several hours after local instillation of RIG, followed by plastic surgery days later.

Prophylaxis (see Table 3.63, p 675). After wound care is completed, concurrent use of passive and active prophylaxis is optimal, with the exceptions of people who previously have received complete vaccination regimens (pre- or postexposure) with a cell culture vaccine or people who have been vaccinated with other types of rabies vaccines and have previously had a documented rabies virus-neutralizing antibody titer; these people should receive only vaccine. Prophylaxis should begin as soon as possible after exposure, ideally within 24 hours. However, a delay of several days or more may not compromise effectiveness, and prophylaxis should be initiated if reasonably indicated, regardless of the interval between exposure and initiation of therapy. In the United States, only human RIG is available for passive immunization. Licensed cell culture rabies vaccine should be used for active immunization. Physicians can obtain expert counsel from their local or state health departments.

Active Immunization (Postexposure). Human diploid cell vaccine (HDCV) and purified chicken embryo cell vaccine (PCECV) are available for use in the United States (see Table 3.64, p 678). For a previously unvaccinated immunocompetent person, a 1.0-mL dose of vaccine is injected intramuscularly in the deltoid area (the anterolateral aspect of the thigh also is acceptable for children) on the first day of postexposure prophylaxis (day 0), and repeated doses are administered on days 3, 7, and 14 after the first dose, for a total of 4 doses,[1] with 1 dose of RIG administered on day 0. The volume of the dose is not decreased for children. For a person with altered immunocompetence, postexposure prophylaxis should include a 5-dose vaccination regimen (ie, 1 dose of vaccine on days 0, 3, 7, 14, and 28), with 1 dose of RIG. Serologic testing to document seroconversion after administration of a rabies vaccine series usually is not necessary but occasionally has been advised for recipients who may be immunocompromised or for people with deviations

---

[1]Centers for Disease Control and Prevention. Use of a reduced (4-dose) vaccine schedule for postexposure prophylaxis to prevent human rabies: recommendations of the Advisory Committee on Immunization Practices. *MMWR Recomm Rep.* 2010;59(RR-02):1–9

from the recommended vaccination schedule. Immune response should be assessed by performing neutralizing antibody testing 7 to 14 days after administration of the final dose in the series. Ideally, a vaccination series should be initiated and completed with 1 vaccine product unless serious adverse reactions occur. Clinical studies evaluating efficacy or frequency of adverse reactions when the series is completed with a second product have not been conducted.

Care should be taken to ensure that the vaccine is administered intramuscularly. Intradermal vaccine is not advised for postexposure prophylaxis in the United States, although for reasons of cost and availability, intradermal regimens are recommended by the World Health Organization and frequently are used in some countries. Because virus-neutralizing antibody responses in adults who received vaccine in the gluteal area sometimes have been less than in those who were injected in the deltoid muscle, the deltoid site always should be used, except in infants and young children, in whom the anterolateral thigh is the appropriate site.

ADVERSE REACTIONS AND PRECAUTIONS WITH HDCV AND PCECV. Reactions are uncommon in children. In adults, mild local reactions, such as pain, erythema, and swelling or itching at the injection site, are reported in 15% to 25%, and mild systemic reactions, such as headache, nausea, abdominal pain, muscle aches, and dizziness, are reported in 10% to 20% of recipients. Immune complex-like reactions in people receiving booster doses of HDCV have been observed, possibly because of interaction between propiolactone contained in the vaccine and human albumin. The reaction, characterized by onset 2 to 21 days after inoculation, begins with generalized urticaria and can include arthralgia, arthritis, angioedema, nausea, vomiting, fever, and malaise. The reaction is not life threatening, occurs in as many as 6% of adults receiving booster doses as part of a preexposure immunization regimen, and is rare in people receiving primary immunization with HDCV. Similar allergic reactions with primary or booster doses have been reported with PCECV. If the patient has a serious allergic reaction to HDCV, PCECV may be administered according to the same schedule as HDCV, and vice-versa. If reactions following vaccine are mild, pretreatment with antihistamines just before the next vaccination can be considered. All suspected serious, systemic, paralytic, or anaphylactic reactions to rabies vaccine should be reported immediately to the Vaccine Adverse Events Reporting System (see p 45).

Although the safety of rabies vaccine during pregnancy has not been studied specifically in the United States, pregnancy should not be considered a contraindication to use of vaccine or RIG after exposure.

NERVE TISSUE VACCINES. Inactivated nerve tissue vaccines are not licensed in the United States and are not recommended by the World Health Organization but still are used in some areas of the world. These preparations induce neuroparalytic reactions in 1 in 2000 to 1 in 8000 recipients. Vaccination with nerve tissue vaccine should be discontinued if meningeal or neuroparalytic reactions develop. Corticosteroids should be used only for life-threatening reactions, because they increase the risk of rabies in experimentally inoculated animals.

Passive Immunization. Human RIG should be used concomitantly with the first dose of vaccine for postexposure prophylaxis to bridge the time between possible infection and antibody production induced by the vaccine (see Table 3.64). If vaccine is not available immediately, RIG should be administered alone, and vaccination should be started as soon as possible. If RIG is not available immediately, vaccine should be administered

Table 3.64. US Food and Drug Administration-Licensed Rabies Vaccines[a] and Rabies Immune Globulin Products

Category	Product	Manufacturer	Dose and Route of Administration
Human rabies vaccine	Human diploid cell vaccine (HDCV) (Imovax)	Sanofi Pasteur	1 mL, IM
	Purified chicken embryo cell vaccine (PCECV) (RabAvert)	Novartis Vaccines and Diagnostics	1 mL, IM
Rabies Immune Globulin	Imogam Rabies-HT	Sanofi Pasteur	20 IU/kg, infiltrate around wound[b]
	HyperRab S/D	Talecris Biotherapeutics	20 IU/kg, infiltrate around wound[b]

IM indicates intramuscular.

[a]Rabies vaccine adsorbed (RVA) is licensed in the United States but no longer is distributed in the United States.

[b]Any remaining volume should be administered intramuscularly.

and RIG should be administered subsequently if obtained within 7 days after initiating vaccination. If administration of both vaccine and RIG is delayed, both should be used regardless of the interval between exposure and treatment, within reason.

The recommended dose of RIG is 20 IU/kg. As much of the dose as possible should be used to infiltrate the wound(s), if present. The remainder is administered intramuscularly into the deltoid muscle. In cases of multiple severe wounds in which RIG is insufficient for infiltration, dilution in saline solution to an adequate volume (twofold or threefold) has been recommended to ensure that all wound areas receive infiltrate. For children with small muscle mass, it may be necessary to administer RIG at multiple sites. Human RIG is supplied in 2-mL (300 IU) and 10-mL (1500 IU) vials. Passive antibody can, in some cases, inhibit the response to rabies vaccines; therefore, the recommended dose should not be exceeded. Vaccine never should be administered in the same parts of the body or with the same syringe used to give RIG. Hypersensitivity reactions to RIG are rare.

Purified equine RIG containing rabies antibodies may be available outside the United States and generally is accompanied by a low rate of serum sickness (less than 1%). Equine RIG is administered at a dose of 40 IU/kg, and desensitization may be required.

Management of Postexposure Prophylaxis in Previously Immunized People. Administration of RIG is not recommended for the following exposed people: (1) people who received postexposure prophylaxis with HDCV, RVA, or PCECV for a previous exposure; (2) people who received a 3-dose, intramuscular, preexposure regimen of HDCV, RVA, or PCECV; (3) people who received a 3-dose, intradermal, preexposure regimen of HDCV with the product used in the United States; and (4) people who have a documented adequate rabies virus antibody titer after previous immunization with any other rabies vaccine. These people should receive two 1.0-mL booster doses of HDCV or PCECV; the first dose ideally is administered on the day of exposure, and the second dose is administered 3 days later.

Preexposure Control Measures, Including Vaccination. The relatively low frequency of reactions to HDCV and PCECV has made provision of preexposure vaccination practical for people in high-risk groups, including veterinarians, animal handlers, certain laboratory workers, and people moving or traveling to areas where canine rabies is common. Others, such as spelunkers (cavers) or animal rehabilitators, who may have frequent exposures to bats and other wildlife, also should be considered for preexposure prophylaxis.

HDCV and PCECV are licensed for intramuscular administration. The preexposure prophylaxis schedule is three 1-mL intramuscular injections each, administered on days 0, 7, and 21 or 28. This series of immunizations has resulted in development of rabies virus-neutralizing antibodies in all people properly immunized. Therefore, routine serologic testing for antibody after primary immunization is not indicated.

Serum antibodies usually persist for 2 years or longer after the primary series is administered intramuscularly. Preexposure booster immunization with 1.0 mL of HDCV or PCEC intramuscularly will produce an effective anamnestic response in most healthy individuals. Rabies virus-neutralizing antibody titers should be determined at 6-month intervals for people at continuous risk of infection (eg, rabies research laboratory workers, rabies biologics production workers). Titers should be determined approximately every 2 years for people with risk of frequent exposure (eg, rabies diagnostic laboratory workers, spelunkers/cavers, veterinarians and staff, animal-control and wildlife workers in areas with enzootic rabies, and all people who frequently handle bats or other wildlife animals). A single booster dose of vaccine should be administered only as appropriate to maintain adequate antibody concentrations. The CDC currently specifies complete viral neutralization at a serum dilution of 1:5 (approximately 0.1 IU/mL or greater) by the rapid fluorescent-focus inhibition test as evidence of an adequate immune response; the World Health Organization specifies a neutralizing antibody titer of 0.5 IU/mL or greater as acceptable. Other people, such as travelers to areas where canine rabies is common, do not need serologic testing and follow-up. If they received preexposure immunization at any time prior to the time they are exposed, then they should receive booster doses of vaccine at days 0 and 3.

Public Health. A variety of approved public health measures, including vaccination of dogs, cats, and ferrets and management of the stray dog population and selected wildlife, are used to control rabies in animals.[1] In regions where oral vaccination of wildlife with recombinant rabies vaccine is undertaken, the prevalence of rabies among foxes, coyotes, and raccoons may be decreased. Unvaccinated dogs, cats, ferrets, or other pets bitten by a known rabid animal should be euthanized immediately. If the owner is unwilling to allow the animal to be euthanized, the animal should be placed in strict isolation for 6 months and immunized at latest 1 month before release. If the exposed animal has been immunized within 1 to 3 years, depending on the vaccine administered and local regulations, the animal should be revaccinated and observed for 45 days.

Case Reporting. All suspected human cases of rabies should be reported promptly to public health authorities.

Rat-Bite Fever

CLINICAL MANIFESTATIONS: Rat-bite fever is caused by *Streptobacillus moniliformis* or *Spirillum minus*. *S moniliformis* infection (streptobacillary fever or Haverhill fever) is characterized by relapsing fever, rash, and migratory polyarthritis. There is an abrupt onset of

---

[1]National Association of State Public Health Veterinarians Inc. Compendium of animal rabies prevention and control, 2011. *MMWR Recomm Rep.* 2011;60(RR-6):1–15

fever, chills, muscle pain, vomiting, headache, and rarely (unlike *S minus*), lymphadenopathy. A maculopapular, purpuric, or petechial rash develops, predominantly on the peripheral extremities including the palms and soles, typically within a few days of fever onset. The skin lesions may become purpuric or confluent and may desquamate. The bite site usually heals promptly and exhibits no or minimal inflammation. Nonsuppurative migratory polyarthritis or arthralgia follows in approximately 50% of patients. Symptoms of untreated infection resolve within 2 weeks, but fever occasionally can relapse for weeks or months. Complications include soft tissue and solid-organ abscesses, septic arthritis, pneumonia, endocarditis, myocarditis, pericarditis, sepsis, and meningitis. The case-fatality rate is 7% to 13% in untreated patients, and fatal cases have been reported in young children.

With *S minus* infection ("sodoku"), a period of initial apparent healing at the site of the bite usually is followed by fever and ulceration, discoloration, swelling, and pain at the site (about 1 to 4 weeks later), regional lymphangitis and lymphadenopathy, and a distinctive rash of red or purple plaques. Arthritis is rare. Infection with *S minus* is rare in the United States.

ETIOLOGY: The causes of rat-bite fever are *S moniliformis,* a microaerophilic, facultatively anaerobic, gram-negative, pleomorphic bacillus, and *S minus,* a small, gram-negative, spiral-shaped bacterium with bipolar flagellar tufts.

EPIDEMIOLOGY: Rat-bite fever is a zoonotic illness. The natural habitat of *S moniliformis* and *S minus* is the upper respiratory tract of rodents. *S moniliformis* is transmitted by bites or scratches from or exposure to oral secretions of infected rats (eg, kissing pet rodents), other rodents (eg, mice, gerbils, squirrels, weasels), and rodent-eating animals, including cats and dogs. Haverhill fever refers to infection after ingestion of unpasteurized milk, water, or food contaminated with *S moniliformis* and may be associated with an outbreak of disease. *S minus* is transmitted by bites of rats and mice. *S moniliformis* infection accounts for most cases of rat-bite fever in the United States; *S minus* infections occur primarily in Asia.

The **incubation period** for *S moniliformis* usually is less than 7 days but can range from 3 days to 3 weeks; for *S minus,* the **incubation period** is 7 to 21 days.

DIAGNOSTIC TESTS: *S moniliformis* is a fastidious, slow-growing organism isolated from specimens of blood, synovial fluid, abscesses, or aspirates from the bite lesion. Growth is best in bacteriologic media enriched with blood (15% rabbit blood seems optimal), serum, and ascitic fluid, and kept in 5% to 10% carbon dioxide atmosphere at 37°C. Cultures should be held for 1 week if *S moniliformis* is suspected. Sodium polyanethol sulfonate (SPS), present in most commercially available aerobic blood culture media, is inhibitory to *S moniliformis.* Therefore, SPS-free media (as is found in anaerobic blood culture bottles) should be used, and the laboratory should be alerted to process the specimen aerobically and hold the culture for a longer period of time. A terminal blind subculture of blood culture broth to enriched media should be performed after the standard incubation time is completed. Alternatively, the addition of fastidious organism supplement (FOS) to standard SPS-containing aerobic blood culture media can improve the yield of *S moniliformis. S moniliformis* also has been detected using a nucleic acid amplification-based assay, available in research laboratories.

S minus has not been recovered on artificial media but can be visualized by darkfield microscopy in wet mounts of blood, exudate of a lesion, and lymph nodes. Blood specimens also should be viewed with Giemsa or Wright stain. *S minus* can be recovered from blood, lymph nodes, or local lesions by intraperitoneal inoculation of mice or guinea pigs.

TREATMENT: Penicillin G procaine administered intramuscularly or penicillin G administered intravenously for 7 to 10 days is the treatment for rat-bite fever caused by either agent; currently in the United States and other countries, intravenous administration is the more acceptable route. Initial intravenous penicillin G therapy for 5 to 7 days followed by oral penicillin V for 7 days also has been successful. Limited experience exists for ampicillin, cefuroxime, and cefotaxime. Doxycycline or streptomycin (limited availability) can be substituted when a patient has a serious allergy to penicillin. Patients with endocarditis should receive intravenous high-dose penicillin G for at least 4 weeks. The addition of streptomycin or gentamicin for initial therapy may be useful in severe infections.

ISOLATION OF THE HOSPITALIZED PATIENT: Standard precautions are recommended.

CONTROL MEASURES: Exposed people should be observed for symptoms. Because the occurrence of *S moniliformis* after a rat bite is approximately 10%, some experts recommend postexposure administration of penicillin. Rat control is important in the control of disease. People with frequent rodent exposure should wear gloves and avoid hand-to-mouth contact during animal handling. Regular hand hygiene should be practiced. Currently, rat bite fever is not a reportable disease to local public health authorities. This practice likely contributes to underestimates of disease incidence.

Respiratory Syncytial Virus

CLINICAL MANIFESTATIONS: Respiratory syncytial virus (RSV) causes acute respiratory tract infections in people of all ages and is one of the most common diseases of early childhood. Most infants infected with RSV experience upper respiratory tract symptoms, and 20% to 30% develop lower respiratory tract disease (eg, bronchiolitis and/or pneumonia) with the first infection. Signs and symptoms of bronchiolitis typically begin with rhinitis and cough, which progress to increased respiratory effort with tachypnea, wheezing, rales, crackles, intercostal and/or subcostal retractions, grunting, and nasal flaring. Infection with RSV during the first few weeks of life, particularly among preterm infants, may produce minimal respiratory tract signs, lethargy, irritability, and poor feeding, sometimes accompanied by apneic episodes. These infants are at particular risk of life-threatening apnea even in the absence of any other severe respiratory symptoms. Most previously healthy infants who develop RSV bronchiolitis do not require hospitalization, and most who are hospitalized improve with supportive care and are discharged after 2 or 3 days. However, approximately 1% to 3% of all children in the first 12 months of life will be hospitalized because of RSV lower respiratory tract disease, with most RSV hospitalizations occurring in the first 6 months of life. RSV hospitalization rates are highest between 30 and 60 days of age. Factors that increase the risk of severe RSV lower respiratory tract illness include prematurity, especially infants born before 29 weeks' gestation; chronic lung disease of prematurity (CLD [formerly called bronchopulmonary dysplasia]); certain types of hemodynamically significant congenital heart disease (CHD), especially conditions associated with pulmonary hypertension; and certain immunodeficiency states. Additional risk factors for severe RSV lower respiratory tract infections in children worldwide include low birth weight, having siblings, maternal smoking during pregnancy, exposure to secondhand smoke in the household, history of atopy, not breastfeeding, and household crowding. Mortality is rare when supportive care is available. Fewer than 125 deaths in children <2 years of age are associated with RSV infection annually in the

United States, and fewer than 50 deaths occur in those with a primary diagnosis of RSV.

The association between RSV infection early in life and subsequent asthma remains poorly understood. Children who experience lower respiratory tract disease (eg, bronchiolitis or pneumonia) from RSV have an increased risk of developing asthma later in life. This association, which also is seen with other viruses including rhinovirus, may reflect an underlying anatomic or genetic predisposition to both severe bronchiolitis and to asthma rather than a direct consequence of RSV infection.

Almost all children are infected by RSV at least once by 24 months of age, and reinfection throughout life is common. Subsequent infections usually are less severe than primary infections. Particularly among older children and adults, recurrent RSV infection manifests as mild upper respiratory tract illness. Serious disease involving the lower respiratory tract may develop in older children and adults, especially in immunocompromised people, people with cardiopulmonary disease, and elderly people, particularly those with comorbidities.

ETIOLOGY: RSV is an enveloped, nonsegmented, negative strand RNA virus of the genus *Pneumovirus* of the family *Paramyxoviridae*. RSV F and G surface proteins likely promote virus attachment, although a virus constructed without the G surface protein was able to infect and replicate in tissue culture. Numerous genotypes have been identified in each RSV subgroup based on the G protein gene, and strains of both subgroups often circulate concurrently in a community. The clinical and epidemiologic significance of strain variation is not clear, although antigenic differences may affect susceptibility to infection. Some RSV strains may be more virulent than others, but severity of disease does not seem more associated to an RSV strains or subgroup.

EPIDEMIOLOGY: Humans are the only source of infection. RSV usually is transmitted by direct or close contact with contaminated secretions, which may occur from exposure to large-particle droplets at short distances (typically <6 feet) or from fomites. Viable RSV can persist on environmental surfaces for several hours and for 30 minutes or more on hands. Infection among health care personnel and others may occur by hand-to-eye or hand-to-nasal epithelium self-inoculation with contaminated secretions. Enforcement of infection-control policies is critical to decrease the risk of health care-associated transmission of RSV. Health care-associated spread of RSV to hematopoietic stem cell or solid organ transplant recipients or to patients with cardiopulmonary abnormalities or immunocompromised conditions has been associated with severe and fatal disease in children and adults. Other immunocompromised children, such as those with human immunodeficiency virus (HIV) infection, experience extended viral shedding and sometimes prolonged illness but usually do not exhibit enhanced disease.

RSV occurs in annual epidemics during winter and early spring in temperate climates. Spread among household and child care contacts, including adults, is common. The period of viral shedding usually is 3 to 8 days but may last longer, especially in young infants and in immunosuppressed people, in whom shedding may continue for 3 to 4 weeks or longer.

The **incubation period** ranges from 2 to 8 days; 4 to 6 days is most common.

DIAGNOSTIC TESTS: Rapid diagnostic assays, including direct fluorescent antibody (DFA) assay and enzyme or chromatographic immunoassay techniques for detection of viral antigen in nasopharyngeal specimens, are available commercially for RSV and generally are reliable in infants and young children. In children, the sensitivity of these assays in comparison with culture varies between 53% and 96%, with most in the 80% to 90%

range. The sensitivity may be lower in older children and is quite poor in adults, because adults typically shed low concentrations of RSV. As with all antigen detection assays, the predictive value is high during the peak season, but false-positive test results are more likely to occur when the incidence of disease is low, such as in the summer in temperate areas. Therefore, antigen detection assays should not be the only basis on which the beginning and end of monthly RSV immunoprophylaxis is determined.

Molecular diagnostic tests using reverse transcriptase-polymerase chain reaction (RT-PCR) are cleared by the US Food and Drug Administration (FDA) and available widely and increase RSV detection rates over viral isolation or antigen detection assays, especially in older children and adults. Many tests are designed as multiplex assays to facilitate testing for multiple respiratory viruses with a single assay. Because of the increased sensitivity of RT-PCR assay, these tests may be preferred. However, results of these tests should be interpreted with caution, especially when a multiplex assay identifies more than one virus, because some viruses (eg, RSV, rhinovirus, adenovirus, and bocavirus) may persist in the airway for many weeks after the acute infection has resolved. As many as 25% of asymptomatic children test positive for respiratory viruses using RT-PCR assays in population-based studies. Up to 30% of children with RSV bronchiolitis may be coinfected with another respiratory tract pathogen, such as human metapneumovirus, rhinovirus, bocavirus, adenovirus, coronavirus, influenza virus, or parainfluenza virus. Whether children with bronchiolitis who are coinfected with more than one virus experience more severe or even less severe disease is not clear.

RSV isolation from respiratory tract secretions in cell culture requires 1 to 5 days (rapid, centrifugation-enhanced, shell vial techniques can produce results within 24–48 hours), but results and sensitivity vary among laboratories; therefore, molecular diagnostic methods are preferred.

Palivizumab may interfere with immunologic-based RSV diagnostic tests, such as some antigen detection-based assays. In addition, palivizumab inhibits virus replication in cell culture and may interfere with viral culture assays. Palivizumab does not interfere with RT-PCR assays. Assay interference could lead to false-negative RSV diagnostic test results. Therefore, diagnostic test results, when obtained in patients receiving palivizumab immunoprophylaxis, should be used in conjunction with clinical findings to guide medical decisions.

Conventional serologic testing of acute and convalescent serum specimens cannot be relied on to diagnose infection in young infants, because sensitivity may be low and the immune response to RSV infection in infants may be limited.

In most outpatient settings for children with bronchiolitis, routine specific respiratory viral testing has little effect on management and testing is not recommended.[1] Specific respiratory viral testing in hospitalized patients has been associated with fewer diagnostic tests in general once RSV or another virus is identified (especially reducing the need for bacterial cultures), use of fewer antibiotics, and in some hospitals, better cohorting and less health care-associated infection.

TREATMENT: No available treatment shortens the course of bronchiolitis or hastens the resolution of symptoms. The variable course of bronchiolitis and the inability to predict whether supportive care will be needed often results in hospital admission, even when

---

[1]Ralston SL, Lieberthal AS, Meissner HC, et al. Clinical practice guideline: the diagnosis, management, and prevention of bronchiolitis. *Pediatrics.* 2014;134(5):e1474–e1502

symptoms are not severe. Management of young children hospitalized with bronchiolitis is supportive and should include hydration, careful assessment of respiratory status, suction of the upper airway, and if necessary, intubation and mechanical ventilation.[1] Clinicians may choose not to administer supplemental oxygen if the oxyhemoglobin saturation exceeds 90% in infants and children hospitalized with bronchiolitis.[1] Clinicians may choose not to use continuous pulse oximetry for children with bronchiolitis.[1] Continuous measurement of oxygen saturation may detect transient fluctuations in oxygenation that are not clinically significant, prolong oxygen use, and delay discharge. Transient desaturation to <90% is a normal occurrence among healthy infants. Among patients with bronchiolitis, pulse oximetry should not be used as a proxy for respiratory distress. The correlation between respiratory distress and oxygen saturation is poor among infants with lower respiratory tract infection. Supplemental oxygen is recommended only when oxyhemoglobin saturation persistently falls below 90% in a previously healthy infant.[1]

Aerosolized ribavirin therapy has been associated with a small but statistically significant increase in oxygen saturation during the acute infection in several small studies. However, a consistent decrease in need for mechanical ventilation, decrease in length of stay in the pediatric intensive care unit, reduction in days of hospitalization, or decrease in mortality among ribavirin recipients has not been demonstrated. The aerosol route of administration, concern about potential toxic effects among exposed health care personnel, conflicting results of efficacy trials, and high cost have led to infrequent use of this drug. Aerosolized ribavirin is not recommended for routine use because of the lack of a clinically significant effect on outcome. Oral ribavirin has been used in a small number of adult hematopoietic stem cell transplant recipients, however, and it may be considered for use in selected patients with severe, life-threatening disease.

Alpha- and Beta-Adrenergic Agents. Beta-adrenergic agents are not recommended for care of first-time wheezing associated with RSV bronchiolitis. Randomized clinical trials have demonstrated that bronchodilators do not affect disease resolution, need for hospitalization, or length of stay. Bronchodilators do not improve oxygen saturation, hospital admission rates after outpatient treatment, or time to resolution of illness at home. For these reasons, a trial of albuterol no longer is included as a recommended option in the management of RSV bronchiolitis.[1] Evidence does not support the use of nebulized epinephrine in children hospitalized with bronchiolitis. Insufficient data are available to recommend routine use of epinephrine for outpatient management of children with bronchiolitis.[1]

Glucocorticoid Therapy. Controlled clinical trials among children with bronchiolitis have demonstrated that corticosteroids do not reduce hospital admissions and do not reduce length of stay for inpatients. Corticosteroid treatment should not be used for infants and children with RSV bronchiolitis. Evidence for potential benefit from combined use of corticosteroids and agents with alpha- or beta-adrenergic activity is insufficient to support a recommendation.[1]

Antimicrobial Therapy. Antimicrobial therapy is not indicated for infants with RSV bronchiolitis or pneumonia unless there is evidence of concurrent bacterial infection. A young child with a distinct viral lower respiratory tract infection (bronchiolitis) has a low risk (<1%) of bacterial infection of the CSF or blood. Bacterial lung infections and bacteremia

---

[1]Ralston SL, Lieberthal AL, Meissner HC, et al. Clinical practice guideline: the diagnosis, management, and prevention of bronchiolitis. *Pediatrics.* 2014;134(5):e1474–e1502

are uncommon in this setting. Acute otitis media (AOM) caused by RSV or bacterial superinfection may occur in infants with RSV bronchiolitis. Oral antimicrobial therapy for treatment of otitis media may be considered if bulging of the tympanic membrane is present.[1]

Other Therapies. Chest physiotherapy should not be used in infants and children with a diagnosis of bronchiolitis. Suctioning of the nasopharynx to remove secretions may provide temporary relief. If indicated, nasogastric or intravenous fluids may be used to maintain hydration.

Nebulized hypertonic saline (3%) appears to be safe and effective at improving the symptoms of mild to moderate bronchiolitis after 24 hours of use and in reducing hospital length of stay in cases in which the duration of stay is likely to exceed 3 days. However, most children hospitalized with bronchiolitis are discharged within 72 hours. Hypertonic saline has not been shown to be effective over the short term for patients managed in the emergency room or when length of hospitalization is brief. Hypertonic saline has not been studied in intensive care settings.

High-flow nasal cannula (HFNC) therapy, nasal continuous positive airway pressure, and heliox have been used for respiratory support in hospitalized infants with bronchiolitis. Only limited data are available on the effectiveness of these therapies in RSV bronchiolitis. Because these therapies typically are used in severely or critically ill infants with bronchiolitis, they should be used only in consultation with a critical care or pulmonary specialist.

Prevention of RSV Infections. Palivizumab is a humanized monoclonal immunoglobulin (Ig) G1K antibody produced by recombinant DNA technology. The antibody is directed against a conserved epitope of an antigenic site of the fusion protein (F), which resides on the viral surface and prevents the conformational change that is necessary for fusion of the viral RSV envelope with the plasma membrane of the respiratory epithelial cell. Without fusion, the virus is unable to enter the cell and unable to replicate.

Palivizumab may be considered to reduce the risk of RSV lower respiratory tract disease in certain children at increased risk of severe disease. Palivizumab is administered intramuscularly at a dose of 15 mg/kg, once every 30 days. Children who qualify for palivizumab prophylaxis should receive the first dose at the onset of the RSV season. For qualifying infants born during the RSV season, fewer than 5 doses will be needed to provide protection until the RSV season ends in their region (maximum of 5 doses). In some reports, palivizumab administration in a home-based program has been shown to improve compliance and to reduce exposure to health care-associated pathogens compared with administration in office- or clinic-based settings. A patient with a history of a severe allergic reaction following a dose of palivizumab should not receive additional doses. Palivizumab is not effective in treatment of RSV disease and is not approved or recommended for this indication.

Cost Considerations. Results of cost-effectiveness analyses of palivizumab prophylaxis depend on several base case assumptions, including baseline RSV hospitalization rates among different groups of high-risk children, the reduction in RSV hospitalization rates among recipients of prophylaxis in different risk groups, the cost of hospitalization (amount saved by avoiding hospitalization), the threshold criteria for hospitalization of a

---

[1]Lieberthal AS, Carroll AE, Chonmaitree T, et al. Clinical practice guideline: the diagnosis and management of acute otitis media. *Pediatrics.* 2013;131(3):e964–e999

child with bronchiolitis (which differs among countries and providers), the number of monthly doses administered, the weight of an infant who receives prophylaxis, variation in the severity of the RSV season, and the acquisition cost of palivizumab. Cost analyses conducted by independent investigators consistently demonstrate the cost of palivizumab prophylaxis far exceeds the economic benefit from a small number of hospitalizations avoided, even among infants at highest risk.

Numerous studies have documented that infants hospitalized with viral lower airway disease are more likely to experience recurrent wheezing compared with infants who do not experience severe bronchiolitis. Data from one trial suggest that avoidance of RSV infection among preterm infants from use of immunoprophylaxis may result in a slight decrease in the incidence of parent-reported wheezing episodes (not medically attended events) in the first years of life. Another study found no reduction in medically attended wheezing events among immunoprophylaxis recipients, despite a reduction in RSV lower respiratory tract disease.

Health care expenditures should not be based only on cost but rather on the assessment of the benefit of the intervention relative to the expenditure. High-cost interventions may be appropriate if highly beneficial. Because the high cost of palivizumab prophylaxis is associated with relatively minimal health benefit, this intervention cannot be considered as high-value health care for any group of infants. To date, there is no study that has shown that palivizumab can reduce RSV-associated mortality or childhood asthma.

Initiation and Termination of Immunoprophylaxis. During the 7 RSV seasons from July 2007 to June 2014, the national median duration of the RSV season ranged from 18 to 21 weeks, with median peak activity from late-December to late January, with the exception of Florida and Alaska. Within the 10 Health and Human Services Regions, in the few regions when the RSV season began in October, the season ended in March. In regions where the RSV season began in December or January, the season ended by April or early May. Because 5 monthly doses of palivizumab at 15 mg/kg/dose will provide more than 6 months of serum palivizumab concentrations above the threshold for protection for most infants, administration of more than 5 monthly doses is not recommended within the continental United States. Children who qualify for palivizumab prophylaxis should receive the first dose at the onset of the RSV season. For qualifying infants born during the RSV season, fewer than 5 doses will be needed to provide protection until the RSV season ends in their region (maximum of 5 doses).

A small number of sporadic RSV hospitalizations will occur before or after the main season in many areas of the United States, but the greatest benefit from prophylaxis is derived during the peak of the season and not when the incidence of RSV hospitalization is low.

Timing of Prophylaxis for American Indian/Alaska Native Infants. Hospitalization rates for all-cause bronchiolitis up to 5 times greater than infants of similar ages have been described in Alaska Native children from the Yukon-Kuskokwim Delta. The rates of RSV hospitalization are at least threefold higher for American Indian/Alaska Native (AI/AN) infants in rural Alaska and southwest Indian Health System regions than for other US infants of similar ages. RSV hospitalization rates for AI/AN infants in these areas are related in part to household crowding and lack of plumbing (Alaska) and are similar to medical high-risk infants in the overall US population. On the basis of epidemiology of RSV in Alaska and Navajo/White Mountain Apache populations, particularly in remote regions where the cost of emergency air transport may alter a cost analysis, the selection of infants eligible for prophylaxis may differ from the remainder of the United States. Because of unique seasonality of RSV in Alaska, clinicians may wish to use RSV laboratory surveillance data generated by the state of Alaska to assist in determining onset and end of the RSV season for appropriate timing of palivizumab administration.

Limited information is available concerning the burden of RSV disease for other American Indian populations, with 2 studies documenting bronchiolitis hospitalization rates in Navajo populations between 91.3 and 96.3/1000 infants younger than 1 year. However, local assessment of the cost-benefit, as occurs for Alaska Native populations, may be prudent for certain American Indian populations. If local data support a high burden of RSV disease in select American Indian populations, selection of infants eligible for prophylaxis may differ from the remainder of the United States for infants in the first year of life.

Timing of Prophylaxis for the State of Florida. Variation in the onset and end of the RSV season in different regions of Florida may affect the timing of palivizumab administration. Florida Department of Health data may be used to determine the appropriate timing for administration of the first dose of palivizumab for qualifying infants. Despite varying onset and end dates of the RSV season in different regions of Florida, a maximum of 5 monthly doses of palivizumab will be adequate for qualifying infants for most RSV seasons in Florida. If the first of 5 monthly doses is administered in July, protective serum concentrations of palivizumab will be present for most infants and young children for more than 6 months (likely into February). More than 5 monthly doses are not recommended, despite the detection of a small number of cases of RSV infection outside this time window.

Eligibility Criteria for Prophylaxis of High-Risk Infants and Young Children.[1,2]

- **Preterm infants with CLD.**
  - Prophylaxis may be considered during the RSV season during the first year of life for preterm infants who develop CLD of prematurity, defined as gestational age <32 weeks, 0 days, and a requirement for >21% oxygen for at least the first 28 days after birth.
  - During the second year, consideration of palivizumab prophylaxis is recommended only for infants who satisfy this definition of CLD of prematurity and continue to require medical support (chronic corticosteroid therapy, diuretic therapy, or supplemental oxygen) during the 6-month period before the start of the second RSV season.
  - For infants with CLD who do not continue to require medical support in the second year of life, prophylaxis is not recommended.

- **Infants with CHD.**
  - Children with hemodynamically significant CHD who are most likely to benefit from immunoprophylaxis include infants with acyanotic heart disease who are receiving medication to control congestive heart failure and will require cardiac

---

[1]American Academy of Pediatrics, Committee on Infectious Diseases, Bronchiolitis Guideline Committee. Technical report: updated guidance for palivizumab prophylaxis among infants and young children at increased risk of hospitalization for respiratory syncytial virus infection. *Pediatrics.* 2014;134(2):e620–e638

[2]American Academy of Pediatrics, Committee on Infectious Diseases, Bronchiolitis Guideline Committee. Policy statement: updated guidance for palivizumab prophylaxis among infants and young children at increased risk of hospitalization for respiratory syncytial virus infection. *Pediatrics.* 2014;134(2):415–420

surgical procedures and infants with moderate to severe pulmonary hypertension.

- ◆ Decisions regarding palivizumab prophylaxis for infants with cyanotic heart defects in the first year of life may be made in consultation with a pediatric cardiologist, as the benefit of prophylaxis in infants with cyanotic heart disease is unknown.
- ◆ These recommendations apply to qualifying infants in their first year.
- ◆ The following groups of infants with CHD are <u>not</u> at increased risk of RSV infection and generally should not receive immunoprophylaxis:
    - – Infants and children with hemodynamically insignificant heart disease (eg, secundum atrial septal defect, small ventricular septal defect, pulmonic stenosis, uncomplicated aortic stenosis, mild coarctation of the aorta, and patent ductus arteriosus);
    - – Infants with lesions adequately corrected by surgery, unless they continue to require medication for congestive heart failure;
    - – Infants with mild cardiomyopathy who are not receiving medical therapy for the condition; and
    - – Children in their second year.
- ◆ Because a mean decrease in palivizumab serum concentration of 58% was observed after surgical procedures that involve cardiopulmonary bypass, for children who are receiving prophylaxis and who continue to require prophylaxis following a surgical procedure, a postoperative dose of palivizumab (15 mg/kg) should be considered after cardiac bypass or at the conclusion of extracorporeal membrane oxygenation (ECMO) for infants and children younger than 2 years.
- ◆ Children younger than 2 years who undergo cardiac transplantation during the RSV season may be considered for palivizumab prophylaxis.

- **Preterm infants without CLD or CHD.**
    - ◆ Palivizumab prophylaxis may be considered for preterm infants born before 29 weeks, 0 days' gestation who are younger than 12 months at the start of the RSV season.
    - ◆ For infants born during the RSV season, fewer than 5 monthly doses will be needed.
    - ◆ Available data for infants born at 29 weeks, 0 days' gestation or later do not identify a gestational age cutoff for which the benefits of prophylaxis are clear. For this reason, otherwise healthy infants born at 29 weeks, 0 days' gestation or later are not recommended to receive palivizumab prophylaxis. Infants born at 29 weeks, 0 days' gestation or later may qualify to receive prophylaxis on the basis of congenital heart disease (CHD), chronic lung disease (CLD), or another condition.
    - ◆ Palivizumab prophylaxis is not recommended in the second year of life on the basis of a history of prematurity alone, regardless of the degree of prematurity.
    - ◆ Some experts believe that on the basis of the data quantifying a small increase in risk of hospitalization, even for infants born earlier than 29 weeks, 0 days' gestation, palivizumab prophylaxis is not justified in the first year of life.

- **Children with anatomic pulmonary abnormalities or neuromuscular disorder.**
    - ◆ No prospective studies or population-based data are available to define the risk of RSV hospitalization in children with pulmonary abnormalities or neuromuscular disease. Infants with neuromuscular disease or a congenital anomaly that impairs

the ability to clear secretions from the upper airway because of ineffective cough are at risk of a prolonged hospitalization related to lower respiratory tract infection and, therefore, may be considered for prophylaxis during their first year.

- **Immunocompromised children.**
  - ◆ No population-based data are available on the incidence of RSV hospitalization in children who undergo hematopoietic stem cell transplantation. An increased risk for RSV disease in pediatric liver transplant recipients was reported in a review of the national transplantation database. Data on the incidence of RSV hospitalizations in other solid organ transplant recipients are not readily available. Severe and even fatal disease attributable to RSV is recognized in children receiving chemotherapy or who are immunocompromised because of other conditions including hematopoietic or solid organ transplantation but the efficacy of prophylaxis in this cohort is not known. Prophylaxis may be considered for children younger than 24 months who will be profoundly immunocompromised during the RSV season.
- **Children with Down syndrome.**
  - ◆ Limited data suggest a slight increase in RSV hospitalization rates among children with Down syndrome.
  - ◆ However, data describing more than a slight increase in hospitalization rates are insufficient to justify a recommendation for routine use of prophylaxis in children with Down syndrome unless qualifying heart disease, CLD, airway clearance issues, or prematurity (<29 weeks, 0 days' gestation) is present.
- **Children with cystic fibrosis.**
  - ◆ Routine use of palivizumab prophylaxis in patients with cystic fibrosis, including neonates diagnosed with cystic fibrosis by newborn screening, is not recommended unless other indications are present.
  - ◆ An infant with cystic fibrosis with clinical evidence of CLD and/or nutritional compromise in the first year may be considered for prophylaxis.
  - ◆ Continued use of palivizumab prophylaxis in the second year may be considered for infants with manifestations of severe lung disease (previous hospitalization for pulmonary exacerbation in the first year or abnormalities on chest radiography or chest computed tomography that persist when stable) or weight-for-length less than the 10th percentile.
- **Preventive measures for all high-risk infants.**
  - ◆ Infants, especially those at high risk, never should be exposed to tobacco smoke. Tobacco smoke exposure is a known risk factor for many adverse health-related outcomes, and studies have shown increased severity of RSV infection in hospitalized children exposed to secondhand smoke. In addition, smoke exposure may increase the risk of developing wheezing after RSV infection. Families with infants, especially with infants who are at increased risk of RSV disease, should be advised to control exposure to tobacco smoke, and referrals for smoking cessation are appropriate.
  - ◆ In contrast to the well-documented beneficial effect of breastfeeding against many viral illnesses, existing data are conflicting regarding the specific protective effect of breastfeeding against RSV infection. Breastfeeding should be encouraged for all infants in accordance with recommendations of the American Academy of Pediatrics.

♦ High-risk infants should be kept away from crowds and from situations in which exposure to infected people cannot be controlled. Participation in group child care should be restricted during the RSV season for high-risk infants whenever feasible.

♦ Parents should be instructed on the importance of careful hand hygiene.

♦ In addition, all infants (beginning at 6 months of age) and their contacts (beginning when the child is born) should receive influenza vaccine as well as other recommended age-appropriate immunizations.

- **Special situations.**
  - ♦ Discontinuation of palivizumab prophylaxis among children who experience breakthrough RSV hospitalization:
    - – If any infant or young child receiving monthly palivizumab prophylaxis experiences a breakthrough RSV hospitalization, monthly prophylaxis should be discontinued because of the extremely low likelihood of a second RSV hospitalization in the same season (<0.5%).
  - ♦ Use of palivizumab in the second year:
    - – Hospitalization rates attributable to RSV decline during the second RSV season for all children.
    - – A second season of palivizumab prophylaxis is recommended only for preterm infants with CLD who continue to require supplemental oxygen, chronic systemic corticosteroid therapy, or diuretic therapy within 6 months of the start of the second RSV season.
  - ♦ Prevention of health care-associated RSV disease:
    - – No rigorous data exist to support palivizumab use in controlling outbreaks of health care-associated disease, and palivizumab use is not recommended for this purpose. Strict adherence to infection control practices is the basis for reducing health care-associated RSV disease.
    - – Infants in a neonatal unit who qualify for prophylaxis because of CLD, prematurity, or CHD may receive the first dose 48 to 72 hours before discharge to home or promptly after discharge.

ISOLATION OF THE HOSPITALIZED PATIENT: In addition to standard precautions, contact precautions are recommended for the duration of RSV-associated hospitalization among infants and young children, including patients treated with ribavirin. The effectiveness of these precautions depends on compliance and necessitates scrupulous adherence to appropriate hand hygiene practices. Patients with RSV infection should be cared for in single rooms or placed in a cohort.

CONTROL MEASURES: The control of health care-associated RSV transmission is complicated by the continuing chance of introduction through infected patients, staff, and visitors. During the peak of the RSV season, many infants and children hospitalized with respiratory tract symptoms will be infected with RSV and should be cared for with contact precautions (see Isolation of the Hospitalized Patient, discussed previously). During community outbreaks of RSV, a variety of measures have been demonstrated to reduce the risk of health care-associated transmission, including: (1) cohorting of symptomatic patients and staff; (2) excluding visitors with current or recent respiratory tract infections; (3) excluding staff with respiratory tract illness or RSV infection from caring for susceptible infants; (4) using gowns and gloves and possibly goggles or masks for protecting health care personnel; (5) emphasizing hand hygiene before and after direct contact with patients, after contact with inanimate objects in the direct vicinity of patients, and after glove removal; and (6) limiting young sibling visitation during the RSV season.

A critical aspect of RSV prevention among high-risk infants is education of parents and other caregivers about the importance of decreasing exposure to and transmission of RSV. Preventive measures include limiting, where feasible, exposure to contagious settings (eg, child care centers); emphasis on hand hygiene in all settings, including the home, especially during periods when contacts of high-risk children have respiratory tract infections; and limiting exposure to secondhand smoke.

Rhinovirus Infections

CLINICAL MANIFESTATIONS: Rhinoviruses are the most frequent cause of the common cold, or rhinosinusitis. Typical clinical manifestations include sore throat, nasal congestion, and nasal discharge that initially is watery and clear but often becomes mucopurulent and viscous after a few days. Malaise, headache, myalgia, low-grade fever, cough, and sneezing may occur. Symptoms typically peak in severity after 3 to 4 days and have a median duration of 7 days, but may persist for more than 10 days in approximately 25% of illnesses. Rhinoviruses also cause otitis media and lower respiratory tract infections (eg, bronchiolitis, pneumonia) in infants, and they are increasingly recognized as an important cause of community-acquired pneumonia in both children and adults. Rhinoviruses also are associated with 60% to 70% of acute exacerbations of asthma in school-aged children.

ETIOLOGY: Human rhinoviruses (HRVs) are small, nonenveloped, single, positive-stranded RNA viruses classified into 3 species (HRV-A, HRV-B, and HRV-C) in the family *Picornaviridae*, genus *Enterovirus*. More than 150 rhinovirus types have been identified by immunologic and molecular methods. Infection confers type-specific immunity, but this protection is limited and temporary.

EPIDEMIOLOGY: Rhinovirus infection is ubiquitous in human populations. Children have an average of 2 rhinovirus infections each year, and 93% of people experience at least 1 rhinovirus infection, which may be either symptomatic or asymptomatic, each year. Rhinoviruses are detected commonly in adults and children with upper and lower respiratory infections and usually are self-limited. Rhinoviruses are the most common cause of pneumonia in immunocompromised people.

Transmission occurs predominantly by person-to-person contact via self-inoculation by contaminated secretions on hands or by large-particle aerosol spread. Infections occur throughout the year, but peak activity occurs during autumn and spring. Multiple serotypes circulate simultaneously, and the prevalent serotypes circulating in a given population change from season to season. HRV-A and HRV-C induce more severe illnesses than HRV-B. In addition, HRV-C infections are more commonly associated with wheezing and lower respiratory illnesses compared with the other 2 serotypes. Viral shedding in nasopharyngeal secretions is most abundant during the first 2 to 3 days of infection and usually ceases by 7 to 10 days. However, virus shedding detectable by polymerase chain reaction testing may continue for as long as 7 weeks or more.

The **incubation period** is usually is 2 to 3 days.

DIAGNOSTIC TESTS: Rhinovirus infection is diagnosed by detection of virus in respiratory secretions, although a specific viral diagnosis generally is not useful clinically. Isolation of virus in cell culture is insensitive. Because of the lack of common group antigen among the various serotypes, antigen detection is not practical for clinical diagnosis. Therefore, reverse transcriptase-polymerase chain reaction (RT-PCR) assays are the preferred way to identify rhinovirus infections, with several commercial assays available and cleared by the US Food and Drug Administration. Most of these assays are designed as multiplexed tests that detect a wide variety of viral and, in some cases, bacterial respiratory pathogens. In general, these assays cannot clearly distinguish human rhinoviruses from enteroviruses because of the genetic similarity of the 2 groups and primers that target genetically conserved regions. Given the prevalence of rhinovirus infection and the occurrence of shedding following infection, rhinovirus detected, even in symptomatic patients, may not be causal. Serologic diagnosis of rhinovirus infection is impractical because of the large number of antigenic types and the absence of a common antigen.

TREATMENT: Treatment is supportive. No specific antiviral therapies are available for treatment of rhinovirus infections. Antimicrobial agents should not be used for prevention of secondary bacterial infection, because their use may promote the emergence of resistant bacteria and subsequently complicate treatment for a bacterial infection, and because of the risk of antibiotic-associated side effects (eg, *Clostridium difficile* disease; see Antimicrobial Resistance and Antimicrobial Stewardship: Appropriate and Judicious Use of Antimicrobial Agents, p 906).

ISOLATION OF THE HOSPITALIZED PATIENT: In addition to standard precautions, droplet precautions are recommended for symptomatic hospitalized infants and children for the duration of illness. Contact precautions should be added if copious moist secretions and close contact are likely to occur (eg, young infants). In symptomatic immunocompromised patients, the duration of contact precautions should be extended because of possible prolonged shedding.

CONTROL MEASURES: Appropriate respiratory hygiene and cough etiquette should be followed. Routine hand washing and ethanol-based hand sanitizers are effective for removal of rhinovirus from the hands.

Rickettsial Diseases

Rickettsial diseases comprise infections caused by bacterial species of the genera *Rickettsia* (endemic and epidemic typhus and spotted fever group rickettsioses), *Orientia* (scrub typhus), *Ehrlichia* (ehrlichiosis), *Anaplasma* (anaplasmosis), *Neoehrlichia*, and *Neorickettsia*.

CLINICAL MANIFESTATIONS: The early signs and symptoms can be nonspecific and often mimic viral illness. Rickettsial infections have many features in common, including the following:

- Fever, rash (especially in spotted fever and typhus group rickettsiae), headache, myalgia, and respiratory tract symptoms are prominent features. The classic rash in Rocky Mountain spotted fever (RMSF) may not appear for 1 week after onset of symptoms, and 10% to 15% of patients do not present with the rash.
- One or more inoculation eschars occur with many rickettsial diseases, especially most spotted fever group rickettsioses, rickettsialpox, and scrub typhus.
- Systemic endothelial damage of small blood vessels resulting in increased vascular permeability is the hallmark pathologic feature of most severe spotted fever and typhus group rickettsial infections.
- Some rickettsial diseases, particularly RMSF and Mediterranean spotted fever, can become life-threatening rapidly. Risk factors for severe disease include glucose-6-

phosphate dehydrogenase deficiency, male gender, and antecedent exposure to sulfonamides.

Immunity against reinfection by the same agent after natural infection is not well studied, but some anecdotal information suggests that prior infection confers immunity for at least 1 year. Documented reinfections with *Rickettsia* and *Ehrlichia* species have been described only rarely.

ETIOLOGY: Currently recognized rickettsial pathogens of humans include more than 20 species of *Rickettsia*, 5 species of *Ehrlichia*, *Anaplasma phagocytophilum*, *Orientia tsutsugamushi*, and *Neorickettsia sennetsu*. Tickborne neoehrlichiosis caused by *Candidatus Neoehrlichia mikurensis*, which features rodents as the primary host, is an emerging disease in Asia and Europe. Rickettsiae are small, coccobacillary gram-negative bacteria that are obligately intracellular pathogens and cannot be grown in cell-free media. *Orientia* and *Rickettsia* organisms reside free within the cytoplasm and *Anaplasmataceae* organisms in phagosomes.

EPIDEMIOLOGY: Rickettsial diseases have various hematophagous arthropod vectors that include ticks, fleas, mites, and lice. Except in the case of *Rickettsia prowazekii*, the cause of epidemic typhus, humans are incidental hosts for rickettsial pathogens. Rickettsial life cycles typically involve one or more arthropod species as well as various mammalian reservoir or amplifying hosts, and transmission to humans occurs during environmental or occupational exposures to infected arthropods. Geographic and seasonal occurrences of each rickettsial disease are related directly to the distributions and life cycles of the specific vector.

Incubation periods vary according to organism (see disease-specific chapters in Section 3).

Other Global Rickettsial Spotted Fever Infections. A number of other epidemiologically distinct fleaborne and tickborne spotted fever infections caused by rickettsiae have been recognized (also see **www.cdc.gov/otherspottedfever/index.html**). These diseases are of importance among people traveling to or returning from areas where these agents are endemic and among people living in these areas. These infections have clinical and pathologic features that vary widely in severity. Many present with an eschar at the site of the tick bite and without rash. The causative agents of some of these infections share the same group antigen as *R rickettsii* and include the following:

- *Rickettsia africae*, the causative agent of African tick bite fever that is endemic in sub-Saharan Africa, Oceania, and some Caribbean islands.
- *Rickettsia conorii* and subspecies, the causative agents of Mediterranean spotted fever, India tick typhus, Marseilles fever, Israeli tick typhus, and Astrakhan spotted fever, that are endemic in southern Europe, Africa, the Middle East, and the Indian subcontinent.
- *Rickettsia parkeri*, a causative agent of eschar-associated infections in the Americas.
- *Rickettsia sibirica*, the causative agent of Siberian tick typhus (or North Asian tick typhus), endemic in central Asia.
- *Rickettsia australis*, the causative agent of North Queensland tick typhus, endemic in eastern Australia.
- *Rickettsia japonica*, the causative agent of Japanese spotted fever, endemic in Japan.
- *Rickettsia honei*, the causative agent of Thai tick typhus and Flinders Island spotted fever, endemic throughout Southeast Asia.
- *Rickettsia slovaca*, the causative agent of tickborne lymphadenopathy (TIBOLA), also known as *Dermacentor*-borne necrosis-erythema-lymphadenopathy (DEBONEL) or the

more overarching term scalp eschars and neck lymphadenopathy (SENLAT), endemic in European countries; *Rickettsia raoultii* infections have a similar presentation and distribution.

- *Rickettsia felis,* the causative agent of cat flea rickettsiosis that occurs worldwide; reports on the severity of illness vary widely.
- *Rickettsia aeschlimannii,* a causative agent of disease with an eschar-associated illness reported from Africa and Europe.
- *Rickettsia heilongjiangensis,* reported from the Russian Far East and China.
- *Rickettsia sibirica* subspecies *mongolitimonae,* reported from Europe, Africa, and Asia, which causes a rickettsiosis with eschar and lymphangitis.
- *Rickettsia massiliae* is widespread in Africa and Europe; the Bar 29 type agent has been found in the United States and is implicated as a cause of illness in Argentina.
- *Rickettsia* species 364D causes eschar, headache, and fever on the US Pacific coast.
- *Rickettsia monacensis* causes a syndrome similar to that caused by *R conorii* and is found in Spain and southern Italy.

DIAGNOSTIC TESTS: Group-specific antibodies are detectable in the serum of most patients by 7 to 14 days after onset of illness, but slower antibody responses may occur, particularly in some diseases of lesser severity. The utility of serologic testing during the acute illness is generally of limited value, and a negative serologic test result during the initial stage of the illness should never be used to exclude a diagnosis of rickettsial disease. Nonetheless, serologic assays provide an excellent method of retrospective confirmation when paired serum samples collected during the illness and approximately 2 to 4 weeks later are tested in tandem. The indirect immunofluorescent antibody assay is recommended in most circumstances but cannot determine the causative agent to the species level. Treatment early in the course of illness can blunt or delay serologic responses. Polymerase chain reaction (PCR) assays can detect rickettsiae in whole blood or tissues collected during the acute stage of illness and before administration of antimicrobial agents; availability of these tests often is limited to reference and research laboratories. In laboratories with experienced personnel, immunohistochemical staining and PCR testing of skin biopsy specimens from patients with rash or eschar lesions can help to diagnose rickettsial infections early in the course of disease. PCR assays and sequencing of DNA collected during acute infection provide more accurate identification of the etiologic agent than serologic testing.

TREATMENT: Prompt initiation of treatment is indicated for all patients in all age groups with suspected RMSF or ehrlichiosis, without waiting for confirmative diagnostic testing. The drug of choice for all rickettsioses, including RMSF and ehrlichiosis, is doxycycline, and the treatment course generally is 7 to 14 days. Antimicrobial treatment is most effective when people are treated appropriately during the first week of illness. If the disease remains untreated during the second week, therapy is less effective in preventing complications. Because confirmatory laboratory test results primarily return during convalescence, treatment decisions should be made on the basis of clinical findings and epidemiologic data and never should be delayed until test results are known.

CONTROL MEASURES: Control measures primarily involve prevention of vector transmission of rickettsial agents to humans (see Prevention of Mosquitoborne and Tickborne Infections, p 195).

Several rickettsial diseases, including spotted fevers, ehrlichiosis, and anaplasmosis, are nationally notifiable diseases and should be reported to state and local health departments.

For more details, the following chapters in Section 3 on rickettsial diseases should be consulted:

- *Ehrlichia* and *Anaplasma* Infections, p 323 (or **www.cdc.gov/ehrlichiosis/**).
- Rickettsialpox, p 696.
- Rocky Mountain Spotted Fever, p 697 (or **www.cdc.gov/rmsf/**).
- Endemic Typhus (Murine Typhus), p 864.
- Epidemic Typhus (Louseborne or Sylvatic Typhus), p 865.

Rickettsialpox

CLINICAL MANIFESTATIONS: Rickettsialpox is a febrile, eschar-associated illness that is characterized by generalized, relatively sparse, erythematous, papulovesicular eruptions on the trunk, face, and extremities (less often on palms and soles) or on mucous membranes of the mouth. The rash develops 1 to 4 days after onset of fever and 3 to 10 days after appearance of an eschar at the site of the bite of a house mouse mite. Regional lymph nodes in the area of the primary eschar typically become enlarged. Without specific antimicrobial therapy, systemic disease lasts approximately 7 to 10 days; manifestations include fever, headache, malaise, and myalgia. Less frequent manifestations include anorexia, vomiting, conjunctivitis, hepatitis, nuchal rigidity, and photophobia. The disease is mild compared with Rocky Mountain spotted fever, and no rickettsialpox-associated deaths have been described; however, disease occasionally is severe enough to warrant hospitalization.

ETIOLOGY: Rickettsialpox is caused by *Rickettsia akari*, a gram-negative intracellular bacillus, which is classified with the spotted fever group rickettsiae and related antigenically to other members of that group.

EPIDEMIOLOGY: The natural host for *R akari* in the United States is *Mus musculus*, the common house mouse. The organism is transmitted by the house mouse mite, *Liponyssoides sanguineus*. Disease risk is heightened in areas infested with mice and rats. The disease can occur wherever the hosts, pathogens, and humans coexist but most frequently is reported in large urban settings. In the United States, rickettsialpox has been described predominantly in northeastern metropolitan centers, especially in New York City. It also has been confirmed in many other countries, including the Netherlands, Croatia, Ukraine, Turkey, Russia, South Korea, South Africa, and Mexico. All age groups can be affected. No seasonal pattern of disease occurs. The disease is not communicable but occurs occasionally among families or people cohabiting a house mouse mite-infested dwelling.

The **incubation period** is 6 to 15 days.

DIAGNOSTIC TESTS: *R akari* can be isolated in cell culture from blood and eschar biopsy specimens during the acute stage of disease, but culture is not attempted routinely. Because antibodies to *R akari* have extensive cross-reactivity with antibodies against *Rickettsia rickettsii* (the cause of Rocky Mountain spotted fever) and other spotted fever-group rickettsiae, an indirect immunofluorescence antibody assay for *R rickettsii* can be used to demonstrate a fourfold or greater change in antibody titers between acute and convalescent serum specimens taken 2 to 6 weeks apart. Use of *R akari* antigen is recommended for a more accurate serologic diagnosis but may be available only in specialized research laboratories. Immunoglobulin (Ig) M and IgG are detected 7 to 15 days after illness onset.

Immunohistochemical testing of formalin-fixed, paraffin-embedded eschars or papulovesicle biopsy specimens can detect rickettsiae in the samples and are useful diagnostic techniques, but because of cross-reactivity, these assays are not able to confirm the etiologic agent. A species-specific real-time polymerase chain reaction assay for detection of rickettsial DNA with subsequent sequence identification can confirm *R akari* infection but currently is not cleared by the US Food and Drug Administration for use in the United States.

TREATMENT: Doxycycline is the drug of choice in all age groups and is effective when administered for 5 to 7 days. Doxycycline shortens the course of disease, and symptoms typically resolve within 12 to 48 hours after initiation of therapy. Chloramphenicol is an alternative drug but carries a risk of serious adverse events and is not available as an oral formulation in the United States. Use of chloramphenicol should be considered only in rare cases, such as for patients with severe doxycycline allergies, because rickettsialpox usually is mild and self-limited. Untreated rickettsialpox usually will resolve within 2 to 3 weeks.

ISOLATION OF THE HOSPITALIZED PATIENT: Person-to-person spread of rickettsialpox has not been reported. Standard precautions are recommended.

CONTROL MEASURES: Application of residual acaricides can be used in heavily mite-infested environments to eliminate the vector. Rodent-control measures are important in limiting or eliminating spread of rickettsialpox; however, they should be conducted only in conjunction with acaricide application to ensure vector control. No specific management of exposed people is necessary.

Rocky Mountain Spotted Fever

CLINICAL MANIFESTATIONS: Rocky Mountain spotted fever (RMSF) is a systemic, small-vessel vasculitis that often involves a characteristic rash. Fever, myalgia, severe headache (less common in young children), photophobia, nausea, vomiting, and anorexia are typical presenting symptoms. Abdominal pain and diarrhea often are present and can obscure the diagnosis. The rash usually begins within the first 2 to 4 days of symptoms as erythematous macules or maculopapules. The rash usually appears first on the wrists and ankles, often spreading within hours proximally to the trunk and distally to the palms and soles. Although early development of a rash is a useful diagnostic sign, the rash can be atypical or absent altogether in a small portion of patients. It may be difficult to visualize in patients with dark skin. A petechial rash typically is a late finding and indicates progression to severe disease. Lack of a typical rash is a risk factor for misdiagnosis and poor outcome. Hepatomegaly and splenomegaly occur in 10% to 20% of patients and may be reported more frequently in children. Meningeal signs with a positive Kernig and Brudzinski sign may occur. Pediatric cases may additionally experience peripheral or periorbital edema. Thrombocytopenia, hyponatremia (serum sodium concentrations <130 mg/dL are observed in 20%–50% of cases), and elevated liver transaminase concentrations develop in many cases, are frequently mild in the early stages of disease, and worsen as disease progresses. White blood cell count typically is normal, but leukopenia and anemia can occur. If not treated, the illness can be severe, with prominent central nervous system, cardiac, pulmonary, gastrointestinal tract, and renal involvement; disseminated intravascular coagulation; and shock leading to death. RMSF can progress rapidly, even in previously healthy people. Delay in appropriate antimicrobial treatment past the fifth day of symptoms is associated with severe disease and poor outcomes. Case-fatality rates of untreated RMSF range from 20% to 80%, with a median time to death of 8 days. Significant long-term sequelae are common in patients with severe RMSF, including neurologic (paraparesis; hearing loss; peripheral neuropathy; bladder and bowel incontinence; and cerebellar, vestibular, and motor dysfunction) and nonneurologic (disability from limb or digit amputation) sequelae. Patients treated early in the course of symptoms may have a mild illness, with fever resolving in the first 48 hours of treatment.

ETIOLOGY: The family *Rickettsiaceae* compromises 2 genera, *Rickettsia* and *Orientia*. *Rickettsia rickettsii*, an obligate, intracellular, gram-negative bacillus and a member of the spotted fever group of rickettsiae, is the causative agent. The primary targets of infection in mammalian hosts are endothelial cells lining the small blood vessels of all major tissues and organs. Diffuse small vessel vasculitis leads to increased permeability.

EPIDEMIOLOGY: The pathogen is transmitted to humans by the bite of a tick of the *Ixodidae* family (hard ticks). Ticks and their small mammal hosts serve as reservoirs of the pathogen in nature. Other wild animals and dogs have been found with antibodies to *R rickettsii*, but their role as natural reservoirs is not clear. People with occupational or recreational exposure to the tick vector (eg, pet owners, animal handlers, and people who spend more time outdoors) are at increased risk of exposure to the organism. People of all ages can be infected. The period of highest incidence in the United States is from April to September, although RMSF can occur year-round in certain areas with endemic disease. Laboratory-acquired infection rarely has resulted from accidental inoculation and aerosol contamination. Transmission has occurred on rare occasions by blood transfusion. RMSF is the most frequently fatal rickettsial illness in the United States; the case-fatality rate in the preantibiotic era was approximately 25%. Present-day case-fatality rates, estimated at 5% to 10% overall, depend in part on the timing of initiation of appropriate treatment; case-fatality rates of 40% to 50% among patients treated on days 8 or 9 of illness have been described. Mortality is highest in males, people older than 50 years, children younger than 10 years, and people with no recognized tick bite or attachment. In approximately half of pediatric RMSF cases, there is no recall of a recent tick bite. Delay in disease recognition and initiation of antirickettsial therapy after the fifth day of symptoms increase the risk of death. Factors contributing to delayed diagnosis include absence of rash or difficulty in its recognition, especially in individuals with darker complexions; initial presentation before the fourth day of illness; and onset of illness during months of low incidence.

RMSF is widespread in the United States, with a reported annual incidence that has increased sixfold, from 1.8 cases per million people in 2000 to 13.0 cases per million in 2015, or approximately 3700 cases per year between 2011 and 2015. Despite its name, RMSF is not common in the Rocky Mountain area. Most cases are reported in the south Atlantic, southeastern, and south central states, although most states in the contiguous United States record cases each year. The principal recognized vectors of *R rickettsii* are *Dermacentor variabilis* (the American dog tick) in the eastern and central United States and *Dermacentor andersoni* (the Rocky Mountain wood tick) in the western United States. Another common tick throughout the world that feeds on dogs, *Rhipicephalus sanguineus* (the brown dog tick) has been confirmed as a vector of *R rickettsii* in Arizona and Mexico and may play a role in other regions. Transmission parallels periods of tick host-seeking activity in a given geographic area. RMSF also occurs in Canada, Mexico, Central America, and South America.

The **incubation period** is approximately 1 week (typical range, 3–12 days).

DIAGNOSTIC TESTS[1]**:** The diagnosis of RMSF must be made on the basis of clinical signs and symptoms and can be confirmed later using confirmatory diagnostic tests. Treatment should never be delayed while awaiting laboratory confirmation. The gold standard for serologic diagnosis of RMSF is the indirect immunofluorescence antibody (IFA) test. A negative serologic test result from the acute phase does not rule out a diagnosis of RMSF in any case. Both immunoglobulin (Ig) G and IgM antibodies begin to increase around day 7 to 10 after onset of symptoms; however, an elevated acute titer may represent prior infection rather than acute infection. Low-level elevated antibody titers can be an incidental finding in a significant proportion of the general population in some regions. IgM antibodies may remain elevated for months and are not highly specific for acute RMSF. A fourfold or greater increase in antigen-specific IgG between acute and convalescent sera obtained 2 to 4 weeks apart confirms the diagnosis (6 weeks for convalescent serum for *Rickettsia africae*). Cross-reactivity may be observed between antibodies to other spotted fever group rickettsiae, including *Rickettsia parkeri* and *R africae*. Enzyme-linked immunosorbent assays also can be used for assessing antibody presence in acute and convalescent sera but are less useful for quantifying changes in titer.

RMSF may be diagnosed by the detection of *R rickettsii* DNA in acute whole blood and serum specimens by polymerase chain reaction (PCR) assay, but there currently are no PCR tests for *R rickettsia* cleared for use by the US Food and Drug Administration. *R rickettsii* typically do not circulate in the whole blood until advanced stages of disease; therefore, detection of *R rickettsii* DNA in whole blood by PCR testing is possible, but it may be considered a less sensitive diagnostic assay in the absence of advanced illness. The specimen should be obtained preferably before (or within 24 hours of) doxycycline administration, and a negative result does not rule out RMSF infection. Diagnosis may be confirmed by the detection of rickettsial DNA in biopsy or autopsy specimens by PCR assay or immunohistochemical (IHC) visualization of rickettsiae in tissues.

R rickettsii also may be isolated from acute blood specimens by animal passage or through tissue culture, but this can be hazardous, and culture is restricted to specialized procedures (not routine blood culture) at reference laboratories with at minimum Biosafety level 3 containment facilities. Cell culture cultivation of the organism must be confirmed by molecular methods.

TREATMENT[1]**:** Doxycycline is the drug of choice for treatment of RMSF in patients of any age and should be started as soon as RMSF is suspected (see Tetracyclines, p 905). Use of antimicrobial agents other than doxycycline increases the risk of mortality. The doxycycline dose for RMSF is 2.2 mg/kg of body weight per dose, twice per day, orally or intravenously (maximum 100 mg per dose). Treatment is most effective if initiated in the first few days of symptoms, and treatment started after the fifth day of symptoms is less likely to prevent death or other adverse outcomes. Therefore, physicians always should treat empirically even when suspicion of the disease is low and should not postpone treatment while awaiting laboratory confirmation or classic symptoms, such as petechiae, to appear. Chloramphenicol sometimes is listed as an alternative treatment; however, its

---

[1]Biggs HM, Behravesh CB, Bradley KK, et al. Diagnosis and management of tickborne rickettsial diseases: Rocky Mountain spotted fever and other spotted fever group rickettsioses, ehrlichioses, and anaplasmosis—United States. A practical guide for health care and public health professionals. *MMWR Recomm Rep*. 2016; 65(RR-2):1–44. Available at: **www.cdc.gov/mmwr/volumes/65/rr/rr6502a1.htm**

use is associated with a higher risk of fatal outcome. In addition, chloramphenicol carries a risk of serious adverse events and is not available as an oral formulation in the United States. Use of chloramphenicol may be considered only in rare cases, such as severe doxycycline allergies. This should be considered on a case-by-case basis, and the risks and benefits should be discussed with the patient and parents. Antimicrobial treatment should be continued until the patient has been afebrile for at least 3 days and has demonstrated clinical improvement; the usual duration of therapy is 5 to 7 days.

ISOLATION OF THE HOSPITALIZED PATIENT: Standard precautions are recommended.

CONTROL MEASURES: Control of ticks in their natural habitat is difficult. Avoidance of tick-infested areas (eg, grassy areas, areas that border wooded regions) is the best preventive measure. If a tick-infested area is entered, people should wear protective clothing and apply tick or insect repellents to clothes and exposed body parts for added protection. All pets should be treated for ticks according to veterinary guidelines. Adults should be taught to inspect themselves, their children (bodies and clothing), and pets thoroughly for ticks after spending time outdoors during the tick season and to remove ticks promptly and properly (see Prevention of Mosquitoborne and Tickborne Infections, p 195).

Prophylactic antimicrobial agents have no role in preventing RMSF, even in children with a documented tick bite who have not developed symptoms. Patients should not be tested or treated for RMSF until at least 1 symptom of illness is present. No licensed *R rickettsii* vaccine is available in the United States. Additional information is available on the Centers for Disease Control and Prevention's Web site (**www.cdc.gov/rmsf/**).

Rotavirus Infections

CLINICAL MANIFESTATIONS: The clinical manifestations vary and depend on whether it is the first infection or reinfection. After 3 months of age, the first infection generally is the most severe. Infection begins with acute onset of vomiting followed 24 to 48 hours later by watery diarrhea; up to one third of the patients will have high fevers. Symptoms generally persist for 3 to 7 days. In moderate to severe cases, dehydration, electrolyte abnormalities, and acidosis may occur. In certain immunocompromised children, including children with congenital cellular immunodeficiencies or severe combined immunodeficiency (SCID) and children who are hematopoietic stem cell or solid organ transplant recipients, severe, prolonged, and sometimes fatal rotavirus diarrhea may occur. The presence of rotavirus RNA in cerebrospinal fluid (CSF) has been detected in children with rotavirus-associated seizures.

ETIOLOGY: Rotaviruses are segmented, nonenveloped, double-stranded RNA viruses belonging to the family *Reoviridae*, with at least 8 distinct groups (A through H). Group A viruses are the major causes of rotavirus diarrhea worldwide in humans, although rotaviruses of groups B and C have been associated with acute gastroenteritis. Genotyping is based on the 2 outer capsid proteins, VP7 glycoprotein (G) and VP4 protease-cleaved hemagglutinin (P). Before introduction of the rotavirus vaccine, genotypes G1P[8], G2P[4], G3P[8], G4P[8], and G9P[8] were the most common genotypes circulating in the United States. However, in 2012 and 2013, G12P[8] was the most common genotype identified.

EPIDEMIOLOGY: Rotavirus is present in high titer in stools of infected patients several days before and several days after onset of clinical disease. Transmission occurs via the fecal-oral route. Rotavirus is very stable and may remain infectious in the environment for weeks to months. Rotavirus can be found on toys and hard surfaces in child care centers, indicating that fomites may serve as a mechanism of transmission. Respiratory transmission may play a minor role in disease transmission. Spread within families and institutions is common. Rarely, common-source outbreaks from contaminated water or food have been reported.

In temperate climates, rotavirus disease is most prevalent during the cooler months. Before licensure of rotavirus vaccines in North America in 2006 and 2008, the annual rotavirus epidemic usually started during the fall in Mexico and the southwest United States and moved eastward, reaching the northeast United States and Maritime Provinces by spring. The seasonal pattern of disease is less pronounced in tropical climates, with rotavirus infection being more common during the cooler, drier months.

The epidemiology and burden of rotavirus disease in the United States has changed dramatically following the introduction of rotavirus vaccines in 2006 and 2008. Before widespread use of these vaccines, rotavirus was the most common cause of gastroenteritis in young children, the most common cause of health care-associated diarrhea in young children, and an important cause of acute gastroenteritis in children attending child care. Since the introduction of rotavirus vaccines in the United States, a biennial pattern has emerged, with small, short seasons beginning in late winter/early spring (eg, 2009, 2011, 2013, 2015) alternating with years with extremely low circulation (eg, 2008, 2010, 2012, 2014). Beginning in 2008, annual hospitalizations for rotavirus disease among US children younger than 5 years declined by approximately 75%, with an estimated 40 000 to 50 000 fewer rotavirus hospitalizations nationally each year. In case-control evaluations in the United States, the rotavirus vaccines (full series) have been found to be approximately 80% to 90% effective against rotavirus disease resulting in hospitalization. The vaccines also are highly effective against rotavirus disease resulting in emergency department care, and substantial reductions in emergency department visits for rotavirus disease have occurred in the years since the vaccines were introduced. During a 4-year period after vaccine introduction, an estimated 177 000 hospitalizations, 242 000 emergency department visits, and 1.1 million outpatient visits for diarrhea were averted among US children younger than 5 years.

The **incubation period** for rotavirus is short, usually less than 48 hours.

DIAGNOSTIC TESTS: It is not possible to diagnose rotavirus infection by clinical presentation or nonspecific laboratory tests. Enzyme immunoassays (EIAs), chromatographic immunoassays, and latex agglutination assays for group A rotavirus antigen detection in stool are available commercially. EIAs are used most widely because of their high sensitivity and specificity and ease of use. A variety of multiplex nucleic acid-based assays for the detection of gastrointestinal pathogens, including rotavirus, are approved by the US Food and Drug Administration (FDA) for in vitro diagnostic use. The major advantages of molecular diagnostic methods are increased sensitivity and the ability to detect viruses, including rotavirus, that are difficult to isolate in cell culture. Interpretation of assay results may be complicated by the frequent detection of viruses in fecal samples from asymptomatic children and the detection of multiple gastrointestinal pathogens in a single sample. A number of standard or real-time reverse transcriptase-polymerase chain reaction (RT-PCR) assays for detection of rotaviral-specific genomic RNA also are available but are not approved by the US Food and Drug Administration.

The following tests are available in some research and reference laboratories: electron microscopy, polyacrylamide gel electrophoresis (PAGE) of viral RNA with silver staining, and viral culture. However, these tests generally are not used for rapid, acute diagnosis of rotaviral disease.

TREATMENT: No specific antiviral therapy is available. Oral or parenteral fluids and electrolytes are given to prevent or correct dehydration. Orally administered Human Immune Globulin, administered as an investigational therapy in immunocompromised patients with prolonged infection, has decreased viral shedding and shortened the duration of diarrhea.

ISOLATION OF THE HOSPITALIZED PATIENT: In addition to standard precautions, contact precautions are indicated for diapered or incontinent children for the duration of illness.

CONTROL MEASURES: Breastfeeding is associated with milder rotavirus disease and should be encouraged.

Child Care. General measures for interrupting enteric transmission in child care centers are available (see Children in Out-of-Home Child Care, p 122). Surfaces should be washed with soap and water. Few commercially available cleaning products have confirmed virucidal activity against rotavirus. Bleach solutions or other products with confirmed virucidal activity against rotavirus can be used to inactivate rotavirus and may help prevent disease transmission resulting from contact with environmental surfaces (**www.cdc. gov/infectioncontrol/guidelines/disinfection/disinfection-methods/ chemical.html**). Infants and children with rotavirus infection should be excluded from child care centers until stools are contained in the diaper or when toilet-trained children no longer have accidents using the toilet and when stool frequency becomes no more than 2 stools above that child's normal frequency for the time the child is in the program, even if the stools remain loose.

Vaccines. Two rotavirus vaccines are licensed for use among infants in the United States. In February 2006, a live, oral human-bovine reassortant pentavalent rotavirus (RV5 [RotaTeq, Merck & Co Inc, Whitehouse Station, NJ]) vaccine was licensed as a 3-dose series for use among infants in the United States. In April 2008, a live, oral human attenuated monovalent rotavirus (RV1 [Rotarix, GlaxoSmithKline, Research Triangle Park, NC]) vaccine was licensed as a 2-dose series for infants in the United States. The products differ in composition and schedule of administration. The American Academy of Pediatrics and the Centers for Disease Control and Prevention do not express a preference for either vaccine.

In 2010, porcine circovirus or porcine circovirus DNA was detected in both rotavirus vaccines. There is no evidence that this virus is a safety risk or causes illness in humans.

Postmarketing surveillance data from the United States, Australia, Mexico, and Brazil indicate that there is a small risk of intussusception from the currently licensed rotavirus vaccines. In the United States, the data currently available suggest the attributable risk is between approximately 1 excess intussusception case per 20 000 to 100 000 vaccinated infants. The risk appears to be primarily during the first week following the first or second dose; data from Australia suggest some risk may extend up to 21 days following the first dose. In the United States as well as other parts of the world, the benefits of rotavirus vaccination in preventing severe rotavirus disease outweigh the risk of intussusception. Parents should be informed of the risk, the early signs and symptoms of intussusception, and the need for prompt care if these develop.

Postmarketing strain surveillance in the United States and other countries has revealed that RV5 vaccine reassortant strains have been detected occasionally in stool samples of children with diarrhea. In some of the reports, the reassortant virus seemed to cause diarrheal illness. An RV1 vaccine wild-type reassortant strain has also been reported outside the United States.

Following are recommendations for use of the currently licensed rotavirus vaccines[1,2] (see Table 3.65):

- Infants in the United States routinely should be immunized with 3 doses of RV5 vaccine administered orally at 2, 4, and 6 months of age or with 2 doses of RV1 vaccine administered orally at 2 and 4 months of age.
- The first dose of rotavirus vaccine should be administered from 6 weeks through 14 weeks, 6 days of age (the maximum age for the first dose is 14 weeks, 6 days).
- Immunization should not be initiated for infants 15 weeks, 0 days of age or older. For infants to whom the first dose of rotavirus vaccine is administered inadvertently at 15 weeks, 0 days of age or older, the remainder of the rotavirus immunization series should be completed according to the schedule.
- The minimum interval between doses of rotavirus vaccine is 4 weeks.
- All doses of rotavirus vaccine should be administered by 8 months, 0 days of age.
- The rotavirus vaccine series should be completed with the same product whenever possible. However, immunization should not be deferred if the product used for previous doses is not available or is unknown. In this situation, the health care professional should continue or complete the series with the product available.
- If any dose in the series was RV5 vaccine or the product is unknown for any dose in the series, a total of 3 doses of rotavirus vaccine should be administered.
- Rotavirus vaccine can be administered concurrently with other childhood vaccines.
- Infants with transient, mild illness, with or without low-grade fever, may receive rotavirus vaccine.
- Preterm infants may be immunized if the infant is at least 6 weeks of postnatal age and

Table 3.65. Recommended Schedule for Administration of Rotavirus Vaccine

Recommendation	RV5 (RotaTeq[a])	RV1 (Rotarix[b])
Number of doses in series	3	2
Recommended ages for doses	2, 4, and 6 months of age	2 and 4 months of age
Minimum age for first dose	6 weeks of age	6 weeks of age
Maximum age for first dose	14 weeks, 6 days of age	14 weeks, 6 days of age
Minimum interval between doses	4 weeks	4 weeks
Maximum age for last dose	8 months, 0 days of age	8 months, 0 days of age

[a]Merck & Co Inc, Whitehouse Station, NJ.
[b]GlaxoSmithKline, Research Triangle Park, NC.

[1]American Academy of Pediatrics, Committee on Infectious Diseases. Prevention of rotavirus disease: updated guidelines for use of rotavirus vaccine. *Pediatrics.* 2009;123(5):1412–1420

[2]Centers for Disease Control and Prevention. Prevention of rotavirus gastroenteritis among infants and children. Recommendations of the Advisory Committee on Immunization Practices (ACIP). *MMWR Recomm Rep.* 2009; 58(RR-2):1–25

is clinically stable. Preterm infants should be immunized on the same schedule and with the same precautions as recommended for full-term infants. The first dose of vaccine should be administered at the time of discharge or after the infant has been discharged from the nursery.

- Infants living in households with immunocompromised people can be immunized. Highly immunocompromised patients should avoid handling diapers of infants who have been vaccinated with rotavirus vaccine for 4 weeks after vaccination.
- Infants living in households with pregnant women should be immunized.
- Rotavirus vaccine should not be administered to infants who have a history of a severe allergic reaction (eg, anaphylaxis) after a previous dose of rotavirus vaccine or to a vaccine component. The tip caps of the prefilled oral applicators of the RV1 vaccine may contain natural rubber latex, so infants with a severe (anaphylactic) allergy to latex should not receive RV1. The RV5 vaccine dosing tube is latex free.
- SCID and history of intussusception are contraindications for use of both rotavirus vaccines. Gastroenteritis, including severe diarrhea and prolonged shedding of vaccine virus, has been reported in infants who were administered live, oral rotavirus vaccines and later identified as having SCID.
- Precautions for administration of rotavirus vaccine include manifestations of altered immunocompetence (other than SCID, which is a contraindication); moderate to severe illness, including gastroenteritis; preexisting chronic intestinal tract disease; and spina bifida or bladder exstrophy (this precaution for RV1 is because of the risk of latex allergy, because the tip caps of the prefilled oral applicators of the RV1 vaccine may contain natural rubber latex).
- Rotavirus vaccine may be administered at any time before, concurrent with, or after administration of any blood product, including antibody-containing blood products.
- Breastfeeding infants should be immunized according to the same schedule as non-breastfed infants.
- If an infant regurgitates, spits out, or vomits during or after vaccine administration, the vaccine dose should not be repeated.
- If a recently immunized infant is hospitalized for any reason, no precautions other than standard precautions need to be taken to prevent spread of vaccine virus in the hospital setting.
- Infants who have had rotavirus gastroenteritis before receiving the full series of rotavirus immunization should begin or complete the schedule following the standard age and interval recommendations.
- Infants exposed in utero to maternally administered biologic response modifiers can have detectable drug concentrations for many months following delivery, resulting in concern for immunosuppression among infants in the 12 months after the last maternal dose during pregnancy. Some of the biologic response modifiers are more efficiently passaged transplacentally in the second and third trimesters compared with the first trimester. Until further data are available, and considering that rotavirus disease is rarely life threatening in the United States, rotavirus vaccines should be avoided in US infants for the first 12 months after the final in utero exposure to a biologic response modifier (see Biologic Response Modifying Drugs Used to Decrease Inflammation, p 85). Catch-up rotavirus vaccination is not recommended once this 12-month interval is reached, because the maximum age for first dose of rotavirus vaccine is 14 weeks, 6 days.

Rubella

CLINICAL MANIFESTATIONS:

Postnatal Rubella. Many cases of postnatal rubella are subclinical. Clinical disease usually is mild and characterized by a generalized erythematous maculopapular rash, lymphadenopathy, and slight fever. The rash starts on the face, becomes generalized in 24 hours, and lasts a median of 3 days. Lymphadenopathy, which may precede rash, often involves posterior auricular or suboccipital lymph nodes, can be generalized, and lasts between 5 and 8 days. Conjunctivitis and palatal enanthema have been noted. Transient polyarthralgia and polyarthritis rarely occur in children but are common in adolescents and adults, especially among females. Encephalitis (1 in 6000 cases) and thrombocytopenia (1 in 3000 cases) are complications.

Congenital Rubella Syndrome. Maternal rubella during pregnancy can result in miscarriage, fetal death, or a constellation of congenital anomalies (congenital rubella syndrome [CRS]). The most commonly described anomalies/manifestations associated with CRS are ophthalmologic (cataracts, pigmentary retinopathy, microphthalmos, congenital glaucoma), cardiac (patent ductus arteriosus, peripheral pulmonary artery stenosis), auditory (sensorineural hearing impairment), or neurologic (behavioral disorders, meningoencephalitis, microcephaly, mental retardation). Neonatal manifestations of CRS include growth restriction, interstitial pneumonitis, radiolucent bone disease, hepatosplenomegaly, thrombocytopenia, and dermal erythropoiesis (so-called "blueberry muffin" lesions); death may occur. Mild forms of the disease can be associated with few or no obvious clinical manifestations at birth. Congenital defects occur in up to 85% if maternal infection occurs during the first 12 weeks of gestation, 50% if infection occurs during the first 13 to 16 weeks of gestation, and 25% if infection occurs during the end of the second trimester. CRS is one of the few known causes of autism.

ETIOLOGY: Rubella virus is an enveloped, positive-stranded RNA virus classified as a *Rubivirus* in the *Togaviridae* family.

EPIDEMIOLOGY: Humans are the only source of infection. Postnatal rubella is transmitted primarily through direct or droplet contact from nasopharyngeal secretions. The peak incidence of infection is during late winter and early spring. Approximately 25% to 50% of infections are asymptomatic. Immunity from wild-type or vaccine virus usually is lifelong, but reinfection on rare occasions has been demonstrated and rarely has resulted in CRS. Although volunteer studies have demonstrated rubella virus in nasopharyngeal secretions from 7 days before to a maximum of 14 days after onset of rash, the period of maximal communicability extends from a few days before to 7 days after onset of rash. Rubella virus has been recovered in high titer from lens aspirates in children with congenital cataracts for several years, and a small proportion of infants with congenital rubella continue to shed virus in nasopharyngeal secretions and urine for 1 year or more, with transmission to susceptible contacts. Rubella also has been associated with Fuchs heterochromic uveitis, sometimes decades after the initial infection.

Before widespread use of rubella vaccine, rubella was an epidemic disease, occurring in 6- to 9-year cycles, with most cases occurring in children. In the postvaccine era, most cases in the mid-1970s and 1980s occurred in young unimmunized adults in outbreaks on college campuses and in occupational settings. More recent outbreaks have occurred in people born outside the United States or among underimmunized populations. The incidence of rubella in the United States has decreased by more than 99% from the prevaccine era.

The United States was determined no longer to have endemic rubella in 2004, and from 2004 through 2014, 94 cases of rubella and 9 cases of CRS were reported in the United States; all of the cases were import associated or from unknown sources.[1] A national serologic survey from 1999–2004 indicated that among children and adolescents 6 through 19 years of age, seroprevalence was approximately 95%. However, approximately 10% of adults 20 through 49 years of age lacked antibodies to rubella, although 92% of women were seropositive. In addition, epidemiologic studies of rubella and CRS in the United States have identified that seronegativity is higher among people born outside the United States or from areas with poor vaccine coverage. The risk of CRS is highest in infants of women born outside the United States, because these women are more likely to be susceptible to rubella.

In 2003, the Pan American Health Organization (PAHO) adopted a resolution calling for elimination of rubella and CRS in the Americas by the year 2010. The strategy consisted of achieving high levels of measles-rubella vaccination coverage in the routine immunization program and in the supplemental vaccination campaigns to rapidly reduce the number of people in the country susceptible to acute infection. This was accomplished while simultaneously strengthening epidemiologic surveillance to monitor impact. The last confirmed endemic rubella case in the Americas was diagnosed in Argentina in February 2009. The last confirmed endemic CRS case was diagnosed in Brazil in August 2009. In April 2015, the PAHO International Expert Committee for Verification of Measles and Rubella Elimination verified and announced that the region of the Americas had achieved the rubella and CRS elimination goals.

The **incubation period** for postnatally acquired rubella ranges from 14 to 21 days, usually 16 to 18 days.

DIAGNOSTIC TESTS:

Rubella. Detection of rubella-specific immunoglobulin (Ig) M antibody usually indicates recent postnatal infection, but both false-negative and false-positive results occur, requiring additional specialized testing in a reference laboratory. Most postnatal cases are IgM-positive by 5 days after symptom onset. For diagnosis of postnatally acquired rubella, a fourfold or greater increase in antibody titer between acute and convalescent periods or seroconversion between acute and convalescent IgG serum titers indicates infection. Acute serum must be collected as close to rash onset as possible.

CRS. CRS can be confirmed by detection of rubella-specific IgM antibody usually within the first 6 months of life. Congenital infection also can be confirmed by stable or increasing serum concentrations of rubella-specific IgG over the first 7 to 11 months of life. Diagnosis of congenital rubella infection in children older than 1 year is difficult because of routine vaccination with measles-mumps-rubella (MMR) vaccine; serologic testing usually is not diagnostic, and viral isolation, although confirmatory, is possible in only the small proportion of congenitally infected children who are still shedding virus at this age.

The most commonly used methods of serologic screening for previous rubella infection are enzyme immunoassays (EIAs) and latex agglutination tests. As a general rule, both IgM and IgG antibody testing should be performed for suspected cases of both congenital and postnatal rubella, because both results may contribute to the diagnosis.

---

[1]Centers for Disease Control and Prevention. Three cases of congenital rubella syndrome in the postelimination era—Maryland, Alabama, and Illinois, 2012. *MMWR Morb Mortal Wkly Rep.* 2013;62(12):226–229

A false-positive IgM test result may be caused by a number of factors including rheumatoid factor, parvovirus IgM, and heterophile antibodies. The use of IgM-capture EIA may reduce the occurrence of false-positive IgM results. The presence of high-avidity IgG or a lack of increase in IgG titers can be useful in identifying false-positive rubella IgM results. Low-avidity IgG is associated with recent primary rubella infection, whereas high-avidity IgG is associated with past infection or reinfection or with previous vaccination. The avidity assay is not a routine test and should be performed at reference laboratories like the Centers for Disease Control and Prevention (CDC).

Rubella virus can be isolated most consistently from throat or nasal swab specimens (and less consistently urine) by inoculation of appropriate cell culture. Detection of rubella virus RNA by real time reverse-transcriptase polymerase chain reaction (RT-PCR) from a throat/nasal swab or urine sample with subsequent genotyping of strains may be valuable for diagnosis and molecular epidemiology. There are currently no RT-PCR assays cleared by the US Food and Drug Administration for rubella, but testing generally is available in commercial and public health laboratories. In most postnatal cases, viral detection is possible by culture or RT-PCR assay on the day of symptom onset, and in most congenital cases, viral detection is possible at birth and in some cases for up to 12 months. Laboratory personnel should be notified immediately that rubella is suspected, because specialized cell culture methods are required to isolate and identify the virus. Blood, urine, and cataract specimens also may yield virus, particularly in infants with congenital infection. With the successful elimination of indigenous rubella and CRS in the Western Hemisphere, molecular typing of viral isolates is critical in defining a source in outbreak scenarios as well as for sporadic cases.

TREATMENT: Supportive.

ISOLATION OF THE HOSPITALIZED PATIENT: In addition to standard precautions, for postnatal rubella, droplet precautions are recommended for 7 days after onset of the rash. Contact isolation is indicated for children with proven or suspected congenital rubella until they are at least 1 year of age, unless 2 cultures of clinical specimens (eg, throat swab and urine specimen) obtained 1 month apart after 3 months of age are negative for rubella virus.

CONTROL MEASURES:

School and Child Care. Children with postnatal rubella should be excluded from school or child care for 7 days after onset of the rash. During an outbreak, children without evidence of immunity should be immunized or excluded for 21 days after onset of rash of the last case in the outbreak. Children with rubella may return to school or child care 7 days after rash onset. Children with CRS should be considered contagious until they are at least 1 year of age, unless 2 clinical specimens obtained 1 month apart are negative for rubella virus after 3 months of age. Infection-control precautions should be considered in children with CRS up to 3 years of age who are hospitalized for congenital cataract extraction. In child care settings, hand hygiene is essential for reducing transmission from the saliva or urine of children with CRS. Caregivers of these infants should be made aware of the potential hazard of the infants to susceptible pregnant contacts.

Surveillance for Congenital Infections. Accurate diagnosis and reporting of CRS are extremely important in assessing control of rubella. All birth defects in which rubella infection is suspected etiologically should be investigated thoroughly and reported to the CDC through local or state health departments.

Care of Exposed People. Evidence of rubella immunity consists of documented receipt of at least 1 dose of rubella-containing vaccine on or after the first birthday or serologic evidence of immunity. People born prior to 1957 can be considered immune. Documented evidence of rubella immunity is especially important for women who could become pregnant. Prenatal serologic screening for rubella immunity should be performed for all pregnant women. Women who have rubella-specific antibody concentrations above the standard positive cutoff value for the assay can be considered to have adequate evidence of rubella immunity. Those without antibody concentrations above the standard positive cutoff or those with equivocal test results should receive rubella vaccine during the immediate postpartum period before discharge. Vaccinated women of childbearing age who have received 1 or 2 doses of rubella-containing vaccine and have rubella serum IgG concentrations that are not clearly positive should receive 1 additional dose of measles-mumps-rubella vaccine (maximum of 3 doses) and do not need to be retested thereafter for serologic evidence of rubella immunity.

When a pregnant woman is exposed to rubella, a blood specimen should be obtained as soon as possible and tested for rubella antibody (IgG and IgM). An aliquot of frozen serum should be stored for possible repeated testing at a later time. The presence of rubella-specific IgG antibody in a properly performed test at the time of exposure indicates that the person most likely is immune. If antibody is not detectable, a second blood specimen should be obtained 2 to 3 weeks later and tested concurrently with the first specimen. If the second test result is negative, another blood specimen should be obtained 6 weeks after the exposure and also tested concurrently with the first specimen; a negative test result in both the second and third specimens indicates that infection has not occurred, and a positive test result in the second or third specimen but not the first (seroconversion) indicates recent infection.

Immune Globulin. Immune Globulin (IG) does not prevent rubella infection after exposure and is not recommended for that purpose. Although administration of IG after exposure to rubella will not prevent infection or viremia, it may modify or suppress symptoms and create an unwarranted sense of security. Therefore, IG is not recommended for routine postexposure prophylaxis of rubella in early pregnancy or any other circumstance. Infants with CRS have been born to women who received IG shortly after exposure. Administration of IG eliminates the value of IgG antibody testing to detect maternal infection. IgM antibody can be used to detect maternal infection after exposure, even after receipt of IG, although false-negative and false-positive results still may occur.

Vaccine. Live-virus rubella vaccine administered after exposure has not been demonstrated to prevent illness. Immunization of exposed nonpregnant people may be indicated, because if the exposure did not result in infection, immunization will protect these people in the future. Immunization of a person who is incubating natural rubella or who already is immune is not associated with an increased risk of adverse effects.

Rubella Vaccine.[1] The live-virus rubella vaccine distributed in the United States is the RA 27/3 strain grown in human diploid cell cultures. Vaccine is administered by subcutaneous injection as a combination vaccine—either MMR or measles-mumps-rubella-varicella (MMRV). Single-antigen rubella vaccine no longer is available in the United States. Vaccine can be administered simultaneously with other vaccines (see

---

[1]Centers for Disease Control and Prevention. Prevention of measles, rubella, congenital rubella syndrome, and mumps, 2013 summary: recommendations of the Advisory Committee on Immunization Practices (ACIP). *MMWR Recomm Rep.* 2013;62(RR-4):1–34

Simultaneous Administration of Multiple Vaccines, p 35). Serum antibody to rubella is induced in more than 95% of recipients after a single dose at 12 months or older. Clinical efficacy and challenge studies have demonstrated that 1 dose confers long-term immunity against clinical and asymptomatic infection in more than 90% of immunized people. However, both symptomatic (rare) and asymptomatic reinfection have occurred.

Because of the 2-dose recommendations for measles- and mumps-containing vaccine (as MMR) and varicella vaccine (as MMRV), 2 doses of rubella vaccine are administered routinely. This provides an added safeguard against primary vaccine failures.

Vaccine Recommendations. At least 1 dose of live attenuated rubella-containing vaccine is recommended for people 12 months or older. In the United States, rubella vaccine is recommended to be administered in combination with measles and mumps vaccines (MMR) or in combination with measles, mumps, and varicella (MMRV), when a child is 12 through 15 months of age, with a second dose of MMR or MMRV at school entry at 4 through 6 years of age or sooner, according to recommendations for routine measles, mumps, rubella, and varicella immunization. People who have not received the dose at school entry should receive their second dose as soon as possible but optimally no later than 11 through 12 years of age (see Measles, p 537).

Special emphasis must continue to be placed on the immunization of at-risk postpubertal males and females, especially college students, military recruits, recent immigrants, health care professionals, teachers, and child care providers. People who were born in 1957 or after and who have not received at least 1 dose of vaccine or who have no serologic evidence of immunity to rubella are considered susceptible and should be immunized with MMR vaccine. Clinical diagnosis of infection is unreliable and should not be accepted as evidence of immunity.

Specific recommendations are as follows:

- Postpubertal females without documentation of presumptive evidence of rubella immunity should be immunized unless they are pregnant. Postpubertal females should be advised not to become pregnant for 28 days after receiving a rubella-containing vaccine (see Precautions and Contraindications, p 710, for further discussion). Routine serologic testing of nonpregnant postpubertal women before immunization is unnecessary and is a potential impediment to protection against rubella, because it requires 2 visits.
- During annual health care examinations, premarital and family planning visits, and visits to sexually transmitted infection clinics, postpubertal females should be assessed for rubella susceptibility and, if deemed susceptible, should be immunized with MMR vaccine.
- Routine prenatal screening for rubella immunity should be performed. If a woman is found to be susceptible, rubella vaccine should be administered during the immediate postpartum period before discharge.
- People who have rubella-specific antibody concentrations above the standard positive cutoff value for the assay can be considered to have adequate evidence of rubella immunity. Except for women of childbearing age, people who have an equivocal serologic test result should be considered susceptible to rubella unless they have documented receipt of 1 dose of rubella-containing vaccine or subsequent serologic test results indicate rubella immunity. Vaccinated women of childbearing age who have received 1 or 2 doses of rubella-containing vaccine and have rubella serum IgG concentrations that are not clearly positive should receive 1 additional dose of MMR vaccine

(maximum of 3 doses) and do not need to be retested thereafter for serologic evidence of rubella immunity.

- Breastfeeding is not a contraindication to postpartum immunization of the mother (for additional information, see Human Milk, p 113).
- All susceptible health care personnel who may be exposed to patients with rubella or who provide care for pregnant women, as well as people who work in educational institutions or provide child care, should be immunized to prevent infection for themselves and to prevent transmission of rubella to pregnant patients.[1]

Adverse Reactions.

- Of susceptible children who receive MMR or MMRV vaccines, fever develops in 5% to 15% from 6 to 12 days after immunization. Rash occurs in approximately 5% of immunized people. Mild lymphadenopathy occurs commonly. Febrile seizures occur slightly more frequently among children 12 through 23 months of age after administration of MMRV vaccine compared with MMR and varicella administered as separate injections during the same visit (see Measles, p 537).
- Joint pain, usually in small peripheral joints, has been reported in approximately 0.5% of young children following vaccination with a rubella-containing vaccine. Arthralgia and transient arthritis tend to be more common in susceptible postpubertal females, occurring in approximately 25% and 10%, respectively, of vaccine recipients. Joint involvement usually begins 7 to 21 days after immunization and generally is transient. The incidence of joint manifestations after immunization is lower than after natural infection at the corresponding age.
- Transient paresthesia and pain in the arms and legs have rarely been reported.
- Central nervous system manifestations have been reported, but no causal relationship with rubella vaccine has been established.
- Other reactions that occur after immunization with MMR or MMRV are associated with the measles, mumps, and varicella components of the vaccine (see Measles, p 537, Mumps, p 567, and Varicella-Zoster Infections, p 869).

Precautions and Contraindications.

- **Pregnancy.** Rubella vaccine should not be administered to pregnant women. If vaccine is administered inadvertently or if pregnancy occurs within 28 days of immunization, the patient should be counseled on the theoretical risks to the fetus. The theoretical maximum risk for CRS after vaccine administration is 0.2%, which is considerably lower than the risk with wild rubella virus or risk of non–CRS-induced congenital defects in pregnancy. Of the 2931 susceptible pregnant women followed globally, 3.3% of offspring had subclinical infection, none had congenital defects, and 96.7% were not infected. In view of these observations, receipt of rubella vaccine during pregnancy is not an indication for termination of pregnancy.
- **Children of pregnant women.** Immunizing susceptible children whose mothers or other household contacts are pregnant does not cause a risk. Most immunized people intermittently shed small amounts of virus from the pharynx 7 to 28 days after immunization, but no evidence of transmission of the vaccine virus from immunized children has been found.
- **Febrile illness.** Children with minor illnesses, such as upper respiratory tract

---

[1]Centers for Disease Control and Prevention. Immunization of health-care personnel: recommendations of the Advisory Committee on Immunization Practices (ACIP). *MMWR Recomm Rep.* 2011;60(RR-7):1–45

infection, may be immunized (see Vaccine Safety, p 41). Fever is not a contraindication to immunization. However, if other manifestations suggest a more serious illness, the child should not be immunized until recovery has occurred.

- **Recent administration of IG.** IG preparations interfere with immune response to measles vaccine and theoretically may interfere with the serologic response to rubella vaccine (see p 39). If rubella vaccine is indicated postpartum for a woman who has received anti-Rho (D) IG or blood products, suggested intervals are the same as used between IG administration and measles immunization (see Table 1.13, p 40).

- **Altered immunity.** Immunocompromised patients with disorders associated with increased severity of viral infections should not receive live-virus rubella vaccine (see Immunization and Other Considerations in Immunocompromised Children, p 72). Exceptions are patients with human immunodeficiency virus infection who are not severely immunocompromised; these patients may be immunized against rubella with MMR vaccine (see Human Immunodeficiency Virus Infection, p 459). If possible, children receiving biologic response modifiers, such as anti-tumor necrosis factor-alpha (see Biologic Response Modifying Drugs Used to Decrease Inflammation, p 85), should be immunized before initiating treatment.

- **Household contacts of immunocompromised people.** The risk of rubella exposure for patients with altered immunity is decreased by immunizing susceptible contacts. Although small amounts of vaccine virus may be isolated from the pharynx, no evidence of transmission of rubella vaccine virus from immunized children to immunocompromised contacts has been found. Precautions and contraindications appropriate for the measles, mumps, and varicella components of MMR or MMRV vaccines also should be reviewed before administration (see Measles, p 537, Mumps, p 567, and Varicella-Zoster Infections, p 869).

Corticosteroids. For patients who have received high doses of corticosteroids (2 mg/kg or greater or more than 20 mg/day) for 14 days or more and who otherwise are not immunocompromised, the recommended interval between stopping the steroids and immunization is at least 4 weeks (see Immunization and Other Considerations in Immunocompromised Children, p 72) after steroids have been discontinued.

Tuberculosis. Tuberculin skin testing is not a prerequisite for MMR immunization. Antituberculosis therapy should be initiated before administering MMR vaccine to people with untreated tuberculosis infection or disease. Tuberculin skin testing, if otherwise indicated, can be performed on the day of immunization with MMR vaccine. Otherwise, tuberculin skin testing should be postponed for 4 to 6 weeks, because measles immunization temporarily may suppress tuberculin skin test reactivity.

Salmonella Infections

CLINICAL MANIFESTATIONS:

Nontyphoidal Salmonella *Infection.* Nontyphoidal *Salmonella* (NTS) infection is associated with a spectrum of illness ranging from asymptomatic gastrointestinal tract carriage to gastroenteritis, urinary tract infection, bacteremia, and focal infections, including meningitis, brain abscess, and osteomyelitis (to which people with sickle cell anemia are predisposed). The most common illness associated with NTS infection is gastroenteritis, with manifestations of diarrhea, abdominal cramps, and fever. The site of infection usually is the distal small intestine as well as the colon. Sustained or intermittent bacteremia can occur, and focal infections are recognized in up to 10% of patients with NTS bacteremia. In the United States, the incidence of invasive *Salmonella* infection is highest among infants. Certain *Salmonella* serovars (eg, Dublin, Typhi, Choleraesuis, Paratyphi A and B), although rare, are more likely to result in invasive infection than gastroenteritis.

Enteric Fever. *Salmonella enterica* serovars Typhi, Paratyphi A, Paratyphi B, and (rarely) Paratyphi C can cause a protracted bacteremic illness referred to, respectively, as typhoid and paratyphoid fever and collectively as enteric fevers. In older children, the onset of enteric fever typically is gradual, with manifestations such as fever, constitutional symptoms (eg, headache, malaise, anorexia, and lethargy), abdominal pain, hepatomegaly, splenomegaly, dactylitis, and rose spots (present in approximately 30%); change in mental status and shock may ensue. Myocarditis or endocarditis occur rarely. In infants and toddlers, invasive infection with enteric fever serovars can manifest as a mild, nondescript febrile illness accompanied by self-limited bacteremia, or invasive infection can occur in association with more severe clinical symptoms and signs, sustained bacteremia, and meningitis. Either diarrhea (resembling pea soup) or constipation can be early features. Gastrointestinal tract bleeding occurs in approximately 10% of hospitalized adults and children with enteric fever. Relative bradycardia (pulse rate slower than would be expected for a given body temperature) has been considered a common feature of typhoid fever in adults but in children is neither a discriminating feature in the assessment of a febrile child from an area where enteric fever is endemic nor a feature of the disease per se.

ETIOLOGY: *Salmonella* organisms are gram-negative bacilli that belong to the family *Enterobacteriaceae*. Current taxonomy recognizes 2 *Salmonella* species: *S enterica* with 6 subspecies and *Salmonella bongori*. *S enterica* subspecies enterica (also called subspecies I) is responsible for the vast majority of infections in humans and other warm-blooded animals; the other *S enterica* subspecies and *S bongori* usually are isolated from cold-blooded animals. More than 2500 *Salmonella* serovars have been described; most serovars causing human disease are classified within O serogroups A through E. *Salmonella* serovar Typhi is classified in O serogroup D, along with many other common serovars including Enteritidis and Dublin. In 2011, the most commonly reported human isolates in the United States were *Salmonella* serovars Enteritidis, Typhimurium, Newport, I 4,[5],12:i:-, and Javiana; these 5 serovars generally account for nearly half of all *Salmonella* infections in the United States **(www.cdc.gov/ncezid/dfwed/pdfs/salmonella-annual-report-2012-508c. pdf)**.

The relative prevalence of other serovars varies by country. Approximately 75% to 95% of the serovars associated with invasive pediatric disease in sub-Saharan Africa are *Salmonella* serovar Typhimurium (mostly of an unusual variant, multilocus sequence type 313, that is distinct genomically), a monophasic variant of ST 313 that does not express phase 2 flagella, or *Salmonella* serovar Enteritidis.

EPIDEMIOLOGY: Every year, NTS organisms are among the most common causes of laboratory-confirmed cases of enteric disease. The principal reservoirs for NTS organisms include birds, mammals, reptiles, and amphibians. The major food vehicles of transmission to humans in industrialized countries include food of animal origin, such as poultry, beef, eggs, and dairy products. Multiple other food vehicles (eg, fruits, vegetables, peanut butter, frozen pot pies, powdered infant formula, cereal, and bakery products) have been implicated in outbreaks in the United States and Europe, presumably when the food was contaminated by contact with an infected animal product or a human carrier. Other modes of transmission include ingestion of contaminated water or contact with infected animals, mainly poultry (eg, chicks, chickens, ducks), reptiles or amphibians (eg, pet turtles, iguanas, geckos, bearded dragons, lizards, snakes, frogs, toads, newts, salamanders), and rodents (eg, hamsters, mice) or other mammals (eg, hedgehogs, guinea pigs). Reptiles and amphibians that live in tanks or aquariums can contaminate the water with bacteria, which can spread to people. Small turtles with a shell length of less than 4 inches are a well-known source of human *Salmonella* infections. Because of this risk, the US Food and Drug Administration (FDA) has banned the interstate sale and distribution of these turtles since 1975. Animal-derived pet foods and treats also have been linked to *Salmonella* infections, especially among young children.

Unlike NTS serovars, the enteric fever serovars (*Salmonella* serovars Typhi, Paratyphi A, Paratyphi B [*sensu stricto*]) are restricted to human hosts, in whom they cause clinical and subclinical infections. Chronic human carriers (mostly involving chronic infection of the gall bladder but occasionally involving infection of the urinary tract) constitute the reservoir in areas with endemic infection. Infection with enteric fever serovars implies ingestion of a food or water vehicle contaminated by a chronic carrier or person with acute infection. Although typhoid fever (300–400 cases annually) and paratyphoid fever (approximately 150 cases annually) are uncommon in the United States, these infections are highly endemic in many resource-limited countries, particularly in Asia. Consequently, most typhoid fever and paratyphoid fever infections in US residents are acquired during international travel.

The incidence of NTS infection is highest in children younger than 4 years. In the United States, rates of invasive infections and mortality are higher in infants, elderly people, and people with hemoglobinopathies (including sickle cell disease) and immunocompromising conditions (eg, malignant neoplasms, human immunodeficiency virus [HIV]) infection). Most reported cases are sporadic, but widespread outbreaks, including health care-associated and institutional outbreaks, have been reported. The incidence of foodborne cases of NTS gastroenteritis has diminished slightly in recent years.

Every year, NTS organisms are one of the most common causes of laboratory-confirmed cases of enteric disease reported by the Foodborne Diseases Active Surveillance Network, or FoodNet (**www.cdc.gov/foodnet**).

A risk of transmission of infection to others persists for as long as an infected person excretes NTS organisms. Twelve weeks after infection with the most common NTS serovars, approximately 45% of children younger than 5 years excrete organisms, compared with 5% of older children and adults; antimicrobial therapy can prolong excretion. Approximately 1% of adults continue to excrete NTS organisms for more than 1 year.

The **incubation period** for NTS gastroenteritis usually is 6 to 48 hours, but incubation periods of a week or more have been reported. For enteric fever, the **incubation period** usually is 7 to 14 days (range, 3–60 days).

DIAGNOSTIC TESTS: Isolation of *Salmonella* organisms from cultures of stool, blood, urine, bile (including duodenal fluid containing bile), and material from foci of infection is diagnostic. Gastroenteritis is diagnosed by stool culture; stool cultures should be obtained in all children with unexplained persistent or severe diarrhea and or those with bloody diarrhea. Optimum recovery of *Salmonella* from stool is achieved with the use of enrichment broth and multiple selective agar plate media. Definitive identification requires confirmation by either phenotypic methods (biochemical profiling) or mass spectrometry of cellular components and O serogroup determination. Serovar (serotype) determination is helpful from an epidemiologic perspective and is usually performed at public health laboratories; hospital-based clinical laboratories generally should save and send isolates to their appropriate public health laboratory.

Diagnostic tests to detect *Salmonella* antigens by enzyme immunoassay, latex agglutination, and monoclonal antibodies have been developed, as have commercial immunoassays that detect antibodies to antigens of enteric fever serovars. The latter tests are more important in areas of the world where typhoid fever is endemic.

Gene-based polymerase chain reaction (PCR) diagnostic tests also are available in research laboratories. A number of multiplex PCR platforms for detection of multiple viral, parasitic, and bacterial pathogens, including *Salmonella*, directly in stool have been cleared for diagnostic use by the FDA, but there is limited clinical experience with these FDA-cleared multiplex assays, and they may not be available locally. In general, laboratories should maintain culture capabilities for *Salmonella* species and other bacterial enteric pathogens, because antimicrobial susceptibility testing and serotyping generally are important for treatment and epidemiologic surveillance. In addition, state public health laboratories require isolates for genomic characterization of strains, which is needed for outbreak detection and investigation.

If enteric fever is suspected, blood, bone marrow, or bile culture is diagnostic, because organisms often are absent from stool. The sensitivity of blood culture and bone marrow culture in children with enteric fever is approximately 60% and 90%, respectively. The combination of a single blood culture plus culture of bile (collected from a bile-stained duodenal string) is 90% sensitive in detecting *Salmonella* serovar Typhi infection in children with clinical enteric fever.

TREATMENT:

- Antimicrobial therapy usually is not indicated for patients with either asymptomatic infection or uncomplicated gastroenteritis caused by NTS serovars, because therapy does not shorten the duration of diarrheal disease and can prolong duration of fecal excretion. Although of unproven benefit, antimicrobial therapy is recommended for gastroenteritis caused by NTS serovars in people at increased risk for invasive disease, including infants younger than 3 months and people with chronic gastrointestinal tract disease, malignant neoplasms, hemoglobinopathies, HIV infection, or other immunosuppressive illnesses or therapies.

- If antimicrobial therapy is initiated in patients in the United States with presumed or proven NTS gastroenteritis, a blood culture should be obtained prior to antibiotic administration and an initial dose of ceftriaxone should be given. The patient who does not appear ill or have evidence of disseminated infection can be discharged with oral azithromycin pending blood culture results. Ampicillin or trimethoprim-sulfamethoxazole may be considered for susceptible strains, once susceptibilities are available. A fluoroquinolone is an alternative option. For those who appear ill or have evidence of disseminated infection, hospitalization is required.

- For bacteremia caused by NTS, disseminated disease (meningitis, osteoarticular infection, endocarditis) should be excluded. Blood cultures should be repeated until negative. Initial therapy with ceftriaxone should be given. Transition from intravenous ceftriaxone to oral azithromycin or a fluoroquinolone may be considered after the blood culture has cleared and focal disease has been excluded, for a total 7- to 10-day course.

- For meningitis, the duration of treatment should be 4 weeks, and for osteomyelitis or other focal metastatic infections, a duration of 4 to 6 weeks is recommended. Evaluation for underlying immunodeficiency (eg, asplenia, human immunodeficiency virus infection) should be considered.

- For enteric fever caused by *Salmonella* serovar Typhi that is known or likely to be multidrug resistant, empiric therapy with azithromycin or a parenteral third-generation cephalosporin should be initiated. A fluoroquinolone is an alternative option depending on the region of acquisition. Drugs of choice, route of administration, and duration of therapy are based on susceptibility of the organism, knowledge of the antimicrobial susceptibility patterns of prevalent strains, site of infection, host, and clinical response. The optimal duration of therapy is unclear, but most experts would treat for at least 7 days for people with uncomplicated disease. Notably, in some highly endemic regions of South and Southeast Asia, the proportion of multidrug-resistant *Salmonella* serovar Typhi strains is diminishing, and strains susceptible to amoxicillin and/or trimethoprim/sulfamethoxazole (TMP/SMX) are becoming increasingly common; if amoxicillin or TMP/SMX is considered on the basis of susceptibility testing, a 14-day course of therapy should be considered. Relapse of typhoidal *Salmonella* infection can occur in up to 17% of patients within 4 weeks and is a particular risk for immunocompromised patients, who may require longer duration of treatment and retreatment. Relapse rates appear to be lower in those treated with azithromycin than with fluoroquinolones or ceftriaxone. Aminoglycosides are not recommended for treatment of invasive *Salmonella* infections, despite in vitro sensitivity of strains, because the clinical effectiveness is poor.

- For enteric fever caused by *Salmonella* serovar Typhi acquired from overseas travel, culture should be performed on stool samples from all people who traveled with the index case(s), and if results are positive, treatment should be initiated with azithromycin or a fluoroquinolone and the patient should be monitored for development of any symptoms. Asymptomatic people in the United States who had contact with the index case(s) but did not travel overseas with them do not require culture of stool samples.

- Blood and stool cultures (positive in 30%) should be obtained for all children who present with unexplained fever after travel to resource poor countries.

- The propensity to become a chronic *Salmonella* serovar Typhi carrier (excretion longer than 1 year) following acute typhoid infection correlates with prevalence of cholelithiasis, increases with age, and is greater in females than males. Chronic carriage in children is uncommon. The chronic carrier state may be eradicated by 4 weeks of oral therapy with ciprofloxacin or norfloxacin, which are antimicrobial agents that are highly concentrated in bile. High-dose parenteral ampicillin also can be used if 4 weeks of oral fluoroquinolone therapy is not well tolerated and if the strain is susceptible. Cholecystectomy followed by another course of antimicrobial agents may be indicated in some adults if antimicrobial therapy alone fails.

- Corticosteroids may be beneficial in children with severe enteric fever, which is characterized by delirium, obtundation, stupor, coma, or shock. These drugs should be reserved for critically ill patients in whom relief of manifestations of toxemia may be lifesaving. The usual regimen is high-dose dexamethasone, administered intravenously at an initial dose of 3 mg/kg, followed by 1 mg/kg, every 6 hours, for a total course of 48 hours.

ISOLATION OF THE HOSPITALIZED PATIENT: In addition to standard precautions, contact precautions should be used for diapered and incontinent children for the duration of illness. In children with enteric fever, precautions should be continued until culture results are negative for 3 consecutive stool specimens obtained at least 48 hours after cessation of antimicrobial therapy.

CONTROL MEASURES: Important measures include proper food hygiene practices; treated water supplies; proper hand hygiene; adequate sanitation to dispose of human fecal waste; exclusion of infected people from handling food or providing health care; education on the risk of *Salmonella* infections from animal contact; prohibiting the sale of pet turtles; limiting exposure of children younger than 5 years and immunocompromised children to reptiles, amphibians, live poultry, and rodents at home, at school, and in child care and public settings (see Diseases Transmitted by Animals [Zoonoses], p 1093); reporting cases to appropriate health authorities; and investigating outbreaks. Eggs and other foods of animal origin should be cooked thoroughly. People should not eat raw eggs or foods containing raw eggs or consume unpasteurized milk or raw milk products.[1] Notification of public health authorities and determination of serovar are of primary importance in detection and investigation of outbreaks.

Child Care. Outbreaks of *Salmonella* illness in child care centers are rare. Specific strategies for controlling infection in out-of-home child care include adherence to hygiene practices, including meticulous hand hygiene, and limiting exposure to certain animals. Animals at higher risk of causing salmonellosis, including reptiles, amphibians, and poultry, are not recommended in schools, child care settings, hospitals, or nursing homes (see Children in Out-of-Home Child Care, p 122).

When NTS serovars are identified in a symptomatic child care attendee or staff member with enterocolitis, older children and staff members do not need to be excluded unless they are symptomatic. Stool cultures are not required for asymptomatic contacts. Likewise, children or staff members with NTS enterocolitis do not require negative culture results from stool samples; children can return to child care facilities if stools are contained in the diaper or when toilet-trained children no longer have accidents using the toilet, and when stool frequency becomes no more than 2 stools above that child's normal frequency for the time the child is in the program, even if the stools remain loose (see Children in Out-of-Home Child Care, p 122). Antimicrobial therapy is not recommended for people with asymptomatic NTS infection or uncomplicated diarrhea or for people who are contacts of an infected person.

When *Salmonella* serovar Typhi infection is identified in a child care staff member, local or state health departments may be consulted regarding regulations for length of exclusion and testing, which may vary by jurisdiction. Because infections with *Salmonella* serovars Typhi or Paratyphi are transmitted easily and can be severe, exclusion of an infected child is warranted until results of 3 stool samples obtained at least 48 hours after cessation of antimicrobial therapy have negative culture results for *Salmonella* serovars Typhi or Paratyphi (see Children in Out-of-Home Child Care, p 122).

Typhoid Vaccine. Protection against *Salmonella* serovar Typhi is enhanced by typhoid immunization, but currently licensed vaccines do not provide complete protection. Two typhoid vaccines are licensed for use in the United States (see Table 3.66), one for use in people 6 years and older and the other in people 2 years and older.

---

[1] American Academy of Pediatrics, Committee on Infectious Diseases and Committee on Nutrition. Consumption of raw or unpasteurized milk and milk products by pregnant women and children. *Pediatrics*. 2014;133(1):175–179

Table 3.66. Commercially Available Typhoid Vaccines in the United States

Typhoid Vaccine	Type	Route	Minimum Age of Receipt, y	No. of Doses[a]	Booster Frequency, y
Ty21a	Live attenuated	Oral	6	4	5
ViCPS	Polysaccharide	Intramuscular	2	1	2

ViCPS indicates Vi capsular polysaccharide vaccine.
[a]Primary immunization. For further information on dosage, schedules, and adverse events, see text.

The demonstrated efficacy of the 2 vaccines licensed by the FDA ranges from 50% to 80%, but the duration of protection differs notably between the vaccines. Vaccine is selected on the basis of age of the child, need for booster doses, and possible contraindications (see Precautions and Contraindications, p 718) and reactions (see Adverse Events, p 718).

Recommended Use. In the United States, immunization is recommended only for the following people:

- **Travelers to areas where risk of exposure to *Salmonella* serovar Typhi is recognized.** Risk is greatest for travelers to the Indian subcontinent; South and Southeast Asia; Latin America, including the Caribbean; the Middle East; and Africa who may have prolonged exposure to contaminated food and drink. Such travelers need to be cautioned that typhoid vaccine is not a substitute for careful selection of food and drink (see **www.cdc.gov/travel**).
- **People with intimate exposure to a documented typhoid fever carrier,** as occurs with continued household contact.
- **Laboratory workers with frequent contact with *Salmonella* serovar Typhi.**

Dosages. For primary immunization, the following dosage is recommended for each vaccine:

- **Typhoid vaccine live oral Ty21a (Vivotif [Crucell Switzerland LTD, Berne, Switzerland).** Children (6 years and older) and adults should take 1 enteric-coated capsule every other day for a total of 4 capsules. Each capsule should be taken with liquid, no warmer than 37°C (98°F), approximately 1 hour before a meal. The capsules should be kept refrigerated, and all 4 doses must be taken to achieve maximal efficacy. Immunization should be completed at least 1 week before possible exposure.
- **Typhoid Vi polysaccharide vaccine (Typhim Vi [Sanofi Pasteur, Lyon, France]).** Primary immunization of people 2 years and older with unconjugated Vi capsular polysaccharide (ViCPS) vaccine consists of one 0.5-mL (25-μg) dose administered intramuscularly. Vaccine should be administered at least 2 weeks before possible exposure.
- **Protection against *Salmonella* serovars Paratyphi A and Paratyphi B.** Neither Ty21a nor ViCPS vaccine provides reliable protection against *Salmonella* serovar Paratyphi A. Results of 2 field trials suggest that Ty21a may provide partial cross-protection against *Salmonella* serovar Paratyphi B.

Booster Doses. In circumstances of continued or repeated exposure to *Salmonella* serovar Typhi, periodic reimmunization is recommended to maintain immunity.

Continued efficacy for 7 years after immunization with the oral Ty21a vaccine has been demonstrated; however, the manufacturer of oral Ty21a vaccine recommends reimmunization (completing the entire 4-dose series) every 5 years if continued or renewed exposure to *Salmonella* serovar Typhi is expected.

ViCPS vaccine is a T-independent antigen that does not elicit immunologic memory to allow boosting of serum Vi antibody titers following an initial immunization. The manufacturer of ViCPS vaccine recommends reimmunization every 2 years if continued or renewed exposure is expected.

Oral Ty21a (which does not express Vi antigen) and ViCPS (which protects by stimulating serum IgG Vi antibody) vaccines mediate protection by distinct mechanisms. No data have been reported concerning use of one vaccine administered after primary immunization with the other.

Adverse Events. The oral Ty21a vaccine is very well tolerated, but mild adverse reactions may occur that include abdominal pain, nausea, diarrhea, vomiting, fever, headache, and rash or urticaria. Reported adverse reactions to ViCPS vaccine also are minimal and include fever, headache, malaise, myalgia, and local reaction of tenderness and pain, erythema, or induration of 1 cm or greater.

Precautions and Contraindications. No data are available regarding efficacy of typhoid vaccines in children younger than 2 years. A contraindication to administration of parenteral ViCPS vaccine is a history of hypersensitivity to any component of the vaccine. No safety data have been reported for typhoid vaccines in pregnant women. The oral Ty21a vaccine is a live attenuated vaccine and should not be administered to immunocompromised people, including people known to be infected with HIV; to have a phagocytic cell defect; or to have chronic granulomatous disease[1]; the parenteral ViCPS vaccine may be an alternative, although the expected immune response may not be achieved. The oral Ty21a vaccine should not be administered during gastrointestinal tract illness. Adequate immune response is achieved when administered simultaneously with either mefloquine or chloroquine; however, if mefloquine is administered, immunization with Ty21a should be delayed for 24 hours. In addition, the antimalarial agent proguanil should not be administered simultaneously with oral Ty21a vaccine but, rather, should be administered 10 or more days after the fourth dose of oral Ty21a vaccine. Atovaquone also can interfere with oral Ty21a immunogenicity. Antimicrobial agents should be avoided for 3 days before the first dose of oral Ty21a vaccine and 7 days after the fourth dose of Ty21a vaccine.

Scabies

CLINICAL MANIFESTATIONS: Scabies is characterized by an intensely pruritic, erythematous eruption that may include papules, nodules, vesicles, or bullae and that is caused by burrowing of adult female mites in upper layers of the epidermis, creating serpiginous burrows. Itching is most intense at night. In older children and adults, the sites of predilection are interdigital folds, flexor aspects of wrists, extensor surfaces of elbows, anterior axillary folds, waistline, thighs, navel, genitalia, areolae, abdomen, intergluteal cleft, and buttocks. In children younger than 2 years, the eruption more often is vesicular and often occurs in areas usually spared in older children and adults, such as the scalp, face, neck,

[1]Rubin LG, Levin MJ, Ljungman P, et al. 2013 IDSA clinical practice guideline for vaccination of the immunocompromised host. *Clin Infect Dis.* 2014;58(3):e44–e100

palms, and soles. The eruption is caused by a hypersensitivity reaction to the proteins of the parasite.

Characteristic scabietic burrows appear as thin, gray or white, serpiginous, thread-like lines. Excoriations are common, and most burrows are obliterated by scratching before a patient seeks medical attention. Occasionally, 2- to 5-mm red-brown nodules are present, particularly on covered parts of the body, such as the genitalia, groin, and axilla. These scabies nodules are a granulomatous response to dead mite antigens and feces; the nodules can persist for weeks and even months after effective treatment. Cutaneous secondary bacterial infection is a frequent complication and usually is caused by *Streptococcus pyogenes* or *Staphylococcus aureus*. Studies have demonstrated a correlation between poststreptococcal glomerulonephritis and scabies.

Crusted (formerly called Norwegian) scabies is an uncommon clinical syndrome characterized by a large number of mites and widespread, crusted, hyperkeratotic lesions. Crusted scabies usually occurs in people with debilitating conditions, people with developmental disabilities, or people who are immunocompromised, including patients receiving biologic response modifiers. Crusted scabies also can occur in otherwise healthy children after long-term use of topical corticosteroid therapy.

Postscabetic pustulosis is a reactive phenomenon that may follow successful treatment of primary infestation with scabies. Affected infants and young children manifest episodic crops of sterile, pruritic papules and pustules predominantly in an acral distribution, but lesions may extend to a lesser degree onto the torso.

ETIOLOGY: The mite *Sarcoptes scabiei* subspecies *hominis* is the cause of scabies. The adult female burrows in the stratum corneum of the skin and lays eggs. Larvae emerge from the eggs in 2 to 4 days and molt to nymphs and then to adults, which mate and produce new eggs. The entire cycle takes approximately 10 to 17 days. *S scabiei* subspecies *canis*, acquired from dogs (with clinical mange), can cause a self-limited and mild infestation in humans usually involving the area in direct contact with the infested animal.

EPIDEMIOLOGY: Humans are the source of infestation. Transmission usually occurs through prolonged close, personal contact. Because of the large number of mites in exfoliating scales, even minimal contact with patients with crusted scabies or their immediate environment can result in transmission. Infestation acquired from dogs and other animals is uncommon, and these mites do not replicate in humans. Scabies of human origin can be transmitted as long as the patient remains infested and untreated, including during the interval before symptoms develop. Scabies is endemic in many countries and occurs worldwide in cycles thought to be 15 to 30 years long. Scabies affects people from all socioeconomic levels without regard to age, gender, or standards of personal hygiene. Scabies in adults often is acquired sexually.[1]

The **incubation period** in people without previous exposure usually is 4 to 6 weeks. People who previously were infested are sensitized and develop symptoms 1 to 4 days after repeated exposure to the mite; however, these reinfestations usually are milder than the original episode.

DIAGNOSTIC TESTS: Diagnosis of scabies typically is made by clinical examination. Diagnosis can be confirmed by identification of the mite or mite eggs or scybala (feces) from scrapings of papules or intact burrows, preferably from the terminal portion where the

---

[1]Centers for Disease Control and Prevention. Sexually transmitted diseases treatment guidelines, 2015. *MMWR Recomm Rep.* 2015;64(RR-3):1–137

mite generally is found. Mineral oil, microscope immersion oil, or water applied to skin facilitates collection of scrapings. A broad-blade scalpel is used to scrape the burrow. Scrapings and oil can be placed on a slide under a glass coverslip and examined microscopically under low power. Adult female mites average 330 to 450 μm in length. Skin scrapings provide definitive evidence of infection but have low sensitivity. Handheld dermoscopy (epiluminescence microscopy) has been used to identify in vivo the pigmented mite parts or air bubbles corresponding to infesting mites within the stratum corneum. Reflectance in vivo microscopy and polymerase chain reaction assays on swabbed skin material are promising techniques with improved sensitivity and specificity.

TREATMENT: Topical permethrin 5% cream or off-label use of oral ivermectin both are effective agents for treatment of scabies (see Drugs for Parasitic Infections, p 985). Most experts recommend starting with topical 5% permethrin cream as the drug of choice, particularly for infants, young children (not approved for children younger than 2 months), and pregnant or nursing women. Permethrin cream should be removed by bathing after 8 to 14 hours. Children and adults with infestation should apply lotion or cream containing this scabicide over their entire body below the head. Permethrin kills the scabies mite and eggs. Two (or more) applications, each about a week apart, may be necessary to eliminate all mites. Because scabies can affect the face, scalp, and neck in infants and young children, treatment of the entire head, neck, and body in this age group is required. Special attention should be given to trimming fingernails and ensuring application of medication to these areas.

A Cochrane review found that oral ivermectin is effective for treating scabies but less effective than topical permethrin. Because ivermectin is not ovicidal, it is given as 2 doses, 7 to 14 days apart. Ivermectin is not approved for treatment of scabies by the US Food and Drug Administration (FDA). Oral ivermectin should be considered for patients who have failed treatment or who cannot tolerate FDA-approved topical medications for the treatment of scabies. Although its use has been reported anecdotally, the safety of ivermectin in children weighing less than 15 kg (33 lb) has not been determined. Ivermectin is not recommended for women who are pregnant or who are lactating and intend to breastfeed.

Alternative drugs include 10% crotamiton cream or lotion, or 5% to 10% precipitated sulfur compounded into petrolatum. Because scabietic lesions are the result of a hypersensitivity reaction to the mite, itching may not subside for several weeks despite successful treatment. The use of oral antihistamines and topical corticosteroids can help relieve this itching. Topical or systemic antimicrobial therapy is indicated for secondary bacterial infections of the excoriated lesions.

Because of safety concerns and availability of other treatments, lindane lotion should not be used in the treatment of scabies.

ISOLATION OF THE HOSPITALIZED PATIENT: In addition to standard precautions, contact precautions are recommended until the patient has been treated with an appropriate scabicide.

CONTROL MEASURES:

- Most experts recommend prophylactic therapy for household members, particularly for household members who have had prolonged direct skin-to-skin contact. Manifestations of scabies infestation can appear as late as 2 months after exposure, during which time patients can transmit scabies. All household members should be treated at the same time to prevent reinfestation. Bedding and clothing worn next to the skin during the 3 days before initiation of therapy should be laundered in a washer with hot water and dried using a hot cycle. Mites do not survive more than 3 days without skin contact. Clothing that cannot be laundered should be removed from the patient and stored for several days to a week to avoid reinfestation.

- Children should be allowed to return to child care or school after treatment has been completed.
- Epidemics and localized outbreaks may require stringent and consistent measures to treat contacts. Health care workers and other caregivers who have had prolonged skin-to-skin contact with patients with infestation may benefit from prophylactic treatment.
- Environmental disinfestation is unnecessary and unwarranted. Thorough vacuuming of environmental surfaces is recommended after use of a room by a patient with crusted scabies.
- People with crusted scabies and their close contacts must be treated promptly and aggressively to avoid outbreaks.

Schistosomiasis

CLINICAL MANIFESTATIONS: Infections are established by skin penetration of infecting larvae (cercariae, shed by freshwater snails). Initial infections often are asymptomatic, but repeat exposures may be accompanied by a hypersensitivity reaction consisting of a transient, pruritic, papular rash (cercarial dermatitis; "swimmer's itch"). After penetration, the parasites enter the bloodstream, migrate through the lungs, and eventually mature into adult worms that reside in the venous plexus that drains the intestines or, in the case of *Schistosoma haematobium*, the urogenital tract. Four to 8 weeks after exposure, worms develop into adults and females begin egg deposition, which can lead to an acute serum sickness-like illness (Katayama syndrome) that manifests as fever, malaise, cough, rash, abdominal pain, hepatosplenomegaly, diarrhea, nausea, lymphadenopathy, and eosinophilia. This syndrome is most common among nonimmune hosts, such as travelers. Adult worms survive 7 to 10 years in the absence of treatment, although several cases have been documented of people having infections decades after leaving an area of endemicity. The severity of symptoms associated with chronic infection is related to the worm burden. People with low to moderate worm burdens may have only subclinical disease or relatively mild manifestations, such as growth stunting or anemia. Higher worm burdens are associated with a range of symptoms caused primarily by inflammation and local fibrosis triggered by the immune response to eggs produced by adult worms. Severe forms of chronic intestinal schistosomiasis (*Schistosoma mansoni* and *Schistosoma japonicum* infections) can result in hepatosplenomegaly, abdominal pain, bloody diarrhea, portal hypertension, ascites, esophageal varices, and hematemesis. Urogenital schistosomiasis (*S haematobium* infections) can result in the bladder becoming inflamed and fibrotic. Urinary tract symptoms and signs include dysuria, urgency, terminal microscopic and gross hematuria, secondary urinary tract infections, hydronephrosis, and nonspecific pelvic pain. *S haematobium* is associated with lesions of the lower genital tract (vulva, vagina, and cervix) in women, prostatitis and hematospermia in men, and certain forms of bladder cancer. Other organ systems can be involved—for example, eggs can embolize to the lungs, causing pulmonary hypertension. Less commonly, eggs can lodge in the central nervous system, causing severe neurologic complications.

Cercarial dermatitis (swimmer's itch) often is caused by larvae of schistosome parasites of birds or other wildlife. These larvae can penetrate human skin but eventually die in the dermis and do not cause systemic disease. Skin manifestations include pruritus at the penetration site a few hours after water exposure, followed in 5 to 14 days by an intermittent pruritic, sometimes papular, eruption. In previously sensitized people, more intense papular eruptions may occur more quickly and last for 7 to 10 days after exposure.

ETIOLOGY: The trematodes (flukes) *S mansoni*, *S japonicum*, *Schistosoma mekongi*, and *Schistosoma intercalatum* cause intestinal schistosomiasis, and *S haematobium* causes urogenital disease. All species have similar life cycles.

EPIDEMIOLOGY: Persistence of schistosomiasis depends on the presence of an appropriate snail as an intermediate host. Eggs excreted in stool (*S mansoni*, *S japonicum*, *S mekongi*, and *S intercalatum*) or urine *(S haematobium)* into fresh water hatch into motile miracidia, which infect snails. After development and asexual replication in snails, cercariae emerge and penetrate the skin of humans in contact with water. Children commonly are first infected when they accompany their mothers to lakes, ponds, and other open fresh water sources. School-aged children typically are the most heavily infected people in the community because of prolonged wading and swimming in infected waters. In addition, children have greater susceptibility to infection than older people because of a lack of high preexisting immunity to these parasites. Children also are important in maintaining transmission through behaviors such as uncontrolled defecation and urination. Communicability lasts as long as infected snails are in the environment or live eggs are excreted in the urine and feces of humans into fresh water sources with appropriate snails. In the case of *S japonicum*, animals play an important zoonotic role (as a source of eggs) in maintaining the life cycle. Infection is not transmissible by person-to-person contact or blood transfusion.

The distribution of schistosomiasis is focal and limited by the presence of appropriate snail vectors, infected human reservoirs, and fresh water sources. *S mansoni* occurs throughout tropical Africa, in parts of several Caribbean islands, and in areas of Venezuela, Brazil, Suriname, and the Arabian Peninsula. *S japonicum* is found in China, the Philippines, and Indonesia. *S haematobium* occurs in Africa and the Middle East; in 2014, local transmission was reported in Corsica. *S mekongi* is found in Cambodia and Laos. *S intercalatum* is found in Central Africa. Adult worms of *S mansoni* usually survive for 5 to 7 years but can live as long as 30 years in the human host. Thus, schistosomiasis can be diagnosed in patients many years after they have left an area with endemic infection. Immunity is incomplete, and reinfection occurs commonly. Swimmer's itch can occur in all regions of the world after exposure to fresh water, brackish water, or salt water.

The **incubation period** is variable but is approximately 4 to 6 weeks for *S japonicum*, 6 to 8 weeks for *S mansoni*, and 10 to 12 weeks for *S haematobium*.

DIAGNOSTIC TESTS: Eosinophilia is common and may be intense in Katayama syndrome (acute schistosomiasis). Infection with *S mansoni* and other species (except *S haematobium*) is determined by microscopic examination of stool specimens to detect characteristic eggs containing fully differentiated larvae, but results may be negative if performed too early in the course of infection. In light infections, several stool specimens examined by a concentration technique may be needed before eggs are found, or eggs may be seen in a biopsy of the rectal mucosa. *S haematobium* is diagnosed by examining urine for eggs, with centrifugation and examination of the urinary sediment required for optimum sensitivity. Egg excretion in urine often peaks between noon and 3 PM. Biopsy of the bladder mucosa may be used to diagnose this infection. Urine reagent dipsticks commonly will be positive for hematuria. Serologic tests, available through the Centers for Disease Control and Prevention and some commercial laboratories, may be helpful for detecting light infections; results of these antibody-based tests remain positive for many years and are not useful in differentiating ongoing infection from past infection or reinfection. Serologic test results are negative during acute infection, turn positive 6 to 12 weeks or more after infection, and may be positive before eggs are detectable. Antibody tests are most useful in travelers from geographic areas where the disease is endemic. Polymerase chain reaction and antigen tests for detection of schistosomes have been developed but are considered to be research tools at present.

Swimmer's itch can be difficult to differentiate from other causes of dermatitis. A skin biopsy may demonstrate larvae, but their absence does not exclude the diagnosis. A history of exposure to water used by waterfowl may be helpful in making the diagnosis.

TREATMENT: The drug of choice for schistosomiasis caused by any species is praziquantel (see Drugs for Parasitic Infections, p 985). The alternative drug for *S mansoni* is oxamniquine, although this drug no longer is available. Praziquantel does not kill developing worms; therapy given within 4 to 8 weeks of exposure should be repeated 1 to 2 months later to improve parasitologic cure. Initial management of acute schistosomiasis and neuroschistosomiasis includes reduction of inflammation with steroids, although optimal dose and duration are uncertain. Initial treatment with praziquantel may exacerbate symptoms. The optimal timing of adding praziquantel is unknown; treating with this drug when inflammation has subsided generally is favored. For acute schistosomiasis, repeating the dose of praziquantel 4 to 6 weeks later may be beneficial. Swimmer's itch is a self-limited disease that may require symptomatic treatment of the rash. More intense reactions may require a course of oral corticosteroids.

ISOLATION OF THE HOSPITALIZED PATIENT: Standard precautions are recommended. Schistosomiasis cannot be transmitted from person to person or by the fecal-oral route.

CONTROL MEASURES: Elimination of the intermediate snail host is difficult to achieve in most areas. Mass or selective treatment of infected populations, sanitary disposal of human waste, water sanitation programs, and education about the source of infection are key elements of current control measures. Travelers to areas with endemic infection should be advised to avoid any contact with freshwater streams, rivers, ponds, or lakes. Swimming and wading should occur only in chlorinated pools. Human schistosomiasis is not transmitted via sea water.

Shigella Infections

CLINICAL MANIFESTATIONS: *Shigella* species primarily infect the large intestine, causing clinical manifestations that range from watery or loose stools with minimal or no constitutional symptoms to more severe symptoms, including high fever, abdominal cramps or tenderness, tenesmus, and mucoid stools with or without blood. *Shigella dysenteriae* serotype 1 often causes a more severe illness than other shigellae with a higher risk of complications, including septicemia, pseudomembranous colitis, toxic megacolon, intestinal perforation, hemolysis, and hemolytic-uremic syndrome (HUS). Infection attributable to *S dysenteriae* type 1 has become rare in industrialized countries. Generalized seizures have been reported among young children with shigellosis attributable to any serotype; although the pathophysiology and incidence are poorly understood, such seizures usually are self-limited and usually are associated with high fever or electrolyte abnormalities. Septicemia is rare during the course of illness and is caused either by *Shigella* organisms or by other gut flora that gain access to the bloodstream through intestinal mucosa damaged during shigellosis. Septicemia occurs most often in neonates, malnourished children, and people with *S dysenteriae* serotype 1 infection but may occur in healthy children with non-dysenteriae shigellosis. Reactive arthritis with possible extraarticular manifestations is a rare complication that can develop weeks or months after shigellosis, especially in patients expressing HLA-B27.

ETIOLOGY: *Shigella* species are facultative aerobic, gram-negative bacilli in the family *Enterobacteriaceae.* Four species (with more than 40 serotypes) have been identified. Among *Shigella* isolates reported in the United States in 2012, approximately 85% were *Shigella sonnei*, 14% were *Shigella flexneri*, 1% were *Shigella boydii*, and less than 1% were other species **(www.cdc.gov/ncezid/dfwed/pdfs/shigella-annual-report-2012-508c. pdf).** In resource-limited countries, especially in Africa and Asia, *S flexneri* predominates, and *S dysenteriae* often causes outbreaks. Shiga toxin, a potent cytotoxin produced by *S dysenteriae* serotype 1, enhances the virulence of this serotype at the colonic mucosa and can cause small blood vessel and renal damage, leading to hemolytic-uremic syndrome (HUS) in some individuals. The genes encoding Shiga toxin are phage encoded and have been found in a small number of strains belonging to other *Shigella* serotypes, including *S flexneri* type 2a, *S dysenteriae* type 4, and *S sonnei*. To date, HUS has not been associated with infections attributable to these serotypes.

EPIDEMIOLOGY: Humans are the natural host for *Shigella* organisms, although other primates can be infected. The primary mode of transmission is the fecal-oral route, although transmission also can occur via contact with a contaminated inanimate object, ingestion of contaminated food or water, or sexual contact. Houseflies also may be vectors through physical transport of infected feces. Ingestion of as few as 10 organisms, depending on the species, is sufficient for infection to occur. Prolonged organism survival in water (up to 6 months) and food (up to 30 days) can occur with *Shigella* species. Children 5 years or younger in child care settings and their caregivers and people living in crowded conditions are at increased risk of infection. Men who have sex with men also are at increased risk of *Shigella*, including infections with multidrug-resistant strains. Infections attributable to *S flexneri*, *S boydii*, and *S dysenteriae* are slightly more common among adults than among children; however, infections attributable to *S sonnei* in the United States predominate among both children and adults. Travel to resource-limited countries with inadequate sanitation can place travelers at risk of infection. Even without antimicrobial therapy, the carrier state usually ceases within 1 to 4 weeks after onset of illness; long-term carriage is uncommon and does not correlate with underlying intestinal dysfunction.

In 2014 in the United States, using the National Antimicrobial Resistance Monitoring System (NARMS), 33.9% of *Shigella* species were resistant to ampicillin, 40.9% were resistant to trimethoprim-sulfamethoxazole, 4.7% were resistant to azithromycin, 2.4% were resistant to ciprofloxacin, and 0.4% were resistant to ceftriaxone **(www.cdc.gov/ narms/reports/index.html).** In 2017, the Centers for Disease Control and Prevention identified an increase in *Shigella* isolates in the United States with minimum inhibitory concentration (MIC) values of 0.12 to 1 µg/mL for ciprofloxacin. Among isolates for which results are available, preliminary data suggest that all *Shigella* isolates with ciprofloxacin MICs in this range harbor at least 1 quinolone resistance gene known to confer reduced susceptibility in enteric bacteria. *Shigella* isolates without a quinolone resistance gene typically have a ciprofloxacin MIC of ≤0.015 µg/mL. Fluoroquinolone resistance is of particular concern, given that NARMS data indicate that many *Shigella* isolates with a quinolone resistance gene also are resistant to many other commonly used treatment agents, such as azithromycin, trimethoprim-sulfamethoxazole, amoxicillin-clavulanic acid, and ampicillin.

The **incubation period** varies from 1 to 7 days but typically is 1 to 3 days.

DIAGNOSTIC TESTS: Isolation of *Shigella* organisms from feces or rectal swab specimens containing feces is diagnostic; sensitivity is improved by testing stool as soon as possible after it is passed, along with the use of enrichment broth media and selective agar plate media. If specimens cannot be transported to the testing laboratory within 2 hours, they should be transferred to appropriate transport media (eg, Cary-Blair or similar media) and transported at 4°C. Definitive identification of the organism requires both biochemical profiling and serogrouping to differentiate *Shigella* from *Escherichia* species. Identification by mass spectrometry of cellular components should not be used, because this method cannot distinguish between the 2 genera. The presence of fecal lactoferrin (or fecal leukocytes) demonstrated on a methylene-blue stained stool smear is fairly sensitive for the diagnosis of colitis but is not specific for shigellosis. Although bacteremia is rare, blood should be cultured in severely ill, immunocompromised, or malnourished children. Multiplex polymerase chain reaction (PCR) platforms for detection of multiple bacterial, viral, and parasitic pathogens including *Shigella* have high sensitivity but may yield false-positive results (eg, detecting nonviable organisms). To guide treatment, if needed, and to improve surveillance and outbreak detection, stool cultures are recommended if shigellosis is diagnosed using multiplex PCR platforms or other nonculture-based diagnostic tests. Other tests for bacterial detection, including qualitative and quantitative PCR assays, are available in research laboratories and some clinical laboratories.

TREATMENT:

- Although severe dehydration is rare with shigellosis, correction of fluid and electrolyte losses, preferably by oral rehydration solutions, is the mainstay of treatment.

- Most clinical infections with *S sonnei* are self-limited (48 to 72 hours), and mild episodes do not require antimicrobial therapy.

- Antimicrobial treatment is recommended for patients with severe disease or with underlying immunosuppressive conditions; in these patients, empiric therapy should be given while awaiting culture and susceptibility results. Available evidence suggests that antimicrobial therapy is somewhat effective in shortening duration of diarrhea and hastening eradication of organisms from feces; however, whether antimicrobial treatment reduces shigellosis transmission is unclear.

- Antimicrobial susceptibility testing of clinical isolates is indicated, because resistance to antimicrobial agents is common and may be increasing and because susceptibility data can guide appropriate therapy. Fluoroquinolones should be avoided if the *Shigella* strain has a minimum inhibitory concentration (MIC) of ≥0.12 µg/mL for ciprofloxacin, even if the laboratory report indicates the strain is "susceptible," until more is known about the clinical effect of ciprofloxacin MICs in the range of 0.12 to 1 µg/mL range. Azithromycin susceptibility testing is not performed widely for *Shigella* species. *Shigella* strains with decreased susceptibility to azithromycin have been reported in the United States, although in a large outbreak among children in 2014 only 2/400 had high-level azithromycin resistance. Ciprofloxacin and ceftriaxone resistance is increasing around the world.

- For cases in which treatment is required and susceptibilities are unknown or an ampicillin- and trimethoprim-sulfamethoxazole–resistant strain is isolated, parenteral ceftriaxone for 2 to 5 days, a fluoroquinolone (eg, ciprofloxacin) for 3 days, or azithromycin for 3 days should be administered. Oral cephalosporins (eg, cefixime) are of unclear efficacy but have been used successfully in treating shigellosis in adults. For susceptible strains, oral ampicillin or trimethoprim-sulfamethoxazole for 5 days is effective; amoxicillin is not effective because of its rapid absorption from the gastrointestinal tract. The oral route of therapy is recommended, except for seriously ill patients.
- Antidiarrheal compounds that inhibit intestinal peristalsis are contraindicated, because they can prolong the clinical and bacteriologic course of disease and can increase the rate of complications.
- Nutritional supplementation, including vitamin A (200 000 IU) and zinc (elemental Zn, orally daily for 10–14 days, 10 mg/day for newborn infants to 6 months of age, and 20 mg/day for those older than 6 months), can be given to hasten clinical resolution in geographic areas where children are at risk of malnutrition.

ISOLATION OF THE HOSPITALIZED PATIENT: In addition to standard precautions, contact precautions are indicated for the duration of illness.

CONTROL MEASURES:

Child Care Centers. General measures for interrupting enteric transmission in child care centers are recommended (see Children in Out-of-Home Child Care, p 122). Meticulous hand hygiene is the single most important measure to decrease transmission. Waterless hand sanitizers may be effective as an adjunct to washing hands with soap and in circumstances where access to soap or clean water is limited. Eliminating access to shared water-play areas and contaminated diapers also can decrease infection rates. Child care staff members should follow all standard infection control recommendations, specifically enhancing hand hygiene and ensuring that those who change diapers are not responsible for food preparation.

When *Shigella* infection is identified in a child care attendee or staff member, stool specimens from symptomatic attendees and staff members should be cultured. The local health department should be notified to evaluate and manage potential outbreaks. Infected people should be excluded until treatment is complete and a test result from at least 1 stool sample is negative (some states may require >1 negative stool sample); following this, children can return to child care facilities if stools are contained in the diaper or when toilet-trained children no longer have accidents using the toilet and when stool frequency becomes no more than 2 stools above that child's normal frequency for the time the child is in the program, even if the stools remain loose (see Children in Out-of-Home Child Care, p 122).

Institutional Outbreaks. The outbreaks that are most difficult to control are those that involve children not yet or only recently toilet-trained, adults who are unable to care for themselves (mentally disabled people or skilled nursing facility residents), or an inadequate supply of chlorinated water. A cohort system, combined with appropriate antimicrobial therapy, and a strong emphasis on hand hygiene should be considered until stool cultures no longer yield *Shigella* species. In residential institutions, ill people and newly admitted patients should be housed in separate areas.

General Control Measures. Strict attention to hand hygiene is essential to limit spread. Other important control measures include improved sanitation, appropriately chlorinating the water supply, proper cooking and storage of food, excluding infected people as food handlers, and measures to decrease contamination of food and surfaces by house-flies. People should refrain from recreational water venues (eg, swimming pools, water parks) while they have diarrhea, and those who are incontinent should continue to avoid recreational water activities for 1 additional week after symptoms resolve. Breastfeeding provides some protection for infants. Case reporting to appropriate health authorities (eg, hospital infection control personnel and public health departments) is essential.

Smallpox (Variola)

The last naturally occurring case of smallpox occurred in Somalia in 1977, followed by 2 cases in 1978 after a photographer was infected during a laboratory exposure and later transmitted smallpox to her mother in the United Kingdom. In 1980, the World Health Assembly declared that smallpox (variola virus) had been eradicated successfully world-wide, and no subsequent cases have been confirmed. The United States discontinued routine childhood immunization against smallpox in 1972 and routine immunization of health care professionals in 1976. Immunization of US military personnel continued until 1990. Following eradication, 2 World Health Organization reference laboratories were authorized to maintain stocks of variola virus. As a result of terrorism events on September 11, 2001 and concern that the virus might be used as a weapon of bioterrorism, the smallpox immunization policy was revisited. In 2002, the United States resumed immunization of military personnel deployed to certain areas of the world and in 2003 initiated a civilian smallpox immunization program for first responders to facilitate preparedness and response to a possible smallpox bioterrorism event. Such a bioterrorism event has not occurred.

CLINICAL MANIFESTATIONS: People infected with variola major strains develop a severe prodromal illness characterized by high fever (102°F–104°F [38.9°C–40.0°C]) and constitutional symptoms, including malaise, severe headache, backache, abdominal pain, and prostration, lasting for 2 to 5 days. Infected children may suffer from vomiting and seizures during this prodromal period. Most patients with smallpox are severely ill and bedridden during the febrile prodrome. The prodromal period is followed by development of lesions on mucosa of the mouth or pharynx, which may not be noticed by the patient. This stage occurs less than 24 hours before onset of rash, which usually is the first recognized manifestation of smallpox. With onset of oral lesions, the patient becomes infectious and remains so until all skin crust lesions have separated. The rash typically begins on the face and rapidly progresses to involve the forearms, trunk, and legs, with the greatest concentration of lesions on the face and distal extremities. The majority of patients will have lesions on the palms and soles. With rash onset, fever decreases but does not resolve. Lesions begin as macules that progress to papules, followed by firm vesicles and then deep-seated, hard pustules described as "pearls of pus." Each stage lasts 1 to 2 days. By the sixth or seventh day of rash, lesions may begin to umbilicate or become confluent. Lesions increase in size for approximately 8 to 10 days, after which they begin to crust. Once all the crusts have separated, 3 to 4 weeks after the onset of rash, the patient no longer is infectious. Variola major in unimmunized people is associated with case-fatality rates of approximately 30% during epidemics of smallpox. The mortality rate is highest in pregnant women, children younger than 1 year, and adults older than 30 years. The potential for modern supportive therapy to improve outcome is not known.

Variola minor strains cause a disease that is indistinguishable clinically from variola major, except that it causes less severe systemic symptoms and has more rapid rash evolution, reduced scarring, and fewer fatalities.

In addition to the typical presentation of smallpox (90% of cases or greater), there are 2 uncommon forms of variola major: hemorrhagic (characterized either by a hemorrhagic diathesis before onset of the typical smallpox rash [early hemorrhagic smallpox] or by hemorrhage into skin lesions and disseminated intravascular coagulation [late hemorrhagic smallpox]) and malignant or flat type (in which the skin lesions do not progress to the pustular stage but remain flat and soft). Each variant occurs in approximately 5% of cases and is associated with a 95% to 100% mortality rate. Pregnancy is a risk factor for hemorrhagic variola. Defects in cellular immunity may be responsible for flat type variola major, which is seen more commonly in children than adults.

Varicella (chickenpox) is the condition most likely to be mistaken for smallpox. Generally, children with varicella do not have a febrile prodrome, but adults may have a brief, mild prodrome. Although the 2 diseases are confused easily in the first few days of the rash, smallpox lesions develop into pustules that are firm and deeply embedded in the dermis, whereas varicella lesions develop into superficial vesicles. Because varicella erupts in crops of lesions that evolve quickly, lesions on any one part of the body will be in different stages of evolution (papules, vesicles, and crusts), whereas all smallpox lesions on any one part of the body are in the same stage of development. The rash distribution of the 2 diseases differs; varicella most commonly starts on the trunk and moves peripherally with less involvement of the extremities as compared with the trunk. Variola lesions can be found distributed on all parts of the body.

ETIOLOGY: Variola is a member of the *Poxviridae* family (genus *Orthopoxvirus*). Other members of this genus that can infect humans include monkeypox virus, cowpox virus, and vaccinia virus. Cowpox virus was used by Benjamin Jesty in 1774 and by Edward Jenner in 1796 as material for the first smallpox vaccine. Later, cowpox virus was replaced with vaccinia virus. In 2003, an outbreak of monkeypox linked to prairie dogs exposed to rodents imported from Ghana occurred in the United States.

EPIDEMIOLOGY: Humans are the only natural reservoir for variola virus (smallpox). Smallpox is spread most commonly in droplets from the oropharynx of infected people, although rare transmission from aerosol spread has been reported. Infection from direct contact with lesion material or indirectly via fomites, such as clothing and bedding, also has been reported. Because most patients with smallpox are extremely ill and bedridden, spread generally is limited to household contacts, hospital workers, and other health care professionals. Secondary household attack rates for smallpox were considerably lower than for measles and similar to or lower than rates for varicella.

The **incubation period** is 7 to 17 days (mean, 10–12 days).

DIAGNOSTIC TESTS: Variola virus can be detected in vesicular or pustular fluid by a number of different methods, including electron microscopy, immunohistochemistry, culture, or polymerase chain reaction (PCR) assay. Only PCR assay can diagnose infection with variola virus definitively; all other methods simply screen for orthopoxviruses. Screening is available through select state health departments. Final, confirmatory variola-specific laboratory testing is available only at the Centers for Disease Control and Prevention (CDC). Diagnostic work-up includes exclusion of varicella-zoster virus or other common conditions that cause a vesicular/pustular rash illness. Caution is required when collecting specimens from patients in whom a diagnosis of smallpox is considered. Detailed guidelines for safe collection of specimens can be obtained through consultation with the CDC (**www.cdc.gov/smallpox/;** 770-488-7100).

TREATMENT: There is no antiviral therapy licensed by the US Food and Drug Administration (FDA) for the treatment of smallpox. Infected patients should receive supportive care. Cidofovir, a nucleotide analogue of cytosine, has demonstrated antiviral activity against certain orthopoxviruses in vitro and in animal models. Its effectiveness in treatment of variola in humans is unknown. Investigational agents, such as brincidofovir (a lipophilic derivative of cidofovir) and tecovirimat (ST-246, an investigational agent with antiviral activity against orthopoxviruses), are being evaluated in animal models; however, benefit in infected humans cannot be tested in the absence of disease. Vaccinia Immune Globulin (VIG) is reserved for certain complications of immunization and has no role in treatment of smallpox. Physicians at civilian medical facilities may request VIG by calling the CDC Smallpox Vaccine Adverse Events Clinical Information Line at 1-800-232-4636. Physicians at military medical facilities may request VIG by calling the US Army Medical Research Institute of Infectious Diseases (USAMRIID) at 301-619-2257 or 1-888-872-7443 (1-888-USA-RIID). Tecovirimat and brincidofovir have been used for the treatment of disseminated vaccinia through individual patient expanded access requests.

ISOLATION OF THE HOSPITALIZED PATIENT: At the time of admission, a patient suspected of having smallpox should be placed in a private, airborne infection isolation room equipped with negative-pressure ventilation with high-efficiency particulate air filtration. Standard, contact, and airborne precautions should be implemented immediately, and hospital infection control personnel and the state (and/or local) health department should be alerted immediately. After evaluation by the state or local health department, if smallpox laboratory diagnostics are considered necessary, the CDC Emergency Operations Center should be consulted at 770-488-7100.

CONTROL MEASURES:

Care of Exposed People. Cases of febrile rash illness for which smallpox is considered in the differential diagnosis should be reported immediately to local or state health departments.

Use of Vaccine. Postexposure immunization (within 3–4 days of exposure) provides some protection against disease and significant protection against a fatal outcome. Except for severely immunocompromised people who are not expected to benefit from live vaccinia vaccine, any person with a significant exposure to a patient with proven smallpox during the infectious stage of illness requires immunization as soon after exposure as possible ("ring vaccination").

Preexposure Immunization.

Smallpox Vaccine. The only smallpox vaccine licensed in the United States is ACAM2000 (Sanofi Pasteur Biologics Co, Cambridge, MA), a live-virus vaccine.[1] The lyophilized vaccine does not contain variola virus but the related vaccinia virus, different from the cowpox virus initially used for immunization by Jesty and Jenner. ACAM2000 elicits an immune response similar to Dryvax, a previously licensed vaccinia vaccine (no longer available) that was highly effective in preventing smallpox, with protection waning after 5 to 10 years following 1 dose and with longer duration of protection after reimmunization. During the time before smallpox eradication when routine smallpox immunization programs utilized vaccinia vaccines, substantial protection against death

---

[1]Centers for Disease Control and Prevention. Notice to readers: newly licensed smallpox vaccine to replace old smallpox vaccine. *MMWR Morb Mortal Wkly Rep.* 2008;57(8):207–208

from smallpox was observed to persist for more than 30 years after immunization during infancy. The ACAM2000 package insert recommends that people at very high risk of exposure, such as those handling variola virus, be vaccinated every 3 years. ACAM2000 is not available for use in the general population and can only be administered by specially trained providers. In the absence of a smallpox outbreak, preexposure smallpox immunization is not recommended for children. Smallpox vaccine had been recommended for adults participating in smallpox response teams and for people working with orthopoxviruses, and smallpox vaccine continues to be administered to eligible military personnel preparing to deploy to certain regions in the world. Inadvertent transmission of the vaccine virus may occur from vaccine recipients to their household contacts. Children who are immunocompromised or have atopic skin disease are at increased risk of serious complications following contact transmission, including progressive vaccinia and eczema vaccinatum. Smallpox reimmunization recommendations can be found on the CDC Web site (**www.cdc.gov/smallpox/clinicians/index.html**). Information about contraindications to preexposure smallpox immunization and adverse reactions to vaccination[1] can be found in the ACAM2000 package insert and medication guide (**www.fda.gov/ BiologicsBloodVaccines/Vaccines/ApprovedProducts/ucm180810.htm**). An investigational attenuated vaccinia vaccine (Imvamune) is part of the national strategic stockpile and is intended for emergency use during a smallpox event in people who are not at high risk of smallpox exposure and who are at increased risk of serious complications following ACAM2000 vaccination, including individuals with immunocompromising conditions or atopic skin disease. Another investigational vaccinia vaccine similar to ACAM2000 (ASPV) also is part of the strategic national stockpile for emergency use during a smallpox event.

Sporotrichosis

CLINICAL MANIFESTATIONS: There are 3 cutaneous patterns described for sporotrichosis. The classic lymphocutaneous process with multiple nodules is seen most commonly in adults. Inoculation occurs at a site of minor trauma, causing a painless papule that enlarges slowly to become a firm slightly tender subcutaneous nodule that can develop a violaceous hue or can ulcerate. Secondary lesions follow the same evolution and develop along the lymphatic distribution proximal to the initial lesion. A localized cutaneous form of sporotrichosis, also called fixed cutaneous form, is seen most commonly in children and presents as a solitary crusted papule or papuloulcerative or nodular lesion in which lymphatic spread is not observed. The extremities and face are the most common sites of infection. A disseminated cutaneous form with multiple lesions is rare, usually occurring in immunocompromised children.

Extracutaneous sporotrichosis is uncommon, with cases occurring primarily in immunocompromised patients or, in adults, those who are alcoholic or have chronic obstructive pulmonary disease. Osteoarticular infection results from hematogenous spread or local inoculation. The most commonly affected joints are the knees, elbows, wrists, and ankles. Pulmonary sporotrichosis clinically resembles tuberculosis and occurs after inhalation or aspiration of aerosolized conidia. Disseminated disease generally

---

[1]Centers for Disease Control and Prevention. Surveillance guidelines for smallpox vaccine (vaccinia) adverse reactions. *MMWR Recomm Rep.* 2006;55(RR-1):1–16

occurs after hematogenous spread from primary skin or lung infection. Disseminated sporotrichosis can involve multiple foci (eg, eyes, pericardium, genitourinary tract, central nervous system) and occurs predominantly in immunocompromised patients. Pulmonary and disseminated forms of sporotrichosis are uncommon in children.

ETIOLOGY: *Sporothrix schenckii* is a thermally dimorphic fungus that grows as a mold or mycelial form at room temperature and as a budding yeast at 35°C to 37°C and in host tissues. *S schenckii* is a complex of at least 6 species. Within this complex, *S schenckii sensu stricto* is responsible for most infections, but in South America, *Sporothrix brasiliensis* is a major cause of infection.

EPIDEMIOLOGY: *S schenckii* is a ubiquitous organism that has worldwide distribution but is most common in tropical and subtropical regions of Central and South America and parts of North America and Asia. Cases in the United States appear to cluster in the Midwest, particularly along the Mississippi and Missouri river areas. The fungus has been isolated from soil and plant material, including hay, straw, sphagnum moss, and decaying vegetation. Thorny plants, such as rose bushes and pine trees, commonly are implicated, because pricks from their thorns or needles inoculate the organism from the soil or moss around the bush or tree. People who handle contaminated plant matter are at risk of infection. Zoonotic spread from infected cats or scratches from digging animals, such as armadillos, has led to cutaneous disease.

The **incubation period** is 7 to 30 days after cutaneous inoculation but can be as long as 6 months.

DIAGNOSTIC TESTS: Culture of *Sporothrix* species from a tissue, wound drainage, or sputum specimen is diagnostic. The mold phase of the organism can be isolated on a variety of fungal media including Sabouraud dextrose agar at 25°C to 30°C. Filamentous colonies generally appear within 1 week. Definitive identification requires conversion to the yeast phase by subculture to enriched media such as brain-heart infusion agar with 5% blood and incubation at 35°C to 37°C. In some cases, repeated subcultures are required for conversion. Culture of *Sporothrix* species from a blood specimen is definite evidence for the disseminated form of infection associated with immunodeficiency. Histopathologic examination of tissue may be helpful but often is not, because the organism seldom is abundant. Special fungal stains including periodic acid-Schiff and Gomori methenamine silver to visualize the oval or cigar-shaped organism are required. Serologic testing and polymerase chain reaction assay show promise for accurate and specific diagnosis but are available only in research laboratories.

TREATMENT[1]: Sporotrichosis usually does not resolve without treatment. Itraconazole (5 mg/kg per dose, twice daily; maximum dose 200 mg) is the drug of choice for children with lymphocutaneous and localized cutaneous disease; many experts prefer using the oral solution, which has no issues with food and appears to achieve better concentrations. The duration of therapy is 2 to 4 weeks after all lesions have resolved, usually for a total duration of 3 to 6 months. Serum trough concentrations of itraconazole should be 1 to 2 µg/mL. Concentrations should be checked after 1 to 2 weeks of therapy to ensure adequate drug exposure. When measured by high-pressure liquid chromatography, both itraconazole and its bioactive hydroxy-itraconazole metabolite are reported, the sum of

[1]Kauffman CA, Bustamante B, Chapman SW, Pappas PG; Infectious Diseases Society of America. Clinical practice guidelines for the management of sporotrichosis: 2007 update by the Infectious Diseases Society of America. *Clin Infect Dis.* 2007;45(10):1255–1265

which should be considered in assessing drug levels. Saturated solution of potassium iodide (1 drop, 3 times daily, increasing as tolerated to a maximum of 1 drop/kg of body
weight or 40 to 50 drops, 3 times daily, whichever is lowest) is an alternative therapy.
Oral fluconazole, 12 mg/kg daily (maximum dose: 400–800 mg daily), should be used
only if the patient cannot tolerate other agents.

Amphotericin B is recommended as the initial therapy for visceral or disseminated
sporotrichosis in children (see Recommended Doses of Parenteral and Oral Antifungal
Drugs, p 945). After clinical response to amphotericin B therapy is documented, itraconazole can be substituted and should be continued for at least 12 months. Itraconazole may
be required for lifelong therapy in children with human immunodeficiency virus infection. Pulmonary and disseminated infections respond less well than cutaneous infection,
despite prolonged therapy.

ISOLATION OF THE HOSPITALIZED PATIENT: Standard precautions are indicated.

CONTROL MEASURES: Use of protective gloves and clothing for occupational and recreational activities that could lead to exposure to *S schenckii* can decrease risk of disease.

Staphylococcal Food Poisoning

CLINICAL MANIFESTATIONS: Staphylococcal foodborne illness is characterized by
abrupt and sometimes violent onset of severe nausea, abdominal cramps, vomiting, and
prostration, often accompanied by diarrhea. Low-grade fever or mild hypothermia can
occur. The illness typically lasts 1 to 2 days, but symptoms are intense and can require
hospitalization. The short incubation period, brevity of illness, and usual lack of fever
help distinguish staphylococcal from other types of food poisoning, with the exception of
the vomiting syndrome caused by *Bacillus cereus*. Chemical food poisoning usually has a
shorter incubation period, and *Clostridium perfringens* food poisoning usually has a longer
incubation period. Patients with foodborne *Salmonella* or *Shigella* infection are more likely
to have fever and a longer incubation period (see Appendix VII, Clinical Syndromes Associated With Foodborne Diseases, p 1086).

ETIOLOGY: Enterotoxins produced by strains of *Staphylococcus aureus* and, rarely, *Staphylococcus epidermidis* and *Staphylococcus intermedius* elicit the symptoms of staphylococcal food
poisoning.

EPIDEMIOLOGY: Illness is caused by ingestion of food containing heat-stable staphylococcal enterotoxins. The most commonly implicated foods are meats, poultry, pastries, cus-
tards, and other milk- or egg-based products served after inadequate heating or refrigeration. These foods may be contaminated by enterotoxigenic strains of *S aureus* via direct
contact with the hands of food handlers, with the organism sometimes originating from
purulent discharge from an infected finger or abscess or from nasopharyngeal secretions.
When contaminated foods remain at room temperature for several hours, the toxin-
producing staphylococcal organisms multiply and produce toxins that are heat-stable (ie,
not inactivated by reheating). Less commonly, the toxigenic staphylococci are of bovine
origin (eg, from cows with mastitis) from contaminated milk or milk products, especially
cheeses.[1]

---

[1]American Academy of Pediatrics, Committee on Infectious Diseases and Committee on Nutrition. Consumption of raw or unpasteurized milk and milk products by pregnant women and children. *Pediatrics*. 2014;133(1):
175–179

The **incubation period** ranges from 30 minutes to 8 hours after ingestion, typically 2 to 4 hours.

DIAGNOSTIC TESTS: In most cases, given the short duration of illness and rapid recovery with supportive care, diagnostic testing to confirm the diagnosis is not necessary. Recovery of large numbers of staphylococci from stool or vomitus and detection of enterotoxin in foods by commercially available kits support the diagnosis. In an outbreak, demonstration of either one or more enterotoxins or $\geq 10^5$ colony-forming units/g in an epidemiologically implicated food confirms the diagnosis. Identification of the same subtype of *S aureus* from the stool or vomitus of 2 or more ill people also confirms the diagnosis. Strain identification is performed commonly by molecular methods including pulsed field gel electrophoresis or sequence-based typing methods and generally is available through public health laboratories for outbreak investigations. Local public health authorities should be notified to help determine the source of the outbreak.

TREATMENT: Treatment is supportive. Antimicrobial agents are not indicated.

ISOLATION OF THE HOSPITALIZED PATIENT: Staphylococcal food poisoning is not spread from person to person. Standard precautions are recommended.

CONTROL MEASURES: People with boils, abscesses, and other purulent lesions of the hands, eyes, face, or nose should be excluded from food preparation and handling until lesions resolve. Strict hand hygiene before food handling should be enforced. Prepared foods should not be stored for more than 2 hours at room temperature and should be refrigerated in wide, shallow containers. Information on recommended safe food handling practices, including time and temperature requirements during cooking, storage, and reheating, can be found online (**www.foodsafety.gov**).

Staphylococcus aureus

CLINICAL MANIFESTATIONS: *Staphylococcus aureus* causes a variety of **localized and invasive suppurative infections** and 3 toxin-mediated syndromes: **toxic shock syndrome, scalded skin syndrome,** and food poisoning (see Staphylococcal Food Poisoning, p 732). Localized infections include cellulitis, skin and soft tissue abscesses, orbital cellulitis/abscess, pustulosis, impetigo (bullous and nonbullous), paronychia, mastitis, hordeola, furuncles, carbuncles, peritonsillar abscesses (Quinsy), omphalitis, parotitis, lymphadenitis, and wound infections. Bacteremia can be associated with focal complications including osteomyelitis; arthritis; endocarditis; pneumonia; pleural empyema; pericarditis; soft tissue, muscle, or visceral abscesses; and septic thrombophlebitis of small and large vessels. In neutropenic patients, ecthyma gangrenosum may occur. Primary *S aureus* pneumonia also can occur after aspiration of organisms from the upper respiratory tract and typically is associated with mechanical ventilation or viral infections in the community (eg, influenza). Meningitis may occur in preterm infants but otherwise is rare unless accompanied by an intradermal foreign body (eg, ventriculoperitoneal shunt) or a congenital or acquired defect in the dura. *S aureus* also causes invasive infections with bacteremia associated with foreign bodies, including intravascular catheters or grafts, peritoneal catheters, cerebrospinal fluid shunts, spinal instrumentation or intramedullary rods, pressure equalization tubes, pacemakers and other intracardiac devices, and prosthetic joints. *S aureus* infections can be fulminant. Certain chronic diseases, such as diabetes mellitus, malignancy, prematurity, immunodeficiency, nutritional disorders, surgery, and transplantation, increase the risk for severe *S aureus* infections. Metastatic foci and abscess formation need to be drained and foreign bodies should be removed. Prolonged antimicrobial therapy often is necessary to achieve cure.

Staphylococcal toxic shock syndrome (TSS), a toxin-mediated disease, usually is caused by strains producing TSS toxin-1 or possibly other related staphylococcal enterotoxins. Characterized by acute onset of fever, generalized erythroderma, rapid-onset hypotension, and signs of multisystem organ involvement, including profuse watery diarrhea, vomiting, conjunctival injection, and severe myalgia (see Table 3.67, for clinical case definition), TSS can occur in menstruating females using tampons, following childbirth or abortion, after surgical procedures, and in association with cutaneous lesions. TSS also can occur in males and females without a readily identifiable focus of infection. Prevailing clones (eg, USA300) of community-associated methicillin-resistant *S aureus* (MRSA) rarely produce TSS toxin. People with TSS, especially menses-associated illness, are at risk of a recurrent episode.

Table 3.67. *Staphylococcus aureus* Toxic Shock Syndrome: Clinical Case Definition[a]

Clinical Findings
- Fever: temperature 38.9°C (102.0°F) or greater
- Rash: diffuse macular erythroderma
- Desquamation: 1–2 weeks after onset, particularly on palms, soles, fingers, and toes
- Hypotension: systolic pressure 90 mm Hg or less for adults; lower than fifth percentile for age for children younger than 16 years; orthostatic drop in diastolic pressure of 15 mm Hg or greater from lying to sitting; orthostatic syncope or orthostatic dizziness
- Multisystem organ involvement: 3 or more of the following:
  1. Gastrointestinal tract: vomiting or diarrhea at onset of illness
  2. Muscular: severe myalgia or creatinine phosphokinase concentration greater than twice the upper limit of normal
  3. Mucous membrane: vaginal, oropharyngeal, or conjunctival hyperemia
  4. Renal: serum urea nitrogen or serum creatinine concentration greater than twice the upper limit of normal or urinary sediment with 5 white blood cells/high-power field or greater in the absence of urinary tract infection
  5. Hepatic: total bilirubin, aspartate transaminase, or alanine transaminase concentration greater than twice the upper limit of normal
  6. Hematologic: platelet count 100 000/mm³ or less
  7. Central nervous system: disorientation or alterations in consciousness without focal neurologic signs when fever and hypotension are absent

Laboratory Criteria
- *Negative* results on the following tests, if obtained:
  1. Blood, throat, or cerebrospinal fluid cultures; blood culture rarely may be positive for *S aureus*
  2. Serologic tests for Rocky Mountain spotted fever, leptospirosis, or measles

Case Classification
- ***Probable:*** a case that meets the laboratory criteria and in which 4 of 5 clinical findings are present
- ***Confirmed:*** a case that meets laboratory criteria and all 5 of the clinical findings, including desquamation, unless the patient dies before desquamation occurs.

[a]Adapted from Wharton M, Chorba TL, Vogt RL, Morse DL, Buehler JW. Case definitions for public health surveillance. *MMWR Recomm Rep.* 1990;39(RR-13):1–43.

Staphylococcal scalded skin syndrome (SSSS) is a toxin-mediated disease caused by circulation of exfoliative toxins A and B. The manifestations of SSSS are age related and include Ritter disease (generalized exfoliation) in the neonate, a tender scarlatiniform eruption and localized bullous impetigo in older children, or a combination of these with thick white/brown flaky desquamation of the entire skin, especially on the face and neck, in older infants and toddlers. The hallmark of SSSS is the toxin-mediated cleavage of the stratum granulosum layer of the epidermis (ie, Nikolsky sign). Proper pain management is a mainstay of therapy for SSSS. Healing occurs without scarring. Bacteremia is rare, but dehydration and superinfection can occur with extensive exfoliation.

ETIOLOGY: Staphylococci are catalase-positive, gram-positive cocci that appear microscopically as grape-like clusters. Staphylococci are ubiquitous and can survive extreme conditions of drying, heat, and low-oxygen and high-salt environments. *S aureus* has many surface proteins, including the microbial surface components recognizing adhesive matrix molecule (MSCRAMM) receptors, which allow the organism to bind to tissues and foreign bodies coated with fibronectin, fibrinogen, and collagen. This permits a low inoculum of organisms to adhere to sutures, catheters, prosthetic valves, and other devices.

EPIDEMIOLOGY: *S aureus* is the most common cause of skin and soft tissue infections and musculoskeletal infections in otherwise healthy children. *S aureus* colonizes the skin and mucous membranes of 30% to 50% of healthy adults and children. *S aureus* is second only to coagulase-negative staphylococci (CoNS) as a cause of health care-associated bacteremia, is one of the most common causes of health care-associated pneumonia in children, and is responsible for most health care-associated surgical site infections.

S aureus-mediated TSS was recognized in 1978, and many early cases were associated with tampon use. Although changes in tampon composition and use have resulted in a decreased proportion of cases associated with menses, menstrual and nonmenstrual cases of TSS continue to occur and are reported with similar frequency. Risk factors for TSS include absence of antibody to TSS toxin-1 and focal *S aureus* infection with a TSS toxin-1–producing strain. TSS toxin-1 producing strains can be part of normal flora of the anterior nares or vagina, and colonization at these sites is believed to result in protective antibody in more than 90% of adults. Health care-associated TSS can occur and most often follows surgical procedures. In postoperative cases, the organism generally originates from the patient's own flora.

Transmission of S aureus. The anterior nares, throat, axilla, perineum, vagina, or rectum are usual sites of colonization. Rates of skin carriage of more than 50% occur in children with desquamating skin disorders or burns and in people with frequent needle use (eg, diabetes mellitus, hemodialysis, illicit drug use, allergy shots). Although domestic animals can be colonized, data suggest that colonization is acquired from humans. Adults who carry MRSA in the nose preoperatively are more likely to develop surgical site infections after general, cardiac, orthopedic, or solid organ transplant surgery than are patients who are not carriers. Hospitalized children who are colonized with MRSA on admission or acquire MRSA colonization in the hospital are at increased risk for subsequent MRSA infection compared with noncolonized children.

S aureus is transmitted most often by direct contact in community settings and indirectly from patient to patient via transiently colonized hands of health care professionals in health care settings. Health care professionals and family members who are colonized with *S aureus* in the nares or on skin also can serve as a reservoir for transmission. Contaminated environmental surfaces and objects also can play a role in transmission of

S aureus, although their relative contribution for spread is unknown. Although not transmitted by the droplet route routinely, *S aureus* can be dispersed into the air over short distances. Dissemination of *S aureus* from people with nasal carriage, including infants, is related to density of colonization, and increased dissemination occurs during viral upper respiratory tract infections. Additional risk factors for health care-associated acquisition of *S aureus* include illness requiring care in neonatal or pediatric intensive care or burn units, surgical procedures, prolonged hospitalization, local epidemic of *S aureus* infection, and the presence of indwelling catheters or prosthetic devices.

Health Care-Associated MRSA. MRSA has been endemic in most US hospitals since the 1980s and recently accounted for more than 40% of health care-associated *S aureus* infections in inpatients reported to the Centers for Disease Control and Prevention (CDC). Risk factors for nasal carriage of health care-associated MRSA strains include hospitalization within the previous year, recent (within the previous 60 days) antimicrobial use, prolonged hospital stay, frequent contact with a health care environment, presence of an intravascular or peritoneal catheter or endotracheal tube, increased number of surgical procedures, or frequent contact with a person with one or more of the preceding risk factors. Carriage can persist for years.

MRSA, both health care- and community-associated strains, and methicillin-resistant CoNS (see Coagulase-Negative Staphylococcal Infections, p 746) are responsible for a large portion of infections acquired in health care settings. Health care-associated MRSA strains are difficult to treat, because they usually are multidrug resistant and predictably are susceptible only to vancomycin, linezolid, and agents not approved by the US Food and Drug Administration (FDA) for use in children.

Community-Associated MRSA. Community-associated MRSA infections emerged in the 1990s; skin and soft tissue abscesses are noted most commonly. Clinical infections are more common in settings where there is crowding; frequent skin-to-skin contact; sharing of personal items, such as towels and clothing; and poor personal hygiene and among those with body piercings. Outbreaks have been reported among athletic teams, in correctional facilities, and in military training facilities. Community-associated MRSA clones have been implicated as a common cause of health care-associated MRSA infections.

Vancomycin-Intermediately Susceptible S aureus. Strains of MRSA with intermediate susceptibility to vancomycin (minimum inhibitory concentration [MIC], 4–8 µg/mL) have been isolated from people (historically dialysis patients) who had received multiple courses of vancomycin for a MRSA infection. Strains of MRSA can be heterogeneous for vancomycin resistance (see Diagnostic Tests). Extensive vancomycin use allows vancomycin-intermediately susceptible *S aureus* (VISA) strains to develop. These strains may emerge during therapy. Control measures recommended by the CDC have included using proper methods to detect VISA, using appropriate infection-control measures, and adopting measures to ensure appropriate vancomycin use.

Vancomycin-Resistant S aureus (VRSA). VRSA infections (MIC >8 µg/mL) are very rare, and in all cases reported patients had underlying medical conditions, a history of MRSA infections, and prolonged exposure to vancomycin.

The **incubation period** is variable for staphylococcal disease. A long delay can occur between acquisition of the organism and onset of disease. For toxin-mediated SSSS, the **incubation period** usually is 1 to 10 days; for postoperative TSS, it can be as short as 12 hours. Menstrual-related cases can develop at any time during menses.

DIAGNOSTIC TESTS: Gram-stained smears of material from skin lesions or pyogenic foci showing gram-positive cocci in clusters can provide presumptive evidence of infection. Isolation of organisms from culture of otherwise sterile body fluid is the method for definitive diagnosis. Molecular assays have been approved by the FDA for direct detection of *S aureus* from blood culture bottles. Nonamplified molecular assays, such as peptide nucleic acid fluorescent in situ hybridization (PNA-FISH), and nucleic acid amplification tests, such as BD GenOhm Staph SR (BD Molecular diagnostics) and Xpert MRSA/SA BC (Cepheid), are approved for detection and identification of *S aureus*, including MRSA, in positive blood cultures. Matrix-assisted laser desorption ionization time-of-flight mass spectrometry (MALDI-TOF) can rapidly identify *S aureus* colonies on culture plates or from growth in blood cultures. *S aureus* almost never is a contaminant when isolated from a blood culture.

S aureus-mediated TSS is a clinical diagnosis (Table 3.67, p 734). *S aureus* grows in culture of blood specimens from fewer than 5% of patients with TSS. Specimens for culture should be obtained from an identified focal site of infection, because these sites usually will yield the organism. Because approximately one third of isolates of *S aureus* from nonmenstrual cases produce toxins other than TSS toxin-1, and TSS toxin-1–producing organisms can be present as normal flora, TSS toxin-1 production by an isolate is not useful diagnostically.

Quantitative antimicrobial susceptibility testing should be performed for all *S aureus* specimens isolated from normally sterile sites. Laboratory practice includes routine screening (D-testing) to exclude inducible clindamycin resistance. Health care-associated MRSA heterogeneous or heterotypic strains appear susceptible by disk testing. However, when a parent strain is cultured on methicillin-containing media, resistant subpopulations are apparent. When these resistant subpopulations are cultured on methicillin-free media, they can continue as stable resistant mutants or revert to susceptible strains (heterogeneous resistance). Cells expressing heteroresistance grow more slowly than the oxacillin-susceptible cells and can be missed at growth conditions above 35°C (95°F).

S aureus strain genotyping has become a necessary adjunct for determining whether several isolates from one patient or from different patients are the same. Typing, in conjunction with epidemiologic information, can facilitate identification of the source, extent, and mechanism of transmission in an outbreak. Antimicrobial susceptibility testing is the most readily available method for typing by a phenotypic characteristic. A number of molecular typing methods are available for *S aureus*, including pulsed-field gel electrophoresis, spa typing, and whole genome sequencing. Choice of method should consider purpose of typing and available resources.

TREATMENT:
Skin and Soft Tissue Infection. Skin and soft tissue infections, such as diffuse impetigo or cellulitis attributable to methicillin-susceptible *S aureus* (MSSA), optimally are treated with oral penicillinase-resistant beta-lactam drugs, such as a first- or second-generation cephalosporin. For the penicillin-allergic patient and in cases in which MRSA is considered, trimethoprim-sulfamethoxazole, doxycycline, or clindamycin can be used if the isolate is susceptible. Topical mupirocin is recommended for localized impetigo.

The most frequent manifestation of community-associated MRSA infection is skin and soft tissue infection. Fig 3.8 shows the initial management of skin and soft tissue infections suspected to be caused by community-associated MRSA. A randomized placebo-controlled study that included children with simple abscesses ≤3 cm (6–11 months of age), ≤4 cm (1–8 years of age), or ≤5 cm (>8 years of age) in diameter showed that drainage plus systemic oral therapy with clindamycin or trimethoprim-sulfamethoxazole is associated with better outcomes compared with drainage alone, and that treatment with clindamycin was associated with fewer recurrences.

In ill patients and for those with complicated skin and soft tissue infection with abscess, drainage/débridement and systemic antimicrobial therapy are warranted; therapy should be focused on the pathogen identified and based on the results of susceptibility testing.

Invasive Staphylococcal Infections. Empiric therapy for suspected invasive staphylococcal infection, including pneumonia, osteoarticular infection, visceral abscesses, and foreign body-associated infection with bacteremia, is vancomycin plus a semisynthetic beta lactam (eg, nafcillin, oxacillin). Subsequent therapy should be determined by antimicrobial susceptibility results. Clindamycin is bacteriostatic and should not be used for treatment of endovascular infection. Serious MSSA infections require intravenous therapy with a beta-lactamase–resistant beta-lactam antimicrobial agent, such as nafcillin or oxacillin, because most *S aureus* strains produce beta-lactamase enzymes and are resistant to penicillin and ampicillin (see Table 3.68, p 740). The addition of rifampin may be considered for those with invasive disease related to an indwelling foreign body, especially if removal of the infected implant is not feasible. Vancomycin is not recommended for treatment of serious MSSA infections, because outcomes are inferior compared with cases in which antistaphylococcal beta lactams are used and to minimize emergence of vancomycin resistance. First- or second-generation cephalosporins (eg, cefazolin) or vancomycin are less effective than nafcillin or oxacillin for treatment of MSSA endocarditis or meningitis.

A patient with MSSA infection (and no evidence of endocarditis or central nervous system [CNS] infection) who has a nonserious allergy to penicillin can be treated with a first- or second-generation cephalosporin or with clindamycin, if the *S aureus* strain is susceptible. Clindamycin is bacteriostatic and should not be used for treatment of endovascular infection.

Guidelines for management of serious skin/soft tissue infection, complicated pneumonia/empyema, CNS infection, osteomyelitis, and endocarditis caused by MRSA are available (**www.idsociety.org/IDSA_Practice_Guidelines/**).

VISA infection is rare in children. For seriously ill patients with a history of recurrent MRSA infections or for patients failing vancomycin therapy in whom VISA strains are a consideration, initial therapy could include linezolid or trimethoprim-sulfamethoxazole, with or without gentamicin. If antimicrobial susceptibility results document multidrug resistance, alternative agents, such as quinupristin-dalfopristin, daptomycin (not approved for pneumonia), ceftaroline, or tigecycline, could be considered.

Duration of therapy for serious MSSA or MRSA infections depends on the site and severity of infection but usually is 4 weeks or more for endocarditis, osteomyelitis, necrotizing pneumonia, or disseminated infection, assuming a documented clinical and microbiologic response. The duration of bacteremia for pediatric patients with staphylococcal infection can be up to 3 to 4 days for MSSA and 7 to 9 days for MRSA. In assessing whether modification of therapy is necessary, clinicians should consider whether the patient is improving clinically, should identify and drain sequestered foci of infection and remove foreign material (such as a central catheter) when possible, and for MRSA strains, should consider the vancomycin MIC and the achievable vancomycin trough concentrations.

FIG 3.8. ALGORITHM FOR INITIAL MANAGEMENT OF SKIN AND SOFT TISSUE INFECTIONS CAUSED BY COMMUNITY-ASSOCIATED *STAPHYLOCOCCUS AUREUS*

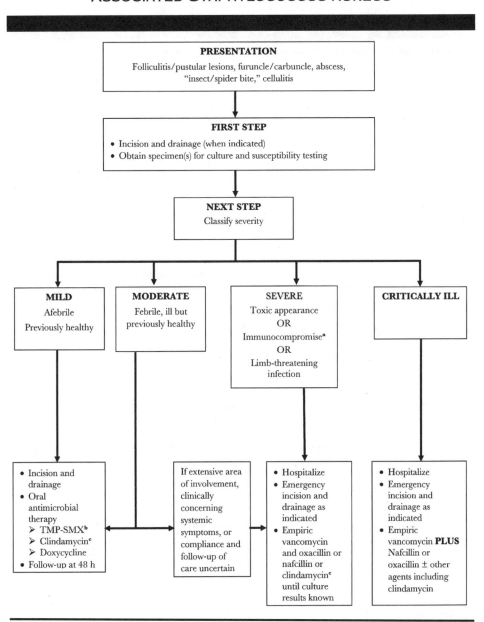

[a]Immunocompromise any chronic condition except asthma or eczema.

[b]TMP-SMX = trimethoprim-sulfamethoxazole, if group A *Streptococcus* unlikely.

[c]Consider prevalence of clindamycin-susceptible methicillin-susceptible *S aureus* and "D" test-negative community-associated methicillin-resistant *S aureus* strains in the community.

Table 3.68. Parenteral Antimicrobial Agent(s) for Treatment of Bacteremia and Other Serious *Staphylococcus aureus* Infections

Susceptibility	Antimicrobial Agents	Comments
I. Initial empiric therapy (organism of unknown susceptibility)		
Drugs of choice:	Vancomycin (15 mg/kg, every 6 h) + nafcillin or oxacillin	For life-threatening infections (ie, septicemia, endocarditis, CNS infection); ceftaroline or linezolid are alternatives, but there are limited efficacy data in children
	Vancomycin (15 mg/kg, every 6–8 h)[a]	For non–life-threatening infection without signs of sepsis (eg, skin infection, cellulitis, osteomyelitis, pyarthrosis) when rates of MRSA colonization and infection in the community are substantial; ceftaroline or linezolid are alternatives
	Clindamycin	For non–life-threatening infection without signs of sepsis when rates of MRSA colonization and infection in the community are substantial and prevalence of clindamycin resistance is <15%
II. Methicillin-susceptible *S aureus* (MSSA)		
Drugs of choice:	Nafcillin or oxacillin[b]	
	Cefazolin	
Alternatives:	Clindamycin	Only for patients with a serious penicillin allergy and clindamycin-susceptible strain
	Vancomycin	Only for patients with a serious penicillin and cephalosporin allergy
	Ampicillin + sulbactam	For patients with polymicrobial infections caused by susceptible isolates.
III. Methicillin-resistant *S aureus* (MRSA; oxacillin MIC, 4 µg/mL or greater)		
A. Health care-associated (multidrug resistant)		
Drugs of choice:	Vancomycin ± gentamicin[b]	
Alternatives: susceptibility testing results available before alternative drugs are used	Trimethoprim-sulfamethoxazole Linezolid[c] Quinupristin-dalfopristin[c]	

Table 3.68. Parenteral Antimicrobial Agent(s) for Treatment of Bacteremia and Other Serious *Staphylococcus aureus* Infections, continued

Susceptibility	Antimicrobial Agents	Comments
B. Community-associated (not multidrug resistant)		
Drugs of choice:	Vancomycin ± gentamicin[b]	For life-threatening infections or endovascular infections including those complicated by venous thrombosis.
	Clindamycin (if strain susceptible)	For pneumonia, septic arthritis, osteomyelitis, skin or soft tissue infections
	Trimethoprim-sulfamethoxazole	For skin or soft tissue infections
	Doxycycline (if strain susceptible)	
Alternative:	Vancomycin	For serious infections
	Linezolid	For serious infections caused by clindamycin resistant isolates in patients with renal dysfunction or those intolerant of vancomycin
IV. Vancomycin-intermediately susceptible *S aureus* (VISA; MIC, 4 to 16 µg/mL)[c]		
Drugs of choice:	Optimal therapy is not known	Dependent on in vitro susceptibility test results
	Linezolid[c]	
	Ceftaroline	
	Daptomycin[d]	
	Quinupristin-dalfopristin[c]	
	Tigecycline	
Alternatives:	Vancomycin + linezolid ± gentamicin	
	Vancomycin + trimethoprim-sulfamethoxazole[b]	

CNS indicates central nervous system; MIC, minimum inhibitory concentration.

[a]Some experts prefer 15 mg/kg every 6 hours for empiric therapy for any invasive infections including osteomyelitis, pyoarthritis, or pneumonia.

[b]Gentamicin and rifampin for the first 2 weeks should be added for endocarditis of a prosthetic device. Addition of rifampin is recommended for other device-related infections (spinal instrumentation, prosthetic joint). Some experts recommend achieving vancomycin trough concentrations between 15 and 20 μg/mL (although this may be associated with increased risk of nephrotoxicity without evidence for improved outcomes) for serious MRSA infections until the patient has improved and blood cultures are sterile. Consultation with an infectious diseases specialist should be considered to determine which agent to use and duration of use.

[c]Linezolid, ceftaroline, quinupristin-dalfopristin, and tigecycline are agents with activity in vitro and efficacy in adults with multidrug-resistant, gram-positive organisms, including *S aureus*. Because experience with these agents in children is limited, consultation with an infectious diseases specialist should be considered before use.

[d]Daptomycin is active in vitro against multidrug-resistant, gram-positive organisms, including *S aureus*. Daptomycin is approved by the US Food and Drug Administration only for treatment of complicated skin and skin structure infections and for *S aureus* bloodstream infections. Daptomycin is ineffective for treatment of pneumonia.

Completion of the course with an oral drug can be considered in children if an endovascular infection (ie, endocarditis or infected thrombus) or CNS infection is not a concern. For endocardiovascular and CNS infections, parenteral therapy is recommended for the entire treatment. Drainage of abscesses and removal of foreign bodies are desirable and almost always are required for medical treatment to be effective. In some cases, multiple débridement procedures are necessary for children with MRSA osteoarticular infection.

Duration of therapy for central line-associated bloodstream infections is controversial and depends on consideration of a number of factors—the type and location of the catheter, the site of infection (exit site vs tunnel vs line), the feasibility of using an alternative vascular access site at a later date, and the presence or absence of a catheter-related thrombus. Infections are more difficult to treat when associated with a thrombus, thrombophlebitis, or intra-atrial thrombus, and a longer course is suggested if the patient is immunocompromised. Experts differ on recommended duration, but many suggest a minimum of 14 days provided there is no evidence of a metastatic focus and the patient responds to antimicrobial therapy with immediate resolution of the *S aureus* bacteremia. If the patient needs a new central line, waiting 48 to 72 hours after bacteremia apparently has resolved before insertion is optimal. If a tunneled catheter is needed for ongoing care, in situ treatment of the infection can be attempted. Vegetations or a thrombus in the heart or great vessels always should be considered when a central line becomes infected and should be suspected more strongly if blood cultures remain positive for more than 2 days on appropriate antimicrobial therapy or if there are other clinical manifestations associated with endocarditis. Transesophageal echocardiography, if feasible, is the most sensitive technique for identifying vegetations, but transthoracic echocardiography generally is adequate for children younger than 10 years and those weighing <60 kg.

Management of S aureus Toxin-Mediated Diseases. The principles of therapy for TSS include aggressive fluid management to maintain adequate venous return and cardiac filling to prevent end organ damage, source control that includes prompt identification and removal of any indwelling foreign body (eg, tampon) or drainable focus, and anticipation and management of the commonly observed multiorgan complications of TSS (eg, acute respiratory distress syndrome, renal dysfunction). Initial antimicrobial therapy should include a parentally administered beta-lactam antistaphylococcal antimicrobial agent and a protein synthesis-inhibiting drug, such as clindamycin, at maximum dosages. Vancomycin should be added to beta lactamase-resistant penicillins or cephalosporins in regions where MRSA infections are common, although MRSA-associated TSS is uncommon in the United States (see Table 3.68, p 740). Once the organism is identified and susceptibilities are known, therapy for *S aureus* should be modified, but an active antimicrobial agent should be continued for 10 to 14 days. Administration of antimicrobial agents can be changed to the oral route once the patient is tolerating oral alimentation. The total duration of therapy is based on the usual duration of established foci of infection (eg, pneumonia, osteomyelitis). Immune Globulin Intravenous (IGIV) can be considered in patients with severe staphylococcal TSS unresponsive to other therapeutic measures, because IGIV may neutralize circulating toxin. Although data on the use of IGIV are not robust, it may be considered for infection refractory to several hours of aggressive therapy or in the presence of an undrainable focus or persistent oliguria with pulmonary edema. The optimal IGIV regimen is unknown, but 150 to 400 mg/kg per day for 5 days or a single dose of 1 to 2 g/kg has been used. SSSS in infants should be treated with a parenteral beta lactamase-resistant beta-lactam antimicrobial agent, or if MRSA is a consideration, vancomycin can be used. Transition to an oral agent can be considered in nonneonates who have demonstrated excellent clinical and microbiologic response to parenteral therapy.

ISOLATION OF THE HOSPITALIZED PATIENT: Contact precautions should be added to standard precautions for patients with abscesses or draining wounds that cannot be covered, regardless of staphylococcal strain, and should be maintained until draining ceases or can be contained by a dressing. Infants and young children with staphylococcal furunculosis and patients with SSSS should be placed on contact precautions for the duration of their illness.

To prevent transmission of VRSA, the CDC has issued specific infection-control recommendations that should be followed (**www.cdc.gov/hai/pdfs/VRSA-Investigation-Guide-05_12_2015.pdf**).

CONTROL MEASURES: Measures to prevent and control *S aureus* infections can be considered separately for people and for health care facilities.

Individual Patient. Community-associated *S aureus* infections in immunocompetent hosts usually cannot be prevented, because the organism is ubiquitous and there is no vaccine. However, strategies focusing on hand hygiene and wound care have been effective at limiting transmission of *S aureus* and preventing spread of infections in community settings. Specific strategies include appropriate wound care, minimizing skin trauma and keeping abrasions and cuts covered, optimizing hand hygiene and personal hygiene practices (eg, shower after activities involving skin-to-skin contact), avoiding sharing of personal items (eg, towels, razors, clothing), cleaning shared equipment between uses, and regular cleaning of frequently touched environmental surfaces. For patients who experience recurrent *S aureus* infections or who are predisposed to *S aureus* infections because of disorders of neutrophil function, chronic skin conditions, or obesity, a variety of techniques have been used to prevent infection, including scrupulous attention to skin hygiene, bleach baths, and the use of clothing and bed linens that minimize sweating, but none have shown definitive effectiveness in preventing recurrent infections with community-associated MRSA. Applying mupirocin to the nares and bathing using chlorhexidine for 5 consecutive days for all family members have been associated with decreased recurrences. Studies in adults have reported success with 7-day course of the combination of oral rifampin and doxycycline plus nasal mupirocin. Household contacts of people with *S aureus* infections do not need to be tested for colonization.

Measures to prevent health care-associated *S aureus* infections in individual patients include strict adherence to recommended infection-control precautions and appropriate intraoperative antimicrobial prophylaxis, and in some circumstances, use of antimicrobial regimens to attempt to eradicate nasal carriage in certain patients can be considered.

Child Care or School Settings. Children with *S aureus* colonization or infection should not be excluded routinely from child care or school settings. Children with draining or open abrasions or wounds should have these covered with a clean, dry dressing. Routine hand hygiene should be emphasized for personnel and children in these facilities.

General Measures. Published recommendations of the CDC Healthcare Infection Control Practices Advisory Committee (HICPAC)[1] for prevention of health care-associated pneumonia should be effective for decreasing the incidence of *S aureus* pneumonia. Careful preparation of the skin before surgery, including cleansing of skin before placement of intravascular catheters using barrier methods, decreases the incidence of *S aureus* wound and catheter-related infections. Meticulous surgical technique with minimal trauma to tissues, maintenance of good oxygenation, and minimal hematoma and dead space formation will minimize risk of surgical site infection. Appropriate hand hygiene, including before and after use of gloves, by health care professionals and strict adherence to contact precautions are of paramount importance.

Intraoperative Antimicrobial Prophylaxis. The benefits of systemic antimicrobial prophylaxis do not justify the potential risks associated with antimicrobial use in most clean surgical procedures, because the risk of overall infection (most commonly caused by *S aureus*) is only 1% to 2%. Some exceptions apply, such as a person undergoing organ transplantation, neurosurgery, or insertion of a major prosthetic device, such as a ventriculoperitoneal shunt or a heart valve, or a known MRSA carrier undergoing a major surgical procedure. If antimicrobial prophylaxis is used, the agent, usually cefazolin, is administered 30 to 60 minutes before the operation (60–120 minutes for vancomycin), and a total duration of therapy of less than 24 hours is recommended.

Eradication of Nasal Carriage. The combination of preoperative chlorhexidine baths with intranasal mupirocin has been demonstrated to be beneficial in reducing deep SSIs in adult MRSA carriers, but data are limited in children. Use of intermittent or continuous intranasal mupirocin for eradication of nasal carriage also has been shown to decrease the incidence of invasive *S aureus* infections in adult patients undergoing long-term hemodialysis or ambulatory peritoneal dialysis. However, eradication of nasal carriage of *S aureus* is difficult, and mupirocin-resistant strains can emerge with repeated or widespread use. Treatment is not recommended for routine use but is considered for those with recurrent skin abscesses and in certain cardiac and orthopedic surgery patients for whom implantable devices are planned.

Institutions. Measures to control spread of *S aureus* within health care facilities involve use

---

[1]Centers for Disease Control and Prevention. Guidelines for preventing health-care–associated pneumonia, 2003: recommendations of CDC and the Healthcare Infection Control Practices Advisory Committee. *MMWR Recomm Rep.* 2004;53(RR-3):1–36

and careful monitoring of HICPAC guidelines.[1,2,3] Strategies for controlling spread of MRSA also are found in recommendations for controlling spread of multidrug-resistant organisms (**www.cdc.gov/drugresistance/index.html**). These include general recommendations for all settings and focus on administrative issues; engagement, education, and training of personnel; judicious use of antimicrobial agents; monitoring of prevalence trends over time; use of standard precautions for all patients; and use of contact precautions when appropriate. When rates of endemicity are not decreasing despite implementation of and adherence to the aforementioned measures, additional interventions, such as use of active surveillance cultures to identify colonized patients and to place them in contact precautions, may be warranted. Decolonization of a health care professional can be considered if the health care professional has been found to be a carrier of *S aureus* and has been epidemiologically linked as a likely source of ongoing transmission to patients. In this situation, attempts to eradicate carriage with topical nasal mupirocin therapy often are made. Both low-level (MIC, 8–256 µg/mL) and high-level (MIC, ≥512 µg/mL) resistance to mupirocin have been identified in *S aureus*, with high-level resistance associated with failure of decolonization therapy.

Recommendations for investigation and control of VRSA have been published by the CDC (**www.cdc.gov/hai/pdfs/VRSA-Investigation-Guide-05_12_2015.pdf**). MRSA isolates with vancomycin MIC of ≥8 µg/mL should be sent to the CDC or to the Antibiotic Regional Laboratory Network (**www.cdc.gov/drugresistance/ solutions-initiative/ar-lab-networks.html**) for confirmatory testing through local or state public health laboratories; notification to the local or state health department is required. Ongoing review and restriction of vancomycin use is critical in attempts to control the emergence of VISA and VRSA (see Antimicrobial Resistance and Antimicrobial Stewardship: Appropriate and Judicious Use of Antimicrobial Agents, p 906). To date, the use of catheters impregnated with various antimicrobial agents or metals to prevent health care-associated infections has not been evaluated adequately in children.

Nurseries. Outbreaks of *S aureus* infections in newborn nurseries require unique measures of control. Hand hygiene should be emphasized to all personnel and visitors. Standard umbilical cord care currently does not include use of topical products (eg, chlorhexidine). Other measures recommended during outbreaks include reinforcement of hand hygiene, alleviating overcrowding and understaffing, colonization surveillance cultures of newborn infants at admission and periodically thereafter, use of contact precautions for colonized or infected infants, and cohorting of colonized or infected infants and their caregivers. For hand hygiene, soaps containing chlorhexidine or alcohol-based hand rubs are preferred during an outbreak. Colonized health care professionals epidemiologically implicated in

[1]Walters M, Lonsway D, Rasheed K, Albrecht V, McAllister S, Limbago B, Kallen A. *Investigation and Control of Vancomycin -Resistant Staphylococcus aureus: A Guide for Health Departments and Infection Control Personnel.* Atlanta, GA: Centers for Disease Control and Prevention; 2015. Available at: **www.cdc.gov/hai/pdfs/VRSA-Investigation-Guide-05_12_2015.pdf**

[2]Siegel JD, Rhinehart E, Jackson M, Chianello L, and the Healthcare Infection Control Practices Advisory Committee. *2007 Guideline for Isolation Precautions: Preventing Transmission of Infectious Agents in Healthcare Settings. Recommendations of the Healthcare Infection Control Practices Advisory Committee.* Atlanta, GA: Centers for Disease Control and Prevention; 2007. Available at: **www.cdc.gov/hicpac/2007IP/2007isolationPrecautions.html**

[3]Siegel JD, Rhinehart E, Jackwson M, Chiarello L; HICPAC. Management of multidrug-resistant organisms in healthcare settings, 2006. Atlanta, GA: Centers for Disease Control and Prevention, 2006. Available at: **www.cdc.gov/infectioncontrol/guidelines/mdro/index.html**

transmission should receive decolonization therapy, but eradication of colonization may not occur.

Coagulase-Negative Staphylococcal Infections

CLINICAL MANIFESTATIONS: Most coagulase-negative staphylococci (CoNS) isolates from patient specimens represent contamination of culture material (see Diagnostic Tests, p 747). Of the isolates that do not represent contamination, most come from infections associated with health care, such as patients with obvious disruptions of host defenses caused by surgery, medical device insertion, immunosuppression, or developmental maturity (eg, very low birth weight infants). CoNS are the most common cause of late-onset bacteremia and septicemia among preterm infants, typically infants weighing less than 1500 g at birth, and of episodes of health care-associated bacteremia in all age groups. CoNS are responsible for bacteremia in children with intravascular catheters, vascular grafts, intracardiac patches, prosthetic cardiac valves, or pacemaker wires. Infection also may occur associated with other indwelling foreign bodies, including cerebrospinal fluid shunts, peritoneal catheters, spinal instrumentation, baclofen pumps, pacemakers, or prosthetic joints. Mediastinitis after open-heart surgery, endophthalmitis after intraocular trauma, and omphalitis and scalp abscesses in preterm neonates have been described. CoNS also can enter the bloodstream from the respiratory tract of mechanically ventilated preterm infants or from the gastrointestinal tract of infants with necrotizing enterocolitis. Some species of CoNS are associated with urinary tract infection, including *Staphylococcus saprophyticus* in adolescent females and young adult women, often after sexual intercourse, and *Staphylococcus epidermidis* and *Staphylococcus haemolyticus* in hospitalized patients with urinary tract catheters. *Staphylococcus lugdunensis* is of particular significance, because it may cause infections resembling *Staphylococcus aureus,* including skin and soft tissue infection and bacteremia with or without endocarditis.

ETIOLOGY: There are more than 40 named coagulase-negative *Staphylococcus* species in the family; *Staphylococcus epidermidis, S haemolyticus, S saprophyticus, Staphylococcus schleiferi,* and *S lugdunensis* most often are associated with human infections. Many CoNS produce an exopolysaccharide slime biofilm that makes these organisms, as they bind to medical devices (eg, catheters), relatively inaccessible to host defenses and antimicrobial agents.

EPIDEMIOLOGY: CoNS are common inhabitants of the skin and mucous membranes. Virtually all infants have colonization at multiple sites by 2 to 4 days of age. The most frequently isolated CoNS organism is *S epidermidis,* which is found widely in most areas of skin. Different species colonize specific areas of the body. *S haemolyticus* is found on areas of skin with numerous apocrine glands, and *Staphylococcus auricularis* is found in the external ear canal. *S lugdunensis* has a predilection for colonization of the inguinal and groin areas. The frequency of health care-associated CoNS infections increased steadily until 2000, when these infections decreased because of rigorous infection control measures. Infants and children in intensive care units, including neonatal intensive care units, have the highest incidence of CoNS bloodstream infections. CoNS can be introduced at the time of medical device placement, through mucous membrane or skin breaks, through loss of bowel wall integrity (eg, necrotizing enterocolitis in very low birth weight neonates), or during catheter manipulation. Less often, health care professionals with environmental CoNS colonization on their hands transmit the organism.

The **incubation period** is variable for CoNS disease. A long delay can occur between acquisition of the organism and onset of disease.

DIAGNOSTICS TESTS: CoNS are nonfastidious organisms readily isolated in culture using the same media and incubation conditions as are used for *S aureus*. Tests for coagulase by traditional methods or by latex agglutination are the same as are used for *S aureus*. CoNS isolated from a single blood culture commonly are classified as skin contaminants introduced into the blood culture bottle during venipuncture, and full identification and antimicrobial susceptibility testing are not performed by most clinical laboratories. Rapid differentiation of CoNS and *S aureus* in positive blood culture can be obtained by using fluorescent in situ hybridization (FISH) probes or multiplex PCR panel assays. In a very preterm neonate, an immunocompromised person, or a patient with an indwelling catheter or prosthetic device, repeated isolation of the same species of CoNS based on identification using biochemical test systems or MALDI-TOF mass spectroscopy from blood cultures or another normally sterile body fluid suggests true infection. This conclusion is further supported by the isolates having comparable antimicrobial susceptibility test patterns. Genotyping of the isolates more strongly supports the diagnosis; however, whereas several molecular typing systems including pulsed field gel electrophoresis have been well-evaluated for *S aureus*, fewer methods are available for the CoNS. For central line-associated bloodstream infection, quantitative blood cultures from the catheter generally will have 5 to 10 times more organisms than cultures from a peripheral blood vessel. This type of analysis requires that both a peripheral and line blood culture be performed at the same time.

Criteria that suggest CoNS as pathogens, rather than contaminants, include the following:

- 2 or more positive blood cultures from different collection sites;
- A single positive culture from blood and another sterile site (eg, cerebrospinal fluid, joint) with identical antimicrobial susceptibility patterns for each isolate;
- Growth in a continuously monitored blood culture system within 15 hours of incubation;
- Clinical findings of infection;
- An intravascular catheter that has been in place for 3 days or more; and
- Similar or identical genotypes among all isolates.

TREATMENT: More than 90% of health care-associated CoNS strains are methicillin resistant. Methicillin-resistant strains are resistant to all beta-lactam drugs, including cephalosporins (except ceftaroline), and usually several other drug classes. Intravenous vancomycin is recommended for treatment of serious infections caused by CoNS strains resistant to beta-lactam antimicrobial agents. An exception to this is *S lugdunensis*, which generally is oxacillin susceptible. Treatment of infected foreign bodies should be continued for 10 to 14 days parenterally. Antimicrobial lock therapy of tunneled central lines may result in a higher rate of catheter salvage in adults with CoNS infections, but experience with this approach is limited in children. If blood cultures remain positive for more than 3 to 5 days after initiation of appropriate antimicrobial therapy for CoNS or if the clinical illness fails to improve, the central line should be removed, parenteral therapy should be continued, and the patient should be evaluated for metastatic foci of infection. If a central line can be removed, there is no demonstrable thrombus, and bacteremia resolves promptly, a 5-day course of therapy seems appropriate for CoNS (other than *S lugdunensis*, which should be managed similarly to *S aureus* catheter-related infections; see *Staphylococcus aureus*, p 733) infections in the immunocompetent host, and for 7 to 10 days in the immunocompromised host.

ISOLATION OF THE HOSPITALIZED PATIENT: Standard precautions are used.

CONTROL MEASURES: Prevention and control of CoNS infections have focused on prevention of intraoperative contamination by skin flora and on sterile insertion of intravascular and intraperitoneal catheters and other prosthetic devices. Catheter-related bloodstream infections can be markedly reduced with a "bundled" preventive approach. Prophylactic administration of an antimicrobial agent intraoperatively lowers the incidence of infection after cardiac surgery and implantation of synthetic vascular grafts and prosthetic devices and often has been used at the time of cerebrospinal fluid shunt placement. Once methicillin resistant CoNS strains become endemic in a hospital, eradication is difficult even when strict infection prevention practices are followed.

Group A Streptococcal Infections

CLINICAL MANIFESTATIONS: The most common group A streptococcal (GAS) infection is acute pharyngotonsillitis (pharyngitis), which is heralded by sore throat with tonsillar inflammation and often tender anterior cervical lymphadenopathy. Pharyngitis may be accompanied by palatal petechiae or a strawberry tongue. Purulent complications of pharyngitis usually occur in patients not treated with antimicrobial agents and include otitis media, sinusitis, peritonsillar or retropharyngeal abscesses, and suppurative cervical adenitis. Nonsuppurative complications include acute rheumatic fever (ARF) and acute glomerulonephritis. The goal of antimicrobial therapy for GAS pharyngitis is to reduce acute morbidity, suppurative and nonsuppurative (ARF) complications, and transmission to close contacts. Antimicrobial therapy for preventing acute poststreptococcal glomerulonephritis after pyoderma or pharyngitis is not effective.

Scarlet fever occurs most often in association with pharyngitis and, rarely, with pyoderma or an infected wound. Scarlet fever usually is a mild disease in the modern era and involves a characteristic confluent erythematous sandpaper-like rash that is caused by one or more of several erythrogenic exotoxins produced by group A streptococci. Other than occurrence of rash, the epidemiologic features, symptoms, signs, sequelae, and treatment of scarlet fever are the same as those of streptococcal pharyngitis.

Acute streptococcal pharyngitis is uncommon in children younger than 3 years. Instead, they may present with rhinitis and then develop a protracted illness with moderate fever, irritability, and anorexia (streptococcal fever or streptococcosis). The second most common site of GAS infection is skin. Streptococcal skin infections (eg, pyoderma or impetigo) can be followed by acute glomerulonephritis, which occasionally occurs in epidemics. ARF has not been proven to be a sequela of GAS skin infection.

Other manifestations of GAS infections include erysipelas, cellulitis (including perianal), vaginitis, bacteremia, sepsis, pneumonia, endocarditis, pericarditis, septic arthritis, necrotizing fasciitis, purpura fulminans, osteomyelitis, myositis, puerperal sepsis, surgical wound infection, mastoiditis, and neonatal omphalitis. Invasive GAS infections often are associated with bacteremia with or without a local focus of infection and can present as streptococcal toxic shock syndrome (STSS), overwhelming sepsis, or necrotizing fasciitis. Necrotizing fasciitis can follow minor or unrecognized trauma, often involves an extremity, and presents as pain out of proportion to examination findings.

STSS is caused by infection of normally sterile body sites (blood, pleura, cerebrospinal fluid, etc) with toxin-producing GAS strains and typically manifests as a severe acute illness characterized by fever, generalized erythroderma, rapid-onset hypotension, and signs of multiorgan involvement, including rapidly progressive renal failure. Evidence of local soft tissue infection (eg, cellulitis, myositis, or necrotizing fasciitis) associated with severe, rapidly increasing pain is common, but STSS can occur without an identifiable focus of infection or with foci such as pneumonia with or without empyema, osteomyelitis, arthritis, or endocarditis.

Rheumatic fever is a nonsuppurative sequela of GAS pharyngitis and is endemic in Africa, Asia, and the Pacific, including the indigenous population in Australia. The United States and Europe are considered low-risk populations, but cases continue to occur sporadically.

An association between GAS infection and sudden onset of obsessive-compulsive behavior, tic disorders, or other unexplained acute neurologic changes—pediatric autoimmune neuropsychiatric disorders associated with streptococcal infections (PANDAS), as a subset of pediatric acute-onset neuropsychiatric syndrome (PANS)—has been proposed. The data for an association with GAS and either PANDAS or PANS rely on a number of small and as yet unduplicated studies. In the absence of acute clinical symptoms and signs of pharyngitis, GAS testing (by culture, antigen detection, or serology) is not recommended for such patients (see Indications for GAS Testing). There also is insufficient evidence to support antibiotic treatment or prophylaxis, Immune Globulin Intravenous, or plasmapheresis for children with symptoms suggestive of PANDAS or PANS. Management is best directed by specialists with experience with the presenting symptoms and signs, which could include child psychiatrists, behavioral and developmental pediatricians, or child neurologists.

ETIOLOGY: More than 240 distinct serotypes or genotypes of group A streptococci *(Streptococcus pyogenes)* have been identified based on M-protein serotype or M-protein gene sequence *(emm* types). Because of a variety of factors, including M nontypability and *emm* sequence variation within given M types, *emm* typing generally is more discriminating than M-protein serotyping. Epidemiologic studies indicate an association between certain serotypes (eg, types 1, 3, 5, 6, 14, 18, 19, and 24) and rheumatic fever, but a specific rheumatogenic factor has not been identified. Several serotypes (eg, types 2, 49, 55, 57, 59, 60, and 61) more commonly are associated with pyoderma and acute glomerulonephritis. Other serotypes (eg, types 1, 6, and 12) are associated with pharyngitis and acute glomerulonephritis. Although many M types can cause STSS, most cases are caused by M types 1 and 3 strains producing at least 1 of several different pyrogenic exotoxins, most commonly streptococcal pyrogenic exotoxin A (SPE A). These toxins act as superantigens that stimulate production of tumor necrosis factor and other inflammatory mediators that cause capillary leak and other physiologic changes, leading to hypotension and multiorgan damage.

EPIDEMIOLOGY: Pharyngitis usually results from contact with the respiratory tract secretions of a person who has GAS pharyngitis. Fomites and household pets, such as dogs, are not vectors of GAS infection. Pharyngitis and impetigo (and their nonsuppurative complications) can be associated with crowding, which often is present in socioeconomically disadvantaged populations. The close contact that occurs in schools, child care centers, contact sports (eg, wrestling), boarding schools, and military installations facilitates transmission. Foodborne outbreaks of pharyngitis occur rarely and are a consequence of human contamination of food in conjunction with improper food preparation or refrigeration procedures.

GAS pharyngitis occurs at all ages but is most common among school-aged children and adolescents, peaking at 7 to 8 years of age. GAS pharyngitis and pyoderma are substantially less common in adults than in children.

Geographically, GAS pharyngitis and pyoderma are ubiquitous. Pyoderma is more common in tropical climates and warm seasons, at least in part because of antecedent insect bites and other minor skin trauma. Streptococcal pharyngitis is more common during late autumn, winter, and spring in temperate climates, in part because of close person-to-person contact in schools. Communicability of patients with streptococcal pharyngitis is highest during acute infection and, when untreated, gradually diminishes over a period of weeks.

Throat culture surveys of healthy asymptomatic children during the streptococcal season and during school outbreaks of pharyngitis have yielded GAS prevalence rates as high as 25%. These surveys identified children who were chronic pharyngeal carriers. Carriage of GAS can persist for many months, but risk of transmission from carriers to others is low.

In streptococcal impetigo, the organism usually is acquired by direct contact from another person. GAS colonization of healthy skin usually precedes development of impetigo, but group A streptococci do not penetrate intact skin. Impetiginous lesions occur at the site of breaks in skin (eg, insect bites, burns, traumatic wounds, varicella lesions). After development of impetiginous lesions, the upper respiratory tract often becomes colonized with GAS. Infection of surgical wounds and postpartum (puerperal) sepsis usually result from transmission through direct contact. Health care workers who are anal or vaginal carriers of GAS and people with skin infection or pharyngeal colonization can transmit GAS organisms to surgical and obstetrical patients, resulting in health care-associated outbreaks. Infections in neonates, uncommon in the United States but common in many developing countries, result from intrapartum or contact transmission; in the latter situation, infection can begin as omphalitis, cellulitis, or necrotizing fasciitis.

In the United States, the incidence of invasive GAS infections is highest in infants and the elderly. Fatal cases in children are not common but when they occur can progress very rapidly (eg, overwhelming sepsis). Before use of varicella vaccine, varicella was the most commonly identified predisposing factor for invasive GAS infection in children. Other factors increasing risk include exposure to other children and household crowding. The portal of entry is unknown in most invasive GAS infections but is presumed to be skin or mucous membranes. Such infections rarely follow symptomatic GAS pharyngitis. An association between use of nonsteroidal anti-inflammatory drugs and invasive GAS infections in children with varicella has been described, but a causal relationship has not been established.

STSS can occur at any age. Fewer than 5% of cases of invasive streptococcal infections in children are associated with STSS. Among children, STSS has been reported with focal lesions (eg, varicella, cellulitis, trauma, osteomyelitis, pneumonia), and with bacteremia without a defined focus. Mortality rates are substantially lower for children than for adults with STSS.

During epidemics of GAS infections on military bases in the 1950s, rheumatic fever developed in 3% of untreated patients with acute GAS pharyngitis; rare cases have occurred in treated patients. The current incidence in the United States is not precisely known but is substantially less than 1%. The incidence of ARF in the United States decreased sharply during the 20th century, and rates of this nonsuppurative sequela are low, with rare exception. Focal outbreaks of ARF in school-aged children occurred in several areas in the 1990s, and small clusters continue to be reported periodically. The highest US rates of ARF are in Utah and Hawaii and are most likely related to circulation of particularly rheumatogenic strains. The occurrence of ARF reemphasizes the importance of diagnosing GAS pharyngitis accurately and treating with a recommended antimicrobial regimen.

The **incubation period** for streptococcal pharyngitis is 2 to 5 days. For impetigo, a 7- to 10-day period between acquisition of GAS on healthy skin and development of lesions has been demonstrated, because GAS organisms do not penetrate intact skin. The **incubation period** for STSS is not known but has been as short as 14 hours in cases associated with subcutaneous inoculation of organisms (eg, childbirth, penetrating trauma).

DIAGNOSTIC TESTS[1]: Children with pharyngitis and obvious viral symptoms (eg, rhinorrhea, cough, hoarseness, oral ulcers) should not be tested or treated for GAS infection; testing also generally is not recommended for children younger than 3 years. Laboratory confirmation before initiation of antimicrobial treatment is required for children with pharyngitis without viral symptoms, because many will not have GAS pharyngitis. A specimen should be obtained by vigorous swabbing using a pair of swabs on both tonsils and the posterior pharynx for rapid antigen testing. It is recommended that a throat swab from a child with a negative rapid antigen test result be submitted to the laboratory for isolation of GAS; the second swab can be used for this purpose. Culture on sheep blood agar can confirm GAS infection, with latex agglutination differentiating GAS from other beta-hemolytic streptococci (group C or G). False-negative culture results occur in fewer than 10% of symptomatic patients when an adequate throat swab specimen is obtained and cultured by trained personnel. Recovery of group A streptococci from the pharynx does not distinguish patients with true acute streptococcal infection from streptococcal carriers who have an intercurrent viral pharyngitis. The number of colonies of group A streptococci on a culture plate also does not reliably differentiate true infection from carriage. Cultures that are negative for group A streptococci after 18 to 24 hours of incubation should be incubated for a second day to optimize recovery of group A streptococci.

Several rapid diagnostic tests for GAS pharyngitis are available. Most are based on nitrous acid extraction of GAS carbohydrate antigen from organisms obtained by throat swab. Specificities of these tests generally are high (very few false-positive results), but the reported sensitivities vary considerably (ie, false-negative results occur). As with throat swab cultures, sensitivity of these tests is highly dependent on the quality of the throat swab specimen, the experience of the person performing the test, and the rigor of the culture method used for comparison. The US Food and Drug Administration (FDA) has cleared a variety of rapid tests for use in home settings. Parents should be informed that home use is discouraged because of the risk of false-positive testing that represents colonization. Clinicians should be aware that home testing likely has an even lower negative predictive value than testing performed in a clinical setting.

Because of the very high specificity of rapid tests, a positive test result does not require throat culture confirmation. Rapid diagnostic tests using techniques such as polymerase

---

[1]Shulman ST, Bisno AL, Clegg HW, et al. Clinical practice guideline for the diagnosis and management of group a streptococcal pharyngitis: 2012 update by the Infectious Diseases Society of America. *Clin Infect Dis.* 2012;55(10):e86–e102

chain reaction (PCR), chemiluminescent DNA probes, and isothermal nucleic acid amplification tests have been developed. The FDA recently approved isothermal nucleic acid amplification tests for detection of group A streptococci from throat swab specimens. Some studies suggest that these tests may be as sensitive as standard throat cultures on sheep blood agar.

Indications for GAS Testing. Factors to be considered in the decision to obtain a throat swab specimen for testing children with pharyngitis are the patient's age, signs and symptoms, season, and family and community epidemiology, including contact with a person with GAS infection or presence in the family of a person with a history of ARF or of poststreptococcal glomerulonephritis.

- Children with manifestations highly suggestive of viral infection, such as coryza, conjunctivitis, hoarseness, cough, anterior stomatitis, discrete ulcerative oral lesions, or diarrhea, are very unlikely to have true GAS pharyngitis and should not be tested.
- Testing children younger than 3 years generally is not indicated. Although small outbreaks of GAS pharyngitis have been reported in young children in child care settings, the risk of ARF is so remote in young children in industrialized countries that diagnostic studies for GAS pharyngitis generally are not indicated for children younger than 3 years.
- In contrast, children with acute onset of sore throat and clinical signs and symptoms such as pharyngeal exudate, pain on swallowing, fever, and enlarged tender anterior cervical lymph nodes, without concurrent viral symptoms and/or exposure to a person with GAS pharyngitis, are more likely to have GAS infection and should have a rapid antigen test and a throat culture if the rapid test result is negative, with treatment initiated if a test result is positive.

Testing Contacts for GAS Infection. Indications for testing contacts for GAS infection vary according to circumstances. Testing asymptomatic household contacts for GAS infection is not recommended except when the contacts are at increased risk of developing sequelae of GAS infection, such as ARF or acute glomerulonephritis; if test results are positive, such contacts should be treated.

In schools, child care centers, or other environments in which a large number of people are in close contact, the prevalence of GAS pharyngeal carriage in healthy children can be as high as 25% in the absence of an outbreak of streptococcal disease. Therefore, classroom or more widespread culture sampling generally is not indicated.

Follow-up Throat Cultures. Post-treatment throat swab cultures are indicated only for patients who are at particularly high risk of ARF (eg, those living in an area with endemic infection). Repeated courses of antimicrobial therapy are not indicated for asymptomatic patients with cultures positive for group A streptococci; the exceptions are people who have personally had or whose family members have had ARF or other uncommon epidemiologic circumstances, such as a community outbreak of ARF or acute poststreptococcal glomerulonephritis.

Patients who have repeated episodes of pharyngitis at short intervals and in whom GAS infection is documented by culture or antigen detection test present a special problem. Most often, these people are chronic GAS carriers who are experiencing frequent viral illnesses and for whom repeated testing and use of antimicrobial agents are unnecessary. In assessing such patients, inadequate adherence to oral treatment also should be considered. Testing asymptomatic household contacts usually is not helpful. However, if multiple household members have pharyngitis or other GAS infections, simultaneous cultures of all household members and treatment of all with positive cultures or rapid antigen test results may be of value.

Testing for Group A Streptococci in Nonpharyngitis Infections. Cultures of impetiginous lesions often yield both streptococci and staphylococci, and determination of the primary pathogen generally is not possible. Culture is performed when it is necessary to determine susceptibility of the *S aureus* organisms. In suspected invasive GAS infections, cultures of blood and of focal sites of possible infection are indicated. In necrotizing fasciitis, imaging studies may delay, rather than facilitate, establishing the diagnosis. Clinical suspicion of necrotizing fasciitis should prompt urgent surgical evaluation with intervention, including débridement of deep tissues with Gram stain and culture of surgical specimens. STSS is diagnosed on the basis of clinical and laboratory findings and isolation of group A streptococci (see Table 3.69). Blood culture results are positive for GAS in approximately 50% of patients with STSS. Culture results from a focal site of infection also usually are positive and can remain so for several days after appropriate antimicrobial agents have been initiated.

Table 3.69. Streptococcal Toxic Shock Syndrome: Clinical Case Definition[a]

I. Isolation of group A *Streptococcus (Streptococcus pyogenes)*
  A. From a normally sterile site (eg, blood, cerebrospinal fluid, peritoneal, joint, pleural, or pericardial fluid)
  B. From a nonsterile site (eg, throat, sputum, vagina, open surgical wound, or superficial skin lesion)
II. Clinical signs of severity
  A. Hypotension: systolic pressure 90 mm Hg or less in adults or lower than the fifth percentile for age in children <16 years of age

AND

  B. Two or more of the following signs of multi-organ involvement:
- Renal impairment: creatinine concentration 177 μmol/L (2 mg/dL) or greater for adults or at least 2 times the upper limit of normal for age[b]
- Coagulopathy: platelet count 100 000/mm³ or less and/or disseminated intravascular coagulation defined by prolonged clotting times, low fibrinogen, and presence of fibrin degradation products
- Hepatic involvement: elevated alanine transaminase, aspartate transaminase, or total bilirubin concentrations at least 2 times the upper limit of normal for age[b]
- Adult respiratory distress syndrome defined by acute onset of diffuse pulmonary infiltrates and hypoxemia in absence of cardiac failure or by evidence of diffuse capillary leak
- A generalized erythematous macular rash that may desquamate
- Soft tissue necrosis, including necrotizing fasciitis or myositis, or gangrene

Adapted from The Working Group on Severe Streptococcal Infections. Defining the group A streptococcal toxic shock syndrome: rationale and consensus definition. *JAMA.* 1993;269(3):390–391.

[a]An illness fulfilling criteria IA and IIA and IIB can be defined as a *confirmed* case. An illness fulfilling criteria IB and IIA and IIB can be defined as a *probable* case if no other cause for the illness is identified. Manifestations need not be detected within the first 48 hours of illness or hospitalization.

[b]In patients with preexisting renal or hepatic disease, concentrations twofold or greater over patient's baseline.

TREATMENT[1]: *S pyogenes* uniformly is susceptible to beta-lactam antimicrobial agents (penicillins and cephalosporins), and susceptibility testing is needed only for non–beta-lactam agents, such as erythromycin, clindamycin, or a macrolide, to which *S pyogenes* can be resistant.

Pharyngitis.

- Penicillin V is the drug of choice for treatment of GAS pharyngitis. A clinical GAS isolate resistant to penicillin or cephalosporin has never been documented. Prompt administration of penicillin shortens the clinical course, decreases risk of suppurative sequelae and transmission, and prevents ARF, even when administered up to 9 days after illness onset. For all patients with ARF, a complete course of penicillin or another appropriate antimicrobial agent for GAS pharyngitis should be administered, even if group A streptococci are not recovered in the initial throat culture.

- Amoxicillin administered orally as a single daily dose (50 mg/kg; maximum, 1000–1200 mg) for 10 days is as effective as penicillin V or amoxicillin administered orally multiple times per day for 10 days, and is available as a more palatable suspension than penicillin V. This regimen has been endorsed by the American Heart Association and the Infectious Disease Society of America in its guidelines for the treatment of GAS pharyngitis and the prevention of ARF.[2] Adherence is particularly important for once-daily dosing regimens.

- The dose of orally administered penicillin V is 400 000 U (250 mg), 2 to 3 times per day, for 10 days for children (250 mg for those <27 kg, and 800 000 U [500 mg], 2 to 3 times per day for those ≥27 kg, including adolescents and adults). To prevent ARF, oral penicillin or amoxicillin should be taken for the full 10 days, regardless of the promptness of clinical recovery. Treatment failures may occur more often with oral penicillin than with intramuscular penicillin G benzathine because of inadequate adherence to oral therapy. In addition, short-course treatment (less than 10 days) for GAS pharyngitis, particularly with penicillin V, is associated with inferior bacteriologic eradication rates.

- Intramuscular penicillin G benzathine is appropriate therapy. It ensures adequate blood concentrations and avoids the problem of adherence, but administration may be painful. For children who weigh less than 27 kg, penicillin G benzathine is administered in a single dose of 600 000 U (375 mg); for heavier children and adults, the dose is 1.2 million U (750 mg). Discomfort is decreased if the preparation of penicillin G benzathine is brought to room temperature before intramuscular injection. Mixtures containing shorter-acting penicillins (eg, penicillin G procaine) in addition to penicillin G benzathine have not been demonstrated to be more effective than penicillin G benzathine alone but are less painful when administered. Although supporting data are limited, the combination of 900 000 U (562.5 mg) of penicillin G benzathine and

[1]Shulman ST, Bisno AL, Clegg HW, et al. Clinical practice guideline for the diagnosis and management of group a streptococcal pharyngitis: 2012 update by the Infectious Diseases Society of America. *Clin Infect Dis.* 2012;55(10):e86–e102

[2]Gerber MA, Baltimore RS, Eaton CB, et al. Prevention of rheumatic fever and diagnosis and treatment of acute streptococcal pharyngitis. A scientific statement from the American Heart Association, Rheumatic Fever, Endocarditis, and Kawasaki Disease Committee, Council on Cardiovascular Disease in the Young, and the Quality of Care and Outcomes Research Interdisciplinary Working Group and endorsed by the American Academy of Pediatrics. *Circulation.* 2009;119(11):1541–1551

300 000 U (187.5 mg) of penicillin G procaine is satisfactory therapy for most children; however, the efficacy of this combination for heavier patients, such as adolescents and adults, has not been demonstrated.

- For patients who have a history of nonanaphylactic allergy to penicillin, a 10-day course of a narrow-spectrum (first-generation) oral cephalosporin (ie, cephalexin) is indicated. Patients with immediate (anaphylactic) or type I hypersensitivity to penicillin should be treated with oral clindamycin (20 mg/kg per day in 3 divided doses; maximum, 900 mg/day for 10 days) rather than a cephalosporin.

- An oral macrolide or azalide (eg, erythromycin, clarithromycin, or azithromycin) also is acceptable for patients who are allergic to penicillins. Therapy for 10 days is indicated, except for azithromycin, which is indicated for 5 days (12 mg/kg/day with on day 1, followed by 6 mg/kg/day for days 2–5; maximum dose, 500 mg/day). Erythromycin is associated with substantially higher rates of gastrointestinal tract adverse effects compared with clarithromycin or azithromycin. GAS strains resistant to macrolides or azalides have been highly prevalent in some areas of the world and have resulted in treatment failures. In recent years, macrolide resistance rates in most areas of the United States have been 5% to 10%, but resistance rates up to 20% have been reported, and continued monitoring is necessary. Susceptibility testing for macrolide resistance may be helpful in deciding which antimicrobial agent to prescribe for specific penicillin-allergic patients.

- Tetracyclines, sulfonamides (including trimethoprim-sulfamethoxazole), and fluoroquinolones should not be used for treating GAS pharyngitis.

Children who have a recurrence of GAS pharyngitis shortly after completing a full course of a recommended oral antimicrobial agent can be retreated with the same antimicrobial agent, an alternative oral drug, or an intramuscular dose of penicillin G benzathine, especially if inadequate adherence to oral therapy is suspected. Alternative drugs include a narrow-spectrum cephalosporin (ie, cephalexin), amoxicillin-clavulanate, clindamycin, a macrolide, or an azalide. Expert opinions differ about the most appropriate therapy in this circumstance.

Management of a patient who has repeated and frequent episodes of acute pharyngitis associated with repeatedly positive laboratory tests for group A streptococci is problematic. To determine whether the patient is a long-term streptococcal pharyngeal carrier who is experiencing repeated episodes of intercurrent viral pharyngitis (which is the situation in most cases), the following should be determined: (1) whether the clinical findings are more suggestive of group A streptococci or a viral infection; (2) whether epidemiologic factors in the household or community support group A streptococci or a virus as the cause; (3) the nature of the clinical response to the antimicrobial therapy (in true GAS pharyngitis, response to therapy usually is 24 hours or less); and (4) whether laboratory test results are positive for GAS infection at times between episodes of acute pharyngitis (suggesting that the patient is a carrier). Measurement of a serial serologic response to GAS extracellular antigens (eg, antistreptolysin O) should be discouraged, because interpretation can be very difficult. Typing (M or *emm* typing) of GAS isolates generally is available only in research laboratories, but if performed, repeated isolation of the same type suggests carriage, and isolation of differing types indicates repeated infections.

Pharyngeal Carriers. Antimicrobial therapy is not indicated for most GAS pharyngeal carriers. The few specific situations in which eradication of carriage may be indicated include the following: (1) a local outbreak of ARF or poststreptococcal glomerulonephritis; (2) an outbreak of GAS pharyngitis in a closed or semiclosed community; (3) a family history of ARF; or (4) multiple ("ping-pong") episodes of documented symptomatic GAS pharyngitis occurring within a family for many weeks despite appropriate therapy.

GAS carriage can be difficult to eradicate with conventional antimicrobial therapy. A number of antimicrobial agents, including clindamycin, cephalosporins, amoxicillin-clavulanate, azithromycin, or a combination that includes either penicillin V or penicillin G benzathine with rifampin for the last 4 days of treatment have been demonstrated to be more effective than penicillin alone in terminating chronic streptococcal carriage. Of these drugs, oral clindamycin, administered as 20 to 30 mg/kg per day in 3 doses (maximum, 900 mg/day) for 10 days has been reported to be most effective. Documented eradication of the carrier state is helpful in the evaluation of subsequent episodes of acute pharyngitis; however, carriage can recur after reacquisition of GAS infection, as some individuals appear to be "carrier prone."

Nonbullous Impetigo. Topical mupirocin or retapamulin ointment may be useful for limiting person-to-person spread of nonbullous impetigo and for eradicating localized disease. With multiple lesions or with nonbullous impetigo in multiple family members, child care groups, or athletic teams, impetigo should be treated with oral antimicrobial agents active against both group A streptococci and *S aureus*.

Toxic Shock Syndrome. As outlined in Tables 3.70 and 3.71, most aspects of management are the same for toxic shock syndrome caused by group A streptococci or by *S aureus*. Paramount are immediate aggressive fluid replacement, management of respiratory and cardiac failure, if present, and aggressive surgical débridement of any deep-seated

Table 3.70. Management of Streptococcal Toxic Shock Syndrome Without Necrotizing Fasciitis

- Fluid management to maintain adequate venous return and cardiac filling pressures to prevent end-organ damage
- Anticipatory management of multisystem organ failure
- Parenteral antimicrobial therapy at maximum doses with the capacity to:
  - Kill organism with bactericidal cell wall inhibitor (eg, beta-lactamase–resistant antimicrobial agent)
  - Decrease enzyme, toxin, or cytokine production with protein synthesis inhibitor (eg, clindamycin)
- IGIV often is used as an adjunct, typically at 1 g/kg on day 1, followed by 0.5 g/kg on 1–2 subsequent days

IGIV indicates Immune Globulin Intravenous.

Table 3.71. Management of Streptococcal Toxic Shock Syndrome With Necrotizing Fasciitis

- Principles outlined in Table 3.70
- Immediate surgical evaluation
  - Exploration or incisional biopsy for diagnosis and culture
  - Resection of all necrotic tissue
- Repeated resection of tissue may be needed if infection persists or progresses

infection. Because *S pyogenes* and *S aureus* toxic shock syndrome are difficult to distinguish clinically, initial antimicrobial therapy should include an antistaphylococcal agent and a protein synthesis-inhibiting antimicrobial agent, such as clindamycin. The addition of clindamycin to penicillin is recommended for serious GAS infections, because the antimicrobial activity of clindamycin is not affected by inoculum size (does not have the Eagle effect that can be observed with the beta-lactam antibiotics), has a long postantimicrobial effect, and acts on bacteria by inhibiting protein synthesis. Inhibition of protein synthesis results in suppression of synthesis of the *S pyogenes* antiphagocytic M-protein and bacterial toxins. Clindamycin should not be used **alone** as initial antimicrobial therapy in life-threatening situations, because in the United States, 1% to 2% of GAS strains are resistant to clindamycin. Higher resistance rates have been reported for strains associated with invasive infection and may be as high as 10%.

Once GAS infection has been confirmed, antimicrobial therapy should be tailored to penicillin and clindamycin. Intravenous therapy should be continued at least until the patient is afebrile and stable hemodynamically and blood is sterile, as evidenced by negative culture results. The total duration of therapy is based on duration established for the primary site of infection.

Aggressive drainage and irrigation of accessible sites of infection should be performed as soon as possible. If necrotizing fasciitis is suspected, immediate surgical exploration or biopsy is crucial to identify and débride deep soft tissue infection.

Immune Globulin Intravenous (IGIV) may be considered as adjunctive therapy for STSS or necrotizing fasciitis if the patient is severely ill, although its use is supported by limited data. An IGIV regimen of 1 g/kg on day 1, followed by 0.5 g/kg on days 2 and 3, has been used, but the optimal regimen is unknown.

Other Infections. Parenteral antimicrobial therapy is required for severe infections, such as endocarditis, pneumonia, empyema, abscess, septicemia, meningitis, arthritis, osteomyelitis, erysipelas, necrotizing fasciitis, and neonatal omphalitis. Treatment often is prolonged (2–6 weeks).

Acute Rheumatic Fever. Jones criteria for diagnosis of ARF were established in 1944, modified in 1992, and revised in 2015[1] as echocardiography has become more widely available globally and studies have confirmed the presence of echocardiographic mitral and aortic regurgitation in patients with ARF who have no auscultatory findings. The 2015 revision of the Jones criteria (Table 3.72) differentiates major and minor criteria on the basis of whether the child is from a population at low risk for ARF (United States and Europe) or a population at moderate/high risk (Africa, Asia-Pacific, indigenous Australian population, any other populations not clearly low risk).

- Laboratory evidence of antecedent GAS infection should be confirmed in all cases of suspected ARF, and evidence includes an increased or rising ASO or anti-DNAase B titer, or a positive rapid antigen or streptococcal throat culture. Because of the long latency between GAS infection and presentation with chorea, such laboratory evidence may be lacking in cases where chorea is the major criteria.

- Major criteria continue to include carditis (clinical and subclinical), arthritis (highly responsive to aspirin or nonsteroidal anti-inflammatory agents), chorea, subcutaneous nodules, and erythema marginatum.

---

[1]Gewitz MH, Baltimore RS, Tani LY, et al. Revision of the Jones criteria for the diagnosis of acute rheumatic fever in the era of Doppler echocardiography. *Circulation.* 2015;131(20):1806–1818

- Echocardiography/Doppler testing should be performed in all cases and specific echocardiographic criteria are available to define subclinical carditis (eg, rheumatic valvulitis). Both clinical and subclinical carditis are major criteria.
- In terms of the major criteria, in low-risk populations, the arthritis that is seen is a migratory polyarthritis usually involving large joints. In moderate/high risk populations, joint involvement may be mono- or polyarthritis or include only polyarthralgia (assuming autoimmune, viral, and reactive arthropathies are excluded).
- Minor criteria in low risk populations include fever ≥38.5°F, polyarthralgia, sedimentation rate ≥60 mm and/or C-reactive protein (CRP) ≥3.0 mg/dL, and prolonged PR interval (unless carditis is a major criterion). In moderate- to high-risk populations, a lower fever ≥38°F is accepted, monoarthralgia is a minor criterion, a lower sedimentation rate ≥30 mm and/or CRP ≥3.0 mg/dL is accepted, and prolonged PR interval (unless carditis is a major criterion) is included.

For a primary episode, 2 major criteria or 1 major and 2 minor criteria are required for diagnosis. Following a primary ARF episode, in patients with documentation of reinfection with group A streptococci, 2 major, 1 major and 2 minor, or 3 minor features are sufficient to confirm the diagnosis of ARF recurrence.

Table 3.72 Revised Jones Criteria (2015)

1. All patients require evidence of antecedent GAS infection for diagnosis of ARF (except in case of chorea, where evidence of antecedent GAS infection is not required).
2. To confirm an initial diagnosis of ARF, need 2 major OR 1 major and 2 minor criteria.
3. To confirm recurrent ARF diagnosis, need 2 major OR 1 major and 2 minor OR 3 minor criteria.
4. Criteria for diagnosis are dependent on whether patient is from a low risk or a moderate/high-risk population. Moderate- and high-risk populations include countries where ARF remains endemic (Africa, Asia-Pacific, indigenous population of Australia). The United States, Canada, and Europe are examples of a low-risk population.
5. Major and minor criteria are listed below, by risk categorization; differences for moderate-/high-risk populations are bolded.

Low-Risk Population	Moderate- and High-Risk Population
Major Criteria	**Major Criteria**
• Carditis (clinical or subclinical)	• Carditis (clinical or subclinical)
• Arthritis (polyarthritis only)	• Arthritis (polyarthritis or **monoarthritis**, or **polyarthralgia**)
• Chorea	• Chorea
• Subcutaneous nodules	• Subcutaneous nodules
• Erythema marginatum	• Erythema marginatum
Minor Criteria	**Minor Criteria**
• Polyarthralgia	• **Monoarthralgia**
• Fever ≥38.5°C	• **Fever ≥38°C**
• ESR ≥60 mm/h and/or CRP ≥3 mg/dL	• **ESR ≥30 mm/h** and/or CRP ≥3 mg/dL
• Prolonged PR interval (in absence of carditis)	• Prolonged PR interval (in absence of carditis)

Modified from Table 7 in Gewitz MH, Baltimore RS, Tani LY, et al. Revision of the Jones criteria for the diagnosis of acute rheumatic fever in the era of Doppler echocardiography: a scientific statement from the American Heart Association. *Circulation*. 2015;131(20):1806–1818.

ESR indicates erythrocyte sedimentation rate; CRP, C-reactive protein.

Treatment for ARF includes eradication of GAS with a standard pharyngitis regimen, treatment of acute manifestations (eg, arthritis or valvulitis associated heart failure), education for parents and patient, and initiation of secondary prophylaxis to prevent against future GAS infection.

Secondary Prophylaxis for Rheumatic Fever. Following initial treatment of ARF, patients who have a well-documented history of ARF (including cases manifested solely as Sydenham chorea) and patients who have documented rheumatic heart disease should be given continuous antimicrobial prophylaxis to prevent recurrent ARF attacks (secondary prophylaxis), because asymptomatic and symptomatic GAS infections can result in a recurrence of ARF. Continuous prophylaxis should be initiated as soon as the diagnosis of ARF or rheumatic heart disease is made.

Duration. Secondary prophylaxis should be long-term, perhaps for life, for patients with rheumatic heart disease (even after prosthetic valve replacement), because these patients remain at risk of recurrence of ARF. The risk of recurrence decreases as the interval from the most recent acute episode increases, and patients without rheumatic heart disease are at a lower risk of recurrence than are patients with residual cardiac involvement. These considerations, as well as the estimate of exposure to GAS infection, influence the duration of secondary prophylaxis in adults but should not alter the practice of secondary prophylaxis for children and adolescents. Secondary prophylaxis for all patients who have had ARF should be continued for at least 5 years or until the person is 21 years of age, whichever is longer (see Table 3.73). Prophylaxis also should be continued if the risk of contact with people with GAS infection is high, such as for parents with school-aged children and for people in professions that bring them into contact with children, such as teachers.

The drug regimens in Table 3.74 are effective for secondary prophylaxis. The intramuscular regimen has been shown to be the most reliable, because the success of oral prophylaxis depends primarily on patient adherence; however, inconvenience and pain of injection may cause some patients to discontinue intramuscular prophylaxis. In non-US populations in which the risk of ARF is particularly high, administration of penicillin G benzathine every 3 weeks is justified and recommended, because drug concentrations in serum can decrease below a protective level before the fourth week after administration of a dose. In the United States, administration every 4 weeks seems adequate, except for people who have developed recurrent ARF despite adherence to an every-4-week regimen. Oral sulfadiazine is as effective as oral penicillin for secondary prophylaxis but may not be available readily in the United States. By extrapolating from data demonstrating effectiveness of sulfadiazine, sulfisoxazole has been deemed an appropriate alternative drug; it is available in combination with erythromycin as a generic version.

Allergic reactions to oral penicillin are less common and usually less severe than reactions to parenteral penicillin and occur much more often in adults than in children. Severe allergic reactions rarely occur in patients receiving intramuscular penicillin G benzathine prophylaxis, but the incidence may be higher in patients older than 12 years with severe rheumatic heart disease. Most severe reactions seem to be vasovagal responses rather than anaphylaxis. A serum sickness-like reaction characterized by fever and joint pains can occur in people receiving prophylaxis and can be mistaken for recurrence of ARF.

Reactions to continuous sulfadiazine or sulfisoxazole prophylaxis are rare and usually minor; evaluation of blood cell counts may be advisable after 2 weeks of prophylaxis,

Table 3.73. Duration of Prophylaxis for People Who Have Had Acute Rheumatic Fever (ARF): Recommendations of the American Heart Association[a]

Category	Duration
Rheumatic fever without carditis	5 years since last episode of ARF or until 21 years of age, whichever is longer
Rheumatic fever with carditis but without residual heart disease (no valvular disease[b])	10 years since last episode of ARF or until 21 years of age, whichever is longer
Rheumatic fever with carditis and residual heart disease (persistent valvular disease[b])	10 years since last episode of ARF or until 40 years of age, whichever is longer; consider lifelong prophylaxis for people with severe valvular disease or likelihood of ongoing exposure to group A streptococcal infection

[a]Modified from Gerber M, Baltimore R, Eaton C, et al. Prevention of rheumatic fever and diagnosis and treatment of acute streptococcal pharyngitis. A scientific statement from the American Heart Association, Rheumatic Fever, Endocarditis, and Kawasaki Disease Committee, Council on Cardiovascular Disease in the Young, and the Quality of Care and Outcomes Research Interdisciplinary Working Group. *Circulation*. 2009;119(11):1541–1551.
[b]Clinical or echocardiographic evidence.

Table 3.74. Chemoprophylaxis for Recurrences of Acute Rheumatic Fever[a]

Drug	Dose	Route
Penicillin G benzathine	1.2 million U, every 4 wk[b]; 600 000 U, every 4 wk for patients weighing less than 27.3 kg (60 lb)	Intramuscular
OR		
Penicillin V	250 mg, twice a day	Oral
OR		
Sulfadiazine or sulfisoxazole	0.5 g, once a day for patients weighing 27 kg (60 lb) or less	Oral
	1.0 g, once a day for patients weighing greater than 27 kg (60 lb)	

For people who are allergic to penicillin and sulfonamide drugs

Macrolide or azalide	Variable (see text)	Oral

[a]Gerber M, Baltimore R, Eaton C, et al. Prevention of rheumatic fever and diagnosis and treatment of acute streptococcal pharyngitis. A scientific statement from the American Heart Association, Rheumatic Fever, Endocarditis, and Kawasaki Disease Committee, Council on Cardiovascular Disease in the Young, and the Quality of Care and Outcomes Research Interdisciplinary Working Group. *Circulation*. 2009;119(11):1541–1551.
[b]In particularly high-risk situations (usually non-US sites), administration every 3 weeks is recommended.

because leukopenia has been reported in people receiving these drugs. Prophylaxis with a sulfonamide during late pregnancy is contraindicated because of interference with fetal bilirubin metabolism. Febrile mucocutaneous syndromes (erythema multiforme, Stevens-Johnson syndrome, or toxic epidermal necrolysis) have been associated with penicillin and with sulfonamides. When an adverse event occurs with any of these prophylactic regimens, the drug should be stopped immediately and an alternative drug should be selected. For the rare patient who is allergic to both penicillins and sulfonamides, erythromycin is recommended. Other macrolides, such as azithromycin or clarithromycin, also are acceptable; they have less risk of gastrointestinal tract intolerance but increased cost.

Poststreptococcal Reactive Arthritis. After an episode of acute GAS pharyngitis, reactive arthritis may develop in the absence of sufficient clinical manifestations and laboratory findings to fulfill the Jones criteria for diagnosis of ARF. This syndrome has been termed poststreptococcal reactive arthritis (PSRA). The precise relationship of PSRA to ARF is unclear. In contrast with the arthritis of ARF, PSRA does not respond dramatically to nonsteroidal anti-inflammatory agents. Because a very small proportion of patients with PSRA have been reported to develop valvular heart disease later, these patients should be observed carefully for 1 to 2 years for evidence of carditis. Some experts recommend secondary prophylaxis for these patients during the observation period. If carditis develops, the patient should be considered to have had ARF, and secondary prophylaxis should be initiated (see Secondary Prophylaxis for Rheumatic Fever, p 759).

ISOLATION OF THE HOSPITALIZED PATIENT: In addition to standard precautions, droplet precautions are recommended for children with GAS pharyngitis or pneumonia until 24 hours after initiation of appropriate antimicrobial therapy. For burns with secondary GAS infection and extensive or draining cutaneous infections that cannot be covered or contained adequately by dressings, contact precautions should be used until at least 24 hours after initiation of appropriate therapy.

CONTROL MEASURES: The most important means of controlling GAS disease and its sequelae is prompt identification and treatment of infections.

School and Child Care. Children with GAS pharyngitis or skin infections should not return to school or child care until well appearing and at least 12 hours after beginning appropriate antimicrobial therapy. Close contact with other children during this time should be avoided.

Care of Exposed People. Symptomatic contacts of a child with documented GAS infection who have recent or current clinical evidence of a GAS infection should undergo appropriate laboratory tests and should be treated if test results are positive. Rates of GAS carriage are higher among sibling contacts of children with GAS pharyngitis than among parent contacts in nonepidemic settings; carriage rates as high as 50% for sibling contacts and 20% for parent contacts have been reported during epidemics. Asymptomatic acquisition of group A streptococci may pose some low risk of nonsuppurative complications; studies indicate that as many as one third of patients with ARF had no history of recent streptococcal infection and another third had minor respiratory tract symptoms that were not brought to medical attention. However, routine laboratory evaluation of asymptomatic household contacts usually is not indicated except during outbreaks or when contacts are at increased risk of developing sequelae of infection (see Indications for GAS Testing, p 752). In rare circumstances, such as a large family with documented, repeated, intrafamilial transmission resulting in frequent episodes of GAS pharyngitis over a prolonged period, physicians may elect to treat all family members identified by laboratory tests as harboring GAS organisms.

Household contacts of patients with severe invasive GAS disease, including STSS, are at some increased risk of developing severe invasive GAS disease compared with the general population. However, the risk is not sufficiently high to warrant routine testing for GAS colonization, and a clearly effective regimen has not been identified to justify routine chemoprophylaxis of all household contacts. However, because of increased risk of sporadic, invasive GAS disease among certain populations (eg, people with human immunodeficiency virus [HIV] infection) and because of increased risk of death in people 65 years and older who develop invasive GAS disease, physicians may choose to offer targeted chemoprophylaxis to household contacts who are 65 years and older or who are members of other high-risk populations (eg, people with HIV infection, varicella, or diabetes mellitus). Because of the rarity of secondary cases and the low risk of invasive GAS infections in children, chemoprophylaxis is not recommended in schools or child care facilities.

Bacterial Endocarditis Prophylaxis.[1] The American Heart Association (AHA) has published updated recommendations regarding use of antimicrobial agents to prevent infective endocarditis (see Prevention of Bacterial Endocarditis, p 1044). The AHA no longer recommends prophylaxis for patients with rheumatic heart disease without a prosthetic valve. However, use of oral antiseptic solutions and maintenance of optimal oral health through daily oral hygiene and regular dental visits remain important components of an overall health care program. For individuals with a prosthetic valve, infective endocarditis prophylaxis still is recommended, and current AHA recommendations should be followed. If penicillin has been used for secondary prevention of rheumatic fever, an agent other than penicillin should be used for infective endocarditis prophylaxis, because penicillin-resistant alpha-hemolytic streptococci are likely to be present in the oral cavity of such patients.

Group B Streptococcal Infections

CLINICAL MANIFESTATIONS: Group B streptococci are a major cause of perinatal infections, including bacteremia, endometritis, intra-amniotic infection (formerly called chorioamnionitis), and urinary tract infections in women during pregnancy and immediately postpartum, and of systemic and focal infections in neonates and young infants. Invasive disease in infants is categorized on the basis of chronologic age at onset. Early-onset disease usually occurs within the first 24 hours of life (range, 0 through 6 days) and is characterized by signs of systemic infection, respiratory distress, apnea, shock, pneumonia, and less often, meningitis (5%–10% of cases). Late-onset disease, which typically occurs at 3 to 4 weeks of age (range, 7 through 89 days), commonly manifests as occult bacteremia or meningitis (approximately 30% of cases); other focal infections, such as osteomyelitis, septic arthritis, necrotizing fasciitis, pneumonia, adenitis, and cellulitis, occur less commonly. Nearly 50% of survivors of early- or late-onset meningitis have long-term neurologic sequelae (encephalomalacia, cortical blindness, cerebral palsy, visual impairment, hearing

---

[1]Wilson W, Taubert KA, Gewitz M, et al. Prevention of infective endocarditis. Recommendations by the American Heart Association. A guideline from the American Heart Association Rheumatic Fever, Endocarditis, and Kawasaki Disease Committee, Council on Cardiovascular Disease in the Young, and the Council on Clinical Cardiology, Council on Cardiovascular Surgery and Anesthesia, and the Quality of Care and Outcomes Research Interdisciplinary Working Group. *Circulation.* 2007;116(15):1736–1754

deficits, or learning disabilities). Late, late-onset disease occurs at 90 days of age and beyond, usually in very preterm infants requiring prolonged hospitalization. Group B streptococci also cause systemic infections in nonpregnant adults with underlying medical conditions, such as diabetes mellitus, obesity, chronic liver or renal disease, malignancy, or other immunocompromising conditions and in adults 65 years and older.

ETIOLOGY: Group B streptococci *(Streptococcus agalactiae)* are gram-positive, aerobic diplococci that typically produce a narrow zone of beta hemolysis on 5% sheep blood agar. These organisms are divided into 10 types on the basis of capsular polysaccharides (Ia, Ib, and II through IX). Types Ia, Ib, II, III, and V account for approximately 95% of cases in infants in the United States, with type IV emerging as an important cause of invasive infections in adults. Type III is the predominant cause of early- and late-onset meningitis and the majority of late-onset infections in infants. Capsular polysaccharides and pilus-like structures are important virulence factors and are potential vaccine candidates.

EPIDEMIOLOGY: Group B streptococci are common inhabitants of the human gastrointestinal and genitourinary tracts. Less commonly, they colonize the pharynx. The colonization rate in pregnant women ranges from 15% to 35%. Colonization during pregnancy can be constant or intermittent. Before recommendations were made for prevention of early-onset group B streptococcal (GBS) disease through maternal intrapartum antimicrobial prophylaxis (see Control Measures, p 765), the incidence was 1 to 4 cases per 1000 live births; early-onset disease accounted for approximately 75% of cases in infants and occurred in approximately 1 to 2 infants per 100 colonized women. Following widespread implementation of maternal intrapartum antimicrobial prophylaxis, the incidence of early-onset disease has decreased by approximately 80% to an estimated 0.25 cases per 1000 live births in 2014. The use of intrapartum chemoprophylaxis has had no measurable effect on late-onset GBS disease. In recent years, the incidence of late-onset disease has nearly equaled that of early-onset disease. The case-fatality ratio in term infants ranges from 1% to 3% but is higher in preterm neonates (estimated to be 20% for early-onset disease and 5% for late-onset disease). Approximately 70% of early-onset and 50% of late-onset cases afflict term neonates.

Transmission from mother to infant occurs shortly before or during delivery. After delivery, person-to-person transmission can occur. Although uncommon, GBS infection can be acquired in the nursery from health care professionals (probably resulting from omissions in hand hygiene) or visitors and more commonly in the community (colonized family members or caregivers). The risk of early-onset disease is increased in preterm infants (less than 37 weeks' gestation), infants born after the amniotic membranes have been ruptured 18 hours or more, and infants born to women with high genital GBS inoculum, intrapartum fever (temperature 38°C [100.4°F] or greater), intra-amniotic infection (formerly called chorioamnionitis), GBS bacteriuria during the current pregnancy, or a previous infant with invasive GBS disease. A low or an undetectable maternal concentration of type-specific serum antibody to capsular polysaccharide of the infecting strain also is a predisposing factor for neonatal infection. Other risk factors are intrauterine fetal monitoring and maternal age younger than 20 years. Black race is an independent risk factor for both early-onset and late-onset disease. Although the incidence of early-onset disease has declined in all racial groups since the 1990s, rates consistently have been higher among black infants (0.54 cases per 1000 live births in 2014) compared with white infants (0.18 cases per 1000 live births), with the highest incidence observed among preterm black infants (0.96 per 1000 live births in 2014). The reason for this racial/ethnic disparity is not known. The period of communicability is unknown but can extend throughout the duration of colonization or disease. Infants can remain colonized for several months after birth and after treatment for systemic infection. Recurrent GBS disease affects an estimated 1% to 3% of appropriately treated infants.

The **incubation period** of early-onset disease is fewer than 7 days. In late-onset and late, late-onset disease, the **incubation period** from GBS acquisition to disease is unknown.

DIAGNOSTIC TESTS: Visualization of Gram-positive cocci in pairs or short chains by Gram stain of body fluids that typically are sterile (eg, cerebrospinal fluid [CSF], pleural fluid, or joint fluid) provides presumptive evidence of infection. Growth of the organism from cultures of blood, CSF, or if present, a suppurative focus is necessary to establish the diagnosis. A meningitis/encephalitis multiplex panel polymerase chain reaction assay cleared by the US Food and Drug Administration (FDA) is approved for direct testing of CSF and detection of GBS along with many other bacterial, viral, and fungal pathogens. Clinical experience with this multiplex assay is limited. For prenatal GBS screening, vaginal and rectal swab maternal specimens are collected and enriched in commercially available selective broth mediums for 18 to 24 hours at 35°C to 37°C in ambient air or 5% carbon dioxide and subsequently plated on tryptic soy blood agar or other selective agars for further 24 to 48 hour incubation and isolation. Alternatively, DNA probe assays, latex agglutination assays, and nucleic acid amplification assays are available to detect GBS from enriched broth specimens. One of these FDA-cleared molecular assays also is approved for intrapartum detection of GBS from vaginal/rectal swab specimens collected from pregnant women presenting in labor if GBS colonization is unknown.

TREATMENT:

- Ampicillin plus an aminoglycoside is the initial treatment of choice for a newborn infant with presumptive early-onset GBS infection. For empirical therapy of late-onset meningitis, ampicillin and an aminoglycoside or cefotaxime are recommended. If the infant is 2 months or older, vancomycin and ceftriaxone are recommended to ensure that therapy would be appropriate for *Streptococcus pneumoniae* meningitis until results of cultures confirm GBS.

- Penicillin G alone is the drug of choice when GBS has been identified as the cause of the infection and when clinical and microbiologic responses have been documented. Ampicillin is an acceptable alternative therapy.

- For infants with meningitis attributable to GBS, the recommended dosage of penicillin G for infants 7 days or younger is 250 000 to 450 000 U/kg per day, intravenously, in 3 divided doses; for infants older than 7 days, 450 000 to 500 000 U/kg per day, intravenously, in 4 divided doses is recommended. For ampicillin, the recommended dosage for infants with meningitis 7 days or younger is 200 to 300 mg/kg per day, intravenously, in 3 divided doses; the recommended dosage for infants older than 7 days is 300 mg/kg per day, intravenously, in 4 divided doses.

- For meningitis, especially in the neonate, some experts recommend a second lumbar puncture be performed approximately 24 to 48 hours after initiation of therapy to assist in management and prognosis. If CSF sterility is not achieved, a complicated course (eg, cerebral infarcts, cerebritis, ventriculitis) can be expected; an increasing protein concentration suggests an intracranial complication (eg, infarction, subdural empyema, ventricular obstruction). Additional lumbar punctures are indicated if response to therapy is in doubt, neurologic abnormalities persist, or focal neurologic deficits occur. Failed hearing screen, abnormal neurologic examination, and certain cranial imaging abnormalities at discharge predict an adverse long-term outcome. Consultation with a specialist in pediatric infectious diseases can assist in treatment of all cases of neonatal meningitis including GBS.

- For infants with bacteremia without a defined focus, treatment should be continued for 10 days. For infants with uncomplicated meningitis, 14 days of treatment is satisfactory, but longer periods of treatment may be necessary for infants with prolonged or complicated courses. Septic arthritis or osteomyelitis requires treatment for 3 to 4 weeks; endocarditis or ventriculitis requires treatment for at least 4 weeks. Treatment should be administered exclusively by the parenteral route.

- Because of the reported increased risk of infection, the birth mates of a multiple birth index case with early- or late-onset disease should be observed carefully and evaluated and treated empirically for suspected systemic infection if signs of illness occur; treatment should be continued for a full course for those with confirmed infection.

ISOLATION OF THE HOSPITALIZED PATIENT: Standard precautions are recommended, except during a nursery outbreak of disease attributable to group B streptococci (see Control Measures, Nursery Outbreak).

CONTROL MEASURES:

Chemoprophylaxis. Recommendations from the Centers for Disease Control and Prevention (CDC)[1] and American Academy of Pediatrics[2] have been incorporated into a smart phone app (**www.cdc.gov/groupbstrep/guidelines/prevention-app.html**) and include the following:

- All pregnant women should have culture screening at 35 to 37 weeks' gestation for vaginal and rectal GBS colonization. For women who present with preterm labor, GBS screening should be performed and parenteral GBS prophylaxis should be initiated. If delivery occurs within 5 weeks and the prior screening result was negative, then no further testing is needed. For those who present >5 weeks after initial preterm labor, then rescreening and management according to the algorithm in the references below is recommended.

- For women who had a previous infant with invasive GBS disease, intrapartum chemoprophylaxis **always** should be administered.

- Women with group B streptococci isolated from urine during the current pregnancy should receive intrapartum chemoprophylaxis, because these women usually have a high inoculum of group B streptococci at vaginal and rectal sites and are at increased risk of delivering an infant with early-onset GBS disease; culture screening at 35 to 37 weeks' gestation is not necessary if GBS is isolated from the urine prior to screening.

- Intrapartum chemoprophylaxis should be given to **all** pregnant women identified as GBS carriers in the index pregnancy. Colonization during a previous pregnancy is *not* an indication for intrapartum chemoprophylaxis.

- If GBS status is not known at onset of labor or rupture of membranes, intrapartum chemoprophylaxis should be administered to **all** women with gestation less than 37 weeks, duration of membrane rupture 18 hours or longer, or intrapartum temperature

[1]Centers for Disease Control and Prevention. Prevention of perinatal group B streptococcal disease. Revised guidelines from CDC, 2010. *MMWR Recomm Rep.* 2010;59(RR-10):1–36

[2]American Academy of Pediatrics, Committee on Infectious Diseases. Recommendations for the prevention of perinatal group B streptococcal (GBS) disease. *Pediatrics.* 2011;128(3):611–616

of 38.0°C (100.4°F) or greater.

- Oral antimicrobial agents should *not* be used to treat women who are found to have GBS colonization during culture screening. If there is GBS bacteriuria, treatment is warranted according to obstetric standards of care. Such treatment is *not* effective in eliminating carriage of group B streptococci or preventing neonatal disease.

- Intrapartum antimicrobial prophylaxis is *not* recommended for cesarean deliveries performed before labor onset in women with intact amniotic membranes. Women expected to undergo cesarean deliveries should undergo routine culture screening, because onset of labor or rupture of membranes can occur before the planned cesarean delivery, and in this circumstance, intrapartum antimicrobial prophylaxis is recommended if the culture screen is positive.

- Intravenous penicillin G (5 million U initially, then 2.5 to 3.0 million U, every 4 hours, until delivery) is the preferred agent for intrapartum chemoprophylaxis because of its efficacy and narrow spectrum of antimicrobial activity. An alternative drug is intravenous ampicillin (2 g initially, then 1 g every 4 hours until delivery).

- Penicillin-allergic women without a history of anaphylaxis, angioedema, respiratory distress, or urticaria following administration of a penicillin should receive intravenous cefazolin (2 g initially, then 1 g every 8 hours). Cefazolin is recommended because of its ability to achieve high amniotic fluid concentrations and effectively prevent early-onset GBS disease.

- Penicillin-allergic women at high risk of anaphylaxis should receive intravenous clindamycin (900 mg every 8 hours) *if* their GBS isolate is documented to be susceptible to clindamycin and erythromycin. If the isolate is sensitive to clindamycin but resistant to erythromycin, clindamycin may be used if testing for inducible clindamycin resistance is negative. Approximately 33% (40% if inducible resistance is included) of GBS isolates in the United States were clindamycin resistant in 2014, and the proportion may vary by country. If clindamycin susceptibility testing has not been performed or if the organism is resistant, intravenous vancomycin (1 g every 12 hours) should be administered. The efficacy of clindamycin or vancomycin in preventing early-onset GBS disease is not established.

- Routine use of antimicrobial agents as chemoprophylaxis for neonates born to mothers who have received adequate intrapartum chemoprophylaxis is *not* recommended. Antimicrobial therapy is appropriate only for infants with clinically suspected systemic infection.

- An algorithm for management of newborn infants is provided in Fig 3.9. The recommendations are intended to help clinicians promptly detect and treat cases of early-onset GBS infections.

- Newborn infants with signs of sepsis should receive a full diagnostic evaluation and initiation of empiric antimicrobial therapy.

- Well-appearing newborn infants whose mothers had suspected intra-amniotic infection (formerly called chorioamnionitis) should undergo a limited evaluation (includes a blood culture and complete blood cell count with differential and platelet counts). Consultation with obstetric providers is important to determine the level of clinical suspicion for intra-amniotic infection. Infants born to women for whom there is a high level of concern for intra-amniotic infection should receive empirical antimicrobial therapy pending culture results.

FIG 3.9. MANAGEMENT OF NEONATES FOR PREVENTION OF EARLY-ONSET GROUP B STREPTOCOCCAL (GBS) DISEASE

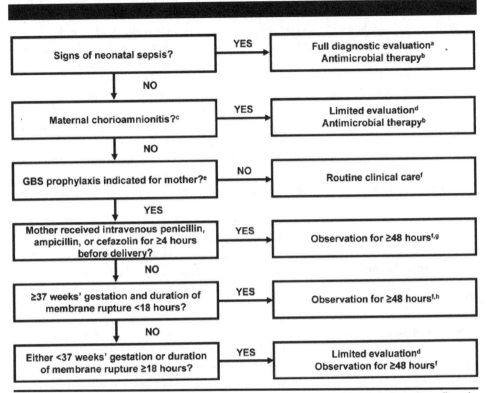

[a]Full diagnostic evaluation includes complete blood cell (CBC) count with differential, platelets, blood culture, chest radiograph (if respiratory abnormalities are present), and lumbar puncture (if patient stable enough to tolerate procedure and sepsis is suspected).

[b]Antimicrobial therapy should be directed toward the most common causes of neonatal sepsis, including GBS and other organisms (including gram-negative pathogens), and should take into account local antimicrobial resistance patterns.

[c]Consultation with obstetric providers is important to determine the level of clinical suspicion for chorioamnionitis (now known as intra-amniotic infection). Intra-amniotic infection is diagnosed clinically, and some of the signs are nonspecific.

[d]Limited evaluation includes blood culture (at birth) and CBC count with differential and platelets (at birth and/or at 6–12 hours of life).

[e]GBS prophylaxis indicated if one or more of the following: (1) mother GBS positive at 35 to 37 weeks' gestation; (2) GBS status unknown with one or more intrapartum risk factors, including <37 weeks' gestation, rupture of membranes ≥18 hours or temperature ≥100.4°F (38.0°C), or intrapartum nucleic acid amplification test results positive for GBS; (3) GBS bacteriuria during current pregnancy; (4) history of a previous infant with GBS disease.

[f]If signs of sepsis develop, a full diagnostic evaluation should be performed and antimicrobial therapy should be initiated.

[g]If ≥37 weeks' gestation, observation may occur at home after 24 hours if other discharge criteria have been met, if there is a knowledgeable observer and ready access to medical care.

[h]Some experts recommend a CBC with differential and platelets at 6 to 12 hours of age.

- Well-appearing infants whose mothers had no intra-amniotic infection and no indication for GBS prophylaxis should receive routine clinical care.
- Well-appearing infants of any gestational age whose mother received adequate intrapartum GBS prophylaxis (defined as ≥4 hours of penicillin, ampicillin, or cefazolin before delivery) should be observed for ≥48 hours; diagnostic testing is *not* recommended.

Observation may occur at home after 24 hours if other discharge criteria have been met and if there is a knowledgeable observer and ready access to medical care. All other maternal antimicrobial agents or durations before delivery are considered inadequate for purposes of neonatal management.

- Well-appearing infants ≥37 weeks' gestation born to mothers who had an indication for GBS prophylaxis but received no or inadequate prophylaxis and in whom duration of membrane rupture before delivery was <18 hours should be observed for ≥48 hours, and *no* diagnostic testing is recommended. Some experts would perform a complete blood count with differential and platelet count at 6 to 12 hours of age in these neonates.

- Well-appearing infants ≥37 weeks' gestation born to mothers who had an indication for GBS prophylaxis but received no or inadequate prophylaxis and in whom duration of membrane rupture before delivery was <18 hours should be observed for ≥48 hours, and *no* diagnostic testing is recommended. Some experts would perform a complete blood count with differential and platelet count at 6 to 12 hours of age in these neonates.

- If the infant was born to a mother who had an indication for GBS prophylaxis but received no or inadequate prophylaxis and is well appearing and either the infant is <37 weeks' gestation or the duration of membrane rupture before delivery was ≥18 hours, then the infant should undergo a limited evaluation and observation for ≥48 hours.

Neonatal Infection Control. Routine cultures to determine whether infants are colonized with GBS are *not* recommended.

Nursery Outbreak. Cohorting of ill and colonized infants and use of contact precautions during an outbreak are recommended. Other methods of control (eg, treatment of asymptomatic carriers with penicillin) are ineffective. Routine hand hygiene by health care professionals and visitors having contact with colonized or infected with GBS is the best way to prevent spread to other infants.

Non-Group A or B Streptococcal and Enterococcal Infections

CLINICAL MANIFESTATIONS: Streptococci other than Lancefield groups A or B can be associated with invasive disease in infants, children, adolescents, and adults. The principal clinical syndromes of groups C and G streptococci (most belong to the *Streptococcus dysgalactiae* group) are bacteremia, septicemia, upper and lower respiratory tract infections (eg, pharyngitis, sinusitis, and pneumonia), skin and soft tissue infections, septic arthritis, osteomyelitis, meningitis with a parameningeal focus, brain abscess, toxic shock syndrome, pericarditis, and endocarditis with various clinical manifestations. Viridans streptococci are the most common cause of bacterial endocarditis in children, especially children with congenital or valvular heart disease, and these organisms are a common cause of bacteremia in neutropenic patients with cancer in the first 2 weeks after hematopoietic stem cell transplantation and as a cause of central line-associated bacteremia. Among the viridans streptococci, group F streptococci (most belong to the *Streptococcus anginosus* group) are implicated in complicated sinus infection but are an infrequent cause of invasive infection. More serious *S anginosus* group infections include brain or dental abscesses or abscesses in other sites, including lymph nodes, liver, pelvis, and lung. These organisms also may cause sinusitis and other head and neck infections, meningitis, spondylodiskitis, spinal epidural abscesses, subdural empyema, peritonitis, appendicitis, abdominal wound infections, and cholangitis. Enterococci are associated with bacteremia in neonates and bacteremia, device-associated infections, intra-abdominal abscesses, and urinary tract infections in those with abnormal anatomy and in older children and adults.

ETIOLOGY: Changes in taxonomy and nomenclature of the *Streptococcus* genus have evolved with advances in molecular technology (see Table 3.75). Among gram-positive organisms that are catalase negative and display chains by Gram stain, the genera associated most often with human disease are *Streptococcus* and *Enterococcus*.

The genus *Streptococcus* has been subdivided into 6 species groups on the basis of 16S rRNA gene sequencing. Members of the genus that are beta-hemolytic on blood agar plates include *Streptococcus pyogenes* (see Group A Streptococcal Infections, p 748), *Streptococcus agalactiae* (see Group B Streptococcal Infections, p 762), and groups C and G streptococci; *S dysgalactiae* subspecies *equisimilis* is the group C subspecies most often associated with human infections. Streptococci that are non-beta–hemolytic (alpha-hemolytic or nonhemolytic) on blood agar plates include: (1) *Streptococcus pneumoniae* (see Pneumococcal Infections, p 639); (2) the *Streptococcus bovis* group; and (3) viridans streptococci clinically relevant in humans, which include 5 *Streptococcus* species groups (*S anginosus* group, *mitis* group, *sanguinis* group, *salivarius* group, and *mutans* group). The *anginosus* group (also known as the *Streptococcus milleri* group) includes *S anginosus*, *Streptococcus constellatus*, and *Streptococcus intermedius*. This group can have variable hemolysis, and approximately one third possess group A, C, F, or G antigens. Nutritionally variant streptococci, once thought to be viridans streptococci, now are classified in the genera *Abiotrophia* and *Granulicatella*.

The genus *Enterococcus* (previously included with Lancefield group D streptococci) contains at least 18 species, with *Enterococcus faecalis* and *Enterococcus faecium* accounting for most human enterococcal infections. Outbreaks and health care-associated spread in association with vancomycin-resistant enterococcal strains including *Enterococcus gallinarum*, *Enterococcus casseliflavus*, or *Enterococcus flavescens* also have occurred occasionally. Nonenterococcal group D streptococci include *S bovis* and *Streptococcus equinus*, both members of the *bovis* group.

Table 3.75. Classification of Streptococci Most Commonly Associated With Disease, by Lancefield Group and by Hemolysis

Species	Lancefield Group	Hemolysis
Streptococcus pyogenes	A	β
Streptococcus agalactiae	B	β
Streptococcus dysgalactiae subspecies *equisimillis*, *Streptococcus equi* subspecies *zooepidemicus*	C	β
Enterococcus faecalis, *Enterococcus faecium*, *Streptococcus bovis*	D	γ
Streptococcus canis	G	β
Streptococcus pneumoniae, viridans streptococci	Not groupable[a]	α

[a] Occasional viridans streptococci have variable hemolysis and can possess Lancefield group A, C, F, or G antigens.

EPIDEMIOLOGY: The habitats that non-group A and B streptococci and enterococci occupy in humans include the skin (groups C and G), oropharynx (groups C and G and the *mutans* group), gastrointestinal tract (groups C and G, *bovis* group, and *Enterococcus* species), and vagina (groups C, D, and G and *Enterococcus* species). Typical human habitats of species of viridans streptococci are the oropharynx, epithelial surfaces of the oral cavity, teeth, skin, and gastrointestinal and genitourinary tracts. Intrapartum transmission is responsible for most cases of early-onset neonatal infection caused by non-group A and B streptococci and enterococci. Environmental contamination or transmission via hands of health care professionals can lead to colonization of patients. Groups C and G streptococci can cause foodborne outbreaks of pharyngitis.

The **incubation period** and the period of communicability are unknown.

DIAGNOSTIC TESTS: Diagnosis is established by culture of usually sterile body sites or abscesses with appropriate biochemical testing and serologic analysis for definitive identification. Mass spectrometry is unreliable in differentiation of *S pneumoniae* from viridians streptococci. Antimicrobial susceptibility testing of isolates from usually sterile sites should be performed to guide treatment of infections caused by viridans streptococci or enterococci. The proportion of vancomycin-resistant enterococci among hospitalized patients can be as high as 30%. Selective agars are available for screening of vancomycin-resistant enterococcus from stool specimens. A rapid automated, molecular assay currently is available for direct detection of *vanA* gene, which confers vancomycin resistance, from rectal swab specimens for screening of vancomycin-resistant enterococci (VRE).

TREATMENT: Penicillin G is the drug of choice for groups C and G streptococci. Other agents with good activity include ampicillin, third- and fourth-generation cephalosporins, vancomycin, and linezolid. The combination of gentamicin with a beta-lactam antimicrobial agent (eg, penicillin or ampicillin) or vancomycin may enhance bactericidal activity needed for treatment of life-threatening infections (eg, endocarditis or meningitis).

Many viridans streptococci remain susceptible to penicillin (minimum inhibitory concentration [MIC], ≤0.12 µg/mL). Infections caused by strains susceptible to penicillin, including endocarditis, can be treated with penicillin or ceftriaxone. Strains with an MIC >0.12 µg/mL and <0.5 µg/mL are considered relatively resistant to penicillin by criteria in the American Heart Association guidelines for treatment of infective endocarditis in childhood.[1] In this situation, penicillin, ampicillin, or ceftriaxone for 4 weeks, combined for the first 2 weeks with gentamicin, is recommended for endocarditis treatment. Strains with a penicillin MIC ≥0.5 µg/mL are considered resistant. Nonpenicillin antimicrobial agents with good activity against viridans streptococci include cephalosporins (especially ceftriaxone), vancomycin, linezolid, daptomycin, and tigecycline, although pediatric experience with tigecycline is limited. *Abiotrophia* and *Granulicatella* organisms can exhibit relative or high-level resistance to penicillin. The combination of high-dose penicillin or vancomycin and an aminoglycoside can enhance bactericidal activity.

Enterococci exhibit uniform resistance to cephalosporins and semisynthetic penicillins, and most are intrinsically resistant to clindamycin. The vast majority of *E faecalis* strains are susceptible to ampicillin. *E faecium* strains may be multidrug resistant. Two types of vancomycin resistance are identified: intrinsic low-level resistance that occurs with *Enterococcus gallinarum* and *Enterococcus casseliflavus*/*Enterococcus flavescens* (these strains

---

[1]Baltimore RS, Gewitz M, Baddour LM, et al. Infective endocarditis in childhood: 2015 update. A scientific statement from the American Heart Association. *Circulation*. 2015;132(15):1487–1515

are ampicillin susceptible), and acquired resistance that has been seen in *Enterococcus faecium* and some *Enterococcus faecalis* strains but also has been recognized in *Enterococcus raffinosus, Enterococcus avium,* and *Enterococcus durans.*

Systemic enterococcal infections, such as endocarditis or meningitis, should be treated with penicillin or ampicillin (if the isolate is susceptible) or vancomycin combined with gentamicin. Gentamicin should be discontinued if in vitro susceptibility testing demonstrates high-level resistance, in which case synergy cannot be achieved. In general, children with a central line-associated bloodstream infection caused by enterococci should have the device removed promptly. The role of combination therapy for treating central line-associated bloodstream infections is uncertain. The combination of ampicillin plus ceftriaxone has been used for endocarditis in adults caused by aminoglycoside nonsusceptible *E faecalis.* VRE can cause endocarditis, but there are insufficient data to determine the most effective treatment. Linezolid or daptomycin are options for treatment of other systemic infections caused by vancomycin-resistant *E faecium.* Linezolid is approved for use in children, including neonates. Isolates of VRE that also are resistant to linezolid have been described, and resistance can develop during prolonged linezolid treatment. Most vancomycin-resistant isolates of *E faecalis* and *E faecium* are daptomycin-susceptible. Data suggest that clearance of daptomycin is more rapid in young children compared with adolescents and adults. Daptomycin should not be used to treat pneumonia, as tissue concentrations are poor and daptomycin is inactivated by surfactants. Quinupristin-dalfopristin is approved for use in adults for treatment of infections attributable to vancomycin-resistant *E faecium* but is not active against *E faecalis;* microbiologic and clinical cure has been reported in children infected with vancomycin-resistant *E faecium* who were treated with quinupristin-dalfopristin. Tigecycline is approved for use in adults with infections caused by vancomycin-susceptible *E faecalis.* Tigecycline is bacteriostatic against both vancomycin-resistant *E faecalis* and vancomycin-resistant *E faecium,* but experience in children is limited.

Endocarditis. Guidelines for treatment of infective endocarditis in children from the American Heart Association should be consulted for regimens that are appropriate for children and adolescents.[1]

ISOLATION OF THE HOSPITALIZED PATIENT: Standard precautions are recommended. For patients with infection or colonization attributable to VRE, contact as well as standard precautions are indicated. Patients harboring vancomycin resistant strains of *Enterococcus gallinarum, E casseliflavus,* or *E flavescens* may be managed using only standard precautions, because these strains generally are susceptible to ampicillin. Common practice is to maintain precautions until the patient no longer harbors the organism or is discharged from the health care facility. Some experts recommend discontinuation of contact precautions if 3 consecutive negative cultures are confirmed from body fluid or tissue specimens from multiple sites (may include stool or rectal swab, perineal area, axilla or umbilicus, wound, and indwelling urinary catheter or colostomy sites, if present). Generally, such cultures should be obtained after cessation of antimicrobial therapy, and each culture is at least 1 week apart from the prior.

CONTROL MEASURES: Patients with a prosthetic valve or prosthetic material used for cardiac valve repair, previous infective endocarditis, or congenital heart disease associated

---

[1]Baltimore RS, Gewitz M, Baddour LM, et al. Infective endocarditis in childhood: 2015 update. A scientific statement from the American Heart Association. *Circulation.* 2015;132(15):1487–1515

with the highest risk of adverse outcome from endocarditis should receive antimicrobial prophylaxis to prevent endocarditis at the time of certain dental procedures (see Prevention of Bacterial Endocarditis, p 1044). For these patients, early instruction in proper diet; oral health, including use of dental sealants and adequate fluoride intake; and prevention or cessation of smoking will aid in prevention of dental caries and potentially will lower their risk of recurrent endocarditis.

Use of vancomycin and treatment with broad-spectrum antimicrobial agents are risk factors for colonization and infection with VRE. Hospitals should develop institution-specific guidelines for the proper use of vancomycin.

Strongyloidiasis
(Strongyloides stercoralis)

CLINICAL MANIFESTATIONS: Most infections with *Strongyloides stercoralis* are asymptomatic. When symptoms occur, they most often are related to larval skin invasion, tissue migration, and/or the presence of adult worms in the intestine. Infective (filariform) larvae are acquired from skin contact with contaminated soil, producing transient pruritic papules at the site of penetration. Larvae migrate to the lungs and can cause a transient pneumonitis or Löffler-like syndrome. After ascending the tracheobronchial tree, larvae are swallowed and mature into adults within the gastrointestinal tract. Symptoms of intestinal infection include nonspecific abdominal pain, malabsorption, vomiting, and diarrhea. Larval migration from defecated stool can result in migratory pruritic skin lesions in the perianal area, buttocks, and upper thighs, which may present as serpiginous, erythematous tracks called "larva currens." Immunocompromised people, most often those receiving glucocorticoids for underlying malignancy or autoimmune disease, solid organ and hematopoietic stem cell transplant recipients (through both reactivation of prior asymptomatic infection in the recipient, or to donor-derived infection), and people infected with human T-lymphotropic virus 1 (HTLV-1), are at risk of *Strongyloides* hyperinfection syndrome and disseminated disease, in which larvae migrate via the systemic circulation to distant organs, including the brain, liver, kidney, heart, and skin. This condition, which frequently is fatal, is characterized by fever, abdominal pain, diffuse pulmonary infiltrates, and septicemia or meningitis caused by enteric gram-negative bacilli.

ETIOLOGY: *S stercoralis* is a nematode (roundworm).

EPIDEMIOLOGY: Strongyloidiasis is endemic in the tropics and subtropics, including the southeastern United States, wherever suitable moist soil and improper disposal of human waste coexist. Because of the capacity for autoinfection, people can remain infected for decades even after leaving an area of endemic infection. Humans are the principal hosts, but dogs, cats, and other animals can serve as reservoirs. Transmission involves penetration of skin by filariform larvae from contact with contaminated soil. Infections rarely can be acquired from intimate skin contact or from inadvertent coprophagy, such as from ingestion of contaminated food or within institutional settings. Adult females release eggs in the small intestine, where they hatch as first-stage (rhabditiform) larvae that are excreted in feces. A small percentage of larvae molt to the infective (filariform) stage during intestinal transit, at which point they can penetrate the bowel mucosa or perianal skin, thus maintaining the life cycle within a single person (autoinfection).

The **incubation period** in humans is unknown.

DIAGNOSTIC TESTS: Strongyloidiasis can be difficult to diagnose in immunocompetent people, because excretion of larvae in feces is highly variable and often of low intensity. At least 3 consecutive stool specimens should be examined microscopically for characteristic larvae (not eggs), but stool concentration techniques may be required to establish the diagnosis. The use of culture methods to visualize tracks of larval migration on agar media may have greater sensitivity than fecal microscopy, but these techniques are not available in all laboratories; examination of duodenal contents obtained using the string test (Entero-Test) or a direct aspirate through a flexible endoscope also may demonstrate larvae. Eosinophilia (blood eosinophil count greater than 500/μL) is common in chronic infection, but its absence does not eliminate infection from consideration. When eosinophilia is absent in hyperinfection syndrome, it may predict poor outcome. Serodiagnosis by enzyme immunoassay is more sensitive, although variable among different commercial assays, and cross-reaction with other nematode species is possible; newer methods such as a luciferase immunoprecipitation system technique with recombinant antigen are even more sensitive and specific but currently only available in reference laboratories. Because infection can persist for decades, a positive serologic test result in the absence of previous treatment should be considered evidence of current infection.

In disseminated strongyloidiasis, filariform larvae may be isolated from other specimens such as sputum or bronchoalveolar lavage fluid, spinal fluid, or in skin biopsies. Gram-negative bacillary meningitis and bacteremia are commonly associated findings in disseminated disease and carry a high mortality rate.

TREATMENT: Ivermectin is the treatment of choice for both chronic (asymptomatic) strongyloidiasis and hyperinfection with disseminated disease. Ivermectin is approved by the US Food and Drug Administration for the treatment of intestinal strongyloidiasis. An alternative agent is albendazole, although it is associated with lower cure rates (see Drugs for Parasitic Infections, p 985). Mebendazole is not recommended. Prolonged or repeated treatment may be necessary in people with hyperinfection and disseminated strongyloidiasis, and relapse can occur.

ISOLATION OF THE HOSPITALIZED PATIENT: Standard precautions are recommended.

CONTROL MEASURES: Sanitary disposal of human waste is effective at interrupting transmission of *S stercoralis*. Serodiagnosis should be considered in all people with unexplained eosinophilia. Any individual at risk epidemiologically for strongyloidiasis who will undergo a solid organ or hematopoietic stem cell transplant or immunosuppressant therapy, particularly with corticosteroids, either should be tested by serology (with treatment if positive), or presumptively treated for strongyloidiasis before the initiation of immunosuppression.

Syphilis

CLINICAL MANIFESTATIONS:

Congenital Syphilis. Intrauterine infection with *Treponema pallidum* can result in stillbirth, hydrops fetalis, or preterm birth or may be asymptomatic at birth. Infected infants can have hepatosplenomegaly; snuffles (copious nasal secretions); lymphadenopathy; mucocutaneous lesions; pneumonia; osteochondritis, periostitis, and pseudoparalysis; edema; rash (maculopapular consisting of small dark red-copper spots that is most severe on the hands and feet); hemolytic anemia; or thrombocytopenia at birth or within the first 4 to 8 weeks of age. Skin lesions or moist nasal secretions of congenital syphilis are highly infectious. However, organisms rarely are found in lesions more than 24 hours after treatment has begun. Untreated infants, regardless of whether they have manifestations in early infancy, may develop late manifestations, which usually appear after 2 years of age and involve the central nervous system (CNS), bones and joints, teeth, eyes, and skin. Some consequences of intrauterine infection may not become apparent until many years after birth, such as interstitial keratitis (5–20 years of age), eighth cranial nerve deafness (10–40 years of age), Hutchinson teeth (peg-shaped, notched central incisors), anterior bowing of the shins, frontal bossing, mulberry molars, saddle nose, rhagades (perioral fissures), and Clutton joints (symmetric, painless swelling of the knees). The first 3 manifestations are referred to as the Hutchinson triad. Late manifestations can be prevented by treatment of early infection.

Acquired Syphilis. Infection with *T pallidum* in childhood or adulthood can be divided into 3 stages. The **primary stage** (or "**primary syphilis**") appears as one or more painless indurated ulcers (chancres) of the skin or mucous membranes at the site of inoculation. Lesions most commonly appear on the genitalia but may appear elsewhere, depending on the sexual contact responsible for transmission (eg, oral, anal). These lesions appear, on average, 3 weeks after exposure (10–90 days) and heal spontaneously in a few weeks. Adjacent lymph nodes frequently are enlarged but are nontender. Chancres sometimes are not recognized clinically and sometimes still are present during the secondary stage of syphilis. The **secondary stage** (or "**secondary syphilis**"), beginning 1 to 2 months later, is characterized by fever, sore throat, muscle aches, rash, mucocutaneous lesions, and generalized lymphadenopathy. The polymorphic maculopapular rash is generalized and typically includes the palms and soles. In moist areas around the vulva or anus, hypertrophic papular lesions (condyloma lata) can occur and can be confused with condyloma acuminata secondary to human papillomavirus (HPV) infection. Malaise, splenomegaly, headache, alopecia, and arthralgia also can be present. Secondary syphilis can be mistaken for other conditions, because its signs and symptoms are nonspecific. This stage also resolves spontaneously without treatment in approximately 3 to 12 weeks, leaving the infected person completely asymptomatic. A variable latent period follows but sometimes is interrupted during the first few years by recurrences of symptoms of secondary syphilis. **Latent syphilis** is defined as the period after infection when patients are seroreactive but demonstrate no clinical manifestations of disease. Latent syphilis acquired within the preceding year is referred to as **early latent syphilis;** all other cases of latent syphilis are **late latent syphilis** (greater than 1 year's duration). Patients who have latent syphilis of unknown duration should be managed clinically as if they have late latent syphilis. The **tertiary stage** of infection occurs 15 to 30 years after the initial infection and can include gumma formation (soft, noncancerous growths that can destroy tissue) or cardiovascular involvement (including aortitis). Neurosyphilis, defined as infection of the central nervous system (CNS) with *T pallidum*, can occur at any stage of infection, especially in people infected with human immunodeficiency virus (HIV) and neonates with congenital syphilis. Manifestations of neurosyphilis include syphilitic meningitis, uveitis, seizures, optic atrophy, and (typically years after infection) dementia and posterior spinal cord degeneration (tabes dorsalis, including a characteristic high-stepping gait with the feet slapping the ground with each step because of loss of proprioception).

ETIOLOGY: *T pallidum* subspecies *pallidum (T pallidum)* is a thin, motile spirochete that is extremely fastidious, surviving only briefly outside the host. The organism has not been cultivated successfully on artificial media. It is the causative agent of venereal syphilis and is very closely related to 3 other organisms causing nonvenereal human disease in distinct geographic regions of the world: *T pallidum* subspecies *pertenue,* which causes yaws; *T pallidum* subspecies *endemica,* which causes endemic syphilis; and *Treponema carateum,* which causes pinta. The genus *Treponema,* along with the genus *Borrelia,* are currently classified in the family *Spirochaetaceae.*

EPIDEMIOLOGY: Syphilis, which is rare in much of the industrialized world, persists in the United States and in resource-limited countries. In 2000 and 2001, the rate of primary and secondary syphilis was the lowest since reporting began in 1941. The rate of primary and secondary syphilis has increased almost every year since then, although initially mostly among men who have sex with men. In 2014, the rate of primary and secondary syphilis increased in every region of the United States in both men and women, with a concomitant increase in cases of congenital syphilis.[1] In adults, infection with HIV is common among individuals with syphilis, particularly among men who have sex with men. Primary and secondary rates of syphilis are highest in black, non-Hispanic people and in males compared with females.

Congenital syphilis is contracted from an infected mother via transplacental transmission of *T pallidum* at any time during pregnancy, or possibly at birth from contact with maternal lesions. Among women with untreated early syphilis, as many as 40% of pregnancies result in spontaneous abortion, stillbirth, or perinatal death. Infection can be transmitted to the fetus at any stage of maternal disease. The rate of transmission is 60% to 100% during primary and secondary syphilis and slowly decreases with later stages of maternal infection (approximately 40% with early latent infection and 8% with late latent infection).

Acquired syphilis almost always is contracted through direct sexual contact with ulcerative lesions of the skin or mucous membranes of infected people. Open, moist lesions of the primary or secondary stages are highly infectious. Relapses of secondary syphilis with infectious mucocutaneous lesions have been observed 4 years after primary infection.

Syphilis acquired beyond the neonatal period should be considered highly suggestive of sexual abuse in infants and prepubertal children once rare vertical transmission is excluded (see Screening Sexually Victimized Children for STIs, p 58). The possibility of nonvenereal endemic syphilis should also be considered in children who have recently emigrated from areas with endemic infection. Health care providers are required to report suspected sexual abuse to the state child protective services agency. This mandate does not require that the provider is certain that abuse has occurred but only that there is "reasonable cause to suspect abuse."

The **incubation period** for acquired primary syphilis typically is 3 weeks but ranges from 10 to 90 days.

DIAGNOSTIC TESTS: Definitive diagnosis is made when spirochetes are identified by microscopic darkfield examination of lesion exudate, nasal discharge, or tissue, such as placenta, umbilical cord, or autopsy specimens. *T pallidum* can be detected by polymerase chain reaction (PCR) assay, but clinical diagnostic PCR assays cleared by the US Food and Drug Administration (FDA) are not yet available. Direct fluorescent antibody (DFA) tests no longer are available in the United States. Specimens should be scraped from moist mucocutaneous lesions or aspirated from a regional lymph node. Specimens from mouth lesions can contain nonpathogenic treponemes that can be difficult to distinguish

[1]Bowen V, Su J, Torrone E, Kidd S, Weinstock H. Increase in incidence of congenital syphilis—United States, 2012–2014. *MMWR Morb Mortal Wkly Rep.* 2015;64(44):1241–1245

from *T pallidum* by darkfield microscopy. Although such testing can provide a definitive diagnosis, serologic testing also is necessary.

Presumptive diagnosis requires the use of both nontreponemal and treponemal serologic tests. Nontreponemal tests for syphilis include the Venereal Disease Research Laboratory (VDRL) slide test and the rapid plasma reagin (RPR) test. These tests are inexpensive, are performed rapidly, and provide semiquantitative results through serial twofold dilutions that can help define disease activity and monitor response to therapy. However, nontreponemal test results may be falsely negative (ie, nonreactive) in early primary syphilis, latent acquired syphilis of long duration, and late congenital syphilis. Occasionally, a nontreponemal test performed on serum samples containing high concentrations of antibody against *T pallidum* will be weakly reactive or falsely negative, a reaction termed the prozone phenomenon; diluting serum results in a positive test. RPR titers generally are higher than VDRL titers; therefore, when nontreponemal tests are used to monitor treatment response, the same test must be used throughout the follow-up period, preferably performed by the same laboratory, to ensure comparability of results.

A reactive nontreponemal test result from a patient with typical lesions indicates a presumptive diagnosis of syphilis but must be confirmed by one of the specific treponemal tests to exclude a false-positive test result. False-positive nontreponemal results can be caused by certain viral infections (eg, Epstein-Barr virus infection, hepatitis, varicella, measles), lymphoma, tuberculosis, malaria, endocarditis, connective tissue disease, pregnancy, abuse of injection drugs, laboratory or technical error, or Wharton jelly contamination when umbilical cord blood specimens are used. Treatment should not be delayed while awaiting the results of the treponemal test results if the patient is symptomatic or at high risk of infection. A sustained fourfold or greater decrease in titer, equivalent to a change of 2 dilutions (eg, from 1:32 to 1:8), of the nontreponemal test result after treatment usually demonstrates adequate therapy, whereas a sustained fourfold or greater increase in titer (eg, from 1:8 to 1:32) after treatment suggests reinfection or relapse. The nontreponemal test titer usually decreases fourfold within 6 to 12 months after therapy for primary or secondary syphilis and usually becomes nonreactive within 1 year after successful therapy if the infection (primary or secondary syphilis) was treated early. The patient usually becomes seronegative within 2 years even if the initial titer was high or the infection was congenital. Some people will continue to have low stable nontreponemal antibody titers (eg, VDRL titer 1:2 or less, RPR titer 1:4 or less) despite effective therapy. This serofast state is more common in patients treated for latent or tertiary syphilis.

Treponemal tests in use include the *T pallidum* particle agglutination (TP-PA) test, *T pallidum* enzyme immunoassay (TP-EIA), *T pallidum* chemiluminescent assay (TP-CIA), and fluorescent treponemal antibody absorption (FTA-ABS) test. Most people who have reactive treponemal test results remain reactive for life, even after successful therapy. However, 15% to 25% of patients treated during the primary stage revert to being serologically nonreactive on treponemal testing after 2 to 3 years. Treponemal tests also are not 100% specific for syphilis; positive reactions occur variably in patients with other spirochetal diseases, such as yaws, pinta, leptospirosis, rat-bite fever, relapsing fever, and Lyme disease. Nontreponemal tests can be used to differentiate Lyme disease from syphilis, because the VDRL test is nonreactive in Lyme disease.

In most cases, if a patient has a positive RPR or VDRL in low titer and has a negative treponemal test result, the nontreponemal antibody test result will be a false positive. However, in patients with early syphilis, the nontreponemal test may become positive before the treponemal test. Therefore, retesting in 2 to 4 weeks and again later if clinically indicated should be considered in persons at increased risk for syphilis, including pregnant women.

The Centers for Disease Control and Prevention (CDC)[1] and the US Preventive Services Task Force (USPSTF)[2] recommend syphilis serologic screening with a nontreponemal test to identify people with possible untreated infection; this screening is followed by confirmation using one of the several available treponemal tests ("conventional diagnostic" approach). However, because of cost issues, some clinical laboratories and blood banks have begun to screen samples using treponemal tests (eg, TP-EIA or TP-CIA) first rather than beginning with a nontreponemal test. This "reverse-sequence screening" approach can be associated with high rates of false-positive results, especially in low-prevalence populations. When the reverse-sequence algorithm is used, people with a positive TP-EIA/TP-CIA result and a negative nontreponemal test result (discordant result) should have a second treponemal test targeting a different *T pallidum* antigen performed to confirm the results of the original test. If the second treponemal test result is negative and the person is at low risk for syphilis, the original treponemal test result likely was a false positive.

All patients who have syphilis should be tested for HIV infection and other sexually transmitted infections (STIs). Point-of-care syphilis tests have been developed, primarily for use in adults in the developing world (**http://apps.who.int/iris/bitstream/ 10665/43590/1/TDR_SDI_06.1_eng.pdf**).

Cerebrospinal Fluid Tests. Cerebrospinal fluid (CSF) abnormalities in patients with neurosyphilis can include increased protein concentration, increased white blood cell (WBC) count, and/or a reactive CSF-VDRL test result. Outside the neonatal period, the CSF-VDRL is highly specific but is insensitive; therefore, a negative CSF-VDRL result does not exclude a diagnosis of neurosyphilis. Conversely, a reactive CSF-VDRL test in a neonate can be the result of nontreponemal IgG antibodies that cross the blood-brain barrier. The CSF leukocyte count usually is elevated in neurosyphilis (>5 WBCs/mm^3). CSF cell counts as high as 25 WBCs/mm^3 and/or protein concentration up to 150 mg/dL may occur among normal, noninfected term neonates and can be even higher in preterm neonates; however, lower values (ie, 5 WBCs/mm^3 and protein of 40 mg/dL) should be considered the upper limits of normal when assessing a term infant for congenital syphilis. A positive CSF FTA-ABS result can support the diagnosis of neurosyphilis but by itself cannot establish the diagnosis. Fewer data exist for the TP-PA or RPR test for CSF, and these tests should not be used for CSF evaluation.

Testing During Pregnancy. Prevention of congenital syphilis depends on the identification and adequate treatment of pregnant women with syphilis. All women should be screened serologically for syphilis early in pregnancy. False-negative test results are possible in recent infection, and syphilis may be acquired later in pregnancy. Therefore, in communities and populations in which the prevalence of syphilis is high, and for women at high risk for infection, serologic testing also should be performed at 28 to 32 weeks' gestation and again at delivery. A nontreponemal test (RPR or VDRL) is recommended for

---

[1]Centers for Disease Control and Prevention. Sexually transmitted diseases treatment guidelines, 2015. *MMWR Recomm Rep.* 2015;64(RR-3):34–51

[2]US Preventive Services Task Force. Screening for syphilis infection in non-pregnant adults and adolescents. *JAMA.* 2016;315(21):2321–2327

screening, followed by a treponemal test if the screening result is positive. In most cases, if the treponemal antibody test result is negative, the nontreponemal test result is falsely positive and no further evaluation is necessary. However, retesting in 2 to 4 weeks, and again later if clinically indicated, should be considered for pregnant women who are at high risk of syphilis.

If the reverse-sequence screening algorithm is used, pregnant women with reactive treponemal EIA/CIA screening test results should have confirmatory testing with a quantitative nontreponemal test. If the nontreponemal test result is negative (discordant result), a second treponemal test using a different *T pallidum* antigen should be obtained to determine whether the initial treponemal test result was a false positive. If the second treponemal test result is positive, it may be attributable to a prior infection adequately treated in the past or to untreated syphilis in a late stage.

For women treated for syphilis during pregnancy, follow-up nontreponemal serologic testing is necessary to assess the effectiveness of therapy. Treated pregnant women with syphilis should have quantitative nontreponemal serologic tests repeated at 28 to 32 weeks of gestation, at delivery, and according to recommendations for the stage of disease. Serologic titers may be repeated monthly in women at high risk of reinfection or in geographic areas where the prevalence of syphilis is high.

Sonographic evaluation of the fetus should be performed when syphilis is diagnosed during the second half of pregnancy. Pathologic examination of the placenta and/or umbilical cord at delivery also should be performed. Any woman who delivers a stillborn infant after 20 weeks' gestation should be tested for syphilis.

Evaluation of Infants for Congenital Infection During the Newborn Period to 1 Month of Age. No newborn infant should be discharged from the hospital without determination of the mother's serologic status for syphilis. All infants born to seropositive mothers require a careful examination and a nontreponemal test obtained from the infant. The test performed on the infant should be the same as that performed on the mother to enable comparison of titer results. A negative maternal RPR or VDRL test result at delivery does not rule out the possibility of the infant having congenital syphilis, although such a situation is rare. The diagnostic approach to infants being evaluated for congenital syphilis is presented in Fig 3.10 (p 781), with treatment recommendations provided in Table 3.76 (p 782). Other causes of elevated CSF laboratory values should be considered when an infant is being evaluated for congenital syphilis. Infants born to mothers who have syphilis and HIV infection do not require different evaluation, therapy, or follow-up for syphilis than is recommended for all infants.[1]

Evaluation of Infants >1 Month of Age and Children. Infants and children identified as having reactive serologic tests for syphilis should have maternal serologic test results and records reviewed to assess whether they have congenital or acquired syphilis. The recommended evaluation for congenital syphilis includes a CSF examination plus other tests as clinically indicated. CSF examination also should be performed in patients with neurologic or

---

[1]Guidelines for prevention and treatment of opportunistic infections in HIV-exposed and HIV-infected children. Recommendations from the National Institutes of Health, Centers for Disease Control and Prevention, the HIV Medicine Association of the Infectious Diseases Society of America, the Pediatric Infectious Diseases Society, and the American Academy of Pediatrics. *Pediatr Infect Dis J.* 2013;32(Suppl 2):i-KK4. Available at: **http://aidsinfo.nih.gov/guidelines/html/5/pediatric-oi-prevention-and-treatment-guidelines/0**

FIG 3.10. ALGORITHM FOR DIAGNOSTIC APPROACH OF INFANTS BORN TO MOTHERS WITH REACTIVE SEROLOGIC TESTS FOR SYPHILIS.

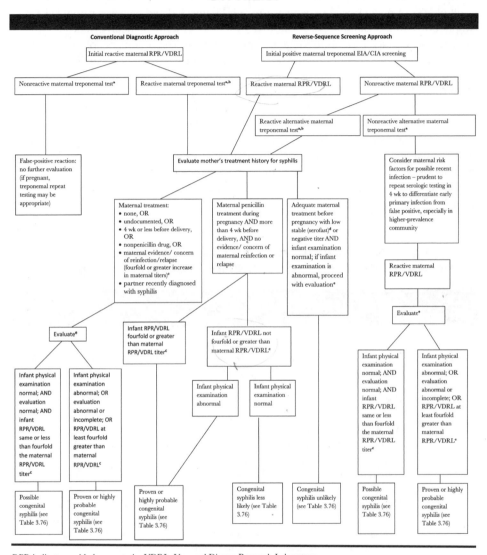

RPR indicates rapid plasma reagin; VDRL, Venereal Disease Research Laboratory.

[a] *Treponema pallidum* particle agglutination (TP-PA) (which is the preferred treponemal test), fluorescent treponemal antibody absorption (FTA-ABS), or microhemagglutination test for antibodies to *T pallidum* (MHA-TP).

[b] Test for human immunodeficiency virus (HIV) antibody. Infants of HIV-infected mothers do not require different evaluation or treatment for syphilis.

[c] A fourfold change in titer is the same as a change of 2 dilutions. For example, a titer of 1:64 is fourfold greater than a titer of 1:16, and a titer of 1:4 is fourfold lower than a titer of 1:16. When comparing titers, the same type of nontreponemal test should be used (eg, if the initial test was an RPR, the follow-up test should also be an RPR).

[d] Stable VDRL titers 1:2 or less or RPR 1:4 or less beyond 1 year after successful treatment are considered low serofast.

[e] Complete blood cell (CBC) and platelet count; cerebrospinal fluid (CSF) examination for cell count, protein, and quantitative VDRL; other tests as clinically indicated (eg, chest radiographs, long-bone radiographs, eye examination, liver function tests, neuroimaging, and auditory brainstem response).

ophthalmic signs or symptoms (eg, iritis, uveitis), evidence of active tertiary syphilis (eg, aortitis, gumma), or treatment failure. Some experts recommend performing a CSF examination on all patients who have latent syphilis and a nontreponemal serologic test result of 1:32 or greater or in patients who are HIV infected and have a serum CD4+ T-lymphocyte count of 350 or less, because the risk of asymptomatic neurosyphilis in these circumstances is increased approximately threefold. However, among people with HIV infection and syphilis, CSF examination has not been associated with improved clinical outcomes in the absence of neurologic signs and symptoms.

TREATMENT[1]: Parenteral penicillin G remains the preferred drug for treatment of syphilis at any stage. Recommendations for penicillin G use and duration of therapy vary, depending on the stage of disease and clinical manifestations. Parenteral penicillin G is the only documented effective therapy for patients who have neurosyphilis, congenital syphilis, or syphilis during pregnancy and is recommended for people with HIV infection.

Penicillin Allergy. Infants and children with a history of penicillin allergy or who develop presumed penicillin allergy during treatment should be desensitized and then treated with penicillin whenever possible.

Table 3.76. Evaluation and Treatment of Infants With Possible, Probable, or Confirmed Congenital Syphilis

Category	Findings	Recommended Evaluation	Treatment
Proven or highly probable congenital syphilis	Abnormal physical examination consistent with congenital syphilis	CSF analysis (CSF VDRL, cell count, and protein)	Aqueous crystalline penicillin G, 50 000 U/kg, IV, every 12 hours (1 wk or younger), then every 8 h for infants older than 1 wk, for a total of 10 days of therapy[a] (**preferred**)
	OR	CBC count with differential and platelet count	
	A serum quantitative nontreponemal serologic titer that is fourfold higher than the mother's titer	Other tests (as clinically indicated): Long-bone radiography Chest radiography Transaminases Neuroimaging	OR
	OR		Procaine penicillin G, 50 000 U/kg, IM, as single daily dose for 10 days
	A positive result of darkfield test or PCR assay of lesions or body fluid(s)	Ophthalmologic examination Auditory brain stem response	

[1]Centers for Disease Control and Prevention. Sexually transmitted diseases treatment guidelines, 2015. *MMWR Recomm Rep.* 2015;64(RR-3):34–51

Table 3.76. Evaluation and Treatment of Infants With Possible, Probable, or Confirmed Congenital Syphilis, continued

Category	Findings	Recommended Evaluation	Treatment
Possible congenital syphilis	Normal infant examination AND A serum quantitative nontreponemal serologic titer equal to or less than fourfold the maternal titer AND ONE OF THE FOLLOWING: Mother was not treated, was inadequately treated, or had no documentation of receiving treatment; OR Mother was treated with erythromycin or a regimen other than those recommended in the guideline (ie, a nonpenicillin regimen) OR Mother received recommended treatment <4 wk before delivery	CSF analysis (CSF VDRL, CBC count, and protein) CBC count with differential and platelet count Long-bone radiography These evaluations may not be necessary if 10 days of parenteral therapy is administered	Aqueous crystalline penicillin G, 50 000 U/kg, IV, every 12 h (1 wk or younger), then every 8 h for infants older than 1 wk, for a total of 10 days of therapy[a] (**preferred**) OR Procaine penicillin G, 50 000 U/kg, IM, as single daily dose for 10 days OR Benzathine penicillin G, 50 000 U/kg, IM, single dose (recommended by some experts, but **only** if all components of the evaluation are obtained and are normal, including normal CSF results[b] and follow-up is certain (some experts)

Table 3.76. Evaluation and Treatment of Infants With Possible, Probable, or Confirmed Congenital Syphilis, continued

Category	Findings	Recommended Evaluation	Treatment
Congenital syphilis less likely	Normal infant examination AND A serum quantitative nontreponemal serologic titer equal to or less than fourfold the maternal titer AND Mother was treated during pregnancy, treatment was appropriate for stage of infection, and treatment was administered >4 wk before delivery AND Mother has no evidence of reinfection or relapse	Not recommended	Benzathine penicillin G, 50 000 U/kg, IM, single dose (**preferred**) Alternatively, infants whose mother's nontreponemal titers decreased at least fourfold after appropriate therapy for early syphilis or remained stable at low titer (eg, VDRL ≤1:2; RPR ≤1:4) may be followed every 2–3 mo without treatment until the nontreponemal test becomes nonreactive Nontreponemal antibody titers should decrease by 3 mo of age and should be nonreactive by 6 mo of age whether the infant was infected and adequately treated or was not infected and initially seropositive because of transplacentally acquired maternal antibody. Patients with increasing titers or with persistent stable titers 6 to 12 mo after initial treatment should be reevaluated, including a CSF examination, and treated with a 10-day course of parenteral penicillin G, even if they were treated previously.

Table 3.76. Evaluation and Treatment of Infants With Possible, Probable, or Confirmed Congenital Syphilis, continued

Category	Findings	Recommended Evaluation	Treatment
Congenital syphilis is unlikely	Normal infant examination AND A serum quantitative nontreponemal serologic titer equal to or less than fourfold the maternal titer AND Mother was treated adequately before pregnancy AND Mother's nontreponemal serologic titer remained low and stable (ie, serofast) before and during pregnancy and at delivery (eg, VDRL ≤1:2; RPR ≤1:4)	Not recommended	No treatment required, but infants with reactive nontreponemal tests should be followed serologically to ensure test result returns to negative Benzathine penicillin G, 50 000 U/kg, IM, single dose can be considered if follow-up is uncertain and infant has a reactive test (some experts) Neonates with a negative nontreponemal test result at birth and whose mothers were seroreactive at delivery should be retested at 3 mo to rule out serologically negative incubating congenital syphilis at the time of birth

PCR indicates polymerase chain reaction; CSF, cerebrospinal fluid; CBC, complete blood cell count; VDRL, Venereal Disease Research Laboratory; IV, intravenously; IM, intramuscularly; RPR, rapid plasma reagin,

Adapted and modified from Centers for Disease Control and Prevention. Sexually transmitted diseases treatment guidelines, 2015. *MMWR Recomm Rep.* 2015;64(RR-3):45–47.

[a]If 24 hours or more of therapy is missed, the entire course must be restarted.

[b]If CSF is not obtained or uninterpretable (eg, bloody tap), a 10-day course is recommended.

Congenital Syphilis: Newborn Period to 1 Month of Age. The management of congenital syphilis is based on whether the infant has proven or probable congenital syphilis, has possible congenital syphilis, or is considered less likely or unlikely to have syphilis. The treatment of infants with congenital syphilis is detailed in Table 3.76 (p 782), with the diagnostic approach to such infants presented in Fig 3.10. If more than 1 day of therapy is missed, the entire course should be restarted. Data supporting use of other antimicrobial agents (eg, ampicillin) for treatment of congenital syphilis are not available. When possible, a full 10-day course of penicillin is preferred, even if ampicillin initially was provided for possible sepsis. Use of agents other than penicillin requires close serologic follow-up to assess adequacy of therapy.

Congenital Syphilis: Infants ≥1 Month of Age and Children. Infants older than 1 month who possibly have congenital syphilis should be treated with intravenous aqueous crystalline penicillin (200 000–300 000 U/kg/day, intravenously, administered as 50 000 U/kg, every 4–6 hours for 10 days). This regimen also should be used to treat children older than 2 years who have late and previously untreated congenital syphilis. Some experts suggest giving such patients a single dose of penicillin G benzathine (50 000 U/kg, intramuscularly, not to exceed 2.4 million U) after the 10-day course of intravenous aqueous crystalline penicillin. If the patient has no clinical manifestations of disease, the CSF examination is normal, and the result of the CSF-VDRL test is negative, some experts would treat with 3 weekly doses of penicillin G benzathine (50 000 U/kg, intramuscularly, not to exceed 2.4 million U).

Syphilis in Pregnancy. Regardless of stage of pregnancy, women should be treated with penicillin according to the dosage schedules appropriate for the stage of syphilis as recommended for nonpregnant patients (see Table 3.77, p 784). For penicillin-allergic patients, no proven alternative therapy has been established. A pregnant woman with a history of penicillin allergy should have skin testing, if available, to evaluate for true allergy, and should be treated with penicillin if allergy is not confirmed; if allergy is confirmed, the woman should undergo desensitization followed by treatment with penicillin. Erythromycin, azithromycin, or any other nonpenicillin treatment of syphilis during pregnancy cannot be considered reliable to cure infection in the fetus. Tetracycline is not recommended for pregnant women because of potential adverse effects on the fetus.

Early Acquired Syphilis (Primary, Secondary, Early Latent Syphilis). A single intramuscular dose of penicillin G benzathine is the preferred treatment for children and adults (see Table 3.77).

For nonpregnant patients who are allergic to penicillin, doxycycline or (if ≥8 years of age) tetracycline should be given for 14 days. Clinical studies (along with biologic and pharmacologic considerations) suggest that ceftriaxone at 1 g, once daily, either intramuscularly or intravenously, for 10 to 14 days (for adolescents and adults) is effective for early-acquired syphilis, but the optimal dose and duration of therapy have not been defined. Single-dose therapy with ceftriaxone is not effective. Azithromycin can be effective as a single oral dose of 2 g; however, azithromycin treatment failures have been reported, and resistance to azithromycin has been documented. Close follow-up of people receiving any alternative therapy is essential. When follow-up cannot be ensured, especially for children younger than 8 years, consideration must be given to hospitalization and desensitization followed by administration of penicillin G.

Syphilis of More Than 1 Year's Duration (Late Latent Syphilis and Late Syphilis). Penicillin G benzathine should be administered intramuscularly, weekly, for 3 successive weeks (see Table 3.77, p 784). In patients who are allergic to penicillin, tetracycline or doxycycline (both if ≥8 years of age) for 4 weeks should be given only with close serologic and clinical follow-up. Doxycycline can be used for short durations (ie, 21 days or less) without regard to patient age, but for the longer treatment durations required for treatment of late latent and late syphilis, doxycycline is not recommended for children younger than 8 years (see Tetracyclines, p 905). Limited clinical studies suggest that ceftriaxone might be effective, but the optimal dose and duration have not been defined.

Table 3.77. Recommended Treatment for Syphilis in People Older Than 1 Month

Status	Children	Adults
Primary, secondary, and early latent syphilis[a]	Penicillin G benzathine,[b] 50 000 U/kg, IM, up to the adult dose of 2.4 million U in a single dose	Penicillin G benzathine, 2.4 million U, IM, in a single dose **OR** *If allergic to penicillin and not pregnant,* Doxycycline, 100 mg, orally, twice a day for 14 days **OR** Tetracycline, 500 mg, orally, 4 times/day for 14 days (≥8 y only)
Late latent syphilis[c]	Penicillin G benzathine, 50 000 U/kg, IM, up to the adult dose of 2.4 million U, administered as 3 single doses at 1-wk intervals (total 150 000 U/kg, up to the adult dose of 7.2 million U)	Penicillin G benzathine, 7.2 million U total, administered as 3 doses of 2.4 million U, IM, each at 1-wk intervals **OR** *If allergic to penicillin and not pregnant,* Doxycycline, 100 mg, orally, twice a day for 4 wk (≥8 y only) **OR** Tetracycline, 500 mg, orally, 4 times/day for 4 wk (≥8 y only)
Tertiary	...	Penicillin G benzathine, 7.2 million U total, administered as 3 doses of 2.4 million U, IM, at 1-wk intervals *If allergic to penicillin and not pregnant, consult an infectious diseases expert*
Neurosyphilis[d]	Aqueous crystalline penicillin G, 200 000–300 000 U/kg/day, IV, administered as 50 000 U/kg every 4–6 h for 10–14 days, in doses not to exceed the adult dose	Aqueous crystalline penicillin G, 18–24 million U per day, administered as 3–4 million U, IV, every 4 h for 10–14 days[e] **OR** Penicillin G procaine,[e] 2.4 million U, IM, once daily **PLUS** probenecid, 500 mg, orally, 4 times/day, both for 10–14 days[e]

IV indicates intravenously; IM, intramuscularly.
[a]Early latent syphilis is defined as being acquired within the preceding year.
[b]Penicillin G benzathine and penicillin G procaine are approved for intramuscular administration only.
[c]Late latent syphilis is defined as syphilis beyond 1 year's duration.
[d]Patients who are allergic to penicillin should be desensitized.
[e]Some experts administer penicillin G benzathine, 2.4 million U, IM, once per week for up to 3 weeks after completion of these neurosyphilis treatment regimens.

Neurosyphilis. For children, intravenous aqueous crystalline penicillin G for 10 to 14 days is recommended. Some experts recommend additional subsequent therapy with intramuscular penicillin G benzathine, 50 000 U/kg per dose (not to exceed 2.4 million U), for up to 3 single weekly doses (see Table 3.77). A patient with a history of penicillin allergy should have skin testing to evaluate for true allergy and treated with penicillin if allergy is not confirmed; if allergy is confirmed, the patient should undergo desensitization followed by treatment with penicillin.

Other Considerations.

- Mothers of infants with congenital syphilis should be tested for other STIs, including *Neisseria gonorrhoeae, Chlamydia trachomatis,* HIV, and hepatitis B. If injection drug use is suspected, the mother also may be at risk of hepatitis C virus infection.
- All patients with syphilis should be tested for other STIs, including *N gonorrhoeae, C trachomatis,* HIV, and hepatitis B. Patients who have primary syphilis should be retested for HIV after 3 months if the first HIV test result is negative. Immunization status for hepatitis B and human papillomavirus (HPV) should be reviewed and vaccines should be administered if not up to date.
- For people with HIV infection and syphilis, careful follow-up is essential. People with HIV infection who have early syphilis may be at increased risk of neurologic complications and higher rates of treatment failure with currently recommended regimens.[1]
- All recent sexual contacts of people with acquired syphilis should be evaluated for other STIs as well as syphilis (see Control Measures, p 788). Partners who were exposed within 90 days preceding the diagnosis of primary, secondary, or early latent syphilis in the index patient should be treated presumptively for syphilis, even if they are seronegative.
- Children with acquired primary, secondary, or latent syphilis should be evaluated for possible sexual assault or abuse.

Follow-up and Management.

Congenital Syphilis. All infants who have reactive serologic tests for syphilis or were born to mothers who were seroreactive at delivery should receive careful follow-up evaluations during regularly scheduled well-child care visits at 2, 4, 6, and 12 months of age. Serologic nontreponemal tests should be performed every 2 to 3 months until the nontreponemal test becomes nonreactive. Nontreponemal antibody titers should decrease by 3 months of age and should be nonreactive by 6 months of age, whether the infant was infected and adequately treated or was not infected and initially seropositive because of transplacentally acquired maternal antibody. The serologic response after therapy may be slower for infants treated after the neonatal period. Patients with increasing titers or with persistent stable titers 6 to 12 months after initial treatment should be reevaluated, including a CSF examination, and treated with a 10-day course of parenteral penicillin G, even if they were treated previously. Neonates with a negative nontreponemal test at birth whose mothers were seroreactive at delivery should be retested at 3 months to rule out seronegative incubating congenital syphilis.

Treponemal tests should not be used to evaluate treatment response, because results for an infected child can remain positive despite effective therapy. Passively transferred

---

[1]Guidelines for prevention and treatment of opportunistic infections in HIV-exposed and HIV-infected children. Recommendations from the National Institutes of Health, Centers for Disease Control and Prevention, the HIV Medicine Association of the Infectious Diseases Society of America, the Pediatric Infectious Diseases Society, and the American Academy of Pediatrics. *Pediatr Infect Dis J.* 2013;32(Suppl 2):i-KK4. Available at: **http://aidsinfo.nih.gov/guidelines/html/5/pediatric-oi-prevention-and-treatment-guidelines/0**

maternal treponemal antibodies can persist in an infant until 15 months of age. A reactive treponemal test after 18 months of age is diagnostic of congenital syphilis. If the nontreponemal test is nonreactive at this time, no further evaluation or treatment is necessary. If the nontreponemal test is reactive at 18 months of age, the infant should be evaluated (or reevaluated) fully and treated for congenital syphilis.

Treated infants with congenital neurosyphilis should undergo repeated clinical evaluation and CSF examination at 6-month intervals until their CSF examination is normal. A reactive CSF VDRL test or abnormal CSF indices that cannot be attributed to another ongoing illness at the 6-month interval are indications for retreatment. Neuroimaging studies, such as magnetic resonance imaging, should be considered in these children.

Acquired Syphilis. People with acquired syphilis should have clinical and serologic evaluations following treatment to evaluate for persistence or recurrence of symptoms or an inadequate serologic response following therapy. People with primary or secondary syphilis should have clinical and serologic evaluations performed at 6 and 12 months after treatment. If signs or symptoms persist or recur, or a fourfold or greater increase in nontreponemal titers occurs, treatment failure or reinfection may be responsible. CSF analysis, HIV testing, and retreatment based on CSF findings are indicated. Failure of nontreponemal titers to decline fourfold within 6 to 12 months may also indicate treatment failure.

Following treatment, people with latent syphilis should experience a fourfold or greater decline in nontreponemal titers within 12 to 24 months. If titers increase at least fourfold or initial high titers fail to fall fourfold, or symptoms of syphilis develop, reevaluation, including a CSF examination, is warranted. Additional guidance can be found in the current CDC guidelines for the management of sexually transmitted diseases.[1]

In all these instances, retreatment should be performed with 3 weekly injections of penicillin G benzathine, 50 000 U/kg up to the adult dose of 2.4 million U, intramuscularly, unless CSF examination indicates that neurosyphilis is present, at which time treatment for neurosyphilis should be initiated. Retreated patients should be treated with the schedules recommended for patients with syphilis for more than 1 year, and only 1 retreatment course is indicated. The possibility of reinfection or concurrent HIV infection should always be considered when retreating patients with early syphilis, and repeat HIV testing should be performed in such cases.

Patients with neurosyphilis associated with acquired syphilis must have periodic serologic testing, clinical evaluation at 6-month intervals, and repeat CSF examinations. If the CSF white blood cell count has not decreased after 6 months or if the CSF white blood cell count or protein concentration is not normal after 2 years, retreatment should be considered. CSF abnormalities may persist for extended periods of time in people with HIV infection with neurosyphilis. Close follow-up is warranted.

ISOLATION OF THE HOSPITALIZED PATIENT: Standard precautions are recommended for all patients, including infants with suspected or proven congenital syphilis. Because moist open lesions, secretions, and possibly blood are contagious in all patients with syphilis, gloves should be worn when caring for patients with congenital, primary, and secondary syphilis with skin and mucous membrane lesions until 24 hours of treatment has been completed.

---

[1]Centers for Disease Control and Prevention. Sexually transmitted diseases treatment guidelines, 2015. *MMWR Recomm Rep.* 2015;64(RR-3):34–51

CONTROL MEASURES:

- Effective prevention of congenital syphilis is predicated on identification and appropriate treatment of pregnant women with syphilis.
- Education of patients and populations about STIs, treatment of sexual contacts, reporting of each case to local public health authorities for contact investigation and appropriate follow-up, and serologic screening of high-risk populations are indicated.
- All recent sexual contacts of a person with acquired syphilis should be identified, examined, serologically tested, and treated appropriately. Sexual contacts of people with primary, secondary, or early latent syphilis who were exposed within the preceding 90 days may be infected even if seronegative and should be treated for early-acquired syphilis. People exposed more than 90 days previously should be treated presumptively if serologic test results are not available immediately and follow-up is uncertain. For identification of at-risk sexual partners, the periods before treatment are as follows: (1) 3 months plus duration of symptoms for primary syphilis; (2) 6 months plus duration of symptoms for secondary syphilis; and (3) 1 year for early latent syphilis.
- All people, including hospital personnel, who have had close unprotected contact with a patient with early congenital syphilis before identification of the disease or during the first 24 hours of therapy should be examined clinically for the presence of lesions 2 to 3 weeks after contact. Serologic testing should be performed and repeated 3 months after contact or sooner if symptoms occur. If the degree of exposure is considered substantial, immediate treatment should be considered.

Tapeworm Diseases

(Taeniasis and Cysticercosis)

CLINICAL MANIFESTATIONS:

Taeniasis. Infection with adult tapeworms often is asymptomatic; however, mild gastrointestinal tract symptoms, such as nausea, diarrhea, and pain, can occur. Tapeworm segments can be seen migrating from the anus or in feces.

Cysticercosis. In contrast, cysticercosis caused by larval pork tapeworm (*Taenia solium*) infection can have serious consequences. Manifestations depend on the location and number of pork tapeworm larval cysts (cysticerci) and on the host response. Cysticerci may be found anywhere in the body. The most common and serious manifestations are caused by cysticerci in the central nervous system. Larval cysts of *T solium* in the brain (neurocysticercosis) can cause seizures, obstructive hydrocephalus, and other neurologic signs and symptoms. Neurocysticercosis is the leading infectious cause of epilepsy in the developing world. The host reaction to degenerating cysticerci can produce signs and symptoms of meningitis or stroke. Cysts in the spinal column can cause gait disturbance, pain, or transverse myelitis. Subcutaneous cysticerci produce palpable nodules, and ocular involvement can cause visual impairment.

ETIOLOGY: Taeniasis is caused by intestinal infection by the adult tapeworm, *Taenia saginata* (beef tapeworm) or *T solium* (pork tapeworm). *Taenia asiatica* causes taeniasis in Asia. Human cysticercosis is caused only by the larvae of *T solium (Cysticercus cellulosae)*.

EPIDEMIOLOGY: These tapeworm diseases have worldwide distribution. Prevalence is high in areas with poor sanitation and human fecal contamination in areas where cattle graze or swine are fed. Most cases of *T solium* infection in the United States are imported from Latin America or Asia, although the disease is prevalent in sub-Saharan Africa as well. High rates of *T saginata* infection occur in Mexico, parts of South America, East Africa, and central Europe. *T asiatica* is common in China, Taiwan, and Southeast Asia. Taeniasis is acquired by eating undercooked beef *(T saginata)*, pork *(T solium)*, or pig viscera *(T asiatica)* that contain encysted larvae.

Cysticercosis in humans is acquired by ingesting eggs of the pork tapeworm *(T solium)* through direct fecal-oral contact with a person harboring the adult tapeworm or through ingestion of fecally contaminated food. Autoinfection is possible. Eggs are found only in human feces, because humans are the obligate definitive host. Eggs liberate oncospheres in the intestine that migrate through the blood and lymphatics to tissues throughout the body, including the central nervous system, where the oncospheres develop into cysticerci. Although most cases of cysticercosis in the United States have been imported, cysticercosis can be acquired in the United States from tapeworm carriers who emigrated from an area with endemic infection and still have *T solium* intestinal-stage infection. *T saginata* and *T asiatica* do not cause cysticercosis.

The **incubation period** for taeniasis (the time from ingestion of the larvae until segments are passed in the feces) is 2 to 3 months. For cysticercosis, the time between infection and onset of symptoms may be several years.

DIAGNOSIS: Diagnosis of taeniasis (adult tapeworm infection) is based on demonstration of the proglottids or ova in feces or the perianal region. However, these techniques are insensitive. Species identification of the parasite is based on the different structures of gravid proglottids and scolex.

Diagnosis of neurocysticercosis typically depends on clinical presentation and imaging of the central nervous system. Serologic testing is also helpful in certain cases. Computed tomography (CT) scanning or magnetic resonance imaging (MRI) of the brain or spinal cord are used to demonstrate lesions compatible with cysticerci. CT scans are helpful in identifying calcifications. MRI is better at identifying extraparenchymal cysts (eg, in ventricles or the subarachnoid space). Antibody assays that detect specific antibodies to larval *T solium* in serum and cerebrospinal fluid (CSF) are useful to confirm the diagnosis and are required in the absence of the identification of a scolex on imaging. Antibody tests can have limited sensitivity if only one cysticercus or only calcified cysticerci are present. In the United States, antibody tests are available through the Centers for Disease Control and Prevention and a few commercial laboratories. In general, antibody tests are more sensitive with serum specimens than with CSF specimens. Serum antibody assay results often are negative in children with solitary parenchymal lesions but usually are positive in patients with multiple lesions. A negative serologic test does not exclude the diagnosis of neurocysticercosis when the clinical suspicion is high. A serologic test could be positive in patients from highly endemic areas and do not have neurocysticercosis.

TREATMENT:
Taeniasis. Praziquantel is highly effective for eradicating infection with the adult tapeworm (see Drugs for Parasitic Infections, p 985). Praziquantel is not approved for this indication, but dosing recommendations are available for children 4 years and older. Niclosamide is not approved for treatment of *T solium* infection but is approved for treatment of *T saginata* infection. However, niclosamide is not available commercially in the United States.

Cysticercosis. Neurocysticercosis treatment should be individualized on the basis of the number, location, and viability of cysticerci as assessed by neuroimaging studies (MRI or CT scan) and the clinical manifestations. Management generally is aimed at symptoms and should include antiseizure medications for patients with seizures and surgery for patients with hydrocephalus. Two antiparasitic drugs—albendazole and praziquantel—are available (see Drugs for Parasitic Infections, p 985). Praziquantel is not approved for this indication, but dosing recommendations are available for children 4 years and older. Although both drugs are cysticercidal and hasten radiologic resolution of cysts, symptoms result from the host inflammatory response and may be exacerbated by treatment. Although not all symptomatic patients with a single cyst within brain parenchyma require antiparasitic medication, controlled studies demonstrate that clinical resolution and seizure recurrence rates are improved with albendazole. Two studies have demonstrated that in those with more than 2 lesions, the response rate was better when albendazole was coadministered with praziquantel and corticosteroids. When a single agent is used, albendazole is preferred over praziquantel because it has fewer drug-drug interactions with anticonvulsants and steroids. Cyst stage is important when considering whether or not to treat with an antiparasitic medication. Patients with viable and colloidal (early degenerating/inflamed) cysts may benefit from an antiparasitic medication. Patients with granular and calcified cysts do not benefit from antiparasitic treatment. Coadministration of corticosteroids during antiparasitic therapy may decrease adverse effects during treatment and is required for some forms of the disease (eg, basilar or subarachnoid, extensive parenchymal, or spinal involvement). Duration of corticosteroid therapy is longer in patients with subarachnoid disease, vasculitis, or encephalitis. Arachnoiditis, vasculitis, or diffuse cerebral edema (cysticercal encephalitis) are treated with corticosteroid therapy until the cerebral edema is controlled. Corticosteroids can affect the tissue concentrations of albendazole. Patients requiring prolonged steroids may need to be screened for strongyloidiasis, latent tuberculosis, and vitamin D deficiency.

The medical and surgical management of cysticercosis can be highly complex and often needs to be conducted in consultation with a neurologist or neurosurgeon and an infectious diseases or tropical medicine expert with experience treating neurocysticercosis. Seizures may recur for months or years. Anticonvulsant therapy is recommended until there is neuroradiologic evidence of resolution and seizures have not occurred for 6 months (for a single lesion) or 1 to 2 years (for multiple lesions). Calcification of cysts may require prolonged or indefinite use of anticonvulsants. Subarachnoid cysticercosis does not respond well to the regimens used for parenchymal disease and generally should be treated with prolonged courses of corticosteroids and antiparasitic drugs. Intraventricular cysticerci and hydrocephalus usually require surgical therapy. Intraventricular cysticerci often can be removed by endoscopic surgery, which is the treatment of choice. If cysticerci cannot be removed easily, hydrocephalus should be corrected with placement of intraventricular shunts. Adjunctive chemotherapy with antiparasitic agents and corticosteroids may decrease the rate of subsequent shunt failure. Ocular cysticercosis is treated by surgical excision of the cysticerci. Ocular cysticercosis generally is not treated with anthelmintic drugs, which can exacerbate inflammation. An ophthalmic examination should be performed before treatment to rule out intraocular cysticerci. Spinal cysticercosis may be treated with medical and/or surgical therapy. There is not adequate evidence to guide the choice of medical versus surgical therapy.

ISOLATION OF THE HOSPITALIZED PATIENT: Standard precautions are recommended.
CONTROL MEASURES: Eating raw or undercooked beef or pork should be avoided. Whole cuts of meat should be cooked to at least 145°F (63°C) and then allowed to rest for 3 minutes before consuming, and ground meat and wild game meat should be cooked to

at least 160°F (71°C). Freezing pork or beef below −5°C (23°F) for more than 4 days kills cysticerci. People known to harbor the adult tapeworm of *T solium* should be treated immediately. Careful attention to hand hygiene and appropriate disposal of fecal material is important.

Examination of stool specimens obtained from food handlers and child care workers who recently have emigrated from countries with endemic infection for detection of eggs and proglottids is advisable. To prevent potential fecal-oral transmission of *T solium* eggs, people traveling to resource-limited countries with high endemic rates of cysticercosis should avoid eating uncooked vegetables and fruits that cannot be peeled. If someone in a household is found to have cysticercosis, household members should be screened for taeniasis, and people with compatible neurologic signs and symptoms should be evaluated for cysticercosis.

Other Tapeworm Infections
(Including Hydatid Disease)

Most tapeworm infections are asymptomatic, but nausea, abdominal pain, and diarrhea have been observed in people who are heavily infected.

ETIOLOGIES, DIAGNOSIS, AND TREATMENT

Hymenolepis nana. This tapeworm, also called the dwarf tapeworm because it is the smallest of the adult human tapeworms, can complete its entire life cycle within humans. New infection may be acquired by ingestion of eggs passed in feces of infected people or by ingestion of infected arthropods (fleas) that have gotten into food. More problematic is autoinfection, which perpetuates infection in the host, because eggs can hatch within the intestine and reinitiate the life cycle, leading to development of new worms and an increasing worm burden. Most infections are asymptomatic. With heavy infection, young children may develop abdominal cramps, diarrhea, and irritability. Anal pruritus and difficulty sleeping also have been reported. Diagnosis is made by recognition of the characteristic eggs passed in stool. Sometimes this infection is mistaken for pinworms. Praziquantel is the treatment of choice, with nitazoxanide as an alternative drug; niclosamide is an alternative therapeutic option but is not available in the United States (see Drugs for Parasitic Infections, p 985). If infection persists after treatment, retreatment with praziquantel is indicated. Praziquantel and nitazoxanide are not approved for this indication, but dosing recommendations are available for children 4 years and older (praziquantel) and 1 year and older (nitazoxanide) for other indications.

Dipylidium caninum. This is the most common tapeworm of dogs and cats and has a wide geographic distribution. Fleas, after a blood meal from an infected dog or cat, serve as intermediate host. Children, who inadvertently swallow a dog or cat flea during close contact with infected pets, then develop infection from *Dipylidium caninum*. Although often asymptomatic, some children have abdominal pain, diarrhea, and anal pruritus. Diagnosis is made by finding the characteristic eggs or motile proglottids in stool. Proglottids resemble rice kernels and may be mistaken for maggots or fly larvae. The infection is self-limiting in the human host and typically spontaneously clears by 6 weeks. Therapy with praziquantel is effective. Niclosamide is an alternative therapeutic option but is not available in the United States (see Drugs for Parasitic Infections, p 985). Praziquantel and niclosamide are not approved for this indication, but dosing recommendations are available for children 4 years and older (praziquantel) and 2 years and older (niclosamide [www.cdc.gov/dpdx/dipylidium/tx.html]).

Diphyllobothrium latum *(and Related Species).* These are the largest tapeworms that can infect humans. Fish are intermediate hosts of the *Diphyllobothrium latum* tapeworm, also called fish tapeworm. Consumption of infected, raw or undercooked freshwater fish (including trout and pike) or anadromous fish (salmon) leads to infection. Three to 6 weeks after ingestion, the adult tapeworm matures and begins to lay eggs. Abdominal pain and diarrhea may occur. The worm may cause mechanical obstruction of the bowel or gallbladder, diarrhea, abdominal pain, or rarely, megaloblastic anemia secondary to vitamin B_{12} deficiency. Diagnosis is made by recognition of the characteristic proglottids or eggs passed in stool. Therapy with praziquantel is effective; niclosamide is an alternative but is not available in the United States (see Drugs for Parasitic Infections, p 985). Praziquantel is not approved for this indication, but dosing recommendations are available for children 4 years and older.

Echinococcus granulosus *and* Echinococcus multilocularis. The larval forms of these tapeworms cause human echinococcosis. *Echinococcus granulosus* causes the disease cystic echinococcosis, also known as hydatid disease. The distribution of *E granulosus* is related to sheep or cattle herding, although dogs are the definitive host. Areas of high prevalence include parts of Central and South America, East Africa, Eastern Europe, the Middle East, the Mediterranean region, China, and Central Asia. The parasite also is endemic in Australia and New Zealand. In the United States, small foci of endemic transmission have been reported in Arizona, California, New Mexico, and Utah, and a strain of the parasite is adapted to wolves, moose, and caribou in Alaska and Canada. Dogs, coyotes, wolves, dingoes, and jackals can become infected by swallowing protoscolices of the parasite within hydatid cysts in the organs of slaughtered sheep or other intermediate hosts. Dogs pass embryonated eggs in their stools, and intermediate hosts become infected by swallowing the eggs. If humans swallow *Echinococcus* eggs, they become inadvertent intermediate hosts, and cysts can develop in various organs, such as the liver, lungs, kidneys, and spleen. Cysts caused by larvae of *E granulosus* usually grow slowly (1 cm in diameter per year) and eventually can contain several liters of fluid. If a cyst ruptures, anaphylaxis and multiple secondary cysts from seeding of protoscolices can result. Clinical diagnosis often is difficult. A history of contact with dogs in an area with endemic infection is helpful. Cystic lesions can be demonstrated by radiography, ultrasonography, or computed tomography of various organs. Serologic testing is helpful, but false-negative results occur. Treatment depends on ultrasonographic staging and may include antiparasitic therapy, PAIR (**p**uncture **a**spiration, **i**njection of protoscolicidal agents, and **r**easpiration), surgical excision, or no treatment but with watchful waiting. In uncomplicated cases, treatment of choice is PAIR. Contraindications to PAIR include communication of the cyst with the biliary tract (eg, bile staining after initial aspiration), superficial cysts, and heavily septated cysts. Surgical therapy is indicated for complicated cases and requires meticulous care to prevent spillage, including preparations such as soaking of surgical drapes in hypertonic saline. In general, the cyst should be removed intact, because leakage of contents is associated with a higher rate of complications. Patients are at risk of anaphylactic reactions to cyst contents. Treatment with albendazole generally should be initiated days to weeks before surgery or PAIR and continued for several weeks to months afterward (see Drugs for Parasitic Infections, p 985).

Echinococcus multilocularis, the causative agent for alveolar echinococcosis, has definitive hosts (foxes, coyotes, other wild canines) and rodents as intermediate hosts. Alveolar echinococcosis is characterized by invasive growth of the larvae in the liver with occasional metastatic spread, most worrisome to the brain. Alveolar echinococcosis is limited to the northern hemisphere and usually is diagnosed in people 50 years or older. The disease has been reported frequently from Western China. Diagnosis can be confirmed by imaging and serologic testing. The preferred treatment is surgical removal of the entire larval mass. In nonresectable cases, continuous treatment with albendazole has been associated with clinical improvement (see Drugs for Parasitic Infections, p 985).

ISOLATION OF THE HOSPITALIZED PATIENT: Standard precautions are recommended.

CONTROL MEASURES: Preventive measures for *Hymenolepis nana* include educating the public about personal hygiene and sanitary disposal of feces.

Infection with *D caninum* is prevented by keeping dogs and cats free of fleas and worms. Children should wash their hands after playing with dogs and cats and after playing in areas heavily soiled with pet feces.

To protect against *D latum*, freshwater fish should be cooked thoroughly to an internal temperature of 63°C (145°F), or should be frozen per the following recommendations:
- At −4°F (−20°C) or below for 7 days (total time), or
- At −31°F (−35°C) or below until solid, and storing at −31°F (−35°C) or below for 15 hours, or
- At −31°F (−35°C) or below until solid and storing at −4°F (−20°C) or below for 24 hours.

Control measures for prevention of *E granulosus* and *E multilocularis* include educating the public about hand hygiene and avoiding exposure to dog and wild canid feces. Prevention and control of infection in dogs (preventing dogs from feeding on rodents or carcasses of sheep) decreases the risk of subsequent human infection.

Tetanus
(Lockjaw)

CLINICAL MANIFESTATIONS: Tetanus is caused by neurotoxin produced by the anaerobic bacterium *Clostridium tetani* in a contaminated wound and can manifest in 4 overlapping clinical forms: generalized, local, neonatal, and cephalic.

Generalized tetanus (lockjaw) is a neurologic disease manifesting as trismus and severe muscular spasms, including risus sardonicus. Onset is gradual, occurring over 1 to 7 days, and symptoms progress to severe painful generalized muscle spasms, which often are aggravated by any external stimulus. Autonomic dysfunction, manifesting as diaphoresis, tachycardia, labile blood pressure, and arrhythmias, often is present. Severe spasms persist for 1 week or more and subside over several weeks in people who recover. Neonatal tetanus is a form of generalized tetanus occurring in newborn infants lacking protective passive immunity because their mothers are not immune.

Local tetanus manifests as local muscle spasms in areas contiguous to a wound. Cephalic tetanus is a dysfunction of cranial nerves associated with infected wounds on the head and neck. Local and cephalic tetanus can precede generalized tetanus.

ETIOLOGY: *C tetani* is a spore-forming, obligate anaerobic, gram-positive bacillus. This organism is a wound contaminant that causes neither tissue destruction nor an inflammatory response. The vegetative form of *C tetani* produces a potent plasmid-encoded exotoxin (tetanospasmin). The heavy chain of tetanospasmin binds to the presynaptic motor neuron and facilitates entry of the light chain, a zinc-dependent protease, into the cytosol.

After retrograde axonal transport to the spinal cord, the toxin enters central inhibitory neurons and cleaves synaptobrevin, which is integral to the binding of neurotransmitter containing vesicles to the cell membrane. As a result, gamma-aminobutyric acid- and glycine-containing vesicles are not released, and inhibitory action on motor and autonomic neurons is lost.

EPIDEMIOLOGY: Tetanus occurs worldwide and is more common in warmer climates and during warmer months, in part because of higher frequency of contaminated wounds associated with those locations and seasons. The organism, a normal inhabitant of soil and animal and human intestines, is ubiquitous in the environment, especially where contamination by excreta is common. Organisms multiply in wounds, recognized or unrecognized, and elaborate toxins in the presence of anaerobic conditions. Contaminated wounds, especially wounds with devitalized tissue and deep-puncture trauma, are at greatest risk. Neonatal tetanus is common in many resource-limited countries where pregnant women are not immunized appropriately against tetanus and nonsterile umbilical cord-care practices are followed. Globally, activities are ongoing to eliminate maternal and neonatal tetanus by improving vaccination coverage among pregnant women and promoting safe delivery practices. Although progress continues to be made, 21 countries had still not reached the maternal and neonatal tetanus elimination status by the end of 2015. The World Health Organization estimates that in 2015 (the latest year for which estimates are available), 34 019 newborn infants died from neonatal tetanus, a 96% reduction from the late 1980s.

Widespread active immunization against tetanus has modified the epidemiology of disease in the United States, where 40 or fewer cases have been reported annually since 1999. Tetanus is not transmissible from person to person.

The **incubation period** ranges from 3 to 21 days, with most cases occurring within 8 days. Shorter incubation periods have been associated with more heavily contaminated wounds, more severe disease, and a worse prognosis. In neonatal tetanus, symptoms usually appear from 4 to 14 days after birth, averaging 7 days.

DIAGNOSTIC TESTS: The diagnosis of tetanus is made clinically by excluding other causes of tetanic spasms, such as hypocalcemic tetany, phenothiazine reaction, strychnine poisoning, and conversion disorder. Attempts to culture *C tetani* are associated with poor yield, and a negative culture does not rule out disease. A protective serum antitoxin concentration should not be used to exclude the diagnosis of tetanus.

TREATMENT: A single dose of human Tetanus Immune Globulin (TIG) is recommended for treatment. However, the optimal therapeutic dose has not been established. Some experts recommend 500 IU, which appears to be as effective as higher doses ranging from 3000–6000 IU and causes less discomfort. Available preparations must be administered intramuscularly. Infiltration of part of the dose locally around the wound is recommended, although the efficacy of this approach has not been proven. Results of studies on the benefit from intrathecal administration of TIG are conflicting. The TIG preparation in use in the United States is not licensed or formulated for intrathecal or intravenous use. If TIG is not available (such as is the case in some countries), Immune Globulin Intravenous (IGIV) can be used at a dose of 200 to 400 mg/kg. IGIV is not approved by the US Food and Drug Administration for this use, and antitetanus antibody concentrations can vary from lot to lot. In some countries, equine tetanus antitoxin may be considered if TIG is not available and the patient is tested for sensitivity and desensitized as necessary.

• All wounds should be cleaned and débrided properly, especially if extensive necrosis is present. In neonatal tetanus, wide excision of the umbilical stump is not indicated.

- Supportive care and pharmacotherapy to control tetanic spasms and autonomic instability are of major importance.

- Oral (or intravenous) metronidazole (30 mg/kg per day, given at 6-hour intervals; maximum, 4 g/day) is effective in decreasing the number of vegetative forms of *C tetani* and is the antimicrobial agent of choice. Parenteral penicillin G (100 000 U/kg per day, given at 4- to 6-hour intervals; maximum 12 million U/day) is an alternative treatment. Therapy for 7 to 10 days recommended.

- Active immunization against tetanus always should be undertaken during convalescence from tetanus. Because of the extreme potency of tiny amounts of toxin, tetanus disease may not result in immunity.

ISOLATION OF THE HOSPITALIZED PATIENT: Standard precautions are recommended.

CONTROL MEASURES:

Care of Exposed People (see Table 3.78). Risk of tetanus disease depends on the type of wound and immune status of the patient. Depending on the clinical scenario, there are 3 potential interventions to prevent tetanus: wound care, active immunization, and passive immunization. Antimicrobial prophylaxis has not been shown to prevent tetanus and is not recommended.

- Wound care: Although any open wound is a potential source of tetanus, wounds contaminated with dirt, feces, soil, or saliva (eg, animal bites) are at increased risk. Punctures and wounds containing devitalized tissue, including necrotic or gangrenous wounds, frostbite, crush and avulsion injuries, and burns, are particularly conducive to *C tetani* infection. Wounds with devitalized tissue should be débrided and have dirt removed. It is not necessary or appropriate to débride puncture wounds extensively.

- Active immunization: Immunization status should be assessed for all wounds, and age-appropriate vaccine should be administered (see Immunization) if not contraindicated on the basis of clinical scenario (Table 3.78). For infants younger than 6 months, maternal tetanus toxoid immunization history at time of delivery should be considered in determining need for infant immunization (and need for TIG, if clinically indicated).

- Passive immunization: Patients with tetanus-prone wounds who have not completed a primary series of tetanus vaccine should be considered nonimmune and receive passive immunization with TIG (in addition to active immunization with tetanus toxoid vaccine, as clinically appropriate). For infants younger than 6 months, maternal tetanus toxoid immunization history at time of delivery should be considered in determining need for TIG (Table 3.78). In patients with HIV or other severe immunodeficiency, TIG should be administered for tetanus-prone wounds regardless of the history of tetanus toxoid immunization. When TIG is required for wound prophylaxis, it is administered intramuscularly in a dose of 250 U (regardless of age or weight). If tetanus toxoid vaccine and TIG are administered concurrently, separate syringes and sites should be used. Administration of TIG (or IGIV) does not preclude initiation of active immunization with adsorbed tetanus toxoid vaccine. Efforts should be made to initiate active immunization and arrange for its completion. Administration of tetanus toxoid vaccine simultaneously with or at an interval after receipt of TIG does not impair development of protective antibody substantially. Following intramuscular administration, the circulating half-life of TIG is approximately 28 days.

Table 3.78. Guide to Tetanus Prophylaxis in Routine Wound Management

History of Adsorbed Tetanus Toxoid (Doses)	Clean, Minor Wounds		All Other Wounds[a]	
	DTaP, Tdap, or Td[b]	TIG[c]	DTaP, Tdap, or Td[b]	TIG[c]
Fewer than 3 or unknown	Yes	No	Yes	Yes
3 or more	No if <10 y since last tetanus-containing vaccine dose	No	No[d] if <5 y since last tetanus-containing vaccine dose	No
	Yes if ≥10 y since last tetanus-containing vaccine dose	No	Yes if ≥5 y since last tetanus-containing vaccine dose	No

Tdap indicates booster tetanus toxoid, reduced diphtheria toxoid, and acellular pertussis vaccine; DTaP, diphtheria and tetanus toxoids and acellular pertussis vaccine; Td, adult-type diphtheria and tetanus toxoids vaccine; TIG, Tetanus Immune Globulin (human).

[a] Such as, but not limited to, wounds contaminated with dirt, feces, soil, and saliva (eg, following animal bites); puncture wounds; avulsions; and wounds resulting from missiles, crushing, burns, and frostbite.

[b] DTaP is used for children younger than 7 years. Tdap is preferred over Td for underimmunized children 7 years and older who have not received Tdap previously.

[c] Immune Globulin Intravenous should be used when TIG is not available.

[d] More frequent boosters are not needed and can accentuate adverse effects.

Immunization. Antibody to tetanus toxoid is detectable 4 to 7 days after a dose of tetanus vaccine, and its concentration peaks at 2 to 4 weeks. Protective antibody is not reliably achieved following a first dose of vaccine to prevent tetanus disease. After completing a vaccination series, circulating antitoxin usually lasts at least 10 years and for a longer time after a booster dose.

Active immunization against tetanus always should be undertaken during convalescence from tetanus, because this exotoxin-mediated disease usually does not confer immunity.

Active immunization with tetanus toxoid vaccine is recommended for all people. For all appropriate indications, tetanus immunization is administered with diphtheria toxoid-containing vaccines or with diphtheria toxoid- and acellular pertussis-containing vaccines. Vaccine is administered intramuscularly and may be administered concurrently with other vaccines (see Simultaneous Administration of Multiple Vaccines, p 35). Conjugate vaccines containing tetanus toxoid (eg, *Haemophilus influenzae* type b) are not substitutes for tetanus toxoid immunization. Recommendations for use of tetanus toxoid-containing vaccines (**http://aapredbook.aappublications.org/site/resources/izschedules.xhtml**) are as follows:

- Immunization for children from 6 weeks through 6 years (up to the seventh birthday) of age:
    - ◆ Recommended schedule: should consist of 5 doses of tetanus and diphtheria toxoid-containing vaccine. All doses are administered as DTaP (or DTaP-containing

vaccines) at 2, 4, and 6 months of age, then a dose at 15 through 18 months of age, and another dose at 4 through 6 years of age (recommended before kindergarten or elementary school entry). DTaP can be administered concurrently with other vaccines (see Simultaneous Administration of Multiple Vaccines, p 35).

♦ Catch up vaccination: the 5-dose DTaP series can be administered with a minimum of 4 weeks between each of the first 3 doses and 6 months between dose 3 and 4 as well as dose 4 and 5. If the fourth dose is administered at 4 years or older, the fifth dose is not needed.

♦ Pertussis vaccination contraindicated (see Pertussis, p 620): DT should be administered (can be administered concurrently with other vaccines). If the vaccine series is initiated at younger than 1 year, 5 doses are administered on a schedule similar to the DTaP schedule. If the DT series is started at or after 1 year of age, DT is administered as a 4-dose series with a minimum of 4 weeks between dose 1 and 2 and 6 months between dose 2 and 3, with a final dose administered at 4 through 6 years of age. With either regimen, the final dose can be omitted if the most recent dose was administered at 4 years or older.

♦ Series was started with DT, but pertussis vaccination is desired and is not contraindicated: doses of DTaP should be administered to complete the recommended pertussis immunization schedule (see Pertussis, p 620); however, the total number of doses of diphtheria and tetanus toxoid vaccines (as DT, DTaP, or DTwP) should not exceed 6 before the seventh birthday.

• Immunization for children ≥7 years (see **http://aapredbook.aappublications. org/site/resources/izschedules.xhtml** and Pertussis [Whooping Cough], p 620)[1]:

♦ Recommended schedule: adolescents 11 years and older should receive a single dose of Tdap instead of Td for booster immunization against tetanus, diphtheria, and pertussis. The preferred age for Tdap immunizations is 11 through 12 years of age. If Td was administered instead of Tdap, then Tdap should be administered regardless of the time since receipt of Td.

♦ Catch up vaccination: Tdap should be substituted for a single dose in the series if pertussis vaccination is needed.

♦ If DTaP is inadvertently administered to a child 7 through 9 years of age, the child may receive an adolescent dose of Tdap.

♦ If more than 5 years have elapsed since the last dose, a booster dose of a tetanus-containing vaccine should be considered for people at risk of occupational exposure in locations where tetanus boosters may not be available readily. Tdap is preferred over Td if the person has not received Tdap previously.

• Pregnant women should receive Tdap during each pregnancy. Pregnant women who have not completed their primary tetanus series should receive 3 vaccinations containing tetanus and reduced diphtheria toxoids, if time permits. The recommended schedule is 0, 4 weeks, and 6 months or later. If there is insufficient time, 2 doses of Td should be administered at least 4 weeks apart, and the second dose should be administered at least 2 weeks before delivery. Tdap should replace 1 of the Td doses,

---

[1]American Academy of Pediatrics, Committee on Infectious Diseases. Additional recommendations for use of tetanus toxoid, reduced-content diphtheria toxoid, and acellular pertussis vaccine (Tdap). *Pediatrics.* 2011;128(4): 809–812

preferably early in the interval between 27 and 36 weeks of gestation (see Pertussis, p 620).

Adverse Events, Precautions, and Contraindications. Severe anaphylactic reactions, Guillain-Barré syndrome (GBS), and brachial neuritis attributable to tetanus toxoid have been reported but are rare. No increased risk of GBS has been observed with use of DTaP in children. For a child with the history of GBS, the decision to administer additional doses of DTaP should be made on the basis of consideration of the benefit of further immunization versus the risk of recurrence of GBS. For example, completion of the primary series is justified.

An immediate anaphylactic reaction to tetanus and diphtheria toxoid-containing vaccines (ie, DTaP, Tdap, DT, Td, or conjugate vaccine containing diphtheria or tetanus toxoid) is a contraindication to further doses unless the patient can be desensitized to these toxoids (see Pertussis, p 620). Injection site pain and erythema are common. Fever may occur, and rarely, whole limb swelling occurs (with or without pain and erythema). Repeat vaccination, as age appropriate, appears to be safe in children who had whole limb swelling. Arthus-type hypersensitivity reaction has been reported in adults who received excessive doses of Td over a short period and usually is associated with high concentrations of tetanus antitoxin. Arthus reactions are rare in children and did not occur in clinical trials of Tdap vaccines.

People who experienced an Arthus-type hypersensitivity reaction after a previous dose of a tetanus toxoid-containing preparation usually have very high serum tetanus antibody concentrations and should not receive dose(s) of tetanus toxoid-containing preparation more frequently than every 10 years, even if they have a wound that is neither clean nor minor.

Other Control Measures. Sterilization of hospital supplies will prevent the rare instances of tetanus that may occur in a hospital from contaminated sutures, instruments, or plaster casts.

For prevention of neonatal tetanus, preventive measures (in addition to maternal immunization) include community immunization programs for adolescent girls and women of childbearing age and appropriate training of midwives in recommendations for immunization and sterile technique.

Tinea Capitis

(Ringworm of the Scalp)

CLINICAL MANIFESTATIONS: Dermatophytic fungal infections of the scalp usually present with an area of localized alopecia and scaling. However, a spectrum can include subtle findings of mild hair loss with faint scaling or a large hairless, boggy erythematous area (kerion). Other manifestations include a common "black dot" pattern reflecting stubs of broken-off hairs at the scalp surface; a less common "grey patch" pattern with prominent, well-demarcated alopecic areas of scaling and erythema; or a vesiculopustular pattern resembling bacterial folliculitis. Regional lymphadenopathy may be present.

The differential diagnosis for tinea capitis depends on the clinical presentation. In the classic scaling presentation, clinicians should consider atopic dermatitis, seborrheic dermatitis, and psoriasis. Alopecia should raise the possibility of trichotillomania and alopecia areata, although these disorders usually are not associated with scaling. When vesiculopustular in nature, lice infestation and bacterial infection should be considered. A boggy fluctuant mass likely represents a kerion, but primary (or secondary) bacterial infection can be considered. Although scalp scarring can result from tinea, particularly when a kerion suppurates, the presence of scalp scarring should raise the possibility of an auto-immune disorder, such as discoid lupus.

An associated skin eruption, known as a dermatophytic or "id" reaction, can occur as a hypersensitivity reaction to the infecting fungus and can manifest as diffuse, pruritic, papular, vesicular, and/or eczematous lesions occurring at sites distant from the fungal infection. Id reactions may have onset following institution of therapy but do not represent a drug allergy.

Tinea capitis can occur in association with tinea corporis. Examination of the body (face, trunk, and limbs) should be performed, particularly in wrestlers and others engaged in contact sports.[1]

ETIOLOGY: Tinea capitis develops when dermatophyte fungal elements invade the scalp hair follicle and shaft. The specific pathogen varies by geographic region and mode of transmission. The primary causes of the disease are fungi of the genus *Trichophyton*, including *Trichophyton tonsurans* and *Trichophyton violaceum*, as well as *Microsporum*, including *Microsporum canis* and *Microsporum audouinii*.

EPIDEMIOLOGY: In the United States, tinea capitis occurs predominantly in young black school-aged children who are infected with *T tonsurans*. However, tinea capitis occurs in all racial and ethnic groups as well as in infants and postmenopausal female caregivers. *T tonsurans* is transmitted person to person. *T violaceum* is more common in Europe and Africa and is seen more frequently in immigrant populations in the United States.

M canis is associated with less than 10% of infections but is more evenly distributed among racial/ethnic groups. *M canis* infection almost always results from contact with infected pets, particularly kittens or puppies. *M canis* outbreaks in schools and child care facilities have followed visits from infected animals.

The dermatophyte organism remains viable for prolonged periods on fomites (eg, brushes, combs, hats, towels), and the rate of asymptomatic carriage and infected individuals among family members of index cases is high. The role of asymptomatic carriers is unclear, but almost certainly carriers may serve as a reservoir of infection within families, schools, and communities.

Immunocompromised people and those with trisomy 21 have an increased susceptibility to dermatophyte infections. Accumulating data also implicate a genetic predisposition to tinea infections in certain individuals.

The **incubation period** is unknown but is thought to be 1 to 3 weeks. However, dermatophyte infections have been reported as early as 3 days of age.

DIAGNOSTIC TESTS: The presence of alopecia, pruritus, scale, and posterior cervical lymphadenopathy makes the diagnosis of tinea capitis almost certain, and most clinicians will choose to treat empirically. Diagnosis can be confirmed by dermatoscopy of the affected area, by microscopic evaluation of a potassium hydroxide wet mount of cutaneous scrapings, or by isolation in culture. Dermatoscopic evaluation of areas of alopecia with a lighted magnifier may show comma- or corkscrew-shaped hairs. Potassium hydroxide wet mount microscopy may be used to examine hairs and scale obtained by gentle scraping of

[1]Davies HD, Jackson MA, Rice SG; American Academy of Pediatrics, Committee on Infectious Diseases, Council on Sports Medicine and Fitness. Infectious diseases associated with organized sports and outbreak control. *Pediatrics.* 2017;140(4):e20172477

a moistened area of the scalp with a blunt scalpel, toothbrush, brush, or plucking with tweezers. Arthroconidia can be visualized within the hair shaft in endothrix infections, such as *T tonsurans*, while ectothrix infections, such as *M canis*, exhibit conidia on the outside of the hair shaft. In both forms, septate hyphae may be visualized in scrapings from the scalp surface. Clinicians may use fungal culture to establish a diagnosis, in conjunction with or instead of microscopy. If fungal culture is desired, a cotton-tipped applicator can be used to gently swab an affected area. The sample is transported to a mycology laboratory for processing; 2 to 4 weeks of incubation on Sabouraud dextrose agar are required for results. Polymerase chain reaction and periodic acid-Schiff stain testing of specimens are available but are expensive and generally are unnecessary. Under Wood lamp, tinea lesions are not fluorescent unless the etiologic agent is of the *Microsporum* genus, in which blue-green fluorescence is noted.

TREATMENT: Tinea capitis always requires systemic medication, because the fungal infection is found at the root of the hair follicles, where topical agents do not reach. Optimal treatment of tinea capitis includes considerations of drug tolerability, availability, and cost. Current treatment options are summarized in Table 3.79. Experts generally use higher doses of griseofulvin than have been approved by the US Food and Drug Administration (FDA) or that were used in clinical trials. Griseofulvin is approved by the FDA for children 2 years or older, is available in either liquid or tablet form, can be administered on a daily basis, and should be taken with fatty foods. Laboratory testing of serum hepatic enzymes is not required if duration of griseofulvin therapy does not exceed 8 weeks. Terbinafine granules (contained in capsules) are approved by the FDA for the treatment of tinea capitis in children 4 years and older for a duration of 6 weeks. To improve palatability, the capsules can be opened and the granules mixed in nonacidic food, such as pudding or peanut butter. Off-label use of terbinafine granules in children younger than 4 years and the use of terbinafine tablets (not FDA approved in pediatric patients), which can be split and mixed with foods, are therapeutic options. The granule dosing is higher than that traditionally recommended for the tablets, reflecting the finding that terbinafine clearance of drug is higher in children.

For *T tonsurans*, most experts consider terbinafine a better choice than griseofulvin because of the possibility of shorter duration of therapy (Table 3.79) and equal or superior effectiveness. The FDA recommends baseline and periodic assessment of serum hepatic enzymes when using terbinafine; some clinicians forego baseline screening in otherwise healthy children but perform follow-up testing 4 to 6 weeks later if therapy is ongoing. Dosing of griseofulvin and terbinafine for tinea capitis (Table 3.79) is based on weight and the formulation used (liquid, capsule, tablet). Fluconazole is the only oral antifungal agent approved by the FDA for children younger than 2 years, albeit not for tinea capitis, but was found to have lower cure rates than other oral agents in a large randomized controlled trial. Itraconazole is not FDA approved for treatment of tinea capitis because of insufficient efficacy and safety data.

For *M canis* infection, high-dose griseofulvin is considered standard of care. Topical treatment, such as with selenium sulfide or ketoconazole or ciclopirox shampoos, may be useful as an adjunct to systemic therapy to decrease carriage of viable conidia. Shampoo can be applied 2 to 3 times per week and left in place for 5 to 10 minutes. Treatments should continue for at least 2 weeks, and some experts recommend continuing topical treatments until clinical and mycologic cure occurs.

Table 3.79. Recommended Therapy for Tinea Capitis

Drug	Dosage	Duration
Griseofulvin microsize (liquid, 125 mg/5 mL)	20–25 mg/kg/day (max 1 g/day)	≥6 wk; continue until clinically clear; approved by US Food and Drug Administration (FDA) for children ≥2 y
Griseofulvin ultramicrosize (tablets of varying size)	10–15 mg/kg/day (max 750 mg/day)	
Terbinafine tablets (250 mg)	4–6 mg/kg/day (max: 250 mg); or 10–20 kg: 62.5 mg 20–40 kg: 125 mg >40 kg: 250 mg	*T tonsurans:* 2–6 wk *M canis:* 8–12 wk
Terbinafine granules (125 mg and 187.5 mg)	<25 kg: 125 mg 25–35 kg: 187.5 mg >35 kg: 250 mg	6 wk for all species; approved by US Food and Drug Administration (FDA) for children ≥4 y
Fluconazole (liquid, 10 mg/mL; tablet, 50 and 100 mg)	6 mg/kg/day (max 400 mg/day)	3–6 wk; FDA approved for the treatment of oral candidiasis in children ≥6 m, but not approved for the treatment of tinea capitis

Kerion is managed by systemic antifungal treatment as outlined above; combined antifungal and corticosteroid therapy (either oral or intralesional) has not been shown to be superior to antifungal therapy alone. Unless secondary bacterial infection has occurred, treatment with antimicrobial agents is unnecessary.

ISOLATION OF THE HOSPITALIZED PATIENT: Standard precautions apply.

CONTROL MEASURES: If discovered while at school, that day's attendance should not be abbreviated. Infected children should receive systemic therapy, with or without adjunctive topical management. They should not be excluded from school once therapy has been instituted. Family members and close contacts should be questioned regarding symptoms, and anyone with symptoms should be evaluated. Some experts recommend topical antifungal shampoo therapy for asymptomatic family members, but evidence is lacking regarding the efficacy of this intervention. Sharing of fomites such as hats and combs/brushes should be avoided in households with an affected person. If pets are suspected as a source of *M canis* infection, evaluation and appropriate treatment of the affected animal should be implemented.

Tinea Corporis
(Ringworm of the Body)

CLINICAL MANIFESTATIONS: Superficial tinea infections of the nonhairy (glabrous) skin, termed tinea corporis, involve the face, trunk, or limbs. The lesions often are ring-shaped or circular (hence, the lay term "ringworm") and are sharply marginated. The involved skin is slightly erythematous and scaly, with color variations from red to brown. The eruption can display a scaly, vesicular, or pustular border (often serpiginous) with central clearing. Small confluent plaques or papules as well as multiple lesions can occur, particularly in wrestlers (tinea gladiatorum).[1]

The differential diagnosis for tinea corporis includes candidiasis, psoriasis, other dermatitides (seborrheic, atopic, irritant or allergic, generally caused by therapeutic agents applied to the area), pityriasis (tinea versicolor), nummular eczema, erythema annulare centrifugum, and erythrasma (an eruption of reddish brown patches resulting from superficial bacterial skin infection caused by *Corynebacterium minutissimum*).

The typical appearance of the lesions is altered in patients who have been treated erroneously with topical corticosteroids. Known as tinea incognito, this altered appearance includes diminished erythema and absence of typical scaling borders. Such patients also can develop Majocchi granuloma, a fungal invasion of the hair shaft and surrounding dermis, which causes a granulomatous dermal reaction that can extend into the surrounding subcutaneous fat. Majocchi granuloma also can occur without prior use of corticosteroids.

An associated dermatophytic or "id" reaction can be present as a hypersensitivity reaction to the infecting fungus, manifesting as diffuse, pruritic, papular, vesicular, or eczematous lesions, which can occur at sites distant from the fungal infection. Sometimes id reactions first appear following institution of therapy, but they do not represent a drug allergy.

In patients with diminished T-lymphocyte function (eg, human immunodeficiency virus infection), skin lesions can occur as grouped papules or pustules without erythema or scaling.

Tinea corporis can occur in association with tinea capitis. The scalp should be examined, particularly in wrestlers and others engaged in contact sports.

ETIOLOGY: Tinea corporis develops when dermatophytic fungi invade the outer skin layers at the affected body region. Primary etiologic agents are *Trichophyton* species, especially *Trichophyton tonsurans*, *Trichophyton rubrum*, and *Trichophyton mentagrophytes*; *Microsporum* species, especially *Microsporum canis*; and *Epidermophyton floccosum*.

EPIDEMIOLOGY: Causative fungi occur worldwide and are transmissible by direct contact with infected humans, animals, soil, or fomites (eg, brushes, combs, hats, towels), where organisms can remain viable for prolonged periods.

Immunocompromised people and those with trisomy 21 have an increased susceptibility to dermatophyte infections. Accumulating data also implicate a genetic predisposition to tinea infections in certain individuals.

The **incubation period** is thought to be 1 to 3 weeks but can be shorter, as reported cases have occurred at 3 days of age.

DIAGNOSTIC TESTS: Tinea corporis is diagnosed by clinical manifestations and can be confirmed by microscopic examination of a potassium hydroxide wet mount of skin scrapings or fungal culture. Skin scrapings are obtained by gentle scraping of a moistened area with a blunt scalpel, toothbrush, or brush or by plucking with tweezers. If fungal culture is desired, a cotton-tipped applicator can be used to gently swab an affected area. The sample is transported to a mycology laboratory for processing; 2 to 4 weeks of

[1]Davies HD, Jackson MA, Rice SG; American Academy of Pediatrics, Committee on Infectious Diseases, Council on Sports Medicine and Fitness. Infectious diseases associated with organized sports and outbreak control. *Pediatrics.* 2017;140(4):e20172477

incubation on Sabouraud dextrose agar are required for results. Polymerase chain reaction and periodic acid-Schiff stain evaluation of specimens are available but are expensive and generally are not necessary. Under Wood lamp, tinea is not fluorescent unless the etiologic agent is of the genus *Microsporum*, in which case a blue-green fluorescence can be seen.

TREATMENT: A myriad of topical options are available for treatment. Some topical agents are approved by the US Food and Drug Administration (FDA) only for certain lesion locations and age groups and with applications specified as once or twice daily (Table 3.80). Any of the following products (applied twice daily) are reasonable first-line therapies if appropriate for age: miconazole, clotrimazole, tolnaftate, or ciclopirox. Any of the following products also can be used (applied once daily) if appropriate for age: ketoconazole, econazole, naftifine, or luliconazole. Oxiconazole and sulconazole can be used (once or twice daily) if appropriate for age (also see Topical Drugs for Superficial Fungal Infections, p 956).

Although clinical resolution may be evident within 2 weeks of therapy, continuing therapy for another 2 to 4 weeks generally is recommended. If significant clinical improvement is not observed after 2 weeks of treatment, an alternate diagnosis and/or systemic therapy should be considered. Topical preparations of antifungal medication combined with a corticosteroid should not be used because of inferior effectiveness, the possibility of leading to Majocchi granuloma, and increase in the rate of relapse, higher cost, and potential for adverse corticosteroid effects.

Table 3.80. Products for Topical Treatment of Tinea Corporis, Cruris, and Pedis

Topical Product	Age for Use	Daily Application
Miconazole	All ages for tinea corporis[a]	Twice
Clotrimazole	All ages	Twice
Tolnaftate	All ages	Twice
Ciclopirox	Age ≥10 y	Twice
Ketoconazole	All ages	Once
Econazole	All ages	Once
Naftifine	Age ≥12 y for tinea corporis[a]	Once
Luliconazole	Adults only	Once
Terbinafine	Age ≥12 y	Once for tinea corporis[b,c]
Butenafine	Age ≥12 y	Once for tinea corporis[b]
Oxiconazole	All ages	Once or twice
Sulconazole	Adults only	Once or twice
Sertaconazole	Age >12 y, for tinea pedis only	Twice

[a] Indication ≥2 y for tinea pedis.
[b] For tinea sites other than corporis, application is twice daily.
[c] Does not have FDA indication for tinea cruris.

If lesions are extensive or unresponsive to topical therapy, griseofulvin (for children ≥2 years) or terbinafine (for children ≥4 years) may be administered orally for 4 to 6 weeks (see Tinea Capitis, p 798). Oral itraconazole does not have FDA indication for treatment of any tinea condition. Oral fluconazole has an FDA indication only for tinea capitis in children 2 to 18 years of age (not adults) but is approved for other indications in children 6 months and older. If a Majocchi granuloma is present, oral antifungal therapy is recommended because topical therapy is unlikely to penetrate adequately to eradicate infection.

Dermatophyte infections in other locations, if present, should be treated concurrently.

ISOLATION OF THE HOSPITALIZED PATIENT: Standard precautions apply. Recent outbreaks of tinea infection in both acute and chronic care facilities among patients and caregivers illustrate the need for education regarding the clinical manifestations of tinea and for infection control procedures in the care of infected individuals.

CONTROL MEASURES[1]: Infections should be treated promptly. Direct contact with known or suspected sources of infection should be avoided. Periodic inspections of contacts for early lesions and prompt therapy are recommended. Athletic mats and equipment should be cleaned frequently, and actively infected athletes in sports with person-to-person contact must be excluded from competitions. Athletes with tinea corporis can participate in matches 72 hours after commencement of topical therapy and when the affected area can be covered. Prophylaxis of wrestling team members is a controversial topic. Fluconazole, 100 mg per day for 3 days, given prophylactically before initiation of competitive interscholastic high school wrestling and given again 6 weeks into the season, has been reported to significantly reduce the incidence of *T corporis* from 67.4% to 3.5%. However, the risk-benefit analysis of giving fluconazole prophylactically in this manner has not been determined, and its use should be in consultation with an infectious diseases expert. Infected pets also should receive antifungal treatment.

Tinea Cruris
(Jock Itch)

CLINICAL MANIFESTATIONS: Tinea cruris is a common superficial fungal disorder of the groin, pubic/perianal area, and upper thighs in adults but is uncommon in children. The lesions often are ring-shaped or circular (hence, the lay term "ringworm"), are sharply marginated, and can be intensely pruritic (jock itch). The involved skin is slightly erythematous and scaly, with color variations from red to brown. Lesions can display a scaly, vesicular, or pustular border (often serpiginous) with central clearing. In chronic infections, the margins can be subtle, and lichenification may be present.

The differential diagnosis for tinea crusis includes intertrigo, candidiasis, psoriasis, other dermatitides (seborrheic, atopic, irritant or allergic, generally caused by therapeutic agents applied to the area), pityriasis (tinea versicolor), nummular eczema, erythema annulare centrifugum, and erythrasma (an eruption of reddish brown patches resulting from superficial bacterial skin infection caused by *Corynebacterium minutissimum*).

An altered appearance known as tinea incognito can occur in patients who have been

---

[1]Davies HD, Jackson MA, Rice SG; American Academy of Pediatrics, Committee on Infectious Diseases, Council on Sports Medicine and Fitness. Infectious diseases associated with organized sports and outbreak control. *Pediatrics.* 2017;140(4):e20172477

treated erroneously with topical corticosteroids, which includes diminished erythema and absence of typical scaling borders. Such patients also can develop Majocchi granuloma when fungi invade the hair shaft and surrounding dermis, causing a granulomatous dermal reaction that can extend into the surrounding subcutaneous fat. Majocchi granuloma also can occur without prior use of topical corticosteroid.

An associated skin eruption, known as a dermatophytic or "id" reaction, can occur as a hypersensitivity reaction to the infecting fungus and manifests as diffuse, pruritic, papular, vesicular, or eczematous lesions at sites distant from the fungal infection. An id reaction can first occur following institution of therapy but does not represent a drug allergy.

Immunocompromised patients and those with trisomy 21 have increased susceptibility to dermatophyte infections. Accumulating data also implicate a genetic predisposition to tinea infections in certain individuals.

Concomitant tinea pedis and tinea unguium have been reported in patients with tinea cruris.

ETIOLOGY: Tinea cruris develops when dermatophyte fungi invade the outer skin layers of the affected body region. The fungi *Epidermophyton floccosum*, *Trichophyton rubrum*, and *Trichophyton mentagrophytes* are the most common causes. *Trichophyton tonsurans*, *Trichophyton verrucosum*, and *Trichophyton interdigitale* also have been identified as causes.

EPIDEMIOLOGY: Tinea cruris occurs predominantly in adolescent and adult males and is acquired principally through indirect contact with desquamated epithelium or hair. Direct person-to-person transmission also occurs. Moisture, close-fitting garments, friction, and obesity are predisposing factors.

In patients with diminished T-lymphocyte function (eg, human immunodeficiency virus infection), skin lesions can appear as grouped papules or pustules unaccompanied by scaling or erythema.

The **incubation period** is unknown but is thought to be approximately 1 to 3 weeks, but can be shorter, as documented cases of dermatophyte infection have occurred at 3 days of age.

DIAGNOSTIC TESTS: Confirmatory diagnostic modalities for tinea cruris are similar to that for tinea corporis (see Tinea Corporis, p 801).

TREATMENT: Treatment is similar to that for tinea corporis (see Tinea Corporis, Table 3.80, p 803). Treatment of concurrent onychomycosis (tinea unguium) and tinea pedis may reduce recurrence. Recurrence is common, particularly if predisposing factors such as moisture and friction are not minimized. Loose-fitting clothing and the use of antifungal powders, such as tolnaftate and miconazole, should aid in recovery and prevent recurrence.

If lesions are unresponsive to topical therapy, griseofulvin, administered orally for 4 to 6 weeks, may be effective (see Tinea Capitis, p 798). Oral terbinafine, itraconazole, and fluconazole are options but do not have a US Food and Drug Administration indication for tinea cruris. If a Majocchi granuloma (deep folliculitis) is present, oral antifungal therapy is recommended because topical therapy is unlikely to penetrate adequately to eradicate infection.

Dermatophyte infections in other locations, if present, should be treated concurrently.

ISOLATION OF THE HOSPITALIZED PATIENT: Standard precautions apply.

CONTROL MEASURES: Infections should be treated promptly. Involved areas should be kept dry to prevent recurrences, and antifungal powders and wearing loose fitting undergarments may be useful. Patients should be advised to dry the groin area before drying their feet to avoid inoculating dermatophytes of tinea pedis into the groin area. When infection is present, towel sharing should be avoided.

Tinea Pedis and Tinea Unguium (Onychomycosis)
(Athlete's Foot, Ringworm of the Feet)

CLINICAL MANIFESTATIONS: Tinea pedis can have a variety of clinical manifestations in children. Lesions can involve all areas of the foot but usually are patchy in distribution, with a predisposition to cause fissures, macerated areas, and scaling between toes, particularly in the third and fourth interdigital spaces. A pruritic, fine scaly, or vesiculopustular eruption is most common. "Moccasin foot" exhibits confluent, hyperkeratotic, dry scaling of the soles. Additionally, toenails can be infected (onychomycosis or tinea unguium) and become distorted, discolored, and thickened with accumulation of subungual debris. A superficial white form of foot and toenail fungal infection can occur in children. Toenails may be the source for recurrent tinea pedis.

Tinea pedis must be differentiated from dyshidrotic eczema, atopic dermatitis, contact dermatitis, juvenile plantar dermatosis, palmoplantar keratoderma, and erythrasma (an eruption of reddish brown patches resulting from superficial bacterial skin infection caused by *Corynebacterium minutissimum*).

An associated skin eruption, known as a dermatophytic or "id" reaction, can occur as a hypersensitivity reaction to the infecting fungus and manifests as diffuse, pruritic, papular, vesicular, or eczematous lesions at sites distant from the fungal infection. An id reaction can first occur following institution of therapy but does not represent a drug allergy.

In patients with diminished T-lymphocyte function (eg, human immunodeficiency virus infection), skin lesions may appear as grouped papules or pustules unaccompanied by erythema or scaling.

Concomitant tinea cruris has been reported in patients with tinea pedis and tinea unguium.

ETIOLOGY: Tinea pedis and unguium develop when dermatophytic fungi invade the skin layers and nails of the affected body region. The fungi *Trichophyton rubrum*, *Trichophyton mentagrophytes,* and *Epidermophyton floccosum* are the most common causes of tinea pedis.

EPIDEMIOLOGY: Tinea pedis is a common infection worldwide in adolescents and adults but is less common in young children. Fungi are acquired by contact with infected skin scales or organisms present in damp areas, such as swimming pools, locker rooms, and showers. Tinea pedis may spread among family members in the household; this may represent enhanced genetic susceptibility as well as increased exposure to the organism. The incidence of onychomycosis increases with age, with worldwide prevalence estimated to be from 0.1 to 0.87%. The increased use of occlusive footwear earlier in childhood and exposure to high-risk areas (eg, swimming pools, gyms) earlier in life may be associated with an increase of tinea pedis in children. Childhood onychomycosis is associated with a history of tinea pedis, a history of family member infection, increased number of siblings, and male sex.

Immunocompromised people and those with trisomy 21 have increased susceptibility to dermatophyte infections. Accumulating data also implicate a genetic predisposition to tinea infections in certain individuals.

The **incubation period** is unknown, thought to be approximately 1 to 3 weeks but can be shorter, as documented cases of dermatophyte infection have occurred at 3 days of age.

DIAGNOSTIC TESTS: Confirmatory diagnostic tests for tinea pedis are similar to those for tinea corporis (see Tinea Corporis, p 801). Fungal infection of the nail (tinea unguium or onychomycosis) can be verified by direct microscopic examination with potassium hydroxide, fungal culture of desquamated subungual material, or fungal stain of a nail clippings fixed in formalin.

TREATMENT: A myriad of topical options are available for treatment of tinea pedis (see Tinea Corporis, Table 3.80, p 803; also see Topical Drugs for Superficial Fungal Infections, p 956). Therapy duration of 2 weeks usually is sufficient for milder cases of tinea pedis in children. Acute vesicular lesions can be treated with intermittent use of open wet compresses (eg, with Burow solution, diluted 1:80). Tinea pedis that is severe, chronic, or refractory to topical treatment can be treated with oral therapy similar to that for tinea corporis (see Tinea Corporis, p 801).

Recurrence of tinea pedis is prevented by proper foot hygiene, which includes keeping the feet dry and cool, cleaning gently, drying between the toes, use of absorbent antifungal foot powder, exposing affected areas to air frequently, and avoidance of occlusive footwear, nylon socks, and other fabrics that interfere with dissipation of moisture. Protective footwear should be worn in common areas such as pools, gyms, and other public facilities.

In the past, onychomycosis (tinea unguium) was believed to require oral therapy; however, topical antifungal lacquers and solutions have been developed that are effective for distal toenail infections that do not involve the nail matrix. Despite lower cure rates, topical agents are preferred because of substantially lower adverse effects, lack of drug-drug interactions, and avoidance of laboratory tests monitoring for toxicity. Topical ciclopirox 8%, with a US Food and Drug Administration (FDA) indication for tinea unguium for patients 12 years and older, can be applied to affected toenail(s) once daily for 4 to 8 weeks, in combination with a comprehensive nail management program. Efinaconazole 10% solution and tavaborole 5% solution (a novel boron-based agent) have an FDA indication for tinea unguium in adults. Topical therapies appear to show a higher cure rate in children than in adults, possibly because of thinner nail plates and faster nail growth rate in children.

Studies in adults have demonstrated the best cure rates for onychomycosis (tinea unguium) are with oral itraconazole or terbinafine. Although oral therapies are more likely to lead to cure, they also require laboratory monitoring and can induce drug–drug interactions. Guidelines for dosing of terbinafine for children are based on studies for treatment of tinea capitis and are weight-based: children weighing 10 to 20 kg, 62.5 mg/day, orally; children weighing 20 to 40 kg, 125 mg/day, orally; and children weighing >40 kg, 250 mg/day, orally; or alternatively dosed as 4 to 6 mg/kg/day, not to exceed 250 mg (Table 3.79, p 801). The duration of therapy is the same as for adults (6 week for fingernail infection, 12 weeks for toenail infection). Pediatric dosing of oral itraconazole is not established for superficial mycoses.

Factors that influence choice of therapy include the severity of the infection, the result of fungal culture or potassium hydroxide preparation (if performed), prior treatments, concomitant drug therapy for other illnesses, patient preference, and cost. Topical and systemic therapy may be used concurrently to increase therapeutic response. Cure rates following oral or combined therapy approach 80% in children. In addition, mechanical débridement and chemical débridement of the nail, using 40% urea ointment daily under occlusion for 10 days, should be performed in refractory cases or when severe thickening of the nail is likely to decrease absorption and response to therapy.

Dermatophyte infections in other locations, if present, should be treated concurrently.

ISOLATION OF THE HOSPITALIZED PATIENT: Standard precautions apply.

CONTROL MEASURES: Treatment of patients with active infections should decrease transmission. Using public areas conducive to transmission (eg, swimming pools) is discouraged in those with active infection. Chemical foot baths can facilitate spread of infection. Because recurrence after treatment is common, proper foot hygiene is important (as described in Treatment). Patients should be advised to dry the groin area before drying the feet to avoid inoculating dermatophytes from tinea pedis into the groin area.

Toxocariasis
(Visceral Toxocariasis [a Form of Visceral Larva Migrans]; Ocular Toxocariasis [a Form of Ocular Larva Migrans])

CLINICAL MANIFESTATIONS: The severity of symptoms associated with toxocariasis correlates roughly with the number of infective eggs ingested and the degree of the host inflammatory response. Although most infected children are asymptomatic, symptoms of visceral toxocariasis include fever, cough, wheezing, abdominal pain, and malaise. Laboratory abnormalities include leukocytosis, eosinophilia, and hypergammaglobulinemia. Ocular invasion (resulting in uveitis, endophthalmitis, or retinal granulomas) most often manifests as unilateral vision loss, often without other systemic signs of infection. Atypical manifestations include myocarditis, seizures and other signs of encephalitis, and hemorrhagic rash.

ETIOLOGY: Toxocariasis is caused by *Toxocara* species, which are nematode parasites (roundworms) of dogs and cats (especially puppies or kittens), specifically *Toxocara canis* and *Toxocara cati* in the United States; most cases are caused by *T canis*.

EPIDEMIOLOGY: On the basis of a nationally representative survey, 14% of the US population older than 5 years has serologic evidence of *Toxocara* infection. Visceral toxocariasis typically occurs in children 2 to 7 years of age but can occur in older children and adults. Ocular toxocariasis usually occurs in older children and adolescents. The highest seroprevalence is found among African American children, children in the southern United States, and some indigenous communities in Canada, as well as populations with low education levels and those living in areas where dog feces are found. Humans are infected by ingestion of soil containing infective eggs of the parasite. Eggs may be found wherever dogs and cats defecate, often in sandboxes and playgrounds. Eggs become infective after 2 to 4 weeks in the environment and may persist long-term in the soil. Direct contact with dogs is not necessary, because eggs are not infective immediately when shed in the feces. Infection risk is highest in hot, humid regions where eggs remain viable in soil.

The **incubation period** cannot be determined accurately.

DIAGNOSTIC TESTS: Laboratory findings include marked leukocytosis with eosinophilia, and occasionally anemia and hypergammaglobulinemia. Patients with visceral disease frequently have increased titers of isohemagglutinin to the A and B blood group antigens. An enzyme-linked immunosorbent assay for *Toxocara* antibodies in serum or vitreous fluid is available through the United States Centers for Disease Control and Prevention as well as commercial laboratories. However, a positive antibody test result does not distinguish between past and current infection, and the test is less sensitive for diagnosis of ocular toxocariasis. For visceral disease, imaging of the liver using ultrasonography, computed tomography, or magnetic resonance imaging may reveal diffuse parenchymal lesions measuring less than 2 cm in diameter. Microscopic identification of larvae in a liver biopsy specimen is diagnostic, but this test is not sensitive or specific and therefore rarely indicated.

TREATMENT: Albendazole (400 mg, twice a day for 5 days) is recommended for treatment of visceral toxocariasis (see Drugs for Parasitic Infections, p 985). The drug has been approved by the US Food and Drug Administration, but not for this indication. Mebendazole is an alternative. In severe cases with myocarditis or involvement of the central nervous system, corticosteroid therapy should be considered.

The benefits of anthelmintic treatment for ocular toxocariasis are not well defined, although positive outcomes have been reported with a 2-week course of albendazole (400 mg per day) and prednisone (1 mg/kg/day). Inflammation may be decreased by topical or systemic corticosteroids, and secondary damage may be decreased with ophthalmologic surgery.

ISOLATION OF THE HOSPITALIZED PATIENT: Standard precautions are recommended. There is no person-to-person spread.

CONTROL MEASURES: Proper disposal of cat and dog feces is essential. Regular veterinary care and periodic deworming of dogs and cats, and especially puppies and kittens, decrease environmental contamination with *Toxocara* eggs. Covering sandboxes when not in use is helpful. No specific management following exposure is recommended.

Toxoplasma gondii Infections
(Toxoplasmosis)

Common syndromes associated with acute infection or reactivation of chronic infection with *Toxoplasma gondii* in immunocompetent or, more commonly, immunocompromised patients include but are not limited to lymphadenopathy with atypical lymphocytosis and hepatic dysfunction, fever, meningoencephalitis, chorioretinitis, myocarditis, pneumonitis, myositis, and myelitis. Toxoplasma infection should be considered in the differential diagnosis of any person presenting with chorioretinitis, especially a pregnant woman or newborn infant, and regardless of lack of previous symptoms compatible with a primary infection.

CLINICAL MANIFESTATIONS:

Asymptomatic Infection. Up to 50% of patients infected with the parasite do not report any recognized risk factors and are asymptomatic.

Congenital Infection. In the United States, mothers are not screened routinely for toxoplasmosis. It is estimated that approximately 12% of infants with congenital infection are born without clinical manifestations at birth; however, visual or hearing impairment, learning disabilities, or mental retardation will later become apparent in a large proportion of these children. Chorioretinitis occurs in 72% of the offspring whose mothers were not treated during gestation and in up to 25% in those whose mothers were treated during pregnancy. In France, where mothers are screened systematically and treated during pregnancy for toxoplasmosis, most infants with congenital infection are asymptomatic (88%), 9% have mild-moderate sequelae, and 3% have severe sequelae.

The classic triad of chorioretinitis, cerebral calcifications, and hydrocephalus is highly suggestive of congenital toxoplasmosis. However, most cases do not have all 3 features, and the complete triad is more likely to be seen in infants whose mothers were not treated for toxoplasmosis during gestation. Additional signs of congenital toxoplasmosis at birth include microcephaly, seizures, hearing loss, strabismus, a maculopapular rash, generalized lymphadenopathy, hepatomegaly, splenomegaly, jaundice, pneumonia, diarrhea, anemia, petechiae, and thrombocytopenia. Chorioretinitis may reactivate later in life and result in vision loss. Meningoencephalitis with cerebrospinal fluid (CSF) abnormalities can be present at birth, often with extremely high protein concentrations (eg, >500 mg/dL) and eosinophilia. Some severely affected fetuses/infants die in utero or within a few days of birth. Cerebral calcifications can be demonstrated by plain radiography, ultrasonography, computed tomography (CT), or magnetic resonance imaging (MRI) of the head. CT is the radiologic technique of choice, because it is the most sensitive for calcifications and can reveal brain abnormalities when plain radiographic and/or ultrasonographic studies are normal.

Postnatally Acquired Primary Infection. *T gondii* infection acquired after birth is asymptomatic in most immunocompetent patients. When symptoms develop, they may be nonspecific and can include malaise, fever, headache, sore throat, arthralgia, and myalgia. Lymphadenopathy, frequently cervical, is the most common sign. Patients occasionally have a mononucleosis-like illness associated with a macular rash, hepatosplenomegaly, hepatic dysfunction, and atypical lymphocytosis. The clinical course usually is benign and self-limited. In a subset of immunocompetent individuals and in immunocompromised patients, primary infection may present with persistent fever, myocarditis, myositis, hepatitis, pericarditis, pneumonia, encephalitis with and without brain abscesses, and skin lesions. These syndromes and a more aggressive clinical course, including life-threatening pneumonia, are especially common in patients who acquired primary toxoplasmosis in certain tropical countries in South America, such as French Guiana, Brazil, and Colombia. Toxoplasmosis should be included in the differential diagnosis of ill travelers who return home with these unexplained syndromes. Occasionally, this more aggressive clinical presentation has been observed in immunocompetent individuals infected in the United States, likely from acute infections associated with high parasite load and/or highly virulent strains.

Toxoplasmic chorioretinitis can occur in the setting of postnatally acquired infection. Most commonly, acute onset of blurred vision, eye pain, decreased visual acuity, floaters, scotoma, photophobia, or epiphora are noted. Ocular disease can reactivate years after the initial infection in both healthy and immunocompromised individuals. The morphology of the retinal lesions with postnatally acquired infection is similar to that of in utero infection. A focal necrotizing retinitis with vitritis and occasionally with anterior uveitis most commonly is described. Often, an atrophic retinochoroidal scar is seen. Complications can include chronic iridocyclitis, cataract formation, secondary glaucoma, band keratopathy, cystoid macular edema, retinal detachment, and if the optic nerve is involved, optic atrophy.

Reactivation of Chronic Infection in Immunocompromised Patients. Reactivation of latent infection may occur in an immunosuppressed patient (eg, organ transplant recipient who is receiving certain monoclonal antibodies, such as alemtuzumab). Reactivation of latent disease can result in life-threatening encephalitis, brain abscesses, seizures, pneumonia, posterior or panuveitis (always with chorioretinitis), fever of unknown origin, disseminated disease, myocarditis, or skin lesions. Toxoplasmic encephalitis (TE) can present as a single brain lesion on MRI or as a diffuse and rapidly progressive process in the setting of apparently normal brain imaging. MRI is superior to CT for the diagnosis of TE and can detect lesions not revealed by CT. In patients with acquired immunodeficiency syndrome (AIDS), TE is the most common cause of space-occupying brain lesions and typically presents with acute to subacute neurologic or psychiatric symptoms and multiple ring-enhancing brain lesions. In these patients, a clear improvement in their neurologic examination within 7 to 10 days of beginning empiric anti-*Toxoplasma* therapy is considered diagnostic of TE.

In the immunosuppressed patient without human immunodeficiency virus (HIV) infection who presents with multiple ring-enhancing brain lesions, brain biopsy should be pursued to establish a tissue diagnosis rather than initiating empiric anti-*Toxoplasma* treatment, because the differential diagnosis is broad and includes a variety of pathogens, such as fungal, mycobacterial, and *Nocardia* infections, as well as neoplasms.

Seropositive hematopoietic stem cell and solid organ transplant recipients are at risk of reactivation. In these patients, toxoplasmosis may manifest as pneumonia, unexplained fever or seizures, myocarditis, hepatosplenomegaly, lymphadenopathy, or skin lesions in addition to brain abscesses and diffuse encephalitis. *T gondii*-seropositive solid organ donors (D+) can transmit the parasite, via the allograft, to seronegative recipients (R−). Thirty percent of D+/R− heart transplant recipients develop toxoplasmosis in the absence of anti-*Toxoplasma* prophylaxis.

ETIOLOGY: *T gondii* is a protozoan and obligate intracellular parasite that exists in nature in relatively few clonal lineages (types I, II, and III, and other lineages including atypical strains). The infectious forms include tachyzoites, tissue cysts containing bradyzoites, and oocysts containing sporozoites. The tachyzoite and the corresponding host immune reaction are responsible for symptoms observed during acute infection or during reactivation of a latent infection in immunocompromised patients. The tissue cyst is responsible for latent infection and usually is present in brain, eye, cardiac tissue, and skeletal muscle of humans and other warm-blooded animals.

EPIDEMIOLOGY: The seroprevalence of *T gondii* infection varies by geographic locale and the socioeconomic strata of the population. The age-adjusted seroprevalence of infection in the United States has been estimated at 9% among women 15 to 44 years of age. *T gondii* is distributed worldwide and can infect most species of warm-blooded animals. Members of the feline family are the definitive host, and they generally acquire the infection by ingestion of tissue cysts present in infected animals (eg, mice) or uncooked household meats or by ingestion of oocysts present in soil organic matter, water, or food. Millions of oocysts are excreted in feline stools 3 to 30 days after primary infection and continue to be shed for 7 to 14 days. After excretion, oocysts require a maturation phase (sporulation) of 1 to 5 days in temperate climates before they are infective by the oral route. Sporulated oocysts can survive for years under most environmental conditions. Intermediate hosts (including sheep, pigs, mice, and cattle) can have tissue cysts in the brain, myocardium, skeletal muscle, and other organs. These cysts remain viable for the lifetime of the host. Humans usually become infected by consumption of raw or undercooked meat that contains cysts or by accidental ingestion of sporulated oocysts from soil or from contaminated food or water. Large outbreaks linked epidemiologically to contamination of municipal drinking water supplies have been reported. The main risk factors associated with acute infection in the United States include eating raw ground beef; eating rare lamb; eating locally produced cured, dried, or smoked meat; working with meat; drinking unpasteurized goat milk; and owning 3 or more kittens. Eating raw oysters, clams, or mussels has also been identified as a novel risk factor. Increased risk of acute infection in those who drink untreated water has also been reported in the United States. There is no evidence of human-to-human transmission except through vertical transmission, blood products, or organ transplantation. Up to 50% of acutely infected people do not report recognized risk factors or symptoms. Therefore, laboratory testing is required to establish or rule out infection.

In most cases, congenital transmission occurs as a result of primary maternal infection during pregnancy. In utero infection rarely occurs as a result of reactivated parasitemia in chronically infected immunocompromised pregnant women. In the United States, the incidence of acute primary *T gondii* infection during pregnancy has been estimated to be between 0.2/1000 and 1.1/1000 pregnant women; the incidence of congenital toxoplasmosis has been estimated to be between 0.5 cases and 0.82 cases per 10 000 live births. Infection rarely has occurred as a result of a laboratory accident or from blood or blood product transfusion.

The **incubation period** of postnatally acquired infection is approximately 7 days, with a range of 4 to 21 days.

DIAGNOSTIC TESTS: Serologic tests are the primary means of diagnosing primary and latent infection. Initial serologic testing for *Toxoplasma* immunoglobulin (Ig) G and IgM can be performed by non-reference laboratories. However, positive *Toxoplasma* IgM test results can be falsely positive, so they should be submitted promptly to reference laboratories with special expertise in *Toxoplasma* serologic assays and their interpretation, such as the Palo Alto Medical Foundation Toxoplasma Serology Laboratory (PAMF-TSL; Palo Alto, CA; **www.pamf.org/serology/**; telephone: (650) 853-4828; e-mail: toxolab@ pamf.org) for additional and confirmatory testing (eg, IgM testing by the double-sandwich enzyme-linked immunosorbent assay [ELISA] using antigen obtained from live parasites, IgA, IgE, avidity, and differential agglutination). Moreover, testing of neonates/infants with congenital toxoplasmosis and of pregnant women with suspected acute primary infection during gestation should be confirmed routinely at reference laboratories with the use of specific panels of tests with high diagnostic accuracy.

IgG-specific antibodies achieve a peak concentration 3 to 5 months after infection and remain positive indefinitely. The vast majority of patients will have low-positive IgG antibody titers 6 months after the acute infection. IgM-specific antibodies can be detected 2 weeks after infection (IgG-specific antibodies usually are negative during this period), achieve peak concentrations in 1 month, decrease thereafter, and usually become undetectable within 6 to 9 months. However, a positive IgM test result may persist for years without apparent clinical significance. Enzyme immunoassays (EIAs) are the most sensitive tests for IgM, and indirect fluorescent antibody tests are the least sensitive tests, but both are less specific than the IgM test offered at PAMF-TSL. To determine the approximate time of infection in IgG-positive adults, specific IgM antibody determinations should be performed. The lack of *T gondii*-specific IgM antibodies in a person with low-positive titers of IgG antibodies (eg, a dye test at PAMF-TSL ≤512) indicates infection of at least 6 months' duration. In contrast, detectable *T gondii*-specific IgM antibodies can indicate recent infection, chronic infection, or a false-positive reaction. If the timing of infection is clinically important (eg, in a pregnant woman), sera with positive *T gondii*-specific IgM test results should be sent to PAMF-TSL to establish acute versus chronic infection. If acute infection is confirmed at PAMF-TSL, further testing can be performed to estimate the timing of the infection. Laboratory tests that have been found to be helpful in determining timing of infection in patients with positive IgM test results include an IgG avidity test, the differential agglutination (AC/HS) test, and IgA- and IgE-specific antibody tests. The presence of high-avidity IgG antibodies indicates that infection occurred at least 12 to 16 weeks previously. However, the presence of low-avidity antibodies is not a reliable indication of more recent infection, and treatment may affect the maturation of IgG avidity and prolong the presence of low-avidity antibodies. A nonacute pattern in the AC/HS test is essentially indicative of an infection that was acquired at least 12 months before the serum was obtained. However, similar to low-avidity IgG test results, an acute AC/HS pattern can last for several months and does not necessarily establish the diagnosis of acute infection. Tests to detect IgA and IgE antibodies, which decrease to undetectable concentrations sooner than do IgM antibodies, also are useful for diagnosis of congenital infections and infections in pregnant women, for whom more precise information about the timing of infection is needed. *T gondii*-specific IgA and IgE antibody tests are available in *Toxoplasma* reference laboratories but generally not in other laboratories. Their presence, particularly at high titers, is indicative of an infection acquired within the past 3 months.

Maternal test results help in the interpretation of test results for a newborn infant. If the mother was not tested during pregnancy, a maternal serum sample should be tested for IgG and IgM, and AC/HS and avidity tests should be performed as soon as possible. Only 2 states (Massachusetts and New Hampshire) routinely screen all newborn infants for antibody to *T gondii*.

Polymerase chain reaction (PCR) detection has been applied to virtually any body fluid or tissue, and *T gondii*-specific immunoperoxidase staining in any tissue, depending on the clinical scenario. Specimens in which PCR assay can be performed include amniotic fluid, CSF, whole blood, bronchoalveolar lavage fluid, vitreous fluid, aqueous humor, peritoneal fluid, ascitic fluid, pleural fluid, bone marrow, and urine. Essentially any tissue can be stained with *T gondii*-specific immunoperoxidase; the presence of extracellular antigens and a surrounding inflammatory response also are diagnostic of toxoplasmosis. A positive PCR test result in tissue must be interpreted with caution, because it may amplify tachyzoite or bradyzoite DNA and, therefore, cannot distinguish between the presence of tachyzoites with acute infection or reactivation or bradyzoites with chronic latent infection.

Isolation of the parasite occasionally is attempted for the purpose of genotyping the infecting strain, although culture is not available in most hospital based clinical laboratories. Correlation of genotype with clinical manifestations may be attempted, but results must be interpreted in the context of each clinical scenario.

Congenital toxoplasmosis. When a neonate is suspected of being congenitally infected with *T gondii*, neonatal peripheral blood for *Toxoplasma* IgG (in parallel with maternal blood for *Toxoplasma* IgG), IgM ISAGA, and IgA ELISA should be sent to a toxoplasmosis reference laboratory. A complete blood cell count and transaminase tests should be performed. Peripheral blood *Toxoplasma* PCR, urine *Toxoplasma* PCR, and CSF *Toxoplasma* PCR should be performed as soon as possible after birth when there is strong suspicion of congenital toxoplasmosis; CSF *Toxoplasma* PCR can be deferred in infants with low suspicion of congenital toxoplasmosis. When CSF is obtained, it should be sent for CSF cell count, differential, protein, and glucose determinations. If there is concern for false-positive *Toxoplasma* IgM or IgA results because of possible contamination of infant's blood with maternal blood during labor, the infant's serologic tests should be repeated at least 10 days after birth (half-life of *Toxoplasma* IgM antibodies is approximately 5 days, and for IgA antibodies is approximately 10 days).

The diagnosis of congenital toxoplasmosis can be confirmed by detection of:

- *T gondii* in umbilical cord blood or in urine, peripheral blood, or CSF of newborn infant, by mouse inoculation;
  - ♦ Examination of the placenta by histologic testing and PCR assay can be helpful, but a positive result does not prove that the newborn also is infected.
- *T gondii* DNA by PCR in amniotic fluid or in peripheral blood, urine, or CSF of newborn infant;
  - ♦ Currently, there are no PCR assays cleared by the US Food and Drug Administration for *T gondii* in the United States.
- IgA and/or IgM antibody to *T gondii* in fetal or newborn blood;
  - ♦ IgA immunosorbent agglutination assay (ISAGA) is more sensitive than enzyme-linked immunosorbent assay (ELISA).
  - ♦ Placental leak occasionally can lead to false-positive IgA or IgM reactions in the newborn infant. Repeat testing after 10 days of life can help confirm the diagnosis, because the half-life of these immunoglobulins is short and the titers in an uninfected infant should rapidly decrease.
  - ♦ If the mother was infected late in gestation, IgA and IgM should be repeated 2 to 4 weeks after birth and then every 4 weeks until 3 months of age (in such cases, the initially negative *Toxoplasma* IgM and IgA in the newborn infant at birth could be because of delayed production of those antibodies).
- IgG and/or IgM antibody to *T gondii* in the CSF of the newborn infant;
- Fetal or newborn *T gondii*-specific IgG 4 times greater than maternal *T gondii*-specific IgG; or
- IgG antibody to *T gondii* that increases or remains positive after 12 months of life in an infant with clinical manifestations consistent with congenital toxoplasmosis but not explained by another diagnosis (eg, Chagas disease, syphilis, rubella, cytomegalovirus, HIV, HTLV, Zika virus, hepatitis B and C).
  - ♦ Follow-up serologic testing is indicated for newborn infants with suspicion for congenital toxoplasmosis who are IgG positive but IgM and IgA negative. IgG testing should be repeated every 4 to 6 weeks until documentation of complete disappearance of IgG.

Evaluation of the infant with congenital toxoplasmosis should include ophthalmologic, auditory, and neurologic examinations; lumbar puncture; and computed tomography of the head. Follow-up ophthalmologic evaluations are necessary, even if the initial evaluation was normal. In a French cohort of children with congenital toxoplasmosis, the initial retinal lesions were first detected after 7 months of age in 75% of the cases, after 3 years in 50%, after 8 years in 25%, after 10 years in 20%, and after 12.5 years in 10%. Long-term neurodevelopmental evaluations are required.

Infants born to women who are infected simultaneously with HIV and *T gondii* and who are not on anti-*Toxoplasma* prophylaxis should be evaluated for congenital toxoplasmosis because of an increased likelihood of maternal reactivation and congenital transmission in this setting. Expert advice is available at the PAMF-TSL (**www.pamf.org/serology**; telephone [650] 853-4828; e-mail toxolab@pamf.org) and the Toxoplasmosis Research Institute and Center; Chicago, IL; **www.toxoplasmosis.org;** telephone

[773] 834-4131; e-mail rmcleod@midway.uchicago.edu).

Immunocompromised Patients. Immunocompromised patients (eg, people with AIDS, hematopoietic stem cell or solid organ transplant recipients, people with cancer, or people taking immunosuppressive drugs) who are infected latently with *T gondii* have variable titers of IgG antibody to *T gondii* but rarely have IgM antibody. Immunocompromised patients should be tested for *T gondii*-specific IgG before commencing immunosuppressive therapy or as soon as possible after their status of immunosuppression is diagnosed to determine whether they are chronically infected with *T gondii* and at risk of reactivation of latent infection. Active disease in immunosuppressed patients may or may not result in seroconversion and a fourfold increase in IgG antibody titers; consequently, serologic diagnosis in these patients often is difficult. Seropositive patients before transplantation may have changes in their IgG titers in any direction (increase, decrease, or no change) posttransplant without any clinical relevance. In these patients, PCR testing, histologic examination, and attempts to isolate the parasite become the laboratory methods of choice to diagnose toxoplasmosis.

In HIV-infected patients who are seropositive for *T gondii* IgG, reactivation of their latent infection usually is manifested by toxoplasmic encephalitis (TE). TE can be diagnosed presumptively on the basis of characteristic clinical and radiographic findings (MRI typically shows multiple ring-enhancing brain lesions). If there is no clinical response to an empiric trial of anti-*T gondii* therapy within 10 days, demonstration of *T gondii* organisms, antigen, or DNA in specimens such as blood, CSF, or bronchoalveolar fluid may be necessary to confirm the diagnosis, and alternative etiologies (eg, chronic Chagas disease) should be considered as the evaluation continues. TE also can present as diffuse encephalitis without space-occupying lesions on brain MRI. Prompt recognition of this syndrome and confirmation of the diagnosis by PCR testing in CSF is crucial, because these patients usually exhibit a rapidly progressive and fatal clinical course if left untreated.

Ocular Toxoplasmosis. Toxoplasmic chorioretinitis usually is diagnosed on the basis of characteristic retinal lesions in conjunction with a positive serum *T gondii*-specific IgG test result. All patients with eye disease also should have an IgM test performed; if a positive IgM test result is confirmed at a reference laboratory and eye lesions are consistent with toxoplasmic chorioretinitis, ocular disease is the result of an acute *T gondii* infection rather than reactivation of a chronic infection. Patients who have atypical retinal lesions or who fail to respond to anti-*T gondii* therapy should undergo examination of vitreous fluid or aqueous humor by PCR, and antibody testing (using the Goldmann-Witmer coefficient, which compares the proportion of *Toxoplasma*-specific IgG in the intraocular sample with that in serum, as measured by ELISA or radioimmunoassay) should be considered. A Goldmann-Witmer coefficient greater than 2 or 3 is considered diagnostic of ocular toxoplasmosis.

TREATMENT:

- Most cases of acquired infection in an immunocompetent host do not require specific antimicrobial therapy unless infection occurs during pregnancy or symptoms are severe or persistent.

- Treatment of primary *T gondii* infection in **pregnant women,** including women with HIV infection who reactivate their chronic *Toxoplasma* infection, is recommended. Appropriate specialists should be consulted for management. Spiramycin treatment of primary infection during gestation is used in an attempt to prevent transmission of *T gondii* from the mother to the fetus in cases in which there is no evidence yet of fetal infection. Spiramycin does not reliably treat the fetus if in utero infection already has occurred, because it does not readily cross the placenta. Spiramycin is available only as an investigational drug in the United States but may be obtained from the manufacturer (compassionately provided), at no cost, following the advice of PAMF-TSL (telephone: [650] 853-4828) or the Toxoplasmosis Research Institute and Center (Chicago, IL; telephone: [773] 834-4131) and with authorization from the US Food and Drug Administration (telephone: [301] 796-1400; fax: [301] 796-9883). If fetal infection is confirmed at or after 18 weeks of gestation or if the mother acquires infection during the third trimester, pyrimethamine plus sulfadiazine and leucovorin should be used, because they cross the placenta. If pyrimethamine cannot be obtained, spiramycin and trimethoprim/sulfamethoxazole double strength (160 mg/800 mg), 1 tablet, 3 times per day, may be initiated until the ideal regimen of pyrimethamine and sulfadiazine can be instituted.

- **Infants with symptomatic congenital toxoplasmosis** should receive oral therapy with:
    - Pyrimethamine at a dose of 1 mg/kg, administered twice daily for 2 days, and then once daily for 6 months, and then 3 times per week to complete a 12-month total course of therapy (maximum 25 mg/dose); PLUS
    - Sulfadiazine at a dose of 50 mg/kg, administered twice daily for a 12-month total course of therapy; PLUS
    - Folinic acid (leucovorin) at a dose of 10 mg, administered 3 times per week to complete a 12-month total course of therapy; folinic acid is used to minimize pyrimethamine toxicity; folic acid may not be substituted for folinic acid.
    - If CSF protein is ≥1 g/dL or patient has severe chorioretinitis: prednisone at a dose of 0.5 mg/kg (maximum 20 mg/dose), administered twice daily until CFS protein <1 g/dL or resolution of severe chorioretinitis; if steroids are to be used, they should be initiated after 72 hours of anti-*Toxoplasma* therapy.
    - In some centers in Europe, the regimen of pyrimethamine/sulfadoxine every 10 to 15 days is used for subclinical/mild forms of congenital toxoplasmosis and/or for poor compliance and/or frequent hematologic adverse effects after the first 2 months of daily therapy with pyrimethamine/sulfadiazine. Some centers in Germany have individualized the duration of the postnatal treatment according to the severity of CT (eg, 3 months' total treatment for asymptomatic infants; 6 months for mildly symptomatic infants and 12 months for severely symptomatic infants).
- For **infants with asymptomatic congenital toxoplasmosis**, the same regimen used for symptomatic infants (pyrimethamine, sulfadiazine, and folinic acid) should be used, but the treatment duration should be for 3 months.
- **Older children with toxoplasmic chorioretinitis** should receive oral therapy with:
    - Pyrimethamine at a dose of 1 mg/kg (max: 25 mg/dose), administered twice daily for 2 days, and then once daily; PLUS
    - Sulfadiazine at a dose of 75 mg/kg for 1 dose, followed by a dose of 50 mg/kg administered twice daily (max: 4 g/day); PLUS
    - Folinic acid (leucovorin) at a dose of 10 to 20 mg, administered daily during and up to 1 week after completion of pyrimethamine.
    - For severe disease, add prednisone at a dose of 0.5 mg/kg twice daily (max: 40 mg/day), with rapid taper.

- ◆ Treatment usually is given for 1 to 2 weeks beyond resolution of clinical manifestations and for approximately 4 to 6 weeks.
- **Immunocompetent and immunocompromised children with severe primary toxoplasmosis** and **immunocompromised children with reactivation of toxoplasmosis** should receive oral therapy with:
  - ◆ Pyrimethamine at a dose of 1 mg/kg, administered twice daily for 2 days (max: 100 mg/day), and then once daily (max: 25 mg/day, but up to 50 mg/day [if <60 kg] or 75 mg/day [if ≥60 kg] in older children with severe disease); PLUS
  - ◆ Sulfadiazine at a dose of 25 to 50 mg/kg, administered 4 times per day (max: 4–6 grams/day for severe disease); PLUS
  - ◆ Folinic acid (leucovorin) at a dose of 10 to 20 mg (up to 50 mg/day), administered daily during and 1 week after pyrimethamine.
- Current treatment recommendations for toxoplasmosis in **HIV-infected children and adolescents** are detailed at **https://aidsinfo.nih.gov/guidelines.** Prevention recommendations are provided in Table 3.81 and at **https://aidsinfo. nih.gov/guidelines.**

Table 3.81. Prophylaxis to Prevent First Episode and Recurrence of Toxoplasmosis in Children

Prevention of	Indication	First Choice	Alternatives
First episode of toxoplasmosis[a]	Severe immuno-suppression and presence of immunoglobulin G antibody to *Toxoplasma*	Trimethoprim-sulfamethoxa-zole, 150–750 mg/m^2/day, orally, once daily	Dapsone (children 1 mo of age or older), 2 mg/kg or 15 mg/m^2 (max 25 mg), orally, once daily; **PLUS** pyrimethamine, 1 mg/kg, orally, once daily (max 25 mg); **PLUS** leucovorin, 5 mg, orally, every 3 days Atovaquone, children 1 through 3 mo or older than 24 mo of age: 30 mg/kg, orally, once daily Atovaquone, children 4 through 24 mo of age: 45 mg/kg, orally, once daily, **with or without** Pyrimethamine, 1 mg/kg or 15 mg/m^2 body surface area (maximum 25 mg), orally, once daily, **PLUS** leucovorin, 5 mg, orally, every 3 days **Acceptable Alternative Dosage Schedules for TMP-SMX:** • TMP-SMX, 150/750 mg/m^2 body surface area per dose, once daily, orally, 3 times weekly on 3 consecutive days per week • TMP-SMX, 75/375 mg/m^2 body surface area per dose, twice daily, orally, every day • TMP-SMX, 75/375 mg/m^2 body surface area per dose, twice daily, orally, 3 times weekly on alternate days

Table 3.81. Prophylaxis to Prevent First Episode and Recurrence of Toxoplasmosis in Children, continued

Prevention of	Indication	First Choice	Alternatives
Recurrence of toxoplasmosis (suppressive therapy)[b]	Prior toxoplasmic encephalitis or toxoplasmosis	Sulfadiazine, 85–120 mg/kg/day (max 2–4 g per day) in 2–4 divided doses, orally, every day, **PLUS** pyrimethamine, 1 mg/kg or 15 mg/m² (maximum, 25 mg), orally, once daily; **PLUS** leucovorin, 5 mg, orally, every 3 days	Clindamycin, 20–30 mg/kg/day in 3 divided doses, orally, every day, **PLUS** pyrimethamine, 1 mg/kg or 15 mg/m² body surface area, orally, once daily (maximum 25 mg); **PLUS** leucovorin, 5 mg, orally, every 3 days Atovaquone, children 1 through 3 mo or older than 24 mo of age: 30 mg/kg, orally, once daily; **PLUS** leucovorin, 5 mg, orally, every 3 days; **PLUS** TMP-SMX, 150/750 mg/m2 body surface area, once daily, orally Atovaquone, children 4 through 24 mo of age: 45 mg/kg, orally, once daily, **with or without** pyrimethamine, 1 mg/kg body weight or 15 mg/m² body surface area (maximum 25 mg), orally, once daily; **PLUS** leucovorin, 5 mg, orally, every 3 days; **PLUS** TMP-SMX, 150/750 mg/m2 body surface area, once daily, orally

[a]Protection against toxoplasmosis is provided by the preferred antipneumocystis regimen (TMP-SMX) and possibly by atovaquone but not by pentamidine. Atovaquone may be used with or without pyrimethamine. Pyrimethamine alone provides little, if any, protection (for information about severe immunosuppression, see Table 3.61, p 655).(**http://aidsinfo.nih.gov/guidelines**).

[b]Only pyrimethamine plus sulfadiazine confers protection against *Pneumocystis jirovecii* pneumonia as well as toxoplasmosis. Although the clindamycin plus pyrimethamine regimen is recommended in adults, this regimen has not been tested in children and has been found to have high rates of relapses in adults. However, these drugs are safe and are used for other infections.

ISOLATION OF THE HOSPITALIZED PATIENT: Standard precautions are recommended.

CONTROL MEASURES: Consideration should be given to testing of household or close family members of individuals diagnosed with acute *Toxoplasma* infection in settings in which individuals at high risk (eg, pregnant women, immunocompromised patients) can be identified, because infections in more than one family member of acutely infected individuals have been documented. All HIV-infected and immunocompromised individuals as well as pregnant women should be counseled about the various sources of toxoplasmic infection and ways to avoid them. Pregnant women and immunocompromised patients whose serostatus for *T gondii* is negative or unknown should avoid activities that potentially expose them to cat feces and be advised of the following:

- Changing litter boxes, gardening, and landscaping should be avoided, or gloves should be worn and hands should be washed if such activities are unavoidable.
- Daily changing of cat litter decreases the chance of infection, because oocysts are not infective during the first 1 to 2 days after passage.
- Domestic cats can be protected from infection by feeding them commercially prepared cat food and preventing them from eating undercooked meat and hunting wild

rodents and birds.

Oral ingestion of viable *T gondii* can be prevented by the following:

- Avoiding consumption of raw or undercooked meat and cooking meat—particularly pork, lamb, and venison—to an internal temperature of 65.5°C to 76.6°C (150°F–170°F [no longer pink]) before consumption;
- Avoiding consumption of smoked meat and meat cured in brine;
- Freezing meat to −12°C (10°F) for 48 hours before consumption;
- Washing fruits and vegetables;
- Washing hands and cleaning kitchen surfaces after handling fruits, vegetables, and raw meat;
- Washing hands after gardening or other contact with soil;
- Preventing contamination of food with raw or undercooked meat or soil;
- Avoiding ingestion of raw shellfish such as oysters, clams, and mussels;
- Avoiding ingestion of raw goat milk; and
- Avoiding ingestion of untreated water, particularly in resource-limited countries.

There currently is no vaccine available for prevention of *T gondii* infection or toxoplasmosis. Additional resources for health care personnel may be found at **www.cdc.gov/parasites/toxoplasmosis/health_professionals/index.html.**

Trichinellosis

(*Trichinella spiralis* and Other Species)

CLINICAL MANIFESTATIONS: The clinical spectrum of *Trichinella* infection ranges from inapparent to fulminant and fatal illness, although most infections are asymptomatic. The severity of disease is proportional to the infective dose. During the first week after ingesting infected meat, a person may experience abdominal discomfort, nausea, vomiting, and/or diarrhea as excysted larvae penetrate the intestinal mucosa. Two to 8 weeks later, as progeny larvae migrate into tissues, fever, myalgia, periorbital edema, urticarial rash, and conjunctival and subungual hemorrhages may develop. In severe infections, myocarditis, neurologic involvement, and pneumonitis can occur in 1 or 2 months. Larvae may remain viable in tissues for years; calcification of some larvae in skeletal muscle usually occurs within 6 to 24 months and may be detected using various imaging modalities.

ETIOLOGY: Infection is caused by nematodes (roundworms) of the genus *Trichinella*. Seven species have been implicated in human disease; worldwide, *Trichinella spiralis* is the most common cause of human infection.

EPIDEMIOLOGY: Infection is enzootic worldwide in carnivores and omnivores, especially scavengers. Infection occurs as a result of ingestion of raw or insufficiently cooked meat containing encysted larvae of *Trichinella* species. Commercial and home-raised pork remain a source of human infections, but meats other than pork, such as venison, horse meat, and particularly meats from wild carnivorous or omnivorous game (especially bear, boar, seal, and walrus) now are the most common sources of infection. The disease is not transmitted from person to person.

The **incubation period** usually is less than 1 month.

DIAGNOSTIC TESTS: Eosinophilia of up to 70%, in conjunction with compatible symptoms and dietary history, suggests the diagnosis. Increases in concentrations of muscle enzymes, such as creatinine phosphokinase and lactic dehydrogenase, occur. Identification of larvae in suspect meat can be the most rapid source of diagnostic information.

Encapsulated larvae in a skeletal muscle biopsy specimen (particularly deltoid and gastrocnemius) can be visualized under light microscopy beginning 2 weeks after infection by examining hematoxylin-eosin stained slides or sediment from digested muscle tissue. Serologic tests are available through the Centers for Disease Control and Prevention as well as commercial and state laboratories. Serum antibody titers generally take 3 or more weeks to become positive and may remain positive for years. Testing paired acute and convalescent serum specimens usually is diagnostic.

TREATMENT: Albendazole and mebendazole both are recommended for treatment of acute trichinellosis (see Drugs for Parasitic Infections, p 985), although anthelmintics typically do not kill larvae that have already encysted within muscles. Neither drug is approved by the US Food and Drug Administration for trichinellosis. Coadministration of corticosteroids with anthelmintics is recommended when systemic symptoms are severe. Corticosteroids can be lifesaving when the central nervous system or heart is involved.

ISOLATION OF THE HOSPITALIZED PATIENT: Standard precautions are recommended. There is no person-to-person spread.

CONTROL MEASURES: Transmission to pigs can be prevented by not feeding them garbage, by preventing cannibalism among animals, and by effective rat control. The public should be educated about the necessity of cooking pork and meat of wild animals thoroughly. Specific recommendations include the following:

- For whole cuts of meat (excluding poultry and wild game): cook to at least 145°F (63°C) as measured with a food thermometer placed in the thickest part of the meat, then allow the meat to rest for 3 minutes before carving or consuming.
- For ground meat (including wild game, excluding poultry): cook to at least 160°F (71°C); ground meats do not require a rest time.
- For all wild game (whole cuts and ground): cook to at least 160°F (71°C).

Freezing pork less than 6 inches thick at 5°F (−15°C) for 20 days kills *T spiralis*. *Trichinella* organisms in wild animals, such as bears and raccoons, are resistant to freezing. People known to have ingested undercooked contaminated meat recently should be treated with albendazole or mebendazole. Case reporting to appropriate health authorities is required (see Appendix IV: Nationally Notifiable Infectious Diseases in the United States, p 1069).

Trichomonas vaginalis Infections

(Trichomoniasis)

CLINICAL MANIFESTATIONS: *Trichomonas vaginalis* infection is asymptomatic in 70% to 85% of infected people. Untreated infections may persist for months to years. Clinical manifestations in symptomatic pubertal or postpubertal females may include a diffuse vaginal discharge, odor, and vulvovaginal pruritus and irritation. Dysuria and, less often, lower abdominal pain can occur. Vaginal discharge may be any color but classically is yellow-green, frothy, and malodorous. The vulva and vaginal mucosa can be erythematous and edematous. The cervix can be inflamed and sometimes is covered with numerous punctate cervical hemorrhages and swollen papillae, referred to as "strawberry" cervix. This finding occurs in less than 5% of infected females but is highly suggestive of trichomoniasis. Clinical manifestations in symptomatic men include urethritis and, rarely, epididymitis or prostatitis. Reinfection is common, and resistance to treatment is uncommon but increasing. Rectal infections are uncommon, and oral infections have not been described.

T vaginalis infections in pregnant females have been associated with premature rupture of the membranes and preterm delivery. Perinatal infection may occur in up to 5% of neonates of infected mothers. *T vaginalis* in female newborn infants may cause vaginal discharge during the first weeks of life but usually is self-limited, resolving as maternal hormones are metabolized. Respiratory infections in newborn infants may occur as well.

ETIOLOGY: *T vaginalis* is a flagellated protozoan approximately the size of a leukocyte. It requires adherence to host cells for survival. The genome of *T vaginalis* has been sequenced.

EPIDEMIOLOGY: Although formal surveillance programs are not in place, several studies suggest that *T vaginalis* infection is the most common nonviral sexually transmitted infection (STI) in the United States and globally. Prevalence in a nationally representative sample of sexually experienced 14- to 19-year-old females in the United States was 2.1% in the early 2000s. It commonly coexists with other conditions, particularly with *Neisseria gonorrhoeae* and *Chlamydia trachomatis* infections and with bacterial vaginosis. Transmission results almost exclusively from sexual contact, and the presence of *T vaginalis* in a child or preadolescent beyond the perinatal period is considered highly suspicious for sexual abuse. *T vaginalis* infection can increase both the acquisition and transmission of human immunodeficiency virus (HIV). The prevalence of trichomoniasis in males who have sex solely with males (MSM) is low.

The **incubation period** averages 1 week but ranges from 5 to 28 days.

DIAGNOSTIC TESTS: The use of highly sensitive and specific tests is recommended for detecting *T vaginalis*. The nucleic acid amplification test (NAAT) is the most sensitive means of diagnosing *T vaginalis* infection. The APTIMA *Trichomonas vaginalis* assay (Hologic Gen-Probe, San Diego, CA), Quidel Amplivue Trich assay (Quidel, San Diego CA), Xpert TV (Cepheid, Sunnyvale, CA), and BD Probe Tec TV Q^x Amplified DNA Assay (Becton Dickinson, Franklin Lakes, NJ) are commercially available assays that are cleared by the US Food and Drug Administration (FDA) for testing vaginal swab, endocervical swab, and urine specimens of females. Analyst-specific *Trichomonas* reagents can be used with urine or urethral swab specimens in laboratories that have met Clinical Laboratory Improvement Amendments (CLIA) requirements and validated their *T vaginalis* NAAT performance on male specimens. Because the duration of persistence of *T vaginalis* nucleic acids in genital specimens is not established, NAAT diagnostic tests within the first few weeks after treatment should not be used routinely to assess therapeutic success or failure.

Culture of *T vaginalis* in Diamond media or other trichomoniasis-specific culture systems (eg, InPouch, BioMed Diagnostics, White City, OR) is a sensitive and specific method of diagnosis in females with a sensitivity of 75% to 96% but has lower sensitivity in males. The most common method for *T vaginalis* diagnosis in a symptomatic female typically is examination of a wet-mount preparation of vaginal discharge. Microscopy sensitivity is only 51% to 65% for *T vaginalis* diagnosis in female vaginal specimens and is less sensitive for male urethral specimens, urine sediment, and semen specimens; test sensitivity declines even further if the microscopic evaluation is delayed.[1]

Two other FDA-cleared tests are available for testing vaginal swab specimens that are more sensitive than microscopy. The OSOM Trichomonas Rapid Test (OSOM, Sekisui

[1]Centers for Disease Control and Prevention. Sexually transmitted diseases treatment guidelines, 2015. *MMWR Recomm Rep.* 2015; 64(RR-3):1–137

Diagnostics, Framingham, MA) is a CLIA-waived, antigen-detection, rapid point-of-care test that uses immunochromatographic capillary flow dipstick technology. Results are available within 10 minutes, with a sensitivity of 82% to 95%. The Affirm VPIII (Becton Dickinson, Sparks, MD) is a DNA hybridization probe test for *T vaginalis*, *Gardnerella vaginalis*, and *Candida albicans*. Results are available in 45 minutes, with a sensitivity of 63% for *T vaginalis* detection. Vaginal swab specimens can be tested as a point-of-care test or sent to a clinical laboratory. Neither the OSOM nor the Affirm VP III test is FDA cleared for use with specimens obtained from males.

TREATMENT[1]: Treatment of adolescents and young adults with metronidazole (2 g, orally, in a single dose) results in cure rates of approximately 84% to 98%. Treatment with tinidazole (2 g, orally, in a single dose) has resulted in cure rates of approximately 92% to 100%. Both drugs are approved for this indication in adolescents and young adults, and metronidazole is approved in children. Tinidazole generally is more expensive, has fewer gastrointestinal adverse effects, and in randomized controlled trials, was found to be equivalent or superior to metronidazole in achieving parasitologic cure and resolution of symptoms. Topical vaginal preparations should not be used, because they do not achieve therapeutic concentrations in the urethra or perivaginal glands. Sexual partners should be treated, even if asymptomatic, because reinfection can occur.

Although most recurrent *T vaginalis* infections result from reinfection, some recurrent infections might be attributed to antimicrobial resistance. Metronidazole resistance occurs in 4% to 10% of cases of vaginal trichomoniasis, and tinidazole resistance occurs in 1%. If treatment failure occurs with a single 2-g dose of metronidazole and reinfection is excluded, metronidazole, 500 mg, orally, twice daily for 7 days, should be used. If treatment failure occurs following this regimen, a course of either metronidazole or tinidazole, 2 g daily, for 7 days, may be used. If several 1-week regimens have failed in a person who is unlikely to have nonadherence or reinfection, testing of the organism for metronidazole and tinidazole susceptibility is recommended. The CDC (**www.cdc.gov/std**) has accumulated experience with testing and treatment of nitroimidazole-resistant *T vaginalis* and can offer susceptibility testing and management assistance. Higher-dose tinidazole (2–3 g for 14 days), often in combination with intravaginal tinidazole, can be considered in cases of nitroimidazole-resistant infections; however, such cases should be managed in consultation with an expert.

Alternative regimens for *T vaginalis* treatment might be effective but have not been evaluated systematically. Metronidazole and tinidazole both are nitroimidazoles. Patients with an immunoglobulin (Ig) E mediated-type allergy to a nitroimidazole can be managed by metronidazole desensitization according to a published regimen in consultation with a specialist.

Pregnancy. *T vaginalis* infection in pregnant females is associated with adverse pregnancy outcomes, particularly premature rupture of membranes, preterm delivery, and delivery of an infant with low birth weight. Although metronidazole treatment produces parasitologic cure, trials have shown no significant difference in perinatal morbidity following metronidazole treatment. Symptomatic pregnant females, regardless of pregnancy stage, should be tested and consideration should be given to treatment with metronidazole (2 g orally, in a single dose). Metronidazole is a pregnancy category B drug (animal studies

[1]Centers for Disease Control and Prevention. Sexually transmitted diseases treatment guidelines, 2015. *MMWR Recomm Rep*. 2015; 64(RR-3):1–137

have revealed no evidence of harm to the fetus, but no adequate and well-controlled studies in pregnant women have been conducted). Tinidazole is a pregnancy category C drug (animal studies have demonstrated an adverse effect, but no adequate and well-controlled studies in pregnant women have been conducted). In lactating females to whom metronidazole is administered, some clinicians advise deferring breastfeeding for 12 to 24 hours following maternal treatment with a single 2-g dose of metronidazole. While using tinidazole, interruption of breastfeeding is recommended during treatment and for 3 days after a single 2-g dose.

People infected with *T vaginalis* should be evaluated for other sexually transmitted infections (STIs), including syphilis, gonorrhea, chlamydia, HIV, human papillomavirus (HPV), and hepatitis B infections. HPV and hepatitis B vaccines should be administered if the person's immunization status for these is not completed. For newborn infants, infection with *T vaginalis* acquired maternally is self-limited, and treatment generally is not recommended.

ISOLATION OF THE HOSPITALIZED PATIENT: Standard precautions are recommended.

CONTROL MEASURES: Measures to prevent STIs, particularly the consistent and correct use of condoms, are indicated. Patients should be instructed to avoid sexual activity until they and their sexual partners are treated and there is resolution of symptoms.

Follow-up. Because of the high rate of trichomoniasis reinfection among females, retesting for *T vaginalis* is recommended for all sexually active females within 3 months following initial treatment regardless of whether they are symptomatic or believe their sex partners were treated. Testing with NAATs can be conducted as soon as 2 weeks after treatment if symptoms recur. Data are insufficient to support retesting men.

Routine Screening Tests[1]: Although routine *T vaginalis* screening of asymptomatic adolescents is not recommended, screening may be considered for people receiving care in high-prevalence settings (eg, STI clinics and correctional facilities) and for asymptomatic people at high risk of infection. Risk factors that may put females at higher risk of *T vaginalis* include new or multiple partners, illicit drug use, or a history of STIs.

Management of Sexual Partners. All people with a known exposure to *T vaginalis* infection should be treated routinely, regardless of a diagnostic test result. Expedited partner therapy might have a role in partner management for trichomoniasis and may be used in states where this approach is permissible.

Trichuriasis
(Whipworm Infection)

CLINICAL MANIFESTATIONS: Disease caused by the whipworm *Trichuris trichiura* generally is proportional to the intensity of the infection. Although most infected children are asymptomatic, those with heavy infestations can develop a colitis that mimics inflammatory bowel disease and can lead to anemia, physical growth restriction, and clubbing. More serious is the condition called *Trichuris* dysentery syndrome, which is characterized by severe abdominal pain, tenesmus, bloody diarrhea, and occasionally rectal prolapse.

ETIOLOGY: *T trichiura*, the human whipworm, is the causative agent of trichuriasis. Adult

---

[1]American Academy of Pediatrics, Committee on Adolescence; Society for Adolescent Health and Medicine. Screening for nonviral sexually transmitted infections in adolescents and young adults. *Pediatrics*. 2014;134(1): e302–e311

worms are 30 to 50 mm long with a large, thread-like anterior end that embeds in the mucosa of the large intestine.

EPIDEMIOLOGY: *T trichiura* is the second most prevalent soil-transmitted helminth in the world, occurring mainly in tropical regions with poor sanitation. It is coendemic with *Ascaris* and hookworm species. Humans are the natural reservoir. Eggs excreted in moist soil require a minimum of 10 days of incubation before they are infectious. Children become infected by accidental ingestion of infective eggs in food or on hands contaminated with soil. The disease is not directly communicable from person to person.

The time between infection and appearance of eggs in the stool (**incubation period**) is approximately 12 weeks.

DIAGNOSTIC TESTS: Eggs may be found on direct examination of stool by the use of the Kato-Katz thick smear method or the McMaster method, although diagnosis of light to moderate infections may require concentration techniques.

TREATMENT: Mebendazole, albendazole, or ivermectin administered for 3 days are recommended for the treatment of whipworm infection (see Drugs for Parasitic Infections, p 985), although the cure rate for any single drug is low. Albendazole and ivermectin are not approved by the US Food and Drug Administration for this indication. Reexamination of stool specimens 2 to 4 weeks after therapy to document cure is recommended, and those who fail therapy should be retreated. Combination therapy with 2 anthelmintics (eg, albendazole or mebendazole with ivermectin) may result in higher cure rates and should be considered in patients who persistently test positive following single-agent treatment. A combination of albendazole and oxantel pamoate recently was noted to have the best efficacy, but oxantel pamoate is not available in the United States.

ISOLATION OF THE HOSPITALIZED PATIENT: Only standard precautions are recommended, because there is no direct person-to-person transmission.

CONTROL MEASURES: Proper disposal of contaminated feces is the most effective means of control for whipworm and other soil-transmitted helminths. Periodic administration of single doses of benzimidazoles (albendazole or mebendazole) provided to high-risk groups is recommended by the World Health Organization for the community-based control of soil-transmitted helminth infections. Evidence of sustained benefit or reductions in prevalence of infections attributable to preventive chemotherapy programs is limited.

African Trypanosomiasis
(African Sleeping Sickness)

CLINICAL MANIFESTATIONS: The clinical course of human African trypanosomiasis has 2 stages: the first is the hemolymphatic stage, in which the parasite multiplies in subcutaneous tissues, lymph, and blood. Once the parasite crosses the blood-brain barrier and infects the central nervous system (CNS), the disease enters the second stage, known as the neurologic stage. The rapidity of disease progression and clinical manifestations vary with the infecting subspecies. With *Trypanosoma brucei gambiense* infection (West African sleeping sickness), initial symptoms may be mild and include fever, muscle aches, and malaise. Pruritus, rash, weight loss, and generalized lymphadenopathy can occur. Posterior cervical lymphadenopathy, known as Winterbottom sign, may be present. CNS involvement typically develops after 1 to 2 years with development of behavioral changes, cachexia, headache, hallucinations, delusions, and daytime somnolence followed by nighttime insomnia. In contrast, *Trypanosoma brucei rhodesiense* infection (East African sleeping sickness) is an acute, generalized illness that develops days to weeks after parasite inoculation, with manifestations including high fever, lymphadenopathy, rash, muscle and joint aches, thrombocytopenia, hepatitis, anemia, myocarditis, and rarely, laboratory evidence of disseminated intravascular coagulopathy. A chancre may develop at the site of the tsetse fly bite. Clinical meningoencephalitis can develop after onset of the untreated systemic illness. Both forms of African trypanosomiasis have high fatality rates; without treatment, infected patients usually die within weeks to months after clinical onset of disease caused by *T brucei rhodesiense* and within a few years from disease caused by *T brucei gambiense*.

ETIOLOGY: Human African trypanosomiasis (sleeping sickness) occurs in sub-Saharan Africa. It is caused by *Trypanosoma brucei* subspecies, which are protozoan parasites transmitted by blood-feeding tsetse flies. The west and central African (Gambian) form progresses more slowly and is caused by *T brucei gambiense*. The east and southern African (Rhodesian) form is more acute and is caused by *T brucei rhodesiense*. Both are extracellular protozoan hemoflagellates that live in blood and tissue of the human host.

EPIDEMIOLOGY: Worldwide, 7106 human cases of African trypanosomiasis were reported annually to World Health Organization in 2012, with 3796 cases reported in 2014. Whereas more than 98% of the total reported cases have been caused by *T brucei gambiense*, the occasional reported cases of African trypanosomiasis in the United States typically have been in returning travelers who became infected with *T brucei rhodesiense* while on safari in East Africa. Transmission of *T brucei* subspecies is confined to an area in Africa between the latitudes of 15° north and 20° south, corresponding precisely with the distribution of the tsetse fly vector (*Glossina* species). In West and Central Africa, humans are the main reservoir of *T brucei gambiense*, although the parasite sometimes can be found in domestic animals, such as dogs and pigs. In East Africa, wild animals, such as antelope, bush buck, and hartebeest, constitute the major reservoirs for sporadic infections with *T brucei rhodesiense*, although cattle serve as reservoir hosts in local outbreaks. In addition to the bite of the tsetse fly, *T brucei* subspecies can also be transmitted congenitally and through blood transfusions or organ transplantation, although these modes are uncommon.

The **incubation period** for *T brucei rhodesiense* infection ranges from 3 to 21 days, and for most cases is 5 to 14 days; for *T brucei gambiense* infection, the incubation period usually is longer but is not well defined.

DIAGNOSTIC TESTS: Diagnosis is made by identification of trypanosomes in specimens of blood, cerebrospinal fluid (CSF), or fluid aspirated from a chancre or lymph node or by inoculation of susceptible laboratory animals (mice) with heparinized blood in the case of *T brucei rhodesiense* infection. Examination of CSF is critical to management, and all patients should undergo lumbar puncture; concentration methods (such as the double-centrifugation technique) typically should be used. Concentration and Giemsa staining of the buffy coat layer of peripheral blood also can be helpful and is easier for *T brucei rhodesiense*, because the density of organisms in circulating blood is higher than for *T brucei gambiense*. *T brucei gambiense* is more likely to be found in lymph node aspirates than in blood. The most widely used criteria for CNS involvement include the identification of trypanosomes in CSF or a CSF white blood cell count of 6 or higher; elevated protein and an increase in immunoglobulin M also may suggest second-stage disease. Serologic testing for antibodies to *T brucei gambiense* is available outside the United States and typically is used only for screening purposes to help identify suspect cases; there is no comparable serologic screening test for *T brucei rhodesiense.*

TREATMENT: The choice of drug(s) used for treatment depends on the type and stage of African trypanosomiasis (**www.cdc.gov/parasites/sleepingsickness/health_professionals/index.html#tx**). When no evidence of CNS involvement is present, the drug of choice for the acute hemolymphatic stage of infection is pentamidine for *T brucei gambiense* infection and suramin for *T brucei rhodesiense* infection. For treatment of infection with CNS involvement, the drug of choice is eflornithine for *T brucei gambiense* infection and melarsoprol for *T brucei rhodesiense* infection (eflornithine is not effective for CNS treatment of *T brucei rhodesiense).* Melarsoprol encephalopathy may be reduced in severity by concomitant administration of corticosteroids. The safety of eflornithine in children has not been established. Eflornithine is not approved by the Food and Drug Administration (FDA) for use in pediatric patients. Suramin, eflornithine, and melarsoprol can be obtained from the Centers for Disease Control and Prevention (phone: [404] 718-4745). In certain cases, nifurtimox is added to eflornithine or melarsoprol. For specific dosing recommendations, see Drugs for Parasitic Infections (p 985). Consultation with a specialist familiar with the disease and its treatment is recommended. Because of the risk of relapse, patients who have had CNS involvement should undergo repeated CSF examinations every 6 months for 2 years. The optimal approach to treatment of relapse is uncertain.

ISOLATION OF THE HOSPITALIZED PATIENT: Standard precautions are recommended.

CONTROL MEASURES: Travelers to areas with endemic infection should avoid known foci of sleeping sickness and tsetse fly infestation and should minimize fly bites by wearing long-sleeved shirts and pants of medium-weight material in neutral colors. Infected patients should not breastfeed or donate blood.

American Trypanosomiasis
(Chagas Disease)

CLINICAL MANIFESTATIONS: The acute phase of *Trypanosoma cruzi* infection lasts 2 to 3 months, followed by the chronic phase that, in the absence of successful antiparasitic treatment, is lifelong. The acute phase commonly is asymptomatic or characterized by mild, nonspecific symptoms. Young children are more likely to exhibit symptoms than are adults. Fever, edema, malaise, lymphadenopathy, and hepatosplenomegaly may develop. Meningoencephalitis and/or acute myocarditis can occur rarely. Unilateral edema of the eyelids, known as the Romaña sign, may occur if the portal of entry is the conjunctiva, but it is usually not present. The edematous skin may be violaceous and associated with conjunctivitis and enlargement of the ipsilateral preauricular lymph node. In some patients, a red, indurated nodule known as a chagoma develops at the site of the original inoculation, usually on the face or arms. The symptoms of acute Chagas disease can resolve without treatment within 3 months, and patients pass into the chronic phase of the infection. Most people with chronic *T cruzi* infection have no signs or symptoms and are said to have the indeterminate form of chronic Chagas disease. In 20% to 30% of cases, serious progressive sequelae affecting the heart and/or gastrointestinal tract develop years to decades after the initial infection (called determinate forms of chronic Chagas disease). Chagas cardiomyopathy is characterized by conduction system abnormalities, especially right bundle branch block and ventricular arrhythmias, and may progress to dilated cardiomyopathy and congestive heart failure. Patients with Chagas cardiomyopathy may die suddenly from ventricular arrhythmias, complete heart block, or embolic phenomena; death also may occur from intractable congestive heart failure. Less commonly, patients with chronic Chagas disease may develop digestive disease with dilatation of the colon and/or esophagus with swallowing difficulties accompanied by severe weight loss. Congenital Chagas disease occurs in 1% to 10% of infants born to infected mothers and may be characterized by low birth weight, hepatosplenomegaly, myocarditis, and/or meningoencephalitis with seizures and tremors, but most infants with congenital *T cruzi* infection have no signs or symptoms of disease. Reactivation of chronic *T cruzi* infection with parasitemia may be life threatening and may occur in immunocompromised people, including people infected with human immunodeficiency virus and those who are immunosuppressed after transplantation.

ETIOLOGY: *T cruzi*, a protozoan hemoflagellate, causes American trypanosomiasis (Chagas disease).

EPIDEMIOLOGY: Parasites are transmitted in feces of infected triatomine insects (sometimes called "kissing bugs," a type of reduviid; local Spanish/Portuguese names include vinchuca, chinche picuda, or barbeiro). When found indoors, they tend to be found in pet areas, under bedding, and in areas of rodent infestation. The bugs defecate during or after taking a blood meal. The bitten person is inoculated through inadvertent rubbing of insect feces containing the parasite into the site of the bite through the harmed skin or mucous membranes of the eye. The parasite also can be transmitted congenitally, during solid organ transplantation, through blood transfusion, and by ingestion of food or drink contaminated by the vector's excreta. Accidental laboratory infections can result from handling parasite cultures or blood from infected people or laboratory animals, usually through needlestick injuries. Vectorborne transmission of the disease, for the most part, is limited to the Western hemisphere, predominantly Mexico and Central and South America. In the United States, 10 species of kissing bugs are known to exist; this results in a distribution of parasites into the southern states from California to Florida and in the East northward to Maryland. Significant numbers of wild animals are infected, including opossums, armadillos, wood rats, and squirrels. Animals usually acquire the parasite by eating the bugs. Rare vectorborne cases of Chagas disease have been noted in the United States. Nevertheless, most *T cruzi*-infected individuals in the United States are immigrants from areas of Latin America with endemic infection.

There are an estimated 300 000 individuals with *T cruzi* infection in the United States. Assuming a 1% to 5% risk of congenital transmission, based on estimates of maternal infection, approximately 63 to 315 infants are born with Chagas disease in the United States every year. Several transfusion- and transplantation-associated cases have been documented in the United States.

The disease is an important cause of morbidity and death in Latin America, where an estimated 8 million people are infected, of whom approximately 30% to 40% either have or will develop cardiomyopathy and/or gastrointestinal tract disorders.

The **incubation period** for the acute phase of disease is 1 to 2 weeks or longer. Chronic manifestations do not appear for years to decades.

DIAGNOSTIC TESTS: During the acute phase of disease, the parasite is demonstrable in blood specimens by Giemsa staining after a concentration technique or in direct wetmount or buffy coat preparations. Molecular detection techniques (available at the Centers for Disease Control and Prevention [CDC]) also have high sensitivity in the acute phase. The chronic phase of *T cruzi* infection is characterized by low-level parasitemia;

the sensitivity of polymerase chain reaction (PCR) assay generally is less than 50%. Diagnosis in the chronic phase relies on serologic tests to demonstrate immunoglobulin (Ig) G antibodies against *T cruzi*. Serologic tests include indirect immunofluorescent and enzyme immunosorbent assays; no single serologic test is sufficiently sensitive or specific to confirm a diagnosis of chronic *T cruzi* infection. The Pan American Health Organization and the World Health Organization recommend that samples be tested using 2 assays of different formats before treatment decisions are made.

The diagnosis of congenital Chagas disease can be made during the first 3 months of life by identification of motile trypomastigotes by direct microscopy of fresh anticoagulated blood specimens or by PCR testing, which is a useful tool in infants and has higher sensitivity than serologic testing. If not diagnosed earlier, serologic testing should be performed after 9 months of age, once serum immunoglobulin (Ig) G measurements are expected to reflect infant response rather than maternal antibody. Some countries have congenital Chagas disease screening programs, which combine maternal screening with microscopic examination of cord blood from infants of seropositive mothers.

Low sensitivity of screening tests and low rates of follow-up likely lead to underestimation of infection rates. Diagnostic testing and consultation are available from the CDC Division of Parasitic Diseases and Malaria (phone: [404] 718-4745; e-mail: parasites@cdc.gov; CDC Emergency Operator [after business hours and on weekends]: [770] 488-7100).

TREATMENT: The only drugs with proven efficacy are benznidazole and nifurtimox (see Drugs for Parasitic Infections, p 985). Benznidazole was approved in 2017 by the US Food and Drug Administration (FDA) for use in children 2 to 12 years of age for the treatment of Chagas disease. Nifurtimox is not approved by the FDA for use in the United States, but can be obtained from the CDC (Division of Parasitic Diseases and Malaria, [404]718-4745) for treatment of patients under a compassionate use protocol.

Antitrypanosomal treatment is recommended for all cases of acute and congenital Chagas disease, reactivated infection attributable to immunosuppression, and chronic *T cruzi* infection in children younger than 18 years. Treatment of chronic *T cruzi* infection in adults without advanced cardiomyopathy generally is recommended.

Trypanocidal therapy with benznidazole in patients with established Chagas cardiomyopathy significantly reduces serum parasite detection but does not significantly reduce cardiac clinical deterioration or death through 5 years of follow-up and is, therefore, not recommended. Both drugs have significant adverse effect profiles. The recommended treatment courses are at least 60 days. Careful consideration of potential risks and benefits in consultation with an expert in treatment of the disease or with CDC may be necessary, especially for patients diagnosed with chronic infection and/or who do not fall under a clearly recommended treatment category.

ISOLATION OF THE HOSPITALIZED PATIENT: Standard precautions should be followed.
CONTROL MEASURES: Risk to travelers is low. Travelers to areas with endemic infection should avoid contact with triatomine bugs by avoiding habitation in buildings vulnerable to infestation, particularly those constructed of mud, palm thatch, or adobe brick. The use of insecticide-impregnated bed nets, tucked under the mattress on all sides, also may be beneficial. Camping or sleeping outdoors in areas with endemic transmission is not recommended. Travelers to regions with endemic infection also should avoid ingestion of unpasteurized juices, such as sugar cane or açaí palm fruit juice, which have been linked to oral transmission of Chagas disease. Diagnostic testing should be performed on

members of households with an infected patient if they have had exposure to the vector similar to that of the patient. All children of women with *T cruzi* infection should be tested for Chagas disease.

Education about the mode of spread and methods of prevention is warranted in areas with endemic infection. Homes should be examined for the presence of the vectors, and if found, measures to eliminate the vector should be taken.

People with known *T cruzi* infection should not donate blood or plan to donate solid organs. Recommendations to all blood collection agencies for the appropriate use of serologic tests to reduce the risk of transfusion-transmitted *T cruzi* infection were issued by the FDA in December 2010.

Tuberculosis

CLINICAL MANIFESTATIONS: Tuberculosis disease is caused by infection with organisms of the *Mycobacterium tuberculosis* complex. Most infections caused by *M tuberculosis* complex in children and adolescents are asymptomatic. When pulmonary tuberculosis occurs, clinical manifestations most often appear 1 to 6 months after infection and include fever, weight loss or poor weight gain, growth delay, cough, night sweats, and chills. Chest radiographic findings rarely are specific for tuberculosis and include lymphadenopathy of the hilar, subcarinal, paratracheal, or mediastinal nodes; atelectasis or infiltrate of a segment or lobe; pleural effusion that can conceal small interstitial lesions; interstitial cavities; or miliary-pattern infiltrates. In selected instances, computed tomography or magnetic resonance imaging of the chest can clarify indistinct radiographic findings, but these methods are not necessary for routine diagnosis. Although cavitation is common in reactivation "adult" tuberculosis, cavitation is uncommon in childhood tuberculosis. Necrosis and cavitation can result from a progressive primary focus in very young or immunocompromised patients and in the setting of lymphobronchial disease. Extrapulmonary manifestations include meningitis and granulomatous inflammation of the lymph nodes, bones, joints, skin, and middle ear and mastoid. Gastrointestinal tract tuberculosis can mimic inflammatory bowel disease. Renal tuberculosis and progression to disease from latent *M tuberculosis* infection ("adult-type pulmonary tuberculosis") are unusual in younger children but can occur in adolescents. In addition, chronic abdominal pain with peritonitis and intermittent partial intestinal obstruction can be present in disease caused by *Mycobacterium bovis*. Congenital tuberculosis can mimic neonatal sepsis, or the infant may come to medical attention in the first 90 days of life with bronchopneumonia and hepatosplenomegaly. Clinical findings in patients with drug-resistant tuberculosis disease are indistinguishable from manifestations in patients with drug-susceptible disease.

ETIOLOGY: The causative agent is *M tuberculosis* complex, a group of closely related acid-fast bacilli, which routinely includes the human pathogens *M tuberculosis*, *M bovis*, *Mycobacterium africanum*, and a few additional species infrequently associated with human infection. *M africanum* is rare in the United States, so clinical laboratories do not distinguish it routinely, and treatment recommendations are the same as for *M tuberculosis*. *M bovis* can be distinguished from *M tuberculosis* in reference laboratories, and although the spectrum of illness caused by *M bovis* is similar to that of *M tuberculosis*, the epidemiology, treatment, and prevention are different, as detailed later in the chapter.

Definitions:

- **Positive tuberculin skin test (TST).** A positive TST result (see Table 3.82) indicates possible infection with *M tuberculosis* complex. Tuberculin reactivity appears 2 to 10 weeks after initial infection; the median interval is 3 to 4 weeks (see The Tuberculin Skin Test, p 833). Bacille Calmette-Guérin (BCG) immunization can produce a positive TST result (see Diagnostic Tests, Testing for *M tuberculosis* Infection).

- **Positive interferon-gamma release assay (IGRA).** A positive IGRA result indicates probable infection with *M tuberculosis* complex. IGRAs measure ex vivo interferon-gamma production from T lymphocytes in response to stimulation with antigens specific to *M tuberculosis* complex, including *M tuberculosis* and *M bovis*. The antigens used in IGRAs are not found in BCG or most pathogenic nontuberculous mycobacteria (eg, are not found in *Mycobacterium avium* complex but are found in *Mycobacterium kansasii*, *Mycobacterium szulgai*, and *Mycobacterium marinum*).

- **Exposed person** refers to a person who has had recent (eg, within 3 months) contact with another person with suspected or confirmed contagious tuberculosis disease (ie, pulmonary, laryngeal, tracheal, or endobronchial disease) and who has a negative TST or IGRA result, normal physical examination findings, and chest radiographic findings that are normal or not compatible with tuberculosis. Some exposed people are or become infected (and subsequently develop a positive TST or IGRA result), and others do not become infected after exposure; the 2 groups cannot be distinguished initially.

Table 3.82. Definitions of Positive Tuberculin Skin Test (TST) Results in Infants, Children, and Adolescents[a]

Induration 5 mm or greater

Children in close contact with known or suspected contagious people with tuberculosis disease

Children suspected to have tuberculosis disease:
- Findings on chest radiograph consistent with active or previous tuberculosis disease
- Clinical evidence of tuberculosis disease[b]

Children receiving immunosuppressive therapy[c] or with immunosuppressive conditions, including human immunodeficiency (HIV) infection

Induration 10 mm or greater

Children at increased risk of disseminated tuberculosis disease:
- Children younger than 4 y
- Children with other medical conditions, including Hodgkin disease, lymphoma, diabetes mellitus, chronic renal failure, or malnutrition (see Table 3.83)

Children with likelihood of increased exposure to tuberculosis disease:
- Children born in high-prevalence regions of the world
- Children who travel to high-prevalence regions of the world
- Children frequently exposed to adults who are HIV infected, homeless, or incarcerated; users of illicit drugs; or residents of nursing homes

Induration 15 mm or greater

Children 4 y or older without any risk factors

[a]These definitions apply regardless of previous bacille Calmette-Guérin (BCG) immunization (see Testing for *M tuberculosis* Infection, p 833); erythema alone at TST site does not indicate a positive test result. Tests should be read at 48 to 72 hours after placement.

[b]Evidence by physical examination or laboratory assessment that would include tuberculosis in the working differential diagnosis (eg, meningitis).

[c]Including immunosuppressive doses of corticosteroids (see Corticosteroids, p 847) or tumor necrosis factor-alpha antagonists or blockers (see Biologic Response Modifying Drugs Used to Decrease Inflammation, p 85).

Table 3.83. Tuberculin Skin Test (TST) and IGRA Recommendations for Infants, Children, and Adolescents[a]

Children for whom immediate TST or IGRA is indicated[b]:
- Contacts of people with confirmed or suspected contagious tuberculosis (contact investigation)
- Children with radiographic or clinical findings suggesting tuberculosis disease
- Children immigrating from countries with endemic infection (eg, Asia, Middle East, Africa, Latin America, countries of the former Soviet Union), including international adoptees
- Children with history of significant travel to countries with endemic infection who have substantial contact with the resident population[c]

Children who should have annual TST or IGRA:
- Children with HIV infection

Children at increased risk of progression of LTBI to tuberculosis disease: Children with other medical conditions, including diabetes mellitus, chronic renal failure, malnutrition, congenital or acquired immunodeficiencies, and children receiving tumor necrosis factor (TNF) antagonists, deserve special consideration. Without recent exposure, these people are not at increased risk of acquiring *M tuberculosis* infection. Underlying immune deficiencies associated with these conditions theoretically would enhance the possibility for progression to severe disease. Initial histories of potential exposure to tuberculosis should be included for all these patients. If these histories or local epidemiologic factors suggest a possibility of exposure, immediate and periodic TST or IGRA should be considered. **A TST or IGRA should be performed before initiation of immunosuppressive therapy, including prolonged systemic corticosteroid administration, organ transplantation, use of TNF-alpha antagonists or blockers, or other immunosuppressive therapy in any child requiring these treatments.**

IGRA indicates interferon-gamma release assay; HIV, human immunodeficiency virus; LTBI, latent *M tuberculosis* infection.
[a]Bacille Calmette-Guérin immunization is not a contraindication to a TST.
[b]Beginning as early as 3 months of age for TST and 2 years of age for IGRAs, for LTBI and disease.
[c]If the child is well and has no history of exposure, the TST or IGRA should be delayed for up to 10 weeks after return.

- **Source case** is defined as the person who has transmitted infection with *M tuberculosis* complex to another person who subsequently develops infection not yet clinically apparent (especially a young child) or develops established latent *M tuberculosis* infection (LTBI) or tuberculosis disease.
- **LTBI** is defined as *M tuberculosis* complex infection in a person who has a positive TST or IGRA result, no physical findings of disease, and chest radiograph findings that are normal or reveal evidence of healed infection (eg, calcification in the lung, the hilar lymph nodes, or both). Note that hilar adenopathy is evidence of tuberculous disease, not LTBI.
- **Tuberculosis disease** is defined as illness in a person with infection in whom symptoms, signs, or radiographic manifestations caused by *M tuberculosis* complex are apparent; disease can be pulmonary, extrapulmonary, or both.
- **Directly observed therapy (DOT)** is defined as an intervention by which medications are administered directly to the patient by a health care professional or trained third party (not a relative or friend) who observes and documents that the patient ingests each dose of medication and assesses for possible adverse drug effects.
- **Multidrug-resistant tuberculosis** is defined as infection or disease caused by a

strain of *M tuberculosis* complex that is resistant to at least isoniazid and rifampin.

- **Extensively drug-resistant tuberculosis** is defined as infection or disease caused by a strain of *M tuberculosis* complex that is resistant to isoniazid and rifampin, at least 1 fluoroquinolone, and at least 1 of the following parenteral drugs: amikacin, kanamycin, or capreomycin.
- **Bacille Calmette-Guérin (BCG)** is a live attenuated vaccine strain of *M bovis*. BCG vaccine rarely is administered to children in the United States but is one of the most widely used vaccines in the world. An isolate of BCG can be distinguished from wild-type *M bovis* only in a reference laboratory.

EPIDEMIOLOGY: Case rates of tuberculosis in all ages are higher in urban, low-income areas and in nonwhite racial and ethnic groups; more than 80% of reported cases in the United States occur in Hispanic and nonwhite people. In recent years, more than 65% of all US cases have been in people born outside the United States. Almost 80% of childhood TB disease is associated with some form of foreign contact of the child, parent, or a household member. Specific groups with greater LTBI and disease rates include immigrants, international adoptees, refugees from or travelers to high-prevalence regions (eg, Asia, Africa, Latin America, and countries of the former Soviet Union), homeless people, people who use alcohol excessively or illicit drugs, and residents of certain correctional facilities and other congregate settings. Secondhand smoke exposure increases the risk of TB disease in infected children.

Infants and postpubertal adolescents are at increased risk of progression of LTBI to tuberculosis disease. Other predictive factors for development of disease include recent infection (within the past 2 years); immunodeficiency, especially from HIV infection; use of immunosuppressive drugs, such as prolonged or high-dose corticosteroid therapy or chemotherapy; intravenous drug use; and certain diseases or medical conditions, including Hodgkin disease, lymphoma, diabetes mellitus, chronic renal failure, and malnutrition. Tuberculosis disease has occurred in adolescents and adults being treated with tumor necrosis factor-alpha (TNF-alpha) antagonists or blocking agents, such as infliximab and etanercept (see Biologic Response Modifying Drugs Used to Decrease Inflammation, p 85). A positive TST or IGRA result should be accepted as indicative of infection in individuals receiving or soon to receive these medications, and the patient should be evaluated and treated accordingly.[1]

A diagnosis of LTBI or tuberculosis disease in a young child is a public health sentinel event often representing recent transmission. Transmission of *M tuberculosis* complex is airborne, with inhalation of droplet nuclei usually produced by an adult or adolescent with contagious pulmonary, endobronchial, or laryngeal tuberculosis disease. Although contagiousness usually lasts only a few days to weeks after initiation of effective drug therapy, it can last longer, especially when the adult patient has a positive acid-fast sputum smear, significant productive cough, pulmonary cavities, does not adhere to medical therapy, or is infected with a drug-resistant strain. If the sputum smear becomes negative for acid-fast bacilli (AFB) on 3 separate specimens at least 8 hours apart after treatment is started and the patient has improved clinically with resolution of cough, the treated person can be considered at low risk of transmitting *M tuberculosis*. Children younger than 10 years with only adenopathy in the chest or small pulmo-

---

[1]Starke JR; American Academy of Pediatrics, Committee on Infectious Diseases. Clinical report: Interferon-γ release assays for diagnosis of tuberculosis infection and disease in children. *Pediatrics.* 2014;134(6):e1763–e1773

nary lesions (paucibacillary disease) and nonproductive cough rarely are contagious. Unusual cases of adult-form pulmonary disease in young children, particularly with lung cavities and positive sputum-smear microscopy for AFB, and cases of congenital tuberculosis can be contagious.

M bovis is transmitted most often by unpasteurized dairy products, but airborne human-to-human transmission can occur.

The **incubation period** from infection to development of a positive TST or IGRA result is 2 to 10 weeks. The risk of developing tuberculosis disease is highest during the 6 months after infection and remains high for 2 years; however, many years can elapse between initial *M tuberculosis* infection and subsequent disease.

DIAGNOSTIC TESTS:

Testing for M tuberculosis Infection

The Tuberculin Skin Test (TST). The TST is an indirect method for detecting *M tuberculosis* infection. It is one of 2 methods for diagnosing LTBI, the other method being IGRA (p 834). Both methods rely on specific cellular sensitization after infection. Conditions that decrease lymphocyte numbers or function can reduce the sensitivity of these tests. The routine (ie, Mantoux) technique of administering the skin test consists of 5 tuberculin units of purified protein derivative (PPD; 0.1 mL) injected intradermally using a 27-gauge needle and a 1.0-mL syringe into the volar aspect of the forearm. Creation of a palpable wheal 6 to 10 mm in diameter is crucial to accurate testing.

Administration of TSTs and interpretation of results should be performed by trained and experienced health care personnel, because administration and interpretation by unskilled people and family members are unreliable. The standardized time for assessing the TST result is 48 to 72 hours after administration. The diameter of **induration,** in millimeters, is measured transversely to the long axis of the forearm and should be recorded as the result. Positive TST results, as defined in Table 3.82 (p 833), can persist for several weeks.

Lack of reaction to a TST does not exclude LTBI or tuberculosis disease. Approximately 10% to 40% of immunocompetent children with culture-documented tuberculosis disease do not react initially to a TST. Host factors, such as young age, poor nutrition, immunosuppression, viral infections (especially measles, varicella, and influenza), recent *M tuberculosis* infection, and disseminated tuberculosis disease, can decrease TST reactivity.

Classification of TST results is based on epidemiologic and clinical factors. Interpretation of the size of induration (mm) as a positive result varies with the person's risk of LTBI and likelihood of progression to tuberculosis disease. Current guidelines from the CDC, the American Thoracic Society, and the American Academy of Pediatrics (AAP) recommend interpretation of TST findings on the basis of an individual's risk stratification and are summarized in Table 3.82 (p 833). Prompt clinical and radiographic evaluation of all children and adolescents with a positive TST result is recommended (see Assessing for *M tuberculosis* Disease, p 837).

Generally, interpretation of TST results in BCG recipients who are known contacts of a person with tuberculosis disease or who are at high risk of tuberculosis disease is the same as for people who have not received BCG vaccine. After BCG immunization, distinguishing between a positive TST result caused by *M tuberculosis* complex infection and that caused by BCG is difficult. Reactivity of the TST after receipt of BCG vaccine does not occur in some patients. The size of the TST reaction (ie, mm of induration) attributable to BCG immunization depends on many factors, including age at BCG immunization, quality and strain of BCG vaccine used, number of doses of BCG vaccine received, nutritional and immunologic status of the vaccine recipient, frequency of TST administration, and time lapse between immunization and TST. Evidence that increases the probability that a positive TST result is attributable to LTBI includes known contact with a person with contagious tuberculosis, a family history of tuberculosis disease, more than 5 years since neonatal BCG immunization, and a TST reaction 15 mm or greater.

Blood-Based Testing With Interferon-Gamma Release Assays (IGRAs).[1,2] QuantiFERON-TB Gold In-Tube (Quest Diagnostics, Madison, NJ) and T-SPOT.*TB* (Oxford Immunotec Inc, Marlborough, MA) are FDA-approved blood tests that measure ex vivo interferon-gamma production from T lymphocytes in response to stimulation with antigens specific to *M tuberculosis* complex, which includes *M tuberculosis* and *M bovis*. However, the IGRA antigens used are not found in BCG. As with TSTs, IGRAs cannot distinguish between latent infection and disease, and a negative result from these tests cannot exclude the possibility of tuberculosis disease in a patient with suggestive clinical findings. The sensitivity of IGRA tests is similar to that of TSTs for detecting infection in adults and children who have untreated culture-confirmed tuberculosis. In many clinical settings, the specificity of IGRAs is higher than that for the TST, because the antigens used are not found in BCG or most pathogenic nontuberculous mycobacteria (eg, are not found in *M avium* complex, but are found in *M kansasii, M szulgai,* and *M marinum*). The published experience testing children with IGRAs demonstrates that IGRAs consistently perform well in children 2 years and older, and some data support their use for even younger children. The negative predictive value of IGRAs is not clear, but in general, if the IGRA result is negative and the TST result is positive in an asymptomatic, unexposed child, the diagnosis of LTBI is unlikely, especially if the child has received a BCG vaccine. A negative result for either a TST or an IGRA should be considered as especially unreliable in infants younger than 3 months.

TST Versus IGRA. For children younger than 2 years, TST is the preferred method for detection of *M tuberculosis* infection. For children 2 years and older, either TST or IGRA can be used, but in people previously vaccinated with BCG IGRA is preferred to avoid a false-positive TST result caused by a previous vaccination with BCG. If a BCG-vaccinated child who is 2 years and older has a positive TST, IGRA can be performed to help determine whether it is attributable to LTBI or to the previous BCG vaccine. Low-grade, false-positive IGRA results occur in some individuals. However:

- Children with a positive result from an IGRA should be considered infected with *M tuberculosis* complex. A negative IGRA result cannot be interpreted universally as evidence of absence of infection.
- Indeterminate or invalid IGRA results have several possible causes that could be related to the patient, the assay itself, or its performance. These results do not exclude *M tuberculosis* infection and may necessitate repeat testing, possibly with a different test. Indeterminate/invalid IGRA results should not be used to make clinical decisions.

---

[1]Centers for Disease Control and Prevention. Updated guidelines for using interferon gamma release assays to detect *Mycobacterium tuberculosis* infection—United States. *MMWR Recomm Rep.* 2010;59(RR-5):1–26

[2]Starke JR; American Academy of Pediatrics, Committee on Infectious Diseases. Clinical report: Interferon-γ release assays for diagnosis of tuberculosis infection and disease in children. *Pediatrics.* 2014;134(6):e1763–e1773

Specific recommendations for TST and IGRA use are provided in Table 3.83 (p 833) and Fig 3.11 (p 838).

Use of Tests for M tuberculosis *Infection.* The most reliable strategies for identifying LTBI and preventing tuberculosis disease in children are based on thorough and expedient contact investigations rather than nonselective testing of large populations. Contact investigations are public health interventions that should be coordinated through the local public health department. Universal testing with TST or IGRA, including programs based at schools, child care centers, and camps that include populations at low risk, is discouraged because it results in either a low yield of positive results or a large proportion of false-positive results, leading to an inefficient use of health care resources. However, using a questionnaire to determine risk factors for LTBI can be effective in health care settings. Simple questionnaires can identify children with risk factors for LTBI (see Table 3.84) who then should have a TST or IGRA performed. Risk assessment for tuberculosis should be performed at the first encounter of a child with a health care provider, and then annually if possible. Household investigation of children for tuberculosis is indicated whenever a TST or IGRA result of a household member converts from a negative to positive result (indicating recent infection).

HIV Infection. Children with HIV infection are considered at high risk for tuberculosis and should be tested annually beginning at 3 through 12 months of age if perinatally infected or at the time of diagnosis of HIV infection in older children or adolescents. Conversely, children who have tuberculosis disease should be tested for HIV infection. The clinical manifestations and radiographic appearance of tuberculosis disease in children with HIV infection tend to be similar to those in immunocompetent children, but manifestations in these children can be more severe and unusual and more often include extrapulmonary involvement of multiple organs. In HIV-infected patients, a TST induration of ≥5 mm is considered a positive result (see Table 3.82, p 830); however, a false-negative TST or IGRA result attributable to HIV-related immunosuppression also can occur. Specimens for culture and, if available, PCR should be obtained from all HIV-infected children with suspected tuberculosis.

Organ Transplant Patients. The risk of tuberculosis in organ transplant patients is several-fold greater than in the general population. A careful history of previous exposure to tuberculosis should be taken from all transplant candidates, including details about previous TST results and exposure to individuals with active TB. All transplant candidates should undergo evaluation by TST or IGRA for LTBI before the initiation of immunosuppressive therapy. A positive result of either test should be taken as evidence of *M tuberculosis* infection.

Table 3.84. Validated Questions for Determining Risk of LTBI in Children in the United States

- Has a family member or contact had tuberculosis disease?
- Has a family member had a positive tuberculin skin test result?
- Was your child born in a high-risk country (countries other than the United States, Canada, Australia, New Zealand, or Western and North European countries)?
- Has your child traveled to a high-risk country? How much contact did your child have with the resident population?

LTBI indicates latent *M tuberculosis* infection.

FIG 3.11. GUIDANCE ON STRATEGY FOR USE OF TST AND IGRA FOR DIAGNOSIS OF LTBI BY AGE AND BCG IMMUNIZATION STATUS

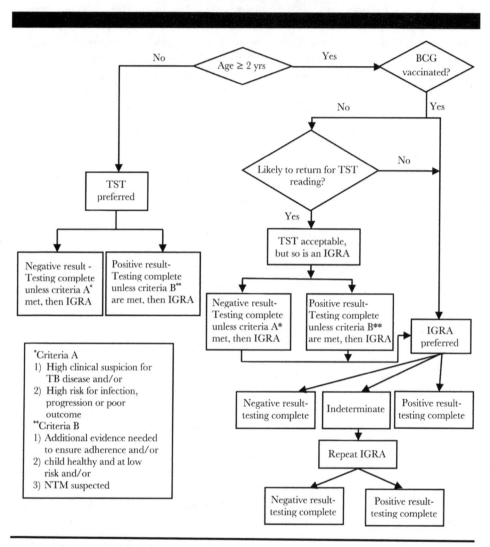

Patients Receiving Immunosuppressive Therapies Including Biologic Response Modifiers. Patients should be questioned for risk factors for *M tuberculosis* complex infection. In the presence or absence of tuberculosis risk factors, a TST or IGRA should be performed before the initiation of therapy with high-dose systemic corticosteroids, antimetabolite agents, and tumor necrosis factor antagonists or blockers (eg, infliximab and etanercept; see Biologic Response Modifying Drugs Used to Decrease Inflammation, p 85). Some experts recommend that if the child has at least 1 tuberculosis risk factor, both a TST and an IGRA should be performed to maximize sensitivity; a positive result of either test should be taken as evidence of *M tuberculosis* infection.

Other Considerations. Testing for tuberculosis at any age is not required before administration of live-virus vaccines. Measles vaccine temporarily can suppress tuberculin reactivity for at least 4 to 6 weeks, but the effect of varicella, yellow fever, and live attenuated influenza vaccines on TST reactivity and IGRA results is not known. If indicated, a TST can be applied or blood drawn for an IGRA at the same visit during which these vaccines are administered (ie, before substantial replication of the vaccine virus). The effects of live-virus vaccination on IGRA characteristics have not been determined; the same precautions as for TST should be followed. There is no evidence that inactivated vaccines, polysaccharide vaccines, or recombinant or subunit vaccines or toxoids interfere with clinical interpretation of TST or IGRAs.

Sensitivity to PPD tuberculin antigen persists for years in most instances, even after effective treatment. The durability of positive IGRA results has not been determined. Repeat testing with either TST or IGRA has no known clinical utility for assessing the effectiveness of treatment or for diagnosing newly acquired infection in patients who previously were infected with *M tuberculosis*.

Assessing for M tuberculosis *Disease*. Although both IGRA and TST testing provide evidence for infection with *M tuberculosis*, they cannot distinguish active from latent tuberculosis. Therefore, patients testing positive for *M tuberculosis* infection by IGRA or TST should be assessed for tuberculous disease before initiating any therapeutic intervention. This assessment should include: (1) assessment for symptoms of active tuberculosis disease, (2) physical examination for signs of active tuberculosis disease, and (3) a chest radiograph. If radiographic signs of active tuberculosis (eg, airspace opacities, pleural effusions, cavities, or changes on serial radiographs) are seen, then sputum or gastric aspirate sampling should then be performed, as described below. Most experts recommend that children younger than 12 months who are suspected of having pulmonary or extrapulmonary tuberculosis disease (eg, have a positive TST and symptoms, physical examination signs, or chest radiograph abnormalities consistent with tuberculosis disease), with or without neurologic symptoms, should have a lumbar puncture to evaluate for tuberculous meningitis. Some experts also recommend performing a lumbar puncture in children 12 through 23 months of age with tuberculosis disease, with or without neurologic symptoms. Children 24 months of age and older with tuberculosis disease require a lumbar puncture only if they have neurologic signs or symptoms.

Laboratory isolation of *M tuberculosis* complex by culture from a specimen of sputum, gastric aspirate, bronchial washing, pleural fluid, cerebrospinal fluid (CSF), urine, or other body fluid or a tissue biopsy specimen confirm the patient has tuberculosis diagnosis. Children older than 2 years and adolescents frequently can produce sputum spontaneously or by induction with aerosolized hypertonic saline. Studies have demonstrated successful collections of induced sputum from infants with pulmonary tuberculosis, but this requires special expertise. The best specimen for diagnosis of pulmonary tuberculosis in any child or adolescent in whom cough is absent or nonproductive and sputum cannot be induced is an early-morning gastric aspirate. Gastric aspirate specimens should be obtained with a nasogastric tube on awakening the child and before ambulation or feeding. Aspirates collected on 3 separate mornings should be submitted for testing by staining and culture.

Fluorescent staining methods for specimen smears are more sensitive than the traditional Kinyoun acid fast smears and are preferred. The overall diagnostic yield of microscopy of gastric aspirates and induced sputum is low in children with clinically suspected pulmonary tuberculosis, and false-positive smear results caused by the presence of nontuberculous mycobacteria occur rarely. Histologic examination for and demonstration of AFB and granulomas in biopsy specimens from lymph node, pleura, mesentery, liver, bone marrow, or other tissues can be useful, but *M tuberculosis* complex organisms cannot be distinguished reliably from other mycobacteria in stained specimens. Regardless of results of the AFB smears, each specimen should be cultured.

Because *M tuberculosis* complex organisms are slow growing, detection of these organisms may take as long as 10 weeks using solid media; use of liquid media and continuous monitoring systems allows detection within 1 to 6 weeks and usually within 3 weeks. Even with optimal culture techniques, *M tuberculosis* complex organisms are isolated from fewer than 75% of infants and 50% of children with pulmonary tuberculosis diagnosed by clinical criteria. Current methods for species identification of isolates from culture include molecular probes, nucleic acid amplification tests (NAATs), genetic sequencing, mass spectrometry, and biochemical tests. *M bovis* usually is suspected because of pyrazinamide resistance, which is characteristic of almost all *M bovis* isolates, but further biochemical or molecular testing is required to distinguish *M bovis* from *M tuberculosis*.

For a child with clinically suspected tuberculosis disease, finding the culture-positive source case supports the child's presumptive diagnosis and provides the likely drug susceptibility of the child's organism. Culture material should be collected from children with evidence of tuberculosis disease, especially when (1) an isolate from a source case is not available; (2) the presumed source case has drug-resistant tuberculosis; (3) the child is immunocompromised or ill enough to require hospital admission; or (4) the child has extrapulmonary disease. Traditional methods of determining drug susceptibility require bacterial isolation. Several new molecular methods of rapidly determining drug resistance directly from clinical samples now are available.

Two NAATs cleared by the US Food and Drug Administration (FDA) are available for detection of *M tuberculosis* complex organisms from smear-positive and smear-negative sputum specimens. One system, Xpert MTB-RIF (Cepheid, Sunnyvale, CA), also can detect the genetic marker for rifampin resistance in specimens within 2 hours. For children, Xpert MTB-RIF is more sensitive than microscopy but is not as sensitive as, and does not replace, culture. It is widely available in countries with a high prevalence of tuberculosis and is increasingly available in the United States. The Centers for Disease Control and Prevention (CDC) recommends a NAAT test on at least 1 respiratory tract specimen in a suspected case of tuberculosis.

TREATMENT (SEE TABLE 3.85):
Specific Drugs. Antituberculosis drugs kill or inhibit multiplication of *M tuberculosis* complex organisms, thereby arresting progression of infection and preventing most complications. Chemotherapy does not cause rapid disappearance of already caseous or granulomatous lesions (eg, mediastinal lymphadenitis). Dosage recommendations and the more commonly reported adverse reactions of major antituberculosis drugs are summarized in Tables 3.85 and 3.86 (p 844). For treatment of tuberculosis disease, these drugs always must be used in recommended combination and dosage to minimize emergence of drug-resistant strains. Use of nonstandard regimens for any reason (eg, drug allergy, drug resistance) should be undertaken only by an expert in treating tuberculosis.

Isoniazid is bactericidal, rapidly absorbed, and well tolerated and penetrates into body fluids, including CSF. Isoniazid is metabolized in the liver and excreted primarily through the kidneys. Hepatotoxic effects are rare in children but can be life threatening.

Table 3.85. Recommended Usual Treatment Regimens for Drug-Susceptible Tuberculosis in Infants, Children, and Adolescents

Infection or Disease Category	Regimen	Remarks
Latent *M tuberculosis* infection (positive TST or IGRA result, no disease)[a]		
• Isoniazid susceptible	12 weeks of isoniazid plus rifapentine, once a week OR 4 mo of rifampin, once a day OR	Continuous daily therapy is required. Intermittent therapy even by DOT is not recommended.
	9 mo of isoniazid, once a day	If daily therapy is not possible, DOT twice a week can be used for 9 mo.
• Isoniazid resistant	4 mo of rifampin, once a day	Continuous daily therapy is required. Intermittent therapy even by DOT is not recommended.
• Isoniazid-rifampin resistant	Consult a tuberculosis specialist	Moxifloxacin or levofloxacin with or without ethambutol or pyrazinamide.
Pulmonary and extrapulmonary (except meningitis)[b]	2 mo of isoniazid, rifampin, pyrazinamide, and ethambutol daily or twice weekly, followed by 4 mo of isoniazid and rifampin[e] by DOT[d] for drug-susceptible *Mycobacterium tuberculosis* 9 to 12 mo of isoniazid and rifampin for drug-susceptible *Mycobacterium bovis*	Some experts recommend a 3-drug initial regimen (isoniazid, rifampin, and pyrazinamide) if the risk of drug resistance is low. DOT is highly desirable. If hilar adenopathy only and the risk of drug resistance is low, a 6-mo course of isoniazid and rifampin is sufficient. Drugs can be given 2 or 3 times/wk under DOT.

Table 3.85. Recommended Usual Treatment Regimens for Drug-Susceptible Tuberculosis in Infants, Children, and Adolescents, continued

Infection or Disease Category	Regimen	Remarks
Meningitis	2 mo of isoniazid, rifampin, pyrazinamide, and an aminoglycoside[e] or ethionamide, once a day, followed by 7–10 mo of isoniazid and rifampin, once a day or twice a week (9–12 mo total) for drug-susceptible *M tuberculosis*	For patients who may have acquired tuberculosis in geographic areas where resistance to streptomycin is common, kanamycin, amikacin, or capreomycin can be used instead of streptomycin.
	At least 12 mo of therapy without pyrazinamide for drug-susceptible *M bovis*	

TST indicates tuberculin skin test; IGRA, interferon-gamma release assay; DOT, directly observed therapy.
[a]See text for comments and additional acceptable/alternative regimens.
[b]Duration of therapy may be longer for human immunodeficiency virus (HIV)-infected people, and additional drugs and dosing intervals may be indicated (see Tuberculosis Disease and HIV Infection, p 847).
[c]Medications should be administered daily for the first 2 weeks to 2 months of treatment and then can be administered 2 to 3 times per week by DOT. (Twice-weekly therapy is not recommended for HIV-infected people.)
[d]If initial chest radiograph shows pulmonary cavities and sputum culture after 2 months of therapy remains positive, the continuation phase is extended to 7 months, for a total treatment duration 9 of months.
[e]Streptomycin, kanamycin, amikacin, or capreomycin.

In children and adolescents who receive recommended doses, peripheral neuritis or seizures caused by inhibition of pyridoxine metabolism are rare, and most do not need pyridoxine supplements. Pyridoxine supplementation is recommended for exclusively breast-fed infants and for children and adolescents who have meat- and milk-deficient diets; children with nutritional deficiencies, including all symptomatic HIV-infected children; and pregnant adolescents and women. For infants and young children, isoniazid tablets can be pulverized or compounded by some pharmacies.

Rifampin is a bactericidal agent in the rifamycin class of drugs that is absorbed rapidly and penetrates into body fluids, including CSF. Other drugs in the rifamycin class approved for treating tuberculosis are rifabutin and rifapentine. Rifampin is metabolized by the liver and can alter the pharmacokinetics and serum concentrations of many other drugs. Rare adverse effects include hepatotoxicity, influenza-like symptoms, pruritus, and thrombocytopenia. Rifampin is excreted in bile and urine and can cause orange urine, sweat, and tears, with discoloration of soft contact lenses. Rifampin can make oral contraceptives ineffective, so nonhormonal birth-control methods should be adopted when rifampin is administered to sexually active female adolescents and adults. For infants and young children, the contents of the capsules can be suspended in flavored syrup or sprinkled on semisoft foods (eg, pudding).

Rifabutin is a suitable alternative to rifampin in HIV-infected children receiving antiretroviral therapy that restricts the use of rifampin because of drug interactions;

however, experience in children is limited, and there is no commercially available pediatric formulation.

Rifapentine is a long-acting rifamycin that permits weekly dosing in selected adults and adolescents with tuberculosis disease and is used for short-course multidrug treatment for LTBI.

Pyrazinamide attains therapeutic CSF concentrations, is detectable in macrophages, is administered orally, and is metabolized by the liver. Administration of pyrazinamide for the first 2 months with isoniazid and rifampin allows for 6-month regimens in immunocompetent patients with drug-susceptible tuberculosis. Almost all isolates of *M bovis* are resistant to pyrazinamide.

Ethambutol is well absorbed after oral administration, diffuses well into tissues, and is excreted in urine. At 20 mg/kg per day, ethambutol is bacteriostatic, and its primary therapeutic role is to prevent emergence of drug resistance. Ethambutol can cause reversible or irreversible optic neuritis, but reports in children with normal renal function are rare.

The less commonly used (eg, "second-line") antituberculosis drugs, their doses, and adverse effects are listed in Table 3.87 (p 845). These drugs have less optimal usefulness because of decreased effectiveness and greater toxicity and should be used only in consultation with a specialist familiar with childhood tuberculosis.

Occasionally, a patient cannot tolerate oral medications. Isoniazid, rifampin, kanamycin and related drugs, linezolid, and fluoroquinolones can be administered parenterally.

Treatment Regimens for LTBI

Several regimens are available. Any of these options is considered adequate, depending on the circumstances for individual patients. When indicated for LTBI, doses are the same as for treatment of tuberculosis (Table 3.86).

Isoniazid-Rifapentine Therapy for LTBI.[1] In 2011, on the basis of a large clinical trial (which included children 2–11 years of age), the CDC recommended a 12-week, once-weekly dose of isoniazid and rifapentine for treatment of LTBI. This regimen was shown to be safe, well tolerated, and at least as efficacious as 9 months of isoniazid given daily by self-supervision. Most experts consider isoniazid-rifapentine to be the preferred regimen for treatment of LTBI for children 5 years and older, and some experts prefer isoniazid-rifapentine therapy for LTBI in children 2 years and older. Isoniazid-rifapentine should not be used in children younger than 2 years because of a lack of pharmacokinetic data or an established dose for rifapentine in this age group.

Rifampin Therapy for LTBI. A 4-month course of rifampin given daily for 4 months also is an acceptable regimen for the treatment of LTBI. Most of the data supporting the efficacy of this regimen come from case control studies in adults and a few trials that included children. The regimen has been as effective as 9 months of daily isoniazid, the rates of adverse effects have been low, and the completion rates of therapy have been much higher than for 9 months of isoniazid. There has been extensive published and unpublished experience with this regimen in children, demonstrating effectiveness, safety, tolerability, and high rates of completion.

---

[1] Centers for Disease Control and Prevention. Recommendations for use of an isoniazid-rifapentine regimen with direct observation to treat latent *Mycobacterium tuberculosis* infection. *MMWR Morb Mortal Wkly Rep.* 2011;60(48):1650–1653

Table 3.86. Commonly Used Drugs for Treatment of Tuberculosis in Infants, Children, and Adolescents

Drugs	Dosage Forms	Daily Dosage (Range), mg/kg	Twice a Week Dosage, mg/kg per Dose	Maximum Dose	Most Common Adverse Reactions
Ethambutol	Tablets 100 mg 400 mg	20 (15–25)	50	Daily, 1 g Twice a week, 2.5 g	Optic neuritis (usually reversible), decreased red-green color discrimination, gastrointestinal tract disturbances, hypersensitivity
Isoniazid[a]	Scored tablets 100 mg 300 mg	10 (10–15)[b]	20–30	Daily, 300 mg Twice a week, 900 mg	Mild hepatic enzyme elevation, hepatitis,[b] peripheral neuritis, hypersensitivity
Pyrazinamide [a]	Scored tablets 500 mg	35 (30–40)	50	2 g	Hepatotoxic effects, hyperuricemia, arthralgia, gastrointestinal tract upset, pruritus, rash
Rifampin[a]	Capsules 150 mg 300 mg Syrup formulated capsules	15–20[c]	15–20[c]	600 mg	Orange discoloration of secretions or urine, staining of contact lenses, vomiting, hepatitis, influenza-like reaction, thrombocytopenia, pruritus; oral contraceptives may be ineffective

[a]Rifamate is a capsule containing 150 mg of isoniazid and 300 mg of rifampin. Two capsules provide the usual adult (greater than 50 kg) daily doses of each drug. Rifater, in the United States, is a capsule containing 50 mg of isoniazid, 120 mg of rifampin, and 300 mg of pyrazinamide. Isoniazid and rifampin also are available for parenteral administration.

[b]When isoniazid in a dosage exceeding 10 mg/kg/day is used in combination with rifampin, the incidence of hepatotoxic effects may be increased.

[c]Many experts recommend using a daily rifampin dose of 20–30 mg/kg/day for infants and toddlers, and for serious forms of tuberculosis such as meningitis and disseminated disease.

Isoniazid Therapy for LTBI. A 9-month course of daily isoniazid therapy in children has an efficacy that approaches 100% if adherence to therapy is high. Unfortunately, many studies have shown the adherence and completion rates to be 50% to 75% over 9 months when families administer isoniazid on their own. Isoniazid should not be used if the child received antituberculosis therapy previously or if resistance to isoniazid is suspected or proven in the source case. Additionally, immigrants who received isoniazid in countries with high rates of isoniazid-resistant tuberculosis may not have been treated adequately.

For infants, children, and adolescents, including those with HIV infection or other immunocompromising conditions, the recommended duration of isoniazid therapy in the United States is 9 months. The World Health Organization recommends a 6-month course of isoniazid, but modeling studies have shown that the efficacy of 6 months of treatment is approximately 30% less than that of a 9-month course. Although there have been no formal trials of interrupted 9-month courses, many experts accept 6 months of uninterrupted treatment as adequate. When adherence with daily therapy with isoniazid cannot be ensured, twice-a-week DOT can be considered, but each dose must be observed directly. Determination of serum transaminase concentrations before or during therapy is not indicated except in patients with underlying liver or biliary disease, during pregnancy or the first 12 weeks postpartum, with concurrent use of other potentially hepatotoxic drugs (eg, anticonvulsant or HIV agents), or if there is clinical concern of possible hepatotoxicity.

Additional Regimens for Treatment of LTBI. Additional possible regimens for treatment of LTBI are: (1) 3 months of daily isoniazid and rifampin, with the isoniazid dosage the same as when used alone and the rifampin dosage of 15 to 20 mg/kg/day (maximum 600 mg); or (2) 2 months of daily rifampin and pyrazinamide when given as part of RIPE (rifampin, isoniazid, pyrazinamide, and ethambutol) therapy for suspected tuberculosis disease that subsequently is determined to be *M tuberculosis* infection only. The rifampin dose is 15 to 20 mg/kg day (maximum 600 mg); and the pyrazinamide dose is 30 to 40 mg/kg/day, maximum 2 g.

Therapy for LTBI and Contacts of Patients With Isoniazid-Resistant M tuberculosis *and When Isoniazid Cannot Be Administered.* The incidence of isoniazid resistance among *M tuberculosis* complex isolates from US patients is approximately 9%. Risk factors for drug resistance are listed in Table 3.88. If the source case is found to have isoniazid-resistant, rifampin-susceptible

Table 3.87. Drugs for Treatment of Drug-Resistant Tuberculosis in Infants, Children, and Adolescents[a]

Drugs	Dosage, Forms	Daily Dosage	Maximum Dose	Adverse Reactions
Amikacin[b]	Vials, 500 mg and 1 g	15–30 mg/kg (intravenous or intramuscular administration)	1 g	Auditory and vestibular toxic effects, nephrotoxic effects
Capreomycin[b]	Vials, 1 g	15–30 mg/kg (intramuscular administration)	1 g	Auditory and vestibular toxicity and nephrotoxic effects
Cycloserine	Capsules, 250 mg	10–20 mg/kg, given in 2 divided doses	1 g	Psychosis, personality changes, seizures, rash
Ethionamide	Tablets, 250 mg	15–20 mg/kg, given in 2–3 divided doses	1 g	Gastrointestinal tract disturbances, hepatotoxic effects, hypersensitivity reactions, hypothyroidism

Table 3.87. Drugs for Treatment of Drug-Resistant Tuberculosis in Infants, Children, and Adolescents,[a] continued

Drugs	Dosage, Forms	Daily Dosage	Maximum Dose	Adverse Reactions
Kanamycin	Vials 75 mg/2 mL 500 mg/2 mL 1 g/3 mL	15–30 mg/kg (intramuscular or intravenous administration)	1 g	Auditory and vestibular toxic effects, nephrotoxic effects
Levofloxacin[c]	Tablets 250 mg 500 mg 750 mg Oral solution 25 mg/mL Vials 5 mg/mL 25 mg/mL	Adults: 750–1000 mg (once daily) Children: 15–20 mg/kg	1 g	Theoretical effect on growing cartilage, tendonitis, gastro-intestinal tract disturbances, cardiac disturbances, peripheral neuropathy, rash, headache, restlessness, confusion
Linezolid		Adults: 600 mg (once daily) Children <10 y: 10 mg/kg/dose, every 12 h Children ≥10 y: 10 mg/kg/dose daily[d]	600 mg	Used for treatment of multidrug-resistant tuberculosis; adverse events include bone marrow suppression
Para-aminosalicyl-ic acid (PAS)	Packets, 3 g	200–300 mg/kg (2–4 times a day)	10 g	Gastrointestinal tract disturbances, hyper-sensitivity, hepatotox-ic effects, hypothy-roidism
Streptomycin[b]	Vials 1 g 4 g	20–40 mg/kg (intramuscular administration)	1 g	Auditory and vestibular toxic effects, nephrotoxic effects (which must be preemptively moni-tored) and rash

[a] These drugs should be used in consultation with a specialist in tuberculosis.
[b] Dose adjustment in renal insufficiency.
[c] Levofloxacin is not approved for use in children younger than 18 years; its use in younger children necessitates assessment of the potential risks and benefits (see Antimicrobial Agents and Related Therapy, p 903).
[d] Linezolid pharmacokinetics have not been well established in children. The doses listed will yield a drug exposure approximate-ly equal to that in adults taking 600 mg daily.

Table 3.88. People at Increased Risk of Drug-Resistant Tuberculosis Infection or Disease

- People with a history of treatment for tuberculosis disease (or whose source case for the contact received such treatment)
- Contacts of a patient with drug-resistant contagious tuberculosis disease
- People from countries with high prevalence of drug-resistant tuberculosis, such as Russia and certain nations of the former Soviet Union, Asia, Africa, and Latin America
- Infected people whose source case has positive smears for acid-fast bacilli or cultures after 2 months of appropriate antituberculosis therapy and patients who do not respond to a standard treatment regimen
- Residence in geographic area with a high percentage of drug-resistant isolates

Source: **wwwnc.cdc.gov/travel/yellowbook/2014/chapter-3-infectious-diseases-related-to-travel/ tuberculosis.**

organisms, isoniazid should be discontinued and rifampin should be administered daily to contacts for a total course of 4 months. Optimal therapy for children with LTBI caused by organisms with resistance to isoniazid and rifampin (ie, multidrug resistance) is not known. In these circumstances, a fluoroquinolone alone and multidrug regimens have been used, but the safety and the efficacy of these empiric regimens have not been assessed in clinical trials. Drugs to consider include levofloxacin, with or without the addition of pyrazinamide or ethambutol, depending on susceptibility of the isolate. Consultation with a tuberculosis specialist is indicated.

Treatment of Tuberculosis Disease. The goal of treatment is to achieve killing of replicating organisms in the tuberculous lesion in the shortest possible time. Achievement of this goal minimizes the possibility of development of resistant organisms. The major problem limiting successful treatment is poor adherence to prescribed treatment regimens. The use of DOT decreases the rates of relapse, treatment failures, and drug resistance; therefore, DOT is recommended strongly for treatment of all children and adolescents with tuberculosis disease in the United States.

Therapy for Presumed or Known Drug-Susceptible Pulmonary Tuberculosis. A 6-month, 4-drug regimen consisting initially of rifampin, isoniazid, pyrazinamide, and ethambutol (RIPE) for the first 2 months and isoniazid and rifampin for the remaining 4 months is recommended for treatment of pulmonary disease, pulmonary disease with hilar adenopathy, and hilar adenopathy disease in infants, children, and adolescents when a multidrug-resistant case is not suspected as the source of infection or when favorable drug-susceptibility results are available from the patient or the likely source case. Some experts administer 3 drugs (isoniazid, rifampin, and pyrazinamide) as the initial regimen if a presumed source case has been identified with known susceptible *M tuberculosis* or has no risk factors for drug-resistant *M tuberculosis*. For children with hilar adenopathy in whom drug resistance is not a consideration, a 6-month regimen of only isoniazid and rifampin is considered adequate by some experts. If the chest radiograph shows one or more pulmonary cavities and sputum culture result remains positive after 2 months of therapy, the duration of therapy should be extended to 9 months.

In the 6-month regimen with 4-drug RIPE therapy, drugs are administered once a day for at least the first 2 weeks by DOT at least 5 days per week. An alternative to daily dosing between 2 weeks and 2 months of treatment is to administer these drugs 2 or 3 times a week by DOT (except in HIV-infected people, in whom intermittent dosing is not recommended). After the initial 2-month period, a DOT regimen of isoniazid and rifampin given 2 or 3 times a week is acceptable (see Table 3.86, p 841, for doses). Several alternative regimens with differing durations of daily therapy and total therapy have been used successfully in adults and children. These alternative regimens should be prescribed and managed by a specialist in pediatric tuberculosis.

Therapy for Drug-Resistant Pulmonary Tuberculosis Disease. Drug resistance is more common in certain groups (Table 3.88). When **resistance to drugs other than isoniazid** is likely (see Table 3.88), initial therapy should be adjusted by adding at least 2 drugs to match the presumed drug susceptibility pattern until drug susceptibility results are available. If an isolate from the pediatric case under treatment is not available, drug susceptibilities can be inferred by the drug susceptibility pattern of isolates from the presumed source case. Data for guiding drug selection may not be available for foreign-born children or in circumstances of international travel or adoption. If this information is not available, a 4- or 5-drug initial regimen should be strongly considered with close monitoring for clinical response.

Most cases of pulmonary tuberculosis in children that are caused by an isoniazid-resistant but rifampin- and pyrazinamide-susceptible strain of *M tuberculosis* complex can be treated with a 6-month regimen of rifampin, pyrazinamide, and ethambutol. For cases of multidrug-resistant tuberculosis disease, the treatment regimen needed for cure should include at least 4 or 5 antituberculosis drugs to which the organism is susceptible. Bedaquiline is approved by the FDA as part of combination therapy in the treatment for adults with multidrug-resistant pulmonary tuberculosis for whom an effective regimen could not be instituted; unfortunately, there currently are no safety, tolerability, efficacy, or pharmacokinetic data on use of bedaquiline in children.[1] Therapy for multidrug-resistant tuberculosis is administered for 12 to 24 months from the time of culture conversion to negativity. An injectable drug, initially administered 5 days per week, such as amikacin, kanamycin, or capreomycin, often is used for the first 4 to 6 months of treatment, as tolerated. Regimens in which drugs are administered intermittently are not recommended for drug-resistant disease; daily DOT is critical to prevent emergence of additional resistance. An expert in drug-resistant tuberculosis should be consulted for all drug-resistant cases.

Extrapulmonary Tuberculosis Disease. In general, extrapulmonary tuberculosis—with the exception of meningitis—can be treated with the same regimens as used for pulmonary tuberculosis. For suspected drug-susceptible tuberculous meningitis, daily treatment with isoniazid, rifampin, pyrazinamide, and ethionamide, if possible, or an aminoglycoside (parenteral streptomycin, kanamycin, amikacin, or capreomycin) should be initiated. When susceptibility to first-line drugs is established, the ethionamide or aminoglycoside can be discontinued. Pyrazinamide is given for a total of 2 months, and isoniazid and rifampin are given for a total of 9 to 12 months. Isoniazid and rifampin can be given daily or 2 or 3 times per week after the first 2 months of treatment if the child has responded well.

Evaluation and Monitoring of Therapy in Children and Adolescents. Careful monthly monitoring

---

[1]Centers for Disease Control and Prevention. Provisional CDC guidelines for the use and safety monitoring of bedaquiline fumarate (Sirturo) for the treatment of multidrug-resistant tuberculosis. *MMWR Recomm Rep.* 2013;62(RR-9):1–11

of clinical and bacteriologic responses to therapy is important. With DOT, clinical evaluation is an integral component of each visit for drug administration. For patients with pulmonary tuberculosis, chest radiographs often are obtained after 2 months of therapy to evaluate response. Even with successful 6-month regimens, hilar adenopathy can persist for 2 to 3 years; normal radiographic findings are not necessary to discontinue therapy. Follow-up chest radiography beyond termination of successful therapy usually is not necessary unless clinical deterioration occurs.

If therapy has been interrupted, the date of completion should be extended. Although guidelines cannot be provided for every situation, factors to consider when establishing the date of completion include the following: (1) length of interruption of therapy; (2) time during therapy (early or late) when interruption occurred; and (3) the patient's clinical, radiographic, and bacteriologic status before, during, and after interruption of therapy. The total doses administered by DOT should be calculated to guide the duration of therapy. Consultation with a specialist in tuberculosis is advised.

Untoward effects of isoniazid therapy, including severe hepatitis in otherwise healthy infants, children, and adolescents, are rare. Routine determination of serum transaminase concentrations is not recommended (see "Isoniazid Therapy for LTBI," p 842). In most other circumstances, monthly clinical evaluations to observe for signs or symptoms of hepatitis and other adverse effects of drug therapy without routine monitoring of transaminase concentrations is appropriate follow-up. Regular physician-patient contact to assess drug adherence, efficacy, and adverse effects is an important aspect of management. Patients should be provided with written instructions and advised to call a physician immediately if symptoms of adverse events, in particular hepatotoxicity (ie, nausea, vomiting, abdominal pain, jaundice), develop.

Other Treatment Considerations

Corticosteroids. The evidence supporting adjuvant treatment with corticosteroids for children with tuberculosis disease is incomplete. Corticosteroids are definitely indicated for children with tuberculous meningitis, because corticosteroids decrease rates of mortality and long-term neurologic impairment. Corticosteroids can be considered for children with pleural and pericardial effusions (to hasten reabsorption of fluid), severe miliary disease (to mitigate alveolocapillary block), endobronchial disease (to relieve obstruction and atelectasis), and abdominal tuberculosis (to decrease the risk of strictures). Corticosteroids should be given only when accompanied by appropriate antituberculosis therapy. Most experts give 2 mg/kg per day of prednisone (maximum, 60 mg/day) or its equivalent for 4 to 6 weeks followed by tapering.

Tuberculosis Disease and HIV Infection.[1] Most HIV-infected adults with drug-susceptible tuberculosis respond well to standard treatment regimens. However, optimal therapy for tuberculosis in children with HIV infection has not been established. Treating tuberculosis in an HIV-infected child is complicated by antiretroviral drug interactions with the rifamycins and overlapping toxicities. Therapy always should include at least 4 drugs initially, should be administered daily via DOT, and should be continued for at least 6 months. Isoniazid, rifampin, and pyrazinamide, usually with ethambutol, should be administered for at least the first 2 months. Ethambutol can be discontinued once

---

[1]Guidelines for the prevention and treatment of opportunistic infections in HIV infected adults and adolescents: Recommendations from CDC, NIH, IDSA. December 2014. Available at: **https://aidsinfo.nih.gov/guidelines**

drug-resistant tuberculosis disease is excluded. Rifampin may be contraindicated in people who are receiving antiretroviral therapy. Rifabutin is substituted for rifampin in some circumstances. Consultation with a specialist who has experience in managing HIV-infected patients with tuberculosis is strongly advised.

Immunizations. Patients who are receiving treatment for tuberculosis can receive measles and other age-appropriate attenuated live-virus vaccines unless they are receiving high-dose systemic corticosteroids, are severely ill, or have other specific contraindications to immunization.

Tuberculosis During Pregnancy and Breastfeeding. Pregnant women who have a positive TST or IGRA result, are asymptomatic, have a normal chest radiograph, and had recent contact with a contagious person should be considered for isoniazid therapy. Therapy in these circumstances should begin after the first trimester and the recommended duration is 9 months. If there has been no recent contact with a contagious case, therapy can be delayed until after delivery. Pyridoxine supplementation is indicated for all pregnant and breastfeeding women receiving isoniazid.

If tuberculosis disease is diagnosed during pregnancy, a regimen of isoniazid, rifampin, and ethambutol is recommended. Pyrazinamide commonly is used in a 3- or 4-drug regimen, but safety during pregnancy has not been established. At least 6 months of therapy is indicated for drug-susceptible tuberculosis disease if pyrazinamide is used; at least 9 months of therapy is indicated if pyrazinamide is not used. Prompt initiation of therapy is mandatory to protect mother and fetus.

Isoniazid, ethambutol, and rifampin are relatively safe for the fetus. The benefit of ethambutol and rifampin for therapy of tuberculosis disease in the mother outweighs the risk to the infant. Because aminoglycosides (streptomycin, kanamycin, amikacin, or capreomycin) can cause ototoxic effects in the fetus, they should not be used unless administration is essential for effective treatment. The effects of other second-line drugs on the fetus are unknown. Ethionamide has been demonstrated to be teratogenic, so its use during pregnancy is contraindicated.

Although isoniazid is secreted in human milk, no adverse effects of isoniazid on nursing infants have been demonstrated. Breastfed infants do not require pyridoxine supplementation unless they are receiving isoniazid. The isoniazid dosage of a breastfed infant whose mother is taking isoniazid does not require adjustment for the small amount of drug in the milk.

Congenital Tuberculosis. Congenital tuberculosis is rare, but in utero infections can occur after maternal bacillemia and have been reported following in vitro fertilization of women from countries with endemic disease in whom infertility likely was related to subclinical maternal genitourinary tract tuberculosis.

If a newborn infant is suspected of having congenital tuberculosis, a TST and IGRA test, chest radiography, lumbar puncture, and appropriate cultures and radiography should be performed promptly. The TST result usually is negative in newborn infants with congenital or perinatally acquired infection. Hence, regardless of the TST or IGRA results, treatment of the infant should be initiated promptly with rifampin, isoniazid, pyrazinamide, and either ethambutol (RIPE) or an aminoglycoside (streptomycin, kanamycin, amikacin, or capreomycin). The placenta should be examined histologically for granulomata and AFB, and a specimen should be cultured for *M tuberculosis* complex. The mother should be evaluated for presence of pulmonary or extrapulmonary disease, including genitourinary tuberculosis. If the physical examination and chest radiographic findings support the diagnosis of tuberculosis disease, the newborn infant should be treated with a regimen recommended for tuberculosis disease. If meningitis is confirmed, corticosteroids should be added (see Corticosteroids, p 847). Drug susceptibility testing of the organism recovered from the mother, infant, or both should be performed. HIV testing of the mother is essential.

Management of the Newborn Infant Whose Mother Has LTBI or Tuberculosis Disease. Management of the newborn infant is based on categorization of the maternal infection. Although protection of the infant from exposure and infection is of paramount importance, contact between infant and mother should be allowed when possible. Differing circumstances and resulting recommendations are as follows:

- **Mother has a positive TST or IGRA result and normal chest radiographic findings.** If the mother is asymptomatic, no separation is required. The mother usually is a candidate for treatment of LTBI after the initial postpartum period. The newborn infant needs no special evaluation or therapy. Because of the young infant's exquisite susceptibility and because the mother's positive TST or IGRA result could be a marker of an unrecognized case of contagious tuberculosis within the household, other household members should have a TST or IGRA and further evaluation; this should not delay the infant's discharge from the hospital. These mothers can breastfeed their infants.

- **Mother has clinical signs and symptoms or abnormal findings on chest radiograph consistent with tuberculosis disease.** Cases of suspected or proven tuberculosis disease in mothers should be reported immediately to the local health department, and investigation of all household members started as soon as possible. If the mother has tuberculosis disease, the infant should be evaluated for congenital tuberculosis (see Congenital Tuberculosis, p 848), and the mother should be tested for HIV infection. The mother and the infant should be separated until the mother has been evaluated and, if tuberculosis disease is suspected, until the mother and infant are receiving appropriate antituberculosis therapy, the mother wears a mask, and the mother understands and is willing to adhere to infection-control measures. During separation, expressed human milk can be fed to the infant unless mother has signs of tuberculous mastitis, which is rare. Once the infant is receiving isoniazid, separation is not necessary unless the mother has possible multidrug-resistant tuberculosis disease or has poor adherence to treatment and DOT is not possible. If the mother is suspected of having multidrug-resistant tuberculosis disease, an expert in tuberculosis disease treatment should be consulted. Women with drug-susceptible tuberculosis disease who have been treated appropriately for 2 or more weeks and who are not considered contagious can breastfeed.

   If congenital tuberculosis is excluded, isoniazid is administered until the infant is 3 or 4 months of age, when a TST should be performed. If the TST result is negative at 3 to 4 months of age and the mother has good adherence and response to treatment and no longer is contagious, isoniazid should be discontinued. If the TST result is positive, the infant should be reassessed for tuberculosis disease. If tuberculosis disease is excluded, isoniazid alone should be continued for a total of 9 months. The infant should be evaluated monthly during treatment for signs of illness or poor growth.

- **Mother has a positive TST or IGRA and abnormal findings on chest radiography but no evidence of tuberculosis disease.** If the chest radiograph of the mother appears abnormal but is not suggestive of tuberculosis disease and the history, physical examination, and sputum smear indicate no evidence of tuberculosis disease, the infant can be assumed to be at low risk of *M tuberculosis* infection and need not be separated from the mother. The mother and her infant should receive follow-up care and the mother should be treated for LTBI. Other household members should have a TST or IGRA and further evaluation.

ISOLATION OF THE HOSPITALIZED PATIENT: Most children with tuberculosis disease, especially children younger than 10 years, are not contagious. Exceptions are the following: (1) children with pulmonary cavities; (2) children with positive sputum AFB smears; (3) children with laryngeal involvement; (4) children with extensive pulmonary infection; or (5) neonates or infants with congenital tuberculosis undergoing procedures that involve the oropharyngeal airway (eg, endotracheal intubation). In these instances, airborne infection isolation precautions for tuberculosis are indicated until effective therapy has been initiated, sputum smears are negative, and coughing has abated. Additional criteria apply to multidrug-resistant tuberculosis. Children with no cough and negative sputum AFB smears can be hospitalized in an open ward. Infection-control measures for hospital personnel and visitors exposed to contagious patients should include the use of personally "fit tested" and "sealed" N-95 particulate respirators for all patient contacts (see Infection Control and Prevention for Hospitalized Children, p 147).

The major concern in infection control relates to adult household members and contacts that can be the source of infection. Visitation should be limited to people who have been evaluated and do not have tuberculosis. Household members and contacts should be managed with tuberculosis precautions when visiting until they are demonstrated not to have contagious tuberculosis.

***Tuberculosis Caused by* M bovis.** Infections with *M bovis* account for approximately 1% to 2% of tuberculosis cases in the United States and higher along the border with Mexico. Children who come from countries where *M bovis* is prevalent in cattle or whose parents come from those countries are more likely to be infected. Most infections in humans are transmitted from cattle by unpasteurized milk and its products, such as fresh cheese,[1] although human-to-human transmission by the airborne route has been documented. In children, *M bovis* more commonly causes cervical lymphadenitis, intestinal tuberculosis disease and peritonitis, and meningitis. In adults, latent *M bovis* infection can progress to advanced pulmonary disease, with a risk of transmission to others.

The TST result typically is positive in a person infected with *M bovis*; IGRAs have not been studied systematically for diagnosing *M bovis* infection in particular, but theoretically they should have acceptable test characteristics (see Blood-Based Testing With Interferon-Gamma Release Assays [IGRAs], p 834). The definitive diagnosis of *M bovis* infection requires a culture isolate. The commonly used methods for identifying a microbial isolate as *M tuberculosis* complex do not distinguish *M bovis* from *M tuberculosis*, *M africanum*, and BCG; *M bovis* is suspected in clinical laboratories by its typical resistance to pyrazinamide. This approach can be unreliable, and species confirmation at a reference laboratory should be requested when *M bovis* is suspected. Molecular genotyping through the state health department may assist in identifying *M bovis*. Resistance to first-line drugs in addition to pyrazinamide has been reported but is uncommon. BCG rarely is isolated from

---

[1]American Academy of Pediatrics, Committee on Infectious Diseases and Committee on Nutrition. Consumption of raw or unpasteurized milk and milk products by pregnant women and children. *Pediatrics*. 2014;133(1): 175–179

pediatric clinical specimens in the United States; however, it should be suspected from localized BCG suppuration or draining lymphadenitis in children who recently (within several months) have received BCG vaccine. Only a reference laboratory can distinguish an isolate of BCG from an isolate of *M bovis*.

Therapy for M bovis *Disease.* Controlled clinical trials for treatment of *M bovis* disease have not been conducted, and treatment recommendations for *M bovis* disease in adults and children are based on results from treatment trials for *M tuberculosis* disease. Although most strains of *M bovis* are pyrazinamide-resistant and resistance to other first-line drugs has been reported, multidrug-resistant strains are rare. Initial therapy for disease caused by *M bovis* should include 3 or 4 drugs, excluding pyrazinamide, that would be used to treat disease attributable to *M tuberculosis*. For isoniazid- and rifampin-susceptible strains, a total treatment course of at least 9 months is recommended.

Parents should be counseled about the many infectious diseases transmitted by unpasteurized milk and its products,[1] and parents who might import traditional dairy products from countries where *M bovis* infection is prevalent in cattle should be advised against giving those products to their children. When people are exposed to an adult who has pulmonary disease caused by *M bovis* infection, they should be evaluated by the same methods as for *M tuberculosis*.

CONTROL MEASURES[2,3]: Reporting of suspected and confirmed cases of tuberculosis disease is mandated by law in all states. LTBI is reportable in only a few states. Control of tuberculosis disease in the United States requires collaboration between health care providers and health department personnel, obtaining a thorough history of exposure(s) to people with contagious tuberculosis, timely and effective contact investigations, proper interpretation of TST or IGRA results, and appropriate antituberculosis therapy, including DOT services. A plan to control and prevent extensively drug-resistant tuberculosis has been published.[4] Eliminating ingestion of unpasteurized dairy products will prevent most *M bovis* infection.[1]

Management of Contacts, Including Epidemiologic Investigation.[3,5] Children with a positive TST or IGRA result or tuberculosis disease ideally should be the starting point for epidemiologic investigation by the local health department. Close contacts of a TST- or IGRA-positive child, if the test was performed because the child has 1 or more risk factors, should have a TST or IGRA, and people with a positive TST or IGRA result or with symptoms consistent with tuberculosis disease should be investigated further. Because

---

[1]American Academy of Pediatrics, Committee on Infectious Diseases and Committee on Nutrition. Consumption of raw or unpasteurized milk and milk products by pregnant women and children. *Pediatrics*. 2014;133(1): 175–179

[2]American Thoracic Society, Centers for Disease Control and Prevention, and Infectious Diseases Society of America. Controlling tuberculosis in the United States. Recommendations from the American Thoracic Society, CDC, and the Infectious Diseases Society of America. *MMWR Recomm Rep*. 2005;54(RR-12):1–81

[3]Starke JR; American Academy of Pediatrics, Committee on Infectious Diseases. Clinical report: interferon-γ release assays for diagnosis of tuberculosis infection and disease in children. *Pediatrics*. 2014;134(6):e1763–e1773

[4]Centers for Disease Control and Prevention. Plan to combat extensively drug-resistant tuberculosis: recommendations of the Federal Tuberculosis Task Force. *MMWR Recomm Rep*. 2009;58(RR-3):1–43

[5]National Tuberculosis Controllers Association and Centers for Disease Control and Prevention. Guidelines for the investigation of contacts of persons with infectious tuberculosis. Recommendations from the National Tuberculosis Controllers Association and CDC. *MMWR Recomm Rep*. 2005;54(RR-15):1–47

children with tuberculosis usually are not contagious unless they have an adult-type multibacillary form of pulmonary or laryngeal disease, their contacts are not likely to be infected unless they also have been in contact with an adult source case. After the presumptive adult source of the child's tuberculosis is identified, other contacts of that adult should be evaluated.

Therapy for Contacts. Children and adolescents recently exposed to a contagious case of tuberculosis disease should have a TST or IGRA test performed and should have an evaluation for tuberculosis disease (history, physical examination, and chest radiography) performed. For exposed contacts with impaired immunity (eg, HIV infection) and all contacts younger than 5 years, treatment for presumptive LTBI should be initiated, even if the initial TST or IGRA result is negative, once tuberculosis disease is excluded (see Treatment Regimens for LTBI, p 841). Infected people can have a negative TST or IGRA result because a cellular immune response has not yet developed or because of anergy. People with a negative TST or IGRA result should be retested 8 to 10 weeks after the last exposure to a source of infection. If the TST or IGRA result still is negative in an immunocompetent person, isoniazid can be discontinued. If the contact is immunocompromised and LTBI cannot be excluded, after an evaluation for TB disease, treatment should be continued to the completion of the regimen. If a TST or IGRA result of a contact becomes positive, the regimen for LTBI should be completed after an evaluation for TB disease.

Child Care and Schools. Children with tuberculosis disease can attend school or child care if they are receiving therapy (see Children in Out-of-Home Child Care, p 122). They can return to regular activities as soon as effective therapy has been instituted, adherence to therapy has been documented, and clinical symptoms have diminished. Children with LTBI can participate in all activities whether they are receiving treatment or not.

BCG Vaccines. BCG vaccine is a live vaccine originally prepared from attenuated strains of *M bovis*. Use of BCG vaccine[1] is recommended by the Expanded Programme on Immunization of the World Health Organization for administration at birth (see Table 1.9, p 14) and is used in more than 100 countries to reduce the incidence of disseminated and other life-threatening manifestations of tuberculosis in infants and young children. Although BCG immunization appears to decrease the risk of serious complications of tuberculosis disease in children, the various BCG vaccines used throughout the world differ in composition and efficacy.

Two meta-analyses of published clinical trials and case-control studies concerning the efficacy of BCG vaccines concluded that BCG vaccine has relatively high protective efficacy (approximately 80%) against meningeal and miliary tuberculosis in children. The protective efficacy against pulmonary tuberculosis differed significantly among the studies, precluding a specific conclusion. Protection afforded by BCG vaccine in one meta-analysis was estimated to be 50%. One BCG vaccine manufactured by Organon Teknika Corp and distributed by Merck/Schering-Plough is licensed in the United States for the prevention of tuberculosis. Comparative evaluations of this and other BCG vaccines have not been performed.

Indications. In the United States, administration of BCG vaccine should be considered only in limited and select circumstances, such as unavoidable risk of exposure to

[1]**www.bcgatlas.org**

tuberculosis and failure or unfeasibility of other control methods. Recommendations for use of BCG vaccine for control of tuberculosis among children and health care personnel have been published by the Advisory Committee on Immunization Practices of the CDC and the Advisory Council for the Elimination of Tuberculosis.[1] For infants and children, BCG immunization should be considered only for people with a negative TST result who are not infected with HIV in the following circumstances:

- The child is exposed continually to a person or people with contagious pulmonary tuberculosis resistant to isoniazid and rifampin and the child cannot be removed from this exposure, OR
- The child is exposed continually to a person or people with untreated or ineffectively treated contagious pulmonary tuberculosis and the child cannot be removed from such exposure or given antituberculosis therapy.

Careful assessment of the potential risks and benefits of BCG vaccine and consultation with personnel in local tuberculosis control programs are recommended strongly before use of BCG vaccine.

Adverse Reactions. Uncommonly (1%–2% of immunizations), BCG vaccine can result in local adverse reactions, such as subcutaneous abscess and regional lymphadenopathy, which generally are not serious. One rare complication, osteitis affecting the epiphysis of long bones, can occur as long as several years after BCG immunization. Disseminated fatal infection occurs rarely (approximately 2 per 1 million people), primarily in people who are severely immunocompromised, such as children with poorly controlled HIV infection or severe combined immunodeficiency. Antituberculosis therapy is recommended to treat osteitis and disseminated disease caused by BCG vaccine. Pyrazinamide is not believed to be effective against BCG and should not be included in treatment regimens.

People with complications caused by BCG vaccine should be referred for management, if possible, to a tuberculosis expert and also should have consideration of evaluation for an immune deficiency.

Contraindications. People with burns, skin infections, and primary or secondary immunodeficiencies, including HIV infection, should not receive BCG vaccine. Because an increasing number of cases of localized and disseminated BCG have been described in infants and children with HIV infection, the World Health Organization no longer recommends BCG in healthy, HIV-infected children. Use of BCG vaccine is contraindicated for people receiving immunosuppressive medications including high-dose corticosteroids (see Corticosteroids, p 847). Although no untoward effects of BCG vaccine on the fetus have been observed, immunization of women during pregnancy is not recommended.

Nontuberculous Mycobacteria

(Environmental Mycobacteria, Mycobacteria Other Than *Mycobacterium tuberculosis*)

CLINICAL MANIFESTATIONS: Several syndromes are caused by nontuberculous mycobacteria (NTM).

---

[1]Centers for Disease Control and Prevention. The role of BCG vaccine in the prevention and control of tuberculosis in the United States: a joint statement by the Advisory Committee for the Elimination of Tuberculosis and the Advisory Committee on Immunization Practices. *MMWR Recomm Rep.* 1996;45(RR-4):1–18

- In children, the most common of these syndromes is cervical lymphadenitis.
- Cutaneous infection may follow soil- or water-contaminated traumatic wounds, surgeries, or cosmetic procedures (eg, tattoos, pedicures, body piercings).
- Less common syndromes include soft tissue infection, osteomyelitis, otitis media, central catheter-associated bloodstream infections, and pulmonary infections, especially in adolescents with cystic fibrosis.
- NTM, especially *Mycobacterium avium* complex (MAC [including *M avium* and *Mycobacterium avium-intracellulare*]) and *Mycobacterium abscessus*, can be recovered from sputum in 10% to 20% of adolescents and young adults with cystic fibrosis and can be associated with fever and declining clinical status.
- Disseminated infections almost always are associated with impaired cell-mediated immunity, as found in children with congenital immune defects (eg, interleukin-12 deficiency, NF-kappa-B essential modulator [NEMO] mutation and related disorders, and interferon-gamma receptor defects), hematopoietic stem cell transplants, or advanced human immunodeficiency virus (HIV) infection. Disseminated NTM infection, most commonly MAC, is rare in HIV-infected children during the first year of life. The frequency of disseminated MAC increases with increasing age and declining CD4+ T-lymphocyte counts, typically less than 50 cells/μL, in children older than 6 years.[1] Manifestations of disseminated NTM infections depend on the species and route of infection but include fever, night sweats, weight loss, abdominal pain, fatigue, diarrhea, and anemia. These signs and symptoms also are found in advanced immunosuppressed HIV-infected children without disseminated MAC. For HIV-infected children who have disseminated MAC, respiratory symptoms and isolated pulmonary disease are uncommon. In HIV-infected patients developing immune restoration with initiation of combination antiretroviral therapy (cART), local NTM symptoms can worsen temporarily. This immune reconstitution syndrome usually occurs 2 to 4 weeks after initiation of cART. Symptoms can include worsening fever, swollen lymph nodes, local pain, and laboratory abnormalities.
- In 2015, an outbreak in Switzerland occurred in which cases of *Mycobacterium chimaera* infection were associated with heater-cooler units (Stöckert 3T, manufactured by Sorin Group Deutschland, now LivaNova) used in open heart surgery and were believed to be caused by aerosolization of contaminated water in the units. Presentation was indolent in all cases, and diagnosis occurred years after exposure. Fever, myalgia, arthralgia, fatigue, and weight loss were initial manifestations. Prosthetic valve endocarditis or vascular graft infection was most commonly identified, but other manifestations have included osteomyelitis, hepatitis, pancytopenia, renal insufficiency, and splenomegaly. Subsequently, patients have been identified internationally and in the United States, and the US Food and Drug Administration (FDA) has determined that all heater-cooler units have common design features that could lead to aerosol formation.

ETIOLOGY: Of the more than 130 species of NTM that have been identified, only a few cause most human infections. However, gene sequencing has led to identification of new

---

[1]Guidelines for prevention and treatment of opportunistic infections in HIV-exposed and HIVinfected children. Recommendations from the National Institutes of Health, Centers for Disease Control and Prevention, the HIV Medicine Association of the Infectious Diseases Society of America, the Pediatric Infectious Diseases Society, and the American Academy of Pediatrics. *Pediatr Infect Dis J*. 2013;32(Suppl 2):i–KK4. Available at: **http://aidsinfo.nih.gov/guidelines/html/5/pediatric-oi-prevention-and-treatment-guidelines/0**

species that cause human disease infrequently. The species most commonly infecting children in the United States are MAC, *Mycobacterium fortuitum*, *M abscessus*, and *Mycobacterium marinum* (see Table 3.89). Several new species, which can be detected by nucleic acid amplification testing but cannot be grown by routine culture methods, have been identified in lymph nodes of children with cervical adenitis. NTM disease in patients with HIV infection usually is caused by MAC. *M fortuitum*, *Mycobacterium chelonae*, *Mycobacterium smegmatis*, and *M abscessus* commonly are referred to as "rapidly growing" mycobacteria, because sufficient growth and identification can be achieved in the laboratory within 3 to 7 days, whereas MAC, *M marinum*, *Mycobacterium szulgai*, and most other NTM usually require several weeks before sufficient growth occurs for identification and are referred to as "slow growing" mycobacteria. Rapidly growing mycobacteria have been implicated in wound, soft tissue, bone, pulmonary, central venous catheter, and middle-ear infections. Other mycobacterial species that usually are not pathogenic have caused infections in immunocompromised hosts or have been associated with the presence of a foreign body.

EPIDEMIOLOGY: Many NTM species are ubiquitous in nature, being found in soil, food, water, and animals. Tap water is the major reservoir for *Mycobacterium kansasii*, *Mycobacterium lentiflavum*, *Mycobacterium xenopi*, *Mycobacterium simiae*, and health care-associated infections attributable to *M abscessus* and *M fortuitum*. Outbreaks have been associated with contaminated water used for acupuncture, pedicures, inks used for tattooing and in children undergoing pulpotomy, which has been associated with improperly maintained dental unit water lines. For *M marinum*, water in a fish tank or aquarium or an injury in a saltwater environment are the major sources of infection. The environmental reservoir for *M abscessus* and MAC causing pulmonary infection is unknown. Although many people are exposed to NTM, it is unknown why some exposures result in acute or chronic infection. Usual portals of entry for NTM infection are believed to be abrasions in the skin, such as cutaneous lesions caused by *M marinum*; penetrating trauma, such as needles and organic material most often associated with *M abscessus* and *M fortuitum*; surgical sites, especially for central vascular catheters; oropharyngeal mucosa, which is the presumed portal of entry for cervical lymphadenitis; tooth eruption, which is the presumed portal of entry for submandibular lymphadenitis; gastrointestinal or respiratory tract, for disseminated MAC; and respiratory tract, including tympanostomy tubes for otitis media. Pulmonary disease and rare cases of mediastinal adenitis and endobronchial disease occur. NTM can be important emerging pathogens in patients with cystic fibrosis and are emerging pathogens in individuals receiving biologic response modifiers, such as antitumor necrosis factor-alpha agents (see Biologic Response Modifying Drugs Used to Decrease Inflammation, p 85). Most infections remain localized at the portal of entry or in regional lymph nodes. Dissemination to distal sites primarily occurs in immunocompromised hosts, except in the case of *M chimaera* infections in those exposed during open-heart surgery, most of whom are immunocompetent. No definitive evidence of person-to-person transmission of NTM exists. Outbreaks of otitis media caused by *M abscessus* have been associated with polyethylene ear tubes and use of contaminated equipment or water. Large clusters of dental infections caused by *M abscessus* have been associated with use of tap water for rinsing and irrigation during procedures. A waterborne route of transmission has been implicated for MAC infection in some immunodeficient hosts. Buruli ulcer disease is a skin and bone infection caused by *Mycobacterium ulcerans*, an emerging disease causing significant morbidity and disability in tropical areas such as Africa, Asia, South America, Australia, and the western Pacific.

Table 3.89. Diseases Caused by Nontuberculous *Mycobacterium* Species

Clinical Disease	Common Species	Less Common Species in the United States
Cutaneous infection	*M marinum, M chelonae, M fortuitum, M abscessus,*	*M ulcerans*[a]
Lymphadenitis	MAC; *M haemophilum; M lentiflavum*	*M kansasii, M fortuitum, M malmoense*[b]
Otologic infection	*M abscessus*	*M fortuitum*
Pulmonary infection	MAC, *M kansasii, M abscessus*	*M xenopi, M malmoense,*[b] *M szulgai, M fortuitum, M simiae*
Catheter-associated infection	*M chelonae, M fortuitum*	*M abscessus*
Prosthetic valve endocarditis	*M chelonae, M fortuitum*	*M chimaera*
Skeletal infection	MAC, *M kansasii, M fortuitum*	*M chelonae, M marinum, M abscessus, M ulcerans*[a]
Disseminated	MAC	*M kansasii, M genavense, M haemophilum, M chelonae*

MAC indicates *Mycobacterium avium* complex.
[a] Not endemic in the United States.
[b] Found primarily in Northern Europe.

The **incubation periods** are variable.

DIAGNOSTIC TESTS: Routine screening of respiratory or gastrointestinal tract specimens for MAC microorganisms is not recommended. Definitive diagnosis of NTM disease requires isolation of the organism. Consultation with the laboratory should occur to ensure that culture specimens are handled correctly. For example, isolation of *Mycobacterium haemophilum* requires that the culture be maintained at 30°C and that heme-containing medium is added for isolation. Because NTM commonly are found in the environment, contamination of cultures or transient colonization can occur. Caution must be exercised in interpretation of cultures obtained from nonsterile sites, such as gastric washing specimens, endoscopy material, a single expectorated sputum sample, or urine specimens, and also when the species cultured usually is nonpathogenic (eg, *Mycobacterium terrae* complex or *Mycobacterium gordonae*). An acid-fast bacilli smear-positive sample and repeated isolation on culture media of a single species from any site are more likely to indicate disease than culture contamination or transient colonization. Diagnostic criteria for NTM lung disease in adults include 2 or more separate sputum samples or 1 bronchial alveolar lavage specimen that grows NTM. These criteria have not been validated in children and apply best to MAC, *M kansasii,* and *M abscessus.* NTM isolates from draining sinus tracts or wounds almost always are significant clinically. Recovery of NTM from sites that usually are sterile, such as cerebrospinal fluid, pleural fluid, bone marrow, blood, lymph node aspirates, middle ear or mastoid aspirates, or surgically excised tissue, are very likely to be significant. However, rare instances of sample or laboratory contamination leading to a false-positive culture result have been reported. With radiometric or nonradiometric broth techniques, blood cultures are highly sensitive in recovery of MAC and other bloodborne

NTM species. If disseminated MAC disease is confirmed, the patient should be evaluated to identify an underlying immunodeficiency condition (eg, HIV, gamma interferon receptor deficiency). Polymerase chain reaction-based assays for some NTM have been developed but are not yet widely available in commercial diagnostic laboratories.

Patients with NTM infection such as *M marinum, M kansasii,* or MAC cervical lymphadenitis can have a positive tuberculin skin test (TST) result, because the purified protein derivative preparation, derived from *M tuberculosis,* shares a number of antigens with these NTM species. These TST reactions usually measure less than 10 mm of induration but can measure more than 15 mm (see Tuberculosis, p 829). The interferon-gamma release assays (IGRAs) use 2 or 3 antigens to detect infection with *M tuberculosis.* Although these antigens are not found on *M avium-intracellulare* and most other NTM species, cross reactions can occur with infection caused by *M kansasii, M marinum,* and *M szulgai* (see Tuberculosis, p 829).

TREATMENT: Many NTM are relatively resistant in vitro to antituberculosis drugs. In vitro resistance to these agents, however, does not necessarily correlate with clinical response, especially with MAC infections. Only limited controlled trials of drug treatment have been performed in patients with NTM infections. The approach to initial therapy should be directed by the following: (1) the species causing the infection; (2) the results of drug-susceptibility testing; (3) the site(s) of infection; (4) the patient's immune status; and (5) the need to treat a patient presumptively for tuberculosis while awaiting culture reports that subsequently reveal NTM.

For NTM lymphadenitis in otherwise healthy children, especially when the disease is caused by MAC, complete surgical excision is curative and limits scar formation. Therapy with clarithromycin or azithromycin combined with ethambutol and/or rifampin or rifabutin may be beneficial for children in whom surgical excision is not possible or is incomplete and for children with recurrent disease (see Table 3.90), although published reports of antimicrobial therapy without surgical incision have had variable success rates. The natural history of NTM lymphadenitis without curative surgical excision is slow resolution but with a high risk of spontaneous drainage through the skin and resulting scarring, even when antimicrobial management is used. Joint decision making with the parent(s) and possibly the child, depending on age, is important in developing the best treatment plan for each patient.

The choice of drugs, dosages, and duration should be reviewed with a consultant experienced in the management of NTM infections (see Table 3.90). Indwelling foreign bodies should be removed, and surgical débridement for serious localized disease is optimal. Clinical isolates of MAC usually are resistant to many of the approved antituberculosis drugs, including isoniazid, but generally are susceptible to clarithromycin and azithromycin and often are susceptible to combinations of ethambutol, rifabutin or rifampin, and amikacin or streptomycin. Secondary agents include moxifloxacin and linezolid. Susceptibility testing to these other agents has not been standardized and, thus, is not recommended routinely. Isolates of rapidly growing mycobacteria (*M fortuitum, M abscessus,* and *M chelonae*) should be tested in vitro against drugs to which they commonly are susceptible and that have been used with some therapeutic success (eg, amikacin, imipenem, sulfamethoxazole or trimethoprim-sulfamethoxazole, cefoxitin, ciprofloxacin, clarithromycin, linezolid, clofazimine, doxycycline, and tigecycline).

Table 3.90. Treatment of Nontuberculous Mycobacteria Infections in Children

Organism	Disease	Initial Treatment
Slowly Growing Species		
Mycobacterium avium complex (MAC); *Mycobacterium haemophilum*; *Mycobacterium lentiflavum*	Lymphadenitis	Complete excision of lymph nodes; if excision incomplete or disease recurs, clarithromycin or azithromycin plus ethambutol and/or rifampin (or rifabutin).
	Pulmonary infection	Clarithromycin or azithromycin plus ethambutol with rifampin or rifabutin (pulmonary resection in some patients who fail to respond to drug therapy). For severe disease, an initial course of amikacin or streptomycin often is included. Clinical data in adults with mild to moderate disease support that 3-times-weekly therapy is as effective as daily therapy, with less toxicity. For patients with advanced or cavitary disease, drugs should be given daily.
Mycobacterium chimaera	Prosthetic valve endocarditis	Valve removal, prolonged antimicrobial therapy based on susceptibility testing.
	Disseminated	See text.
Mycobacterium kansasii	Pulmonary infection	Rifampin plus ethambutol with isoniazid daily. If rifampin resistance is detected, a 3-drug regimen based on drug susceptibility testing should be used.
	Osteomyelitis	Surgical débridement and prolonged antimicrobial therapy using rifampin plus ethambutol with isoniazid.
Mycobacterium marinum	Cutaneous infection	None, if minor; rifampin, trimethoprim-sulfamethoxazole, clarithromycin, or doxycycline[a] for moderate disease; extensive lesions may require surgical débridement. Susceptibility testing not routinely required.

Table 3.90. Treatment of Nontuberculous Mycobacteria Infections in Children, *continued*

Organism	Disease	Initial Treatment
Mycobacterium ulcerans	Cutaneous and bone infections	Daily intramuscular streptomycin and oral rifampin for 8 weeks; excision to remove necrotic tissue, if present; potential response to thermotherapy.

Rapidly Growing Species

Organism	Disease	Initial Treatment
Mycobacterium fortuitum group	Cutaneous infection	Initial therapy for serious disease is amikacin plus meropenem, IV, followed by clarithromycin, doxycycline[a] or trimethoprim-sulfamethoxazole, or ciprofloxacin, orally, on the basis of in vitro susceptibility testing; may require surgical excision. Up to 50% of isolates are resistant to cefoxitin.
	Catheter infection	Catheter removal and amikacin plus meropenem, IV; clarithromycin, trimethoprim-sulfamethoxazole, or ciprofloxacin, orally, on the basis of in vitro susceptibility testing.
Mycobacterium abscessus	Otitis media; cutaneous infection	There is no reliable antimicrobial regimen because of variability in drug susceptibility. Clarithromycin plus initial course of amikacin plus cefoxitin or imipenem/meropenem; may require surgical débridement on the basis of in vitro susceptibility testing (50% are amikacin resistant).
	Pulmonary infection (in cystic fibrosis)	Serious disease, clarithromycin, amikacin, and cefoxitin or imipenem/meropenem on the basis of susceptibility testing; most isolates have very low MICs to tigecycline; may require surgical resection.

Table 3.90. Treatment of Nontuberculous Mycobacteria Infections in Children, continued

Organism	Disease	Initial Treatment
Mycobacterium chelonae	Catheter infection, prosthetic valve endocarditis	Catheter removal; débridement, removal of foreign material; valve replacement; and tobramycin (initially) plus clarithromycin, meropenem, and linezolid.
	Disseminated cutaneous infection	Tobramycin and meropenem or linezolid (initially) plus clarithromycin.

IV indicates intravenously; MIC, minimum inhibitory concentration.

*Doxycycline can be used for short durations (ie, 21 days or less) without regard to patient age, but for longer treatment durations is not recommended for children younger than 8 years (see Tetracyclines, p 905). Only 50% of isolates of *M marinum* are susceptible to doxycycline.

The duration of therapy for NTM infections will depend on host status, site(s) of involvement, and severity. Patients receiving therapy should be monitored. Patients receiving clarithromycin plus rifabutin or high-dose rifabutin (with another drug) should be observed for the rifabutin-related development of leukopenia, uveitis, polyarthralgia, and pseudojaundice.

Most patients who respond ultimately show substantial clinical improvement in the first 4 to 6 weeks of therapy. Elimination of the organisms from blood cultures can take longer, often up to 12 weeks. Most experts recommend a minimum of 3 to 6 months or longer.

For patients with cystic fibrosis and isolation of MAC species, treatment is suggested only for those with clinical symptoms not attributable to other causes, worsening lung function, and chest radiographic progression. The decision to embark on therapy should take into consideration susceptibility testing results and should involve consultation with an expert in cystic fibrosis care.

In patients with acquired immunodeficiency syndrome (AIDS) and in other immunocompromised people with disseminated MAC infection, multidrug therapy is recommended. Treatment of disseminated MAC infection should be undertaken in consultation with an expert because the infections are life threatening and drug-drug interactions may occur between medications used to treat disseminated MAC and HIV infections.

The optimal time to initiate ART in a child in whom HIV and disseminated MAC are newly diagnosed is not established. Many experts provide treatment of disseminated MAC for 2 weeks before initiating ART in an attempt to minimize occurrence of the immune reconstitution syndrome and minimize confusion relating to the cause of drug-associated toxicity.

Chemoprophylaxis. The most effective way to prevent disseminated MAC in HIV-infected children is to preserve their immune function through use of combination cART. HIV-infected children with advanced immunosuppression should be offered prophylaxis against disseminated MAC with azithromycin or clarithromycin. Oral suspensions of clarithromycin and azithromycin are available in the United States. Appropriate doses are: clarithromycin, 7.5 mg/kg (maximum, 500 mg), orally, twice daily; azithromycin,

20 mg/kg (maximum, 1200 mg), orally, weekly; or azithromycin, 5 mg/kg (maximum, 250 mg), orally, daily. No pediatric formulation of rifabutin is available, but a dosage of 5 mg/kg per day (maximum, 300 mg) has been used for children 6 years or older. Rifabutin is a less effective alternative agent that should not be used until tuberculosis disease has been excluded.

Disseminated MAC should be excluded by a negative blood culture result before prophylaxis is initiated. Combination therapy for prophylaxis should be avoided in children, if possible, because it has not been shown to be cost effective and increases rates of adverse events. Children with a history of disseminated MAC and continued immunosuppression should receive lifelong prophylaxis to prevent recurrence. Prophylaxis can be discontinued in some HIV-infected children after immune reconstitution (**https:// aidsinfo.nih.gov/guidelines/html/5/pediatric-opportunistic-infection/ 413/mycobacterium-avium-complex-disease**).

ISOLATION OF THE HOSPITALIZED PATIENT: Standard precautions are recommended.

CONTROL MEASURES: Control measures include chemoprophylaxis for high-risk patients with HIV infection (see Treatment, p 857) and avoidance of tap water contamination of central venous catheters, dental procedures, surgical wounds, skin, or endoscopic equipment.

If heater-cooler units implicated in *M chimaera* infection have been or are to be used in open-heart surgeries, patients should be informed (preferably before their surgery) of the risk and monitored after surgery for signs and symptoms suggestive of infection. If infection is suspected or documented, an FDA medical device report should be filed with MedWatch (see MedWatch – the FDA Safety Information and Adverse Event-Reporting Program, p 1026).

Tularemia

CLINICAL MANIFESTATIONS: There are several common presentations of tularemia in children, with ulceroglandular disease being the most frequently identified. Characterized by a maculopapular lesion at the entry site with subsequent ulceration and slow healing, the ulceroglandular variant is associated with tender regional lymphadenopathy that can drain spontaneously. The glandular variant (regional lymphadenopathy with no ulcer) also is common. Less common disease variants include oculoglandular (severe conjunctivitis and preauricular lymphadenopathy), oropharyngeal (severe exudative stomatitis, pharyngitis, or tonsillitis with cervical lymphadenopathy), vesicular skin lesions that can be mistaken for herpes simplex virus or varicella zoster virus cutaneous infections, typhoidal (high fever, hepatomegaly, splenomegaly, systemic infection including septicemia; pneumonia and or meningitis may be seen as complications), and intestinal (intestinal pain, vomiting, and diarrhea). Respiratory tularemia, characterized by flu-like symptoms often without chest radiograph abnormalities, presents with fever, dry cough, chest pain, and hilar adenopathy and normally is associated with farming or, infrequently, lawn maintenance activities that create aerosols and dust. This would also be the anticipated variant after intentional aerosol release of organisms.

ETIOLOGY: *Francisella tularensis* is a small, weakly staining, gram-negative pleomorphic coccobacillus. Two subspecies cause human infection in North America: *F tularensis* subspecies *tularensis* (type A), and *F tularensis* subspecies *holarctica* (type B). Type A can be further subdivided into 4 distinct genotypes (A1a, A1b, A2a, A2b), with A1b appearing to produce more serious disease in humans. Type A generally is considered more virulent, although either can be lethal, especially if inhaled.

EPIDEMIOLOGY: *F tularensis* can infect more than 100 animal species; the vertebrate species considered most important in enzootic cycles are rabbits, hares, and rodents, especially muskrats, voles, beavers, and prairie dogs. Domestic cats are an additional but rare source of infection. In the United States, a majority of human cases are attributed to tick bites but may also result from bites of other arthropod vectors, such as deer flies, or direct from contact with any of the aforementioned animal species. Infections attributable to tick and deer fly bites usually take the form of ulceroglandular or glandular tularemia. *F tularensis* bacteria can be transmitted to humans via the skin when handling infected animal tissue, as can occur when hunting or skinning infected rabbits, muskrats, prairie dogs, and other rodents. Infection has been reported in commercially traded hamsters and prairie dogs. Infection also can be acquired following ingestion of contaminated water or inadequately cooked meat, inhalation of contaminated aerosols generated during lawn mowing, brush cutting, or certain farming activities (eg, baling contaminated hay). At-risk people have occupational or recreational exposure to infected animals or their habitats; this includes rabbit hunters and trappers, people exposed to certain ticks or biting insects, and laboratory technicians working with *F tularensis,* which is highly infectious and may be aerosolized when grown in culture. In the United States, most cases occur during May through September. Approximately two thirds of cases occur in males, and one quarter of cases occur in children 1 to 14 years of age.

Tularemia has been reported in all US states except Hawaii. Tularemia has been a nationally notifiable disease since 2000. During 2005–2014, 1424 cases were reported (median: 143 cases per year; range: 93–180). Seven states accounted for 66% of reported cases: Missouri (16%), Arkansas (15%), Oklahoma (9%), Kansas (9%), Massachusetts (6%), Nebraska (5%), and South Dakota (5%). Notably, during 2015, sharp increases occurred in the number of cases recorded in Colorado, Nebraska, South Dakota, and Wyoming. Of the 10 states with the highest incidence of tularemia, all but Massachusetts were located in the central or western United States.

Organisms can be present in blood during the first 2 weeks of disease and in cutaneous lesions for as long as 1 month if untreated. Person-to-person transmission has not been reported.

The **incubation period** usually is 3 to 5 days, with a range of 1 to 21 days.

DIAGNOSTIC TESTS: Diagnosis is established most often by serologic testing. Patients do not develop antibodies until the second week of illness. A single serum antibody titer of 1:128 or greater determined by microagglutination (MA) or of 1:160 or greater determined by tube agglutination (TA) is consistent with recent or past infection and constitutes a presumptive diagnosis. In acute infection, an antibody titer of >1:1024 commonly is found. For those with suspected disease and an initial nondiagnostic titer, a repeat titer should be obtained in 2 to 4 weeks. Confirmation by serologic testing requires a fourfold or greater titer change between serum samples obtained at least 2 weeks apart, with 1 of the specimens having a minimum titer of 1:128 or greater by MA or 1:160 or greater by TA. Nonspecific cross-reactions can occur with specimens containing heterophile antibodies, or antibodies to *Brucella* species, *Legionella* species, or other Gram-negative bacteria. However, cross-reactions rarely result in MA or TA titers that are diagnostic. Because of its propensity for causing laboratory-acquired infections, laboratory personnel should be alerted when *F tularensis* infection is suspected.

F tularensis in ulcer exudate or aspirate material can be identified by laboratory developed polymerase chain reaction (PCR) assay or direct fluorescent antibody assay. Immunohistochemical staining is specific for detection of *F tularensis* in fixed tissues; however, this method is not available in most clinical laboratories. Isolation of *F tularensis* from specimens of blood, skin, ulcers, lymph node drainage, gastric washings, or respiratory tract secretions is best achieved by inoculation of cysteine-enriched media, such as that used for clinical isolation of *Legionella* species. *F tularensis* often is isolated on chocolate agar. Because *F tularensis* is a biosafety level 3 agent, if suspected on the basis of clinical and epidemiological history or Gram stain identification of tiny, gram-negative coccobacillus, further work should only be performed in a certified Class II Biosafety Cabinet. All isolates suspected to be *F tularensis* should be forwarded for confirmation to local reference laboratories (usually the state laboratory) that are part of the Laboratory Response Network.

TREATMENT: Gentamicin (5 mg/kg/day, divided twice or 3 times/day, intravenously or intramuscularly, with the dose adjusted to maintain the desired peak serum levels of at least 5 µg/mL) is the drug of choice for the treatment of tularemia in children because of the limited availability of streptomycin (30–40 mg/kg/day, divided twice/day, intramuscularly; maximum 2 g/day) and the fewer adverse effects of gentamicin. Duration of therapy usually is 10 days. A 5- to 7-day course may be sufficient in mild disease, but a longer course is required for more severe illness (eg, meningitis). Ciprofloxacin is an alternative for mild disease. Doxycycline is associated with a higher rate of relapse compared with other therapies and, therefore, is not recommended for definitive treatment. Suppuration of lymph nodes can occur despite antimicrobial therapy. *F tularensis* is not susceptible to beta-lactam drugs, including carbapenems. Because of the difficulty in achieving good CSF levels of gentamicin, combination therapy with doxycycline or ciprofloxacin plus gentamicin may be considered for patients with tularemic meningitis. Because treatment delay is associated with therapeutic failure, treatment should be initiated as soon as tularemia is suspected.

ISOLATION OF THE HOSPITALIZED PATIENT: Standard precautions are recommended.

CONTROL MEASURES:

- People should protect themselves against arthropod bites by wearing protective clothing, by frequent inspection for and removal of ticks from the skin and scalp, and by using insect repellents (see Prevention of Mosquitoborne and Tickborne Infections, p 195).
- Drinking untreated surface water should be avoided.
- Gloves should be worn by those handling the carcasses of wild rabbits, muskrats, prairie dogs, and other potentially infected animals. Children should not handle sick or dead animals, including pets.
- People should avoid mowing over live or dead animals, because this may aerosolize infective material.
- Game meats should be cooked thoroughly.
- Primary clinical specimens may be handled in the laboratory using Biological Safety Level 2 (BSL2) precautions. Work with suspected cultures requires BSL3 precautions. Note that *F tularensis* is a tier 1 select agent and must be handled as such after it has been identified.
- Standard precautions should be used for handling clinical materials.
- A 14-day course of doxycycline or ciprofloxacin is recommended for children and

adults after exposure to an intentional release of tularemia (eg, a bioterrorism attack) and for laboratory workers with inadvertent exposure to *F tularensis*.

- A vaccine that had been available to protect laboratory workers and other high-risk personnel is under review by the US Food and Drug Administration but is not currently available in the United States.

Endemic Typhus

(Murine Typhus)

CLINICAL MANIFESTATIONS: Endemic typhus resembles epidemic (louseborne) typhus but usually has a less abrupt onset with less severe systemic symptoms. In young children, the disease can be mild. Fever, present in almost all patients, can be accompanied by a persistent, usually severe, headache and myalgia. Nausea and vomiting also develop in approximately half of patients. A rash appears in approximately 50% of patients on day 4 to 7 of illness, is macular or maculopapular, lasts 4 to 8 days, and tends to remain discrete, with sparse lesions and no hemorrhage. Illness seldom lasts longer than 2 weeks; visceral involvement is uncommon. Laboratory findings include thrombocytopenia, elevated liver transaminases, and hyponatremia. Fatal outcome is rare except in untreated severe disease.

ETIOLOGY: Endemic typhus is caused by *Rickettsia typhi* and *Rickettsia felis*, which are gram-negative obligate intracellular bacteria.

EPIDEMIOLOGY: Rats, in which infection is unapparent, are the natural reservoirs for *Rickettsia typhi*. Outside the United States, the primary vector for transmission among rats and transmission to humans is the rat flea, *Xenopsylla cheopis*, although other fleas and mites have been implicated. In southern California and Texas, a suburban cycle involving cat fleas (*Ctenocephalides felis*) and opossums (*Didelphis virginiana*) has emerged as an important cause of endemic typhus. Infection occurs when infected flea feces are rubbed into broken skin or mucous membranes or are inhaled. The disease is worldwide in distribution and tends to occur most commonly in adults, in males, and during the months of April to October in the United States; in children, males and females are affected equally. Worldwide, exposure to rats and their fleas is the major risk factor for infection, although a history of such exposure often is absent. Endemic typhus is rare in the United States, although it is likely underdiagnosed, with most cases occurring in southern California, southern Texas, the southeastern Gulf Coast, and Hawaii.

The **incubation period** is 6 to 14 days.

DIAGNOSTIC TESTS: Antibody titers determined with *R typhi* antigen by an indirect fluorescent antibody (IFA) assay are most commonly measured. Enzyme immunoassay or latex agglutination tests are also available. Antibody levels peak at around 4 weeks after infection, but results of these tests may be negative early in the course of illness. A fourfold increase in immunoglobulin (Ig) G titer between acute and convalescent serum specimens taken 2 to 3 weeks apart is diagnostic. Although more prone to false-positive results, immunoassays demonstrating increases in specific IgM antibody can aid in distinguishing clinical illness from previous exposure if interpreted with a concurrent IgG test result; use of IgM assays alone is not recommended. Serologic tests may not differentiate murine typhus caused by *R typhi* or *R felis* from epidemic (louseborne) typhus or from infection with spotted fever rickettsiae, such as *R rickettsii*, without antibody cross-absorption for IFA or western blotting analyses, which are not available routinely. Isolation of the organism in cell culture potentially is hazardous and is best performed by specialized laboratories, such as the Centers for Disease Control and Prevention (CDC). Routine hospital blood cultures are not suitable for culture of *R typhi*. Molecular diagnostic assays on infected whole blood and skin biopsies can distinguish endemic and epidemic typhus and other rickettsioses and are performed at the CDC. Immunohistochemical procedures on formalin-fixed skin biopsy tissues can be performed at the CDC.

TREATMENT: Doxycycline is the treatment of choice for endemic typhus, regardless of patient age. The recommended dosage of doxycycline is 4.4 mg/kg per day, divided every 12 hours, intravenously or orally (maximum 100 mg/dose [see Tetracyclines, p 905]). Early diagnosis should be based on clinical suspicion and epidemiology. In a patient with disease that is clinically compatible with endemic typhus, treatment should not be withheld because of a negative laboratory result or while awaiting laboratory confirmation, because severe or fatal infection can develop when treatment is delayed. Treatment should be continued for at least 3 days after defervescence and evidence of clinical improvement is documented, and the total treatment course usually is 7 to 14 days. Fluoroquinolones or chloramphenicol are alternative medications but may not be as effective; fluoroquinolones are not approved for this use in children younger than 18 years (see Fluoroquinolones, p 904).

ISOLATION OF THE HOSPITALIZED PATIENT: Standard precautions are recommended.

CONTROL MEASURES: Fleas should be controlled by appropriate insecticides before use of rodenticides, because fleas will seek alternative hosts, including humans. Suspected animal populations should be controlled by species-appropriate means. No prophylaxis is recommended for exposed people. The disease should be reported to local or state public health departments.

Epidemic Typhus
(Louseborne or Sylvatic Typhus)

CLINICAL MANIFESTATIONS: Clinically, epidemic typhus should be considered when people in crowded conditions or people with exposure to flying squirrels develop abrupt onset of high fever, chills, and myalgia accompanied by severe headache and malaise. Although patients with epidemic typhus often develop a rash by day 4 to 7 after the start of illness, rash may not always be present and should not be relied on for diagnosis. When present, the rash usually begins on the trunk and axilla, spreads centrifugally to the limbs, and generally spares the face, palms, and soles. The rash typically is macular to maculopapular, but in advanced stages can become petechial or hemorrhagic. There is no eschar, as might be present in many other rickettsial diseases. Abdominal complaints (stomach pain, nausea) and changes in mental status are common, including delirium, seizures, and coma. Myocardial and renal failure can occur when the disease is severe. The fatality rate in untreated people is as high as 30%. Mortality is less common in children, and the rate increases with advancing age. Untreated patients who recover typically have an illness lasting 2 weeks. Brill-Zinsser disease is a relapse of epidemic typhus that can occur years after the initial episode and is generally milder in nature. Factors that reactivate the rickettsiae are unknown, but relapse often is more mild and of shorter duration. Laboratory abnormalities in epidemic typhus may include thrombocytopenia, increased hepatic enzymes, hyperbilirubinemia, and elevated blood urea nitrogen.

ETIOLOGY: Epidemic typhus is caused by *Rickettsia prowazekii*.

EPIDEMIOLOGY: Humans are the primary reservoir of the organism, which is transmitted from person to person by the human body louse, *Pediculus humanus corporis*. Infected louse feces are rubbed into broken skin or mucous membranes or are inhaled. All ages are affected. Poverty, crowding, and poor sanitary conditions contribute to the spread of body lice and, hence, the disease. Cases of epidemic typhus are rare in the United States; however, there is no formal system for epidemic typhus surveillance. The last known epidemic in the United States occurred in 1921. Cases have occurred throughout the world, including the colder, mountainous areas of Asia, Africa, some parts of Europe, and Central and South America, particularly in refugee camps and jails of resource-limited countries. Epidemic typhus is most common during winter, when conditions favor person-to-person transmission of the vector. Rickettsiae are present in the blood and tissues of patients during the early febrile phase but are not found in secretions. Direct person-to-person spread of the disease does not occur in the absence of the louse vector.

In the United States, sporadic human cases associated with close contact with infected flying squirrels (*Glaucomys volans*), their nests, or their ectoparasites occasionally are reported in the eastern United States. Cases have been reported in people who reside or work in flying squirrel-infested dwellings, even when direct contact is not reported. Flying squirrel-associated disease, called sylvatic typhus, typically presents with a similar but generally milder illness to that observed with body louse-transmitted infection. Untreated illness can be severe, although no fatal cases of sylvatic typhus have been reported; the later development of Brill Zinsser disease has been confirmed in at least 1 case of untreated sylvatic typhus. *Amblyomma* ticks in the Americas and in Ethiopia have been shown to carry *R prowazekii*, but their vector potential is unknown.

The **incubation period** is 1 to 2 weeks.

DIAGNOSTIC TESTS: Epidemic typhus may be diagnosed by the detection of *R prowazekii* DNA in acute blood and serum specimens by polymerase chain reaction (PCR) assay. The specimen should preferably be obtained within the first week of symptoms and before (or within 24 hours of) doxycycline administration, and a negative result does not rule out *R prowazekii* infection. Diagnosis may also be attained by the detection of rickettsial DNA in biopsy or autopsy specimens by PCR assay or immunohistochemical (IHC) visualization of rickettsiae in tissues. The gold standard for serologic diagnosis of epidemic typhus is a fourfold increase in immunoglobulin (Ig) G antibody titer by the indirect fluorescent antibody (IFA) test. A negative acute serologic test result does not rule out a diagnosis of epidemic typhus. Both IgG and IgM antibodies begin to increase around day 7 to 10 after onset of symptoms; therefore, an elevated acute titer may represent past infection rather than acute infection. Low-level elevated antibody titers can be an incidental finding in a significant proportion of the general population in some regions. IgM antibodies may remain elevated for months and are not highly specific for acute epidemic typhus. A confirmed case, therefore, is one that shows a fourfold or greater increase in antigen-specific IgG between acute and convalescent sera obtained 2 to 6 weeks apart. Cross-reactivity may be observed to antibodies to *R typhi* (the agent of endemic typhus), *R rickettsii* (the agent of Rocky Mountain spotted fever), and other spotted fever group rickettsiae. Testing of acute and convalescent sera by enzyme immunoassays or dot blot immunoassay tests also can be used for assessing presence of antibody but are less useful for quantifying changes in titer. *R prowazekii* may also be isolated from acute blood specimens by animal passage or through tissue culture, but this can be hazardous and culture is restricted to specialized procedures (not routine blood culture) at reference laboratories with at minimum Biosafety Level 3 containment facilities. Cell culture cultivation of the organism must be confirmed by molecular methods.

TREATMENT: Doxycycline is the drug of choice to treat epidemic typhus, regardless of patient age. The recommended dosage of doxycycline is 4.4 mg/kg per day, divided every 12 hours, intravenously or orally (maximum 100 mg/dose [see Tetracyclines, p 905]). Doxycycline is available in both oral and intravenous formulations. Treatment should be continued for at least 3 days after defervescence and evidence of clinical improvement is documented, and the total treatment course is usually for 5 to 10 days. Other broad-spectrum antimicrobial agents, including ciprofloxacin, are not recommended and may be more likely to result in fatal outcome. Chloramphenicol may be used in cases of absolute contraindication of doxycycline (life-threatening allergy) but also carries significant risks (ie, aplastic anemia). In epidemic situations in which antimicrobial agents may be limited (eg, refugee camps), a single dose of doxycycline may provide effective treatment (4.4 mg/kg, up to 200 mg) and facilitate outbreak control when combined with delousing efforts.

ISOLATION OF THE HOSPITALIZED PATIENT: Standard precautions are recommended. Precautions should be taken to delouse hospitalized patients with louse infestations.

CONTROL MEASURES: Thorough delousing in epidemic situations, particularly among exposed contacts of cases, is recommended. Several applications of pediculicides may be needed, because lice eggs are resistant to most insecticides. Washing clothes in hot water kills lice and eggs. During epidemics, insecticides dusted onto clothes of louse-infested populations are effective. Prevention and control of flying squirrel-associated typhus requires application of insecticides and precautions to prevent contact with these animals and their ectoparasites and to exclude them from human dwellings. No prophylaxis is recommended for people exposed to flying squirrels. In situations involving outbreaks of epidemic typhus in prisons and refugee settings, active surveillance for fever is important to assess efficacy of control measures and to ensure rapid and effective treatment. To halt the spread of disease to other people, louse-infested patients should be treated with cream or gel pediculicides containing pyrethrins or permethrin; malathion is prescribed most often when pyrethroids fail. Cases should be reported to local, state, regional, or national public health departments.

Ureaplasma urealyticum and *Ureaplasma parvum* Infections

CLINICAL MANIFESTATIONS: The role of *Ureaplasma* species in human disease is controversial. There has been an inconsistent association with *Ureaplasma urealyticum* infections and nongonococcal urethritis (NGU). Although 15% to 40% of cases of NGU are caused by *Chlamydia trachomatis* and an additional 15% to 25% by *Mycoplasma genitalium*, *U urealyticum*, but not *Ureaplasma parvum*, has been implicated as an etiologic agent in some cases in the United States. Without treatment, the infection usually resolves within 1 to 6 months, although asymptomatic infection may persist. There also has been an inconsistent relationship of infection by *Ureaplasma* species with prostatitis and epididymitis in men and salpingitis and endometritis in women. *Ureaplasma* organisms commonly are detected in placentas with histologic chorioamnionitis (now known as intra-amniotic infection). Some reports also describe an association between *Ureaplasma* infection with recurrent pregnancy loss and preterm birth.

Although *U urealyticum* and *U parvum* have been isolated from the lower respiratory tract and from lung biopsy specimens of preterm infants, their contribution to intrauterine pneumonia and chronic lung disease of prematurity remains controversial. These organisms also have been recovered from respiratory tract secretions of infants 3 months or younger with pneumonia, but their role in development of lower respiratory tract disease in otherwise healthy young infants is unclear. *Ureaplasma* species have been isolated from the bloodstream of newborn infants with bacteremia and from cerebrospinal fluid of infants with meningitis, intraventricular hemorrhage, and hydrocephalus. The contribution of *U urealyticum* to the outcome of infants with infections of the central nervous system is unclear given the confounding effects of preterm birth and intraventricular hemorrhage. Numerous cases of *U urealyticum* or *U parvum* arthritis, osteomyelitis, pneumonia, pericarditis, meningitis, and progressive sinopulmonary disease, mainly in immunocompromised patients, have been reported.

ETIOLOGY: *Ureaplasma* organisms are small pleomorphic bacteria that lack a cell wall. The genus contains 2 species capable of causing human infection, *U urealyticum* and *U parvum*. At least 14 serotypes have been described, 4 for *U parvum* and 10 for *U urealyticum*.

EPIDEMIOLOGY: The principal reservoir of human *Ureaplasma* species is the genital tract of sexually active adults. Colonization occurs in approximately half of sexually active women; the incidence in sexually active men is lower. Colonization is uncommon in prepubertal children and adolescents who are not sexually active, but a positive genital tract culture is not clearly definitive of sexual abuse. Transmission during delivery is likely from an asymptomatic colonized mother to her newborn infant, and infection also may occur in utero. *Ureaplasma* species may colonize the throat, eyes, umbilicus, and perineum of newborn infants and may persist for several months after birth. *U parvum* generally is more common than *U urealyticum* as a colonizer in pregnant women and their offspring.

Because *Ureaplasma* species commonly are isolated from the female lower genital tract and neonatal respiratory tract in the absence of disease, a positive culture does not establish its causative role in acute infection. However, recovery of these organisms from an upper genital tract or lower respiratory tract specimen is much more indicative of true infection.

The **incubation period** after sexual transmission is 10 to 20 days.

DIAGNOSTIC TESTS: Specimens for culture require specific *Ureaplasma* transport media with refrigeration at 4°C (39°F). Dacron or calcium alginate swabs should be used; cotton swabs should be avoided. Several rapid, sensitive real-time polymerase chain reaction assays for detection of *U urealyticum* and *U parvum* have been developed. Many of these assays have greater sensitivity than culture, but they are not widely available outside of reference laboratories. *Ureaplasma* species can be cultured in urea-containing broth and agar in 2 to 4 days. Serologic testing is of limited value for diagnostic purposes and is not available commercially.

TREATMENT: A positive *Ureaplasma* culture does not indicate need for therapy if the patient is asymptomatic. *Ureaplasma* species generally are susceptible to macrolides, tetracyclines, and quinolones, but because they lack a cell wall, they are not susceptible to penicillins or cephalosporins. They also are not susceptible to trimethoprim-sulfamethoxazole or clindamycin. For symptomatic children, adolescents, and adults, doxycycline can be used for treatment. Doxycycline can be used for short durations (ie, 21 days or less) without regard to patient age (see Tetracyclines, p 905). Persistent urethritis after doxycycline treatment can be attributable to doxycycline-resistant *U urealyticum* or *M genitalium*. Recurrences are common, and tetracycline resistance may occur in up to 50% of *Ureaplasma* isolates in some patient populations. Azithromycin is the preferred antimicrobial agent for people who are allergic to tetracyclines, and people with infections caused by tetracycline-resistant strains. A quinolone would be another option if azithromycin resistance is possible (eg, detection of *Ureaplasma* in a patient who has received azithromycin for prolonged periods). On the basis of very limited data, quinolone and macrolide resistance remain uncommon, less than 5%. Both doxycycline and azithromycin produce similar clinical and microbiologic cure rates.

Antimicrobial treatment with erythromycin has failed to prevent preterm delivery and in preterm infants has failed to prevent pulmonary disease, both in small randomized trials and in reports of cohort studies in pregnant women. Although in vitro efficacy against *Ureaplasma* species is observed with clarithromycin, azithromycin, and fluoroquinolones, lack of evidence of benefit precludes recommendations on treatment for preterm infants. Definitive evidence of efficacy of antimicrobial agents in the treatment of central nervous system infections caused by *Ureaplasma* species in infants and children also is lacking. There are reports of preterm infants with *Ureaplasma* species identified in cerebrospinal fluid who have or have not received antimicrobial therapy and who have had documentation of sterilization of cerebrospinal fluid.

ISOLATION OF THE HOSPITALIZED PATIENT: Standard precautions are recommended.
CONTROL MEASURES: Sexual partners of patients with NGU attributable to *U urealyticum* should be offered treatment.

Varicella-Zoster Virus Infections

CLINICAL MANIFESTATIONS: Primary infection results in varicella (chickenpox), manifesting in unvaccinated people as a generalized, pruritic, vesicular rash typically consisting of 250 to 500 lesions in varying stages of development (papules, vesicles) and resolution (crusting), low-grade fever, and other systemic symptoms. Complications include bacterial superinfection of skin lesions with or without bacterial sepsis, pneumonia, central nervous system involvement (acute cerebellar ataxia, encephalitis, stroke/vasculopathy), thrombocytopenia, and rarer complications such as glomerulonephritis, arthritis, and hepatitis. Primary viral pneumonia is not common among immunocompetent children but is the most common complication in adults. Varicella tends to be more severe in adults and in infants and adolescents than in other children. Before the introduction of routine immunization against varicella, an average of 100 to 125 people died of chickenpox in the United States each year. Breakthrough varicella cases can occur in immunized children, as described in Active Immunization (p 13), but usually are mild and clinically modified. Reye syndrome may follow varicella, although this outcome has become very rare with the recommendation not to use salicylate-containing compounds (eg, aspirin, bismuth-subsalicylate) for children with chickenpox. In immunocompromised children, progressive, severe varicella may occur with continuing eruption of lesions (sometimes including hemorrhagic skin lesions) along with high fever persisting into the second week of illness and visceral dissemination (ie, encephalitis, hepatitis, and pneumonia). Severe and even fatal varicella has been reported in otherwise healthy children on high-dose corticosteroids (greater than 2 mg/kg/day of prednisone or equivalent) for treatment of asthma and other illnesses. The risk is especially high when corticosteroids are administered during the varicella incubation period.

Varicella-zoster virus (VZV) establishes latency in sensory (dorsal root, cranial nerve, and autonomic including enteric) ganglia during primary VZV infection. This latency occurs with wild-type VZV or with the vaccine strain. Reactivation results in herpes zoster (shingles), characterized by grouped vesicular skin lesions in the distribution of 1 to 3 sensory dermatomes, frequently accompanied by pain and/or itching localized to the area. *Postherpetic neuralgia*, pain that persists after resolution of the zoster rash, may last for weeks to months but is very unusual in children. Zoster occasionally becomes disseminated in immunocompromised patients, with lesions appearing outside the primary dermatomes and/or visceral complications. VZV reactivation less frequently occurs in the absence of skin rash (zoster sine herpete); these patients may present with aseptic meningitis, encephalitis, stroke, or gastrointestinal tract involvement (visceral zoster).

Fetal infection after maternal varicella during the first or early second trimester of pregnancy occasionally results in fetal death or varicella embryopathy, characterized by limb hypoplasia, cutaneous scarring, eye abnormalities, and damage to the central nervous system (congenital varicella syndrome). The incidence of the congenital varicella syndrome among infants born to mothers who experience gestational varicella is approximately 2% when infection occurs between 8 and 20 weeks of gestation. Rarely, cases of congenital varicella syndrome have been reported in infants of women infected after 20 weeks of pregnancy, the latest occurring at 28 weeks' gestation. Children infected with VZV in utero may develop zoster early in life without having had extrauterine varicella.

Varicella infection has a higher case-fatality rate in infants when the mother develops varicella from 5 days before to 2 days after delivery, because there is little opportunity for development and transfer of maternal antibody across the placenta prior to delivery and the infant's cellular immune system is immature. When varicella develops in a mother more than 5 days before delivery and gestational age is 28 weeks or more, the severity of disease in the newborn infant is modified by transplacental transfer of VZV-specific maternal immunoglobulin (Ig) G antibody. Neither wild-type VZV nor Oka vaccine strain virus have been shown to be transmitted by human milk; expressed/pumped milk from a mother with varicella or zoster can be given to the infant, provided no lesions are on the breast.

ETIOLOGY: VZV (also known as human herpesvirus 3) is a member of the *Herpesviridae* family, the subfamily *Alphaherpesvirinae*, and the genus *Varicellovirus*.

EPIDEMIOLOGY: Humans are the only source of infection for this highly contagious virus. Infection occurs when the virus comes in contact with the mucosa of the upper respiratory tract or the conjunctiva of a susceptible person. Person-to-person transmission occurs either from direct contact with VZV lesions from varicella or herpes zoster or from airborne spread. Varicella is much more contagious than is herpes zoster. Skin lesions appear to be the major source of transmissible VZV; transmission from infected respiratory tract secretions is possible but probably less common. There is no evidence of VZV spread from fomites; the virus is extremely labile and is unable to survive for long in the environment. In utero infection occurs as a result of transplacental passage of virus during viremic maternal varicella infection. VZV infection in a household member usually results in infection of almost all susceptible people in that household. Children who acquire their infection at home (secondary family cases) often have more skin lesions than the index case. Health care-associated transmission is well documented in pediatric units.

In temperate climates in the prevaccine era, varicella was a childhood disease with a marked seasonal distribution, with peak incidence during late winter and early spring and among children younger than 10 years. High rates of vaccine coverage in the United

States have effectively eliminated discernible seasonality of varicella. In tropical climates, acquisition of varicella often occurs later in childhood, resulting in a significant proportion of susceptible adults. Following implementation of universal immunization in the United States in 1995, varicella incidence declined in all age groups as a result of personal and herd immunity. In areas with active surveillance and high 1-dose vaccine coverage, the rate of varicella disease decreased by approximately 90% between 1995 and 2005. Since recommendation of a routine second dose of vaccine in 2006, varicella outpatient visits have declined by an additional 60%, and varicella hospitalizations have declined by an additional 40%. The age of peak varicella incidence is shifting from children younger than 10 years to children 10 through 14 years of age, although the incidence in all age groups is lower than in the prevaccine era. Immunity to varicella generally is lifelong. Cellular immunity is more important than humoral immunity for limiting the extent of primary infection with VZV and for preventing reactivation of virus with herpes zoster. Symptomatic reinfection is uncommon in immunocompetent people. Asymptomatic primary infection is unusual.

Since 2007, coverage with 1 or more doses of varicella vaccine among 19- through 35-month-old children in the United States has been >90%. As the majority of children are vaccinated against varicella and the incidence of wild-type varicella decreases, a greater proportion of varicella cases are occurring in immunized people as breakthrough disease.

Immunocompromised people with primary (varicella) or recurrent (herpes zoster) infection are at increased risk of severe disease. Severe varicella and disseminated zoster are more likely to develop in children with congenital T-lymphocyte defects or acquired immunodeficiency syndrome than in people with B-lymphocyte abnormalities. Other groups of pediatric patients who may experience more severe or complicated varicella include infants, adolescents, patients with chronic cutaneous or pulmonary disorders, and patients receiving systemic corticosteroids, other immunosuppressive therapy, or long-term salicylate therapy.

Patients are contagious from 1 to 2 days before onset of the rash until all lesions have crusted.

The **incubation period** usually is 14 to 16 days, with a range of 10 to 21 days after exposure to rash. The incubation period may be prolonged for as long as 28 days after receipt of Varicella-Zoster Immune Globulin (VariZIG [Cangene Corp, Winnipeg, Canada]) or Immune Globulin Intravenous (IGIV) and can be shortened in immunocompromised patients. Varicella can develop between 2 and 16 days after birth in infants born to mothers with active varicella around the time of delivery; the usual interval from onset of rash in a mother to onset in her neonate is 9 to 15 days.

DIAGNOSTIC TESTS: Diagnostic tests for VZV are summarized in Table 3.91. Vesicular fluid or a scab can be used to identify VZV using a polymerase chain reaction (PCR) test, which currently is the diagnostic method of choice. During the acute phase of illness, VZV also can be identified by PCR assay of saliva or buccal swabs, although VZV is more likely to be detected in vesicular fluid or scabs. VZV can be demonstrated by direct fluorescent antibody (DFA) assay, using scrapings of a vesicle base early in the eruption or by viral isolation in cell culture from vesicular fluid. Viral culture and DFA assay both are less sensitive than PCR assay, and neither method is capable of distinguishing vaccine-strain from wild-type viruses. PCR testing that discriminates between vaccine and wild type VZV is available free of charge through the specialized reference laboratory at the

Centers for Disease Control and Prevention (CDC [404-639-0066]), through a safety research program sponsored by Merck & Co (1-800-672-6372), and from 4 state public health laboratories serving as vaccine preventable disease reference centers (Wisconsin, Minnesota, California, and New York).

A significant increase (4-fold increase in titer) in serum varicella immunoglobulin (Ig) G antibody between acute and convalescent samples by any standard serologic assay can confirm a diagnosis retrospectively, but this may not reliably occur in immunocompromised people (see Care of Exposed People, p 874). However, diagnosis of VZV infection by serologic testing seldom is indicated. Commercially available enzyme immunoassay (EIA) tests usually are not sufficiently sensitive to demonstrate reliably a vaccine-induced antibody response, and therefore, routine postvaccination serologic testing is not recommended. IgM tests are not reliable for routine confirmation or ruling out of acute infection. All VZV IgM assays are prone to false-negative and false-positive results.

TREATMENT: Nonspecific therapies for varicella includes keeping fingernails short to prevent trauma and secondary bacterial infection from scratching, frequent bathing, application of Calamine lotion to reduce pruritus, and acetaminophen for fever. Children with varicella should not receive salicylates or salicylate-containing products (eg, aspirin, bismuth-subsalicylate), because these products increase the risk of Reye syndrome. Salicylate therapy should be stopped in an unimmunized child who is exposed to varicella. Treatment with ibuprofen is controversial, because it has been associated with life-threatening streptococcal skin infections, perhaps because of delays in recognition, and should be avoided if possible.

Table 3.91. Diagnostic Tests for Varicella-Zoster Virus (VZV) Infection

Test	Specimen	Comments
PCR	Vesicular swabs or scrapings, scabs from crusted lesions, biopsy tissue, CSF	Very sensitive method. Specific for VZV. Methods have been designed that distinguish vaccine strain from wild-type (see text).
DFA	Vesicle scraping, swab of lesion base (must include cells)	Specific for VZV. More rapid and more sensitive than culture, less sensitive than PCR.
Viral culture	Vesicular fluid, CSF, biopsy tissue	Distinguishes VZV from HSV. High cost, limited availability, requires up to a week for result. Least sensitive method.
Serology (IgG)	Acute and convalescent serum specimens for IgG	Specific for VZV. Commercial assays generally have low sensitivity to reliably detect vaccine-induced immunity. gpELISA and FAMA are the only IgG methods that can readily detect vaccine seroconversion, but these tests are not commercially available.
Capture IgM	Acute serum specimens for IgM	Specific for VZV. IgM inconsistently detected. Not reliable method for routine confirmation. Requires special equipment.

PCR indicates polymerase chain reaction; CSF, cerebrospinal fluid; DFA, direct fluorescent antibody; HSV, herpes simplex virus; IgG, immunoglobulin G; gpELISA, glycoprotein enzyme-linked immunoassay; FAMA, fluorescent antibody to membrane antigen (assay); IgM, immunoglobulin M.

The decision to use antiviral therapy and the route and duration of therapy should be determined by host factors and extent of infection. Antiviral drugs have a limited window of opportunity to affect the outcome of VZV infection. In immunocompetent hosts, most virus replication has stopped by 72 hours after onset of rash; the duration of replication may be extended in immunocompromised hosts. Oral acyclovir and valacyclovir are not recommended for routine use in otherwise healthy younger children with varicella, because their use results in only a modest decrease in symptoms. Antiviral therapy should be considered for otherwise healthy people at increased risk of moderate to severe varicella, such as unvaccinated people older than 12 years, and those with chronic cutaneous or pulmonary disorders, those receiving long-term salicylate therapy, or those receiving short or intermittent courses of corticosteroids. Some experts also recommend use of oral acyclovir or valacyclovir for secondary household cases in which the disease usually is more severe than in the primary case. For recommendations on dosage and duration of therapy, see Non-HIV Antiviral Drugs (p 966).

Acyclovir is a category B drug based on US Food and Drug Administration (FDA) Drug Risk Classification in pregnancy. Some experts recommend oral acyclovir or valacyclovir for pregnant women with varicella, especially during the second and third trimesters. Intravenous acyclovir is recommended for pregnant patients with serious complications of varicella.

Intravenous acyclovir therapy is recommended for immunocompromised patients, including patients being treated with high-dose corticosteroid therapy for more than 14 days. Therapy initiated early in the course of the illness, especially within 24 hours of rash onset, maximizes benefit. Oral acyclovir should not be used to treat immunocompromised children with varicella because of poor oral bioavailability. Valacyclovir (20 mg/kg per dose, with a maximum dose of 1000 mg, administered orally 3 times daily for 5 days) is licensed for treatment of varicella in children 2 through 17 years of age. Some experts have used valacyclovir, with its improved bioavailability compared with oral acyclovir, in selected immunocompromised patients perceived to be at low to moderate risk of developing severe varicella, such as human immunodeficiency virus (HIV)-infected patients with relatively normal concentrations of CD4+ T-lymphocytes and children with leukemia in whom careful follow-up is ensured. Famciclovir is available for treatment of VZV infections in adults, but its efficacy and safety have not been established for children. Although VariZIG or, if not available, IGIV, administered shortly after exposure, can prevent or modify the course of disease, Immune Globulin preparations are not effective treatment once disease is established (see Care of Exposed People).

Infections caused by acyclovir-resistant VZV strains, which generally are rare and limited to immunocompromised hosts, should be treated with parenteral foscarnet.

ISOLATION OF THE HOSPITALIZED PATIENT: In addition to standard precautions, airborne and contact precautions are recommended for patients with varicella until all lesions are dry and crusted, typically at least 5 days after onset of rash but a week or longer in immunocompromised patients. In patients with varicella pneumonia, precautions are prolonged for the duration of illness. For immunized patients with breakthrough varicella with only maculopapular lesions, isolation is recommended until no new lesions appear within a 24-hour period, even if lesions have not resolved completely. For exposed patients without evidence of immunity (see Evidence of Immunity to Varicella, p 874), airborne and contact precautions from 8 until 21 days after exposure to the index patient also are indicated; these precautions should be maintained until 28 days after exposure for those who received VariZIG or IGIV.

Airborne and contact precautions are recommended for neonates born to mothers with varicella until 21 days of age, or until 28 days of age if VariZIG or IGIV was administered. To minimize the possibility of infection of the infant, the mother and the infant should be isolated separately until the mother's vesicles have dried, even if the infant has received VariZIG. If the infant develops clinical varicella, the mother may care for the infant. If the neonate is born with lesions (eg, congenital varicella), the mother and her newborn should be isolated (they can be isolated together) and discharged home when clinically stable. If the infant is clinically stable for discharge during the incubation period and has not developed varicella, isolation to complete the 21- or 28-day period should continue at home by ensuring that relatives and contacts have evidence of immunity to varicella. If the infant needs to see the health care provider during that period, the office should be notified of the need for airborne and contact precautions.

Infants with varicella embryopathy do not require isolation if they do not have active skin lesions.

Airborne and contact precautions are recommended for both immunocompetent and immunocompromised patients with disseminated zoster for the duration of illness. Immunocompromised patients with localized disease require airborne and contact precautions until disseminated infection is ruled out. For immunocompetent patients with localized zoster, standard precautions and complete covering of the lesions (if possible) are indicated until all lesions are crusted.

CONTROL MEASURES:

Evidence of Immunity to Varicella. Evidence of immunity to varicella includes any of the following:

1. Documentation of age-appropriate immunization
   - Preschool-aged children (ie, ≥12 months of age): 1 dose
   - School-aged children, adolescents, and adults: 2 doses
2. Laboratory evidence of immunity or laboratory confirmation of disease
3. Varicella diagnosed by a physician or verification of history of varicella disease
4. History of herpes zoster diagnosed by a physician

Child Care and School. Children with uncomplicated varicella who have been excluded from school or child care may return when the rash has crusted or, in immunized people without crusts, until no new lesions appear within a 24-hour period.

Exclusion of children with zoster whose lesions cannot be covered is based on similar criteria. Children who are excluded may return after the lesions have crusted. Lesions that are covered pose little risk to susceptible people, although transmission has been reported.

Care of Exposed People. Potential interventions for people without evidence of immunity exposed to a person with varicella or herpes zoster include: (1) varicella vaccine, administered ideally within 3 days but up to 5 days after exposure (followed by a second dose of vaccine at the age-appropriate interval after the first dose); (2) when indicated and available, VariZIG (or IGIV; see Unavailability of Varicella-Zoster Immune Globulin, p 876); or (3) if the child cannot be immunized and VariZIG is not indicated or is unavailable, preemptive oral acyclovir or valacyclovir starting day 7 after exposure. These options are discussed in detail below. When used, VariZIG should be administered as soon as possible following exposure, ideally within 96 hours for greatest effectiveness; limited data suggest benefit when administered up to 10 days after exposure. Preemptive oral acyclovir has only been studied in the normal host but sometimes is used in addition to VariZIG or IGIV in the immunocompromised host.

Hospital Exposure. If an inadvertent exposure occurs in the hospital to an infected person by a patient, health care professional, or visitor, the following control measures are recommended:

- Health care professionals, patients, and visitors who have been exposed (see Fig 3.12, p 879) and who lack evidence of immunity to varicella should be identified.
- Varicella immunization is recommended for people without evidence of immunity, provided there are no contraindications to vaccine use.
- VariZIG should be administered to appropriate candidates (see Fig 3.12, p 877) up to day 10 postexposure. If VariZIG is not available, IGIV should be considered as an alternative (see Unavailability of Varicella-Zoster Immune Globulin, p 876).
- If vaccine cannot be administered and VariZIG/IVIG is not indicated, preemptive oral acyclovir or valaciclovir can be considered.
- All exposed patients without evidence of immunity should be discharged as soon as possible.
- All exposed patients without evidence of immunity who cannot be discharged should be placed in isolation from day 8 to day 21 after exposure to the index patient (see Isolation of the Hospitalized Patient). For people who received VariZIG or IGIV, isolation should continue until day 28.
- Health care professionals who have received 2 doses of vaccine and who are exposed to VZV should be monitored daily during days 8 through 21 after exposure through the employee health program or by an infection-control nurse to determine clinical status. They should be placed on sick leave immediately if symptoms such as fever, headache, other constitutional symptoms, or any suspicious skin lesions occur.
- Health care professionals who have received only 1 dose of vaccine and who are exposed to VZV should receive the second dose with a single-antigen varicella vaccine, preferably within 3 to 5 days of exposure, provided 4 weeks have elapsed after the first dose. After immunization, management is similar to that of 2-dose vaccine recipients. For more information, see the recommendations of the CDC.[1]
- Immunized health care professionals who develop breakthrough infection should be considered infectious until vesicular lesions have crusted or, if they had maculopapular lesions, until no new lesions appear within a 24-hour period.

Postexposure Immunization. Varicella vaccine should be administered to healthy people without evidence of immunity who are 12 months or older, including adults, as soon as possible, preferably within 3 days and possibly up to 5 days after varicella or herpes zoster exposure, if there are no contraindications to vaccine use. This approach may prevent or modify disease. Patients should be counseled that not all close exposures result in infection, so vaccination even after 3 to 5 days following exposure is still warranted. A second vaccine dose should be administered at the age-appropriate interval after the first dose. Physicians should advise parents and their children that the vaccine may not protect against disease in all cases, because some children may have been exposed at the same time as the index case.

Passive Immunoprophylaxis. The decision to administer VariZIG depends on 3 factors:

---

[1]Centers for Disease Control and Prevention. Immunization of health-care personnel: recommendations of the Advisory Committee on Immunization Practices (ACIP). *MMWR Recomm Rep.* 2011;60(RR-7):1–45

(1) the likelihood that the exposed person has no evidence of immunity to varicella; (2) the probability that a given exposure to varicella or zoster will result in infection; and (3) the likelihood that complications of varicella will develop if the person is infected.

Data are not available regarding the sensitivity and specificity of serologic tests in immunocompromised patients. Detection of VZV IgG after one dose of varicella vaccine might not correspond to adequate protection in immunocompromised people, and false-positive results can occur. Therefore, regardless of serologic test results, careful questioning of the child and parents about potential past disease or exposure to disease can be helpful in determining immunity. Administration of VariZIG or IGIV as soon as possible within 10 days to immunocompromised children who are exposed with no history of varicella or vaccination and/or unknown or negative serologic test results is recommended. The degree and type of immunosuppression should be considered in making this decision. VariZIG is administered intramuscularly at the recommended dose of 62.5 units (0.5 vial) for children weighing ≤2.0 kg; 125 units (1 vial) for children weighing 2.1 to 10 kg; 250 units (2 vials) for children weighing 10.1 to 20 kg; 375 units (3 vials) for children weighing 20.1 to 30 kg; 500 units (4 vials) for children weighing 30.1 to 40 kg; and 625 units (5 vials) for all people weighing >40 kg. IGIV is administered intravenously at the dose of 400 mg/kg.

Patients receiving monthly high-dose IGIV (400 mg/kg or greater) at regular intervals are likely to be protected if the last dose of IGIV was administered 3 weeks or less before exposure.

Where to Obtain VariZIG. VariZIG can be obtained from FFF Enterprises (Temecula, CA; telephone 800-843-7477; **www.fffenterprises.com**) and ASD Healthcare (Frisco, TX; telephone 800-746-6273; **www.asdhealthcare.com**).

Recommended Use of Varicella-Zoster Immune Globulin. Fig 3.12 identifies people without evidence of immunity who should receive VariZIG if exposed, including immunocompromised people, pregnant women, and certain newborn infants.

For healthy term infants exposed postnatally to varicella, including infants whose mother's rash developed more than 48 hours after delivery, VariZIG is not indicated. However, some experts advise use of VariZIG for exposed newborn infants within the first 2 weeks of life whose mothers do not have evidence of immunity to varicella.

Subsequent Exposures and Follow-up of Varicella-Zoster Immune Globulin Recipients. Any patient to whom VariZIG is administered to prevent varicella subsequently should receive age-appropriate varicella vaccine, provided that receipt of live vaccines is not contraindicated. Varicella immunization should be delayed until 5 months after VariZIG administration. Varicella vaccine is not needed if the patient develops varicella despite VariZIG.

Unavailability of Varicella-Zoster Immune Globulin. If VariZIG is not available, IGIV can be used (Fig 3.12). The recommendation for use of IGIV is based on "best judgment of experts" and is supported by reports comparing VZV IgG antibody titers measured in both IGIV and VariZIG preparations and patients receiving IGIV or VariZIG. Although licensed IGIV preparations contain antivaricella antibodies, the titer of any specific lot of IGIV is uncertain, because IGIV is not tested routinely for antivaricella antibodies. No clinical data demonstrating effectiveness of IGIV for postexposure prophylaxis of varicella are available. The recommended IGIV dose for postexposure prophylaxis of varicella is 400 mg/kg, administered once intravenously.

FIG 3.12. MANAGEMENT OF EXPOSURES TO VARICELLA-ZOSTER VIRUS

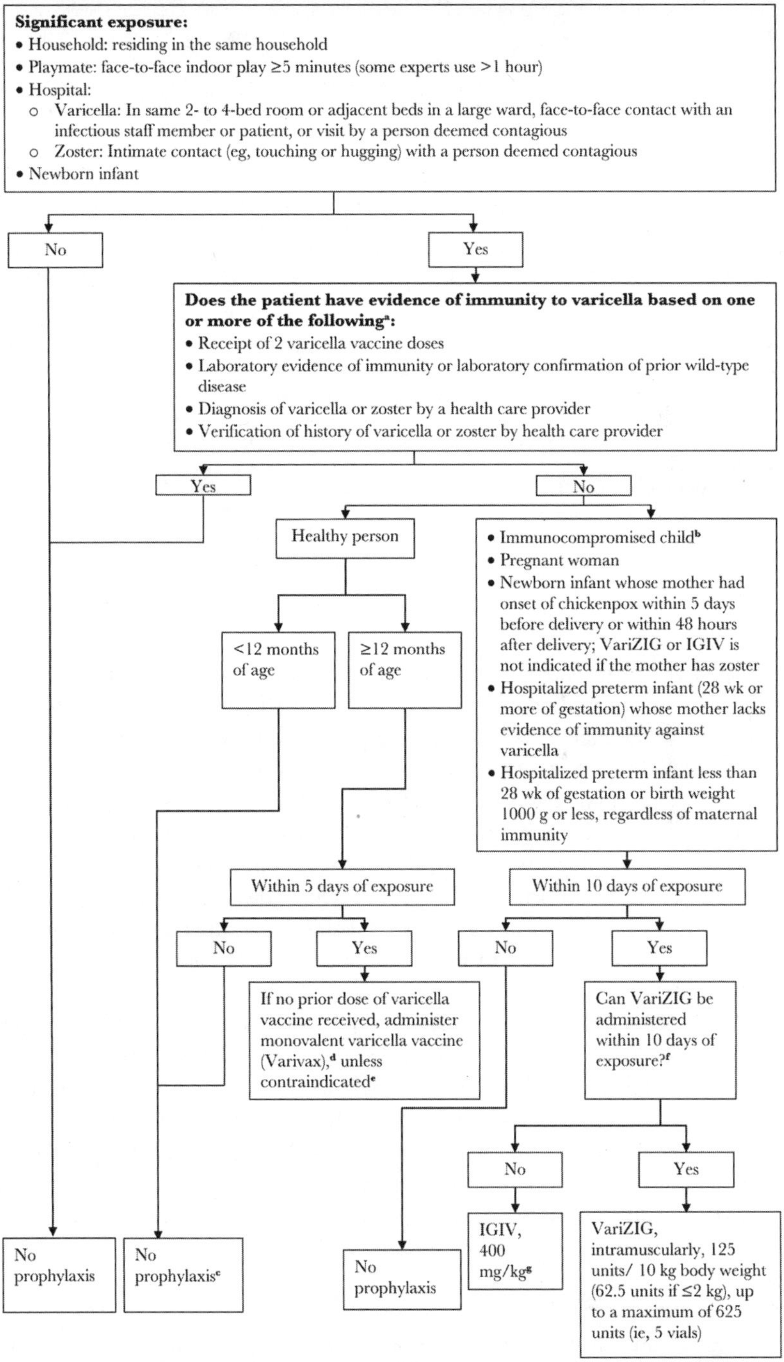

Significant exposure:
- Household: residing in the same household
- Playmate: face-to-face indoor play ≥5 minutes (some experts use >1 hour)
- Hospital:
  - Varicella: In same 2- to 4-bed room or adjacent beds in a large ward, face-to-face contact with an infectious staff member or patient, or visit by a person deemed contagious
  - Zoster: Intimate contact (eg, touching or hugging) with a person deemed contagious
- Newborn infant

No / Yes

Does the patient have evidence of immunity to varicella based on one or more of the following[a]:
- Receipt of 2 varicella vaccine doses
- Laboratory evidence of immunity or laboratory confirmation of prior wild-type disease
- Diagnosis of varicella or zoster by a health care provider
- Verification of history of varicella or zoster by health care provider

Yes / No

Healthy person

- Immunocompromised child[b]
- Pregnant woman
- Newborn infant whose mother had onset of chickenpox within 5 days before delivery or within 48 hours after delivery; VariZIG or IGIV is not indicated if the mother has zoster
- Hospitalized preterm infant (28 wk or more of gestation) whose mother lacks evidence of immunity against varicella
- Hospitalized preterm infant less than 28 wk of gestation or birth weight 1000 g or less, regardless of maternal immunity

<12 months of age / ≥12 months of age

Within 5 days of exposure

No / Yes

If no prior dose of varicella vaccine received, administer monovalent varicella vaccine (Varivax),[d] unless contraindicated[e]

Within 10 days of exposure

No / Yes

Can VariZIG be administered within 10 days of exposure?[f]

No / Yes

No prophylaxis

No prophylaxis[e]

No prophylaxis

No prophylaxis

IGIV, 400 mg/kg[g]

VariZIG, intramuscularly, 125 units/ 10 kg body weight (62.5 units if ≤2 kg), up to a maximum of 625 units (ie, 5 vials)

VariZIG indicates Varicella-Zoster Immune Globulin; IGIV, Immune Globulin Intravenous.

[a]People who receive hematopoietic stem cell transplants should be considered nonimmune regardless of previous history of varicella disease or varicella vaccination in themselves or in their donors.

[b]Immunocompromised children include those with congenital or acquired T-lymphocyte immunodeficiency, including leukemia, lymphoma, and other malignant neoplasms affecting the bone marrow or lymphatic system; children receiving immunosuppressive therapy, including ≥2 mg/kg/day of systemic prednisone (or its equivalent) for ≥14 days; all children with human immunodeficiency virus (HIV) infection regardless of CD4+ T-lymphocyte percentage; and all hematopoietic stem cell transplant patients regardless of pretransplant immunity status.

[c]If the exposed person is an adolescent or adult, has chronic illness, or there are other compelling reasons to try to avert varicella, some experts recommend preemptive therapy with oral acyclovir (20 mg/kg per dose administered 4 times per day, with a maximum daily dose of 3200 mg) or oral valacyclovir (if ≥3 months of age; 20 mg/kg per dose administered 3 times per day, with a maximum daily dose of 3000 mg) beginning 7 to 10 days after exposure and continuing for 7 days. If the child is ≥12 months of age, age-appropriate vaccination still is recommended for protection against subsequent exposures, but vaccine should not be administered while antiviral therapy is being administered; if the exposure occurred during an outbreak, 2-dose vaccination is recommended for preschool-aged children younger than 4 years for outbreak control.

[d]If 1 prior dose of varicella vaccine has been received, a second dose should be administered at ≥4 years of age. If the exposure occurred during an outbreak, a second dose is recommended for preschool-aged children younger than 4 years for outbreak control if at least 3 months have passed after the first dose.

[e]Contraindications include patients who are allergic to a vaccine component, or who are immunocompromised (see above footnote), or pregnant. Caution should be used in patients receiving salicylates. Vaccine may not be as effective if patient has recently received Immune Globulin Intravenous, whole blood, or plasma transfusions, and for this reason, it is recommended that varicella vaccine be withheld for 3 to 11 months, depending on the dose, after administration of these products.

[f]VariZIG is manufactured by Cangene Corporation (Winnipeg, Canada) and distributed in the United States by FFF Enterprises (Temecula, California; 800-843-7477; **www.fffenterprises.com**) and ASD Healthcare (Frisco, Texas; 800-746-6273; **www.asdhealthcare.com**).

[g]If VariZIG and IGIV are not available, some experts recommend preemptive therapy with oral acyclovir (20 mg/kg per dose, administered 4 times per day, with a maximum daily dose of 3200 mg) or oral valacyclovir (if ≥3 months of age; 20 mg/kg per dose, administered 3 times per day, with a maximum daily dose of 3000 mg) beginning 7 to 10 days after exposure and continuing for 7 days. Preemptive oral acyclovir has only been studied in the normal host but sometimes is used in addition to VariZIG or IGIV in the immunocompromised host.

Chemoprophylaxis. Some experts recommend preemptive antiviral therapy in select circumstances for mildly immunocompromised patients without evidence of immunity or for immunocompetent patients for whom varicella prevention is desired (eg, healthy older adolescent or adult contacts for whom vaccination is not possible) who have been exposed to varicella or herpes zoster (Fig 3.12). Acyclovir (20 mg/kg per dose, administered orally 4 times per day, with a maximum daily dose of 3200 mg) or valacyclovir (20 mg/kg per dose, administered orally 3 times per day, with a maximum daily dose of 3000 mg) beginning 7 to 10 days after exposure and continuing for 7 days can be used. Limited data on acyclovir as postexposure prophylaxis are available for healthy children, and no studies have been performed for adults or immunocompromised people.

Active Immunization.[1]

Vaccine. Varicella vaccine is a live attenuated preparation of the serially propagated and attenuated Oka strain, originally isolated from a boy with the last name of Oka who had wild-type varicella. The product contains gelatin and trace amounts of neomycin. The monovalent vaccine was developed in the early 1970s by Professor Michiaki Takahashi and was licensed in March 1995 by the FDA for use in healthy people 12 months or older who have not had varicella illness. Quadrivalent measles-mumps-rubella-varicella (MMRV) vaccine was licensed in September 2005 by the FDA for use in healthy children 12 months through 12 years of age.

---

[1]Centers for Disease Control and Prevention. Prevention of varicella: recommendations of the Advisory Committee on Immunization Practices (ACIP). *MMWR Recomm Rep.* 2007;56(RR-4):1–40

Dose and Administration. The recommended dose of vaccine is 0.5 mL, administered subcutaneously.

Immunogenicity. Approximately 76% to 85% of immunized healthy children older than 12 months develop a humoral immune response to VZV at levels considered associated with protection after a single dose of varicella vaccine. Seroprotection rates and cell-mediated immune responses approach 100% after 2 doses.

Effectiveness. The effectiveness of 1 dose of varicella vaccine is about 82% against any clinical varicella and 98% against severe disease. Two doses of vaccine demonstrated 92% effectiveness against any clinical varicella.

Simultaneous Administration With Other Vaccines or Antiviral Agents. Varicella-containing vaccines may be administered simultaneously with other childhood immunizations recommended for children 12 through 15 months of age and 4 through 6 years of age **(http://aapredbook.aappublications.org/site/resources/izschedules. xhtml).** If not administered at the same visit or as MMRV vaccine, the interval between administration of a varicella-containing vaccine and measles-mumps-rubella (MMR) vaccine should be at least 28 days. The minimal interval between MMRV vaccine doses is 3 months. Because of susceptibility of vaccine virus to acyclovir, valacyclovir, or famciclovir, these antiviral agents usually should be avoided from 1 day before to 21 days (the outer limit of the incubation period) after receipt of a varicella-containing vaccine.

Adverse Events. Varicella vaccine is safe; reactions generally are mild and occur with an overall frequency of approximately 5% to 35%. Approximately 20% to 25% of immunized people will experience minor injection site reactions (eg, pain, redness, swelling). In approximately 1% to 3% of immunized children, a localized rash develops, and in an additional 3% to 5%, a generalized varicella-like rash develops. These rashes typically consist of 2 to 5 lesions and may be maculopapular rather than vesicular; lesions usually appear 5 to 26 days after immunization. However, not all observed postimmunization rashes can be attributable to vaccine. After MMRV or monovalent varicella vaccine plus MMR, a measles-like rash was reported in 2% to 3% of recipients. Fever was reported in a higher proportion after the first dose of MMRV than after the first dose of monovalent varicella vaccine plus MMR (22% vs 15%) in young children. Both fever and measles-like rash usually occurred within 5 to 12 days of immunization, were of short duration, and resolved without sequelae.

A slightly increased risk of febrile seizures is associated with the higher likelihood of fever following the first dose of MMRV compared with MMR and monovalent varicella. One additional febrile seizure is expected to occur per approximately 2300 to 2600 young children immunized with a first dose of MMRV compared with a first dose of MMR and monovalent varicella. After the second vaccine dose administered in older children (4 to 6 years of age), there were no differences in incidence of fever, rash, or febrile seizures among recipients of MMRV vaccine compared with recipients of simultaneous MMR and varicella vaccines.[1]

Breakthrough Disease. Breakthrough disease is defined as a case of infection with wild-type VZV occurring more than 42 days after immunization. Varicella in vaccine recipients usually is very mild, with rash frequently atypical (predominantly maculopapular

---

[1]Centers for Disease Control and Prevention. Use of combination measles, mumps, rubella, and varicella vaccine: recommendations of the Advisory Committee on Immunization Practices (ACIP). *MMWR Recomm Rep.* 2010;59(RR-3):1–12

with a median of fewer than 50 lesions), a lower rate of fever, and faster recovery than disease in unimmunized children. It may be mistaken for other conditions, such as insect bites or poison ivy. Vaccine recipients with mild breakthrough disease are approximately one third as contagious as unimmunized children. However, approximately 25% to 30% of breakthrough cases are not mild, with clinical features similar to those in unvaccinated people.

Herpes Zoster After Immunization. Vaccine-strain VZV can cause herpes zoster in immunocompetent and immunocompromised people. However, data from postlicensure surveillance indicate that the age-specific risk of herpes zoster is lower among immunocompetent children immunized with varicella vaccine than among children who have had natural varicella infection. Wild-type VZV has been identified in skin lesion specimens in people with herpes zoster after immunization, indicating that herpes zoster in immunized people also may result from unrecognized natural VZV infection that occurred before or after immunization.

Transmission of Vaccine-Strain VZV. Vaccine-strain VZV transmission to contacts is rare (documented from only 9 vaccinees, resulting in 11 secondary cases). In all cases, the immunized person had a rash following vaccine. Postexposure prophylaxis with VariZIG, IGIV, acyclovir, or valacyclovir in high-risk people exposed to immunized people with varicella lesions has not been studied. Some experts believe that immunocompromised people with skin lesions that are presumed to be attributable to vaccine virus should receive acyclovir or valacyclovir treatment. Attempts to confirm the presence of VZV should be made in these patients usually via PCR assay.

Recommendations for Immunization.

Children 12 Months Through 12 Years of Age. Both monovalent varicella vaccine and MMRV have been licensed for use for healthy children 12 months through 12 years of age.[1] Children in this age group should receive two 0.5-mL doses of monovalent varicella vaccine or MMRV administered subcutaneously, separated by at least 3 months. However, provided the second dose is administered a minimum 28 days after the first dose, it does not need to be repeated.

All healthy children should receive the first dose of varicella-containing vaccine at 12 through 15 months of age. The second dose of vaccine is recommended routinely when children are 4 through 6 years of age (ie, before a child enters kindergarten or first grade) but can be administered at an earlier age. Because of the minimal potential for increased febrile seizures after the first dose of MMRV vaccine in children 12 through 15 months of age, the American Academy of Pediatrics recommends a choice of either MMR plus monovalent varicella vaccine or MMRV for toddlers receiving their first immunization of this kind. Parents should be counseled about the rare possibility of their child developing a febrile seizure 1 to 2 weeks after immunization with MMRV for the first immunizing dose. For the second dose at 4 through 6 years of age, MMRV generally is preferred over MMR plus monovalent varicella to minimize the number of injections. A catch-up second dose of varicella vaccine should be offered to all children 7 years and older who have received only 1 dose.

If the first dose of varicella-containing vaccine is administered 5 or more days before

---

[1]Centers for Disease Control and Prevention. Use of combination measles, mumps, rubella, and varicella vaccine: recommendations of the Advisory Committee on Immunization Practices (ACIP). *MMWR Recomm Rep.* 2010;59(RR-3):1–12

the first birthday, the dose does not count toward the 2 doses needed for evidence of immunity to varicella. In such a circumstance, the varicella dose should be repeated at 12 through 15 months, as long as at least 28 days have elapsed from the invalid dose. For example, if the first dose of varicella vaccine were inadvertently administered at age 10 months, the repeat dose would be administered no earlier than the child's first birthday (the minimum age for the first dose). If the first dose of varicella vaccine were administered at age 11 months and 2 weeks, the repeat dose should be administered no earlier than 28 days thereafter, which would occur after the first birthday.

People 13 Years or Older. Immunocompetent individuals 13 years or older without evidence of immunity should receive two 0.5-mL doses of monovalent varicella vaccine, separated by at least 28 days. The recommendation for at least a 28-day interval between doses is based on the design of the studies evaluating 2 doses in this age group. For people who previously received only 1 dose of varicella vaccine, a second dose is necessary. Only monovalent varicella vaccine is licensed for use in this age group.

Contraindications and Precautions.

Intercurrent Illness. As with other vaccines, varicella vaccine should not be administered to people who have moderate or severe illnesses, with or without fever.

Immunization of Immunocompromised Patients.

GENERAL RECOMMENDATIONS.[1] Varicella vaccine (as a 2-dose regimen if there is sufficient time) should be administered to immunocompetent patients without evidence of varicella immunity, if it can be administered ≥4 weeks before initiating immunosuppressive therapy. Varicella vaccine should not be administered to highly immunocompromised patients. Certain categories of patients (eg, patients with HIV infection without severe immunosuppression or with a primary immune deficiency disorder without defective T-cell–mediated immunity, such as primary complement component deficiency disorder or chronic granulomatous disease [CGD]) should receive varicella vaccine. Children with impaired humoral immunity alone may be immunized. Immunodeficiency should be excluded before immunization in children with a family history of hereditary immunodeficiency.

In people with possible altered immunity, only monovalent varicella vaccine (not MMRV) should be used for immunization against varicella. The Oka vaccine strain remains susceptible to acyclovir, and if a high-risk patient develops vaccine-related varicella, then acyclovir or valacyclovir should be used as treatment.

MALIGNANCY.[1] The interval until immune reconstruction varies with the intensity and type of immunosuppressive therapy, radiation therapy, underlying disease, and other factors, complicating the ability to make a definitive recommendation for an interval after cessation of immunosuppressive therapy when live-virus vaccines can be administered safely and effectively. Current recommendations are for patients to be vaccinated with varicella vaccine when in remission and at least three months after cancer chemotherapy, with evidence of restored immunocompetence. In regimens that included anti–B-cell antibodies, vaccinations should be delayed at least 6 months.

HEMATOPOIETIC STEM CELL TRANSPLANT.[1] A 2-dose series of varicella vaccine should be administered a minimum of 24 months after hematopoietic stem cell transplant to varicella-seronegative patients who do not have graft versus host disease, are considered

---

[1]Rubin LG, Levin MJ, Ljungman P, et al. 2013 IDSA clinical practice guideline for vaccination of the immunocompromised host. *Clin Infect Dis.* 2014;58(3):e44–e100

immunocompetent, and whose last dose of IGIV was 8 to 11 months previously. Nonimmune family members, close contacts, and health care workers associated with the patient should be immunized before that time. Immunized people in whom a postimmunization rash develops should avoid direct contact with an immunocompromised host who lacks evidence of immunity for the duration of the rash.

HIV INFECTION.[1] The live-virus measles-mumps-rubella (MMR) vaccine and monovalent varicella vaccine can be administered to asymptomatic HIV-infected children and adolescents without severe immunosuppression (that is, can be administered to children 1 through 13 years of age with a CD4+ T-lymphocyte percentage $\geq 15\%$ and to adolescents ≥ 14 years with a CD4+ T-lymphocyte count ≥ 200 lymphocytes/mm^3). Severely immunocompromised HIV-infected infants, children, adolescents, and young adults (eg, children 1 through 13 years of age with a CD4+ T-lymphocyte percentage $< 15\%$ and adolescents ≥ 14 years with a CD4+ T-lymphocyte count < 200 lymphocytes/mm^3) should not receive measles virus-containing vaccine, because vaccine-related pneumonia has been reported. The quadrivalent measles-mumps-rubella-varicella (MMRV) vaccine should not be administered to any HIV-infected infant, regardless of degree of immunosuppression, because of lack of safety data in this population. Parents and guardians should be instructed to return for evaluation if the child experiences a postimmunization varicella-like rash. Varicella vaccine has been shown to decrease the incidence of both varicella and herpes zoster in children with HIV infection.

CHILDREN RECEIVING CORTICOSTEROIDS. Varicella vaccine should not be administered to people who are receiving high doses of systemic corticosteroids (2 mg/kg per day or more of prednisone or its equivalent or 20 mg/day of prednisone or its equivalent) for 14 days or more. The recommended interval between discontinuation of high dose corticosteroid therapy and immunization with varicella vaccine is at least 1 month. Varicella vaccine may be administered to individuals receiving only inhaled, nasal, or topical steroids.

CHILDREN WITH NEPHROTIC SYNDROME. The results of one small study indicate that 2 doses of varicella vaccine in 29 children between 12 months and 18 years of age generally were well tolerated and immunogenic, including in children receiving low-dose, alternate-day prednisone.

HOUSEHOLDS WITH POTENTIAL CONTACT WITH IMMUNOCOMPROMISED PEOPLE. Household contacts of immunocompromised people should be immunized if they have no evidence of immunity to decrease the likelihood that wild-type VZV will be introduced into the household. No precautions are needed following immunization of healthy people who do not develop a rash. Immunized people in whom a postimmunization rash develops should avoid direct contact with an immunocompromised host who lacks evidence of immunity for the duration of the rash.

Pregnancy and Lactation. Varicella vaccine should not be administered to pregnant women, because the possible effects on fetal development are unknown, although no cases of

---

[1] Guidelines for prevention and treatment of opportunistic infections in HIV-exposed and HIV-infected children. Recommendations from the National Institutes of Health, Centers for Disease Control and Prevention, the HIV Medicine Association of the Infectious Diseases Society of America, the Pediatric Infectious Diseases Society, and the American Academy of Pediatrics. *Pediatr Infect Dis J.* 2013;32(Suppl 2):i-KK4. Available at: **http://aidsinfo.nih.gov/guidelines/html/5/pediatric-oi-prevention-and-treatment-guidelines/0**

congenital varicella syndrome or patterns of malformation have been identified after inadvertent immunization of pregnant women. Pregnancy should be avoided for at least 1 month after immunization. A pregnant mother or other household member is not a contraindication for immunization of a child in the household.

Varicella vaccine should be administered to nursing mothers who lack evidence of immunity. A study of breastfeeding mothers and their infants showed no evidence of excretion of vaccine strain in human milk or of transmission to infants.

Immune Globulin. Whether Immune Globulin (IG) can interfere with varicella vaccine-induced immunity is unknown, although IG can interfere with immunity induction by measles vaccine. Pending additional data, varicella vaccine should be withheld for the same intervals after receipt of any form of IG or other blood product as measles vaccine (see Measles, p 537; and Table 1.13, p 40). Conversely, IG should be withheld for at least 2 weeks after receipt of varicella vaccine. Transplacental antibodies to VZV do not interfere with the immunogenicity of varicella vaccine administered at 12 months or older.

Salicylates. No cases of Reye syndrome have been reported following varicella vaccination with >140 million doses distributed in the United States. However, because use of salicylates during varicella infection is associated with Reye syndrome, the vaccine manufacturer recommends that salicylates be avoided for 6 weeks after administration of varicella vaccine. Physicians need to weigh the theoretical risks associated with varicella vaccine against the known risks of wild-type virus in children receiving long-term salicylate therapy.

Allergy to Vaccine Components. Varicella vaccine should not be administered to people who have had an anaphylactic-type reaction to any component of the vaccine, including gelatin and neomycin. Most people with allergy to neomycin have resulting contact dermatitis, a reaction that is not a contraindication to immunization. Monovalent varicella vaccine does not contain preservatives or egg protein, and although the measles and mumps vaccines included in MMRV vaccine are produced in chick embryo culture, the amounts of egg cross-reacting proteins are not significant. Therefore, children with egg allergy may receive MMRV without previous skin testing or special precautions.

VIBRIO INFECTIONS

Cholera
(Vibrio cholerae)

CLINICAL MANIFESTATIONS: Cholera is characterized by voluminous watery diarrhea and rapid onset of life-threatening dehydration. Hypovolemic shock may occur within hours of the onset of diarrhea. Stools have a characteristic rice-water appearance, are white-tinged and contain small flecks of mucus, and contain high concentrations of sodium, potassium, chloride, and bicarbonate. Vomiting is a common feature of cholera. Fever and abdominal cramps usually are absent. In addition to dehydration and hypovolemia, common complications of cholera include hypokalemia, metabolic acidosis, and hypoglycemia, particularly in children. Although severe cholera is a distinctive illness characterized by profuse diarrhea and rapid dehydration, people infected with toxigenic *Vibrio cholerae* O1 may have either no symptoms or mild to moderate diarrhea lasting 3 to

7 days.

ETIOLOGY: *V cholerae* is a curved or comma-shaped motile gram-negative rod. There are more than 200 *V cholerae* serogroups, some of which carry the cholera toxin (CT) gene. Although those serogroups with the CT gene and others without the CT gene can cause acute watery diarrhea, only toxin-producing serogroups O1 and O139 cause epidemic cholera, with O1 causing the vast majority of cases of cholera. *V cholerae* O1 is classified into 2 biotypes, classical and El Tor, and 2 major serotypes, Ogawa and Inaba. Since 1992, toxigenic *V cholerae* serogroup O139 has been recognized as a cause of epidemic cholera in Asia. Aside from the substitution of the O139 for the O1 antigen, the organism is almost identical to *V cholerae* O1 El Tor. All other serogroups of *V cholerae* are known collectively as *V cholerae* non-O1/non-O139. Toxin-producing strains of *V cholerae* non-O1/non-O139 can cause sporadic cases of severe dehydrating diarrheal illness but have not caused large outbreaks of cholera. Non–toxin-producing strains of *V cholerae* non-O1/non-O139 are associated with sporadic cases of gastroenteritis, sepsis, and rare cases of wound infection (discussed in Other Vibrio Infections, p 887).

EPIDEMIOLOGY: Since the early 1800s, there have been 7 cholera pandemics. The current pandemic began in 1961 and is caused by *V cholerae* O1 El Tor. Molecular epidemiology shows that this pandemic has occurred in 3 successive waves, with each one spreading from South Asia to other regions in Asia, Africa, and the Western Pacific Islands (Oceania). In 1991, epidemic cholera caused by toxigenic *V cholerae* O1 El Tor appeared in Peru and spread to most countries in South, Central, and North America, causing more than 1 million cases of cholera before subsiding. In 2010, *V cholerae* O1 El Tor was introduced into Haiti, on the island of Hispaniola, initiating a massive epidemic of cholera. In the United States, sporadic cases resulting from travel to or ingestion of contaminated food transported from regions with endemic cholera are reported, including several cases imported from Hispaniola since 2010. Domestically acquired cases in the United States have been reported from eating Gulf coast seafood.

Humans are the only documented natural host, but free-living *V cholerae* organisms can persist in the aquatic environment. Infection primarily is acquired by ingestion of large numbers of organisms from contaminated water or food (particularly raw or undercooked shellfish, raw or partially dried fish, or moist grains or vegetables held at ambient temperature). People with low gastric acidity and with blood group O are at increased risk of severe cholera infection.

The **incubation period** usually is 1 to 3 days, with a range of a few hours to 5 days.

DIAGNOSTIC TESTS: *V cholerae* can be cultured from fecal specimens (preferred) or vomitus plated on thiosulfate citrate bile salts sucrose agar. Because most laboratories in the United States do not culture routinely for *V cholerae* or other *Vibrio* organisms, clinicians should request appropriate cultures for clinically suspected cases. Isolates of *V cholerae* should be sent to a state health department laboratory for confirmation and then forwarded to the Centers for Disease Control and Prevention (CDC) for confirmation, serogrouping, and detection of the cholera toxin gene (**www.cdc.gov/laboratory/ specimen-submission/detail.html?CDCTestCode=CDC-10119).** Tests to detect serum antibodies to *V cholerae,* such as the vibriocidal assay and an anticholera toxin enzyme-linked immunoassay, are available at the CDC subject to preapproval. Both assays require submission of acute and convalescent serum specimens and, thus, provide a retrospective diagnosis. Although not diagnostic, a fourfold increase in vibriocidal antibody titers between acute and convalescent sera suggests the diagnosis of cholera. Several commercial tests for rapid antigen detection of *V cholerae* O1 and O139 in stool specimens have been developed. These *V cholerae* O1 and O139 rapid diagnostic tests (RDTs) have sensitivities ranging from approximately 80% to 97% and specificities of approximately 70% to 90% compared with culture on thiosulfate citrate bile salts sucrose agar. RDTs are not a substitute for stool culture but potentially provide a rapid presumptive indication of a suspect cholera outbreak in regions where stool culture is not immediately available. Multiplex PCR panels have been cleared by the US Food and Drug Administration for detection of various bacteria, parasites, and viruses associated with gastrointestinal tract infections and can specifically detect *V cholera* directly from stool specimens.

TREATMENT: Timely and appropriate rehydration therapy is the cornerstone of management of cholera and reduces the mortality of severe cholera to less than 0.5%. Rehydration therapy should be based on World Health Organization (WHO) standards, with the goal of replacing the estimated fluid deficit within 3 to 4 hours of initial presentation. In patients with severe dehydration, isotonic intravenous fluids should be used, and lactated Ringer solution is the preferred commercially available option.[1] For patients without severe dehydration, oral rehydration therapy using the WHO's reduced-osmolality oral rehydration solution (ORS) has been the standard, but data suggest that rice-based ORS or amylase-resistant starch ORS are more effective.

Prompt initiation of antimicrobial therapy decreases the duration and volume of diarrhea and decreases the shedding of viable bacteria. Antimicrobial therapy should be considered for people who are moderately to severely ill. The choice of antimicrobial therapy should be made on the basis of the age of the patient (Table 3.92) as well as prevailing patterns of antimicrobial resistance. In cases in which prevailing patterns of resistance are unknown, antimicrobial susceptibility testing should be performed and monitored. Zinc supplementation should be considered as an adjunct to rehydration in children (**www. cdc.gov/cholera/treatment/zinc-treatment.html**).

ISOLATION OF THE HOSPITALIZED PATIENT: In addition to standard precautions, contact precautions are indicated for diapered children or incontinent people for the duration of illness.

CONTROL MEASURES:

Hygiene. Disinfection of drinking water through chlorination or boiling prevents waterborne transmission of V cholerae. Thoroughly cooking crabs, oysters, and other shellfish from the Gulf Coast before eating is recommended to decrease the likelihood of transmission. Foods such as fish, rice, or grain gruels should be refrigerated promptly and thoroughly reheated before eating, and fruits and vegetables should be peeled before eating. The use of latrines or burying feces is recommended, and defecation should be avoided near any body of water. Appropriate hand hygiene after defecating and before preparing or eating food is important for preventing transmission.

Treatment of Contacts. Although administration of appropriate antimicrobial agents within 24 hours of identification of the index case may prevent additional cases of cholera among household contacts, chemoprophylaxis of contacts currently is not recommended by the WHO, except in special circumstances in which the probability of fecal exposure is high and medication can be delivered rapidly.

---

[1]World Health Organization. *The Treatment of Diarrhoea, a Manual for Physicians and Other Senior Health Workers.* 4th Rev. WHO/FCH/CAH/05.1. Geneva, Switzerland: World Health Organization; 2005

Table 3.92. Antibiotics for Suspected Cholera

Antibiotic	Pediatric Dose[a]	Adult Dose	Comment(s)
Doxycycline	4.4 mg/kg, single dose	300 mg, single dose	Use should be in epidemics caused by susceptible isolates. Can be used for short durations (ie, 21 days or less) without regard to patient age. Not recommended for pregnant women.
Ciprofloxacin[b]	15 mg/kg, twice daily for 3 days (single dose 20 mg/kg has been used)	500 mg, twice daily for 3 days	Decreased susceptibility to fluoroquinolones is associated with treatment failure. Ciprofloxacin is not recommended in children and pregnant women.
Azithromycin	20 mg/kg, single dose	1 g, single dose	
Erythromycin	12.5 mg/kg, 4 times/day for 3 days	250 mg, 4 times/day for 3 days	
Tetracycline[c]	12.5 mg/kg, 4 times/day for 3 days	500 mg, 4 times/day for 3 days	

[a] Not to exceed adult dose.

[b] Fluoroquinolones are not approved for children for children younger than 18 years for this indication.

[c] For use in children ≥8 y.

Vaccine. A single-dose, live attenuated monovalent oral vaccine, (Vaxchora [PaxVax Inc, Redwood City, CA]), has been approved by the US Food and Drug Administration and is available in the United States for use for travelers 18 through 64 years of age who are traveling to areas where cholera is a risk.[1] In addition to following safe food and water precautions, the Advisory Committee on Immunization Practices of the CDC recommends cholera vaccine for adult travelers (18 through 64 years old) to an area of active cholera transmission. A pediatric study of this vaccine in children and adolescents 2 through 17 years of age began in July 2017 and is expected to enroll over 3 years. An area of active cholera transmission is defined as a province, state, or other administrative subdivision within a country with endemic or epidemic cholera caused by toxigenic *V cholerae* O1 and includes areas with cholera activity within the last 1 year that are prone to recurrence of cholera epidemics; it does not include areas where rare sporadic cases only have been reported. Information about destinations with active cholera transmission is available at **wwwnc.cdc.gov/travel/**.

Three inactivated oral vaccines exist currently, 2 of which are approved by the WHO, that are available in a number of countries outside of the United States. Dukoral (Crucell, Leiden, The Netherlands/SBL Vaccin AB, Sweden) is a WHO-approved monovalent inactivated vaccine based on heat-killed whole cells of serogroup O1 plus recombinant cholera toxin B subunit and is 85% protective against cholera. The vaccine also may provide some protection against heat-labile enterotoxigenic *E coli* infection. Children between 2 and 6 years of age require 3 doses, and adults and children 6 years and older

---

[1] Wong KK, Burdette E, Mahon BE, Mintz ED, Ryan ET, Reingold AL. Recommendations of the Advisory Committee on Immunization Practices for use of cholera vaccine. *MMWR Morb Mortal Wkly Rep.* 2017;66:482–485. Available at: **http://dx.doi.org/10.15585/mmwr.mm6618a6**

require 2 doses at least 1 week apart. Bivalent (O1 and O139) vaccine, available as ORC-Vax and mORC-Vax (VaBiotech, Vietnam) and Shanchol (Shantha Biotechnics/Sanofi Pasteur, India [WHO approved]), also are licensed for use. In 2011, the WHO initiated a global oral cholera vaccine stockpile to allow for its rapid deployment during cholera epidemics and other emergencies. Instructions regarding access to the stockpile are available at **www.who.int/cholera/vaccines/ocv_stockpile_2013/en/**.

Cholera immunization is not required for travelers entering the United States from cholera-affected areas, and the WHO no longer recommends immunization for travel to or from areas with cholera infection. No country requires cholera vaccine for entry.

Public Health Reporting. Confirmed cases of cholera must be reported to health authorities in any country in which they occur and were contracted. Local and state health departments should be notified immediately of presumed or known cases of cholera.

Other *Vibrio* Infections

CLINICAL MANIFESTATIONS: Illness attributable to the following (mostly nontoxigenic species) of the *Vibrionaceae* family is known as vibriosis: (1) *Vibrio parahaemolyticus, Vibrio vulnificus,* and other *Vibrio* species; (2) nontoxigenic *Vibrio cholerae;* (3) toxigenic *V cholerae* O75 and O141; and (4) members of the *Vibrionaceae* family that are not in the genus *Vibrio* (eg, *Grimontia hollisae*). Associated clinical syndromes include gastroenteritis, wound infection, and septicemia. Gastroenteritis is the most common syndrome and is characterized by acute onset of watery nonbloody stools and crampy abdominal pain. Approximately half of affected people will have low-grade fever, headache, and chills; approximately 30% will have vomiting. Spontaneous recovery follows in 2 to 5 days. Wound infections typically start as cellulitis with vesicles and can progress to hemorrhagic bullae, necrosis, and/or necrotizing fasciitis. Septicemia can be primary or follow gastroenteritis or wound infection and often is fulminant and accompanied by development of metastatic skin lesions within 36 hours. Risk factors for severe wound infections and for septicemia include liver disease, iron overload, hemolytic anemia, chronic renal failure, diabetes mellitus, low gastric acidity, and immunosuppression. Various otolaryngologic manifestations attributable to *Vibrio alginolyticus* have been linked to swimming in salt water.

ETIOLOGY: *Vibrio* organisms are facultatively anaerobic, motile, gram-negative bacilli that are tolerant of salt. The most commonly reported nontoxigenic *Vibrio* species associated with diarrhea are *V parahaemolyticus* and *V cholerae* non-O1/non-O139. *V vulnificus* typically causes primary septicemia and severe wound infections, but the other species also can cause these syndromes. *V alginolyticus* typically causes wound infections.

EPIDEMIOLOGY: *Vibrio* species are natural inhabitants of marine and estuarine environments. In temperate climates, most noncholera *Vibrio* infections occur during summer and autumn months, when *Vibrio* populations in seawater are highest. Gastroenteritis usually follows ingestion of raw or undercooked seafood, especially oysters, clams, crabs, and shrimp. Wound infections usually are attributable to *V vulnificans* and can result from exposure of a preexisting wound to contaminated seawater or from punctures resulting from handling of contaminated fish or shellfish. Exposure to contaminated water during natural disasters, such as hurricanes, has resulted in wound infections. Person-to-person transmission has not been reported. Infections associated with noncholera *Vibrio* organisms became nationally notifiable in January 2007.

The **incubation period** for gastroenteritis is typically 24 hours (with a range of 5 to

92 hours) and is 1 to 7 days for wound infections and septicemia.

DIAGNOSTIC TESTS: Depending on the clinical syndrome, *Vibrio* organisms can be isolated from stool, wound exudates, or blood. Because identification of the organism requires special techniques, laboratory personnel should be notified when infection with *Vibrio* species is suspected. Molecular diagnostics are useful if available.

TREATMENT: Diarrhea typically is mild and self-limited and requires only oral rehydration. Wound infections require surgical débridement of necrotic tissue, if present. Antimicrobial therapy is indicated for severe diarrhea, wound infection, and septicemia. Septicemia with or without hemorrhagic bullae and wound infections should be treated with a third-generation cephalosporin plus either doxycycline or ciprofloxacin. Severe diarrhea should be treated with doxycycline or ciprofloxacin. Doxycycline can be used for short durations (ie, 21 days or less) without regard to patient age (see Tetracyclines, p 905). A combination of trimethoprim-sulfamethoxazole and an aminoglycoside is an alternative regimen.

ISOLATION OF THE HOSPITALIZED PATIENT: In addition to standard precautions, contact precautions are recommended for diapered or incontinent children.

CONTROL MEASURES: Seafood should be cooked fully and refrigerated if not consumed immediately. Cross-contamination of cooked seafood by contact with surfaces and containers contaminated by raw seafood should be avoided. Uncooked mollusks and crustaceans should be handled with care, and gloves can be worn during preparation. Abrasions suffered by ocean bathers should be rinsed with clean fresh water. All children, immunocompromised people, and people with chronic liver disease should avoid eating raw oysters or clams, and all individuals should be advised of risks associated with seawater exposure if a wound is present or likely to occur. Vibriosis is a nationally notifiable disease, and cases should be reported to local or state health departments.

West Nile Virus

CLINICAL MANIFESTATIONS: An estimated 70% to 80% of people infected with West Nile virus (WNV) are asymptomatic. Most symptomatic people experience an acute systemic febrile illness that often includes headache, myalgia, arthralgia, vomiting, diarrhea, or a transient maculopapular rash. Less than 1% of infected people develop neuroinvasive disease, which typically manifests as meningitis, encephalitis, or acute flaccid myelitis. WNV meningitis is indistinguishable clinically from aseptic meningitis caused by other viruses. Patients with WNV encephalitis usually present with fever, headache, seizures, mental status changes, focal neurologic deficits, or movement disorders. WNV acute flaccid myelitis often is clinically and pathologically identical to poliovirus-associated poliomyelitis, with damage of anterior horn cells, and may progress to respiratory paralysis requiring mechanical ventilation. WNV-associated Guillain-Barré syndrome also has been reported and can be distinguished from WNV acute flaccid myelitis by clinical manifestations, findings on cerebrospinal fluid analysis, and electrophysiologic testing. Cardiac dysrhythmias, myocarditis, rhabdomyolysis, optic neuritis, uveitis, chorioretinitis, orchitis, pancreatitis, and hepatitis have been described rarely after WNV infection.

Routine clinical laboratory results generally are nonspecific in WNV infections. In patients with neuroinvasive disease, cerebrospinal fluid (CSF) examination generally shows lymphocytic pleocytosis, but neutrophils may predominate early in the illness. Brain magnetic resonance imaging frequently is normal, but signal abnormalities may be seen in the basal ganglia, thalamus, and brainstem with WNV encephalitis and in the spinal cord with WNV acute flaccid myelitis.

Most patients with WNV nonneuroinvasive disease or meningitis recover completely, but fatigue, malaise, and weakness can linger for weeks or months. Recovery from WNV encephalitis or acute flaccid myelitis often takes weeks to months, and patients commonly have residual neurologic deficits. Among patients with neuroinvasive disease, the overall case-fatality rate is approximately 10% but is significantly higher in WNV encephalitis and myelitis than in WNV meningitis.

Most women known to have been infected with WNV during pregnancy have delivered infants without evidence of infection or clinical abnormalities; only a few cases of WNV in newborn infants have been confirmed. In the best-documented case of confirmed congenital WNV infection, the mother developed WNV encephalitis during week 27 of gestation, and the infant was born with cystic lesions of cerebral tissue and chorioretinitis. In a case of likely early human milk-transmitted infection, a woman developed encephalitis following postpartum transfusion, and 3 weeks later her breastfed infant had documented infection, although the infant remained healthy. If WNV disease is diagnosed during pregnancy, a detailed examination of the fetus and of the newborn infant should be performed.[1]

ETIOLOGY: WNV is an RNA virus of the *Flaviviridae* family (genus *Flavivirus*) that is related antigenically to St. Louis encephalitis and Japanese encephalitis viruses.

EPIDEMIOLOGY: WNV is an arthropodborne virus (arbovirus) that is transmitted in an enzootic cycle between mosquitoes and amplifying vertebrate hosts, primarily birds. WNV is transmitted to humans primarily through bites of infected *Culex* mosquitoes. Humans usually do not develop a level or duration of viremia sufficient to infect mosquitoes, and therefore are dead-end hosts. However, person-to-person WNV transmission can occur through blood transfusion and solid organ transplantation. Intrauterine and probable breastfeeding transmission have been described rarely. Transmission through percutaneous and mucosal exposure has occurred in laboratory workers and occupational settings.

WNV transmission has been documented on every continent except Antarctica. Since the 1990s, the largest outbreaks of WNV neuroinvasive disease have occurred in the Middle East, Europe, and North America. WNV first was detected in the Western Hemisphere in New York City in 1999 and subsequently spread across the continental United States and Canada. From 1999 through 2015, a total of 20 265 cases of WNV neuroinvasive disease were reported in the United States. The national incidence of WNV neuroinvasive disease peaked in 2002 (2946 cases and 278 deaths; 1.02 cases per 100 000 persons per year) and 2003 (2866 cases and 232 deaths; 0.98 cases per 100 000), and again in 2012 (2873 cases, 270 deaths; 0.92 cases per 100 000). Although incidence has declined from 2012 to 2015, WNV remains the leading cause of neuroinvasive arboviral disease in the United States. In 2015, a total of 1455 WNV neuroinvasive disease cases were reported—more than 10 times the number of neuroinvasive disease cases reported for all other domestic arboviruses combined (eg, Eastern equine encephalitis, La Crosse, Powassan, and St. Louis encephalitis viruses). California (1.5 per 100 000), North Dakota (1.3 per

[1]Centers for Disease Control and Prevention. Interim guidelines for the evaluation of infants born to mothers infected with West Nile virus during pregnancy. *MMWR Morb Mortal Wkly Rep.* 2004;53(7):154–157. Available at: **www.cdc.gov/mmwr/preview/mmwrhtml/mm5307a4.htm**

100 000), South Dakota (1.3 per 100 000), Oklahoma (1.3 per 100 000), Colorado (1.0 per 100 000), and Nebraska (1.0 per 100 000) had the highest incidence of reported neuroinvasive disease in 2015. Alaska and Hawaii are the only states that have not reported local transmission of WNV. A map of the distribution of WNV neuroinvasive disease across the United States can be found on the Centers for Disease Control and Prevention (CDC) Web site (**www.cdc.gov/westnile/statsMaps**).

In temperate and subtropical regions, most human WNV infections occur in summer or early autumn. Although all age groups and both genders are susceptible to WNV infection, the incidence of severe disease (eg, encephalitis and death) is highest among older adults. In 2015, the incidence of neuroinvasive disease was 1.71 per 100 000 in adults 70 years or older compared with 0.03 per 100 000 in children younger than 10 years. Chronic renal failure, history of cancer, history of alcohol abuse, diabetes, and hypertension have been associated with developing severe WNV disease.

The **incubation period** usually is 2 to 6 days but ranges from 2 to 14 days and can be up to 21 days in immunocompromised people.

DIAGNOSTIC TESTS: Detection of anti-WNV immunoglobulin (Ig) M antibodies in serum or CSF is the most common way to diagnose WNV infection. The presence of anti-WNV IgM usually is good evidence of recent WNV infection but may indicate infection with another closely related *Flavivirus*. Because anti-WNV IgM can persist in the serum of some patients for longer than 1 year, a positive test result occasionally may reflect past infection. Detection of WNV IgM in CSF generally is indicative of recent neuroinvasive infection. WNV IgM antibodies are detectable in most WNV-infected patients within 3 to 8 days of symptom onset and remain detectible for 30 to 90 days, although in some people it may persist for longer than 1 year. For patients in whom serum collected within 8 days of illness lacks detectable IgM, testing should be repeated on a convalescent-phase sample. IgG antibody generally is detectable shortly after IgM and can persist for years. Plaque-reduction neutralization tests can be performed to measure virus-specific neutralizing antibodies and to discriminate between cross-reacting antibodies from closely related flaviviruses. A fourfold or greater increase in virus-specific neutralizing antibodies between acute- and convalescent-phase serum specimens collected 2 to 3 weeks apart may be used to confirm recent WNV infection.

Viral culture and WNV nucleic acid amplification tests (including reverse transcriptase-polymerase chain reaction) can be performed on acute-phase serum, CSF, or tissue specimens. However, by the time most immunocompetent patients present with clinical symptoms, WNV RNA usually no longer is detectable; therefore, polymerase chain reaction assay is not recommended for diagnosis in immunocompetent hosts. The sensitivity of these tests is likely higher in immunocompromised patients. Immunohistochemical staining can detect WNV antigens in fixed tissue, but negative results are not definitive.

WNV disease should be considered in the differential diagnosis of febrile or acute neurologic illnesses associated with recent exposure to mosquitoes, blood transfusion, or solid organ transplantation and of illnesses in neonates whose mothers were infected with WNV during pregnancy or while breastfeeding. In addition to other more common causes of aseptic meningitis and encephalitis (eg, herpes simplex virus and enteroviruses), WNV and other arboviruses should also be considered in the differential diagnosis (see Arboviruses, p 220). The CDC has developed a comprehensive Web site for assessing and managing patients with acute flaccid myelitis as part of its emerging infection surveillance efforts (eg, WNV, enterovirus D68) and in preparation for the final efforts to eradicate

polioviruses worldwide (**www.cdc.gov/acute-flaccid-myelitis/hcp/index.html**).
TREATMENT: No specific therapy is available; management of WNV disease is supportive. Although various therapies have been evaluated or used for WNV disease, none has
shown specific benefit thus far. A review summarizing potential treatments (including
Immune Globulin Intravenous with or without a high titer of WNV antibody, WNV recombinant humanized monoclonal antibody, interferon, corticosteroid, ribavirin) is available online at **www.cdc.gov/westnile/resources/pdfs/WNV-therapeutics-
summary.pdf.** Updated information about ongoing or completed clinical trials is available online (**http://clinicaltrials.gov/ct2/results?term=west+nile+virus&
Search=Search**).
ISOLATION OF THE HOSPITALIZED PATIENT: Standard precautions are recommended.
CONTROL MEASURES: Candidate WNV vaccines are being evaluated, but none are licensed for use in humans. In the absence of a vaccine, prevention of WNV disease depends on community-level mosquito control programs to reduce vector densities, on personal protective measures to decrease exposure to infected mosquitoes, and on screening
of blood and organ donors. Personal protective measures include use of mosquito repellents, wearing long-sleeved shirts and long pants, and limiting outdoor exposure from
dusk to dawn (see Prevention of Mosquitoborne and Tickborne Infections, p 195). Using
air conditioning, installing window and door screens, and reducing peridomestic mosquito breeding sites can further decrease the risk of WNV exposure. Blood donations in the
United States are screened for WNV infection, but physicians should remain vigilant for
the possible transmission of WNV through blood transfusion or organ transplantation.
Any suspected WNV infections temporally associated with blood transfusion or organ
transplantation should be reported promptly to the appropriate state health department.

Pregnant women should take the aforementioned precautions to avoid mosquito
bites. Products containing N,N-diethyl-meta-toluamide (DEET) can be used in pregnancy
without adverse effects. Pregnant women who develop meningitis, encephalitis, acute
flaccid myelitis, or unexplained fever in areas of ongoing WNV transmission should be
tested for WNV infection. Confirmed WNV infections should be reported to the local or
state health department, and women should be followed to determine the outcomes of
their pregnancies. Although WNV probably has been transmitted through human milk,
such transmission appears rare, and no adverse effects on infants have been described.
Because the benefits of breastfeeding outweigh the risk of WNV disease in breastfeeding
infants, mothers should be encouraged to breastfeed even in areas with ongoing WNV
transmission.

Yersinia enterocolitica and *Yersinia pseudotuberculosis* Infections
(Enteritis and Other Illnesses)

CLINICAL MANIFESTATIONS: *Yersinia enterocolitica* causes several age-specific syndromes
and a variety of other less commonly reported clinical illnesses. Infection with *Y enterocolitica* typically manifests as fever, diarrhea, and abdominal pain in children younger than 5
years; stool often contains leukocytes, blood, and mucus. Diarrhea commonly persists for
more than 2 weeks. Relapsing disease and, rarely, necrotizing enterocolitis also have been
described. In older children and adults, a pseudoappendicitis syndrome attributable to

mesenteric lymphadenitis (fever, abdominal pain, tenderness in the right lower quadrant of the abdomen, and leukocytosis) predominates. Bacteremia is the major complication of *Y enterocolitica*-associated enteric infection occurring mostly in children younger than 1 year and in older children with predisposing conditions, such as excessive iron storage (eg, deferoxamine use, sickle cell disease, and beta-thalassemia) and immunosuppressive states. Extraintestinal manifestations of *Y enterocolitica* are uncommon and include pharyngitis, meningitis, osteomyelitis, pyomyositis, conjunctivitis, pneumonia, empyema, endocarditis, acute peritonitis, abscesses of the liver and spleen, urinary tract infection, and primary cutaneous infection. Postinfectious sequelae with *Y enterocolitica* infection include erythema nodosum, reactive arthritis, and proliferative glomerulonephritis. These sequelae occur most often in older children and adults, particularly people with HLA-B27 antigen.

Major manifestations of *Yersinia pseudotuberculosis* infection include fever, scarlatiniform rash, acute gastroenteritis, and abdominal symptoms. Acute pseudoappendiceal abdominal pain is common, resulting from ileocecal mesenteric adenitis or terminal ileitis. Other uncommon findings reported have been intestinal intussusception, erythema nodosum, septicemia mainly among individuals with underlying conditions, acute renal failure with nephritis, and sterile pleural and joint effusions. Clinical features can mimic those of Kawasaki disease; in Hiroshima, Japan, nearly 10% of children with a diagnosis of Kawasaki disease have serologic or culture evidence of *Y pseudotuberculosis* infection.

ETIOLOGY: The genus *Yersinia* consists of 17 species of gram-negative bacilli belonging to the family *Enterobacteriaceae*. *Y enterocolitica*, *Y pseudotuberculosis*, and *Yersinia pestis* (see Plague, p 637) are the 3 most recognized human pathogens; however, other *Yersinia* species also have been isolated from clinical specimens. *Y enterocolitica* bioserotypes most often associated with human illness are 1B/O:8, 2/O:5,27, 2/O:9, 3/O:3, and 4/O:3, with bioserotype 4/O:3 now predominating as the most common type in the United States. The 3 *Yersinia* species have in common a tropism for lymphoid tissue and share factors that promote serum resistance, coordinate gene expression, and facilitate iron acquisition. Differences in virulence gene distribution exist among *Yersinia* species; for example, *Y enterocolitica* has a chromosomal gene encoding for an enterotoxin, and *Y pseudotuberculosis* produces a superantigen toxin among other factors. Virulence can be attributed to adhesion/invasion genes, enterotoxins, iron-scavenging genomic islands, and secretion systems. Highly pathogenic *Yersinia* are known to carry a 70 kb pYV virulence plasmid, which encodes a type III secretion system that is activated at human body temperatures and promotes entry into lymph tissues and subsequent evasion of host defense mechanisms.

EPIDEMIOLOGY: *Yersinia* infections are reported uncommonly in the United States, and infection is not nationally notifiable. *Y enterocolitica* and *Y pseudotuberculosis* are isolated most often during the cool months of temperate climates. The Foodborne Disease Active Surveillance Network (FoodNet) conducts active surveillance for infections caused by 9 pathogens, including *Yersinia*. According to data gathered by FoodNet, during 2012, 3.3 laboratory-confirmed infections per 1 million people were reported to surveillance sites. During FoodNet surveillance from 1996–2009, the average annual incidence of *Y enterocolitica* was 0.5 per 100 000 people and was highest in black people (0.9 per 100.000); there is a clear declining trend over the years from 3.9 to 0.4 per 100.000; 47% of infections were in children younger than 5 years; 28% were hospitalized, and 1% died. Most isolates were recovered from stool. In comparison, the average annual incidence in

Germany during 2001–2008 was 7.2 per 100 000 people. In contrast, the average annual incidence of *Y pseudotuberculosis* was 0.04 cases per 1 million people; the median age was 47 years, 72% were hospitalized, and 11% died. Two-thirds of *Y pseudotuberculosis* isolates were recovered from blood.

The principal reservoir of *Y enterocolitica* is swine, although it can be isolated from a variety of domestic and wildlife animals; *Y pseudotuberculosis* has been isolated from ungulates (deer, elk, goats, sheep, cattle), rodents (rats, squirrels, beaver), rabbits, and many bird species. Infection with *Y enterocolitica* is believed to be transmitted by ingestion of contaminated food (raw or incompletely cooked pork products, tofu, and unpasteurized or inadequately pasteurized milk[1]), by contaminated surface or well water, by direct or indirect contact with animals, and rarely by transfusion with contaminated packed red blood cells and by person-to-person transmission. Cross-contamination has been documented to lead to infection in infants if their caregivers handle raw pork intestines (ie, chitterlings) and do not cleanse their hands adequately before handling the infant or the infant's toys, bottles, or pacifiers. *Y pseudotuberculosis* can follow exposure to well and mountain waters contaminated with animal feces. Household pets can be source of infection for children. Infections in Finland have been associated with eating fresh produce, presumably contaminated by wild animals carrying the organism.

The **incubation period** typically is 4 to 6 days, with a range of 1 to 14 days. Organisms typically are excreted for 2 to 3 weeks and up to 2 to 3 months in untreated cases. Prolonged asymptomatic carriage is possible.

DIAGNOSTIC TESTS: *Y enterocolitica* and *Y pseudotuberculosis* can be recovered from stool, throat swab specimens, mesenteric lymph nodes, peritoneal fluid, and blood. *Y enterocolitica* also has been isolated from synovial fluid, bile, urine, cerebrospinal fluid, sputum, pleural fluid, and wounds. Stool cultures generally yield bacteria during the first 2 weeks of illness, regardless of the nature of gastrointestinal tract manifestations. *Yersinia* organisms are not sought routinely in stool specimens by most laboratories in the United States. Laboratory personnel should be notified when *Yersinia* infection is suspected so that stool can be cultured on suitable media (eg, CIN agar); however, strains of *Y enterocolitica* 3/O:3 and *Y pseudotuberculosis* may be inhibited on CIN agar, and MacConkey is preferred. DNA-based gastrointestinal syndrome panels that can reliably detect *Yersinia* are commercially available. Biotyping and serotyping for further identification of pathogenic strains is available through public health reference laboratories. Infection also can be confirmed by demonstrating increases in serum antibody titer after infection, but these tests generally are available only in reference or research laboratories. Cross-reactions of these antibodies with *Brucella, Vibrio, Salmonella*, and *Rickettsia* organisms and *Escherichia coli* can lead to false-positive *Y enterocolitica* and *Y pseudotuberculosis* titers. In patients with thyroid disease, persistently increased *Y enterocolitica* antibody titers can result from antigenic similarity of the organism with antigens of the thyroid epithelial cell membrane. Characteristic ultrasonographic features demonstrating edema of the wall of the terminal ileum and cecum with normal appendix help to distinguish pseudoappendicitis from appendicitis and can help avoid exploratory surgery. Several DNA-based methods have been developed for both *Y enterocolitica* and *Y pseudotuberculosis* for use in clinical, food, and environmental

---

[1]American Academy of Pediatrics, Committee on Infectious Diseases and Committee on Nutrition. Consumption of raw or unpasteurized milk and milk products by pregnant women and children. *Pediatrics.* 2014;133(1):175–179

samples. Results from nonsterile sites should be interpreted with caution.

TREATMENT: Neonates, immunocompromised hosts, and all patients with septicemia or extraintestinal disease require treatment for *Yersinia* infection. Parenteral therapy with a third-generation cephalosporin is appropriate, and evaluation of cerebrospinal fluid should be performed for infected neonates. Otherwise healthy nonneonates with enterocolitis can be treated symptomatically. Antimicrobial therapy decreases the duration of fecal excretion of *Y enterocolitica* and *Y pseudotuberculosis*. Although a clinical benefit of antimicrobial therapy for immunocompetent patients with enterocolitis, pseudoappendicitis syndrome, or mesenteric adenitis has not been established, treatment also is unlikely to cause any detrimental clinical effects and can be considered because of its favorable effect on shedding of the organism. In addition to third-generation cephalosporins, *Y enterocolitica* and *Y pseudotuberculosis* usually are susceptible to trimethoprim-sulfamethoxazole, aminoglycosides, fluoroquinolones, chloramphenicol, tetracycline, or doxycycline. *Y enterocolitica* isolates usually are resistant to first-generation cephalosporins and most penicillins.

ISOLATION OF THE HOSPITALIZED PATIENT: In addition to standard precautions, contact precautions are indicated for diapered or incontinent children for the duration of diarrheal illness.

CONTROL MEASURES: Ingestion of uncooked or undercooked meat, unpasteurized milk, or contaminated water should be avoided. People who handle raw meat products should minimize contact with young children and their possessions while handling raw products. Meticulous hand hygiene should be practiced before and after handling and preparation of uncooked products.

Zika

CLINICAL MANIFESTATIONS: Most Zika virus infections are asymptomatic. In situations in which infection is symptomatic, the clinical disease usually is mild and symptoms last for a few days to a week. Commonly reported signs and symptoms include fever, pruritic maculopapular rash, arthralgia, and conjunctival hyperemia. Other findings include myalgia, headache, edema of the extremities, vomiting, retroorbital pain, and lymphadenopathy. Clinical laboratory abnormalities are observed uncommonly in symptomatic patients but can include thrombocytopenia, leukopenia, and increased liver transaminase concentrations. Severe disease requiring hospitalization and deaths are rare. However, Guillain-Barré syndrome and rare reports of other neurologic complications (eg, meningoencephalitis, myelitis, and uveitis) have been associated with Zika virus infection.

Congenital Zika virus infection can cause fetal loss as well as microcephaly and other serious neurologic anomalies. Clinical findings reported in infants with confirmed congenital Zika virus infection include brain anomalies (eg, subcortical calcifications, ventriculomegaly, abnormal gyral patterns, corpus callosum agenesis, and cerebellar hypoplasia), ocular anomalies (eg, microphthalmia, cataracts, chorioretinal atrophy, and optic nerve hypoplasia), congenital contractures (eg, clubfoot and arthrogryposis), and neurologic sequelae (eg, hypertonia, hypotonia, irritability, tremors, swallowing dysfunction, hearing loss, and visual impairment).

At least 2 cases of perinatal transmission from mothers who were viremic at delivery have been reported. One infant was asymptomatic; the other infant developed mild thrombocytopenia and a transient diffuse rash 4 days after delivery.

ETIOLOGY: Zika virus is a single-stranded, RNA virus in the genus *Flavivirus* that is related antigenically to dengue, yellow fever, West Nile, St. Louis encephalitis, and Japanese encephalitis viruses. Two major lineages, African and Asian, have been identified through phylogenetic analyses.

EPIDEMIOLOGY: Zika virus is transmitted to humans primarily by *Aedes aegypti* mosquitoes and less commonly by other *Aedes* (*Stegomyia*) species (eg, *Aedes albopictus, Aedes polynesiensis,* and *Aedes hensilli).* In the United States, *Ae aegypti* mosquitoes are found primarily in southern states. *Ae albopictus* mosquitoes have a wider distribution, including not only the southern United States but also extending north into the Ohio Valley and west to a number of the plains states. *Ae aegypti* and *Ae albopictus* mosquitoes can be found in small areas of the southwest and parts of California. Both *Aedes* species of mosquitoes bite humans during the daytime. These are the same vectors that transmit dengue, chikungunya, and yellow fever viruses. Human and nonhuman primates are the main reservoirs of the virus, with humans acting as the primary host in which the virus multiplies, allowing spread to additional mosquitoes and then other humans. Additional modes of transmission have been identified, including perinatal, in utero, sexual, blood transfusion, and laboratory exposure. Although Zika virus has been detected in human milk, transmission through breastfeeding has not yet been demonstrated.

Zika virus first was identified in the Zika forest of Uganda in 1947. Prior to 2007, only sporadic human disease cases were reported from countries in Africa and Asia. In 2007, the first documented Zika virus disease outbreak was reported in the Federated States of Micronesia. In subsequent years, outbreaks of Zika virus disease were identified in countries in Southeast Asia and the Western Pacific. In 2015, Zika virus was identified for the first time in the Western hemisphere, with large outbreaks reported in Brazil. Since then, the virus has spread throughout much of the Americas, with 48 countries and territories in the Americas reporting local transmission. During 2016 in the United States, large outbreaks occurred in Puerto Rico and the US Virgin Islands, and limited local transmission was identified in parts of Florida and Texas. Current information on Zika virus transmission and travel guidance can be found at **www.cdc.gov/zika/geo/index. html** and **wwwnc.cdc.gov/travel/page/zika-travel-information,** respectively.

The **incubation period** is 3 to 14 days after the bite of an infected mosquito, with 50% of cases developing symptoms 1 week after exposure.

DIAGNOSTIC TESTS: Zika virus infection should be considered in patients with acute onset of fever, maculopapular rash, arthralgia, or conjunctivitis who live in or have traveled to an area with ongoing transmission in the 2 weeks preceding illness onset. Because dengue and chikungunya virus infections share a similar geographic distribution and symptomology with Zika virus infection, patients with suspected Zika virus infection also should be evaluated and managed for possible dengue or chikungunya virus infection. Other considerations in the differential diagnosis include malaria, rubella, measles, parvovirus, adenovirus, enterovirus, leptospirosis, rickettsiosis, and group A streptococcal infections.

Laboratory testing for Zika virus has a number of limitations. Zika virus RNA is only transiently present in body fluids; thus, a negative real-time reverse transcriptase-polymerase chain reaction (RT-PCR) result does not rule out infection. Likewise, a negative immunoglobulin (Ig) M serologic test result does not rule out infection because the serum specimen might have been collected before the development or after waning of IgM antibodies. Alternatively, IgM antibodies might be detectable for months after the initial infection, making it difficult to distinguish the timing of Zika acquisition. Cross-reactivity of the Zika virus IgM antibody tests with other flaviviruses can result in a false-positive test result. Recent epidemiologic data indicate a declining prevalence of Zika virus infection in the Americas; this lower prevalence will result in a lower pretest probability of infection and a higher probability of false-positive test results.

Zika Laboratory Testing in Nonpregnant Symptomatic Individuals. For people with suspected Zika virus disease, Zika virus RT-PCR assay should be performed on serum and urine specimens collected <14 days after onset of symptoms. Serum immunoglobulin (Ig) M antibody testing should be performed if the RT-PCR result is negative or when ≥14 days have passed since illness onset.

Zika Laboratory Testing in Pregnant Women. Current recommendations from the Centers for Disease Control and Prevention (CDC) take into account the decreasing prevalence of Zika virus disease cases in the Americas that occurred in 2017.[1] Zika virus testing is not routinely recommended for asymptomatic pregnant women who have possible recent but not ongoing Zika virus exposure. Zika virus RT-PCR testing should be offered as part of routine obstetric care to asymptomatic pregnant women with ongoing possible Zika virus exposure; however, because of the potential for persistence of IgM antibodies over several months, serologic testing is no longer routinely recommended to screen asymptomatic women.

Zika Laboratory Testing for Congenital Infection. Zika virus testing is recommended for infants with clinical findings consistent with congenital Zika syndrome and possible maternal Zika virus exposure during pregnancy, regardless of maternal testing results, and for infants without clinical findings consistent with congenital Zika syndrome who are born to women with laboratory evidence of possible infection during pregnancy. Recommended laboratory testing for possible congenital Zika virus infection includes evaluation for Zika virus RNA in infant serum and urine and Zika virus IgM antibodies in serum. In addition, if cerebrospinal fluid (CSF) is obtained for other purposes, RT-PCR and IgM antibody testing should be performed on CSF, because CSF was the only sample that tested positive in a limited number of infants with congenital Zika virus infection.

Laboratory testing of infants should be performed as soon as possible after birth (within the first few days of life), although testing specimens within the first few weeks to months after birth might still be useful. If CSF was not collected for other reasons, testing CSF for Zika virus RNA and Zika virus IgM should be considered to improve the likelihood of diagnosis, especially if serum and urine testing are negative and another etiology has not been identified. Diagnosis of congenital Zika virus infection is confirmed by a positive Zika virus RT-PCR, or by a positive Zika virus IgM and neutralizing antibody result. If neither Zika virus RNA nor Zika IgM antibodies are detected on the appropriate specimens obtained within the first few days after birth, congenital Zika virus infection is unlikely.

The plaque reduction neutralization test (PRNT), which measures virus-specific neutralizing antibodies, can be used to help identify false-positive results. If the infant's initial sample is IgM nonnegative (non-negative serology terminology varies by assay and might include "positive," "equivocal," "presumptive positive," or "possible positive") and

[1]Oduyebo T, Polen KD, Walke HT, et al. Update: Interim guidance for health care providers caring for pregnant women with possible zika virus exposure—United States (including U.S. territories), July 2017. *MMWR Morb Mortal Wkly Rep*. 2017;66(29):781–793

RT-PCR negative, and PRNT was not performed on the mother's sample, PRNT for Zika and dengue viruses should be performed on the infant's initial sample. If the Zika virus PRNT result is negative, this suggests that the infant's Zika virus IgM test result is a false positive. For infants with clinical findings consistent with congenital Zika syndrome or maternal evidence of possible Zika virus infection during pregnancy who were not tested near birth, PRNT at age ≥18 months (after maternal antibodies have dissipated from the infant's system) might help confirm or rule out congenital Zika virus infection. If the PRNT result is negative at age ≥18 months, congenital Zika virus infection is unlikely.

TREATMENT: No specific antiviral treatment currently is available for Zika virus disease. Only supportive care is indicated, including rest, fluids, and symptomatic treatment (acetaminophen to relieve fever and antihistamines to treat pruritus). Aspirin and nonsteroidal anti-inflammatory drugs (NSAIDs) should be avoided until dengue can be ruled out to reduce the risk of hemorrhagic complications.

Guidance is updated as new information is obtained; for the most recent guidance, visit: **www.cdc.gov/Zika.** Fig 3.13 (p 900) outlines the current recommended evaluation of infants with possible maternal and congenital Zika virus exposure during pregnancy.[1]

Clinical Management of Infants With Clinical Findings Consistent With Congenital Zika Infection. Zika virus testing is recommended (see Zika Laboratory Testing for Congenital Infection, p 896), ultrasonography of the head should be performed, and a comprehensive ophthalmologic examination should be performed by age 1 month by an ophthalmologist experienced in assessment of infants. Referrals to a developmental specialist and early intervention are recommended. Additional consultation should be considered by infectious disease (for evaluation of other congenital infections and assistance with Zika virus diagnosis and testing), clinical genetics (for evaluation for other causes of microcephaly or congenital anomalies), and neurology by age 1 month (for comprehensive neurologic examination and consideration for other evaluations, such as advanced neuroimaging and electroencephalography [EEG]). The initial clinical evaluation, including subspecialty consultations, can be performed before hospital discharge or as an outpatient. Ophthalmologic follow-up after the initial examination should be based on ophthalmology recommendations. Infants should be referred for automated brainstem response (ABR) testing by age 1 month if the newborn hearing screen was passed using only otoacoustic emissions (OAE) methodology.

Clinical Management of Infants Without Clinical Findings Consistent With Congenital Zika Infection but Maternal Laboratory Evidence of Possible Zika Virus Infection During Pregnancy. Zika virus testing is recommended (see Zika Laboratory Testing for Congenital Infection, p 896), and ultrasonography of the head should be performed by age 1 month to detect subclinical brain findings. All infants should have a comprehensive ophthalmologic examination by age 1 month to detect subclinical eye findings; further follow-up visits with an ophthalmologist after the initial examination should be based on ophthalmology recommendations. Infants should be referred for automated ABR testing by 1 month of age if newborn screen was passed using only OAE methodology. Infants should be monitored for findings consistent with congenital Zika syndrome that could develop over time

[1]Adebanjo T, Godfred-Cato S, Viens L, et al. Update: interim guidance for the diagnosis, evaluation, and management of infants with possible congenital Zika virus infection—United States, October 2017. *MMWR Morb Mortal Wkly Rep.* 2017;66(41):1089–1099

Fig 3.13. Recommendations for the Evaluation of Infants with Possible Congenital Zika Virus Infection Based on Infant Clinical Findings,[a,b] Maternal Testing Results,[c,d] and Infant Testing Results[e,f]—United States, October 2017[1]

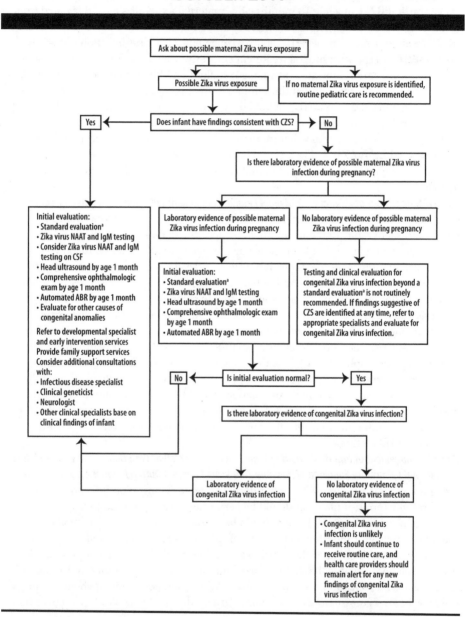

[1]Adebanjo T, Godfred-Cato S, Viens L, et al. Update: interim guidance for the diagnosis, evaluation, and management of infants with possible congenital Zika virus infection—United States, October 2017. *MMWR Morb Mortal Wkly Rep.* 2017;66(41):1089–1099

CZS indicates congenital Zika syndrome; NAAT, nucleic acid amplification test; IgM, immunoglobulin M; CSF, cerebrospinal fluid; ABR, auditory brainstem response; PRNT, plaque reduction neutralization test.

[a] All infants should receive a standard evaluation at birth and at each subsequent well-child visit by their health care providers, including (1) comprehensive physical examination, including growth parameters; and 2) age-appropriate vision screening and developmental monitoring and screening using validated tools. Infants should receive a standard newborn hearing screen at birth, preferably using auditory brainstem response.

[b] Automated ABR by age 1 month if newborn hearing screen passed but performed with otoacoustic emission methodology.

[c] Laboratory evidence of possible Zika virus infection during pregnancy is defined as (1) Zika virus infection detected by a Zika virus RNA NAAT on any maternal, placental, or fetal specimen (referred to as NAAT-confirmed), or (2) diagnosis of Zika virus infection, timing of infection cannot be determined or unspecified *Flavivirus* infection, timing of infection cannot be determined by serologic tests on a maternal specimen (ie, positive/equivocal Zika virus IgM and Zika virus PRNT titer ≥10, regardless of dengue virus PRNT value; or negative Zika virus IgM, and positive or equivocal dengue virus IgM, and Zika virus PRNT titer ≥10, regardless of dengue virus PRNT titer). The use of PRNT for confirmation of Zika virus infection, including in pregnant women, is not routinely recommended in Puerto Rico (**www.cdc.gov/zika/laboratories/lab-guidance.html**).

[d] This group includes women who were never tested during pregnancy as well as those whose test result was negative because of issues related to timing or sensitivity and specificity of the test. Because the latter issues are not easily discerned, all mothers with possible exposure to Zika virus during pregnancy who do not have laboratory evidence of possible Zika virus infection, including those who tested negative with currently available technology, should be considered in this group.

[e] Laboratory testing of infants for Zika virus should be performed as early as possible, preferably within the first few days after birth, and includes concurrent Zika virus NAAT in infant serum and urine, and Zika virus IgM testing in serum. If CSF is obtained for other purposes, Zika virus NAAT and Zika virus IgM testing should be performed on CSF.

[f] Laboratory evidence of congenital Zika virus infection includes a positive Zika virus NAAT or a nonnegative Zika virus IgM with confirmatory neutralizing antibody testing, if PRNT confirmation is performed.

(eg, impaired visual acuity/function, hearing problems, developmental delay, delay in head growth).

Clinical Management of Infants Without Clinical Findings Consistent With Congenital Zika Infection Born to Mothers With Possible Zika Virus Infection During Pregnancy but Without Laboratory Evidence of Zika Virus During Pregnancy. Zika virus testing is not routinely recommended, and specialized clinical evaluation or follow-up is not routinely indicated. Health care providers can consider additional evaluation in consultation with families. If findings suggestive of congenital Zika syndrome are identified at any time, referrals to the appropriate specialists should be made.

ISOLATION OF THE HOSPITALIZED PATIENT: Standard precautions are recommended, with attention to the potential for bloodborne transmission. People infected with Zika virus, as well as other arboviruses, should be protected from further mosquito exposure, especially during the first week of illness, to reduce the risk of local transmission to others.

CONTROL MEASURES: Vaccines to prevent Zika virus infection currently are not available. Prevention and control measures rely on personal prevention measures to avoid mosquito bites, and community-level programs to reduce vector densities in areas with endemic infection. Personal measures include using insect repellent; wearing long pants, socks, and long-sleeved shirts while outdoors; staying in air-conditioned buildings or buildings with window and door screens; and limiting outdoor activities during peak vector feeding times. Permethrin-treated clothing and gear can repel mosquitoes. Bed nets are advised for travel to areas where accommodations are not adequately screened or air conditioned. Travelers returning to the United States from an area with risk of Zika, even if asymptomatic, should take steps to prevent mosquito bites for 3 weeks to minimize spread to local mosquito populations (**www.cdc.gov/zika/prevention/plan-for-travel.html**).

Insect repellents registered by the US Environmental Protection Agency (EPA) can be used according to directions on the product labels. Products containing N,N-diethyl-meta-toluamide (DEET), picaridin, oil of lemon eucalyptus, or IR3535 provide protection

from mosquito bites. Products containing up to 50% DEET for adults (including pregnant and lactating women) and up to 30% DEET for infants and children are recommended. Insect repellents containing oil of lemon eucalyptus (para-menthane-3,8-diol)
should not be used in children younger than 3 years. All travelers should take precautions
to avoid mosquito bites to prevent Zika virus infection and other mosquitoborne diseases
(see Prevention of Mosquitoborne and Tickborne Infections, p 195).

Sexual Transmission. Zika virus can be transmitted sexually. Couples in whom the man
or woman has had possible Zika virus exposure who want to maximally reduce their risk
for sexually transmitting Zika virus to the uninfected partner should use condoms or abstain from sex for at least 6 months for men or 8 weeks for women after symptom onset (if
symptomatic) or last possible Zika virus exposure (if asymptomatic). Men should not donate sperm for at least 6 months from infection or last exposure.

Women Who Are Pregnant or Seeking to Become Pregnant. Pregnant women should postpone travel to any area where local Zika virus transmission is ongoing. Pregnant women
who do travel to one of these areas should talk to their health care provider before traveling and should strictly follow steps to avoid mosquito bites during travel. There is no restriction on the use of insect repellents by pregnant women if used in accordance with the
instructions on the product label. Male partners of pregnant women who have traveled to
areas with local transmission of Zika virus should abstain from sex or use condoms for the
duration of the pregnancy to avoid sexual transmission to their pregnant partners.

For couples who have possible Zika virus exposure and who are considering pregnancy, the CDC recommends postponing pregnancy for 6 months following potential exposure or diagnosis of Zika infection. These recommendations for couples considering pregnancy are likely to change as more data become available concerning the duration of
viremia and persistence of virus in semen for symptomatic and asymptomatic people.

Pregnant women who develop a clinically compatible illness during or within 2 weeks
of returning from an area with Zika virus transmission should be tested for Zika virus
infection. Fetuses and infants of women with possible Zika virus exposure or known Zika
virus infection during pregnancy should be evaluated for possible congenital infection (Fig
3.13).

Blood and Tissue Donation. The US Food and Drug Administration (FDA) recommends
temporary deferral of blood donors who recently were infected with Zika virus infection,
as well as testing of all blood donations collected in the United States and its territories to
reduce the risk for transfusion-associated transmission of Zika virus. Because of universal
Zika virus testing of blood donors, people who traveled to areas with local Zika virus
transmission and who did not exhibit any evidence of infection may donate blood.

The CDC also has developed guidance to reduce potential Zika virus transmission
from human cells, tissues, and cellular and tissue-based products (HCT/Ps). The guidance addresses donation of HCT/Ps from both living and deceased donors, including
donors of umbilical cord blood, placenta tissue, or other gestational tissues. The guidance
recognizes the potential risk of transmission of Zika virus from HCT/Ps. Living donors
should be considered ineligible to donate HCT/Ps if they had a diagnosis of Zika virus
infection, were in an area with Zika virus transmission, or had sex with a male with either
of these risk factors, within the past 6 months. Donors of umbilical cord blood, placenta
tissue, or other gestational tissues should be considered ineligible if any of the aforementioned risk factors occurred at any point during pregnancy. This guidance likely will
change as more evidence becomes available about persistence of Zika virus in human

tissues and fluids.

REPORTING: Health care professionals should report suspected Zika virus infection to their state or local health departments to facilitate diagnosis and mitigate the risk of local transmission. Zika virus disease and congenital infections were added to the list of nationally notifiable diseases in 2016 (see Appendix IV: Nationally Notifiable Infectious Diseases in the United States, p 1069). State health departments should then report cases to the CDC through ArboNET, the national surveillance system for arboviral diseases.

Antimicrobial Agents and Related Therapy

INTRODUCTION

The product label (package insert) approved by the US Food and Drug Administration (FDA) for a given antimicrobial drug provides information on indications (the clinical infections that require antimicrobial treatment, such as "complicated urinary tract infection") based on clinical trial data reviewed by the FDA. Virtually all current antimicrobial product labels are available at **http://dailymed.nlm.nih.gov/dailymed/about. cfm.** The FDA also maintains a general Web site (**www.accessdata.fda.gov/ scripts/cder/ob/default.cfm**) of approved drug products with therapeutic equivalence evaluations that can be searched by active ingredient or proprietary names.

An FDA-approved indication usually means that statistically adequate and well-controlled studies were conducted (usually by the drug's manufacturer), presented to, and reviewed by the FDA and, if appropriate, approved for use in the populations in which the drug was investigated. However, accepted medical practice (ie, when to use which antimicrobial agent for a specific infection or "indication") often includes use of drugs that are not reflected in approved indications found in the drug label. These additional uses of antimicrobial agents usually are based on studies that may or may not have been supported by the drug's original manufacturer, particularly for generic drugs. These studies are not always presented formally to the FDA by the clinical investigators or the sponsor for review because of the substantial cost of conducting the clinical trials, collecting and analyzing the data, and presenting the data to the FDA for approval for that specific indication. Lack of FDA approval for an indication, therefore, does not necessarily mean lack of effectiveness, but may signify either that FDA-required studies have not been performed or that they have not been submitted to the FDA for approval for that specific indication. Therefore, unapproved use does not imply improper use, provided that reasonable supporting medical evidence exists and that use of the drug is deemed to be in the best interest of the patient. Conversely, many vaccines or drugs are not recommended for use by the American Academy of Pediatrics (AAP) or Centers for Disease Control and Prevention (CDC), despite licensed indications noted in the package label. The decision to prescribe a drug is the responsibility of the medical provider, who must weigh the risks and benefits of using the drug for a specific situation.

Manufacturing of drugs is the responsibility of the pharmaceutical industry, which is regulated by the FDA. On occasion, drug shortages can occur. The pharmaceutical company may share information about the shortage with the FDA (**www.fda.gov/cder/ drug/shortages/default.htm**). Alternative, nonstandard therapy may be required when drug shortages occur.

Some antimicrobial agents with proven therapeutic benefit in adults are not approved by the FDA for use in pediatric patients or, more rarely, are considered contraindicated in children because of possible toxicity. The following information delineates general principles for use of fluoroquinolones, tetracyclines, and other agents that are approved for adults with serious bacterial infections.

Fluoroquinolones

Fluoroquinolones (eg, ciprofloxacin, levofloxacin, gemifloxacin, moxifloxacin) should not be used routinely as first-line agents in children younger than 18 years except when specific indications exist or in specific conditions for which there are no alternative agents (including oral agents) and the drug is known to be effective for the specific situation. Current information on the safety of fluoroquinolones for children was reviewed and published by the AAP.[1]

Although generally well tolerated, transient arthralgia has been reported in patients treated with fluoroquinolones; however, these reported symptoms have not been confirmed by clinical examination. Arthralgia also has been noted in some children in the control groups in these studies, making it difficult to assess the fluoroquinolone-attributable contribution to this adverse effect. For some fluoroquinolones, cartilage damage in animal models occurs at doses that approximate therapeutic doses in humans. The mechanism of damage remains speculative. In some pediatric studies, an increased incidence of reversible adverse events involving joints or surrounding tissues has been observed with fluoroquinolones compared with other agents. Long-term safety data have been reported for both levofloxacin and moxifloxacin. To date, there is no compelling evidence of long-term sequelae related to fluoroquinolone bone or joint toxicity in children.

There is a risk of *Clostridium difficile* disease in patients treated with fluoroquinolone-class antibiotic agents. Certain fluoroquinolones (moxifloxacin, levofloxacin, ciprofloxacin) have been shown to potentially prolong the QT interval and should be avoided in patients with long QT syndrome, those with hypokalemia or hypomagnesemia, those with organic heart disease including congestive heart failure, those receiving an antiarrhythmic agent from class Ia (particularly quinidine), and those who are receiving a concurrent drug that prolongs the QTc interval independently.

Two black box warnings have been issued by the FDA related to fluoroquinolones. First, fluoroquinolones are associated in adults with an increased risk of tendon rupture (with a predilection for the Achilles tendon) and tendonitis, with further increased risk in people older than 60 years; in those who have received renal, heart, or lung transplants; and with concurrent use of corticosteroids. To date there have been no reports of Achilles tendon rupture in children in association with quinolone use. Additionally, a black box warning states that fluoroquinolones may worsen muscle weakness in people with myasthenia gravis. Neurologic complications associated with fluoroquinolone use include peripheral neuropathy, dizziness, and headaches. In 2016, the FDA released a Drug Safety Communication for the fluoroquinolone class, advising that health care providers should not prescribe systemic fluoroquinolones to patients who have other treatment options for acute bacterial sinusitis, acute bacterial exacerbation of chronic bronchitis, and uncom-

---

[1]Jackson MA, Schutze GE, American Academy of Pediatrics Committee on Infectious Diseases. The use of systemic and topical fluoroquinolones. *Pediatrics*. 2016;138(5):e20162706

plicated urinary tract infections, because the risks outweigh the benefits in these patients.[1]

Although ciprofloxacin is approved for complicated urinary tract infection or pyelonephritis in children, other agents should be used preferentially if the pathogens are susceptible. The other approved indications in children are for postexposure prophylaxis for inhalation anthrax (ciprofloxacin primarily, with levofloxacin and moxifloxacin considered equivalent alternatives) and treatment of plague (levofloxacin, which achieves higher cerebrospinal fluid concentrations). Circumstances in which use of systemic fluoroquinolones may be justified in children include the following: (1) parenteral therapy is not practical and no other safe and effective oral agent is available; and (2) infection is caused by a multidrug-resistant pathogen, such as certain *Pseudomonas* or *Mycobacterium* strains, for which there is no other effective intravenous or oral agent available.

Potential uses of fluoroquinolones for pediatric patients include the following:

- Urinary tract infections caused by *Pseudomonas aeruginosa* or other multidrug-resistant, gram-negative bacteria;
- Multidrug-resistant (beta-lactam, macrolide, and trimethoprim-sulfamethoxazole) pneumococcal infections;
- Chronic suppurative otitis media or malignant otitis externa caused by *P aeruginosa*;
- Chronic or acute osteomyelitis or osteochondritis caused by *P aeruginosa*, or other multidrug-resistant, gram-negative bacterial infection caused by isolates known to be susceptible to fluoroquinolones but resistant to standard, nonfluoroquinolone agents;
- Gram-negative bacterial infections in immunocompromised hosts in which oral therapy is desired or antibacterial resistance to alternative agents is present;
- Gastrointestinal tract infection caused by suspected or documented multidrug-resistant *Shigella* species, *Salmonella* species, *Vibrio cholerae*, *Campylobacter jejuni*, or *Campylobacter coli*.
- Serious infections attributable to fluoroquinolone-susceptible pathogen(s) in children with severe allergy to alternative agents.
- Topical fluoroquinolone-containing agents are preferred as safer alternatives to aminoglycoside-containing agents for treatment of otorrhea associated with tympanic membrane perforation, and tympanostomy tube otorrhea.

Inappropriate use of fluoroquinolones in children and adults is likely to be associated with increasing resistance to these agents.

Tetracyclines

Use of tetracyclines in pediatric patients historically has been limited because of reports that this class of antimicrobial drugs could cause permanent dental discoloration in children younger than 8 years. Studies have documented that tetracyclines and their colored degradation products are incorporated in enamel. The period of odontogenesis to completion of formation of enamel in permanent teeth appears to be the critical time for effects of these drugs and virtually ends by 8 years of age, at which time the drug can be given without concern for dental staining. The degree of staining appears to depend on dosage, duration of therapy, and which drug in the tetracycline class is used.

Doxycycline binds less readily to calcium compared with other members of the

---

[1]US Food and Drug Administration. FDA Drug Safety Communication: FDA advises restricting fluoroquinolone antibiotic use for certain uncomplicated infections; warns about disabling side effects that can occur together. Available at: **www.fda.gov/Drugs/DrugSafety/ucm500143.htm**

tetracycline class, but because of concern for a drug class effect with tetracyclines, its use previously has been limited largely to patients 8 years and older, and these older children have been studied more thoroughly than younger children. Recent comparative data in younger children, however, suggest that doxycycline is not likely to cause visible teeth staining or enamel hypoplasia in children younger than 8 years. These reassuring data support the revised recommendation by the American Academy of Pediatrics, reflected throughout the 2018 *Red Book*, that doxycycline can be administered for short durations (ie, 21 days or less) without regard to the patient's age. When used, patients should be careful to avoid excess sun exposure due to the photosensitivity associated with doxycycline.

Other Agents

Other antimicrobial agents in a variety of classes have been studied and approved by the FDA for use in adults for certain indications but still are under investigation for pharmacokinetics, safety, and efficacy in children. These agents include but are not limited to daptomycin, dalbavancin, oritavancin, telavancin, tedizolid, ceftolozane/tazobactam, and tigecycline. These drugs should be used in children only when no other safe and effective agents that are FDA approved for use in children are available and when benefits are expected to exceed risks for that patient. For these agents with relatively undefined safety and efficacy in pediatrics, consultation with an expert in pediatric infectious diseases should be considered.

....

ANTIMICROBIAL RESISTANCE AND ANTIMICROBIAL STEWARDSHIP: APPROPRIATE AND JUDICIOUS USE OF ANTIMICROBIAL AGENTS[1]

Antimicrobial Resistance

The Centers for Disease Control and Prevention (CDC), World Health Organization (WHO), and other international agencies have identified antimicrobial resistance as one of the world's most pressing public health threats. In the United States, it is estimated that more than 2 million people are infected with antimicrobial-resistant bacteria, and at least 23 000 people die each year as a direct result of these infections. Highly resistant gram-negative pathogens (*Pseudomonas aeruginosa, Acinetobacter* species, extended-spectrum beta-lactamase–producing *Escherichia coli,* carbapenemase-producing *Klebsiella pneumoniae,* and *Burkholderia cepacia)* and gram-positive pathogens (methicillin-resistant *Staphylococcus aureus,* and *Enterococcus* species resistant to ampicillin and vancomycin) increasingly are associated with invasive infections.

---

[1]Barlam TF, Cosgrove SE, Abbo LM, et al. Implementing an antibiotic stewardship program: guidelines from the Infectious Diseases Society of America and the Society for Healthcare Epidemiology of America. *Clin Infect Dis.* 2016;62(10):e51–e77

The presence of resistant pathogens complicates patient management, increases morbidity and mortality, and increases medical expenses for patients and the health care system. Studies have estimated that antimicrobial resistance in the United States adds as much as $20 billion in excess costs to the health care system each year, and costs to society as a result of lost productivity are as high as $35 billion.

Factors Contributing to Resistance

The use of antimicrobial agents is the single most important factor leading to the development of resistance. Antimicrobial agents are among the most commonly prescribed drugs used in human medicine. However, at least 30% of all US outpatient antibiotic prescriptions are unnecessary,[1] and 30% to 50% of antibiotic agents used in US hospitals are unnecessary or inappropriate in selection, dose, or duration (**www.cdc.gov/ getsmart/healthcare/implementation/core-elements.html**).

The number of antibiotic-resistant bacteria and the diversity of molecular mechanisms of resistance have increased sharply in recent years, but the development of newer, effective antimicrobial agents has not kept pace. The loss of effective antimicrobial agents will hamper clinicians' efforts to treat potentially life-threatening infections. At the same time, many advances in medical treatment involve immunosuppression; subsequently, patients' ability to control infections depends even more on the receipt of effective antimicrobial agents. When first-line and second-line treatment options are limited by resistance or are unavailable, health care providers are forced to use antimicrobial agents that may be more toxic, more expensive, and/or less effective.

The overuse of antimicrobial agents in animal agriculture also contributes substantially to the problem of antimicrobial resistance. The vast majority of antimicrobial use in animals is not to treat infections; rather, animals are fed antibiotic agents to speed growth and to compensate for unsanitary and crowded conditions. The CDC has determined that antimicrobial use in animals is linked to resistance in humans. The US Food and Drug Administration recently described a pathway toward reducing inappropriate antimicrobial use in animals, and many major medical and public health organizations, including the American Academy of Pediatrics (AAP), have called for stronger action.

Antimicrobial Resistance Threats

The CDC released a landmark report, "Antibiotic Resistance Threats in the United States, 2013" (**www.cdc.gov/drugresistance/threat-report-2013/**), that describes the burden and threats posed by antimicrobial resistance and outlines immediate actions that must be taken to address the problem. The CDC report ranked the antimicrobial-resistant bacteria (and fungi) that have the most impact on human health in categories of urgent, serious, and concerning threats (Table 4.1). The threats were assessed according to 7 factors associated with resistant infections: health impact, economic impact, incidence of the infection, 10-year projection of incidence, ease of transmission, availability of effective antimicrobial agents, and barriers to prevention.

---

[1]Fleming-Dutra KE, Hersh AL, Shapiro DJ, et al. Prevalence of inappropriate antibiotic prescriptions among US ambulatory care visits, 2010-2011. *JAMA*. 2016;315(17):1864–1873

Table 4.1. Antibiotic-Resistant Bacteria Posing Health Threats

Urgent Threats	Serious Threats	Concerning Threats
Carbapenem-resistant *Enterobacteriaceae*	Methicillin-resistant *Staphylococcus aureus*	Vancomycin-resistant *Staphylococcus aureus*
Antibiotic-resistant *Neisseria gonorrhoeae*	Drug-resistant tuberculosis	Erythromycin-resistant group A streptococci
	Drug-resistant *Streptococcus pneumoniae*	Clindamycin-resistant group B streptococci
	Extended-spectrum betalactamase-producing *Enterobacteriaceae*	
	Multidrug-resistant *Acinetobacter* species	
	Drug-resistant *Campylobacter* species	
	Fluconazole-resistant *Candida* species (a fungus)	
	Vancomycin-resistant *Enterococcus* species	
	Multidrug-resistant *Pseudomonas aeruginosa*	
	Drug-resistant nontyphoidal *Salmonella*	
	Drug-resistant *Salmonella* Typhi	
	Drug-resistant *Shigella*	

Adapted from Zaoutis T. CDC highlights threats posed by antibiotic resistance, calls for action. *AAP News.* 2013;34(11):11. See the CDC Web site for further details (**www.cdc.gov/drugresistance/threat-report-2013/**).

Actions to Prevent or Slow Antimicrobial Resistance

Antimicrobial resistance can be addressed only through concerted and collaborative efforts. To combat the threat posed by antimicrobial resistance, the CDC has identified 4 core actions that must be taken[1]:

1. **Prevent infections and prevent the spread of resistance.** Antimicrobial-resistant infections can be prevented by immunization, infection prevention in health care settings, safe food preparation and handling, and handwashing.

2. **Track antimicrobial resistant infections.** The CDC gathers data on antimicrobial-resistant infections to help inform strategies and interventions for prevention.

3. **Improve antimicrobial use and promote antimicrobial stewardship.** The most important action is to modify the way antimicrobial agents are used in humans and animals. Unnecessary and inappropriate use of antimicrobial agents is common in outpatients and hospitalized patients. Inappropriate use of antimicrobial agents often is a result of errors in antimicrobial selection, dosing, or duration of therapy. Unnecessary exposure to antimicrobial agents results in adverse drug reactions, complications including *C difficile* infections, and subsequent treatment challenges related to the development of antimicrobial resistance. *Clostridium difficile* infection, the most common cause of diarrhea acquired in a health care facility and an infection that usually results from antimicrobial exposure, causes approximately 250 000 hospitalizations and at least 15 000 deaths annually.[2] Although *C difficile* infection often is considered to affect

[1]Sanchez GV, Fleming-Dutra KE, Roberts RM, Hicks LA. Core elements of outpatient antibiotic stewardship. *MMWR Recomm Rep.* 2016;11:65(6):1–12

[2]Lessa FC, Mu Y, Bamberg WM, et al. Burden of *Clostridium difficile* infection in the United States. *N Engl J Med.* 2015;372(9):825–834

predominately adults, recent evidence suggests an increase in infection rates and mortality in children. Every hospital should have a formal antimicrobial stewardship program built on validated core elements (see next section). The standard practice of outpatient antimicrobial stewardship also is important to combat inappropriate antibiotic prescribing and antibiotic resistance.

4. **Develop drugs and improved diagnostic tests.** Discovery of new antimicrobial agents is needed to keep pace with the emergence of pathogen resistance. Unfortunately, the number of antimicrobial agents in late-phase clinical development is low; in particular, few agents are being developed with a new mechanism of action to treat resistant gram-negative infections. In addition, new diagnostic tests are needed to guide antimicrobial therapy and to track the development of resistance.

Antimicrobial Stewardship

The primary goal of antimicrobial stewardship is to optimize antimicrobial use with the aim of decreasing inappropriate use that leads to unwarranted toxicity and to selection and spread of resistant organisms. The CDC describes 7 core elements to successful inpatient stewardship programs: leadership support, accountability (physician leader), drug expertise (pharmacy leader), action to support optimal antibiotic use, tracking, reporting, and education. (**www.cdc.gov/getsmart/healthcare/implementation/ core-elements.html**). Hospital administration should support and provide dedicated time to a physician director and clinical pharmacist(s) as well as financial and technologic resources needed to accomplish the programmatic goals. Core members of an inpatient antimicrobial stewardship program include infectious diseases specialists, clinical pharmacists, clinical microbiologists, hospital epidemiologists, infection prevention professionals, and information systems specialists.[1,2] Actions of antimicrobial stewardship in the inpatient setting include the implementation of core strategies such as antibiotic "time outs," prospective audit and feedback, and/or prior authorization. Additional actions include education, development of clinical practice guidelines, conversion from intravenous to oral agents, dose optimization, and implementation of electronic decision support. The program should provide tracking of antimicrobial usage and resistance patterns, hospital-acquired *C difficile* infections rates, and patient outcomes such as readmission rates. The stewardship program should implement interventions to improve use, followed by direct reporting to and education of staff. All medical providers can help stewardship programs protect patients and preserve the therapeutic effectiveness of antimicrobial agents.

Although inpatients frequently are exposed to broad-spectrum and potentially toxic antimicrobial agents, the vast majority of antibiotic exposure occurs in the outpatient setting. Many different strategies have been used to improve antimicrobial use in the outpatient setting. Common approaches include patient education, provider education, communications training, provider audit and feedback with peer comparisons, and clinical decision support. Interventions that incorporate a combination of approaches tend to be most effective. Additionally, pediatricians should seek understanding of parents'

---

[1]Bryant KA, Harris AD, Gould CV, et al. Necessary infrastructure of infection prevention and healthcare epidemiology programs: a review. *Infect Cont Hosp Epidemiol.* 2016;37(4):371–380

[2]Newland JG, Banerjee R, Gerber JS, Hersh AL, Steinke L, Weissman SJ. Antimicrobial stewardship in pediatric care: strategies and future directions. *Pharmacotherapy.* 2012;32(8):735–743

expectations for antibiotic agents, because prescribing significantly increases when clinicians believe a parent is expecting an antibiotic agent.

Role of the Medical Provider

Medical providers can integrate key recommendations that focus on antibiotic prescribing for common infections in children. These include the following:

1. Confirm urinary tract infection by documenting that the patient is symptomatic and has a properly obtained urinalysis and quantitative culture with each clinical episode, with a positive result based on the specific bacteria isolated and the colony count. When the infection is confirmed and susceptibility tests are completed, choose an appropriate agent with the narrowest spectrum of activity.

2. Before treating a patient for bacterial pneumonia, ensure that there is not an alternate diagnosis or explanation for radiologic findings. The vast majority of respiratory syncytial virus infections in infants are not complicated by bacterial infection, but migratory atelectasis is common. For infants with bronchiolitis, antimicrobial agents are not indicated, unless a concomitant bacterial infection is present.[1]

3. Standardize processes to ensure that appropriate cultures and other diagnostic tests are obtained before antimicrobial agents are administered.

4. Know how to access local antibiograms and be aware of antimicrobial resistance patterns.

5. Initiate antimicrobial therapy promptly for suspected or proven infection, and document indication, dose, timing, and anticipated duration.

6. Perform an "antibiotic timeout" in hospitalized patients. Reassess response to therapy within 48 hours, taking into account new clinical and laboratory data. Focus definitive therapy to use the most appropriate agent with the narrowest spectrum and to discontinue antibiotic therapy when a treatable bacterial infection is excluded.

7. Collaborate with the local antibiotic stewardship team and request formal infectious diseases consultation for cases in which the patient has comorbidities or a severe illness or if the diagnosis is uncertain.

Additional information for health care professionals and parents on judicious use of antimicrobial agents (The Get Smart Campaign) and antimicrobial resistance is available on the CDC Web site (**www.cdc.gov/getsmart/** and **www.cdc.gov/drugresistance**).

Principles of Appropriate Use of Antimicrobial Therapy for Upper Respiratory Tract Infections[2]

More than half of all outpatient prescriptions for antimicrobial agents for children are given for 5 conditions: otitis media, sinusitis, cough illness/bronchitis, pharyngitis, and nonspecific upper respiratory tract infection (the common cold). Antimicrobial agents

---

[1]Ralston SL, Lieberthal AS, Meissner HC, et al. Clinical practice guideline: the diagnosis, management, and prevention of bronchiolitis. *Pediatrics*. 2015;136(4):2015–2862

[2]Hersh AL, Jackson MA, Hicks LA; American Academy of Pediatrics, Committee on Infectious Diseases. Clinical report: Principles of judicious antibiotic prescribing for upper respiratory tract infections in pediatrics. *Pediatrics* 2013;132(6):1146–1154

often are prescribed, even though many of these illnesses are caused by viruses, which are unresponsive to antibiotic therapy. Children treated with an antimicrobial agent for respiratory tract infections are at increased risk of becoming colonized with resistant respiratory tract flora, including *Streptococcus pneumoniae* and *Haemophilus influenzae*. These same children, who may experience future respiratory tract infections, are more likely to experience failure of subsequent antimicrobial therapy and are likely to spread resistant bacteria to close contacts. The following principles, with supporting evidence, are published by the AAP and CDC to assist pediatricians in using antibiotic agents appropriately and only when needed for these common pediatric conditions.

OTITIS MEDIA

- Antimicrobial therapy versus observation for children diagnosed with acute otitis media (AOM) needs to account for illness severity, laterality of infection, age of patient, and assurance of follow-up.[1] Children 6 months and older with otorrhea or severe signs and symptoms (temperature ≥39°F [102.2°F], ear pain for ≥48 hours, or moderate to severe ear pain) and children 6 through 23 months of age with bilateral AOM (regardless of severity) should receive immediate antibiotic treatment. Children 6 to 23 months of age without severe symptoms and unilateral AOM and children 24 months and older without severe symptoms (with unilateral or bilateral AOM) can be offered observation for 48 to 72 hours with close follow-up, based on shared-decision making with the parent or caregiver.
- When antimicrobial agents are used for AOM, a narrow-spectrum antimicrobial agent (eg, amoxicillin, 80–90 mg/kg per day in 2 divided doses) should be used for most children. For children younger than 24 months or with severe symptoms at any age, a 10-day course should be used. For children 2 through 5 years of age without severe symptoms, a 7-day course may be used. For children 6 years and older without severe symptoms, a 5- to 7-day course may be used. Microbiologic and clinical failure with high-dose amoxicillin has been associated with highly penicillin-resistant pneumococci (uncommon currently with widespread use of the 13-valent pneumococcal conjugate vaccine [PCV13]) and with beta-lactamase–producing *Haemophilus* species and *Moraxella* species (an increasing problem as the proportion of cases of AOM caused by pneumococci decreases). Additional β-lactamase coverage for AOM using amoxicillin-clavulanate is indicated if the child has received amoxicillin in the last 30 days, has concurrent purulent conjunctivitis, or has a history of recurrent AOM unresponsive to amoxicillin.[2]
- Children with underlying medical conditions, craniofacial abnormalities, chronic or recurrent otitis media, or perforation of the tympanic membrane represent a more complicated and diverse population. Initial therapy with a 10-day course of an antimicrobial agent is likely to be more effective than shorter courses for many of these children.
- Persistent middle ear effusion (MEE) is common and can be detected by pneumatic otoscopy (with or without verification by tympanometry) after resolution of acute symptoms. Two weeks after successful antibiotic treatment of AOM, 60% to 70% of

---

[1]Lieberthal AS, Carroll AE, Chonmaitree T, et al. Clinical practice guideline: the diagnosis and management of acute otitis media. *Pediatrics*. 2013;131(3):e964–e999

children have MEE, decreasing to 40% at 1 month and 10% to 25% at 3 months after successful antibiotic treatment. The presence of MEE without clinical symptoms is defined as otitis media with effusion (OME). OME must be differentiated clinically from AOM and requires infrequent additional monitoring and no antibiotic therapy. Assuring families that OME resolves is particularly important for children with cognitive or developmental delay that may be affected adversely by transient hearing loss associated with MEE.

ACUTE SINUSITIS

- Sinusitis is the diagnosis most identified with outpatient antibiotic prescriptions in the United States. Clinical practice guidelines from the AAP[1] and the Infectious Diseases Society of America[2] delineate evidence-based criteria for the diagnosis and treatment of acute bacterial sinusitis. Clinical diagnosis of acute bacterial sinusitis requires the presence of one of the following criteria: (1) persistent nasal discharge (of any quality) or daytime cough (which may be worse at night) without evidence of clinical improvement for ≥10 days; (2) a worsening course (worsening or new onset of nasal discharge, daytime cough, or fever after initial improvement); or (3) body temperature of ≥39°C (≥102°F) with either purulent nasal discharge and/or facial pain concurrently for at least 3 consecutive days in a child who seems ill. Most diagnoses are made by criteria 1 and 2. Findings on sinus imaging correlate poorly with disease and should not be used for acute uncomplicated bacterial sinusitis or to distinguish acute bacterial sinusitis from viral upper respiratory infection. Computed tomography and/or magnetic resonance imaging of sinuses is indicated when complications (eg, orbital or central nervous system complications) are suspected.
- Antimicrobial therapy is indicated for children with severe onset or a worsening course. For children with nonsevere, persistent illness with ≥10 days of symptoms, either observation for an additional 3 days or antimicrobial therapy is indicated.
- When antibiotic therapy is initiated, amoxicillin alone or with clavulanate is preferred. Amoxicillin may be used in standard dose (45 mg/kg/day in 2 divided doses) or in high dose (80–90 mg/kg/day in 2 divided doses) in areas with high prevalence (>10%) of nonsusceptible *S pneumoniae*. Amoxicillin-clavulanate (80–90 mg/kg/day of amoxicillin with 6.4 mg/kg/day of clavulanate [14:1 formulation] in 2 divided doses) may be indicated for children with moderate-to-severe illness, children younger than 2 years, or children attending child care or when antimicrobial resistance is likely (eg, recent treatment with antibiotic agents). Treatment duration typically is 10 days.
- As noted in the guidelines from the Infectious Diseases Society of America,[2] existing clinical criteria are limited in their ability to differentiate bacterial from viral acute rhinosinusitis. The guidelines also highlight the changing prevalence and antimicrobial susceptibility profiles of bacterial isolates associated with sinusitis and the impact of pneumococcal conjugate vaccines on the microbiology of sinusitis.

---

[1]Wald ER, Applegate KE, Bordley C, et al; American Academy of Pediatrics. Clinical practice guideline for the diagnosis and management of acute bacterial sinusitis in children aged 1 to 18 years. *Pediatrics*. 2013;132(1):e262–e280

[2]Chow AW, Benninger MS, Brook I, et al; Infectious Disease Society of America. IDSA clinical practice guideline for acute bacterial rhinosinusitis in children and adults. *Clin Infect Dis*. 2012;54(8):e72–e112

COUGH ILLNESS/BRONCHITIS

- Nonspecific cough illness/bronchitis in children does not warrant antimicrobial treatment.
- Prolonged cough (10–14 days or more) may be caused by *Bordetella pertussis, Bordetella parapertussis, Mycoplasma pneumoniae,* or *Chlamydia pneumoniae.* When infection caused by one of these organisms is suspected clinically or is confirmed, appropriate antimicrobial therapy is indicated (see Pertussis, p 620, *Mycoplasma pneumoniae* and Other *Mycoplasma* Species Infections, p 573, and Chlamydial Infections, p 273).

PHARYNGITIS

(See Group A Streptococcal Infections, p 748.)
- Diagnosis of group A streptococcal pharyngitis should be made on the basis of results of appropriate laboratory tests in conjunction with clinical and epidemiologic findings.
- Group A streptococcal testing should only be performed in patients with signs and symptoms of pharyngitis without evidence of a viral upper respiratory infection.
- Most cases of pharyngitis are viral in origin. Antimicrobial therapy should not be given to a child with pharyngitis in the absence of positive group A streptococcal testing. Rarely, other bacteria may cause pharyngitis (eg, *Arcanobacterium haemolyticum, Corynebacterium diphtheriae, Francisella tularensis,* groups G and C hemolytic streptococci, *Neisseria gonorrhoeae*), and treatment should be provided according to recommendations in disease-specific chapters in section 3.
- Penicillin remains the drug of choice for treating group A streptococcal pharyngitis. Amoxicillin suspension may be more acceptable to children in taste than penicillin and is equally as effective.

THE COMMON COLD

- Antimicrobial agents should not be given for the common cold.
- Mucopurulent rhinitis (thick, opaque, or discolored nasal discharge that begins a few days into a viral upper respiratory tract infection) commonly accompanies the common cold and is not an indication for antimicrobial treatment.

DRUG INTERACTIONS

Use of multiple drugs for treatment increases the probability of adverse drug-drug interactions. Complete drug interaction software programs are used by most hospital and health care system pharmacies. Mobile device-based software applications are available for physicians to check drug-drug interactions. Detailed description of drug interactions can be found on the Food and Drug Administration Web site (**www.fda.gov/ Drugs/DevelopmentApprovalProcess/DevelopmentResources/ DrugInteractionsLabeling/ucm080499.htm**). Labels for individual drugs often include information about clinically significant drug interactions. Individual drug labels can be found online through two websites: the DailyMed (**https://dailymed.nlm. nih.gov/dailymed/about.cfm**) or Drugs@FDA (**www.accessdata.fda.gov/ scripts/cder/drugsatfda/**).

TABLES OF ANTIBACTERIAL DRUG DOSAGES

Recommended dosages for antibacterial agents commonly used for neonates (see Table 4.2, p 915) and for infants and children (see Table 4.3, p 920) are provided separately because of the pharmacokinetic and dosing differences between these 2 groups.

Table 4.2 is organized by variables such as gestational age (GA), postnatal age (PNA), and postmenstrual age (PMA), that best guide neonatal dosing for a given group of agents. Aminoglycosides and vancomycin are listed in separate tables to highlight their target serum concentration. For agents used to treat *Bacillus anthracis*, see Fluoroquinolones (p 904) and Anthrax (p 214).

Recommended dosages are not absolute and are intended only as a guide. When a dosage range is provided, the high dose generally is intended for severe infections. Clinical judgment about the disease, alterations in renal or hepatic function, drug interactions, patient response, and laboratory results may dictate modifications of these recommendations in an individual patient. In some cases, monitoring of serum drug concentrations is recommended to avoid toxicity and to achieve concentrations associated with therapeutic efficacy.

Product label information or a pediatric pharmacist should be consulted for details such as the appropriate methods of preparation and administration, measures to be taken to avoid drug interactions, and other precautions. US Food and Drug Administration (FDA)-approved drug labels can be found online at DailyMed (**www.dailymed. nlm.nih.gov**) and at Drugs@FDA (**www.accessdata.fda.gov/scripts/cder/ drugsatfda/**).

For antimicrobial agents not yet approved for children by the FDA but under study, the infections and dosages used for investigational treatments may be found at **http:// clinicaltrials.gov.**

Table 4.2. Antibacterial Drugs for Neonates (≤28 Postnatal Days of Age). (Adapted from American Academy of Pediatrics. *2018 Nelson's Pediatric Antimicrobial Therapy*. 24th ed. Itasca, IL: American Academy of Pediatrics; 2018)

Penicillins

Drug	Route	GA ≤34 wk		GA >34 wk	
		PNA ≤7 days	PNA >7 days	PNA ≤7 days	PNA >7 days
Ampicillin[a]	IV, IM	50 mg/kg every 12 h	75 mg/kg every 12 h	50 mg/kg every 8 h	
Nafcillin, oxacillin[b]	IV, IM	25 mg/kg every 12 h	25 mg/kg every 8 h	25 mg/kg every 8 h	25 mg/kg every 6 h

Drug	Route	GA ≤34 wk		GA >34 wk	
		PNA ≤7 days	PNA >7 days	PNA ≤7 days	PNA >7 days
Penicillin G aqueous[c]	IV, IM	50 000 U/kg every 12 h		50 000 U/kg every 8 h	
Penicillin G procaine	IM only	50 000 U/kg every 24 h		50 000 U/kg every 24 h	
Amoxicillin	PO	15 mg/kg every 12 h		15 mg/kg every 12 h	

Drug	Route	PMA ≤30 wk	PMA >30 wk
Piperacillin-tazobactam	IV	100 mg/kg every 8 h	80 mg/kg every 6 h

Cephalosporins

Drug	Route	GA <32 wk		GA ≥32 wk	
		PNA <14 days	PNA ≥14 days	PNA ≤7 days	PNA >7 days
Cefazolin	IV, IM	50 mg/kg every 12 h	50 mg/kg every 8 h	50 mg/kg every 12 h	50 mg/kg every 8 h
Cefotaxime	IV, IM	50 mg/kg every 12 h	50 mg/kg every 8 h	50 mg/kg every 12 h	50 mg/kg every 8 h
Ceftazidime	IV, IM	50 mg/kg every 12 h	50 mg/kg every 8 h	50 mg/kg every 12 h	50 mg/kg every 8 h
Cefuroxime	IV, IM	50 mg/kg every 12 h	50 mg/kg every 8 h	50 mg/kg every 12 h	50 mg/kg every 8 h

Drug	Route	GA <32 wk		GA ≥32 wk
		PNA ≤7 days	PNA >7 days	
Cefoxitin	IV, IM	35 mg/kg every 12 h	35 mg/kg every 8 h	35 mg/kg every 8 h

Table 4.2. Antibacterial Drugs for Neonates (≤28 Postnatal Days of Age). (Adapted from American Academy of Pediatrics. 2018 Nelson's Pediatric Antimicrobial Therapy. 24th ed. Itasca, IL: American Academy of Pediatrics; 2018), continued

Drug	Route	All neonates
Ceftriaxone[d]	IV, IM	50 mg/kg every 24 h

Drug	Route	GA <36 wk	GA ≥36 wk
Cefepime	IV	30 mg/kg every 12 h	50 mg/kg every 12 h[e]

Carbapenems

Drug	Route	GA <32 wk PNA <14 days	GA <32 wk PNA ≥14 days	GA ≥32 wk PNA <14 days	GA ≥32 wk PNA ≥14 days
Meropenem[b]	IV	20 mg/kg every 12 h	20 mg/kg every 8 h	20 mg/kg every 8 h	30 mg/kg every 8 h

Drug	Route	PNA ≤7 days	PNA >7 days
Imipenem-cilastatin	IV	25 mg/kg every 12 h	25 mg/kg every 8 h

Other agents

Drug	Route	All neonates
Azithromycin[f]	IV, PO	10 mg/kg every 24 h[g]
Erythromycin[f]	IV, PO	10 mg/kg every 6 h
Rifampin[h]	IV, PO	10 mg/kg every 24 h

Table 4.2. Antibacterial Drugs for Neonates (≤28 Postnatal Days of Age). (Adapted from American Academy of Pediatrics. 2018 Nelson's Pediatric Antimicrobial Therapy. 24th ed. Itasca, IL: American Academy of Pediatrics; 2018), continued

Drug	Route	GA <34 wk		GA ≥34 wk	
		PNA ≤7 days	PNA >7 days	PNA ≤7 days	PNA >7 days
Aztreonam[b]	IV	30 mg/kg every 12 h	30 mg/kg every 8 h	30 mg/kg every 8 h	30 mg/kg every 6 h

Drug	Route	PMA ≤32 wk	PMA 33–40 wk	PMA >40 wk
Clindamycin	IV, PO	5 mg/kg every 8h	7 mg/kg every 8 h	9 mg/kg every 8 h

Drug	Route	GA <34 wk		GA ≥34 wk	
		PNA ≤7 days	PNA >7 days	PNA ≤7 days	PNA >7 days
Linezolid	IV, PO	10 mg/kg every 12 h	10 mg/kg every 8 h	10 mg/kg every 8 h	10 mg/kg every 8 h

Drug	Route	PMA ≤34 wk	PMA 35–40 wk	PMA >40 wk
Metronidazole[i]	IV	7.5 mg/kg every 12 h	7.5 mg/kg every 8 h	10 mg/kg every 8 h

Table 4.2. Antibacterial Drugs for Neonates (≤28 Postnatal Days of Age). (Adapted from American Academy of Pediatrics. 2018 Nelson's Pediatric Antimicrobial Therapy. 24th ed. Itasca, IL: American Academy of Pediatrics; 2018), continued

Aminoglycosides

Drug	Route	GA <30 wk		GA 30–34 wk		GA ≥35 wk	
		PNA ≤14 days	>14 days	≤14 days	>14 days	≤7 days	>7 days
Amikacin[j]	IV, IM	15 mg/kg every 48 h	15 mg/kg every 24 h	15 mg/kg every 36 h	15 mg/kg every 24 h	15 mg/kg every 24 h	18 mg/kg every 24 h
Gentamicin[k]	IV, IM	5 mg/kg every 48 h	5 mg/kg every 36 h	5 mg/kg every 36 h	5 mg/kg every 24 h	4 mg/kg every 24 h	5 mg/kg every 24 h
Tobramycin[k]	IV, IM	5 mg/kg every 48 h	5 mg/kg every 36 h	5 mg/kg every 36 h	5 mg/kg every 24 h	4 mg/kg every 24 h	5 mg/kg every 24 h

Vancomycin

Begin with a 20-mg/kg loading dose followed by a maintenance dose, according to the table

GA ≤28 wk		GA >28 wk	
Serum Creatinine[l]	Dosage	Serum Creatinine[l]	Dosage
<0.5	15 mg/kg every 12 h	<0.7	15 mg/kg every 12 h
0.5–0.7	20 mg/kg every 24 h	0.7–0.9	20 mg/kg every 24 h
0.8–1	15 mg/kg every 24 h	1–1.2	15 mg/kg every 24 h
1.1–1.4	10 mg/kg every 24 h	1.3–1.6	10 mg/kg every 24 h
>1.4	15 mg/kg every 48 h	>1.6	15 mg/kg every 48 h

GA indicates gestational age; PNA, postnatal age; IV, intravenous; IM, intramuscular; GBS, Guillain-Barré syndrome; CNS, central nervous system; PO, oral; MIC, minimum inhibitory concentration.

a For GBS meningitis, 100 mg/kg every 8 hours when PNA ≤7 days and 75 mg/kg every 6 h when PNA >7 days. See Group B Streptococcal Infections, p 762.

b Higher doses than those listed may be required for meningitis, although safety and efficacy data for dosing of neonates with CNS infection are lacking for these agents.

c For GBS meningitis, 125 000 units/kg every 6 h. See Group B Streptococcal Infections, p 762.

d Neonates should not receive IV ceftriaxone if they also are receiving IV calcium in any form, including parenteral nutrition (see *Pediatrics* 2009;123(4):e609–613). Hyperbilirubinemic neonates, especially those that are premature, should not be treated with ceftriaxone for injection because in vitro studies have shown that ceftriaxone can displace bilirubin from its binding to serum albumin, leading to a possible risk of bilirubin encephalopathy in these patients.

e May give 30 mg/kg every 12 h if target pathogen MIC <8 mg/L.

f An association between orally administered erythromycin and azithromycin and infantile hypertrophic pyloric stenosis (IHPS) has been reported in infants younger than 6 weeks. Infants treated with either of these antimicrobials should be followed for signs and symptoms of IHPS.

g 20 mg/kg every 24 hours is recommended for infants with chlamydial pneumonia.

h See *Haemophilus influenzae* Infections, p 367, and Meningococcal Infections, p 550, for alternate dosing in special situations.

i Begin with a 15 mg/kg loading dose.

j Desired serum concentrations: 24–40 mg/L (peak), <7 mg/L (trough).

k Desired serum concentrations: 6–12 mg/L (peak), <2 mg/L (trough).

l mg/dL. The maintenance dose should begin at the same number of hours after the loading dose as the maintenance interval. Serum creatinine concentrations normally fluctuate and are partly influenced by transplacental maternal creatinine in the first week of postnatal age. Cautious use of creatinine-based dosing strategy with frequent reassessment of renal function and vancomycin serum concentrations is recommended in neonates ≤7 days old. For invasive methicillin-resistant *S aureus* infections, a 24-hour area under the curve (AUC) to MIC ratio of ≥400 mg·h/L is recommended based on adult studies. The AUC is best calculated from 2 (eg, peak and trough) rather than 1 trough serum concentration measurement. In situations where AUC calculation is not feasible, a trough concentration 10–12 mg/L is very highly likely (>90%) to achieve the AUC target in neonates when the MIC is 1 mg/L.

Table 4.3. Antibacterial Drugs for Pediatric Patients Beyond the Newborn Period[a]

Drug Generic (Trade Name)	Generic Available	Route	Dosage per kg per Day (absolute maximum dosage provided if known)	Comments
Aminoglycosides[b]				
Amikacin	Y	IV, IM	15–22.5 mg divided in 2–3 doses or in 1 dose	See Table 4.2 for serum concentration targets. Higher doses than those given are appropriate for cystic fibrosis.
Gentamicin	Y	IV, IM	6–7.5 mg divided in 3 doses, or 5–7.5 mg in 1 dose	
Neomycin	Y	PO	100 mg divided in 4 doses, max 12 g per day	For some enteric infections.
Tobramycin	Y	IV, IM	6–7.5 mg divided in 3–4 doses, or 5–7.5 mg in 1 dose	Higher doses than those given are appropriate for cystic fibrosis.
Aztreonam (Azactam)	Y	IV, IM	90–120 mg divided in 3 or 4 doses, max 8 g per day	A monobactam antibiotic.
Carbapenems[c]				
Imipenem/cilastatin (Primaxin)	Y	IV	60–100 mg divided in 4 doses, max 4 g per day	Caution in use for treatment of CNS infections because of increased risk of seizures. Higher dose should be used for *Pseudomonas aeruginosa* infections.
Meropenem (Merrem)	Y	IV	60 mg divided in 3 doses, max 3 g per day 120 mg divided in 3 doses for meningitis, max 6 g per day	Extended infusion may be needed for susceptible dose-dependent infections.
Ertapenem (Invanz)	N	IV/IM	30 mg divided in 2 doses, max 1 g per day ≥13 y and adults, 1 g once daily	Poor activity against *Pseudomonas* and *Acinetobacter* species.

Table 4.3. Antibacterial Drugs for Pediatric Patients Beyond the Newborn Period,[a] continued

Drug Generic (Trade Name)	Generic Available	Route	Dosage per kg per Day (absolute maximum dosage provided if known)	Comments
Cephalosporins[c]				The generation of each agent is listed as a guide to antimicrobial spectrum.
Cefaclor (Ceclor)	Y	PO	20–40 mg divided in 2 or 3 doses, max 1 g per day	Second generation.
Cefadroxil (Duricef)	Y	PO	30 mg divided in 2 doses, max 2 g per day	First generation.
Cefazolin (Ancef)	Y	IV, IM	25–75 mg divided in 3 doses, max 6 g per day Up to 150 mg divided in 3–4 doses for bone/joint infections, max 12 g per day	First generation. Limited data on dosages above 100 mg/kg/day.
Cefdinir (Omnicef)	Y	PO	14 mg divided in 1 or 2 doses, max 600 mg/day	Third generation. Inadequate activity against penicillin-resistant pneumococci.
Cefepime (Maxipime)	Y	IV, IM	100 mg divided in 2 doses, max 4 g per day 150 mg divided in 3 doses for *Pseudomonas* infections or febrile neutropenia	Fourth generation. Max 6 g per day. Extended infusion may be needed for susceptible dose-dependent infections.
Cefixime (Suprax)	Y	PO	8 mg divided in 1 or 2 doses, max 400 mg per day	Third generation. Inadequate activity against penicillin-resistant pneumococci.
Cefotaxime (Claforan)	Y	IV, IM	150–180 mg divided in 3 doses, max 8 g per day 200–225 mg divided in 4 doses for meningitis, max 12 g per day	Third generation. Up to 300 mg divided in 4 or 6 doses may be used for meningitis.

Table 4.3. Antibacterial Drugs for Pediatric Patients Beyond the Newborn Period,[a] continued

Drug Generic (Trade Name)	Generic Available	Route	Dosage per kg per Day (absolute maximum dosage provided if known)	Comments
Cefotetan (Cefotan)	Y	IV, IM	60–100 mg divided in 2 doses, max 6 g per day	Second generation. A cephamycin, active against anaerobes.
Cefoxitin (Mefoxin)	Y	IV, IM	80–160 mg divided in 3–4 doses, max 12 g per day	Second generation. A cephamycin, active against anaerobes.
Cefpodoxime (Vantin)	Y	PO	10 mg divided in 2 doses, max 400 mg per day 400 mg/dose twice daily effective in adults with severe non-MRSA SSTI.	Third generation.
Cefprozil (Cefzil)	Y	PO	15–30 mg divided in 2 doses, max 1 g per day	Second generation.
Ceftaroline (Teflaro)	N	IV	2 mo to <2 y: 24 mg divided in 3 doses 2 y to <18 y of age: ≤33 kg: 36 mg divided in 3 doses >33 kg: Adult dose For complicated CABP, including MRSA: 2 mo to <6 mo of age: 30 mg divided in 3 doses ≥6 mo of age: 45 mg divided in 3 doses, max single dose 600 mg	Fifth generation with anti-MRSA activity. No activity against *Pseudomonas* species. Adult dose: 400 mg/dose every 8 h or 600 mg/dose every 12 h (max 1200 mg/day).
Ceftazidime (Fortaz)	Y	IV, IM	90–150 mg divided in 3 doses, max 6 g per day 200–300 mg divided in 3 doses for serious *Pseudomonas* infections	Third generation. Max 6 g per day (12 g per day for serious *Pseudomonas* infections).
Ceftibuten (Cedax)	Y	PO	9 mg once daily, max 400 mg per day	Third generation. Inadequate activity against penicillin-resistant pneumococci.

Table 4.3. Antibacterial Drugs for Pediatric Patients Beyond the Newborn Period,[a] continued

Drug Generic (Trade Name)	Generic Available	Route	Dosage per kg per Day (absolute maximum dosage provided if known)	Comments
Ceftriaxone (Rocephin)	Y	IV, IM	50–75 mg once daily, max 1 g per day 100 mg divided in 1 or 2 doses, max 4 g per day 50 mg/kg IM once daily for 1–3 days for AOM, max 1 g per day	Third generation. Larger dosage appropriate for meningitis or penicillin-resistant pneumococcal pneumonia.
Cefuroxime (Zinacef)	Y	IV, IM	100–150 mg divided in 3 doses, max 6 g per day	Second-generation. Limited activity against penicillin-resistant pneumococcus.
Cefuroxime axetil (Ceftin)	Y	PO	20–30 mg divided in 2 doses, max 1 g per day Up to 100 mg divided in 3 doses for bone or joint infections, max 3 g per day	Second-generation. Limited activity against penicillin-resistant pneumococcus.
Cephalexin (Keflex)	Y	PO	25–50 mg divided in 2 doses 75–100 mg divided in 3–4 doses for bone or joint infections, max 4 g per day	First-generation.
Chloramphenicol	Y	IV	50–100 mg divided in 4 doses Adjust based on target serum concentrations (15–25 mg/L)	Reserved for serious infections because of rare risk of aplastic anemia. IV is preferred over PO, because PO may increase risk of aplastic anemia.
Clindamycin (Cleocin)	Y	IM, IV	20–40 mg divided in 3–4 doses, max 2.7 g per day	Active against pneumococci, CA-MRSA, anaerobes.
	Y	PO	10–25 mg divided in 3 doses 30–40 mg divided in 3–4 doses for AOM or CA-MRSA, max 1.8 g per day	

Table 4.3. Antibacterial Drugs for Pediatric Patients Beyond the Newborn Period,[a] continued

Drug Generic (Trade Name)	Generic Available	Route	Dosage per kg per Day (absolute maximum dosage provided if known)	Comments
Daptomycin (Cubicin)	N	IV	4–6 mg once daily 10 mg once daily if <6 y of age	Neuromuscular toxicity in neonatal and juvenile canine model. FDA warns to avoid use in infants <12 mo of age.
Fluoroquinolones see also p 904.				
Ciprofloxacin (Cipro)	Y	PO	20–40 mg divided in 2 doses, max 1.5 g per day	FDA recommends restricting use for certain uncomplicated infections (sinusitis, uncomplicated UTIs, or acute exacerbations of chronic bronchitis) because of serious adverse reactions.
		IV	20–30 mg divided in 2 or 3 doses, max 0.8–1.2 g per day	
Levofloxacin (Levaquin)	Y	IV, PO	≥6 mo and <50 kg: 16 mg divided in 2 doses, max 500 mg per day for *Bacillus anthracis* exposure >50 kg: 500 mg total daily dose (not per kg) once daily	FDA recommends restricting use for certain uncomplicated infections (sinusitis, uncomplicated UTIs, or acute exacerbations of chronic bronchitis) because of serious adverse reactions.
Macrolides				
Azithromycin (Zithromax, Zmax)	Y	PO	5–10 mg once daily for the immediate release products, 60 mg as a single dose for the extended-release (ER) formulation Respiratory tract infection dosages (per kg, interval is once daily):	Per dose max 250 mg for 6 mg/kg, 500 mg for 10–12 mg/kg, 1.5 g for 30 mg/kg. Normal adult total course is 1.5–2 g. Total course max 2.5 g. ER suspension for infants and children >6 mo of age, max 2 g.

Table 4.3. Antibacterial Drugs for Pediatric Patients Beyond the Newborn Period,[a] continued

Drug Generic (Trade Name)	Generic Available	Route	Dosage per kg per Day (absolute maximum dosage provided if known)	Comments
			AOM: 10 mg for 3 days; or 30 mg for 1 day; or 10 mg for 1 day then 5 mg for 4 days	Multiple additional indications. See relevant chapters in Section 3.
			Pharyngitis: 12 mg for 1 day, then 6 mg for 4 days	
			Sinusitis: 10 mg for 3 days, or 10 mg for 1 day, then 5 mg for 4 days	
			CABP: 10 mg for 1 day then 5 mg for 4 days, or 60 mg one time of the ER suspension	
	Y	IV	10 mg once daily, max 500 mg per day	
Clarithromycin (Biaxin)	Y	PO	15 mg divided in 2 doses, max 1 g per day	Similar activity to erythromycin; more activity against *Mycobacterium avium* and *Helicobacter pylori*.
Erythromycin (numerous)	Y	PO	40–50 mg divided in 3–4 doses, max 4 g per day	Available in base, stearate, and ethylsuccinate preparations.
	N	IV	20 mg divided in 4 doses, max 4 g per day	Administer over at least 60 minutes to potentially prevent cardiac arrhythmias.
Fidaxomicin (Dificid)	N	PO	Adults: 400 mg total daily dose (not per kg) divided in 2 doses	For treatment of *Clostridium difficile* infection. Not yet FDA approved for children, but under investigation.

Table 4.3. Antibacterial Drugs for Pediatric Patients Beyond the Newborn Period,[a] continued

Drug Generic (Trade Name)	Generic Available	Route	Dosage per kg per Day (absolute maximum dosage provided if known)	Comments
Metronidazole (Flagyl)	Y	PO	15–50 mg divided in 3 doses, max 2.25 g per day	30 mg divided in 4 doses for *C difficile* infection. 15–25 mg divided in 3 doses for bacterial vaginosis. 45 mg divided in 3 doses for *Trichomonas vaginalis*.
	Y	IV	22.5–40 mg divided in 3 or 4 doses, max 4 g per day	
Nitrofurantoin (Furadantin, Macrodantin)	Y	PO	5–7 mg divided in 4 doses, max 400 mg per day UTI prophylaxis: 1–2 mg once daily	For treatment of cystitis; not appropriate for pyelonephritis.
Oxazolidinones				
Linezolid (Zyvox)	Y	PO, IV	≤11 y of age: 30 mg divided in 3 doses >11 y of age: 1200 mg (not per kg) divided in 2 doses	5–11 y: 20 mg divided in 2 doses for SSTI. Myelosuppression increases with duration of therapy over 10 days.
Tedizolid (Sivextro)	N	PO, IV	Adults: 200 mg (not per kg) once daily	Not yet FDA approved for children, but under investigation.
Penicillins[c]				
Amoxicillin (Amoxil)	Y	PO	Standard dose: 40–45 mg divided in 3 doses High dose: 80–90 mg divided in 2 doses ≥12 y of age: 775 mg (not per kg) once daily of ER formulation	90 mg/kg/day divided in 2 doses for AOM. 50 mg/kg once daily for streptococcal pharyngitis (see Group A Streptococcal Infections p 748).

Table 4.3. Antibacterial Drugs for Pediatric Patients Beyond the Newborn Period,[a] continued

Drug Generic (Trade Name)	Generic Available	Route	Dosage per kg per Day (absolute maximum dosage provided if known)	Comments
Amoxicillin-clavulanic acid (Augmentin)	Y	PO	14:1 Formulation: 90 mg divided in 2 doses 7:1 Formulation: 25–45 mg divided in 2 doses, max 1750 mg per day 4:1 Formulation: 20–40 mg divided in 3 doses, max 1500 mg per day	Dosed on amoxicillin component. Max 4 g per day based on XR formulation for ≥40 kg.
Ampicillin	Y	IV, IM	50–200 mg divided in 4 doses, max 8 g per day 300–400 mg divided in 6 doses for meningitis, endocarditis, max 12 g per day	
	Y	PO	50–100 mg divided in 4 doses, max 2 g per day	
Ampicillin-sulbactam (Unasyn)	Y	IV	100–200 mg divided in 4 doses, max 8 g per day 200–400 mg divided in 4 doses for meningitis or severe infections attributable to resistant *Streptococcus pneumoniae*	Dosed on ampicillin component.
Dicloxacillin (Dynapen)	Y	PO	12–25 mg divided in 4 doses, max 1 g per day 100 mg divided in 4 doses for bone or joint infections, max 2 g per day	
Nafcillin (Nallpen)	Y	IV, IM	100–200 mg divided in 4–6 doses, max 12 g per day	Use high end of dosage for meningitis.
Oxacillin (Bactocill)	Y	IV, IM	100–200 mg divided in 4–6 doses, max 12 g per day	Oxacillin is FDA approved for children.

Table 4.3. Antibacterial Drugs for Pediatric Patients Beyond the Newborn Period,[a] continued

Drug Generic (Trade Name)	Generic Available	Route	Dosage per kg per Day (absolute maximum dosage provided if known)	Comments
Penicillin G, crystalline potassium or sodium	Y	IV, IM	100 000–300 000 units divided in 4–6 doses, 300 000–400 000 units divided in 6 doses for meningitis	Max 24 million units per day.
Penicillin G procaine	Y	IM	50 000 units divided in 1–2 doses, max 1.2 million units	Not safe for IV administration.
Penicillin G benzathine (Bicillin LA)	N	IM	Group A streptococcal pharyngitis (see p 748): ≤27 kg (60 lb) 600 000 units (not per kg) one time >27 kg (60 lb) 1.2 million units (not per kg) one time	Not safe for IV administration. See Group A Streptococcal Infections, p 748.
Penicillin G benzathine/ procaine (Bicillin CR)	N	IM	<14 kg (30 lb) 600 000 units (not per kg) one time 14–27 kg (30–60 lb) 1.2 million units (not per kg) one time ≥27 kg (60 lb) 2.4 million units (not per kg) one time	Not safe for IV administration. Major use is treatment of Group A Streptococcal infections (see p 748).
Penicillin V	Y	PO	25–50 mg divided in 4 doses, max 2 g per day	50–75 mg divided in 4 doses for Group A streptococcal pneumonia.

Table 4.3. Antibacterial Drugs for Pediatric Patients Beyond the Newborn Period,[a] continued

Drug Generic (Trade Name)	Generic Available	Route	Dosage per kg per Day (absolute maximum dosage provided if known)	Comments
Piperacillin-tazobactam (Zosyn)	Y	IV	240–300 mg divided in 3–4 doses, max 16 g per day	Dosed on piperacillin component. Extended infusion may be needed for susceptible-dose dependent infections. 400–600 mg divided in 6 doses, max 24 g per day may be appropriate in some patients with cystic fibrosis.
Polymyxins				
Colistimethate (Colymycin M)	Y	IV, IM	2.5–5 mg base divided in 2–4 doses	Up to 7 mg base/kg/day may be required. 1 mg base = 2.7 mg colistimethate.
Polymyxin B	Y	IV	2.5 mg divided in 2 doses	>3 mg/kg/day not well studied. 1 mg = 10 000 units.
Quinupristin + Dalfopristin (Synercid)	N	IV	15 mg divided in 2 doses	Moderate activity against *Staphylococcus aureus*. Limited experience in children.

Table 4.3. Antibacterial Drugs for Pediatric Patients Beyond the Newborn Period,[a] continued

Drug Generic (Trade Name)	Generic Available	Route	Dosage per kg per Day (absolute maximum dosage provided if known)	Comments
Rifamycins				
Rifampin (Rifadin)	Y	IV, PO	15–20 mg divided in 1–2 doses, max 600 mg per day See p 838–841 for *M tuberculosis* dosing	Should not be used routinely as monotherapy because of rapid emergence of resistance. Many experts recommend using a daily rifampin dose of at least 20 mg/kg/day for infants and toddlers, and for serious forms of tuberculosis such as meningitis and disseminated disease.
Rifaximin (Xifaxan)	N	PO	≥12 y of age: 600 mg/day (not per kg) divided in 3 doses Used off-label for primary gastrointestinal tract indications (eg, SBBO, IBD) in younger children at similar dosages; consult pediatric gastroenterologist	Treatment of travelers' diarrhea caused by noninvasive *Escherichia coli*.
Sulfonamides				
Sulfadiazine	Y	PO	120–150 mg divided in 4–6 doses, max 6 g per day Rheumatic fever secondary prevention: 500 mg (not per kg) once daily in children <30 kg, 1 g once daily in bigger children and adults	

Table 4.3. Antibacterial Drugs for Pediatric Patients Beyond the Newborn Period,[a] continued

Drug Generic (Trade Name)	Generic Available	Route	Dosage per kg per Day (absolute maximum dosage provided if known)	Comments
Trimethoprim - Sulfamethoxazole (TMP-SMX) (Bactrim, Septra)	Y	PO, IV	8–10 mg divided in 2 doses 2 mg once daily for UTI prophylaxis 15–20 mg divided in 3–4 doses for *Pneumocystis jiroveci* treatment, no max 5 mg divided in 2 doses 3 times/wk for prophylaxis, max 160 mg per dose	Dosed on TMP component. See also *Pneumocystis jiroveci* Infections, p 651.
Tetracyclines see also p 905				
Doxycycline (Vibramycin)	Y	PO, IV	2.2–4.4 mg divided in 2 doses, max 200 mg per day	
Minocycline (Minocin)	Y	PO, IV	4 mg divided in 2 doses, max 200 mg per day	
Tetracycline (Sumycin)	Y	PO	25–50 mg divided in 4 doses, max 2 g per day	Tetracycline limited to ≥8 y of age. See p 905 for exceptions.
Vancomycin (Vancocin)	Y	IV	45–60 mg divided in 3–4 doses	Measured serum concentrations should guide ongoing therapy. See Table 4.2, p 915
		PO	40 mg divided in 4 doses, up to 500 mg per day	For *C difficile* infection (CDI). Up to 2 g per day divided in 4 doses for severe, complicated CDI.

AOM indicates acute otitis media; CABP, community-acquired bacterial pneumonia; CA-MRSA, community associated methicillin-resistant *Staphylococcus aureus*; CDI, *Clostridium difficile* infection; CNS, central nervous system; ER, extended-release; FDA, US Food and Drug Administration; IBD, inflammatory bowel disease; IM, intramuscular; IV, intravenous; MRSA, methicillin-resistant *Staphylococcus aureus*; PO, oral; SBBO, small bowel bacterial overgrowth; SSTI, skin and soft tissue infection; UTI, urinary tract infection; XR, extended release.

[a] Adapted from; American Academy of Pediatrics. *2018 Nelson's Pediatric Antimicrobial Therapy.* 24th ed. Itasca, IL: American Academy of Pediatrics; 2018.

[b] Extended interval ("once daily") dosing may provide equal efficacy with reduced toxicity. See *Pediatrics.* 2004;114(1):e111–e118, and *Pediatr Infect Dis J.* 2011;30(10):827–832.

[c] Children with a history of an IgE-mediated, immediate hypersensitivity reaction to penicillins (urticaria, angioedema, bronchospasm, anaphylaxis) who require treatment with an alternate β-lactam should be considered for skin testing (if available) to confirm the allergy, and/or undergo supervised graded clinical challenge or desensitization with the alternate β-lactam agent under the supervision of an expert in drug allergy and desensitization.

···

SEXUALLY TRANSMITTED INFECTIONS

Table 4.4. Guidelines for Treatment of Sexually Transmitted Infections in Children ≥45 kg, Adolescents, and Young Adults According to Syndrome

Preferred regimens are listed. For further information concerning other acceptable regimens and diseases not included, see recommendations in disease-specific chapters in Section 3. In addition, recommendations on treatment of sexually transmitted infections have been issued by the Centers for Disease Control and Prevention at **www.cdc.gov/std/treatment.**[a]

Syndrome	Organisms/ Diagnoses	Treatment of Children Weighing ≥45 kg, Adolescents, and Young Adults[a]
Urethritis and Cervicitis: Inflammation of urethra and/or cervix with erythema and/or mucoid, mucopurulent, or purulent discharge	*Neisseria gonorrhoeae, Chlamydia trachomatis* Other causes include *Mycoplasma genitalium* and possibly *Ureaplasma urealyticum,* and sometimes *Trichomonas vaginalis* and herpes simplex virus (HSV)	Ceftriaxone, 250 mg, IM, in a single dose[b] **PLUS EITHER** Azithromycin, 1 g, orally, in a single dose **OR** Doxycycline, 100 mg, orally, twice a day for 7 days
Persistent and Recurrent Nongonococcal Urethritis: persistent symptoms after treatment with objective signs of urethral inflammation	Noncompliance with treatment regimen or reexposed to untreated sex partner	Retreat with the initial regimen
	M genitalium	Males initially treated with doxycycline: Azithromycin, 1 g, orally, in a single dose Males who fail azithromycin therapy: Moxifloxacin, 400 mg, orally, once daily for 7 days
	T vaginalis (in males who have sex with females)	Metronidazole, 2 g, orally, in a single dose[c,d] **OR** Tinidazole, 2 g, orally, in a single dose[c,d]
Vulvovaginitis	*T vaginalis*	Metronidazole, 2 g, orally, in a single dose[c,d] **OR** Tinidazole, 2 g, orally, in a single dose[c,d]

Table 4.4. Guidelines for Treatment of Sexually Transmitted Infections in Children ≥45 kg, Adolescents, and Young Adults According to Syndrome, continued

Syndrome	Organisms/ Diagnoses	Treatment of Children Weighing ≥45 kg, Adolescents, and Young Adults[a]
	Bacterial vaginosis	Metronidazole, 500 mg, orally, twice daily for 7 days[c,d] **OR** Metronidazole gel 0.75%, 1 full applicator (5 g), intravaginally, once a day for 5 days[c,d] **OR** Clindamycin cream 2%, 1 full applicator (5 g), intravaginally at bedtime, for 7 days
	C albicans (and occasionally other *Candida* species or yeasts	See Table 4.6, Recommended Regimens for Vulvovaginal Candidiasis (p 938)
Pelvic inflammatory disease (PID)	*N gonorrhoeae, C trachomatis,* polymicrobial infection (eg, *M genitalium*, anaerobes, coliform bacteria, and *Streptococcus* species)	See Pelvic Inflammatory Disease (Tables 3.50, p 618, and 3.51, p 618)
Genital ulcer disease	*Treponema pallidum* (primary syphilis)	Penicillin G benzathine, 2.4 million U, IM, in a single dose
	Genital HSV—1st clinical episode[e]	Acyclovir, 400 mg, orally, 3 times/day for 7–10 days **OR** Acyclovir, 200 mg, orally, 5 times/day for 7–10 days **OR** Valacyclovir, 1 g, orally, twice daily for 10 days **OR** Famciclovir, 250 mg, orally, 3 times/day for 7–10 days
	Recurrent genital HSV	See Herpes Simplex (p 437)
	Haemophilus ducreyi (chancroid)	Azithromycin, 1 g, orally, in a single dose **OR** Ceftriaxone, 250 mg, IM, in a single dose **OR** Ciprofloxacin, 500 mg, orally, twice daily for 3 days[f] **OR** Erythromycin base, 500 mg, orally, 3 times/day for 7 days
	Klebsiella granulomatis (granuloma inguinale [Donovanosis])	Azithromycin, 1 g, orally, once/wk or 500 mg, daily, for at least 3 wk and until all lesions have healed completely

Table 4.4. Guidelines for Treatment of Sexually Transmitted Infections in Children ≥45 kg, Adolescents, and Young Adults According to Syndrome, *continued*

Syndrome	Organisms/ Diagnoses	Treatment of Children Weighing ≥45 kg, Adolescents, and Young Adults[a]
	C trachomatis serovars L1, L2, or L3 (Lymphogranuloma venereum)	Doxycycline, 100 mg, orally, twice a day for 21 days
Epididymitis	*C trachomatis, N gonorrhoeae*	Ceftriaxone, 250 mg, IM, in a single dose **PLUS** Doxycycline, 100 mg, orally, twice daily for 10 days
	Enteric organisms (eg, *Escherichia coli*) among males who practice insertive anal sex	Ceftriaxone, 250 mg, IM, in a single dose **PLUS EITHER** Levofloxacin, 500 mg, orally, once a day for 10 days **OR** Ofloxacin, 300 mg, orally, twice a day for 10 days
External anogenital warts (ie, penis, groin, scrotum, vulva, perineum, external anus, and perianus)	Human papillomavirus	*Patient-applied:* Imiquimod 5% cream, applied once at bedtime, 3 times/wk for up to 16 wk[f,g] **OR** Imiquimod 3.75% cream, applied once at bedtime every night for up to 16 wk[f,g] **OR** Podofilox 0.5% solution or gel applied to anogenital warts twice a day for 3 days, followed by 4 days of no therapy. Can repeat for up to 4 cycles[f] **OR** Sinecatechins 15% ointment applied 3 times daily for up to 16 wk[f] *Provider-administered:* Cryotherapy with liquid nitrogen or cryoprobe **OR** Surgical removal either by tangential scissor excision, tangential shave excision, curettage, laser, or electrosurgery **OR** Trichloroacetic acid or bichloroacetic acid 80%–90% applied only to warts and allow to dry; can repeat weekly

IM indicates intramuscularly; STI, sexually transmitted infection.

[a]For additional information and recommendations, see Centers for Disease Control and Prevention. Sexually transmitted diseases treatment guidelines, 2015. *MMWR Recomm Rep.* 2015;64(RR-3):1–137. Available at: **www.cdc.gov/std/treatment**

[b]If ceftriaxone is not feasible, may substitute cefixime, 400 mg, orally, in a single dose.

[c]In areas where *T vaginalis* is prevalent, males who have sex with females and have persistent or recurrent urethritis should be presumptively treated for *T vaginalis*.

[d]Alcohol consumption should be avoided during treatment with metronidazole or tinidazole; breastfeeding should be deferred for 72 hours after mother has received a 2-g dose of tinidazole.

[e]Treatment can be extended if healing is incomplete after 10 days of therapy.

[f]Avoid in pregnancy.

[g]Wash treatment area with soap and water 6–10 hours after application.

Adapted from Centers for Disease Control and Prevention. Sexually transmitted diseases treatment guidelines, 2015. *MMWR Recomm Rep.* 2015;64(RR-3):1–137.

Table 4.5. Guidelines for Treatment of Sexually Transmitted Infections in Infants and Children <45 kg According to Syndrome

Preferred regimens are listed. For further information concerning other acceptable regimens and diseases not included, see recommendations in disease-specific chapters in Section 3. In addition, recommendations on treatment of sexually transmitted infections have been issued by the Centers for Disease Control and Prevention in 2015[a] (**www.cdc. gov/std/treatment**).

Syndrome	Organisms/ Diagnoses	Treatment of Infants and Children <45 kg[a,b]
Urethritis: Inflammation of urethra with erythema and/or mucoid, mucopurulent, or purulent discharge Note: Cervicitis occurs rarely in prepubertal girls	*Neisseria gonorrhoeae, Chlamydia trachomatis* Other causes include *Mycoplasma genitalium,* possibly *Ureaplasma urealyticum,* and sometimes *Trichomonas vaginalis* and herpes simplex virus (HSV)	Ceftriaxone, 125 mg, IM, in a single dose[c] **PLUS EITHER** Erythromycin base or ethylsuccinate, 50 mg/kg per day, orally, in 4 divided doses (maximum 2 g/day) for 14 days **OR** Azithromycin, 60/mg/kg, orally in a single dose, maximum of 1 g[d]
Prepubertal vaginitis (STI related):	*N gonorrhoeae*	Ceftriaxone, 25–50 mg/kg, IV or IM, in a single dose, not to exceed 125 mg, IM, in a single dose[c]
	C trachomatis	Erythromycin base or ethylsuccinate, 50 mg/kg per day, orally, in 4 divided doses (maximum 2 g/day) for 14 days
	T vaginalis	Metronidazole, 45 mg/kg per day, orally, in 3 divided doses (maximum 2 g/day) for 7 days

Table 4.5. Guidelines for Treatment of Sexually Transmitted Infections in Infants and Children <45 kg According to Syndrome, continued

Syndrome	Organisms/ Diagnoses	Treatment of Infants and Children <45 kg[a,b]
	Bacterial vaginosis	Metronidazole, 45 mg/kg per day, orally, in 3 divided doses (maximum 2 g/day) for 7 days
Genital ulcer disease	T pallidum (primary syphilis)[e]	Benzathine penicillin G, 50 000 U/kg IM, up to the adult dose of 2.4 million U in a single dose
	HSV—1st clinical episode	Acyclovir, 80 mg/kg per day, orally, in 4 divided doses (maximum 3.2 g/day) for 7–10 days **OR** Valacyclovir, 40 mg/kg per day (maximum 2 g/day), orally, in 2 divided doses for 7–10 days
	Haemophilus ducreyi (chancroid)	Ceftriaxone, 50 mg/kg, IM, in a single dose (maximum 250 mg)[c] **OR** Azithromycin, 20 mg/kg, orally, in a single dose (maximum 1 g)
Anogenital warts	Human papillomavirus	Same as for adolescents. See Table 4.4.

IM indicates intramuscularly; STI, sexually transmitted infection.

[a]For additional information and recommendations, see Centers for Disease Control and Prevention. Sexually transmitted diseases treatment guidelines, 2015. *MMWR Morb Mortal Wkly Rep.* 2015;64(RR-3):1–137. Available at: **www.cdc.gov/std/treatment**

[b]Infants and children aged ≥1 month with a sexually transmitted infection should be evaluated for sexual abuse (eg, through consultation with child-protection services).

[c] If ceftriaxone is not feasible, may substitute cefixime, 8 mg/kg, up to 400 mg, orally, in a single dose, for a child weighing <45 kg, or 4 mg/kg x2 doses, every 12 hours, up to 400 mg. Providers treating patients with a severe cephalosporin allergy should consult an infectious disease specialist.

[d]Data are limited on the effectiveness and optimal dose of azithromycin for the treatment of chlamydial infection in infants and children who weigh <45 kg.

[e]Infants and children >1 mo of age who receive a diagnosis of syphilis should have birth and maternal medical records reviewed to assess whether they have congenital or acquired syphilis. Infants and children ≥1 mo of age with primary syphilis should be managed by a pediatric infectious disease specialist.

Table 4.6. Recommended Treatment Regimens for Vulvovaginal Candidiasis[a]

Over-the-Counter Intravaginal Agents[b]
Clotrimazole 1% cream, 5 g, intravaginally, for 7–14 days
OR
Clotrimazole 2% cream, 5 g, intravaginally, for 3 days
OR
Miconazole 2% cream, 5 g, intravaginally, for 7 days
OR
Miconazole 4% cream, 5 g, intravaginally, for 3 days
OR
Miconazole, 100-mg vaginal suppository, 1 suppository for 7 days
OR
Miconazole, 200-mg vaginal suppository, 1 suppository for 3 days
OR
Miconazole, 1200-mg vaginal suppository, 1 suppository for 1 day
OR
Tioconazole, 6.5% ointment, 5 g, intravaginally, in a single application
Prescription Intravaginal Agents[b]
Butoconazole 2% cream (single-dose bioadhesive product), 5 g intravaginally in a single
  application
OR
Terconazole 0.4% cream, 5 g, intravaginally, daily for 7 days
OR
Terconazole 0.8% cream, 5 g, intravaginally, for 3 days
OR
Terconazole, 80-mg vaginal suppository, 1 suppository for 3 days
Oral Agent
Fluconazole, 150-mg oral tablet, 1 tablet in single dose

[a]Adapted from the Centers for Disease Control and Prevention. Sexually transmitted diseases treatment guidelines, 2015. *MMWR Recomm Rep.* 2015;64(RR-3):1–137.
[b]These creams and suppositories are oil-based and might weaken latex condoms and diaphragms.

....

ANTIFUNGAL DRUGS FOR SYSTEMIC FUNGAL INFECTIONS

Polyenes

Amphotericin B is a fungicidal agent that is effective against a broad array of fungal species. Amphotericin B, especially the "conventional" deoxycholate formulation, is associated with multiple adverse reactions, particularly renal toxicity, so its use is limited in certain patients. Lipid-associated formulations of amphotericin B, especially liposomal amphotericin B, limit renal toxicity but also are associated with multiple other adverse effects and do not achieve optimal concentrations in some sites of infection (eg, kidneys).

Amphotericin B deoxycholate is the preferred formulation for treatment of neonates with systemic candidiasis because of better penetration into the central nervous system, urinary tract, and eye, which often are involved in neonatal *Candida* infections; lipid-associated formulations do not penetrate as well into these body sites. Amphotericin B deoxycholate is administered intravenously in a single daily dose of 1 mg/kg or up to 1.5 mg/kg when administered on alternate days (maximum, 1.5 mg/kg/day). Amphotericin B is administered in 5% dextrose in water at a concentration of 0.1 mg/mL and delivered through a central or peripheral venous catheter. Infusion times of 1 to 2 hours have been shown to be well tolerated in adults and older children and theoretically increase the blood-to-tissue gradient, thereby improving drug delivery. After completing 1 week of daily therapy, adequate serum concentrations of the drug usually can be maintained by administering 1.5 mg/kg on alternate days because of the long half-life. The total duration of therapy depends on the type and extent of the specific fungal infection.

Amphotericin B deoxycholate is eliminated by a renal mechanism for approximately 2 weeks after therapy is discontinued. No adjustment in dose is required for neonates or for children with impaired renal function, because serum concentrations are not increased significantly in these patients. If renal toxicity occurs, alternate-day dosing is preferred to a decrease in daily dose. Neither hemodialysis nor peritoneal dialysis significantly decreases serum concentrations of the drug.

Infusion-related reactions to amphotericin B deoxycholate include fever, chills, and sometimes nausea, vomiting, headache, generalized malaise, hypotension, and arrhythmias; these reactions are rare in neonates. Onset usually is within 1 to 3 hours after starting the infusion; duration typically is less than an hour. Hypotension and arrhythmias are idiosyncratic reactions that are unlikely to occur if not observed after the initial dose but also can occur in association with rapid infusion. Multiple regimens have been used to prevent infusion-related reactions, but few have been studied in controlled clinical trials. Pretreatment with acetaminophen, alone or combined with diphenhydramine, may alleviate febrile reactions; these reactions appear to be less common in children than in adults. Hydrocortisone (25–50 mg in adults and older children) also can be added to the infusion to decrease febrile and other systemic reactions. Tolerance to febrile reactions develops with time, allowing tapering and eventual discontinuation of the hydrocortisone and often diphenhydramine and antipyretic agents. Meperidine and ibuprofen have been effective in preventing or treating fever and chills in some patients who are refractory to the conventional premedication regimen.

Toxicity from amphotericin B deoxycholate can include nephrotoxicity, hepatotoxicity, anemia, or neurotoxicity. Nephrotoxicity is caused by decreased renal blood flow and can be prevented or ameliorated by hydration, saline solution loading (0.9% saline solution over 30 minutes) before infusion of amphotericin B, and avoidance of diuretic drugs. Hypokalemia is common and can be exacerbated by sodium loading. Renal tubular acidosis can occur but usually is mild. Permanent nephrotoxicity is related to cumulative dose. Nephrotoxicity is increased by concomitant administration of amphotericin B and aminoglycosides, cyclosporine, tacrolimus, cisplatin, nitrogen mustard compounds, or acetazolamide. Anemia is secondary to inhibition of erythropoietin production. Neurotoxicity occurs rarely and can manifest as confusion, delirium, obtundation, psychotic behavior, seizures, blurred vision, or hearing loss.

Lipid preparations of amphotericin B have a role in children who are intolerant of or refractory to amphotericin B deoxycholate or who have renal insufficiency or are at risk of significant renal toxicity from concomitant medications. Amphotericin B lipid formulations approved by the US Food and Drug Administration (FDA) for treatment of invasive fungal infections in children and adults who are refractory to or intolerant of amphotericin B deoxycholate therapy are amphotericin B lipid complex (ABLC, Abelcet) and liposomal amphotericin B (L-AmB, AmBisome). Acute infusion-related reactions occur with both formulations but are less frequent with AmBisome. Nephrotoxicity is less common with lipid-associated products than with amphotericin B deoxycholate. Liver toxicity, which generally is not associated with amphotericin B deoxycholate, has been reported with the lipid formulations.

Pyrimidines

Among pyrimidine antifungal agents, only flucytosine (5-fluorocytosine) is approved by the FDA for use in children. Flucytosine has a limited spectrum of activity against fungi (*Cryptococcus* and *Candida* species) and has potential for toxicity and should be avoided in the setting of renal dysfunction. When flucytosine is used as a single agent, resistance often emerges rapidly. Flucytosine can be used in combination with amphotericin B for cryptococcal meningitis. It is important to monitor serum concentrations of flucytosine to avoid bone marrow toxicity. Flucytosine is only available in oral formulation in the United States.

Azoles

Six oral azoles are available in the United States: ketoconazole, fluconazole, itraconazole, voriconazole, posaconazole, and isavuconazonium sulfate (the prodrug for isavuconazole). All have relatively broad activity against common fungi but differ in their in vitro activity (see Table 4.7, p 942), bioavailability, adverse effects, and potential for drug interactions. Fewer data are available regarding the safety and efficacy of azoles in pediatric than in adult patients, and trials comparing these agents with amphotericin B have been limited. Azoles are easy to administer and have little toxicity, but their use can be limited by the frequency of their interactions with coadministered drugs. These drug interactions can result in decreased serum concentrations of the azole (ie, poor therapeutic activity) or unexpected toxicity from the coadministered drug (caused by increased serum concentrations of the coadministered drug). When considering use of azoles, the patient's concurrent medications should be reviewed to avoid potential adverse clinical outcomes. Another potential limitation of azoles is emergence of resistant fungi, especially *Candida* species resistant to fluconazole. *Candida krusei* intrinsically are resistant to fluconazole, and strains of *Candida glabrata* increasingly are resistant to both fluconazole and voriconazole. Itraconazole is approved by the FDA for treatment of blastomycosis, histoplasmosis (nonmeningeal), and aspergillosis in patients who are intolerant to amphotericin B, and for empiric therapy of febrile neutropenic patients with suspected fungal infection. Itraconazole does not cross the blood-brain barrier and should not be used for infections of the central nervous system. Voriconazole has been approved by the FDA for primary treatment of invasive *Aspergillus* species, for candidemia in nonneutropenic patients, for esophageal candidiasis, and for refractory infection with *Fusarium* species and some *Scedosporium* species, such as *Scedosporium apiospermum*. Intravenous and oral formulations are available. Posaconazole is approved for use in adults for prophylaxis of invasive aspergillosis and candidiasis and treatment of oropharyngeal candidiasis. Intravenous and oral formulations are available, and strategies to enhance absorption are necessary (eg, administration with high-fat meal, avoidance of proton pump inhibitors) when using the oral suspension. Isavuconazole, available in oral and intravenous forms, has been approved by the FDA for patients 18 years or older for invasive aspergillosis and invasive mucormycosis. Keto-conazole seldom is used, because other azoles have fewer adverse effects and other agents provide better coverage for common pathogens. Therapeutic monitoring of azole drugs with measurement of serum trough concentrations is critical in patients with serious infections.

Echinocandins

Caspofungin, micafungin, and anidulafungin are the only echinocandins approved by the FDA. Caspofungin is approved for treatment of pediatric patients 3 months of age and older with esophageal candidiasis, empiric therapy for presumed fungal infections in febrile neutropenic patients, invasive candidiasis, and aspergillosis in adults who are refractory to or intolerant of other antifungal drugs. Clinical trials have demonstrated safety and efficacy in pediatric patients as young as 3 months of age; noncomparative anecdotal experience in neonatal infections also is reported. Micafungin is approved by the FDA for intravenous treatment of pediatric patients 4 months and older with candidemia, acute disseminated candidiasis, *Candida* peritonitis and abscesses, esophageal candidiasis and prophylaxis of invasive *Candida* infections in patients undergoing hematopoietic stem cell transplantation. Although micafungin is not FDA approved for aspergillosis, data are available to support its use in the treatment of refractory disease. Anidulafungin is not approved by the FDA for use in children but is FDA approved for the treatment of candidemia, *Candida* infections, and esophageal candidiasis in adults. Table 4.7 provides data on the relative in vitro susceptibilities of specific fungal species with amphotericin B, azoles, echinocandins, and flucytosine.

Table 4.7. Fungal Species, Antifungal Drugs, Activity, Route, Clearance, CSF Penetration, Drug Monitoring Targets, and Adverse Events

Fungal Species	Amphotericin B Formulations	Fluconazole	Itraconazole	Voriconazole	Posaconazole	Isavuconazole	Flucytosine	Echinocandins[a]
Candida albicans	+	++	+	++	+	+/-	+	++
Candida tropicalis	+	++	+	++	+	+/-	+	++
Candida parapsilosis	++	++	+	++	+	+/-	+	+
Candida glabrata	+	-	-	-	+/-	+/-	+	+/-
Candida krusei	+	-	-	+	+	+/-	+	++
Candida lusitaniae	-	++	+	++	+	+/-	+	+
Candida guilliermondii	+	+	+	+	+	+/-	+	+/-
Candida auris	+/-	-	+/-	+/-	+	+/-	+/-	++
Cryptococcus species	++	++	+	+	+	+	++	-
Trichosporon species	+	+	+	++	+	+	-	-
Aspergillus fumigatus[b]	+	-	+	++	+	++	-	+
Aspergillus terreus[b]	-	-	+	++	+	++	-	+
Aspergillus calidoustus[b]	++	-	-	-	-		-	++
Fusarium species[b]	+	-	-	++	+	+	-	-
Mucor species[b]	++	-	+/-	-	+	+	-	-
Rhizopus species[b]	++	-	-	-	+	+	-	-
Scedosporium apiospermum[b]	-	-	+	++	+	+	-	-
Scedosporium prolificans[b]	-	-	+/-	+/-	+/-	+/-	-	-
Penicillium (Talaromyces) species[b]	+/-	-	++	+	+	+	-	-

Table 4.7. Fungal Species, Antifungal Drugs, Activity, Route, Clearance, CSF Penetration, Drug Monitoring Targets, and Adverse Events, continued

Fungal Species	Amphotericin B Formulations	Fluconazole	Itraconazole	Voriconazole	Posaconazole	Isavuconazole	Flucytosine	Echinocandins[a]
Histoplasma capsulatum[c]	++	+	++	+	+	+	–	–
Coccidioides immitis[c]	++	++	++	+	+	+	–	–
Blastomyces dermatitidis[c]	++	+	++	+	+	+	–	–
Paracoccidioides species[c]	+	+	++	+	+	+	–	–
Sporothrix species[c]	+	+	++	+	+	+	–	–
IV/PO	IV only	IV and PO	PO only	IV and PO	IV and PO	IV and PO[b]	PO only	IV only
Clearance	Renal	Renal/hepatic	Hepatic	Hepatic	Hepatic	Hepatic	Renal	Hepatic (micafungin)
CSF penetration	Good	Good	Limited	Good	Minimal	Good	Good	Minimal
Therapeutic drug monitoring (treatment)	No	No	Trough 1–2 µg/mL (when measured by high-pressure liquid chromatography, both itraconazole and its bioactive hydroxy-itraconazole metabolite are reported, the sum of which should be considered in assessing drug levels)	Trough 2–6 µg/mL	Trough >0.7 µg/mL; higher rate of adverse effects when trough levels exceed 1 µg/mL	Unknown	Peak 40–80 µg/mL	No

Table 4.7. Fungal Species, Antifungal Drugs, Activity, Route, Clearance, CSF Penetration, Drug Monitoring Targets, and Adverse Events, continued

Fungal Species	Amphotericin B Formulations	Flucona-zole	Itraconazole	Voriconazole	Posacona-zole	Isavucon-azole	Flucyto-sine	Echi-nocandins[a]
Common adverse reactions	Infusion reaction, nephrotoxicity (watch potassium, magnesium); liposomal: hepatoxicity	Hepatotoxicity, increased QTc, headache, gastrointestinal tract effects	Hepatotoxicity, increased QTc; negative inotrope (avoid in congestive heart failure)	Hepatotoxicity, increased QTc, central nervous system effects, vision changes, phototoxicity	Hepatotoxicity, increased QTc, headache, gastrointestinal tract effects	Abdominal pain, nausea, diarrhea, conjunctivitis, flu-like illness	Neutropenia, hepatotoxicity (avoid in decreased renal function), gastrointestinal	Usually well tolerated; gastrointestinal tract effects, headache, hepatotoxicity

CSF, cerebrospinal fluid; IV, intravenous; PO, oral.

NOTE: ++, more active, scenario dependent; +, usually active; +/−, variably active; −, usually not active.

[a] Caspofungin, anidulafungin, and micafungin.

[b] Mold.

[c] Endemic fungi where mold/yeast phase is temperature-dependent.

RECOMMENDED DOSES OF PARENTERAL AND ORAL ANTIFUNGAL DRUGS

Table 4.8. Recommended Doses of Parenteral and Oral Antifungal Drugs

Drug	Route	Dose (per day)	Adverse Reactions[a,b]
Amphotericin B deoxycholate (see Antifungal Drugs for Systemic Fungal Infections, p 938, for detailed information)	IV	1.0–1.5 mg/kg per day; infuse as a single dose over 2–4 h.	Fever, chills, phlebitis, gastrointestinal tract symptoms, headache, hypotension, renal dysfunction, hypokalemia, anemia, cardiac arrhythmias, neurotoxicity, anaphylaxis.
	IT	0.025 mg, slow increase to 0.5 mg, twice/wk.	Headache, gastrointestinal tract symptoms, arachnoiditis/radiculitis.
Amphotericin B lipid complex (Abelcet)[c]	IV	3–5 mg/kg per day, infused over 2 h.	Fever, chills, other reactions associated with amphotericin B deoxycholate, but less nephrotoxicity; hepatotoxicity has been reported with lipid complex.
Liposomal amphotericin B (AmBisome)[c]	IV	3–5 mg/kg, infused over 1–2 h. IFI prophylaxis*: 1 mg/kg/dose every other day or 2.5 mg/kg/dose twice/wk.	Fever, chills, less infusion reactions and nephrotoxicity than associated with amphotericin B deoxycholate; hepatotoxicity has been reported.
Anidulafungin[c,d]	IV	For adults and adolescents 13 y and older: Candidemia and other forms of *Candida* infections: 200 mg on day 1, followed by 100-mg daily dose thereafter for at least 14 days after the last positive culture. Esophageal candidiasis: 100 mg on day 1, followed by 50-mg daily dose thereafter for a minimum of 14 days and for at least 7 days following resolution of symptoms. The rate of infusion should not exceed 1.1 mg/minute.	Fever, headache, nausea, vomiting, diarrhea, leukopenia, hypokalemia, hepatitis, hepatic enzyme elevations, hypersensitivity, and phlebitis.

Table 4.8. Recommended Doses of Parenteral and Oral Antifungal Drugs, continued

Drug	Route	Dose (per day)	Adverse Reactions[a,b]
Caspofungin[e]	IV	Dosage in adults (18 y and older): 70 mg loading dose on day 1, followed by 50 mg once daily for all indications except esophageal candidiasis. For esophageal candidiasis, 50 mg once daily without loading dose. Dosage in pediatric patients (3 months through 17 y of age): For all indications, 70 mg/m^2 loading dose on day 1, followed by 50 mg/m^2 once daily thereafter. Maximum loading dose and daily maintenance dose should not exceed 70 mg, regardless of the patient's calculated dose. Dose adjustment is needed for patients with severe hepatic impairment and in patients receiving concomitant inducers of hepatic CYP enzymes.	Adults: Diarrhea, pyrexia, hepatic enzymes elevations, and hypokalemia. Pediatric: Pyrexia, diarrhea, rash, hepatic enzymes elevations, hypokalemia, hypotension, and chills. Isolated cases of hepatic dysfunction, hepatitis, or hepatic failure have been reported.
Clotrimazole	PO	10-mg lozenge, 5 times per day (dissolved slowly in mouth).	Gastrointestinal tract symptoms, hepatotoxicity.

Table 4.8. Recommended Doses of Parenteral and Oral Antifungal Drugs, continued

Drug	Route	Dose (per day)	Adverse Reactions[a,b]
Fluconazole[f]	IV, PO	Oropharyngeal candidiasis: 6 mg/kg (adult dose: 200 mg) on the first day, followed by 3–6 mg/kg (adult dose: 100 mg) once daily. Treatment should be given for at least 2 wk to decrease the likelihood of relapse. Esophageal candidiasis: 6 mg/kg (adult dose: 200 mg) on the first day, followed by 6 mg/kg (adult dose: 100 mg) once daily. Doses up to 12 mg/kg/day may be used, based on medical judgment of the patient's response to therapy. Treatment for a minimum of 3 wk and for at least 2 wk following the resolution of symptoms. Systemic *Candida* infections: 12 mg/kg/day. Cryptococcal meningitis (children): Following induction therapy with amphotericin B plus flucytosine for 2–6 wk, initiate consolidation therapy with fluconazole 12 mg/kg in 2 divided doses (maximum 800 mg) once daily. Duration of fluconazole consolidation treatment is a minimum of 8 wk after the CSF becomes culture negative; for suppression of relapse in children with AIDS, use 6 mg/kg once daily. Cryptococcal meningitis (adults): 400 mg on the first day, followed by 200 mg once daily. A dosage of 400 mg once daily may be used, based on medical judgment of the patient's response to therapy. The recommended duration of fluconazole consolidation treatment is a minimum of 8 wk after the CSF fluid becomes culture negative; 200 mg once daily is used for suppression of relapse of cryptococcal meningitis in patients with AIDS. Prophylaxis in patients undergoing bone marrow transplantation: 400 mg, once daily.	Rash, gastrointestinal tract symptoms, hepatotoxicity, Stevens-Johnson syndrome, anaphylaxis.

Table 4.8. Recommended Doses of Parenteral and Oral Antifungal Drugs, continued

Drug	Route	Dose (per day)	Adverse Reactions[a,b]
Flucytosine	PO	100 mg/kg/day divided dosing every 6 h (adjust dose for renal dysfunction and neonatal age); follow 2-h post peak levels closely (therapeutic range 25–100 µg/mL).	Bone marrow suppression, hepatotoxicity, renal dysfunction, gastrointestinal tract symptoms, rash, neuropathy, confusion, hallucinations. Cytosine arabinoside, a cytostatic agent, has been reported to inactivate the antifungal activity of flucytosine by competitive inhibition; drugs that impair glomerular filtration may prolong the biological half-life of flucytosine. The hematologic parameters should be monitored frequently; liver and kidney function should be carefully monitored during therapy. Flucytosine should be used in combination with amphotericin B for the treatment of cryptococcosis because of the emergence of resistance to flucytosine.
Griseofulvin	PO	Ultramicrosize: 10–15 mg/kg, single dose; maximum dose, 750 mg. Microsize: 20–25 mg/kg per day divided in 2 doses; maximum dose, 1000 mg.	Rash, paresthesias, leukopenia, gastrointestinal tract symptoms, proteinuria, hepatotoxicity, mental confusion, headache.

Table 4.8. Recommended Doses of Parenteral and Oral Antifungal Drugs, continued

Drug	Route	Dose (per day)	Adverse Reactions[a,b]
Isavuconazole (prodrug is isavuconazonium sulfate)[g]	IV, PO	Adults: 200 mg, every 8 h for 6 doses, then 200 mg, once daily (corresponding to 372 mg of the sulfate compound every 8 h for 6 doses, then 372 mg daily), starting 12 to 24 h after the last loading dose. Pediatrics: No data or dosage regimen available.	Most frequent adverse reactions are nausea, vomiting, diarrhea, headache, elevated transaminases, hypokalemia, constipation, dyspnea, cough, peripheral edema, and back pain. CYP3A4 inhibitors or inducers may alter the plasma concentrations of isavuconazole. Appropriate therapeutic drug monitoring and dose adjustment of immunosuppressants (ie, tacrolimus, sirolimus, and cyclosporine) may be necessary when coadministered with isavuconazole. Drugs with a narrow therapeutic window that are P-gp substrates, such as digoxin, may require dose adjustment coadministered concomitantly with isavuconazole.

Table 4.8. Recommended Doses of Parenteral and Oral Antifungal Drugs, continued

Drug	Route	Dose (per day)	Adverse Reactions[a,b]
Itraconazole[e]	IV, PO	Children: 10 mg/kg per day divided into 2 doses; acid stomach pH for better absorption; oral solution supplies more reliable bioavailability; confirm therapeutic trough level after several days of therapy to ensure adequate drug exposure (1–2 µg/mL; when measured by high-pressure liquid chromatography, both itraconazole and its bioactive hydroxy-itraconazole metabolite are reported, the sum of which should be considered in assessing drug levels); IFI prophylaxis[e]: 2.5 mg/kg twice a day, with minimum therapeutic level of 0.5 µg/mL. Adults: 200–400 mg/day once or twice a day for treatment of blastomycosis, histoplasmosis, and aspergillosis; 100–200 mg once daily for oropharyngeal and esophageal candidiasis.	Gastrointestinal tract symptoms, rash, edema, headache, hypokalemia, hepatotoxicity, tremor, thrombocytopenia, leukopenia, systolic hypotension with IV administration in critically ill children; strong P450 CYP3A4 inhibitor; can heighten risk of QT prolongation via metabolism interference with drugs having that adverse effect.
Ketoconazole[e]	PO	Children[h]: 3.3–6.6 mg/kg per day, single dose (maximum 400 mg). Adults: 200 mg, twice a day for 4 doses, then 200 mg, once a day.	Hepatotoxicity, gastrointestinal tract symptoms, rash, anaphylaxis, thrombocytopenia, hemolytic anemia, gynecomastia, adrenal insufficiency; cardiac toxicity is possible in patients also taking terfenadine or astemizole.

Table 4.8. Recommended Doses of Parenteral and Oral Antifungal Drugs, continued

Drug	Route	Dose (per day)	Adverse Reactions[a,b]
Micafungin[c]	IV	Adults: 100 mg daily for treatment of candidemia, acute disseminated candidiasis, candida peritonitis and abscesses; 150 mg daily for esophageal candidiasis; and 50 mg daily for prophylaxis of candida infections in HSCT recipients. Pediatric: 2 mg/kg/day (maximum 100 mg daily) for candidemia, and acute disseminated candidiasis; 1 mg/kg/day (maximum 50 mg daily) for prophylaxis of *Candida* infections; for treatment of esophageal candidiasis, 3 mg/kg/day is used for children ≤30 kg and 2.5 mg/kg/day with a maximum 150 mg daily is used for children ≥30 kg; neonatal dosing is 10 mg/kg/day.	Fever, headache, nausea, vomiting, diarrhea, rash, leukopenia, thrombocytopenia, hepatic enzyme elevations (greater risk at doses >4 mg/kg), hypokalemia, and phlebitis; histamine-mediated symptoms including rash, pruritus, facial swelling, and vasodilatation can occur.
Nystatin	PO	Infants: 200 000 U, 4 times a day, after meals. Children and adults: 400 000–600 000 U, 3 times a day, after meals.	Gastrointestinal tract symptoms, rash.

Table 4.8. Recommended Doses of Parenteral and Oral Antifungal Drugs, continued

Drug	Route	Dose (per day)	Adverse Reactions[a,b]
Posaconazole[e]	PO, IV[i]	Adults and adolescents[j]: for IFI prophylaxis[e] and *Candida* infections: IV formulation is approved only for use in patients 18 y or older. 300 mg IV twice a day on first day, followed by 300 mg IV once daily starting on second day. Oral suspension and delayed-release tablets can be used in the age group 13 y and older; 300-mg delayed-release tablets twice a day on the first day followed by 300 mg once daily, starting on second day; 200-mg (5-mL) oral solution 3 times a day; duration of therapy for both IV and oral is based on recovery from neutropenia or immunosuppression; tablet and liquid forms are not interchangeable given bioavailability and dosing differences. For oropharyngeal candidiasis: oral suspension 100 mg (2.5 mL) twice a day on first day followed by 100 mg once daily for 13 days. For oropharyngeal candidiasis refractory to Itraconazole and/or fluconazole: oral suspension 400 mg (10 mL) twice a day; duration of therapy is based on the severity of the patient's underlying disease and clinical response. Children: Non–FDA-approved labeling used by St. Jude's Children's Research Hospital suggested treatment dose range in those weighing <34 kg is 18–24 mg/kg/day and in those weighing ≥34 kg is 800 mg/day, all divided into 4 doses; minimum target trough concentrations for efficacy of 0.7 μg/mL, progressing to ≥1.25 μg/mL if poor response; IFI prophylaxis[e]: 4 mg/kg/dose (max 200 mg) 3 times daily with target trough ≥0.7 μg/mL (patients with GVHD may achieve lower levels); large variability in resultant trough levels particularly in children <12 y of age.	Diarrhea, nausea, fever, vomiting, headache, coughing, hypokalemia, rash, edema, headache, anemia, neutropenia, thrombocytopenia, fatigue, thrombophlebitis, arthralgia, myalgia, fever; interactions with P450 CYP3A4 substrate drugs and can potentiate QT prolongation; posaconazole injection should be avoided in patients with moderate or severe renal impairment (creatinine clearance <50 mL/min), higher rate of adverse effects when trough levels exceed 1 μg/mL.

Table 4.8. Recommended Doses of Parenteral and Oral Antifungal Drugs, continued

Drug	Route	Dose (per day)	Adverse Reactions[a,b]
Terbinafine	PO	Children: once daily dosing Onychomycosis: 10–20 kg: 62.5 mg/day; 21–40 kg: 125 mg/day; >40 kg: 250 mg/day; treatment course of 12 wk for toenails, 6 wk for fingernails. Tinea capitis: <25 kg: 125 mg/day, 25–35 kg: 187.5 mg/day; >35 kg: 250 mg once daily; treatment course of 6 wk. Adults: 250 mg, once daily.	Common adverse events include headache, diarrhea, rash, dyspepsia, liver enzyme abnormalities, pruritus, taste disturbance, nausea, abdominal pain, and flatulence; liver failure, sometimes leading to liver transplant or death, has been reported with the use of oral terbinafine. Terbinafine is an inhibitor of CYP450 2D6 isozyme and has an effect on metabolism of desipramine. Drug interactions with cimetidine, fluconazole, cyclosporine, rifampin, and caffeine have also been reported.

Table 4.8. Recommended Doses of Parenteral and Oral Antifungal Drugs, continued

Drug	Route	Dose (per day)	Adverse Reactions[a,b]
Voricona-zole[c,k]	IV	FDA-approved dosage regimen in adolescents is 6 mg/kg/dose, IV, every 12 h on day 1, followed by 4 mg/kg/dose, IV, every 12 h; however, recommendations for higher doses in immunosuppressed patients is based on need to achieve trough levels commensurate with clinical response. Limited safety and efficacy data in pediatric patients <12 y. Treatment or IFI prophylaxis[e] in children: if 2–<12 y of age or 12–14 y of age and weight <50 kg: 9 mg/kg, IV, twice daily on day 1 of treatment; thereafter 8 mg/kg, IV, twice daily or 9 mg/kg, PO, twice daily; if ≥15 y of age or 12–14 y of age and weight ≥50 kg: 6 mg/kg, IV, on day 1 of treatment; thereafter 4 mg/kg, IV, twice daily or 200 mg, PO, twice daily; therapeutic drug monitoring is needed to ensure trough levels 2–6 μg/mL. A simpler proposed oral regimen for IFI prophylaxis[e]: 200 mg, PO, twice daily if weight is ≥40 kg and 100 mg, PO, twice daily if weight is <40 kg; if IV needed, then 4 mg/kg every 12 h is administered.	Concentration- or dose-related toxicities: hepatic toxicity, arrhythmias/QT prolongation, dermatologic reactions, visual disturbance, hallucinations, increased liver enzymes and bilirubin, encephalopathy; phototoxicity, rash; cutaneous squamous cell carcinoma associated with prolonged voriconazole use in lung transplant patients; there have been postmarketing reports of pancreatitis in pediatric patients; drug interactions or genetic polymorphisms involving P450 CYP2C19 can markedly alter voriconazole pharmacokinetics and enhance toxicity risk; pharmacogenetic testing may lead to optimized dosing earlier in the treatment course.

CYP indicates cytochrome P; GVDH, graft versus host disease; IFI, Invasive fungal infection; IT, intrathecal; IV, intravenous; PO, oral.

[a] See package insert or listing in current edition of the *Physicians' Desk Reference* or **www.pdr.net** (for registered users only).

[b] Interactions with other drugs are common. Consult **www.fda.gov/Drugs/DevelopmentApprovalProcess/DevelopmentResources/ DrugInteractionsLabeling/default.htm?utm_campaign=Google2&utm_source=fdaSearch&utm_medium=website&utm_term= drug%20interactions&utm_content=1** and the *Physicians' Desk Reference* (a drug interaction reference or database) or a pharmacist before prescribing these medications.

[c] Limited or no information about use in newborn infants is available.

[d] Safety and effectiveness of anidulafungin in patients ≤16 years old has not been established.

[e] Invasive fungal infection prophylaxis in at-risk pediatric patients with immunosuppression attributable to cancer or hematopoietic stem cell transplant.

[f] Experience with fluconazole in neonates is limited to pharmacokinetic studies in preterm newborn infants. Based on the prolonged half-life seen in preterm newborn infants (gestational age 26 to 29 weeks), these children, in the first 2 weeks of life, should receive the same dosage (mg/kg) as in older children, but administered every 72 hours. After the first 2 weeks, these children should be dosed once daily.

[g] Safety and effectiveness of isavuconazole in patients younger than 12 years have not been established.

[h] For children 2 years and younger, the daily dose of ketoconazole has not been established.

[i] IV formulation of posaconazole is recommended only for 18 years or older. For systemic *Candida* infections including candidemia, disseminated candidiasis, and pneumonia, optimal therapeutic dosage and duration of therapy have not been established. In open, noncomparative studies of small numbers patients, doses of up to 400 mg daily have been used.

[j] Safety and effectiveness of posaconazole have been established in the age groups 13 years and older.

[k] Voriconazole has now been identified as an independent risk factor for development of cutaneous malignancies in lung transplant patients.

Table 4.9. Topical Drugs for Superficial Fungal Infections

TOPICAL DRUGS FOR SUPERFICIAL FUNGAL INFECTIONS

Drug	Strength	Formula-tion	Trade Name Examples	Application(s) per Day	Adverse Reactions/Notes
Amorolfine HCl (OTC)	5%	NL	Loceryl; Cura-nail; Locetar; Odenil; Omicur	1–2 weekly (mild ony-chomycosis)	Well tolerated; minor local; not FDA approved.
Basic fuchsin, phenol, resor-cinol, and ace-tone (Rx)		S	Castellani Paint Modified	1	Excellent for intertriginous areas. Stains everything. Also available as a colorless solution with alcohol and without basic fuchsin. This is an alternative if the patient cannot tolerate other topical antifungals. Not FDA approved. Must be compounded.
Butenafine HCl (Rx and OTC)	1%	C	Mentax; Lotri-min Ultra	1–2, typically for 2 wk; Lotrimin Ultra may be used 2/day for 1 wk or 1/day for 4 wk	Safety and efficacy in patients young-er than 12 y of age have not been established. Do not occlude. Sensi-tivity to allylamines. Not to be used on scalp or nails.

Table 4.9. Topical Drugs for Superficial Fungal Infections, continued

Drug	Strength	Formulation	Trade Name Examples	Application(s) per Day	Adverse Reactions/Notes
Ciclopirox olamine (Rx)	0.77%	C, L, S, P, G, NL	Loprox; Penlac nail lacquer; Ciclodan	2	Irritant dermatitis, hair discoloration; shake lotion vigorously before application; safety and efficacy in children younger than 10 y of age have not been established. Precautions: diabetes mellitus; immune compromise; seizures. Do not occlude.
Clioquinol (Rx and OTC)		C, O (F available in Canada)	Vioform	2–4/day for 2–8 wk; 2 wk (tinea cruris)	Irritant dermatitis. Can stain skin, hair, nails, and clothing yellow in color.
Clotrimazole (Rx and OTC)	1%	C, L, S, P, Com, SpP, SpL; check with pharmacist	Topical solution (more than 10 preparations); Lotrimin, Mycelex, Desenex, Cruex, FungiCURE, Fungoid, Pedesil, Trivagizole, Femcare	1 (Rx) 2 (OTC) for 2–4 wk	Irritant dermatitis. Avoid topical steroid combinations.[a]

Table 4.9. Topical Drugs for Superficial Fungal Infections, continued

Drug	Strength	Formulation	Trade Name Examples	Application(s) per Day	Adverse Reactions/Notes
Clotrimazole and betamethasone dipropionate (Rx)	1%/0.05%	C, L	Lotrim and Fungizid spray; Lotrisone[b]	2[a]	Irritant dermatitis: Not generally intended for patients younger than 17 y or for diaper dermatitis. In 2 studies in pediatric subjects, 39.5% of tinea pedis patients and 47.1% of tinea cruris patients demonstrated adrenal suppression as determined by cosyntropin testing. If used in the groin area, patients should use medication for 2 wk only and use sparingly. Do not occlude. Contraindication: avoid steroid in varicella.
Econazole nitrate (Rx)	1%	C, L, P, S, F	Spectazole, Pevaryl-Ecreme	1 (dermatophyte) 2 (candidiasis)	Irritant dermatitis; safety and efficacy in children have not been established.
Efinaconazole (Rx)	10%	S	Jublia	1, for 48 wk (*Trichophyton rubrum* and *Trichophyton mentagrophytes*)	Application site dermatitis; application site vesicles; application site pain. Safety and efficacy have not been established in children.

Table 4.9. Topical Drugs for Superficial Fungal Infections, continued

Drug	Strength	Formulation	Trade Name Examples	Application(s) per Day	Adverse Reactions/Notes
Iodoquinol and 2% hydrocortisone acetate (Rx)	1%	G	Alcortin A	3–4	Burning/itching sensation. Local allergic reaction. Can stain skin and clothes. Can interfere with results of thyroid function tests. Not to be used under occlusion in the diaper area. Not intended for use on infants. Not FDA approved.
Iodoquinol and 1% aloe polysaccharides (Rx)	1.25%	G	Aloquin	3–4	Can interfere with thyroid function tests. False-positive ferric chloride test (used for PKU) if present in the diaper or urine. Discoloration of skin, hair, and fabric, which can be removed with normal cleansing. Not intended for use on infants, under occlusions or in the diaper area. Safety and efficacy in pediatric patients younger than 12 y not established. Not FDA approved.

Table 4.9. Topical Drugs for Superficial Fungal Infections, continued

Drug	Strength	Formulation	Trade Name Examples	Application(s) per Day	Adverse Reactions/Notes
Ketoconazole (Rx and OTC)	1%, 2%	C, Sh, G, F, S	Nizoral, Nizoral AD, Sebizol, Ex-Xolegel, Ex-tina, Ketodan, KetoKuric, Keto-derm	1 (tinea dermato-phyte) for 2–6 wk 2 (candidiasis) Once to treat (Rx S) Every 3–4 days (OTC S)	Potential sulfite reaction with anaphylactic or asthmatic reaction; shampoo can cause dry or oily hair and increase hair loss; irritant dermatitis. May interfere with permanent waving or changes in hair texture. Intended for patients 12 y and older; safety and efficacy not established for younger than 12 y. Foam must not be applied directly to hands, but onto a cool surface and applied using fingertips. OTC shampoo may be used for up to 8 wk to treat, and then used as needed to control dandruff.
Miconazole nitrate (Rx and OTC)	2%	O, C, P, S, SpP, SpL; check with pharmacist[c]	More than 10 preparations; Monistat-Derm, Zeasorb AF, Micatin, Daktarin tinc-ture	2 (seborrhea), apply 2–3 times/day for several months 2 (C, L) 2 (P, L) 1 (Pityriasis versicolor)	Irritant and allergic contact dermatitis. Generally not recommended for children younger than 2 y.

Table 4.9. Topical Drugs for Superficial Fungal Infections, continued

Drug	Strength	Formulation	Trade Name Examples	Application(s) per Day	Adverse Reactions/Notes
Miconazole nitrate and 15% Zinc oxide (Rx)	0.25%	O	Vusion	Every diaper change for 1 wk	Skin irritation. Can be used in children 4 wk and older. Do not routinely use for more than 7 days. Do not use in infants or children who do not have a normal immune system.
Naftifine HCl (Rx)	1%, 2% gel	C, G	Naftin	1 (C) 1–2 (Gel) for 2 wk	Burning/stinging, irritant dermatitis. Safety and efficacy in children have not been established. Do not occlude.
Nystatin (Rx and OTC	100 000 U/mL or 100 000 U/g	C, P, O, Com	Nystatin, Nystop powder, Pedi-Dri powder, Mycostatin, Nyamyc	2 (C) 2–3 (P)	Nontoxic except with topical steroid combinations.[d]

Table 4.9. Topical Drugs for Superficial Fungal Infections, continued

Drug	Strength	Formulation	Trade Name Examples	Application(s) per Day	Adverse Reactions/Notes
Nystatin and triamcinolone acetonide (Rx)	100 000 USP nystatin and 1 mg triamcinolone acetonide	C, O	Mytrex cream, Mytrex ointment, Mycolog-II, Mycogen II	2	Pediatric patients may demonstrate greater susceptibility to topical corticosteroid-induced hypothalamic-pituitary-adrenal (HPA) axis suppression and Cushing syndrome than mature patients because of a larger ratio of skin surface area to body weight. Contraindications: Hypersensitivity to component drug. Avoid steroid use in varicella or vaccinia. Do not occlude. Use lowest effective dose. Do not routinely use for more than 2 wk.
Oxiconazole (Rx)	1%	C, L	Oxistat	1–2 (tinea dermatophyte)	Pruritus, burning, irritant dermatitis. Do not occlude.
Sertaconazole nitrate (Rx)	2%	C	Ertaczo	2 for 4 wk	Dry skin, skin tenderness, contact dermatitis, local hypersensitivity. Safety and efficacy in children younger than 12 y have not been established.
Sulconazole (Rx)	1%	C, S	Exelderm	1–2 (tinea versicolor) 2 (tinea pedis)	Irritant dermatitis. Safety and efficacy in children have not been established.

Table 4.9. Topical Drugs for Superficial Fungal Infections, continued

Drug	Strength	Formulation	Trade Name Examples	Application(s) per Day	Adverse Reactions/Notes
Tavaborole (Rx)	5%	S	Kerydin	1, for 48 wk (*Trichophyton rubrum* and *Trichophyton mentagrophytes*)	Application site exfoliation; application site erythema; application site dermatitis. Safety and efficacy have not been established in children.
Terbinafine (Rx and OTC)	1%	C, G, S, Sp	Lamisil, Lamisil AT	1–2	Irritant dermatitis. Avoid use of occlusive clothing or dressings. Do not apply spray to face. Safety and efficacy in children younger than 12 y have not been established.
Tolnaftate (OTC)	1%	C, P, S, G, SpP, SpL; check with pharmacist[e]	>10 preparations; Tinactin, Fungicure	1–2	Irritant and allergic contact dermatitis. Not recommended if younger than 2 y of age.
Undecylenic acid and derivatives (OTC)	8%–25%	C, O, S, F, SpP, P, soap (See pharmacist for formulations and applications[e])	Blis-To-Sol; Caldesene; Cruex	2 (tincture); spray 1–2 sec	Irritant dermatitis. Generally not recommended for children younger than 2 y.

Table 4.9. Topical Drugs for Superficial Fungal Infections, continued

Drug	Strength	Formulation	Trade Name Examples	Application(s) per Day	Adverse Reactions/Notes
Undecylenic acid and chloroxylenol	25% 3%	S	Gordochom solution	2 for 4 wk	Local hypersensitivity. Generally not recommended for children younger than 2 y. Not effective on scalp or nails.
Other Remedies					
Benzoic acid and salicylic acid (OTC)	12%	O	Whitfields Ointment, Bensal HP	2	Warm, burning sensation. Avoid eyes, mouth, and nose. Keep out of the reach of children. Safety and efficacy in children not established. Not FDA approved.
Gentian violet (OTC)	2%	S	…	1–3 for 3 days	Staining. Keep out of the reach of children. Safety and efficacy in children not established. OTC monograph not final.

Table 4.9. Topical Drugs for Superficial Fungal Infections, continued

Drug	Strength	Formulation	Trade Name Examples	Application(s) per Day	Adverse Reactions/Notes
Selenium sulfide (Rx and OTC)	2.5%	Sh, L	Selsun 2.5%	Use twice weekly for 2 wk (Sh) 1 for 7 days (L)	Irritant dermatitis and ulceration. For tinea capitis, to decrease spore formation and to decrease the potential spread of the dermatophyte. Hair loss, discoloration of hair, oiliness or dryness of scalp. Safety and efficacy in children not established. May damage jewelry. Not to be used when inflammation or exudation is present.
	1%	Sh, L	Head & Shoulders, Selsun Blue	Use twice weekly for at least 2 wk	For tinea capitis, to decrease spore formation and to decrease the potential spread of the dermatophyte.
Sodium thiosulfate		L	Versiclear Lotion	2	Safety and effectiveness in children younger than 12 y has not been established.

OTC indicates over the counter; NL, nail lacquer; FDA, US Food and Drug Administration; Rx, prescription; S, solution; C, cream; L, lotion; P, powder; G, gel; O, ointment; F, foam; Com, combinations; SpP, spray powder; SpL, spray lotion; PKU, phenylketonuria; Sh, shampoo; Sp, spray.

ᵃTopical steroids must be used with caution in young children and in areas of thin skin (eg, diaper area). In these circumstances, high systemic exposure may occur, resulting in endogenous synthesis suppression with the potential for serious adverse effects. Potential adverse effects include irritant dermatitis, folliculitis, hypertrichosis, acneform eruptions, hypopigmentation, perioral dermatitis, allergic contact dermatitis, maceration, secondary infection, skin atrophy, striae, and miliaria.

ᵇLotrisone cream no longer is available; lotion is available.

ᶜPharmacists are an excellent resource to verify formulations that are available and new (they use *Facts and Comparisons* reference products).

ᵈAny topical preparation has the potential to irritate the skin and cause itching, burning, stinging, erythema, edema, vesicles, and blister formation.

For more information on individual drugs, see *Physician's Desk Reference* or **www.pdr.net** (for registered users only).

NON-HIV ANTIVIRAL DRUGS

Table 4.10. Non-HIV Antiviral Drugs[a]

Generic (Trade Name)	Indication	Route	Age	Usually Recommended Dosage
Acyclovir[b,c,d,e] (Zovirax)	Neonatal herpes simplex virus (HSV) infection	IV	Birth to ≤4 mo	Treatment dosing: 60 mg/kg per day, in 3 divided doses for 14–21 days (durations >21 days are necessary if CSF PCR remains positive near end of treatment course)
		Oral	2 wk to 8 mo	Oral suppressive dosing following completion of IV treatment; dosing: 300 mg/m², 3 times per day for 6 mo
	HSV encephalitis	IV	>4 mo to 12 y	30–45 mg/kg per day, in 3 divided doses for 14–21 days; FDA-approved dose of 60 mg/kg per day for this age range and indication is not recommended, as risk of acute kidney injury may increase at incremental doses exceeding 500 mg/m² or 15 mg/kg; dosing per m² causes excessive weight-based dosing in younger children[f]; concomitant ceftriaxone may enhance nephrotoxicity risk; neurotoxicity (agitation, myoclonus, delirium, altered consciousness, etc) can occur with accumulated high acyclovir levels, often a result of renal dysfunction and unadjusted dosage

Table 4.10. Non-HIV Antiviral Drugs,ᵃ continued

Generic (Trade Name)	Indication	Route	Age	Usually Recommended Dosage
		IV	≥12 y	30 mg/kg per day, in 3 divided doses for 14–21 days
	Varicella in immunocompetent hostᵍ	Oral	≥2 y	≤40 kg: 80 mg/kg per day, in 4 divided doses for 5 days; maximum daily dose, 3200 mg/day >40 kg: 3200 mg, in 4 divided doses for 5 days
	Varicella in immunocompetent host requiring hospitalization	IV	≥2 y	30 mg/kg per day for 7–10 days or 1500 mg/m² per day, in 3 divided doses for 7–10 days
	Varicella in immunocompromised host	IV	<2 y	30 mg/kg per day, in 3 divided doses for 7–10 days
		IV	≥2 y	1500 mg/m² per day, in 3 divided doses for 7–10 days; some experts recommend the 30 mg/kg per day dose
	Zoster in immunocompetent host	IV (if requiring hospitalization)	All ages	Same as for varicella in immunocompromised host
		Oral	≥12 y	4000 mg/day, in 5 divided doses for 5–7 days
	Zoster in immunocompromised host	IV	All ages	30 mg/kg per day, in 3 divided doses, for 7–10 days

Table 4.10. Non-HIV Antiviral Drugs,ᵃ continued

Generic (Trade Name)	Indication	Route	Age	Usually Recommended Dosage
	HSV infection in immunocompromised host (localized, progressive, or disseminated)	IV	All ages	30 mg/kg per day, in 3 divided doses for 7–14 days
		Oral	≥2 y	1000 mg/day, in 3–5 divided doses for 7–14 days
	Prophylaxis of HSV in immunocompromised hosts who are HSV seropositive	Oral	≥2 y	600–1000 mg/day, in 3–5 divided doses during period of risk
		IV	All ages	15 mg/kg, in 3 divided doses during period of risk
	Genital HSV infection: first episode	Oral	≥12 y	1000–1200 mg/day, in 3–5 divided doses for 7–10 days. Oral pediatric dose: 40–80 mg/kg per day, divided in 3–4 doses (maximum 1.0 g/day)
		IV	≥12 y	15 mg/kg per day, in 3 divided doses for 5–7 days
	Genital HSV infection: recurrence	Oral	≥12 y	1000 mg in 5 divided doses for 5 days, or 1600 mg in 2 divided doses for 5 days, or 2400 mg in 3 divided doses for 2 days

Table 4.10. Non-HIV Antiviral Drugs,[a] continued

Generic (Trade Name)	Indication	Route	Age	Usually Recommended Dosage
	Chronic suppressive therapy for recurrent genital and cutaneous (ocular) HSV episodes	Oral	≥12 y	800 mg/day, in 2 divided doses for as long as 12 continuous mo
Adefovir[b] (Hepsera)	Chronic hepatitis B	Oral	≥12 y	10 mg, once daily, in patients with creatinine clearance ≥50 mL/min; optimal duration of therapy unknown, although minimum of 1 y + additional 12 mo after HBeAg seroconversion has been suggested; monitor for hepatic exacerbation and renal dysfunction
		Oral	2–12 y	≥7–12 y: 0.25 mg/kg, 2–<7y: 0.3 mg/kg once daily (both to a maximum of 10 mg) gives similar systemic exposure as in adults
Cidofovir (Vistide)	Cytomegalovirus (CMV) retinitis	IV	Adult dose[h] and adolescents (off label)	Induction: 5 mg/kg, once weekly, × 2 doses with probenecid 25–40 mg/kg (maximum 2 g) and hydration with each dose Maintenance: 5 mg/kg, once every 2 wk, with probenecid and hydration with each dose

Table 4.10. Non-HIV Antiviral Drugs,ᵃ continued

Generic (Trade Name)	Indication	Route	Age	Usually Recommended Dosage
Daclatasir (Daklinza)	Chronic hepatitis C (genotype 1 and 3)	Oral	Adult	60 mg, once daily, together with sofosbuvir for 12 wk, with or without ribavirin Need for ribavirin is based on HCV genotype, cirrhosis status, and liver transplant status
Elbasvir and Grazoprevir (Zepatier)	Chronic hepatitis C (genotype 1 and 4)	Oral	≥18 y	50 mg elbasvir and 100 mg grazoprevir, once daily, for 12–16 wk, with or without ribavirin Need for ribavirin is based on HCV genotype and prior treatment status
Entecavir (Baraclude)	Chronic hepatitis B	Oral	≥16 yʰ	0.5 mg, once daily, in nucleoside-therapy-naïve patients; 1 mg once daily in patients who were previously treated with a nucleoside (not first choice in this setting); optimum duration of therapy unknown
		Oral	2 to <16 y, naïve to treatment (normal renal function)	10–11 kg: 0.15 mg oral solution once daily >11–14 kg: 0.2 mg oral solution once daily >14–17 kg: 0.25 mg oral solution once daily >17–20 kg: 0.3 mg oral solution once daily >20–23 kg: 0.35 mg oral solution once daily >23–26 kg: 0.4 mg oral solution once daily >26–30 kg: 0.45 mg oral solution once daily >30 kg: 0.5 mg oral solution or tablet once daily
			Lamivudine-treated	Double the dosage in each above weight bracket

Table 4.10. Non-HIV Antiviral Drugs,[a] continued

Generic (Trade Name)	Indication	Route	Age	Usually Recommended Dosage
Famciclovir[b]	Genital HSV infection, acute recurrent episodes	Oral	Adult dose,[h] adolescents	Immunocompetent: 2000 mg/day, in 2 divided doses for 1 day; CDC regimens featuring smaller incremental doses and greater number of treatment days are available. HIV-infected patients: 1000 mg, in 2 divided doses for 7 days (CDC and NIH guidelines provide range of 5–14 days)
	Daily suppressive therapy	Oral	Adult dose,[h] adolescents and children	Immunocompetent: 500 mg/day, in 2 divided doses for 1 y, then reassess for recurrence of HSV infection; HIV: 1000 mg/day, in 2 divided doses for minimum of 1 y; same dosage for children and adolescents old enough to receive adult doses
	Recurrent herpes labialis	Oral	Adult dose,[h] adolescents	Immunocompetent: 1500 mg as a single dose HIV-infected patients: 1000 mg/day, in 2 divided doses for 7 days (CDC and NIH guidelines provide range of 5–10 days); comparatively slower resolution seen in adolescent patients
	Herpes zoster	Oral	Adult dose,[h] adolescents	1500 mg/day, in 3 divided doses for 7 days (7–10 days in HIV patients with localized lesions, longer if lesions resolving slowly, or 10–14 days total course with initial IV acyclovir if more severe skin or visceral infection)

Table 4.10. Non-HIV Antiviral Drugs,ᵃ continued

Generic (Trade Name)	Indication	Route	Age	Usually Recommended Dosage
Foscarnet[b] (Foscavir)	CMV retinitis in HIV infected patients (alternative in ganciclovir-resistant disease)	IV	Adult dose[h] and infants, children, and adolescents (off label)	180 mg/kg per day, in 2–3 divided doses for 14–21 days, then 90–120 mg/kg once a day for maintenance therapy; IV infused no faster than 1 mg/kg/minute
	HSV infection resistant to acyclovir in immunocompromised host	IV	Adult dose[h] and adolescents (off label)	80–120 mg/kg per day, in 2–3 divided doses for 3 wk or until infection resolves
	VZV infection resistant to acyclovir	IV	Adult dose[h] and adolescents (off label)	Patients with HIV: 90 mg/kg per dose every 12 h
			Infants and children	40–60 mg/kg per dose every 8 h for 7–10 days or until no new lesions have appeared for 48 h
Ganciclovir[b] (Cytovene)	Symptomatic congenital CMV disease	IV	Birth to 2 mo	12 mg/kg per day, divided every 12 h; duration of treatment is 6 mo, but most or all of the treatment should be accomplished with oral valganciclovir, as detailed below (there is no benefit to using ganciclovir instead of valganciclovir) for improved long-term developmental and hearing outcomes; dosage adjustment if neutropenia develops

Table 4.10. Non-HIV Antiviral Drugs,[a] continued

Generic (Trade Name)	Indication	Route	Age	Usually Recommended Dosage
	Acquired CMV retinitis in immuno-compromised host[i]	IV	Adult dose[h]	Treatment: 10 mg/kg per day, in 2 divided doses for 14–21 days; long-term suppression 5 mg/kg per day for 7 days/wk or 6 mg/kg per day for 5 days/wk; HIV: duration of maintenance treatment is for at least 3–6 mo, with lesions inactive, and with CD4+ T-lymphocyte count >100 cells/mm³ for 3 to 6 mo in response to cART
		IV	Infants, children, and adolescents	10 mg/kg per day, in 2 divided doses for 14–21 days; increase to 15 mg/kg/day in 2 divided doses if needed, then 5 mg/kg body weight once daily for 5–7 days per wk for chronic suppression; discontinuation after 6 mo may be considered in children 1–5 y if CD4+ T-lymphocyte count >500/m³ (or CD4+ T-lymphocyte percentage ≥15%); may add foscarnet if vision at risk, or ganciclovir intravitreal injection or implant in children 9–12 y and adolescents
	Prophylaxis of CMV in high-risk host	IV	All ages	10 mg/kg per day, in 2 divided doses for 5–7 days, then 5 mg/kg per day, in 1 dose for 100 days, or 6 mg/kg per day for 5 days/wk for 100 days 10 mg/kg per day, in 2 divided doses for 1–2 wk

Table 4.10. Non-HIV Antiviral Drugs,[a] continued

Generic (Trade Name)	Indication	Route	Age	Usually Recommended Dosage
	Preemptive therapy of CMV in high-risk host	IV	All ages	10 mg/kg per day, in 2 divided doses for 7–14 days, then 5 mg/kg once daily if CMV is still detectable and declining and continue until the indicator test is negative
Interferon alfa-2b (Intron A)	Chronic hepatitis B	SC	1–18 y	Initial dosing of 3 million IU/m², SC, during first wk, then 6 million IU/m², SC (maximum dose 10 million IU), 3 times/wk for 16–24 wk; 50% dose reduction if severe adverse reactions
			>18 y	5 million IU/day; or 10 million IU, IM or SC, 3 times/wk, for 16 wk
	Chronic hepatitis C	SC, IM	>18 y	3 million IU, IM or SC, 3 times/wk, for 24–48 wk; length of treatment depending on HCV genotype Note: pegylated interferon preferred over interferon alfa-2b
		SC, IM	≥3 y and >61 kg	3 million IU, IM or SC, 3 times/wk plus daily ribavirin, for 24–48 wk; length of treatment depending on HCV genotype
		SC, IM	≥3 y and 25–61 kg	3 million IU/m², SC 3 times/wk plus daily ribavirin, for 24–48 wk; length of treatment depending on HCV genotype

Table 4.10. Non-HIV Antiviral Drugs,ᵃ continued

Generic (Trade Name)	Indication	Route	Age	Usually Recommended Dosage
Lamivudineᵇ (Epivir-HBV)	Treatment of chronic hepatitis B	Oral	Infants and children (HIV positive)	4 mg/kg/dose (maximum 150 mg/dose) twice daily, or 8 mg/kg/dose (maximum 300mg/dose), once daily; children coinfected with HIV and hepatitis B should use the approved dose and combination products for HIV.
		Oral	Adolescents (HIV positive)	300 mg, once daily, or 150 mg, twice daily
		Oral	Infants and children (HIV negative)	3 mg/kg/dose, once daily (maximum of 100 mg per day); use oral solution for doses <100 mg
		Oral	Adolescents (HIV negative)	100 mg, once daily
Ombitasvir, paritaprevir, and ritonavir (Technivie), in combination with ribavirin	Chronic hepatitis C (genotype 4)	Oral	≥18 y	12.5 mg ombitasvir, 75 mg paritaprevir, 50 mg ritonavir per tablet Dose is 2 tablets, once daily, plus ribavirin, for 12 wk

Table 4.10. Non-HIV Antiviral Drugs,[a] continued

Generic (Trade Name)	Indication	Route	Age	Usually Recommended Dosage
Ombitasvir, paritaprevir, and ritonavir tablets; dasabuvir tablets, copackaged for oral use (Viekira Pak)	Chronic hepatitis C (genotype 1)	Oral	≥18 y	Two ombitasvir, paritaprevir, ritonavir 12.5/75/50-mg tablets, once daily (in the morning), and 1 dasabuvir 250-mg tablet, twice daily (morning and evening), for 12–24 wk
Oseltamivir[b,j] (Tamiflu)	Influenza A and B: treatment (see Influenza, p 476)	Oral (suspension)	Birth to <9 mo[k]	3 mg/kg twice daily for 5 days[k]
		Oral (suspension)	9–11 mo	3.5 mg/kg twice daily for 5 days
		Oral (suspension and tablets)	1–12 y	≤15 kg: 30 mg, twice daily; 15.1–23 kg: 45 mg, twice daily; 23.1–40 kg: 60 mg, twice daily; >40 kg: 75 mg, twice daily for 5 days
		Oral (tablets)	≥13 y	75 mg, twice daily for 5 days

Table 4.10. Non-HIV Antiviral Drugs,[a] continued

Generic (Trade Name)	Indication	Route	Age	Usually Recommended Dosage
	Influenza A and B: prophylaxis	Oral	3 mo–12 y	Same as the above treatment doses for patients 3 mo–12 y of age, except dose given once rather than twice daily, and given for 10 days rather than 5 (following known exposure) or for up to 6 wk (preexposure during community outbreak); not routinely recommended for infants <3 mo given lack of efficacy data
		Oral	≥13 y	75 mg, once daily for 10 days (following known exposure) or for up to 6 wk (preexposure during community outbreak)
Pegylated interferon alfa-2a (Pegasys)	Chronic hepatitis B	SC	>18 y[h]	180 μg, once weekly for 48 wk
	Chronic hepatitis C	SC	≥5 to 18 y	180 μg/1.73 m² (or 104 μg/m²; maximum 180 μg), once weekly for 24–48 wk; length of treatment depending on HCV genotype; given concomitantly with oral ribavirin[i]
				Dosage regimens adjusted based on any of the following: psychiatric sequelae, neutrophil count, platelet count, or hepatic function
		SC	>18 y[h]	180 μg, once weekly for 24–48 wk; length of treatment depending on HCV genotype

Table 4.10. Non-HIV Antiviral Drugs,[a] continued

Generic (Trade Name)	Indication	Route	Age	Usually Recommended Dosage
Pegylated interferon-alfa-2b (PegIntron)	Chronic hepatitis C	SC	>18 y	1.5 µg/kg, once weekly for 24–48 wk; length of treatment depending on HCV genotype; patient weight ranges used to round to nearest 0.1-mL injection volume
		SC	>3 to 18 y	60 µg/m^2, once weekly for 24–48 wk; length of treatment depending on HCV genotype; AASLD recommends 48 wk of treatment regardless of HCV genotype
Peramivir[b] (Rapivab)	Influenza A and B	IV	≥2 y	2–12 y: 12 mg/kg, once (maximum dose: 600 mg) ≥13 y: 600 mg, once
Ribavirin (Rebetol or Copegus)	Treatment of hepatitis C in combination with pegylated interferon alfa-2a	Oral	≥3 y	15 mg/kg per day, in 2 divided doses (fixed dose by weight is suggested) for 24–48 wk; length of treatment depending on HCV genotype 25–36 kg: 200 mg in AM and PM >36–49 kg: 200 mg in AM and 400 mg in PM >49–61 kg: 400 mg in AM and PM >61–75 kg: 400 mg in AM and 600 mg in PM >75 kg: 600 mg in AM and PM

Table 4.10. Non-HIV Antiviral Drugs,[a] continued

Generic (Trade Name)	Indication	Route	Age	Usually Recommended Dosage
Simeprevir (Olysio)	Chronic hepatitis C (genotype 1 and 4)	Oral	Adult dose[h]	150 mg, taken once daily with food, as a component of combination therapy with sofosbuvir, or both pegylated interferon alfa and ribavirin; not recommended if moderate or severe hepatic impairment
Sofosbuvir (Sovaldi)	Chronic hepatitis C (genotype 1, 2, 4, 5, 6)	Oral	Adolescents ≥12 y (or ≥35 kg), adults	400 mg, taken once daily with or without food, as a component of combination therapy with other direct-acting antivirals (eg, simeprevir, daclatasvir), ribavirin, or with ribavirin plus pegylated interferon; length of treatment depending on HCV genotype and concomitant therapy used Available in a fixed-dose combination tablet with 90 mg ledipasvir (marketed as Harvoni) for use in adolescents ≥12 y (or ≥35 kg) and adults Available in a fixed-dose combination tablet with 100 mg velpatasvir (marketed as EPCLUSA) for use in adults
Telbivudine[b] (Tyzeka)	Chronic hepatitis B	Oral	Adult and adolescent (≥16 y) dose[h]	600 mg, once daily

Table 4.10. Non-HIV Antiviral Drugs,[a] continued

Generic (Trade Name)	Indication	Route	Age	Usually Recommended Dosage
Tenofovir[b] (Viread)	Chronic hepatitis B	Oral	Adolescents ≥12 y and weighing ≥ 35 kg, with or without HIV coinfection, adults	300 mg, once daily; adjustment of dosing interval recommended for creatinine clearance <50 mL/min
			2 to 11 y with HIV (off label)	8 mg/kg (maximum 300 mg), once daily
Valacyclovir[b] (Valtrex)	Varicella	Oral	2 to <18 y	20 mg/kg, 3 times daily for 5 days, not to exceed 1 g per dose 3 times daily; same dose for up to 6 wk after IV acyclovir treatment of acute retinal necrosis
	Genital HSV infection, first episode	Oral	Adult and adolescent dose	2 g/day, in 2 divided doses for 10 days (5–14 days in HIV infected patients)
			Children	<45 kg: 40 mg/kg/day in 2 divided doses ≥45 kg: 1 g every 12 h 7–10 days of treatment
	Episodic recurrent genital HSV infection	Oral	Adult and adolescent dose	1 g/day, in 2 divided doses for 3 days; HIV-infected patients should receive 2 g/day for 5–14 days

Table 4.10. Non-HIV Antiviral Drugs,ᵃ continued

Generic (Trade Name)	Indication	Route	Age	Usually Recommended Dosage
	Daily suppressive therapy for recurrent genital HSV infection	Oral	Adult doseʰ	Immunocompetent patients: 1000 mg, once daily for 1 y or assess history of recurrences (eg, 500 mg, once daily, in patients with ≤9 recurrences/y) HIV-infected patients (CD4+ T-lymphocyte count ≥100 cells/mm³): 500 mg, twice daily for at least 6 mo
			Adolescent	500 mg or 1 g, once daily (the lower dose is less effective if frequent recurrences)
	Recurrent herpes labialis	Oral	≥12 y	4 g/day, in 2 divided doses for 1 day
	Herpes zoster	Oral	Adult and adolescent doseʰ	3 g/day, in 3 divided doses for 7 days
Valganciclovirᵇ (Valcyte)	Symptomatic congenital CMV disease	Oral	Birth through 6 mo	32 mg/kg per day, in 2 divided doses, started within the first mo of life and continued for a total of 6 mo of treatment; for improved long-term developmental and hearing outcomes; dosage adjustment if neutropenia develops

Table 4.10. Non-HIV Antiviral Drugs,[a] continued

Generic (Trade Name)	Indication	Route	Age	Usually Recommended Dosage
	Acquired CMV retinitis in immuno-compromised host	Oral	Adult and adolescent dose[h]	Treatment: 900 mg, twice daily for 2–3 wk Long-term suppression: 900 mg, once daily; HIV: duration of maintenance treatment is for at least 3–6 mo, with lesions inactive, and with CD4+ T-lymphocyte count >100 cells/mm^3 for 3 mo to 6 mo in response to ART
	Prevention of CMV disease in kidney, liver, or heart transplant patients	Oral	4 mo–16 y	Dose once a day within 10 days of transplantation according to dosage algorithm based on body surface area and creatinine clearance: Dose (mg) = 7 × body surface area × creatinine clearance (calculated using the Schwartz equation; see drug package insert; maximum 900 mg/day); round dose to the nearest 10-mg increment; duration: 200 days after renal transplant, 100 days after heart or liver transplant
		Oral	Adolescents ≥17 y	900 mg, once daily, for post-transplant patients; duration as above in children depends on type of transplant
	Prevention of CMV disease in HIV-infected patients	Oral	4 mo–16 y	Same calculated dose regimen as above; duration: stopping primary prophylaxis can be considered when the CD4+ T-lymphocyte cell count is >100 cells/mm^3 for children ≥6 y, or CD4+ T-lymphocyte percentage is >10% in children <6 y

Table 4.10. Non-HIV Antiviral Drugs,[a] continued

Generic (Trade Name)	Indication	Route	Age	Usually Recommended Dosage
Zanamivir (Relenza)	Influenza A and B: treatment (see Influenza, p 476)	Inhalation	≥7 y (treatment)	10 mg (one 5-mg blister per inhalation), twice daily for 5 days; first 2 doses can be separated by as little as 2 h; only use diskhaler device
	Influenza A and B: prophylaxis	Inhalation	≥5 y (prophylaxis)	10 mg, once daily for as long as 28 days (community outbreaks) or 10 days (household setting)

AASLD indicates American Association for the Study of Liver Diseases; ART, antiretroviral therapy; CDC, Centers for Disease Control and Prevention; CSF, cerebrospinal fluid; FDA, US Food and Drug Administration; IV, intravenous; HBeAg, hepatitis B e antigen; HCV, hepatitis C virus; HIV, human immunodeficiency virus; IM, intramuscular; mo, month; NIH, National Institutes of Health; PCR, polymerase chain reaction; SC, subcutaneous; VZV, varicella-zoster virus; y, year.

[a]Drugs for human immunodeficiency virus infection are not included. See **http://aidsinfo.nih.gov** for current information on HIV drugs and treatment recommendations.

[b]Dose should be decreased in patients with impaired renal function.

[c]Oral dosage of acyclovir in children should not exceed 80 mg/kg per day (3200 mg/day).

[d]Acyclovir doses listed in this table are based on clinical trials and clinical experience and may not be identical to doses approved by the FDA.

[e]In times of shortage of intravenous acyclovir, the American Academy of Pediatrics Committee on Infectious Diseases recommends that existing supplies of intravenous acyclovir be conserved to improve availability for neonatal HSV infections, herpes simplex encephalitis, or HSV and varicella-zoster virus infections in immunocompromised patients, including more ill pregnant women with visceral dissemination of either virus. If acyclovir is not available, intravenous ganciclovir should be substituted. Alternative regimens to the use of intravenous acyclovir and other options for priority and nonpriority conditions are outlined in an exclusive *Red Book* Online Intravenous Acyclovir Shortage Table **(http://redbook.solutions.aap.org/selfserve/ ssPage.aspx?SelfServeContentId=acyclovir-shortage).**

[f]Monitor for nephrotoxicity and neurologic irritation. Consider involving an infectious diseases or pharmacology specialist if weight-based dosing exceeds 800 mg per dose or if being administered with other nephrotoxic medications.

[g]Selective indications; see Varicella-Zoster Infections (p 869).

[h]There are not sufficient clinical data to identify the appropriate dose for use in children.

[i]Some experts use ganciclovir in immunocompromised hosts with CMV gastrointestinal tract disease and CMV pneumonitis (with or without CMV Immune Globulin Intravenous).

[j]See Influenza (p 476) and **www.cdc.gov/flu/professionals/antivirals/index.htm** for specific recommendations, which may vary on the basis of most recent influenza virus susceptibility patterns.

[k]Preterm, <38 weeks' postmenstrual age, oseltamivir, 1.0 mg/kg/dose, orally, twice daily; preterm, 38 through 40 weeks' postmenstrual age, 1.5 mg/kg/dose, orally, twice daily; preterm >40 weeks' postmenstrual age through 8 months' chronologic age, 3.0 mg/kg/dose, orally, twice daily.

[l]See approved product label for PEGASYS (pegylated interferon alfa-2a).

For more information on individual drugs, see *Physician's Desk Reference* or **www.pdr.net** (for registered users only).

DRUGS FOR PARASITIC INFECTIONS

Table 4.11. Drugs for Parasitic Infections[1]

Disease	Drug	Adult Dosage	Pediatric Dosage	CDC Web Site[2] (includes listings of adverse events)
African trypanosomiasis (African sleeping sickness)				**www.cdc.gov/parasites/ sleepingsickness/health_ professionals/index.html**
Trypanosoma brucei rhodesiense, hemolymphatic stage	Suramin[3]	1 g, IV, on days 1, 3, 7, 14, and 21[4]	20 mg/kg/day (max 1 g), IV, on days 1, 3, 7, 14, and 21[5]	
T brucei rhodesiense, CNS involvement	Melarsoprol[6]	2.2 mg/kg/day, IV, for 10 days[7]	2.2 mg/kg/day, IV, for 10 days[7]	
T brucei gambiense, hemolymphatic stage	Pentamidine[8]	4 mg/kg/day, IV or IM, for 7–10 days	4 mg/kg/day, IV or IM, for 7–10 days	
T brucei gambiense, CNS involvement	Eflornithine[9]	400 mg/kg/day, IV, in 4 divided doses for 14 days	400 mg/kg/day, IV, in 4 divided doses for 14 days	

Table 4.11. Drugs for Parasitic Infections,[1] continued

Disease	Drug	Adult Dosage	Pediatric Dosage	CDC Web Site[2] (includes listings of adverse events)
American trypanoso-miasis (Chagas disease; *Trypanosoma cruzi* infection)	Benznida-zole[10]	5–7 mg/kg/day, orally, in 2 (or 3) divided doses for 60 days	Age <12 y: 5–7.5 mg/kg/day, orally, in 2 (or 3) divided doses for 60 days	www.cdc.gov/parasites/chagas/health_professionals/index.html
			Age ≥12 y: 5–7 mg/kg/day, orally, in 2 (or 3) divided doses for 60 days	
	OR			
	Nifurtimox[10]	8–10 mg/kg/day (max 720 mg), orally, in 3 or 4 divided doses for 90–120 days	Age ≤10 y: 15–20 mg/kg/day (max 720 mg), orally, in 3 or 4 divided doses for 90 days	
			Age 11–16 y: 12.5–15 mg/kg/day (max 720 mg), orally, in 3 or 4 divided doses for 90 days	
			Age ≥17 y: 8–10 mg/kg/day (max 720 mg), orally, in 3 or 4 divided doses for 90–120 days	
Ascariasis (*Ascaris lumbricoides*; intestinal roundworm)	Albendazole[11]	400 mg, orally, once		www.cdc.gov/parasites/ascariasis/health_professionals/index.html
	OR			
	Meben-dazole[12]	100 mg, orally, twice daily for 3 days OR 500 mg, orally, once		
	OR			
	Ivermectin[13]	150–200 µg/kg, orally, once		

Table 4.11. Drugs for Parasitic Infections,[1] continued

Disease	Drug	Adult Dosage	Pediatric Dosage	CDC Web Site[2] (includes listings of adverse events)
	OR			
	Pyrantel pamoate[14]	11 mg/kg (up to a maximum of 1 g), orally, daily for 3 days		
	OR			
	Nitazoxanide	500 mg, orally, twice daily for 3 days	Age 1–3 y: 100 mg, orally, twice daily for 3 days Age 4–11 y: 200 mg, orally, twice daily for 3 days Age ≥12 y: 500 mg, orally, twice daily for 3 days	
Babesiosis[15]	Atovaquone PLUS	750 mg, orally, twice daily for at least 7–10 days	40 mg/kg/day, orally, in 2 doses (max 750 mg/dose) for at least 7–10 days	**www.cdc.gov/parasites/ babesiosis/health_ professionals/index.html**
	Azithromycin[16]	On the first day, give a total dose in the range of 500–1000 mg, orally; on subsequent days, give a total daily dose in the range of 250–500 mg, for a total duration of therapy of at least 7–10 days	10 mg/kg (max 500 mg/dose), orally, on day 1; then 5 mg/kg/day (max 250 mg/dose), orally, on subsequent days, for a total duration of therapy of at least 7–10 days	
	OR			

Table 4.11. Drugs for Parasitic Infections,[1] continued

Disease	Drug	Adult Dosage	Pediatric Dosage	CDC Web Site[2] (includes listings of adverse events)
	Clindamycin	600 mg, orally, 3 times daily, **or** 300–600 mg, IV, 4 times daily, for at least 7–10 days	20–40 mg/kg/day, orally, in 3 doses (max 600 mg/dose), for at least 7–10 days	
	PLUS			
	Quinine	650 mg, orally, 3 times daily, for at least 7–10 days	30 mg/kg/day, orally, in 3 doses (max 650 mg/dose), for at least 7–10 days	
Balantidiasis (*Balantidium coli*)	Tetracycline	500 mg, orally, 4 times daily for 10 days	Age ≥8 y: 40 mg/kg/day (max 2 g per day), orally, in 4 doses for 10 days	www.cdc.gov/parasites/ balantidium/health_ professionals/index.html
	OR			
	Metronidazole	500–750 mg, orally, 3 times daily for 5 days	35–50 mg/kg/day, orally, in 3 doses for 5 days	
	OR			
	Iodoquinol	650 mg, orally, 3 times daily for 20 days	30–40 mg/kg/day (max 2 g per day), orally, in 3 doses for 20 days	
	OR			
	Nitazoxanide	500 mg, orally, twice daily for 3 days	Age 1–3 y: 100 mg, orally, twice daily for 3 days Age 4–11 y: 200 mg, orally, twice daily for 3 days Age ≥12 y: 500 mg, orally, twice daily for 3 days	

Table 4.11. Drugs for Parasitic Infections,[1] continued

Disease	Drug	Adult Dosage	Pediatric Dosage	CDC Web Site[2] (includes listings of adverse events)
Baylisascariasis (raccoon roundworm infection)	Albendazole[11]	25–50 mg/kg/day, orally, for 10–20 days[17]		www.cdc.gov/parasites/baylisascaris/health_professionals/index.html
Blastocystis hominis infection[18]	Metronidazole	250 mg to 750 mg, orally, 3 times daily for 10 days OR 1500 mg, orally, once daily for 10 days	35–50 mg/kg/day, orally, in 3 doses for 10 days	www.cdc.gov/parasites/blastocystis/health_professionals/index.html
	OR			
	Trimethoprim (TMP)/sulf amethoxa-zole (SMX)	160 mg TMP, 800 mg SMX, orally, twice daily for 7 days	Age >2 mo: 8 mg/kg TMP and 40 mg/kg SMX per day, orally, in 2 divided doses for 7 days	
	OR			
	Nitazoxanide	500 mg, orally, twice daily for 3 days	Age 1–3 y: 100 mg, orally, twice daily for 3 days Age 4–11 y: 200 mg, orally, twice daily for 3 days Age ≥12 y: 500 mg, orally, twice daily for 3 days	
	OR			
	Tinidazole	2 g, orally, once	Age ≥3 y: 50 mg/kg (max 2 g) once	

Table 4.11. Drugs for Parasitic Infections,[1] continued

Disease	Drug	Adult Dosage	Pediatric Dosage	CDC Web Site[2] (includes listings of adverse events)
Capillariasis	Mebendazole[12]	200 mg, orally, twice daily for 20–30 days		www.cdc.gov/parasites/capillaria/health_professionals/index.html
	OR			
	Albendazole[11]	400 mg, orally, once daily for 10–30 days		
Chilomastix mesnili	No treatment is necessary; this protozoan is considered nonpathogenic but may be an indicator of ingestion of fecally contaminated food or water			www.cdc.gov/parasites/nonpathprotozoa/health_professionals/index.html
Clonorchiasis	Praziquantel[19]	75 mg/kg/day, orally, in 3 doses for 2 days		www.cdc.gov/parasites/clonorchis/health_professionals/index.html
	OR			
	Albendazole[11]	10 mg/kg/day, orally, for 7 days		
	OR			
	Mebendazole[12]	30 mg/kg/day, orally, for 20–30 days		
Cryptosporidiosis	Nitazoxanide[20]	500 mg, orally, twice a day for 3 days	Age 1–3 y: 100 mg, orally, twice a day for 3 days Age 4 to 11 y: 200 mg, orally, twice a day for 3 days Age ≥12 y: 500 mg, orally, twice a day for 3 days	www.cdc.gov/parasites/crypto/health_professionals/index.html
Cutaneous larva migrans (zoonotic hookworm)	Albendazole[11]	400 mg/day, orally, once daily for 3–7 days	Age >2 y: 15 mg/kg/day (max 400 mg/day), orally, for 3 days	www.cdc.gov/parasites/zoonotichookworm/health_professionals/index.html
	OR			
	Ivermectin[13]	200 µg/kg, orally, once daily for 1–2 days	Weight >15 kg: 200 µg/kg, orally, once daily for 1–2 days	

Table 4.11. Drugs for Parasitic Infections,[1] continued

Disease	Drug	Adult Dosage	Pediatric Dosage	CDC Web Site[2] (includes listings of adverse events)
Cyclosporiasis	Trimethoprim (TMP)/ sulfamethoxazole (SMX)	160 mg TMP/800 mg SMX, orally, 2 times/day for 7–10 days[21]	Age >2 mo: 8–10 mg/kg TMP and 40–50 mg/kg SMX per day, orally, in 2 divided doses for 7–10 days[21]	www.cdc.gov/parasites/ cyclosporiasis/health_ professionals/index.html
Cystoisosporiasis (*Cystoisospora* infection; formerly isosporiasis)[22]	Trimethoprim (TMP)/ sulfamethoxazole (SMX)	160 mg TMP/800 mg SMX, IV or orally, 2 times/day for 10 days	Age >2 mo: 8–10 mg/kg TMP and 40–50 mg/kg SMX per day, IV or orally, in 2 divided doses for 10 days	www.cdc.gov/parasites/ cystoisospora/health_ professionals/index.html
	OR			
	Pyrimethamine PLUS leucovorin (first-line alternative)	50–75 mg per day of pyrimethamine, either once daily or divided into 2 separate doses 10–25 mg per day of leucovorin	--	
	OR			
	Ciprofloxacin (second-line alternative)	500 mg, orally, 2 times/day for 7 days	--	

Table 4.11. Drugs for Parasitic Infections,[1] continued

Disease	Drug	Adult Dosage	Pediatric Dosage	CDC Web Site[2] (includes listings of adverse events)
Dientamoeba fragilis infection	Iodoquinol	650 mg, orally, 3 times/day for 20 days	30–40 mg/kg/day (max 2 g), orally, divided 3 times/day for 20 days	www.cdc.gov/parasites/dientamoeba/health_professionals/index.html
	OR			
	Paromomycin	25–35 mg/kg/day, orally, divided 3 times/day for 7 days		
	OR			
	Metronidazole	500–750 mg, orally, 3 times/day for 10 days	35–50 mg/kg/day, orally, in 3 divided doses (max 500–750 mg/dose) for 10 days	
Diphyllobothrium infection	Praziquantel[19]	5–10 mg/kg, orally, in a single dose		www.cdc.gov/parasites/diphyllobothrium/health_professionals/index.html
	OR			
	Niclosamide[23]	2 g, orally, once	50 mg/kg (max 2 g), orally, once	
Dipylidium caninum infection (dog or cat flea tapeworm)	Praziquantel[19]	5–10 mg/kg, orally, in a single dose		www.cdc.gov/parasites/dipylidium/health_professionals/index.html
	OR			
	Niclosamide[23]	2 g, orally, once	50 mg/kg (max 2 g), orally, once	
Echinococcosis[24]	Albendazole[11]	400 mg, orally, twice daily for 1–6 mo	10–15 mg/kg/day (max 800 mg/day), orally, in 2 doses for 1–6 mo	www.cdc.gov/parasites/echinococcosis/health_professionals/index.html
Endolimax nana	No treatment is necessary; this protozoan is harmless			www.cdc.gov/parasites/nonpathprotozoa/
Entamoeba coli	No treatment is necessary; this protozoan is harmless			www.cdc.gov/parasites/nonpathprotozoa/

Table 4.11. Drugs for Parasitic Infections,[1] continued

Disease	Drug	Adult Dosage	Pediatric Dosage	CDC Web Site[2] (includes listings of adverse events)
Entamoeba dispar	No treatment is necessary; this protozoan is harmless			**www.cdc.gov/parasites/ nonpathprotozoa/**
Entamoeba hartmanni	No treatment is necessary; this protozoan is harmless			**www.cdc.gov/parasites/ nonpathprotozoa/**
Entamoeba histolytica (amebiasis)[25] Asymptomatic	Iodoquinol	650 mg, orally, 3 times/day for 20 days	30–40 mg/kg/day (max 2 g), orally, divided 3 times/day for 20 days	**www.cdc.gov/parasites/ amebiasis/index.html**
	OR			
	Paromomycin	25–35 mg/kg/day, orally, divided 3 times/day for 7 days		
	OR			
	Diloxanide furoate[26]	500 mg, orally, 3 times/day for 10 days	20 mg/kg/day, orally, divided 3 times a day for 10 days	
Entamoeba histolytica (amebiasis)[25] Mild to moderate intestinal disease	Metronidazole	500 to 750 mg, orally, 3 times/day for 7–10 days	35–50 mg/kg/day, orally, divided 3 times/day for 7–10 days	**www.cdc.gov/parasites/ amebiasis/index.html**
	OR			
	Tinidazole	2 g, orally, once daily for 3 days	Age ≥3 y: 50 mg/kg (max 2 g), orally, once daily for 3 days	
	FOLLOWED EITHER BY			
	Iodoquinol	650 mg, orally, 3 times/day for 20 days	30–40 mg/kg/day (max 2 g), orally, divided 3 times/day for 20 days	
	OR BY			
	Paromomycin	25–35 mg/kg/day, orally, divided 3 times/day for 7 days		

Table 4.11. Drugs for Parasitic Infections,[1] continued

Disease	Drug	Adult Dosage	Pediatric Dosage	CDC Web Site[2] (includes listings of adverse events)
Entamoeba histolytica (amebiasis)[25] Severe intestinal and extraintestinal disease	Metronidazole	500 to 750 mg, orally, 3 times/day for 7–10 days	35–50 mg/kg/day, orally, divided 3 times/day for 7–10 days	**www.cdc.gov/parasites/ amebiasis/index.html**
	OR			
	Tinidazole	2 g, orally, once daily for 5 days	Age ≥3 y: 50 mg/kg (max 2 g), orally, once daily for 5 days	
	FOLLOWED EITHER BY			
	Iodoquinol	650 mg, orally, 3 times/day for 20 days	30–40 mg/kg/day (max 2 g), orally, divided 3 times/day for 20 days	
	OR BY			
	Paromomycin	25–35 mg/kg/day, orally, divided 3 times/day for 7 days		
Entamoeba polecki	No treatment is necessary; this protozoan is harmless			**www.cdc.gov/parasites/ nonpathprotozoa/health_ professionals/index.html**
Enterobiasis (pinworm)	Mebendazole[12]	100 mg, orally, once; repeat in 2 wk		**www.cdc.gov/parasites/ pinworm/health_ professionals/index.html**
	OR			
	Pyrantel pamoate[14]	11 mg/kg base, orally, once (max 1 g); repeat in 2 wk		
	OR			
	Albendazole[11]	400 mg orally once; repeat in 2 wk	Age ≥2 y: 400 mg orally once; repeat in 2 wk	
Fascioliasis (*Fasciola hepatica*; sheep liver fluke)	Triclabenda-zole[27]	10 mg/kg, orally, once or twice		**www.cdc.gov/parasites/fasciola/ health_professionals/index.html**
	OR			

Table 4.11. Drugs for Parasitic Infections,[1] continued

Disease	Drug	Adult Dosage	Pediatric Dosage	CDC Web Site[2] (includes listings of adverse events)
	Nitazoxanide	500 mg, orally, 2 times/day for 7 days	Age 1–3 y: 100 mg, orally, 2 times/day for 7 days Age 4–11 y: 200 mg, orally, 2 times/day for 7 days Age ≥12 y: 500 mg, orally, 2 times/day for 7 days	
Fasciolopsiasis (*Fasciolopsis buski*; intestinal fluke)	Praziquantel[19]	75 mg/kg/day, orally, in 3 divided doses for 1 day		**www.cdc.gov/parasites/ fasciolopsis/health_ professionals/index.html**
	Metronidazole	250 mg, orally, 3 times/day for 5–7 days	15 mg/kg/day (max 250 mg/dose), orally, divided 3 times/day for 5–7 days	
	OR			
Giardiasis[28]	Nitazoxanide	500 mg, orally, 2 times/day for 3 days	Age 1–3 y: 100 mg, orally, 2 times/day for 3 days Age 4–11 y: 200 mg, orally, 2 times/day for 3 days Age ≥12 y: 500 mg, orally, 2 times/day for 3 days	**www.cdc.gov/parasites/ giardia/audience-health- professionals.html**
	OR			
	Tinidazole	2 g, orally, once	Age ≥3 y: 50 mg/kg, orally, once (max 2 g)	
Gnathostomiasis (cutaneous)	Albendazole[11]	400 mg, orally, 2 times/day for 21 days		**www.cdc.gov/parasites/ gnathostoma/health_ professionals/index.html**
	OR			
	Ivermectin[13]	200 µg/kg, orally, once daily for 2 days		

Table 4.11. Drugs for Parasitic Infections,[1] continued

Disease	Drug	Adult Dosage	Pediatric Dosage	CDC Web Site[2] (includes listings of adverse events)
Heterophyiasis	Praziquantel[19]	75 mg/kg/day, orally, divided 3 times/day for 1 day		www.cdc.gov/dpdx/heterophyiasis/index.html
Hymenolepiasis (*Hymenolepis nana*; dwarf tapeworm)	Praziquantel[19]	25 mg/kg in a single-dose therapy, orally; some experts recommend a second dose 10 days later		www.cdc.gov/parasites/hymenolepis/health_professionals/index.html
	OR			
	Niclosamide[23]	2 g in a single dose for 7 days, orally	Weight 11–34 kg: 1 g in a single dose on day 1; then 500 mg per day, orally, for 6 days. Weight >34 kg: 1.5 g in a single dose on day 1; then 1 g per day, orally, for 6 days	
	OR			
	Nitazoxanide	500 mg, orally, 2 times/day for 3 days	Age 1–3 y: 100 mg, orally, 2 times/day for 3 days. Age 4–11 y: 200 mg, orally, 2 times/day for 3 days. Age ≥12 y: 500 mg, orally, 2 times/day for 3 days	
Hookworm (Human; *Ancylostoma duodenale, Necator americanus*)	Albendazole[11]	400 mg, orally, once		www.cdc.gov/parasites/hookworm/health_professionals/index.html
	OR			
	Mebendazole[12]	100 mg, orally, twice daily for 3 days; OR 500 mg, orally, once		
	OR			
	Pyrantel pamoate[14]	11 mg/kg (up to a maximum of 1 g), orally, daily for 3 days		

Table 4.11. Drugs for Parasitic Infections,[1] continued

Disease	Drug	Adult Dosage	Pediatric Dosage	CDC Web Site[2] (includes listings of adverse events)
Iodamoeba buetschlii	No treatment is necessary; this protozoan is harmless			www.cdc.gov/parasites/nonpathprotozoa/health_professionals/index.html
Leishmaniasis[29]	Liposomal amphotericin B	3 mg/kg/day, IV, on days 1–5, 14, and 21		www.cdc.gov/parasites/leishmaniasis/health_professionals/index.html[30]
	OR			
	Sodium stibogluconate	20 mg pentavalent antimony (Sb)/kg/day, IV or IM, for 28 days		
	OR			
Visceral (kala-azar)	Miltefosine	30 through 44 kg: 50 mg, orally, twice daily, for 28 consecutive days ≥45 kg: 50 mg, orally, 3 times daily, for 28 consecutive days		
	OR			
	Amphotericin B deoxycholate	1 mg/kg, IV, daily or every second day (cumulative total usually ~15–20 mg/kg)		
Cutaneous	Sodium stibogluconate	20 mg Sb/kg/day, IV or IM, for 20 days		
	OR			

Table 4.11. Drugs for Parasitic Infections,[1] continued

Disease	Drug	Adult Dosage	Pediatric Dosage	CDC Web Site[2] (includes listings of adverse events)
	Miltefosine	30 through 44 kg: 50 mg, orally, twice daily, for 28 consecutive days ≥45 kg: 50 mg, orally, 3 times daily, for 28 consecutive days	30 through 44 kg: 50 mg, orally, twice daily, for 28 consecutive days ≥45 kg: 50 mg, orally, 3 times daily, for 28 consecutive days	
	Sodium stibogluconate	20 mg Sb/kg/day, IV or IM, for 28 days	20 mg Sb/kg/day, IV or IM, for 28 days	
	OR			
Mucosal	Amphotericin B deoxycholate	0.5–1 mg/kg, IV, daily or every second day for a cumulative total of ~20–45 mg/kg	0.5–1 mg/kg, IV, daily or every second day for a cumulative total of ~20–45 mg/kg	
	OR			
	Miltefosine	30 through 44 kg: 50 mg, orally, twice daily, for 28 consecutive days ≥45 kg: 50 mg, orally 3 times daily, for 28 consecutive days	30 through 44 kg: 50 mg, orally, twice daily, for 28 consecutive days ≥45 kg: 50 mg, orally 3 times daily, for 28 consecutive days	
Lice infestation (*Pediculus humanus*, *P capitis*, *Phthirus pubis*)[31]	Pyrethrins with piperonyl butoxide[32]	Topically, twice, 9–10 days apart	Topically, twice, 9–10 days apart	www.cdc.gov/parasites/lice/body/health_professionals/index.html www.cdc.gov/parasites/lice/head/health_professionals/index.html www.cdc.gov/parasites/lice/pubic/health_professionals/index.html
	OR			
	0.5% Ivermectin[13] lotion[33]	Topically, once	Topically, once	
	OR			

Table 4.11. Drugs for Parasitic Infections,[1] continued

Disease	Drug	Adult Dosage	Pediatric Dosage	CDC Web Site[2] (includes listings of adverse events)
	0.9% Spinosad suspension[34]	Topically, twice (if crawling lice present, 7 days apart	Topically, twice (if crawling lice present), 7 days apart	
	OR			
	1% Permethrin[32]	Topically, twice, 9–10 days apart	Topically, twice, 9–10 days apart	
	OR			
	5% Benzyl alcohol lotion[35]	Topically, twice, 9–10 days apart	Topically, twice, 9–10 days apart	
	OR			
	0.5% Malathion[36]	Topically, twice (if needed), 7–9 days apart	Topically, twice (if needed), 7–9 days apart	
	OR			
	Ivermectin[13,37]	200 µg/kg, orally, twice, 9–10 days apart OR 400 µg/kg, orally, twice, 9–10 days apart	200 µg/kg, orally, twice, 9–10 days apart OR 400 µg/kg, orally, twice, 9–10 days apart	
Loiasis (*Loa loa*)	Diethylcarbamazine (DEC)[38]	(Symptomatic loiasis with microfilariae of *L loa* (MF)/mL <8000) 8–10 mg/kg/day, orally, in 3 divided doses for 21 days		**www.cdc.gov/parasites/loiasis/ health_professionals/index.html**

Table 4.11. Drugs for Parasitic Infections,[1] continued

Disease	Drug	Adult Dosage	Pediatric Dosage	CDC Web Site[2] (includes listings of adverse events)
	Albendazole[11]	(Symptomatic loiasis, with MF/mL <8000 and failed 2 rounds of DEC) OR (Symptomatic loiasis, with MF/mL ≥8000 to reduce level to <8000 prior to treatment with DEC) 200 mg, orally, twice daily for 21 days		
	Apheresis followed by DEC Note: Apheresis should be performed at an institution with experience in using this therapeutic modality for loiasis.	(Symptomatic loiasis, with MF/mL ≥8000)		
Lymphatic filariasis (elephantiasis; *Wuchereria bancrofti, Brugia malayi, Brugia timori*)	Diethylcarbamazine (DEC)[38]	Treatment of lymphatic filariasis[39]: Adults and children ≥18 mo: 6 mg/kg/day, orally, in 3 divided doses for 12 consecutive days; OR 6 mg/kg as a single oral dose Treatment of tropical pulmonary eosinophilia (TPE): Adults and children ≥18 mo: 6 mg/kg/day, orally, in 3 divided doses for 14–21 days		**www.cdc.gov/parasites/ lymphaticfilariasis/health_ professionals/index.html**

Table 4.11. Drugs for Parasitic Infections,[1] continued

Disease	Drug	Adult Dosage	Pediatric Dosage	CDC Web Site[2] (includes listings of adverse events)
Malaria (*Plasmodium* species)	Region infection acquired			**www.cdc.gov/malaria/ resources/pdf/ treatmenttable.pdf** CDC Malaria Hotline: (770) 488-7788 or (855) 856-4713 toll-free Monday–Friday 9 am to 5 pm EST; (770) 488-7100 after hours, weekends, and holidays
Uncomplicated malaria *P falciparum* or species not identified If "species not identified" subsequently diagnosed as *P vivax* or *P ovale*, see below re: treatment with primaquine	Chloroquine-resistant or unknown resistance[40,41] (All malarious regions except those specified as chloroquine-sensitive listed below.)			
	Atovaquone-proguanil[42]	1000 mg atovaquone/400 mg proguanil, orally, once daily for 3 days	Weight 5–8 kg: 2 pediatric tablets, orally, once daily for 3 days Weight 9–10 kg: 3 pediatric tablets, orally, once daily for 3 days Weight 11–20 kg: 1 adult tab, orally, once daily for 3 days Weight 21–30 kg: 2 adult tablets, orally, once daily for 3 days Weight 31–40 kg: 3 adult tablets, orally, once daily for 3 days Weight >40 kg: 4 adult tablets, orally, once daily for 3 days	
	OR			

Table 4.11. Drugs for Parasitic Infections,[1] continued

Disease	Drug	Adult Dosage	Pediatric Dosage	CDC Web Site[2] (includes listings of adverse events)
	Artemether-lumefantrine[42] 1 tablet = 20 mg artemether and 120 mg lumefantrine	A 3-day treatment schedule with a total of 6 oral doses is recommended for both adult and pediatric patients based on weight. The patient should receive the initial dose, followed by the second dose 8 h later, then 1 dose, orally, 2 times/day, for the following 2 days. Weight 5–<15 kg: 1 tablet per dose Weight 15–<25 kg: 2 tablets per dose Weight 25–<35 kg: 3 tablets per dose Weight ≥35 kg: 4 tablets per dose		
	OR			
	Quinine sulfate[43,44] PLUS ONE OF THE FOLLOWING: Doxycycline,[45] Tetracycline,[45] or Clindamycin	Quinine sulfate: 542 mg base (=650 mg salt), orally, 3 times/day for 3 or 7 days[44] Doxycycline: 100 mg, orally, 2 times/day for 7 days Tetracycline: 250 mg, orally, 4 times/day for 7 days Clindamycin: 20 mg base/kg/day, orally, divided 3 times/day for 7 days	Quinine sulfate: 8.3 mg base/kg (=10 mg salt/kg), orally, 3 times/day for 3 or 7 days[44] Doxycycline: 2.2 mg/kg, orally, every 12 h for 7 days Tetracycline: 25 mg/kg/day, orally, divided 4 times/day for 7 days Clindamycin: 20 mg base/kg/day, orally, divided 3 times/day for 7 days	
	OR			

Table 4.11. Drugs for Parasitic Infections,[1] continued

Disease	Drug	Adult Dosage	Pediatric Dosage	CDC Web Site[2] (includes listings of adverse events)
	Mefloquine[46]	684 mg base (=750 mg salt), orally, as initial dose, followed by 456 mg base (=500 mg salt), orally, given 6–12 h after initial dose Total dose = 1250 mg salt	13.7 mg base/kg (=15 mg salt/kg), orally, as initial dose, followed by 9.1 mg base/kg (=10 mg salt/kg), orally, given 6–12 h after initial dose Total dose = 25 mg salt/kg	
	Chloroquine-sensitive (Central America west of Panama Canal, Haiti, the Dominican Republic, and most of the Middle East)			
Uncomplicated malaria *P falciparum* or species not identified	Chloroquine phosphate[47]	600 mg base (=1000 mg salt), orally, immediately, followed by 300 mg base (=500 mg salt), orally, at 6, 24, and 48 h Total dose: 1500 mg base (=2500 mg salt)	10 mg base/kg, orally, immediately, followed by 5 mg base/kg, orally, at 6, 24, and 48 h Total dose: 25 mg base/kg	
	OR			

Table 4.11. Drugs for Parasitic Infections,[1] continued

Disease	Drug	Adult Dosage	Pediatric Dosage	CDC Web Site[2] (includes listings of adverse events)
	Hydroxychloroquine	620 mg base (=800 mg salt), orally, immediately, followed by 310 mg base (=400 mg salt), orally, at 6, 24, and 48 h Total dose: 1550 mg base (=2000 mg salt)	10 mg base/kg, orally, immediately, followed by 5 mg base/kg, orally, at 6, 24, and 48 Total dose: 25 mg base/kg	
Uncomplicated malaria *P malariae or P knowlesi*	All regions			
	Chloroquine phosphate[47]	600 mg base (=1000 mg salt), orally, immediately, followed by 300 mg base (=500 mg salt), orally, at 6, 24, and 48 h Total dose: 1500 mg base (=2500 mg salt)	10 mg base/kg, orally, immediately, followed by 5 mg base/kg, orally, at 6, 24, and 48 h Total dose: 25 mg base/kg	
	OR			

Table 4.11. Drugs for Parasitic Infections,[1] continued

Disease	Drug	Adult Dosage	Pediatric Dosage	CDC Web Site[2] (includes listings of adverse events)
	Hydroxychloroquine	620 mg base (=800 mg salt), orally, immediately, followed by 310 mg base (=400 mg salt), orally, at 6, 24, and 48 h Total dose: 1550 mg base (=2000 mg salt)	10 mg base/kg, orally, immediately, followed by 5 mg base/kg, orally, at 6, 24, and 48 h Total dose: 25 mg base/kg	
Uncomplicated malaria *P vivax* or *P ovale*	All regions Note: for suspected chloroquine-resistant *P vivax*, see row below			
	Chloroquine phosphate[47] PLUS	600 mg base (=1000 mg salt), orally, immediately, followed by 300 mg base (=500 mg salt), orally, at 6, 24, and 48 h Total dose: 1500 mg base (=2500 mg salt)	10 mg base/kg, orally, immediately, followed by 5 mg base/kg, orally, at 6, 24, and 48 h Total dose: 25 mg base/kg	
	Primaquine phosphate[48]	30 mg base, orally, once daily for 14 days	0.5 mg base/kg, orally, once daily for 14 days	
	OR			

Table 4.11. Drugs for Parasitic Infections,[1] continued

Disease	Drug	Adult Dosage	Pediatric Dosage	CDC Web Site[2] (includes listings of adverse events)
	Hydroxychloroquine	620 mg base (=800 mg salt), orally, immediately, followed by 310 mg base (=400 mg salt), orally, at 6, 24, and 48 h Total dose: 1550 mg base (=2000 mg salt)	10 mg base/kg, orally, immediately, followed by 5 mg base/kg, orally, at 6, 24, and 48 h Total dose: 25 mg base/kg	
	PLUS			
	Primaquine phosphate[48]	30 mg base, orally, once daily for 14 days	0.5 mg base/kg, orally, once daily for 14 days	
Uncomplicated malaria *P vivax*	Chloroquine-resistant[49] (Papua New Guinea and Indonesia)			

Table 4.11. Drugs for Parasitic Infections,[1] continued

Disease	Drug	Adult Dosage	Pediatric Dosage	CDC Web Site[2] (includes listings of adverse events)
	Quinine sulfate[43] PLUS EITHER Doxycycline or Tetracy-cline[45] PLUS Primaquine phosphate[48]	Quinine sulfate: 542 mg base (=650 mg salt), orally, 3 times/day for 3 or 7 days[44] Doxycycline: 100 mg, orally, 2 times/day for 7 days Tetracycline: 250 mg, orally, 4 times/day for 7 days Primaquine phosphate: 30 mg base, orally, once daily for 14 days	Quinine sulfate: 8.3 mg base/kg (=10 mg salt/kg), orally, 3 times/day for 3 or 7 days[44] Doxycycline: 2.2 mg/kg, orally, every 12 h for 7 days Tetracycline: 25 mg/kg/day, orally, divided 4 times/day for 7 days Primaquine phosphate: 0.5 mg base/kg, orally, once daily for 14 days	
	OR			

Table 4.11. Drugs for Parasitic Infections,[1] continued

Disease	Drug	Adult Dosage	Pediatric Dosage	CDC Web Site[2] (includes listings of adverse events)
	Atovaquone-proguanil PLUS Primaquine phosphate[48]	Atovaquone-proguanil: 1000 mg atovaquone/400 mg proguanil, orally, once daily for 3 days Primaquine phosphate: 30 mg base, orally, once daily for 14 days	Atovaquone-proguanil: 5–8 kg: 2 pediatric tablets, orally, once daily for 3 days 9–10 kg: 3 pediatric tablets, orally, once daily for 3 days 11–20 kg: 1 adult tablet, orally, once daily for 3 days 21–30 kg: 2 adult tablets, orally, once daily for 3 days 31–40 kg: 3 adult tablets, orally, once daily for 3 days >40 kg: 4 adult tablets, orally, once daily for 3 days Primaquine phosphate: 0.5 mg base/kg, orally, once daily for 14 days	
OR				

Table 4.11. Drugs for Parasitic Infections,[1] continued

Disease	Drug	Adult Dosage	Pediatric Dosage	CDC Web Site[2] (includes listings of adverse events)
	Mefloquine PLUS Primaquine phosphate[48]	Mefloquine: 684 mg base (=750 mg salt), orally, as initial dose, followed by 456 mg base (=500 mg salt), orally, given 6–12 h after initial dose Total dose= 1250 mg salt Primaquine phosphate: 30 mg base, orally, once daily for 14 days	Mefloquine: 13.7 mg base/kg (=15 mg salt/kg), orally, as initial dose, followed by 9.1 mg base/kg (=10 mg salt/kg), orally, given 6–12 h after initial dose Total dose = 25 mg salt/kg Primaquine phosphate: 0.5 mg base/kg, orally, once daily for 14 days	
Uncomplicated malaria: alternatives for pregnant women[50,51,52]	Chloroquine-sensitive (see uncomplicated malaria sections above for chloroquine-sensitive species by region)			

Table 4.11. Drugs for Parasitic Infections,[1] continued

Disease	Drug	Adult Dosage	Pediatric Dosage	CDC Web Site[2] (includes listings of adverse events)
	Chloroquine phosphate[47]	600 mg base (=1000 mg salt), orally, immediately, followed by 300 mg base (=500 mg salt), orally, at 6, 24, and 48 h Total dose: 1500 mg base (=2500 mg salt)	Not applicable	
	OR			
	Hydroxychloroquine	620 mg base (=800 mg salt), orally, immediately, followed by 310 mg base (=400 mg salt), orally, at 6, 24, and 48 h Total dose: 1550 mg base (=2000 mg salt)	Not applicable	
	Chloroquine-resistant (see sections above for regions with chloroquine-resistant *P falciparum* and *P vivax*)			

Table 4.11. Drugs for Parasitic Infections,[1] continued

Disease	Drug	Adult Dosage	Pediatric Dosage	CDC Web Site[2] (includes listings of adverse events)
	Quinine sulfate[43] PLUS Clindamycin	Quinine sulfate: 542 mg base (=650 mg salt), orally, 3 times/day for 3 or 7 days[44] Clindamycin: 20 mg base/kg/day, orally, divided 3 times/day for 7 days	Not applicable	
	OR			
	Mefloquine	684 mg base (=750 mg salt), orally, as initial dose, followed by 456 mg base (=500 mg salt), orally, given 6–12 h after initial dose Total dose= 1250 mg salt	Not applicable	
Severe malaria[53,54,55]	All regions			

Table 4.11. Drugs for Parasitic Infections,[1] continued

Disease	Drug	Adult Dosage	Pediatric Dosage	CDC Web Site[2] (includes listings of adverse events)
	Quinidine gluconate[54] PLUS ONE OF THE FOLLOWING: Doxycycline, Tetracycline,[45] or Clindamycin	Quinidine gluconate: 6.25 mg base/kg (=10 mg salt/kg) loading dose, IV over 1–2 h, then 0.0125 mg base/kg/min (=0.02 mg salt/kg/min) continuous infusion for at least 24 h. An alternative regimen is 15 mg base/kg (=24 mg salt/kg) loading dose, IV infused over 4 h, followed by 7.5 mg base/kg (=12 mg salt/kg) infused over 4 h every 8 h, starting 8 h after the loading dose (see package insert). Once parasite density <1% and patient can take oral medication, complete treatment with oral quinine, dose as above.[43] Quinidine/quinine course = 7 days in Southeast Asia; = 3 days in Africa or South America.	Quinidine gluconate: Same mg/kg dosing and recommendations as for adults. Doxycycline: 2.2 mg/kg, orally, every 12 h for 7 days. If patient not able to take oral medication, may give IV. For children <45 kg, give 2.2 mg/kg, IV, every 12 h and then switch to oral doxycycline (dose as above) as soon as patient can take oral medication. For children >45 kg, use same dosing as for adults. For IV use, avoid rapid administration. Treatment course = 7 days. Tetracycline: 25 mg/kg/day, orally, divided 4 times/day for 7 days.	

Table 4.11. Drugs for Parasitic Infections,[1] continued

Disease	Drug	Adult Dosage	Pediatric Dosage	CDC Web Site[2] (includes listings of adverse events)
		Doxycycline: 100 mg, orally, 2 times/day for 7 days. If patient not able to take oral medication, give 100 mg, IV, every 12 h and then switch to oral doxycycline (as above) as soon as patient can take oral medication. For IV use, avoid rapid administration. Treatment course = 7 days. Tetracycline: 250 mg, orally, 4 times/day for 7 days. Clindamycin: 20 mg base/kg/day, orally, divided 3 times/day for 7 days. If patient not able to take oral medication, give 10 mg base/kg loading dose, IV, followed by 5 mg base/kg, IV, every 8 h. Switch to oral clindamycin (oral dose as above) as soon as patient can take oral medication. For IV use, avoid rapid administration. Treatment course = 7 days.	Clindamycin: 20 mg base/kg/day, orally, divided 3 times/day for 7 days. If patient not able to take oral medication, give 10 mg base/kg loading dose, IV, followed by 5 mg base/kg, IV, every 8 h. Switch to oral clindamycin (oral dose as above) as soon as patient can take oral medication. For IV use, avoid rapid administration. Treatment course = 7 days. *Investigational new drug (contact CDC for information):* Artesunate followed by one of the following: atovaquone-proguanil, clindamycin, or mefloquine	

Table 4.11. Drugs for Parasitic Infections,[1] continued

Disease	Drug	Adult Dosage	Pediatric Dosage	CDC Web Site[2] (includes listings of adverse events)
		Investigational new drug (contact CDC for information): Artesunate followed by one of the following: atovaquone-proguanil, doxycycline (clindamycin in pregnant women), or mefloquine		
Microsporidiosis				
Ocular				www.cdc.gov/dpdx/ microsporidiosis/ tx.html
Encephalitozoon helem,, E cuniculi, Vittaforma [Nosema] corneae	Fumagillin[56] PLUS for management of systemic infection: Albendazole[11]	Fumagillin in saline equivalent to fumagillin 70 µg/mL eye drops 2 drops every 2 h for 4 days, then 2 drops 4 times per day 400 mg, orally, twice a day	15 mg/kg/day, orally, divided 2 times/day (max 400 mg/dose)	
Intestinal				
E bieneusi	Fumagillin[57]	20 mg, orally, 3 times/day for 14 days		
E intestinalis	Albendazole[11]	400 mg, orally, twice a day for 21 days	15 mg/kg/day in 2 doses (max 400 mg/dose)	

Table 4.11. Drugs for Parasitic Infections,[1] continued

Disease	Drug	Adult Dosage	Pediatric Dosage	CDC Web Site[2] (includes listings of adverse events)
Disseminated[58]				
E hellem, E cuniculi, E intestinalis, Pleistophora species, *Trachipleistophora* species, and *Anncaliia* [*Brachiola*] *vesicularum*	Albendazole[11]	Immunocompromised: 400 mg, orally, twice per day for 14 to 28 days. Continue treatment until CD4+ T-lymphocyte count >200 cells/μL for >6 mo after initiation of antiretroviral therapy Immunocompetent: 400 mg, orally, twice a day for 7 to 14 days	15 mg/kg/day, orally, divided 2 times/day (max 400 mg/dose)	
Neurocysticercosis[59]	Albendazole[11]	≥60 kg: 400 mg, orally, 2 times/day for 8–30 days <60 kg: 15 mg/kg/day (max 800 mg), orally, divided 2 times/day for 8–30 days	15 mg/kg/day (max 800 mg), orally, in 2 divided doses for 8–30 days	www.cdc.gov/parasites/cysticercosis/health_professionals/index.html
	OR			
	Praziquantel[19]	50 mg/kg/day, orally, for 10–15 days[60]		
Onchocerciasis (*Onchocerca volvulus*; River Blindness)[61]	Ivermectin[13]	150 μg/kg, orally, in 1 dose every 6 mo until asymptomatic		www.cdc.gov/parasites/onchocerciasis/health_professionals/index.html
	OR			
	Doxycycline[62]	200 mg, orally, daily for 6 wk		
Opisthorchis Infection (Southeast Asian liver fluke)	Praziquantel[19]	75 mg/kg/day, orally, divided 3 times/day for 2 days		www.cdc.gov/parasites/opisthorchis/health_professionals/index.html
	OR			
	Albendazole[11]	10 mg/kg/day, orally, for 7 days		

Table 4.11. Drugs for Parasitic Infections,[1] continued

Disease	Drug	Adult Dosage	Pediatric Dosage	CDC Web Site[2] (includes listings of adverse events)
Paragonimiasis (lung fluke)	OR			www.cdc.gov/parasites/paragonimus/health_professionals/index.html
	Mebendazole[12]	30 mg/kg/day, orally, for 20–30 days		
	Praziquantel[12]	75 mg/kg/day, orally, divided 3 times/day for 2–3 days		
	OR			
	Triclabendazole[2] [7]	10 mg/kg, orally, once or twice		
Scabies (Mite Infestation)	Permethrin cream 5%	Topically, twice, at least 7 days apart		www.cdc.gov/parasites/scabies/health_professionals/meds.html
	OR			
	Crotamiton lotion 10% and Crotamiton cream 10%	Topically, overnight, on days 1, 2, 3, and 8		
	OR			
	Ivermectin[13]	200 µg/kg, orally, twice, at least 7 days apart		
Schistosomiasis (Bilharzia)	Schistosoma mansoni, S haematobium, S intercalatum			www.cdc.gov/parasites/schistosomiasis/health_professionals/index.html
	Praziquantel[19]	40 mg/kg/day, orally, divided 2 times/day for 1 day		
	S japonicum, S mekongi			
	Praziquantel[19]	60 mg/kg/day, orally, divided 3 times/day for 1 day		

Table 4.11. Drugs for Parasitic Infections,[1] continued

Disease	Drug	Adult Dosage	Pediatric Dosage	CDC Web Site[2] (includes listings of adverse events)
Strongyloidiasis (*Strongyloides stercoralis*)	Ivermectin[13]	200 µg/kg, orally, daily for 1–2 days; for patients unable to take ivermectin orally, a subcutaneous formulation is available commercially for veterinary use and may be used under a single-patient investigational new drug (IND) protocol on request to FDA		www.cdc.gov/parasites/ strongyloides/ health_professionals/ index.html
	OR			
	Albendazole[11]	400 mg, orally, 2 times/day for 7 days		
Taeniasis [*Taenia saginata* (beef tapeworm), *Taenia solium* (pork tapeworm), and *Taenia asiatica* (Asian tapeworm)]	Praziquantel[19]	5–10 mg/kg, orally, once		www.cdc.gov/parasites/ taeniasis/ health_professionals/ index.html
	OR			
	Niclosamide[23]	2 g, orally, once	50 mg/kg (max 2 g), orally, once	
Toxocariasis (Ocular Larva Migrans, Visceral Larva Migrans)	Albendazole[11]	400 mg, orally, 2 times/day for 5 days		www.cdc.gov/parasites/ toxocariasis/ health_professionals/ index.html
	OR			
	Mebendazole[12]	100–200 mg, orally, 2 times/day for 5 days		

Table 4.11. Drugs for Parasitic Infections,[1] continued

Disease	Drug	Adult Dosage	Pediatric Dosage	CDC Web Site[2] (includes listings of adverse events)
Toxoplasmosis CNS disease (*Toxoplasma gondii*)[63]	Pyrimethamine[64] PLUS Sulfadiazine	200 mg, orally, once, then 50–75 mg/day, orally, for 3–6 wk 1.0–1.5 g, orally, 4 times/day for 3–6 wk	2 mg/kg/day, orally, for 2 days, then 1 mg/kg/day (max 25 mg/day) for 3–6 wk 100–200 mg/kg/day, orally, divided every 6 h for 3–6 wk	www.cdc.gov/parasites/ toxoplasmosis/ health_professionals/ index.html
	OR			
	Pyrimethamine[64] PLUS Clindamycin	200 mg, orally, once; then 50–75 mg/day, orally, for 3–6 wk 1.8–2.4 g/day, IV or orally, divided 3 or 4 times/day for 3–6 wk	2 mg/kg/day, orally, for 2 days; then 1 mg/kg/day (max 25 mg/day) for 3–6 wk 5–7.5 mg/kg/dose (max 600 mg/dose), IV or orally, 3 or 4 times/day for 3–6 wk	
	OR			
	Pyrimethamine[64] PLUS Atovaquone	200 mg, orally, once, then 50–75 mg/day, orally, for 3–6 wk 1500 mg, orally, 2 times/day	2 mg/kg/day, orally, for 2 days, then 1 mg/kg/day (max 25 mg/day) for 3–6 wk See footnote 63	
	OR			
	Trimethoprim (TMP)/ Sulfamethoxazole (SMX)	5 mg/kg TMP and 25 mg/kg SMX, IV or orally, 2 times daily for 3–6 wk	Age >2 mo: 5 mg/kg TMP and 25 mg/kg SMX, IV or orally, 2 times daily for 3–6 wk	

Table 4.11. Drugs for Parasitic Infections,[1] continued

Disease	Drug	Adult Dosage	Pediatric Dosage	CDC Web Site[2] (includes listings of adverse events)
Toxoplasmosis in pregnancy and neonates (*Toxoplasma gondii*)	See Toxoplasmosis chapter			www.cdc.gov/parasites/ toxoplasmosis/ health_professionals/ index.html
Trichinellosis (trichinosis; *Trichinella* species)[65]	Albendazole[11]	10 mg/kg (max 400 mg), orally, twice daily for 8 to 14 days		www.cdc.gov/parasites/ trichinellosis/ health_professionals/ index.html
	OR			
	Mebendazole[12]	200–400 mg, orally, 3 times daily for 3 days; then 400–500 mg, orally, 3 times daily for 10 days		
Trichuriasis (whipworm infection; *Trichuris trichiura*)	Albendazole[11]	400 mg, orally, for 3 days		www.cdc.gov/parasites/ whipworm/ health_professionals/ index.html
	OR			
	Mebendazole[12]	100 mg, orally, twice daily for 3 days		
	OR			
	Ivermectin[13]	200 µg/kg/day, orally, for 3 days		

CDC indicates Centers for Disease Control and Prevention; IV, intravenous; CNS, central nervous system; IM, intramuscular; FDA, US Food and Drug Administration.

[1] The contents of this table are provided to assist in decision making for patient management, but are not a substitute for clinical judgment or expert consultation. The table may not address issues pertinent to some special populations (eg, patients with HIV/AIDS). Recommendations in the table may not represent all potential treatment or dosage options.

[2] See CDC Web site for additional information on each disease and the treatment thereof. Not all recommended therapies and dosages included in this table match the recommendations on the pathogen-specific CDC web pages. Inclusion of the links to the CDC Web site does not suggest endorsement of the content of this table by CDC.

[3] Pentamidine is also effective against *T b rhodesiense* in the hemolymphatic stage, but suramin may have higher efficacy. Suramin is not approved by the FDA but is available through the CDC Drug Service under an investigational new drug (IND) protocol. Questions should be directed to Parasitic Diseases Inquiries (404-718-4745; e-mail **parasites@cdc.gov**).

[4] A suramin test dose of 100 mg should be given before the first dose, and the patient should be monitored for hemodynamic stability.

[5] A suramin test dose of 2 mg/kg (max 100 mg) should be given before the first dose, and the patient should be monitored for hemodynamic stability.

[6] Corticosteroids have been used to prevent melarsoprol encephalopathy. Melarsoprol is not approved by the FDA but is available through the CDC Drug Service under an IND protocol. Questions should be directed to Parasitic Diseases Inquiries (404-718-4745; e-mail **parasites@cdc.gov**).

[7] The traditional regimens of melarsoprol typically entailed 3 courses of drug (each of which consisted of 3 consecutive days of therapy) that were separated by a 7-day rest period. The daily dose of melarsoprol was progressively increased during the first course.

[8] Suramin also is effective against *T b gambiense* in the hemolymphatic stage but should be used only in patients in whom onchocerciasis has been excluded. Suramin is not approved by the FDA but is available through the CDC Drug Service under an IND protocol. Questions should be directed to Parasitic Diseases Inquiries (404-718-4745; e-mail **parasites@cdc.gov**).

[9] Eflornithine (400 mg/kg/day, IV, in 2 divided doses for 7 days) given in combination with oral nifurtimox (15 mg/kg/day, in 3 divided doses for 10 days) is also highly effective against *T b gambiense* with CNS involvement; eflornithine is available through the CDC Drug Service; questions should be directed to Parasitic Diseases Inquiries (404-718-4745; e-mail **parasites@cdc.gov**). Nifurtimox is not FDA approved, nor is this use covered by CDC's IND protocol for nifurtimox, which solely covers treatment of Chagas disease; permission for other uses would need to be obtained.

[10] The 2 drugs used to treat infection with *Trypanosoma cruzi* are benznidazole and nifurtimox. Benznidazole was approved in 2017 by the US Food and Drug Administration (FDA) for use in children 2–12 years of age for the treatment of Chagas disease. Nifurtimox is not approved by the FDA for use in the United States but can be obtained from the CDC (Division of Parasitic Diseases and Malaria, 404-718-4745; e-mail **parasites@cdc.gov**) for treatment of patients under a compassionate use protocol. For both drugs, adverse effects are common and are more frequent and more severe with increasing age.

[11] The safety of albendazole in children younger than 6 years is not certain. Studies of the use of albendazole in children as young as 1 year suggest that its use is safe.

[12] The safety of mebendazole in children has not been established. There are limited data in children 2 years and younger.

[13] The safety of ivermectin in treating children who weigh less than 15 kg has not been established.

[14] The safety of pyrantel pamoate in children has not been established. According to WHO guidance on preventive chemotherapy, pyrantel may be used in children age 1 year and older during mass treatment programs without diagnosis.

15 The combination of clindamycin plus quinine is the standard of care for babesiosis in patients who are severely ill.

16 Some immunocompromised adults with babesiosis have been treated with doses of azithromycin in the range of 600–1000 mg/day, in combination with atovaquone (750 mg twice per day).

17 In cases in which suspicion of exposure is high, immediate treatment with albendazole (25–50 mg/kg/day, orally, for 10–20 days) may be appropriate. Treatment is successful when administered soon after exposure to abort the migration of larvae. Treatment should be initiated as soon as possible after ingestion of infectious material, ideally within 3 days. For clinical baylisascariasis, treatment with albendazole with concurrent corticosteroids to help reduce the inflammatory reaction is indicated to attempt to control the disease.

18 The clinical significance of *Blastocystis* species is controversial.

19 Praziquantel is not approved for treatment of children younger than 4 years, but this drug has been used successfully to treat cases of *D caninum* infection in children as young as 6 months.

20 There are no drug regimens with proven efficacy for the treatment of cryptosporidiosis in immunosuppressed patients.

21 HIV-infected patients may need longer courses of therapy for cyclosporiasis.

22 Expert consultation for treatment of cystoisosporiasis is recommended if the patient is immunosuppressed.

23 Niclosamide is unavailable in the United States.

24 Treatment of cystic echinococcosis depends on the World Health Organization classification of the cysts. Albendazole is not appropriate for all forms of the infection.

25 Mild-to-moderate intestinal disease as well as severe intestinal and extraintestinal disease require different treatment regimens.

26 Dioxanide furoate is not commercially available in the United States.

27 Triclabendazole is not approved by the FDA but is available through the CDC Drug Service; questions should be directed to Parasitic Diseases Inquiries (404–718-4745; e-mail **parasites@cdc.gov**). Release of the drug by CDC requires an individual IND from the FDA. The safety of triclabendazole in children has not been established.

28 Alternative treatments for giardiasis include paromomycin, quinacrine, and furazolidone.

29 Sodium stibogluconate is not approved by the FDA but is available through the CDC Drug Service under an IND protocol; questions should be directed to Parasitic Diseases Inquiries (404–718-4745; e-mail **parasites@cdc.gov**). Only selected antileishmanial agents and regimens are listed in the table. Expert consultation about these and other potential treatment options for leishmaniasis is encouraged. For some cases of cutaneous leishmaniasis, no therapy may be needed or local (vs systemic) therapy may suffice or other systemic treatments may be considered. Miltefosine (IMPAVIDO) was approved in March 2014 by the FDA—for treatment of visceral leishmaniasis caused by *L donovani*; mucosal leishmaniasis caused by *L (Viannia) braziliensis*; and cutaneous leishmaniasis caused by *L (V) braziliensis*, *L (V) guyanensis*, and *L (V) panamensis* (ie, some New World cutaneous leishmaniasis species but no Old World cutaneous leishmaniasis species)—for patients who are at least 12 years of age, weigh at least 30 kg, and are not pregnant or breastfeeding during or for 5 months after the treatment course.

30 IDSA leishmaniasis guidelines are also available at **www.idsociety.org/Guidelines/Patient_Care/IDSA_Practice_Guidelines/ Infections_by_Organism/Parasites/Leishmaniasis/**.

31 Pediculicides should not be used for infestations of the eyelashes. Such infestations are treated with petrolatum ointment applied 2 to 4 times/day for 10 days. For pubic lice, treat with 1% permethrin, pyrethrins with piperonyl butoxide, or ivermectin.

[32] Permethrin and pyrethrin are pediculicidal; retreatment in 9–10 days is needed to eradicate the infestation. Some lice are resistant to pyrethrins and permethrin. Pyrethrins with piperonyl butoxide are recommended for use in children ≥2 years of age; permethrin for children ≥2 months of age.

[33] Ivermectin is not ovicidal, but lice that hatch from treated eggs die within 48 hours after hatching. Recommended for use in children ≥6 months of age.

[34] Spinosad causes neuronal excitation in insects leading to paralysis and death. The formulation also includes benzyl alcohol, which is pediculicidal. Two applications 7 days apart are needed. Recommended for children ≥6 months of age.

[35] Benzyl alcohol prevents lice from closing their respiratory spiracles and the lotion vehicle then obstructs their airway causing them to asphyxiate. It is not ovicidal. Two applications 9–10 days apart are needed. Recommended for use in children ≥6 months of age. Resistance, which is a problem with other drugs, is unlikely to develop.

[36] Malathion is both ovicidal and pediculicidal; 2 applications 7–9 days apart are generally necessary to kill all lice and nits. Recommended for children ≥6 years of age, and contraindicated in children <24 months of age.

[37] Ivermectin is pediculicidal but not ovicidal; more than 1 dose is generally necessary to eradicate the infestation. The number of doses and the interval between doses have not been established; animal studies have shown adverse effects on the fetus. A single oral dose of 200 μg/kg, repeated in 9–10 days, has been shown to be effective against head lice. Most recently, a single oral dose of 400 μg/kg, repeated in 9–10 days, has been shown to be more effective than 0.5% malathion lotion.

[38] Diethylcarbamazine (DEC) is not approved by the FDA but is available through the CDC Drug Service under an IND protocol; questions should be directed to Parasitic Diseases Inquiries (404-718-4745; e-mail **parasites@cdc.gov**). DEC is contraindicated in patients who may also have onchocerciasis. Before DEC therapy for lymphatic filariasis or loiasis, onchocerciasis should be excluded in all patients with a consistent exposure history because of the possibility of severe exacerbations of skin and eye involvement (Mazzotti reaction). People coinfected with *L loa* and *O volvulus* should not be treated with DEC until the onchocerciasis is treated; their onchocerciasis should not be treated with ivermectin if it is unsafe to treat their loiasis.

[39] Doxycycline is not standard treatment for lymphatic filariasis. However, some studies have shown adult-worm killing with doxycycline therapy (200 mg/day for 4–6 weeks).

[40] If a person develops malaria despite taking chemoprophylaxis, that particular medicine should not be used as a part of his or her treatment regimen. Use one of the other options instead.

[41] There are 4 options available for treatment of uncomplicated malaria caused by chloroquine-resistant *P falciparum*. The first 3 options are equally recommended. Because of a higher rate of severe neuropsychiatric reactions seen at treatment doses, mefloquine is not recommended unless the other options cannot be used. For the third option, because there are more data on the efficacy of quinine in combination with doxycycline or tetracycline, these treatment combinations are generally preferred to quinine in combination with clindamycin.

[42] Atovaquone-proguanil or artemether-lumefantrine should be taken with food or whole milk. If patient vomits within 30 minutes of taking a dose, the dose should be repeated. Adult tablet = 250 mg atovaquone/100 mg proguanil. Pediatric tablet = 62.5 mg atovaquone/25 mg proguanil.

[43] The US-manufactured quinine sulfate capsule is in a 324-mg dosage; therefore, 2 capsules should be sufficient for adult dosing. Pediatric dosing may be difficult because of unavailability of noncapsule forms of quinine.

[44] For infections acquired in Southeast Asia, quinine treatment should continue for 7 days. For infections acquired elsewhere, quinine treatment should continue for 3 days.

[45] Tetracycline is not indicated for use in children younger than 8 years. Doxycycline can be administered for short durations (ie, 21 days or less) without regard to the patient's age (see Tetracyclines, p 905). For children younger than 8 years with chloroquine-resistant *P falciparum*, atovaquone-proguanil and artemether-lumefantrine are recommended treatment options; mefloquine is the recommended treatment. If it is not available or is not being tolerated and if the treatment benefits outweigh the risks, atovaquone-proguanil or artemether-lumefantrine should be used instead.

[46] Treatment with mefloquine is not recommended in people who have acquired infections from Southeast Asia because of drug resistance.

[47] When treating chloroquine-sensitive infections, chloroquine and hydroxychloroquine are recommended options. However, regimens used to treat chloroquine-resistant infections may also be used if available, more convenient, or preferred.

[48] Primaquine is used to eradicate any hypnozoites that may remain dormant in the liver and, thus, prevent relapses in *P vivax* and *P ovale* infections. Because primaquine can cause hemolytic anemia in glucose-6-phosphate dehydrogenase (G6PD)-deficient people, G6PD screening must occur prior to starting treatment with primaquine. For people with borderline G6PD deficiency or as an alternate to the above regimen, primaquine, 45 mg, orally, once per week for 8 weeks may be given; consultation with an expert in infectious disease and/or tropical medicine is advised if this alternative regimen is considered in G6PD-deficient people. Primaquine must not be used during pregnancy.

[49] There are 3 options available for treatment of uncomplicated malaria caused by chloroquine-resistant *P vivax*. High treatment failure rates attributable to chloroquine-resistant *P vivax* have been well documented in Papua New Guinea and Indonesia. Rare case reports of chloroquine-resistant *P vivax* have also been documented in Burma (Myanmar), India, and Central and South America. People acquiring *P vivax* infections outside of Papua New Guinea or Indonesia should be started on chloroquine. If the patient does not respond, the treatment should be changed to a chloroquine-resistant *P vivax* regimen and the CDC should be notified (Malaria Hotline number listed previously). For treatment of chloroquine-resistant *P vivax* infections, the 3 options are equally recommended.

[50] For pregnant women diagnosed with uncomplicated malaria caused by chloroquine-resistant *P falciparum* or chloroquine-resistant *P vivax* infection, treatment with doxycycline or tetracycline is generally not indicated. However, doxycycline or tetracycline may be used in combination with quinine (as recommended for nonpregnant adults) if other treatment options are not available or are not being tolerated, and the benefit is judged to outweigh the risks.

[51] Atovaquone-proguanil and artemether-lumefantrine are generally not recommended for use in pregnant women, particularly in the first trimester, because of lack of sufficient safety data. For pregnant women diagnosed with uncomplicated malaria caused by chloroquine-resistant *P falciparum* infection, atovaquone-proguanil or artemether-lumefantrine may be used if other treatment options are not available or are not being tolerated, and if the potential benefit is judged to outweigh the potential risks.

[52] For *P vivax* and *P ovale* infections, primaquine phosphate for radical treatment of hypnozoites should not be given during pregnancy. Pregnant patients with *P vivax* and *P ovale* infections should be maintained on chloroquine prophylaxis for the duration of their pregnancy. The chemoprophylactic dose of chloroquine phosphate is 300 mg base (=500 mg salt), orally, once per week. After delivery, pregnant patients who do not have G6PD deficiency should be treated with primaquine.

[53] People with a positive blood smear OR history of recent possible exposure and no other recognized pathologic abnormality who have 1 or more of the following clinical criteria (impaired consciousness/coma, severe normocytic anemia, renal failure, pulmonary edema, acute respiratory distress syndrome, circulatory shock, disseminated intravascular coagulation, spontaneous bleeding, acidosis, hemoglobinuria, jaundice, repeated generalized convulsions, and/or parasitemia of >5%) are considered to have manifestations of more severe disease. Severe malaria is most often caused by *P falciparum*.

[54] Patients with a diagnosis of severe malaria should be treated aggressively with parenteral antimalarial therapy. Treatment with IV quinidine should be initiated as soon as possible after the diagnosis has been made. Patients with severe malaria should be given an intravenous loading dose of quinidine unless they have received more than 40 mg/kg of quinine in the preceding 48 hours or if they have received mefloquine within the preceding 12 hours. Consultation with a cardiologist and a physician with experience treating malaria is advised when treating malaria patients with quinidine. During administration of quinidine, blood pressure monitoring (for hypotension) and cardiac monitoring (for widening of the QRS complex and/or lengthening of the QTc interval) should be monitored continuously and blood glucose (for hypoglycemia) should be monitored periodically. Cardiac complications, if severe, may warrant temporary discontinuation of the drug or slowing of the intravenous infusion. The manufacturer of intravenous quinidine is ceasing production, and it will no longer be available after March 2019. Please consult the CDC malaria website for therapeutic options thereafter, including intravenous artesunate.

[55] Pregnant women diagnosed with severe malaria should be treated aggressively with parenteral antimalarial therapy.

[56] Available as an investigational agent (non–FDA approved) in the United States from Leiter's Park Avenue Pharmacy (a custom compounding pharmacy), San Jose, CA; 800-292-6773; **www.leiterrx.com**. For lesions attributable to *V corneae*, topical therapy is generally not effective and keratoplasty may be required (RM Davis, Font RL, Keisler MS, Shadduck JA. Corneal microsporidiosis. A case report including ultrastructural observations. *Ophthalmology*. 1990;97[7]:953-957). Data are insufficient to make recommendations on the use of fumagillin in children (see "Guidelines for the Prevention and Treatment of Opportunistic Infection in HIV-Exposed and HIV-Infected Children," 2013; **https://aidsinfo.nih.gov/guidelines/html/5/pediatric-oi-prevention-and-treatment-guidelines/412/microsporidiosis**).

[57] For gastrointestinal infections caused by *Enterocytozoon bieneusi*, fumagillin, 20 mg, orally 3 times daily, is the only drug with proven efficacy. However, its use is associated with severe thrombocytopenia in 30% to 50% of patients, which is reversible on discontinuation of treatment, and the drug is not currently available in the United States.

[58] There is no established treatment for *Pleistophora*. For disseminated disease attributable to *Trachipleistophora* or *Anncaliia*, itraconazole, 400 mg, orally, once per day, plus albendazole may also be tried.

[59] Although not all symptomatic patients with a single cyst of neurocysticercosis within brain parenchyma require antiparasitic medication, controlled studies demonstrate that clinical resolution and seizure recurrence rates are improved with albendazole. Two studies have demonstrated that in those with more than 2 lesions, the response rate was better when albendazole was coadministered with praziquantel and corticosteroids. When a single agent is used, albendazole is preferred over praziquantel because it has fewer drug-drug interactions with anticonvulsants and steroids. Longer courses may be needed for subarachnoid disease. Corticosteroid therapy is almost always required when albendazole or praziquantel is used.

[60] A 10-day course of praziquantel has been used in combination therapy with albendazole.

[61] People coinfected with *O volvulus* and *L loa* should not be treated with diethylcarbamazine (DEC) until the onchocerciasis is treated; their onchocerciasis should not be treated with ivermectin if it is unsafe to treat their loiasis. Patients should only be treated with doxycycline if they no longer live in areas with endemic infection unless there is a contraindication for ivermectin.

[62] Doxycycline is not standard therapy, but several studies support its use and safety. Treatment with a single oral dose of ivermectin (150 μg/kg) should be given 1 week before treatment with doxycycline to provide symptom relief to the patient. If the patient cannot tolerate the dosage of 200 mg, orally, daily of doxycycline, 100 mg, orally, daily is sufficient to sterilize female *Onchocerca* organisms.

[63]For treatment and chronic suppression of toxoplasmosis in human immunodeficiency virus (HIV) infected children, see Guidelines for the Prevention and Treatment of Opportunistic Infections Among HIV-Exposed and HIV-Infected Children, 2013 at **http://aidsinfo.nih.gov/contentfiles/lvguidelines/oi_guidelines_pediatrics.pdf.**

[64]Plus leucovorin, 10–25 mg, with each dose of pyrimethamine.

[65]In addition to antiparasitic medication, treatment with corticosteroids sometimes is required in more severe cases of trichinellosis.

MEDWATCH–THE FDA SAFETY INFORMATION AND ADVERSE EVENT-REPORTING PROGRAM

Adverse drug events can cause direct harm to patients, can negatively affect clinical practice, and can be economically costly for patients and the healthcare system. MedWatch, the Food and Drug Administration (FDA) Safety Information and Adverse Event Reporting Program, serves as a gateway for clinically important safety information and reporting of adverse events for human medical products, including FDA-regulated prescription and over-the-counter drugs, biologics (including human cells, tissues, and cellular and tissue-based products), medical devices (including in vitro diagnostics), special nutritional products, and cosmetics. MedWatch collects reports of drug side effects, product use errors, product quality problems, and therapeutic failures. Although reporting to MedWatch by health care professionals and consumers is voluntary, manufacturers of prescription medical products are required to submit adverse event reports to the FDA.

As many prelicensure clinical trials are not large enough to reveal rare adverse events, postlicensure safety surveillance is used to identify and evaluate new safety concerns with drugs and devices after they are approved and widely used in clinical practice. MedWatch reports are used by the FDA as a pharmacovigilance data source. If a potential safety concern is identified through analysis of MedWatch reports, FDA's further evaluation might include conducting studies using other databases. Based on information from postmarketing safety surveillance, the FDA may take regulatory actions, such as revising and strengthening warnings, precautions, contraindications, and adverse reaction descriptions in medication package inserts; issuing "Dear Health Care Professional" letters; and posting safety alerts on the agency's Web site.

Health care professionals and consumers are encouraged to report adverse events associated with medical products. The MedWatch voluntary form is a 1-page, postage-paid form (see Fig 4.1). The MedWatch form can be sent by fax (800-FDA-0178) or mail. Adverse events can also be reported online at **www.fda.gov/MedWatch/report. htm.** A toll-free number (800-FDA-1088) is available to report by phone or request blank forms with instructions.

Vaccine-related adverse events should be reported to the Vaccine Adverse Event Reporting System (**http://vaers.hhs.gov/**) (see p 45).

FIG 4.1 MEDWATCH VOLUNTARY REPORTING FORM

Reset Form

U.S. Department of Health and Human Services

MEDWATCH
The FDA Safety Information and
Adverse Event Reporting Program

For VOLUNTARY reporting of
adverse events, product problems and
product use errors

Page 1 of 3

Form Approved: OMB No. 0910-0291, Expires: 9/30/2018
See PRA statement on reverse.

FDA USE ONLY
Triage unit sequence #
FDA Rec. Date

PLEASE TYPE OR USE BLACK INK

Note: For date prompts of "dd-mmm-yyyy" please use 2-digit day, 3-letter month abbreviation, and 4-digit year; for example, 01-Jul-2015.

A. PATIENT INFORMATION

1. Patient Identifier	2. Age ☐ Year(s) ☐ Month(s) ☐ Week(s) ☐ Days(s) or Date of Birth (e.g., 08 Feb 1925) In Confidence	3. Sex ☐ Female ☐ Male	4. Weight ☐ lb ☐ kg

5.a. Ethnicity (Check single best answer)
☐ Hispanic/Latino
☐ Not Hispanic/Latino

5.b. Race (Check all that apply)
☐ Asian ☐ American Indian or Alaskan Native
☐ Black or African American ☐ White
☐ Native Hawaiian or Other Pacific Islander

B. ADVERSE EVENT, PRODUCT PROBLEM

1. Check all that apply
☐ Adverse Event ☐ Product Problem (e.g., defects/malfunctions)
☐ Product Use Error ☐ Problem with Different Manufacturer of Same Medicine

2. Outcome Attributed to Adverse Event (Check all that apply):
☐ Death Include date (dd-mmm-yyyy):
☐ Life-threatening
☐ Hospitalization – initial or prolonged
☐ Other Serious (Important Medical Events)
☐ Required Intervention to Prevent Permanent Impairment/Damage (Devices)
☐ Disability or Permanent Damage
☐ Congenital Anomaly/Birth Defects

3. Date of Event (dd-mmm-yyyy)   4. Date of this Report (dd-mmm-yyyy)

5. Describe Event, Problem or Product Use Error

(Continue on page 3)

6. Relevant Tests/Laboratory Data, Including Dates

(Continue on page 3)

7. Other Relevant History, Including Preexisting Medical Conditions (e.g., allergies, pregnancy, smoking and alcohol use, liver/kidney problems, etc.)

(Continue on page 3)

C. PRODUCT AVAILABILITY

2. Product Available for Evaluation? (Do not send product to FDA)
☐ Yes ☐ No ☐ Returned to Manufacturer on (dd-mmm-yyyy)

D. SUSPECT PRODUCTS

1. Name, Manufacturer/Compounder, Strength (from product label)

#1 – Name and Strength	#1 – NDC # or Unique ID
#1 – Manufacturer/Compounder	#1 – Lot #
#2 – Name and Strength	#2 – NDC # or Unique ID
#2 – Manufacturer/Compounder	#2 – Lot #

3. Dose or Amount   Frequency   Route
#1
#2

4. Dates of Use (From/To for each) (If unknown, give duration, or best estimate) (dd-mmm-yyyy)
#1
#2

5. Diagnosis or Reason for Use (indication)
#1
#2

6. Is the Product Compounded?
#1 ☐ Yes ☐ No
#2 ☐ Yes ☐ No

7. Is the Product Over-the-Counter?
#1 ☐ Yes ☐ No
#2 ☐ Yes ☐ No

8. Expiration Date (dd-mmm-yyyy)
#1   #2

9. Event Abated After Use Stopped or Dose Reduced?
#1 ☐ Yes ☐ No ☐ Doesn't apply
#2 ☐ Yes ☐ No ☐ Doesn't apply

10. Event Reappeared After Reintroduction?
#1 ☐ Yes ☐ No ☐ Doesn't apply
#2 ☐ Yes ☐ No ☐ Doesn't apply

E. SUSPECT MEDICAL DEVICE

1. Brand Name

2. Common Device Name   2b. Procode

3. Manufacturer Name, City and State

4. Model #	Lot #	5. Operator of Device ☐ Health Professional ☐ Lay User/Patient ☐ Other
Catalog #	Expiration Date (dd-mmm-yyyy)	
Serial #	Unique Identifier (UDI) #	

6. If Implanted, Give Date (dd-mmm-yyyy)   7. If Explanted, Give Date (dd-mmm-yyyy)

8. Is this a single-use device that was reprocessed and reused on a patient? ☐ Yes ☐ No

9. If Yes to Item 8, Enter Name and Address of Reprocessor

F. OTHER (CONCOMITANT) MEDICAL PRODUCTS

Product names and therapy dates (Exclude treatment of event)

(Continue on page 3)

G. REPORTER (See confidentiality section on back)

1. Name and Address

Last Name:	First Name:
Address:	
City:	State/Province/Region:
Country:	ZIP/Postal Code:
Phone #:	Email:

2. Health Professional? ☐ Yes ☐ No

3. Occupation

4. Also Reported to:
☐ Manufacturer/Compounder
☐ User Facility
☐ Distributor/Importer

5. If you do NOT want your identity disclosed to the manufacturer, please mark this box: ☐

FORM FDA 3500 (10/15)   Submission of a report does not constitute an admission that medical personnel or the product caused or contributed to the event.

Available for download at **www.fda.gov/downloads/AboutFDA/ReportsManualsForms/Forms/UCM163919.pdf.**

Antimicrobial Prophylaxis

ANTIMICROBIAL PROPHYLAXIS

Antimicrobial prophylaxis is defined as the use of antimicrobial drugs in the absence of suspected or documented infection to prevent development of infection or disease and is a common practice in pediatrics. The efficacy of antimicrobial prophylaxis has been documented for some conditions but not for many more for which it is used. "Antibiotic solutions" for irrigation or instillation should not be considered prophylaxis and generally are unproven as efficacious for prevention of infection.

Effective chemoprophylaxis should be directed at pathogens common in the infection-prone body sites (Table 5.1). When using prophylactic antimicrobial therapy, the risk of emergence of antimicrobial-resistant organisms and the possibility of an adverse event from the drug must be weighed against potential benefits. Ideally, prophylactic agents should have a narrow spectrum of activity and should be used for as brief a period as possible.

Infection-Prone Body Sites

Antibiotic prophylaxis in vulnerable body sites is most successful if: (1) the period of risk is defined and brief; (2) the expected pathogens have predictable antimicrobial susceptibility; and (3) the site is accessible to adequate antimicrobial concentrations.

ACUTE OTITIS MEDIA

Studies performed decades ago demonstrated that amoxicillin prophylaxis was modestly effective in reducing the frequency of recurrent episodes of otitis media in otitis-prone children. However, antimicrobial prophylaxis often alters the nasopharyngeal flora and fosters colonization with resistant organisms, compromising long-term efficacy and complicating treatment options if disease occurs despite prophylaxis. The use of pneumococcal conjugate vaccines (eg, PCV13) has been effective in reducing episodes and recurrences of acute otitis media (AOM). Use of continuous (eg, 3 to 6 months) orally administered antimicrobial prophylaxis should be reserved for the infrequent patient with ≥3 episodes of AOM in 6 months or ≥4 episodes in the preceding 12 months and after weighing benefits and risks. Antimicrobial prophylaxis is an alternative to tympanostomy tube placement for children with recurrent otitis media with persistent middle ear effusion. Tympanostomy tubes have been associated with a modest benefit of reducing episodes of AOM, by an average 1.5 episodes per child in the first 6 months after placement.

Table 5.1. Antimicrobial Chemoprophylaxis[a]

Anatomic Site-Related Infections	Exposed Host; Time-Limited Exposure	Vulnerable Host (Pathogen); Ongoing Exposure
Otitis media Urinary tract infection Endocarditis	*Bordetella pertussis* exposure *Neisseria meningitidis* exposure Traveler's diarrhea (*Escherichia coli,* *Shigella* species, *Salmonella* species, *Campylobacter* species) Perinatal group B *Streptococcus* (mother/infant) exposure Bite wound (human, animal, reptile) Infants born to HIV-infected mothers, to decrease the risk of HIV transmission. Influenza virus, following close family exposure in those unimmunized Susceptible contacts of index cases of invasive *Haemophilus influenzae* type b disease Exposure to aerosolized spores of *Bacillus anthracis* *Borrelia burgdorferi*[c]	Immunosuppressed patients because of treatment of conditions, eg, oncologic, rheumatologic (*Pneumocystis jirovecii,* fungi) Solid organ and stem cell transplant patients (CMV, *P jirovecii,* fungi) HIV-infected children (*P jirovecii;* polysaccharide-encapsulated bacteria) Preterm neonates (*Candida* species) Anatomic or functional asplenia (polysaccharide-encapsulated bacteria)[b] Chronic granulomatous disease (*Staphylococcus aureus* and certain other catalase-positive bacteria and fungi) Congenital immune deficiencies (various pathogens) Rheumatic fever (group A *Streptococcus*) Infant with neonatal HSV disease[d]

HIV indicates human immunodeficiency virus; CMV, cytomegalovirus; HSV, herpes simplex virus.

[a] Antimicrobial prophylactic regimens for exposed hosts and vulnerable hosts (pathogens) are described in each pathogen or disease-specific chapter in Section 3. Immune globulin prophylaxis is not discussed in this Section but should be considered for specific bacteria (eg, *Clostridium tetani*) or viruses (eg, respiratory syncytial virus).

[b] See Immunization and Other Considerations in Immunosuppressed Children (p 72).

[c] Doxycycline prophylaxis of Lyme disease following tick bites may be considered in specific circumstances (see Lyme Disease [p 515]).

[d] 6-month post-treatment suppressive therapy to prevent reactivation within the brain or on the skin.

URINARY TRACT INFECTION[1]

The role of chemoprophylaxis for urinary tract infection (UTI) is a balance between the impact of modest reduction of recurrent UTI versus the emergence of resistant organisms. Resistance usually will develop to any agent used for prophylaxis. The anatomic abnormalities of the urinary tract, the consequences of recurrent infection, the risks of infection caused by a resistant pathogen, and the anticipated duration of prophylaxis need to be carefully assessed for each patient. Data do not support use of antimicrobial prophylaxis to prevent febrile recurrent UTIs in infants without vesicoureteral reflux (VUR).[1] Among children with grade I through grade IV VUR, chemoprophylaxis with

[1] American Academy of Pediatrics, Subcommittee on Urinary Tract Infections, Steering Committee on Quality Improvement and Management. Urinary tract infection: clinical practice guideline for the diagnosis and management of the initial UTI in febrile infants and children 2 to 24 months. *Pediatrics.* 2011;128(3):595-610

trimethoprim-sulfamethoxazole compared with placebo decreased recurrent UTI following a first or second febrile or symptomatic UTI from 27% to 15%, albeit with an increase in resistance of causative organisms from 25% to 68%.[1,2] The proportion of children with renal scarring after 2 years was not affected by prophylaxis.

Exposure to Specific Pathogens

Prophylaxis may be appropriate or indicated if an increased risk of serious infection with a specific pathogen exists and a specific antimicrobial agent has been demonstrated to decrease the risk of infection by that pathogen. Pathogen-specific prophylaxis is addressed in Section 3. It is assumed that the benefit of prophylaxis is greater than the risk of adverse effects of the antimicrobial agent or the risk of subsequent infection by antimicrobial-resistant organisms. For some pathogens that colonize the upper respiratory tract, elimination of the carrier state can be difficult and may require use of a specific antimicrobial agent that achieves microbiologically effective concentrations in nasopharyngeal secretions (eg, rifampin).

Vulnerable Hosts

Attempts to prevent serious infections in specific populations of vulnerable patients with antimicrobial prophylaxis have been successful in some carefully defined populations that are known to be at risk of infection caused by defined pathogens. In some situations, such as prophylaxis of pneumococcal bacteremia in asplenic children, resistance to beta-lactam agents may lead to decreased effectiveness of continuous prophylaxis. In other situations, such as prophylaxis of *Pneumocystis* infection in immune-compromised children with trimethoprim-sulfamethoxazole, resistance has not appeared to develop despite years of continuous prophylaxis.

···

ANTIMICROBIAL PROPHYLAXIS IN PEDIATRIC SURGICAL PATIENTS

Surgical site infections (SSIs) complicate 2% to 5% of inpatient surgeries, prolong the length of hospitalization, and increase the risk of death. Prevention of SSIs should be a priority for children's hospitals. Active surveillance targeting high-risk, high-volume procedures should be in place and requires education of surgeons and perioperative personnel, technological infrastructure, and use of a multidisciplinary team of trained personnel who are knowledgeable regarding SSI criteria. Institutions should monitor compliance with basic process measures and provide regular feedback to surgical personnel and hospital leadership.

---

[1]Craig JC, Simpson JM, Williams GJ, et al; Prevention of Recurrent Urinary Tract Infection in Children with Vesicoureteric Reflux and Normal Renal Tracts (PRIVENT) Investigators. Antibiotic prophylaxis and recurrent urinary tract infection in children. *N Engl J Med*. 2009;361(18):1748–1759

[2]The RIVUR Trial Investigators. Antimicrobial prophylaxis for children with vesicoureteral reflux. *N Engl J Med*. 2014;370(25):2367–2376

Prevention of postoperative wound infections through perioperative prophylaxis is recommended for procedures with moderate or high infection rates, such as appendectomy for a ruptured appendix, and for procedures in which the consequences of infection are likely to be serious, such as implantation of prosthetic material. Consensus recommendations for prevention of SSIs in adults and children have been developed. Although few data exist specifically for pediatric surgical prophylaxis, the principles of antimicrobial agent selection and exposure at surgical sites in adults should apply to children. Consequences of inappropriate use of prophylactic antimicrobial agents include increased costs, adverse events, and emergence of resistant organisms. The emergence of drug-resistant organisms poses a risk not only to the recipient but to other hospitalized patients in whom a health care-associated infection could develop.

Guidelines for Appropriate Use

Guidelines for prevention of SSIs have been published.[1,2] General principles include that agents used for antimicrobial prophylaxis should prevent SSIs and related morbidity and mortality, reduce the duration and cost of care, produce no adverse effects, and minimize adverse consequences on the microbial flora. Published guidelines address indications, appropriate drug selection, dosing, preoperative timing and need for intraoperative redosing, and duration of prophylaxis.

Indications for Prophylaxis

Major determinants of SSIs include the number of microorganisms in the wound during the procedure, the virulence of the microorganisms, the presence of foreign material in the wound, and host risk factors, including preoperative health status. The classification of surgical procedures is based on an estimation of bacterial contamination and, thus, risk of subsequent infection. The 4 classes are: (1) clean wounds; (2) clean-contaminated wounds; (3) contaminated wounds; and (4) dirty and infected wounds. Additional risk factors for SSIs include the operative site and the duration of the procedure. A patient risk index, which incorporates the American Society of Anesthesiologists' preoperative physical status assessment score, the duration of the operation, and the aforementioned wound classification, has been demonstrated to be a good predictor of SSIs.[3] Others have summarized patients at "high risk" of surgical site infection.[2] Although a high-risk pediatric patient is not clearly defined, high-risk factors in adult patients include obesity, coexistent infections at a remote body site, altered immune response, colonization with pathogenic microorganisms, and diabetes mellitus.

[1]Antimicrobial prophylaxis for surgery. *Treat Guidel Med Lett.* 2012;10(122):73-78

[2]Bratzler DW, Dellinger EP, Olsen KM, et al; American Society of Health-System Pharmacists; Infectious Disease Society of America; Surgical Infection Society; Society for Healthcare Epidemiology of America. Clinical practice guidelines for antimicrobial prophylaxis in surgery. *Am J Health Syst Pharm.* 2013;70(3):195-283; **www.ajhp.org/content/ajhp/70/3/195.full.pdf?sso-checked=true**

[3]Gaynes RP, Culver DH, Horan TC, Edwards JR, Richards C, Tolson JS. Surgical site infection (SSI) rates in the United States, 1992–1998: the National Nosocomial Surveillance System basic SSI risk index. *Clin Infect Dis.* 2001;33(Suppl 2):S69–S77

CLEAN WOUNDS

Clean wounds are uninfected operative wounds in which no inflammation is encountered; the respiratory, alimentary, and genitourinary tracts or oropharyngeal cavity are not entered; and no break in aseptic technique occurred. The operative procedures usually are elective, and wounds are closed primarily and, if necessary, drained with closed drainage. Operative incisional wounds that follow nonpenetrating (blunt) trauma are included in this category, provided that the surgical procedure does not involve entry into the gastrointestinal or genitourinary tracts. The benefits of systemic antimicrobial prophylaxis do not justify the potential risks associated with antimicrobial use in most clean wound procedures, because the risk of infection is low (1%–2%). Some exceptions exist in which prophylaxis is administered because the risks or consequences of infection are high. Examples include implantation of intravascular prosthetic material (eg, insertion of a prosthetic heart valve or a prosthetic joint), open-heart surgery for repair of structural defects, body cavity exploration in neonates, and most neurosurgical operations.

CLEAN-CONTAMINATED WOUNDS

In clean-contaminated wounds, the respiratory, alimentary, or genitourinary tracts are entered under controlled conditions without significant contamination. Operations involving the gastrointestinal tract, the biliary tract, appendix, vagina, or oropharynx, and urgent or emergency surgery in an otherwise clean procedure, are included in this category, provided that no evidence of infection is encountered and no major break in aseptic technique occurs. Prophylaxis is limited to procedures in which a substantial amount of wound contamination is expected. The overall risk of infection for these surgical sites is 3% to 15%. On the basis of data from adults, procedures for which prophylaxis is indicated for pediatric patients include: (1) all gastrointestinal tract procedures in which there is obstruction, when the patient is receiving H_2 receptor antagonists or proton pump blockers, or when the patient has a permanent foreign body; (2) selected biliary tract operations (eg, when there is obstruction from common bile duct stones); and (3) urinary tract surgery or instrumentation in the presence of bacteriuria or obstructive uropathy.

CONTAMINATED WOUNDS

Contaminated wounds are previously sterile tissue sites that are likely to be heavily contaminated with bacteria and include open, fresh wounds; operative wounds in the setting of major breaks in aseptic technique or gross spillage from the gastrointestinal tract; exposed viscera at birth from congenital anomalies; penetrating trauma of fewer than 4 hours' duration; and incisions in which acute nonpurulent inflammation is encountered. The estimated rate of infection for these surgical sites is 15%. In contaminated wound procedures, antimicrobial prophylaxis is appropriate for some patients with acute nonpurulent inflammation isolated to, and contained within, an inflamed viscus (such as acute, nonperforated appendicitis or cholecystitis). For wounds in which contaminating bacteria have had an opportunity to establish inflammation and ongoing infection, antimicrobial use should be considered as treatment rather than prophylaxis.

DIRTY AND INFECTED WOUNDS

Dirty and infected wounds include penetrating trauma of more than 4 hours' duration from time of occurrence (the prolonged period assumes that the infection is already established), wounds with retained devitalized tissue, and wounds involving existing clinical infection or perforated viscera. This definition suggests that the organisms causing postoperative infection were present in the operative field before surgery, and antimicrobial use should be considered as treatment rather than prophylaxis. The estimated rate of infection for these surgical sites is 40%. In dirty and infected wound procedures, such as procedures for a perforated abdominal viscus (eg, ruptured appendix), a compound fracture, a laceration attributable to an animal or human bite >12 hours after injury, or when a major break in sterile technique occurs, antimicrobial agents are given as treatment rather than prophylaxis.

Surgical Site Infection Criteria

Specific classification criteria for SSIs have been developed by the National Healthcare Safety Network (NHSN), and are updated yearly (**www.cdc.gov/nhsn/index.html**).

SUPERFICIAL INCISIONAL SSI

A superficial incisional SSI is an infection that involves only the skin and subcutaneous layers of the incision and occurs within 30 days of the operation, and from which the patient presents with one of the following: (1) purulent drainage from the superficial incision; (2) an organism(s) that is (are) identified from an aseptically obtained specimen from the superficial incision or subcutaneous tissue by culture or molecular analysis; (3) surgical wound exploration (in the absence of laboratory results) when the patient presents with one of the following signs or symptoms: pain or tenderness, localized swelling, erythema, or pain; or (4) diagnosis of superficial incisional SSI by a physician, nurse practitioner, or physician assistant.

DEEP INCISIONAL SSI

A deep incisional SSI occurs within 30 or 90 days after the operative procedure, depending on the surgery, if no implant is left in place or within 1 year if an implant is in place; involves only the fascial or muscle layers; and results in at least 1 of the following: (1) purulent drainage from the deep incision but not from the organ/space component of the surgical site; (2) a deep incision that spontaneously dehisces or is deliberately opened by a physician, nurse practitioner, or physician assistant and at least 1 of the following signs or symptoms: fever (>38°C), localized pain, or localized tenderness; or (3) an abscess or other evidence of infection involving the deep incision that is found on direct examination, during reoperation, or by histopathologic or radiologic examination.

ORGAN/SPACE SSI

An organ or space SSI is defined by the specific site of infection that is opened and manipulated during the procedure (eg, endocarditis, mediastinitis, osteomyelitis) and excludes the superficial, subcutaneous, fascia, or muscle layers that have been manipulated during the procedure. Organ/space SSI must occur within 30 or 90 days of the surgery or within 1 year if an implant is in place, and the patient must have 1 or more of the following: (1) purulent drainage from a drain that is placed through a stab wound into the organ/space; (2) organisms isolated from an aseptically obtained culture of fluid or tissue in the organ/space; or (3) an abscess or other evidence of infection involving the organ/space that is found on direct examination, during reoperation, or by histopathologic or radiologic examination.

Timing of Administration of Prophylactic Antimicrobial Agents

Effective chemoprophylaxis occurs only when the appropriate antimicrobial drug is present in tissues at sufficient local concentrations at the time of intraoperative bacterial contamination. Administration of an antimicrobial agent within 1 or 2 hours before surgery has been demonstrated to decrease the risk of wound infection. Accordingly, administration of the prophylactic agent is recommended within 60 minutes before surgical incision to ensure adequate tissue concentrations at the start of the procedure. When antimicrobial agents require longer administration times, such as glycopeptides (eg, vancomycin) or fluoroquinolones, administration should begin within 120 minutes before the surgery begins.

Dosing and Duration of Administration of Antimicrobial Agents

Weight-based dosing for pediatric patients is routine, but preoperative doses should not exceed the usual dose for adults.

Adequate antimicrobial concentrations should be maintained throughout the surgical procedure; in most instances, a single dose of an antimicrobial agent is sufficient, and the duration of prophylaxis after any procedure should not exceed 24 hours. Intraoperative dosing is required if the duration of the procedure is greater than 2 times the half-life of the antimicrobial agent or if there is excessive blood loss (eg, >1500 mL in adults). For example, cefazolin may be administered every 3 to 4 hours during a prolonged surgical procedure or one that involves large-volume blood loss. Postoperative doses after closure generally are not recommended.

Preoperative Screening and Decolonization

The use of preoperative surveillance to identify carriers of methicillin-susceptible *Staphylococcus aureus* (MSSA) or methicillin-resistant *S aureus* (MRSA) has been explored in the adult population. Use of preoperative nasal mupirocin and chlorhexidine baths for *S aureus* carriers may reduce the risk of deep SSI and is recommended as an adjunct to intravenous prophylaxis in adult cardiac and orthopedic surgery patients. Similar studies have not been performed in children.

Recommended Antimicrobial Agents

An antimicrobial agent is chosen on the basis of bacterial pathogens most likely to cause infectious complications during and after the specific procedure, the antimicrobial susceptibility pattern of these pathogens, and the safety and efficacy of the drug. Newer, more broad-spectrum, and more costly antimicrobial agents are not recommended unless prophylactic efficacy has been proven to be superior to drugs of established benefit or there is a shift in organisms and/or their antimicrobial resistance patterns causing SSIs. Antimicrobial agents administered prophylactically do not have to be active in vitro against every potential organism to be effective, because it is unlikely that all potential organisms are actually contaminating the wound. Doses are determined on the basis of the need to achieve therapeutic blood and tissue concentrations throughout the procedure. Antimicrobial prophylaxis for most surgical procedures, including gastric, biliary, thoracic (noncardiac), vascular, neurosurgical, and orthopedic operations, can be achieved effectively using an agent such as a first-generation cephalosporin (eg, cefazolin) unless the risk for MRSA infection is high, in which case vancomycin may be indicated. For colorectal surgery or appendectomy, effective prophylaxis requires antimicrobial agents that are active against aerobic and anaerobic intestinal flora. Table 5.2 provides recommendations for drugs to be used in children undergoing surgical manipulation or invasive procedures. Physicians should be aware of potential interactions and adverse effects associated with prophylactic antimicrobial agents and other medications the patient may be receiving. Routine use of broad-spectrum agents (extended-spectrum cephalosporins and carbapenems) for surgical prophylaxis generally is not necessary or desirable. Hospital systems should be evaluated regularly to ensure that the process for provision, delivery, and maintenance of appropriate antimicrobial prophylaxis is in place. There are no data to support the practice of continuing antibiotic prophylaxis until all invasive lines, drains, and indwelling catheters have been removed.

Routine use of vancomycin for prophylaxis is not recommended. However, vancomycin prophylaxis may be considered for patients with congenital heart disease who undergo cardiac surgery, patients who undergo certain orthopedic procedures (eg, spinal procedures, implantation of foreign materials), children known to be colonized or previously infected by MRSA, or children living in a community with a high rate of MRSA infections.

The use of local antibiotic delivery (eg antibiotic-impregnated polymethylmethacrylate [PMMA] cement beads, vancomycin powder) into the surgical space has increased in practice. The advantage of locally delivered antibiotic is the high concentration at the applied site, with avoidance of systemic adverse effects. The lack of standardization of these local antibiotic preparations renders comparisons among published studies difficult. There is no high-quality evidence to support these practices of locally delivered antibiotic agents as an adjunct or the sole prophylaxis against SSIs in pediatric patients.

Table 5.2. Recommendations for Preoperative Antimicrobial Prophylaxis

Operation	Likely Pathogens	Recommended Drugs	Preoperative Dose
Neonatal (≤72 h of age)—all major procedures	Group B streptococci, enteric gram-negative bacilli,[a] enterococci, coagulase-negative staphylococci	Ampicillin **PLUS** Gentamicin	50 mg/kg 4 mg/kg
Neonatal (>72 h of age)—all major procedures	Prophylaxis targeted to colonizing organisms, nosocomial organisms, and operative site		
Cardiac (cardiac surgical procedures, prosthetic valve or pacemaker, ventricular assist devices)	*Staphylococcus epidermidis, Staphylococcus aureus, Corynebacterium* species, enteric gram-negative bacilli[a]	Cefazolin **OR** (if MRSA or MRSE is likely) Vancomycin	30 mg/kg (max 2 g) 15 mg/kg
Gastrointestinal			
Esophageal and gastroduodenal	Enteric gram-negative bacilli,[a] gram-positive cocci	Cefazolin (high risk only[b])	30 mg/kg (max 2 g)
Biliary tract	Enteric gram-negative bacilli,[a] enterococci	Cefazolin[c]	30 mg/kg (max 2 g)

Table 5.2. Recommendations for Preoperative Antimicrobial Prophylaxis, continued

Operation	Likely Pathogens	Recommended Drugs	Preoperative Dose
Colorectal or appendectomy (uncomplicated, nonperforated)	Enteric gram-negative bacilli,[a] enterococci, anaerobes (*Bacteroides* species)[d]	Cefoxitin	40 mg/kg (max 3 g)
		OR	
		Metronidazole **PLUS**	15 mg/kg (max 1 g)
		Gentamicin	2.5 mg/kg
		OR	
		Cefazolin **PLUS**	30 mg/kg (max 2 g)
		Metronidazole	15 mg/kg (max 1 g)
		OR	
		Clindamycin **PLUS**	10 mg/kg (max 600 mg)
		Gentamicin **OR** Ciprofloxacin	2.5 mg/kg (gentamicin); 10 mg/kg (ciprofloxacin)

Table 5.2. Recommendations for Preoperative Antimicrobial Prophylaxis, continued

Operation	Likely Pathogens	Recommended Drugs	Preoperative Dose
Ruptured viscus (regarded as treatment, not prophylaxis)	Enteric gram-negative bacilli,[a] enterococci, anaerobes (*Bacteroides* species)[d]	Cefoxitin	40 mg/kg (max 3 g)
		WITH OR WITHOUT	
		Gentamicin	2.5 mg/kg
		OR	
		Gentamicin	2.5 mg/kg
		PLUS	
		Metronidazole	15 mg/kg (max 1 g)
		PLUS	
		Ampicillin	50 mg/kg (max 2 g)
		OR	
		Meropenem	20 mg/kg (max 1 g)
		OR	
		Other regimens for complicated appendicitis[e]	

Table 5.2. Recommendations for Preoperative Antimicrobial Prophylaxis, continued

Operation	Likely Pathogens	Recommended Drugs	Preoperative Dose
Genitourinary	Enteric gram-negative bacilli,[a] enterococci	Cefazolin	30 mg/kg (max 2 g)
		OR	
		Ampicillin **PLUS**	50 mg/kg (max 2 g)
		Gentamicin	2.5 mg/kg
Head and neck surgery (incision through oral or pharyngeal mucosa)	Anaerobes, enteric gram-negative bacilli,[a] S aureus	Clindamycin **WITH OR WITHOUT** Gentamicin	10 mg/kg (max 600 mg) 2.5 mg/kg
		OR	
		Cefazolin **PLUS**	30 mg/kg (max 2 g)
		Metronidazole	15 mg/kg (max 1 g)
Neurosurgery (craniotomy, intrathecal baclofen shunt or ventricular shunt placement)	S epidermidis, S aureus	Cefazolin	30 mg/kg (max 2 g)
		OR	
		(if MRSA or MRSE is likely) Vancomycin	15 mg/kg

Table 5.2. Recommendations for Preoperative Antimicrobial Prophylaxis, continued

Operation	Likely Pathogens	Recommended Drugs	Preoperative Dose
Ophthalmic	*S epidermidis*, *S aureus*, streptococci, enteric gram-negative bacilli,[a] *Pseudomonas* species	Gentamicin, ciprofloxacin, ofloxacin, moxifloxacin, tobramycin	Multiple drops topically for 2–24 h before procedure
		OR	
		Neomycin-gramicidin-polymyxin B	Multiple drops topically for 2–24 h before procedure
		OR	
		Cefazolin	100 mg, subconjunctivally
Orthopedic (internal fixation of fractures, implantation of materials including prosthetic joint and spinal procedures with and without instrumentation)	*S epidermidis*, *S aureus*	Cefazolin	30 mg/kg (max 2 g)
		OR	
		(if MRSA or MRSE is likely) Vancomycin	15 mg/kg
Thoracic (noncardiac)	*S epidermidis*, *S aureus*, streptococci, gram-negative enteric bacilli[a]	Cefazolin	30 mg/kg (max 2 g)
		OR	
		(if MRSA is likely) Vancomycin	15 mg/kg

Table 5.2. Recommendations for Preoperative Antimicrobial Prophylaxis, continued

Operation	Likely Pathogens	Recommended Drugs	Preoperative Dose
Traumatic wound (exceptionally varied pathogens, based on the anatomic site injured, and the instrument causing the trauma, particularly for penetrating injuries such as motor vehicle accidents or farm injuries)	Skin: *S aureus*, group A streptococci, *S epidermidis*	Cefazolin	30 mg/kg (max 2 g)
	Perforated viscus: gram-negative enteric bacilli, *Clostridium* species	Cefoxitin **WITH OR WITHOUT** Gentamicin	40 mg/kg (max. 3 g) 2.5 mg/kg
		OR	
		Gentamicin **PLUS** Metronidazole **PLUS** Ampicillin	2.5 mg/kg 10 mg/kg (max 1 g) 50 mg/kg (max 2 g)
		OR	
		Meropenem	20 mg/kg (max 1 g)
		OR	
		Other regimens for complicated appendicitis[e]	

MRSA indicates methicillin-resistant *Staphylococcus aureus*; MRSE, methicillin-resistant *Staphylococcus epidermidis*.

[a]Selection of antibiotics should take into consideration the susceptibility patterns of isolates found in the patient and at the institution.

[b]Esophageal obstruction, decreased gastric acidity, or gastrointestinal motility; see text for additional high risk factors.

[c]Acute cholecystitis, nonfunctioning gallbladder, obstructive jaundice, common duct stones.

[d]High rates of resistance to clindamycin (~30%) now reported for *Bacteroides fragilis*. Lowest rates of resistance to carbapenems, ampicillin/sulbactam, and piperacillin/tazobactam. Resistance to cefoxitin reported at 3.5% to 9.4% (Snydman DR, Jacobus NV, McDermott LA, et al. Update on resistance of *Bacteroides fragilis* group and related species with special attention to carbapenems 2006-2009. *Anaerobe*. 2011;17[4]:147-151).

[e]Solomkin JS, Mazuski JE, Bradley JS, et al. Diagnosis and management of complicated intra-abdominal infection in adults and children: guidelines by the Surgical Infection Society and the Infectious Diseases Society of America (erratum in *Clin Infect Dis*. 2010;50(12):1695; dosage error in article text). *Clin Infect Dis*. 2010;50(2):133-164.

PREVENTION OF BACTERIAL ENDOCARDITIS

The Committee on Rheumatic Fever, Endocarditis, and Kawasaki Disease of the American Heart Association periodically issues detailed recommendations on the rationale, indications, and antimicrobial regimens for prevention of bacterial endocarditis for people at increased risk. In recommendations published in 2007,[1] the committee noted that data had cast doubt on benefits of episodic antimicrobial prophylaxis at the time of dental procedures to prevent endocarditis, because bacteremia associated with most dental procedures represents only a very small fraction of bacteremia episodes that occur with events of daily living, such as brushing teeth, chewing, and other oral hygiene measures. The committee has restricted recommendations for endocarditis prophylaxis to a considerably narrower group of people who have certain cardiac abnormalities and for fewer procedures than in the past. Although previous recommendations stressed endocarditis prophylaxis for people undergoing procedures most likely to induce bacteremia, the 2007 revision stresses only those cardiac conditions in which an episode of infective endocarditis has a high risk of an adverse outcome. Furthermore, prophylaxis is recommended only for certain dental procedures. Prophylaxis no longer is recommended for procedures involving the gastrointestinal and genitourinary tracts solely to prevent endocarditis.

In 2015, the American Heart Association issued updated guidance on the epidemiology, clinical findings, pathogenesis, diagnosis, and treatment of bacterial endocarditis.[2] At the end of that document is included a short section on endocarditis prevention, which reiterates the 2007 published recommendations.[1] The 2007 document is the more comprehensive discussion of bacterial endocarditis prophylaxis.

The cardiac conditions and procedures for which endocarditis prophylaxis is recommended are discussed in this section, and specific prophylactic regimens are presented in Table 5.3. Antibiotic prophylaxis is reasonable for the patients with cardiac conditions listed below who undergo an invasive procedure of the respiratory tract that involves incision or biopsy of the respiratory tract mucosa. Physicians should consult the published recommendations for further details (**http://circ.ahajournals.org/cgi/content/full/116/15/1736**).

Cardiac conditions associated with the highest risk of an adverse outcome from endocarditis for which prophylaxis with dental procedures is reasonable include the following[3]:

- Prosthetic cardiac valve or prosthetic material used for repair of valve.
- Previous infective endocarditis.

---

[1]Wilson W, Taubert KA, Gewitz M, et al. Prevention of Infective Endocarditis. Guidelines from the American Heart Association. A Guideline From the American Heart Association Rheumatic Fever, Endocarditis, and Kawasaki Diseases Committee, Council on Cardiovascular Disease in the Young, and the Council on Clinical Cardiology, Council on Cardiovascular Surgery and Anesthesia, and the Quality of Care and Outcomes Research Interdisciplinary Working Group. *Circulation.* 2007;116(15):1736–1754

[2]Baltimore RS, Gewitz M, Baddour LM, et al; American Heart Association Rheumatic Fever, Endocarditis, and Kawasaki Disease Committee of the Council on Cardiovascular Disease in the Young and the Council on Cardiovascular and Stroke Nursing. Infective endocarditis in childhood: 2015 update: a scientific statement from the American Heart Association. *Circulation.* 2015;132(15):1487-1515

[3]Except for the conditions listed, antimicrobial prophylaxis no longer is recommended for any other form of CHD.

- Congenital heart disease (CHD):
  - ◆ Unrepaired cyanotic CHD, including palliative shunts and conduits.
  - ◆ Completely repaired congenital heart defect with prosthetic material or device, whether placed by surgery or by catheter intervention, during the first 6 months after the procedure.[1]
  - ◆ Repaired CHD with residual defect(s) at the site or adjacent to the site of a prosthetic patch or prosthetic device (which inhibits endothelialization).
- Cardiac transplantation with subsequent cardiac valvulopathy.

Dental procedures for which endocarditis prophylaxis is reasonable for patients with a cardiac condition listed above include the following:

- All dental procedures that involve manipulation of gingival tissue or the periapical region of teeth or perforation of the oral mucosa. This includes procedures such as biopsies, suture removal, and placement of orthodontic bands.
- The following procedures and events do not require prophylaxis: routine anesthetic injections through noninfected tissue, taking dental radiographs, placement of removable prosthodontic or orthodontic appliances, adjustment of orthodontic appliances, placement of orthodontic brackets, shedding of deciduous teeth, and bleeding from trauma to the lips or oral mucosa.

Table 5.3. Regimens for Antimicrobial Prophylaxis for a Dental Procedure[a]

| Situation | Agent | Regimen: Single Dose 30 to 60 min Before Procedure | |
		Children	Adults
Oral	Amoxicillin	50 mg/kg	2 g
Unable to take oral medication	Ampicillin	50 mg/kg, IM or IV	2 g, IM or IV
Allergic to penicillins or oral ampicillin	Cephalexin[b,c]	50 mg/kg	2 g
	OR		
	Clindamycin	20 mg/kg	600 mg
	OR		
	Azithromycin or clarithromycin	15 mg/kg	500 mg
Allergic to penicillins or ampicillin and unable to take oral medication	Cefazolin or ceftriaxone[c]	50 mg/kg, IM or IV (cefazolin); 50 mg/kg, IM or IV (ceftriaxone)	1 g, IM or IV
	OR		
	Clindamycin	20 mg/kg, IM or IV	600 mg, IM or IV

IM, indicates intramuscular; IV, intravenous.

[a]Pediatric dosage should not exceed recommended adult dosage.

[b]Or other first- or second-generation oral cephalosporin in equivalent pediatric or adult dosage.

[c]Cephalosporins should not be used in a person with a history of anaphylaxis, angioedema, or urticaria with penicillins or ampicillin.

---

[1]Prophylaxis is recommended, because endothelialization of prosthetic material occurs within 6 months after the procedure.

PREVENTION OF NEONATAL OPHTHALMIA

Ophthalmia neonatorum is defined as conjunctivitis occurring within the first 4 weeks of life. Infection usually is transmitted during passage through the birth canal, although ascending infection can occur. The causes of ophthalmia neonatorum are presented in Table 5.4 (p 1048). Neonates with ophthalmia neonatorum require clinical evaluation with appropriate laboratory testing, and prompt initiation of therapy if an infectious etiology is identified. The Centers for Disease Control and Prevention (CDC) recommends routine first-trimester screening for chlamydia and gonorrhea in all high-risk pregnant women (24 years or younger, having new or multiple sex partners, having a sex partner with concurrent partners, having a sex partner with a sexually transmitted infection, or living in an area in which the prevalence of *Chlamydia trachomatis* or *Neisseria gonorrhoeae* is high). Because determining high-risk status in pregnant women with the exception of age may be difficult, consideration of screening all women for *C trachomatis* and *N gonorrhoeae* at the first prenatal visit is reasonable, especially in areas of high prevalence of either pathogen (**www.cdc.gov/std/Gonorrhea/; www.cdc.gov/std/chlamydia/default. htm**). Additionally, the CDC advises rescreening for chlamydia and gonorrhea during the third trimester for all women at high risk as defined above. Women in whom chlamydial infection is diagnosed during the first trimester should receive a test to document chlamydial eradication 3 to 4 weeks after treatment and should be tested 3 months after treatment as well as in the third trimester (see Chlamydial Infections, p 273, and Gonococcal Infections, p 355). Those diagnosed with gonorrhea should be treated immediately and retested in 3 months as well as in the third trimester. If a pregnant woman has not been tested for *C trachomatis* and/or *N gonorrhoeae* prior to labor/delivery, she should be tested during labor/delivery or immediately postpartum for *C trachomatis* and *N gonorrhoeae* infections. If either pathogen is identified, the infant should receive therapy as outlined in the following sections on gonococcal ophthalmia or chlamydial ophthalmia.

Gonococcal Ophthalmia

Healthy infants born to women with untreated (no treatment or inadequate treatment) gonococcal infection should receive 1 dose of ceftriaxone (25–50 mg/kg, intravenously [IV] or intramuscularly [IM], not to exceed 125 mg IM). Topical antimicrobial therapy alone is inadequate for *N gonorrhoeae*-exposed or infected infants and is not necessary when systemic antimicrobial therapy is administered.

Infants with gonococcal ophthalmia disease should be hospitalized, evaluated for disseminated infection, and treated (see Gonococcal Infections, p 355). Appropriate chlamydial testing should be performed simultaneously. Frequent eye irrigations with saline solution should be performed until resolution of the discharge. One dose of ceftriaxone is adequate therapy for gonococcal conjunctivitis in the absence of dissemination. Evaluation by a pediatric ophthalmologist should be considered.

Note that neonates with hyperbilirubinemia, especially those born preterm, should not be treated with ceftriaxone for injection, because in vitro studies have shown that ceftriaxone can displace bilirubin from its binding to serum albumin, leading to a possible risk of bilirubin encephalopathy in these patients.

Chlamydial Ophthalmia

Recommended topical prophylaxis with erythromycin for all newborn infants for prevention of gonococcal ophthalmia will not prevent neonatal chlamydial conjunctivitis or extraocular infection, and it does not eliminate nasopharyngeal colonization by *C trachomatis*. Neonatal ophthalmia attributable to *C trachomatis* is not as clinically severe as gonococcal conjunctivitis. Chlamydial conjunctivitis in the neonate is characterized by a mucopurulent discharge, eyelid swelling, a propensity to form membranes on the palpebral conjunctiva, and lack of a follicular response. Chlamydial conjunctivitis should be in the differential diagnosis for infants younger than 30 days who have conjunctivitis, especially if the mother has a history of treated chlamydia infection. Most sensitive and specific non-culture tests, such as nucleic acid amplification tests (NAATs), are not cleared by the US Food and Drug Administration for detection of chlamydia from conjunctival swab specimens. However, laboratories that have met Clinical Laboratory Improvement Amendment (CLIA) requirements and validated chlamydia NAAT performance on conjunctival swab specimens may offer these tests. Infants with chlamydial conjunctivitis are treated with oral erythromycin base or ethylsuccinate (50 mg/kg/day in 4 divided doses daily) for 14 days or with azithromycin (20 mg/kg as a single daily dose) for 3 days. Because the efficacy of erythromycin therapy is approximately 80% for both of these conditions, a second course may be required, and follow-up of infants is recommended. A diagnosis of *C trachomatis* infection in an infant should prompt treatment of the mother and her sexual partner(s).

Infants born to mothers known to have untreated chlamydial infection are at high risk of infection; however, prophylactic antimicrobial treatment is not indicated, because the efficacy of such treatment is unknown. Infants should be monitored clinically to ensure appropriate treatment if infection develops. If adequate follow-up cannot be ensured, preemptive therapy should be considered.

An association between orally administered erythromycin and infantile hypertrophic pyloric stenosis (IHPS) has been reported in infants younger than 6 weeks, and particularly in infants younger than 2 weeks. The risk of IHPS after treatment with other macrolides (eg, azithromycin and clarithromycin) is unknown, although IHPS has been reported after use of azithromycin. Because confirmation of azithromycin as a contributor to cases of IHPS will require additional investigation and because alternative therapies are not as well studied, the American Academy of Pediatrics continues to recommend use of erythromycin for treatment of diseases caused by *C trachomatis* in infants. Physicians who prescribe macrolides to newborn infants should inform parents about the signs and potential risks of developing IHPS. Cases of pyloric stenosis after use of macrolides should be reported to MedWatch (see MedWatch, p 1026). Topical therapy is redundant and is inadequate on its own to prevent development of chlamydial pneumonia (see Chlamydial Infections, p 273).

Pseudomonal Ophthalmia

Neonatal ophthalmia attributable to *Pseudomonas aeruginosa* is infrequent but may now be at least as common as gonococcal ophthalmia. This form of neonatal ophthalmia has a predilection for preterm infants and presents with eyelid edema and erythema, purulent discharge, and pannus formation. Because superficial infection can progress rapidly to corneal perforation, endophthalmitis, blindness, serious systemic infection (sepsis, meningitis), and death, this is the third form of bacterial neonatal ophthalmia that urgently requires a combination of systemic and topical therapy, as systemic antibiotics alone have poor penetration in the anterior chamber of the eye. The diagnosis should be suspected when Gram-stained specimens of exudate contain gram-negative bacilli and should be confirmed by culture. Until *Pseudomonas* infection is excluded, evaluation for systemic infection and topical and systemic therapy with an aminoglycoside is required; systemic therapy with an antipseudomonal β-lactam also may be indicated. Ophthalmology consultation is recommended.

Other Nongonococcal, Nonchlamydial Ophthalmia

Neonatal ophthalmia can be caused by many other bacterial pathogens (see Table 5.4). Once gonococcal, chlamydial, and pseudomonal infections have been excluded, uncomplicated resolution can be expected with topical treatment with antimicrobial ointments or solutions.

Table 5.4. Major and Minor Etiologies in Ophthalmia Neonatorum

Etiology of Ophthalmia Neonatorum	Proportion of Cases	Incubation Period (Days)	Severity of Conjunctivitis[a]	Associated Problems
Chlamydia trachomatis	2%–40%	5–12	+	Pneumonitis 3 wk–3 mo (see Chlamydial Infections, p 273)
Neisseria gonorrhoeae	Less than 1%	2–5	+++	Disseminated infection (see Gonococcal Infections, p 355)
Pseudomonas aeruginosa	Less than 1%	5–28	+++	Sepsis, meningitis
Other bacterial microbes[b]	30%–50%	5–14	+	Variable
Herpes simplex virus	Less than 1%	6–14	+	Disseminated infection, meningoencephalitis (see Herpes simplex, p 437); keratitis and ulceration also possible
Chemical	Varies with silver nitrate use	1	+	…

[a] + indicates mild; +++, severe.
[b] Includes skin, respiratory, vaginal and gastrointestinal tract pathogens such as *Staphylococcus aureus; Streptococcus pneumoniae; Haemophilus influenzae*, nontypeable; group A and B streptococci; *Corynebacterium* species; *Moraxella catarrhalis; Escherichia coli;* and *Klebsiella pneumoniae*.

Herpes simplex keratoconjunctivitis should be considered in neonates with conjunctival inflammation and discharge, particularly when tests for bacterial and chlamydial infection are negative. The diagnosis should be suspected if there are also cutaneous vesicles or oral ulcers, or vesicles and can be confirmed by demonstration of dendritic keratitis (requiring ophthalmological consultation for examination with fluorescein staining), or by virologic testing (eg, PCR or culture). Specific treatment is indicated (see Herpes Simplex, p 437). Conjunctivitis caused by other viruses generally resolves without specific treatment.

Administration of Neonatal Ophthalmic Prophylaxis

In a case in which gonorrhea is prevalent in the region and prenatal treatment cannot be ensured, or where required by law, a prophylactic agent of 0.5% erythromycin ointment should be instilled into the eyes of all newborn infants (including those born by cesarean delivery) to prevent sight-threatening gonococcal ophthalmia. Efficacy is unlikely to be influenced by delaying prophylaxis for as long as 1 hour to facilitate parent-infant bonding. Longer delays have not been studied for efficacy. Hospitals should establish processes to ensure that infants are given prophylaxis appropriately. Before administering local prophylaxis, each eyelid should be wiped gently with sterile cotton. A 1-cm ribbon of 0.5% erythromycin ointment should then be placed in each lower conjunctival sac. The eyelids should then be massaged gently to spread the ointment. After 1 minute, ointment may be wiped away with sterile cotton. The ointment should not be flushed from the eyes after instillation, because flushing can decrease efficacy.

If erythromycin ointment is not available, azithromycin ophthalmic solution 1% is recommended as an acceptable substitute. One to 2 drops of this product are placed in each conjunctival sac. Because it is a solution rather than an ointment, care must be taken to ensure the drops are placed properly. The CDC recommends that 2 people provide the prophylaxis—1 to hold the lids open and the other to instill the drops. If azithromycin ophthalmic solution 1% is not available, gentamicin or tobramycin ointments are recommended for consideration. Lastly, if none of the previously mentioned alternatives are available, ciprofloxacin ophthalmic ointment 0.3% can be considered as a less suitable but acceptable alternative. In most cases, potential resistance of *N gonorrhoeae* to ciprofloxacin will be overcome by the high concentrations of ciprofloxacin achieved.

Legal Mandates for Topical Prophylaxis for Neonatal Ophthalmia

Since Credé demonstrated the efficacy of topical silver nitrate solution for prevention of gonococcal ophthalmia neonatorum in 1881, interruption of maternal-neonatal transmission has been the mainstay strategy for prevention of neonatal ophthalmia. Silver nitrate was displaced by less noxious topical antibiotics, including erythromycin ointment, which now is the only product available for this indication in the United States. Because prophylaxis with topical antimicrobial agents is highly effective in preventing blindness from gonococcal neonatal ophthalmia, it was mandated by law in many jurisdictions. These mandates have been abandoned in many countries over the last several decades but remain in force in nearly all of the United States. The necessity for mandatory eye prophylaxis in this country has been questioned, primarily because rates of intrapartum exposure to gonorrhea have been greatly reduced by prenatal screening and treatment of maternal disease. Increasing resistance of gonococcal isolates has cast doubt on the continued efficacy of erythromycin, which is not effective for prevention of ophthalmia of other etiologies, including *Chlamydia*. When neonatal ophthalmia does develop, effective therapies are readily available, and sequelae (including loss of vision) now are exceedingly rare. Countries with well-organized systems of prenatal care, including Canada, have recommended elimination of eye prophylaxis. Resurgence either of cases of gonococcal ophthalmia neonatorum or of blindness from that condition has not been reported. The American Academy of Pediatrics believes it is now time to reevaluate the continued necessity of legislative mandates in the United States for eye prophylaxis and instead to advocate for states to adopt strategies to prevent neonatal ophthalmia based on the following steps:

- Diligent compliance with CDC recommendations for prenatal screening for and treatment of *N gonorrhoeae* and *C trachomatis*, to prevent intrapartum exposures.
- Testing of unscreened women for *N gonorrhoeae* and *C trachomatis* infection at the time of labor or delivery, with treatment of infected women and their babies.
- Counseling of parents to bring conjunctival discharge and inflammation to immediate medical attention resulting in optimal treatment of neonatal ophthalmia.
- Continuation of mandatory reporting of cases of gonococcal ophthalmia neonatorum to identify patterns of failure of primary prevention measures.

In regions where gonorrhea remains prevalent and prenatal screening and treatment is not routinely achievable, neonatal topical prophylaxis remains appropriate. Data from countries where neonatal prophylaxis no longer is practiced can inform this transition.

APPENDIX I

Directory of Resources[a]

Organization	Telephone/Fax Number	Web Site
AIDSinfo	1-800-HIV-0440 (1-800-448-0440, US) 1-301-315-2816 (Outside US) TTY: 1-888-480-3739 Fax: 1-301-315-2818	www.aidsinfo.nih.gov
American Academy of Pediatrics (AAP)	1-630-626-6000 or 1-800-433-9016 Fax: 1-847-434-8000 Publications/Customer Service: 1-866-THEAAP1 (1-866-843-2271)	www.aap.org
American Sexual Health Association	1-919-361-8400 Fax: 919-361-8425	www.ashastd.org
Canadian Paediatric Society (CPS)	1-613-526-9397 Fax: 1-613-526-3332	www.cps.ca
Centers for Disease Control and Prevention (CDC)	1-800-232-4636 TTY: 888-232-6348	www.cdc.gov
24-Hour Service	1-770-488-7100	
Advisory Committee on Immunization Practices	1-404-639-8836	www.cdc.gov/vaccines/acip

Directory of Resources,[a] continued

Organization	Telephone/Fax Number	Web Site
Botulism case consultation and antitoxin	1-770-488-7100	
Division of Foodborne, Waterborne, and Environmental Diseases	1-404-639-1603	www.cdc.gov/ncezid/dfwed/
Division of Healthcare Quality Promotion	1-404-639-4000	www.cdc.gov/ncezid/dhqp/index.html
Division of Tuberculosis Elimination	1-404-639-8120	www.cdc.gov/tb
Division of Vector-Borne Diseases	1-970-221-6400	www.cdc.gov/ncezid/dvbd
Division of Viral Hepatitis	1-888-4-HEP-CDC (1-888-443-7232)	www.cdc.gov/hepatitis/index.htm
Division of High-Consequence Pathogens and Pathology	1-404-639-3574	www.cdc.gov/ncezid/dhcpp/
Contact Center	1-800-CDC-INFO (1-800-232-4636)	www.cdc.gov/netinfo.htm
Drug Service	1-404-639-3670 (business hours) 1-770-488-7100 (after hours)	www.cdc.gov/laboratory/drugservice/
Influenza		www.cdc.gov/flu
Malaria Hotline	1-770-488-7788 1-855-856-4713 1-770-488-7100 (after hours)	www.cdc.gov/malaria
National Prevention Information Network	1-800-458-5231	https://npin.cdc.gov/
Parasitic Diseases Branch	1-404-718-4745	www.cdc.gov/parasites
Public Inquiries	1-404-639-3534	
Publications	1-800-232-2522	www.cdc.gov/publications.htm#pubs

Directory of Resources,[a] continued

Organization	Telephone/Fax Number	Web Site
Travelers' Health	1-800-232-4636	www.cdc.gov/travel
Vaccines and Immunizations	1-800-232-4636	www.cdc.gov/vaccines
Vaccine Safety		www.cdc.gov/vaccinesafety/index.html
Vaccine Information Statements		www.cdc.gov/vaccines/hcp/vis/index.html
Vaccines for Children Program		www.cdc.gov/vaccines/programs/vfc/index.html
Food and Drug Administration (FDA)	1-888-INFO-FDA (1-888-463-6332)	www.fda.gov
Center for Biologics Evaluation and Research	1-800-835-4709	www.fda.gov/AboutFDA/CentersOffices/OfficeofMedicalProductsandTobacco/CBER/default.htm
Center for Drug Evaluation and Research	1-888-463-6332 or 1-855-543-3784	www.fda.gov/AboutFDA/CentersOffices/OfficeofMedicalProductsandTobacco/CDER/default.htm
Drugs		www.fda.gov/Drugs/default.htm
Safety Report on products presented to the Pediatric Advisory Committee		www.fda.gov/scienceresearch/specialtopics/pediatrictherapeuticsresearch/ucm123229.htm
New Pediatric Labeling Information Database		www.accessdata.fda.gov/scripts/sda/sdNavigation.cfm?sd=labelingdatabase

Directory of Resources,[a] continued

Organization	Telephone/Fax Number	Web Site
Pediatric Studies Characteristics Database		www.accessdata.fda.gov/scripts/sda/ sdNavigation.cfm?sd=fdaaadescriptors sortablewebdatabase
Vaccines, Blood, and Biologics		www.fda.gov/BiologicsBloodVaccines/ default.htm
MedWatch	1-800-FDA-1088 (1-800-332-1088) Fax: 1-800-FDA-0178 (1-800-332-0178)	www.fda.gov/Safety/MedWatch/ default.htm
Vaccine Adverse Event Reporting System (VAERS)	1-800-822-7967	https://vaers.hhs.gov/index.html
Vaccine Package Inserts		www.fda.gov/BiologicsBloodVaccines/Vacci nes/ApprovedProducts/ucm093833.htm
Immunization Action Coalition (IAC)	1-651-647-9009 Fax: 1-651-647-9131	www.immunize.org
Infectious Diseases Society of America (IDSA)	1-703-299-0200 Fax: 1-703-299-0204	www.idsociety.org
Institute for Vaccine Safety		www.vaccinesafety.edu
National Academy of Medicine (formerly the Institute of Medicine)	1-202-334-2352	https://nam.edu
National Institutes of Health (NIH)	1-301-496-4000	www.nih.gov
National Institute of Allergy and Infectious Diseases (NIAID)	1-301-496-5717 or toll-free: 1-866-284-4107	www.niaid.nih.gov

Directory of Resources,[a] continued

Organization	Telephone/Fax Number	Web Site
AIDS Therapies Resource Guide		www.niaid.nih.gov/research/aids-therapies-resource-guide
National Library of Medicine	1-888-346-3656	www.nlm.nih.gov
National Resource Center for Health and Safety in Child Care and Early Education		www.nrckids.org
National Vaccine Injury Compensation Program (for information on filing claims)	1-800-338-2382	www.hrsa.gov/vaccinecompensation/index.html
National Vaccine Program Office (NVPO)	1-202-690-5566	www.hhs.gov/nvpo/
Parents of Kids with Infectious Diseases (PKIDS)		www.pkids.org
Pediatric Oncology Branch, Center for Cancer Research, National Cancer Institute	1-301-496-4256 1-877-624-4878	https://ccr.cancer.gov/Pediatric-Oncology-Branch
Pediatric Infectious Diseases Society	1-703-299-6764 Fax: 1-703-299-0473	www.pids.org
Sociedad Latinoamericana de Infectología Pediátrica (SLIPE)		www.slipe.org

Directory of Resources,[a] continued

Organization	Telephone/Fax Number	Web Site
Vaccine Education Center of the Children's Hospital of Pennsylvania		http://vaccine.chop.edu/centers-programs/vaccine-education-center
Voices for Vaccines		www.voicesforvaccines.org
Women, Children, and HIV		www.womenchildrenhiv.org/
World Health Organization (WHO)	(+41 22) 791 21 11 Fax: (+41 22) 791 31 11 Regional Office for the Americas: 1-202-974-3000 Fax: 1-202-974-3663	www.who.int

[a]Internet addresses and telephone/fax numbers are current at the time of publication.

....

APPENDIX II

Codes for Commonly Administered Pediatric Vaccines/Toxoids and Immune Globulins

Vaccine, toxoid, and Immune Globulin codes use a specific vaccine *Current Procedural Terminology* (CPT) code to indicate which immunization product was administered to the patient. A regularly updated listing of CPT product codes for commonly administered pediatric vaccines can be found at **www.aap.org/en-us/Documents/coding_vaccine_coding_table.pdf.**

CPT codes for vaccine administrations are reported in addition to the CPT codes for specific vaccines and toxoid products. 90460 and 90461 are only reported when the physician or other qualified health care professional provides face-to-face counseling during the encounter when a vaccine is administered to a patient through 18 years of age. Otherwise, the administration codes 90471–90474 are used, depending on the number of vaccines administered and the route of administration. The 90460 code should be used for each vaccine administered. For vaccines with multiple components, code 90460 should be reported in conjunction with 90461 for each additional component in a given vaccine (eg, DTaP administration would include 90460 + 90461 x 2). Multivalent antigens or multiple serotypes of antigens against a single organism are considered a single component of vaccines (eg, PCV-13 administration should use only one 90460). Immune Globulin products are not considered vaccines, and the administration code 96372, therapeutic injection given intramuscularly or subcutaneously, should be used.

Unlike ICD-9, ICD-10-CM has only a single diagnosis code for reporting vaccines, Z23. When reporting vaccines administered, ICD-10 requires use of Z23 regardless of the reason for the encounter. For example, if vaccines are given as part of a childhood preventive care visit, Z23 should be reported in addition to Z00.121 (encounter for routine child health examination).

For Rabies Immune Globulin and rabies vaccine administration, Z20.3 (contact with and [suspected] exposure to rabies) should be reported as well as the ICD-10-CM codes describing the nature of the injuries and circumstances surrounding the injury, including type of animal involved (ie, codes found in the V-Y categories). For RSV Immune Globulin, palivizumab, the appropriate ICD-10-CM diagnoses of gestational age and/or other medical condition(s) that support the need to administer palivizumab should be reported.

····································

APPENDIX III

Vaccine Injury Table

Applies Only to Petitions for Compensation Filed under the National Vaccine Injury Compensation Program on or after March 21, 2017

(a) In accordance with section 312(b) of the National Childhood Vaccine Injury Act of 1986 (NCVIA), Title III of Public Law 99-660, 100 Stat. 3779 (42 USC 300aa-1 note) and section 2114(c) of the Public Health Service Act, as amended (PHS Act) (42 USC 300aa-14(c)), the following is a table of vaccines, the injuries, disabilities, illnesses, conditions, and deaths resulting from the administration of such vaccines, and the time period in which the first symptom or manifestation of onset or of the significant aggravation of such injuries, disabilities, illnesses, conditions, and deaths is to occur after vaccine administration for purposes of receiving compensation under the Program. Paragraph (b) of this section sets forth additional provisions that are not separately listed in this Table but that constitute part of it. Paragraph (c) of this section sets forth the qualifications and aids to interpretation for the terms used in the Table. Conditions and injuries that do not meet the terms of the qualifications and aids to interpretation are not within the Table. Paragraph (d) of this section sets forth a glossary of terms used in paragraph (c).

Vaccine	Illness, Disability, Injury, or Condition Covered	Time Period for First Symptom or Manifestation of Onset or of Significant Aggravation After Vaccine Administration
I. Vaccines containing tetanus toxoid (eg, DTaP, DTwP, DT, Td, or TT)	A. Anaphylaxis	≤4 hours
	B. Brachial neuritis	2–28 days (not less than 2 days and not more than 28 days)
	C. Shoulder injury related to vaccine administration	≤48 hours
	D. Vasovagal syncope	≤1 hour
II. Vaccines containing whole cell pertussis bacteria, extracted or partial cell pertussis bacteria, or specific pertussis antigen(s) (eg, DTwP, DTaP, P, DTP-Hib)	A. Anaphylaxis	≤4 hours
	B. Encephalopathy or encephalitis	≤72 hours
	C. Shoulder injury related to vaccine administration	≤48 hours
	D. Vasovagal syncope	≤1 hour
III. Vaccines containing measles, mumps, and rubella virus or any of its components (eg, MMR, MM, MMRV)	A. Anaphylaxis	≤4 hours
	B. Encephalopathy or encephalitis	5–15 days (not less than 5 days and not more than 15 days)
	C. Shoulder injury related to vaccine administration	≤48 hours
	D. Vasovagal syncope	≤1 hour

Vaccine	Illness, Disability, Injury, or Condition Covered	Time Period for First Symptom or Manifestation of Onset or of Significant Aggravation After Vaccine Administration
IV. Vaccines containing rubella virus (eg, MMR, MMRV)	A. Chronic arthritis	7–42 days (not less than 7 days and not more than 42 days)
V. Vaccines containing measles virus (eg, MMR, MM, MMRV)	A. Thrombocytopenic purpura	7–30 days (not less than 7 days and not more than 30 days)
	B. Vaccine-strain measles viral disease in an immunodeficient recipient	
	—Vaccine-strain virus identified	Not applicable
	—If strain determination is not performed or if laboratory testing is inconclusive	≤12 months
VI. Vaccines containing polio live virus (OPV)	A. Paralytic polio	
	—in a nonimmunodeficient recipient	≤30 days
	—in an immunodeficient recipient	≤6 month
	—in a vaccine-associated community case	Not applicable
	B. Vaccine-strain polio viral infection	
	—in a nonimmunodeficient recipient	≤30 days
	—in an immunodeficient recipient	≤6 months
	—in a vaccine-associated community case	Not applicable
VII. Vaccines containing polio inactivated virus (eg, IPV)	A. Anaphylaxis	≤4 hours
	B. Shoulder injury related to vaccine administration	≤48 hours
	C. Vasovagal syncope	≤1 hour
VIII. Hepatitis B vaccines	A. Anaphylaxis	≤4 hours
	B. Shoulder injury related to vaccine administration	≤48 hours
	C. Vasovagal syncope	≤1 hour
IX. *Haemophilus influenzae* type b (Hib) vaccines	A. Shoulder injury related to vaccine administration	≤48 hours
	B. Vasovagal syncope	≤1 hour
X. Varicella vaccines	A. Anaphylaxis	≤4 hours
	B. Disseminated varicella vaccine-strain viral disease	

Vaccine	Illness, Disability, Injury, or Condition Covered	Time Period for First Symptom or Manifestation of Onset or of Significant Aggravation After Vaccine Administration
	—Vaccine-strain virus identified	Not applicable
	—If strain determination is not performed or if laboratory testing is inconclusive	7–42 days (not less than 7 days and not more than 42 days)
	C. Varicella vaccine-strain viral reactivation	Not applicable
	D. Shoulder injury related to vaccine administration	≤48 hours
	E. Vasovagal syncope	≤1 hour
XI. Rotavirus vaccines	A. Intussusception	1–21 days (not less than 1 day and not more than 21 days)
XII. Pneumococcal conjugate vaccines	A. Shoulder injury related to vaccine administration	≤48 hours
	B. Vasovagal syncope	≤1 hour
XIII. Hepatitis A vaccines	A. Shoulder injury related to vaccine administration	≤48 hours
	B. Vasovagal syncope	≤1 hour
XIV. Seasonal influenza vaccines	A. Anaphylaxis	≤4 hours
	B. Shoulder injury related to vaccine administration	≤48 hours
	C. Vasovagal syncope	≤1 hour
	D. Guillain-Barré syndrome	3–42 days (not less than 3 days and not more than 42 days)
XV. Meningococcal vaccines	A. Anaphylaxis	≤4 hours
	B. Shoulder injury related to vaccine administration	≤48 hours
	C. Vasovagal syncope	≤1 hour
XVI. Human papillomavirus (HPV) vaccines	A. Anaphylaxis	≤4 hours
	B. Shoulder injury related to vaccine administration	≤48 hours
	C. Vasovagal syncope	≤1 hour
XVII. Any new vaccine recommended by the Centers for Disease Control and Prevention for routine administration to children, after publication by the Secretary of a notice of coverage	A. Shoulder injury related to vaccine administration	≤48 hours
	B. Vasovagal syncope	≤1 hour

(b) Provisions that apply to all conditions listed.

(1) Any acute complication or sequela, including death, of the illness, disability, injury, or

condition listed in paragraph (a) of this section (and defined in paragraphs (c) and (d) of this section) qualifies as a Table injury under paragraph (a) except when the definition in paragraph (c) requires exclusion.

(2) In determining whether or not an injury is a condition set forth in paragraph (a) of this section, the Court shall consider the entire medical record.

(3) An idiopathic condition that meets the definition of an illness, disability, injury, or condition set forth in paragraph (c) of this section shall be considered to be a condition set forth in paragraph (a) of this section.

(c) Qualifications and aids to interpretation. The following qualifications and aids to interpretation shall apply to, define and describe the scope of, and be read in conjunction with paragraphs (a), (b), and (d) of this section:

(1) Anaphylaxis. Anaphylaxis is an acute, severe, and potentially lethal systemic reaction that occurs as a single discrete event with simultaneous involvement of two or more organ systems. Most cases resolve without sequela. Signs and symptoms begin minutes to a few hours after exposure. Death, if it occurs, usually results from airway obstruction caused by laryngeal edema or bronchospasm and may be associated with cardiovascular collapse. Other significant clinical signs and symptoms may include the following: cyanosis, hypotension, bradycardia, tachycardia, arrhythmia, edema of the pharynx and/or trachea and/or larynx with stridor and dyspnea. There are no specific pathological findings to confirm a diagnosis of anaphylaxis.

(2) Encephalopathy. A vaccine recipient shall be considered to have suffered an encephalopathy if an injury meeting the description below of an acute encephalopathy occurs within the applicable time period and results in a chronic encephalopathy, as described in paragraph (d) of this section.

(i) Acute encephalopathy. (A) For children younger than 18 months of age who present:

(1) Without a seizure, an acute encephalopathy is indicated by a significantly decreased level of consciousness that lasts at least 24 hours.

(2) Following a seizure, an acute encephalopathy is demonstrated by a significantly decreased level of consciousness that lasts at least 24 hours and cannot be attributed to a postictal state—from a seizure or a medication.

(B) For adults and children 18 months of age or older, an acute encephalopathy is one that persists at least 24 hours and is characterized by at least two of the following:

(1) A significant change in mental status that is not medication related (such as a confusional state, delirium, or psychosis);

(2) A significantly decreased level of consciousness which is independent of a seizure and cannot be attributed to the effects of medication; and

(3) A seizure associated with loss of consciousness.

(C) The following clinical features in themselves do not demonstrate an acute encephalopathy or a significant change in either mental status or level of consciousness: Sleepiness, irritability (fussiness), high-pitched and unusual screaming, poor feeding, persistent inconsolable crying, bulging fontanelle, or symptoms of dementia.

(D) Seizures in themselves are not sufficient to constitute a diagnosis of encephalopathy and in the absence of other evidence of an acute encephalopathy seizures shall not be viewed as the first symptom or manifestation of an acute encephalopathy.

(ii) Exclusionary criteria for encephalopathy. Regardless of whether or not the specific cause of the underlying condition, systemic disease, or acute event (including an infectious organism) is known, an encephalopathy shall not be considered to be a condition set forth in the Table if it is shown that the encephalopathy was caused by:

(A) An underlying condition or systemic disease shown to be unrelated to the vaccine (such as malignancy, structural lesion, psychiatric illness, dementia, genetic disorder, prenatal or perinatal central nervous system [CNS] injury); or

(B) An acute event shown to be unrelated to the vaccine such as a head trauma, stroke, transient ischemic attack, complicated migraine, drug use (illicit or prescribed) or an infectious disease.

(3) Encephalitis. A vaccine recipient shall be considered to have suffered encephalitis if an injury meeting the description below of acute encephalitis occurs within the applicable time period and results in a chronic encephalopathy, as described in paragraph (d) of this section.

(i) Acute encephalitis. Encephalitis is indicated by evidence of neurologic dysfunction, as described in paragraph (c)(3)(i)(A) of this section, plus evidence of an inflammatory process in the brain, as described in paragraph (c)(3)(i)(B) of this section.

(A) Evidence of neurologic dysfunction consists of either:

(1) One of the following neurologic findings referable to the CNS: Focal cortical signs (such as aphasia, alexia, agraphia, cortical blindness); cranial nerve abnormalities; visual field defects; abnormal presence of primitive reflexes (such as Babinski sign or sucking reflex); or cerebellar dysfunction (such as ataxia, dysmetria, or nystagmus); or

(2) An acute encephalopathy as set forth in paragraph (c)(2)(i) of this section.

(B) Evidence of an inflammatory process in the brain (central nervous system or CNS inflammation) must include cerebrospinal fluid (CSF) pleocytosis (>5 white blood cells (WBC)/mm3 in children >2 months of age and adults; >15 WBC/mm3 in children <2 months of age); or at least two of the following:

(1) Fever (temperature ≥100.4°F);

(2) Electroencephalogram findings consistent with encephalitis, such as diffuse or multifocal nonspecific background slowing and periodic discharges; or

(3) Neuroimaging findings consistent with encephalitis, which include, but are not limited to brain/spine magnetic resonance imaging (MRI) displaying diffuse or multifocal areas of hyperintense signal on T2-weighted, diffusion-weighted image, or fluid-attenuation inversion recovery sequences.

(ii) Exclusionary criteria for encephalitis. Regardless of whether or not the specific cause of the underlying condition, systemic disease, or acute event (including an infectious organism) is known, encephalitis shall not be considered to be a condition set forth in the Table if it is shown that the encephalitis was caused by:

(A) An underlying malignancy that led to a paraneoplastic encephalitis;

(B) An infectious disease associated with encephalitis, including a bacterial, parasitic, fungal or viral illness (such as herpes viruses, adenovirus, enterovirus, West Nile Virus, or human immunodeficiency virus), which may be demonstrated by clinical signs and symptoms and need not be confirmed by culture or serologic testing; or

(C) Acute disseminated encephalomyelitis (ADEM). Although early ADEM may have laboratory and clinical characteristics similar to acute encephalitis, findings on MRI are distinct with ADEM displaying evidence of acute demyelination (scattered, focal, or multifocal areas of inflammation and demyelination within cerebral subcortical and deep cortical white matter; gray matter involvement may also be seen but is a minor component); or

(D) Other conditions or abnormalities that would explain the vaccine recipient's symptoms.

(4) Intussusception. (i) For purposes of paragraph (a) of this section, intussusception means the invagination of a segment of intestine into the next segment of intestine, resulting in bowel obstruction, diminished arterial blood supply, and blockage of the venous blood flow. This is characterized by a sudden onset of abdominal pain that may be manifested by anguished crying, irritability, vomiting, abdominal swelling, and/or passing of stools mixed with blood and mucus.

(ii) For purposes of paragraph (a) of this section, the following shall not be considered to be a Table intussusception:

(A) Onset that occurs with or after the third dose of a vaccine containing rotavirus;

(B) Onset within 14 days after an infectious disease associated with intussusception, including viral disease (such as those secondary to non-enteric or enteric adenovirus, or other enteric viruses such as Enterovirus), enteric bacteria (such as Campylobacter jejuni), or enteric parasites (such as Ascaris lumbricoides), which may be demonstrated by clinical signs and symptoms and need not be confirmed by culture or serologic testing;

(C) Onset in a person with a preexisting condition identified as the lead point for intussusception such as intestinal masses and cystic structures (such as polyps, tumors, Meckel diverticulum, lymphoma, or duplication cysts);

(D) Onset in a person with abnormalities of the bowel, including congenital anatomic abnormalities, anatomic changes after abdominal surgery, and other anatomic bowel abnormalities caused by mucosal hemorrhage, trauma, or abnormal intestinal blood vessels (such as Henoch Schonlein purpura, hematoma, or hemangioma); or

(E) Onset in a person with underlying conditions or systemic diseases associated with intussusception (such as cystic fibrosis, celiac disease, or Kawasaki disease).

(5) Chronic arthritis. Chronic arthritis is defined as persistent joint swelling with at least two additional manifestations of warmth, tenderness, pain with movement, or limited range of motion, lasting for at least 6 months.

(i) Chronic arthritis may be found in a person with no history in the 3 years prior to vaccination of arthropathy (joint disease) on the basis of:

(A) Medical documentation recorded within 30 days after the onset of objective signs of acute arthritis (joint swelling) that occurred between 7 and 42 days after a rubella vaccination; and

(B) Medical documentation (recorded within 3 years after the onset of acute arthritis) of the persistence of objective signs of intermittent or continuous arthritis for more than 6 months following vaccination; and

(C) Medical documentation of an antibody response to the rubella virus.

(ii) The following shall not be considered as chronic arthritis: Musculoskeletal disorders such as diffuse connective tissue diseases (including but not limited to rheumatoid arthritis, juvenile idiopathic arthritis, systemic lupus erythematosus, systemic sclerosis, mixed connective tissue disease, polymyositis/dermatomyositis, fibromyalgia, necrotizing vasculitis and vasculopathies and Sjögren syndrome), degenerative joint disease, infectious agents other than rubella (whether by direct invasion or as an immune reaction), metabolic and endocrine diseases, trauma, neoplasms, neuropathic disorders, bone and cartilage disorders, and arthritis associated with ankylosing spondylitis, psoriasis, inflammatory bowel disease, Reiter syndrome, blood disorders, or arthralgia (joint pain), or joint stiffness without swelling.

(6) Brachial neuritis. This term is defined as dysfunction limited to the upper extremity nerve plexus (ie, its trunks, divisions, or cords). A deep, steady, often severe aching pain in the shoulder and upper arm usually heralds onset of the condition. The pain is typically followed in days or weeks by weakness in the affected upper extremity muscle groups. Sensory loss may accompany the motor deficits, but is generally a less notable clinical feature. Atrophy of the affected muscles may occur. The neuritis, or plexopathy, may be present on the same side or on the side opposite the injection. It is sometimes bilateral, affecting both upper extremities. A vaccine recipient shall be considered to have suffered brachial neuritis as a Table injury if such recipient manifests all of the following:

(i) Pain in the affected arm and shoulder is a presenting symptom and occurs within the specified time-frame;

(ii) Weakness;

(A) Clinical diagnosis in the absence of nerve conduction and electromyographic studies requires weakness in muscles supplied by more than one peripheral nerve.

(B) Nerve conduction studies (NCS) and electromyographic (EMG) studies localizing the injury to the brachial plexus are required before the diagnosis can be made if weakness is limited to muscles supplied by a single peripheral nerve.

(iii) Motor, sensory, and reflex findings on physical examination and the results of NCS and EMG studies, if performed, must be consistent in confirming that dysfunction is attributable to the brachial plexus; and

(iv) No other condition or abnormality is present that would explain the vaccine recipient's symptoms.

(7) Thrombocytopenic purpura. This term is defined by the presence of clinical manifestations, such as petechiae, significant bruising, or spontaneous bleeding, and by a serum platelet count less than 50 000/mm^3 with normal red and white blood cell indices. Thrombocytopenic purpura does not include cases of thrombocytopenia associated with other causes such as hypersplenism, autoimmune disorders (including alloantibodies from previous transfusions) myelodysplasias, lymphoproliferative disorders, congenital thrombocytopenia, or hemolytic uremic syndrome. Thrombocytopenic purpura does not include cases of immune (formerly called idiopathic) thrombocytopenic purpura that are mediated, for example, by viral or fungal infections, toxins, or drugs. Thrombocytopenic purpura does not include cases of thrombocytopenia associated with disseminated intravascular coagulation, as observed with bacterial and viral infections. Viral infections include, for example, those infections secondary to Epstein Barr virus, cytomegalovirus, hepatitis A and B, human immunodeficiency virus, adenovirus, and dengue virus. An antecedent viral infection may be demonstrated by clinical signs and symptoms and need not be confirmed by culture or serologic testing. However, if culture or serologic testing is performed, and the viral illness is attributed to the vaccine-strain measles virus, the presumption of causation will remain in effect. Bone marrow examination, if performed, must reveal a normal or an increased number of megakaryocytes in an otherwise normal marrow.

(8) Vaccine-strain measles viral disease. This term is defined as a measles illness that involves the skin and/or another organ (such as the brain or lungs). Measles virus must be isolated from the affected organ or histopathologic findings characteristic for the disease must be present. Measles viral strain determination may be performed by methods such

as polymerase chain reaction test and vaccine-specific monoclonal antibody. If strain determination reveals wild-type measles virus or another nonvaccine-strain virus, the disease shall not be considered to be a condition set forth in the Table. If strain determination is not performed or if the strain cannot be identified, onset of illness in any organ must occur within 12 months after vaccination.

(9) Vaccine-strain polio viral infection. This term is defined as a disease caused by poliovirus that is isolated from the affected tissue and should be determined to be the vaccine-strain by oligonucleotide or polymerase chain reaction. Isolation of poliovirus from the stool is not sufficient to establish a tissue specific infection or disease caused by vaccine-strain poliovirus.

(10) Shoulder injury related to vaccine administration (SIRVA). SIRVA manifests as shoulder pain and limited range of motion occurring after the administration of a vaccine intended for intramuscular administration in the upper arm. These symptoms are thought to occur as a result of unintended injection of vaccine antigen or trauma from the needle into and around the underlying bursa of the shoulder resulting in an inflammatory reaction. SIRVA is caused by an injury to the musculoskeletal structures of the shoulder (tendons, ligaments, bursae, etc). SIRVA is not a neurological injury and abnormalities on neurological examination or nerve conduction studies (NCS) and/or electromyographic (EMG) studies would not support SIRVA as a diagnosis (even if the condition causing the neurological abnormality is not known). A vaccine recipient shall be considered to have suffered SIRVA if such recipient manifests all of the following:

(i) No history of pain, inflammation, or dysfunction of the affected shoulder prior to intramuscular vaccine administration that would explain the alleged signs, symptoms, examination findings, and/or diagnostic studies occurring after vaccine injection;

(ii) Pain occurs within the specified time-frame;

(iii) Pain and reduced range of motion are limited to the shoulder in which the intramuscular vaccine was administered; and

(iv) No other condition or abnormality is present that would explain the patient's symptoms (eg, NCS/EMG or clinical evidence of radiculopathy, brachial neuritis, mononeuropathies, or any other neuropathy).

(11) Disseminated varicella vaccine-strain viral disease. Disseminated varicella vaccine-strain viral disease is defined as a varicella illness that involves the skin beyond the dermatome in which the vaccination was given and/or disease caused by vaccine-strain varicella in another organ. For organs other than the skin, the disease must be demonstrated in the involved organ and not just through mildly abnormal laboratory values. If there is involvement of an organ beyond the skin, and no virus was identified in that organ, the involvement of all organs must occur as part of the same, discrete illness. If strain determination reveals wild-type varicella virus or another, nonvaccine-strain virus, the viral disease shall not be considered to be a condition set forth in the Table. If strain determination is not performed or if the strain cannot be identified, onset of illness in any organ must occur 7–42 days after vaccination.

(12) Varicella vaccine-strain viral reactivation disease. Varicella vaccine-strain viral reactivation disease is defined as the presence of the rash of herpes zoster with or without concurrent disease in an organ other than the skin. Zoster, or shingles, is a painful, unilateral, pruritic rash appearing in one or more sensory dermatomes. For organs other than the skin, the disease must be demonstrated in the involved organ and not just through mildly

abnormal laboratory values. There must be laboratory confirmation that the vaccine-strain of the varicella virus is present in the skin or in any other involved organ, for example by oligonucleotide or polymerase chain reaction. If strain determination reveals wild- type varicella virus or another, nonvaccine-strain virus, the viral disease shall not be considered to be a condition set forth in the Table.

(13) Vasovagal syncope. Vasovagal syncope (also sometimes called neurocardiogenic syncope) means loss of consciousness (fainting) and postural tone caused by a transient decrease in blood flow to the brain occurring after the administration of an injected vaccine. Vasovagal syncope is usually a benign condition but may result in falling and injury with significant sequela. Vasovagal syncope may be preceded by symptoms such as nausea, lightheadedness, diaphoresis, and/or pallor. Vasovagal syncope may be associated with transient seizure-like activity, but recovery of orientation and consciousness generally occurs simultaneously with vasovagal syncope. Loss of consciousness resulting from the following conditions will not be considered vasovagal syncope: organic heart disease, cardiac arrhythmias, transient ischemic attacks, hyperventilation, metabolic conditions, neurological conditions, and seizures. Episodes of recurrent syncope occurring after the applicable time period are not considered to be sequela of an episode of syncope meeting the Table requirements.

(14) Immunodeficient recipient. Immunodeficient recipient is defined as an individual with an identified defect in the immunological system which impairs the body's ability to fight infections. The identified defect may be attributable to an inherited disorder (such as severe combined immunodeficiency resulting in absent T lymphocytes), or an acquired disorder (such as acquired immunodeficiency syndrome resulting from decreased CD4 cell counts). The identified defect must be demonstrated in the medical records, either preceding or postdating vaccination.

(15) Guillain-Barré Syndrome (GBS). (i) GBS is an acute monophasic peripheral neuropathy that encompasses a spectrum of 4 clinicopathological subtypes described below. For each subtype of GBS, the interval between the first appearance of symptoms and the nadir of weakness is between 12 hours and 28 days. This is followed in all subtypes by a clinical plateau with stabilization at the nadir of symptoms, or subsequent improvement without significant relapse. Death may occur without a clinical plateau. Treatment related fluctuations in all subtypes of GBS can occur within 9 weeks of GBS symptom onset and recurrence of symptoms after this time-frame would not be consistent with GBS.

(ii) The most common subtype in North America and Europe, comprising more than 90% of cases, is acute inflammatory demyelinating polyneuropathy (AIDP), which has the pathologic and electrodiagnostic features of focal demyelination of motor and sensory peripheral nerves and nerve roots. Another subtype called acute motor axonal neuropathy (AMAN) is generally seen in other parts of the world and is predominated by axonal damage that primarily affects motor nerves. AMAN lacks features of demyelination. Another less common subtype of GBS includes acute motor and sensory neuropathy (AMSAN), which is an axonal form of GBS that is similar to AMAN, but also affects the sensory nerves and roots. AIDP, AMAN, and AMSAN are typically characterized by symmetric motor flaccid weakness, sensory abnormalities, and/or autonomic dysfunction caused by autoimmune damage to peripheral nerves and nerve roots. The diagnosis of AIDP, AMAN, and AMSAN requires:

(A) Bilateral flaccid limb weakness and decreased or absent deep tendon reflexes in weak limbs;

(B) A monophasic illness pattern;

(C) An interval between onset and nadir of weakness between 12 hours and 28 days;

(D) Subsequent clinical plateau (the clinical plateau leads to either stabilization at the nadir of symptoms, or subsequent improvement without significant relapse; however, death may occur without a clinical plateau); and,

(E) The absence of an identified more likely alternative diagnosis.

(iii) Fisher syndrome (FS), also known as Miller Fisher syndrome, is a subtype of GBS characterized by ataxia, areflexia, and ophthalmoplegia, and overlap between FS and AIDP may be seen with limb weakness. The diagnosis of FS requires:

(A) Bilateral ophthalmoparesis;

(B) Bilateral reduced or absent tendon reflexes;

(C) Ataxia;

(D) The absence of limb weakness (the presence of limb weakness suggests a diagnosis of AIDP, AMAN, or AMSAN);

(E) A monophasic illness pattern;

(F) An interval between onset and nadir of weakness between 12 hours and 28 days;

(G) Subsequent clinical plateau (the clinical plateau leads to either stabilization at the nadir of symptoms, or subsequent improvement without significant relapse; however, death may occur without a clinical plateau);

(H) No alteration in consciousness;

(I) No corticospinal track signs; and

(J) The absence of an identified more likely alternative diagnosis.

(iv) Evidence that is supportive, but not required, of a diagnosis of all subtypes of GBS includes electrophysiologic findings consistent with GBS or an elevation of cerebral spinal fluid (CSF) protein with a total CSF white blood cell count below 50 cells/μL. Both CSF and electrophysiologic studies are frequently normal in the first week of illness in otherwise typical cases of GBS.

(v) To qualify as any subtype of GBS, there must not be a more likely alternative diagnosis for the weakness.

(vi) Exclusionary criteria for the diagnosis of all subtypes of GBS include the ultimate diagnosis of any of the following conditions: chronic immune demyelinating polyradiculopathy (CIDP), carcinomatous meningitis, brain stem encephalitis (other than Bickerstaff brainstem encephalitis), myelitis, spinal cord infarct, spinal cord compression, anterior horn cell diseases such as polio or West Nile virus infection, subacute inflammatory demyelinating polyradiculoneuropathy, multiple sclerosis, cauda equina compression, metabolic conditions such as hypermagnesemia or hypophosphatemia, tick paralysis, heavy metal toxicity (such as arsenic, gold, or thallium), drug-induced neuropathy (such as vincristine, platinum compounds, or nitrofurantoin), porphyria, critical illness neuropathy, vasculitis, diphtheria, myasthenia gravis, organophosphate poisoning, botulism, critical illness myopathy, polymyositis, dermatomyositis, hypokalemia, or hyperkalemia. The above list is not exhaustive.

(d) Glossary for purposes of paragraph (c) of this section:

(1) Chronic encephalopathy.

(i) A chronic encephalopathy occurs when a change in mental or neurologic status, first manifested during the applicable Table time period as an acute encephalopathy or encephalitis, persists for at least 6 months from the first symptom or manifestation of onset or of significant aggravation of an acute encephalopathy or encephalitis.

(ii) Individuals who return to their baseline neurologic state, as confirmed by clinical findings, within less than 6 months from the first symptom or manifestation of onset or of significant aggravation of an acute encephalopathy or encephalitis shall not be presumed to have suffered residual neurologic damage from that event; any subsequent chronic encephalopathy shall not be presumed to be a sequela of the acute encephalopathy or encephalitis.

(2) Injected refers to the intramuscular, intradermal, or subcutaneous needle administration of a vaccine.

(3) Sequela means a condition or event that was actually caused by a condition listed in the Vaccine Injury Table.

(4) Significantly decreased level of consciousness is indicated by the presence of one or more of the following clinical signs:

(i) Decreased or absent response to environment (responds, if at all, only to loud voice or painful stimuli);

(ii) Decreased or absent eye contact (does not fix gaze upon family members or other individuals); or

(iii) Inconsistent or absent responses to external stimuli (does not recognize familiar people or things).

(5) Seizure includes myoclonic, generalized tonic-clonic (grand mal), and simple and complex partial seizures, but not absence (petit mal), or pseudo seizures. Jerking movements or staring episodes alone are not necessarily an indication of seizure activity.

(e) Coverage provisions.

(1) Except as provided in paragraph (e)(2), (3), (4), (5), (6), (7), or (8) of this section, this section applies only to petitions for compensation under the program filed with the United States Court of Federal Claims on or after February 21, 2017.

(2) Hepatitis B, Hib, and varicella vaccines (Items VIII, IX, and X of the Table) are included in the Table as of August 6, 1997.

(3) Rotavirus vaccines (Item XI of the Table) are included in the Table as of October 22, 1998.

(4) Pneumococcal conjugate vaccines (Item XII of the Table) are included in the Table as of December 18, 1999.

(5) Hepatitis A vaccines (Item XIII of the Table) are included on the Table as of December 1, 2004.

(6) Trivalent influenza vaccines (Included in item XIV of the Table) are included on the Table as of July 1, 2005. All other seasonal influenza vaccines (Item XIV of the Table) are included on the Table as of November 12, 2013.

(7) Meningococcal vaccines and human papillomavirus vaccines (Items XV and XVI of the Table) are included on the Table as of February 1, 2007.

(8) Other new vaccines (Item XVII of the Table) will be included in the Table as of the effective date of a tax enacted to provide funds for compensation paid with respect to such vaccines. An amendment to this section will be published in the Federal Register to announce the effective date of such a tax.

APPENDIX IV

Nationally Notifiable Infectious Diseases in the United States

Nationally notifiable infectious diseases are those that public health officials from local, state, and territorial public health departments voluntarily report to the Centers for Disease Control and Prevention (CDC). Surveillance for nationally notifiable infectious diseases helps public health agencies monitor the occurrence and spread of disease across the nation and evaluate prevention and control measures, among other purposes. To ensure consistency in how the data are classified and enumerated, national surveillance case definitions are established and used for each disease. The Council of State and Territorial Epidemiologists (CSTE), with advice from the CDC, reviews the list of nationally notifiable infectious diseases on an annual basis and may recommend that a disease be added or deleted from the list or that a case definition be revised. Provisional nationally notifiable infectious disease data are published weekly (for selected nationally notifiable diseases) and quarterly (for tuberculosis) in the *Morbidity and Mortality Weekly Report (MMWR)* data tables; finalized data are published annually in the *MMWR* series "Summary of Notifiable Infectious Diseases and Conditions, United States." The 2018 list of nationally notifiable infectious diseases is included in Table 1. Should a more current list of such diseases be needed, visit **wwwn.cdc.gov/nndss/conditions/**.

Nationally notifiable infectious disease reports are based on data collected at the local, state, and territorial levels as a result of legislation and regulations in those jurisdictions that require health care providers, clinical laboratories, hospitals, and other entities to submit health-related data on reportable diseases to public health departments. Case reporting to local, state, or territorial public health officials provides them the information needed to investigate these diseases and to implement prevention and control strategies, among other purposes. Because the list of reportable infectious diseases is determined by local, state, and territorial law and varies by jurisdiction, health care providers, clinical laboratories, hospitals, and other required reporters are strongly encouraged to obtain specific reporting requirements from the appropriate public health department, including the timeliness required for case reporting.

If a reportable disease meets the criteria for a nationally notifiable infectious disease, the local, state, or territorial public health department will submit a case notification to the CDC. The timeliness of such notifications varies by disease, with some requiring notification within 4 hours.

Table 1. Infectious Diseases and Conditions Designated as Notifiable at the National Level—United States, 2018[1,2]

- Anthrax
- Arboviral diseases, neuroinvasive and nonneuroinvasive
  - California serogroup virus diseases
  - Chikungunya virus disease
  - Eastern equine encephalitis virus disease
  - Powassan virus disease
  - St. Louis encephalitis virus disease
  - West Nile virus disease
  - Western equine encephalitis virus disease
- Babesiosis
- Botulism
  - Botulism, foodborne
  - Botulism, infant
  - Botulism, other
  - Botulism, wound
- Brucellosis
- Campylobacteriosis
- Carbapenemase-producing carbapenem-resistant *Enterobacteriaceae* (CP-CRE)
  - CP-CRE, *Enterobacter* species
  - CP-CRE, *Escherichia coli*
  - CP-CRE, *Klebsiella* species
- Chancroid
- *Chlamydia trachomatis* infection
- Cholera
- Coccidioidomycosis
- Congenital syphilis
  - Syphilitic stillbirth
- Cryptosporidiosis
- Cyclosporiasis
- Dengue virus infections
  - Dengue
  - Dengue-like illness
  - Severe dengue
- Diphtheria
- Ehrlichiosis and Anaplasmosis
  - *Anaplasma phagocytophilum* infection
  - *Ehrlichia chaffeensis* infection
  - *Ehrlichia ewingii* infection
  - Undetermined human ehrlichiosis/anaplasmosis
- Giardiasis
- Gonorrhea

- *Haemophilus influenzae*, invasive disease
- Hansen disease
- Hantavirus infection, non-Hantavirus pulmonary syndrome
- Hantavirus pulmonary syndrome (HPS)
- Hemolytic uremic syndrome, postdiarrheal
- Hepatitis A, acute
- Hepatitis B, acute
- Hepatitis B, chronic
- Hepatitis B, perinatal infection
- Hepatitis C, acute
- Hepatitis C, chronic
- Hepatitis C, perintal infection
- HIV infection (AIDS has been reclassified as HIV Stage III)
- Influenza-associated pediatric mortality
- Invasive pneumococcal disease
- Legionellosis
- Leptospirosis
- Listeriosis
- Lyme disease
- Malaria
- Measles
- Meningococcal disease
- Mumps
- Novel influenza A virus infections
- Pertussis
- Plague
- Poliomyelitis, paralytic
- Poliovirus infection, nonparalytic
- Psittacosis
- Q fever, acute and chronic
- Rabies, animal
- Rabies, human
- Rubella
- Rubella, congenital syndrome
- Salmonellosis
- Severe acute respiratory syndrome-associated Coronavirus disease
- Shiga toxin-producing *Escherichia coli*
- Shigellosis
- Smallpox
- Spotted fever rickettsiosis

- Streptococcal toxic shock syndrome
- Syphilis
  - Syphilis, primary
  - Syphilis, secondary
  - Syphilis, early nonprimary nonsecondary
  - Syphilis, unknown duration or late
- Tetanus
- Toxic shock syndrome (other than streptococcal)
- Trichinellosis
- Tuberculosis
- Tularemia
- Typhoid fever
- Vancomycin-intermediate *Staphylococcus aureus* and Vancomycin-resistant *Staphylococcus aureus* (VISA/VRSA)
- Varicella
- Varicella deaths
- Vibriosis
- Viral hemorrhagic fever (VHF)
  - Crimean-Congo hemorrhagic fever virus
  - Ebola virus
  - Lassa virus
  - Lujo virus
  - Marburg virus
  - New World arenavirus – Guanarito virus
  - New World arenavirus – Junin virus
  - New World arenavirus – Machupo virus
  - New World arenavirus – Sabia virus
- Yellow fever
- Zika virus disease and Zika virus infection
  - Zika virus disease, congenital
  - Zika virus disease, noncongenital
  - Zika virus infection, congenital
  - Zika virus infection, noncongenital

[1] wwwn.cdc.gov/nndss/conditions/notifiable/2017/infectious-diseases/

[2] wwwn.cdc.gov/nndss/data-and-statistics.html

....

APPENDIX V

Guide to Contraindications and Precautions to Immunizations, 2018

A contraindication to vaccination is a condition in a patient that increases the risk of a serious adverse reaction and for whom this increased risk of an adverse reaction outweighs the benefit of the vaccine. A vaccine should not be administered when a contraindication is present. The only contraindication applicable to all vaccines is a history of anaphylaxis to a previous dose or to a vaccine component, unless the patient has undergone desensitization. Refer to the Description section of manufacturer's package inserts for components of each vaccine; package inserts are available at **www.fda.gov/ BiologicsBloodVaccines/Vaccines/ApprovedProducts/ucm093833.htm.** A precaution is a condition in a recipient that might increase the risk or seriousness of an adverse reaction or complicate making another diagnosis because of a possible vaccine-related reaction. A precaution also may exist for conditions that might compromise the ability of the vaccine to produce immunity (eg, administering measles vaccine to a person with passive immunity to measles from a blood product transfusion). People who administer vaccines should screen recipients for contraindications and precautions before administering vaccines, and this screening should be documented (eg, in the electronic medical record). This information is based on recommendations of the Committee on Infectious Diseases of the American Academy of Pediatrics (AAP) and the Advisory Committee on Immunization Practices (ACIP) of the Centers for Disease Control and Prevention (CDC). Sometimes, these recommendations differ from information in the manufacturers' package inserts. For more detailed information, physicians should consult published recommendations of the ACIP and AAP, manufacturers' package inserts, and **www.cdc. gov/vaccines/hcp/admin/contraindications.html.** These guidelines, originally issued in 1993, have been updated to give recommendations as of 2017 (on the basis of information available as of December 2016).

Guide to Contraindications and Precautions to Immunizations, 2018

Vaccine	Contraindications	Precautions[a]	Conditions in Which Vaccines Should Be Given if Indicated
General for all routinely administered vaccines (eg, DTaP, DT, Td, Tdap, IPV, MMR, MMRV, Hib, pneumococcal, meningococcal, hepatitis B, varicella, hepatitis A, influenza, zoster, rotavirus, HPV)	Severe allergic reaction (eg, anaphylaxis) to a vaccine contraindicates further doses of that vaccine Severe allergic reaction (eg, anaphylaxis) to a vaccine constituent contraindicates the use of vaccines containing that substance	Current moderate or severe illnesses with or without fever Latex allergy[b]	Mild to moderate local reaction (soreness, redness, swelling) after a dose of an injectable antigen Low-grade or moderate fever after a previous vaccine dose Current mild acute illness with or without low-grade fever Current antimicrobial therapy Convalescent phase of illnesses Preterm birth (same dosage and indications as for healthy, full-term infants); hepatitis B is the exception[c] (see Hepatitis B, p 401) Recent exposure to an infectious disease History of penicillin or other nonspecific allergies or fact that relatives have such allergies Pregnancy of mother or household contact Unimmunized household contact Immunodeficient household contact Breastfeeding (nursing infant OR lactating mother) Lack of a physical examination

Guide to Contraindications and Precautions to Immunizations, 2018, continued

Vaccine	Contraindications	Precautions[a]	Conditions in Which Vaccines Should Be Given if Indicated
DTaP	Severe allergic reaction (eg, anaphylaxis) after a previous dose or to a vaccine component Encephalopathy (eg, coma, decreased level of consciousness, or prolonged seizures) not attributable to another identifiable cause, within 7 days of administration of previous dose of DTaP/DTwP	Current moderate or severe illnesses with or without fever Progressive neurologic disorder, including infantile spasms, uncontrolled epilepsy, progressive encephalopathy, generally have DTaP immunization deferred temporarily until neurologic status clarified and stabilized. Temperature of 40.5°C (105°F) or greater within 48 h after immunization with a previous dose of DTaP/DTwP Guillain-Barré syndrome (GBS) within 6 wk after a dose[e] History of Arthus-type hypersensitivity reaction after a previous dose of a tetanus- or diphtheria toxoid- containing vaccine (defer for 10 years after last tetanus toxoid-containing vaccine)	Family history of seizures[d] Family history of sudden infant death syndrome Family history of an adverse event after DTaP/DTwP administration Fever <105°F (<40°C), fussiness, or mild drowsiness after a previous dose of DTwP/DTaP Stable neurologic conditions (eg, cerebral palsy, well-controlled seizures, or developmental delay)

Guide to Contraindications and Precautions to Immunizations, 2018, continued

Vaccine	Contraindications	Precautions[a]	Conditions in Which Vaccines Should Be Given if Indicated
DT, Td	Severe allergic reaction (eg, anaphylaxis) after a previous dose or to a vaccine component	Current moderate or severe acute illness with or without fever GBS within 6 wk after previous dose of tetanus toxoid-containing vaccine History of Arthus-type hypersensitivity reaction after a previous dose of tetanus or diphtheria toxoid-containing vaccine; defer vaccination until at least 10 years have elapsed since the last tetanus toxoid-containing vaccine (see DTaP)	
Hepatitis A	Severe allergic reaction (eg, anaphylaxis) after a previous dose or to a vaccine component	Current moderate or severe acute illness with or without fever	Pregnancy Autoimmune disease (eg, systemic lupus erythematosis or rheumatoid arthritis).
Hepatitis B	Severe allergic reaction (eg, anaphylaxis) after a previous dose or to a vaccine component Hypersensitivity to yeast	Current moderate or severe acute illness with or without fever Preterm birth[c]	
Hib	Severe allergic reaction (eg, anaphylaxis) after a previous dose or to a vaccine component	Current moderate or severe acute illness with or without fever	

Guide to Contraindications and Precautions to Immunizations, 2018, continued

Vaccine	Contraindications	Precautions[a]	Conditions in Which Vaccines Should Be Given if Indicated
HPV	Severe allergic reaction (eg, anaphylaxis) after a previous dose or to a vaccine component	Current moderate or severe acute illness with or without fever Pregnancy	Administration to people with minor acute illnesses Immunosuppression Equivocal or abnormal Papanicolaou test HPV infection, anogenital warts, or HPV-associated lesions Breastfeeding
Influenza (inactivated)[f]	Severe allergic reaction (eg, anaphylaxis) to a previous dose or vaccine component	Current moderate or severe acute illness with or without fever GBS within 6 wk after a previous influenza immunization	Pregnancy Nonsevere allergy to thimerosal Current administration of warfarin or theophylline All children with egg allergy can receive influenza vaccine with no additional precautions from those of routine vaccinations[g]

Guide to Contraindications and Precautions to Immunizations, 2018, continued

Vaccine	Contraindications	Precautions[a]	Conditions in Which Vaccines Should Be Given if Indicated
Influenza (live attenuated)[h]	An interim recommendation that intranasal quadrivalent live attenuated influenza vaccine (LAIV4) **not** be used in any setting in the United States was made in 2016 and continues through the 2017–2018 influenza season, although it is still licensed by the FDA for healthy people 2 through 49 years of age (see Influenza, p 476). Severe allergic reaction (eg, anaphylaxis) to a previous dose or vaccine component Pregnancy Receipt of specific antivirals (ie, zanamivir, oseltamivir, peramivir) 48 hours before vaccination. Avoid use of these antiviral drugs for 5–7 days after vaccination Children 2 through 4 y of age whose parents or caregivers report that a health care provider has told them during the preceding 12 mo that their child had wheezing or asthma or whose medical record indicates a wheezing episode has occurred during the preceding 12 mo Children with the diagnosis of asthma Receiving aspirin or other salicylates	Current moderate or severe acute illness with or without fever GBS within 6 wk after a previous influenza immunization Conditions for which the ACIP lists as precautions but which are not contraindications in the vaccine package insert: immune suppression, certain chronic medical conditions such as: asthma, diabetes, heart or kidney disease	Health care providers that see patients with chronic diseases or altered immunocompetence (an exception is providers for severely immunocompromised patients requiring care in a protected environment, such as a bone marrow transplant unit) Breastfeeding Contacts of people with chronic disease or altered immunocompetence (an exception is contacts of severely immunocompromised patients requiring care in a protected environment) All children with egg allergy can receive influenza vaccine with no additional precautions from those of routine vaccinations[g]

Guide to Contraindications and Precautions to Immunizations, 2018, continued

Vaccine	Contraindications	Precautions[a]	Conditions in Which Vaccines Should Be Given if Indicated
IPV	Severe allergic reaction (eg, anaphylaxis) after a previous dose or to a vaccine component	Current moderate or severe acute illness with or without fever	Previous receipt of one or more doses of oral poliovirus vaccine.
Meningococcal conjugate (MenACWY)	Severe allergic reaction (eg, anaphylaxis) after a previous dose or to a vaccine component or to diphtheria toxoid	Current moderate or severe acute illness with or without fever	
Meningococcal B (MenB)	Severe allergic reaction (eg, anaphylaxis) after a previous dose or to a vaccine component	Current moderate or severe acute illness with or without fever	
MMR[f,h]	Severe allergic reaction (eg, anaphylaxis) after a previous dose or to a vaccine component	Current moderate or severe acute illness with or without fever	Simultaneous tuberculin skin testing or IGRA[m]
	Pregnancy	Recent (within 11 mo, depending on product and dose) Immune Globulin administration (see Table 1.13, p 40)	Breastfeeding
	Known severe immunodeficiency (eg, from hematologic and solid tumors, receipt of chemotherapy, long-term immunosuppressive therapy,[i] receipt of biologic response modifiers,[j] congenital immunodeficiency, or patients with HIV infection who are severely immunocompromised[k]	Thrombocytopenia or history of thrombocytopenic purpura, in isolation or after prior MMR vaccination (see Measles, p 537)	Pregnancy of mother of recipient
		Tuberculosis or positive PPD or interferon gamma release assay (IGRA)[l]	Immunodeficient family member or household contact
		Personal or family history of seizure if provided as MMRV (consider giving as separate administrations [MMR+V])	Nonanaphylactic reactions to gelatin or neomycin
			Allergy to egg
			Recipient is a female of childbearing age

Guide to Contraindications and Precautions to Immunizations, 2018, continued

Vaccine	Contraindications	Precautions[a]	Conditions in Which Vaccines Should Be Given if Indicated
PCV13 and PPSV23	For PCV13, severe allergic reaction (eg, anaphylaxis) after a previous dose of PCV7 or PCV13 or to a vaccine component, or to diphtheria toxoid For PPSV23, severe allergic reaction (eg, anaphylaxis) after a previous dose or to a vaccine component	Current moderate or severe acute illness with or without fever	History of invasive pneumococcal disease or pneumonia
Rotavirus	Severe allergic reaction (eg, anaphylaxis) after a previous dose or to a vaccine component Severe combined immune deficiency (SCID) History of previous episode of intussusception Avoid use in infants exposed in utero to biologic response modifiers such as anti-TNF agents	Current moderate or severe acute illness, with or without fever Altered immunocompetence other than SCID Chronic gastrointestinal disease Spina bifida or bladder exstrophy	Breastfeeding Immunodeficient family member or household contact Preterm infants Pregnant household contacts

Guide to Contraindications and Precautions to Immunizations, 2018, continued

Vaccine	Contraindications	Precautions[a]	Conditions in Which Vaccines Should Be Given if Indicated
Tdap	Severe allergic reaction (eg, anaphylaxis) to a previous dose or vaccine component History of encephalopathy (eg, coma, prolonged seizures) within 7 days of administration of a pertussis vaccine that is not attributable to another identifiable cause	Current moderate or severe acute illness, with or without fever GBS 6 wk or less after previous dose of a tetanus toxoid vaccine Progressive neurologic disorder, uncontrolled epilepsy, or progressive encephalopathy until the condition has stabilized History of Arthus-type hypersensitivity reaction (see DTaP)	Temperature 105°F (40.5°C) or greater within 48 h after DTwP/DTaP immunization not attributable to another cause Collapse or shock-like state (hypotonic hyporesponsive episode) within 48 h after DTwP/DTaP immunization Persistent crying lasting 3 h or longer, occurring within 48 h after DTwP/DTaP immunization Convulsions with or without fever, occurring within 3 days after DTwP/DTaP immunization History of extensive limb swelling reaction after pediatric DTwP/DTaP or Td immunization that was not an Arthus-type hypersensitivity reaction Stable neurologic disorder, including well-controlled seizures, history of seizure disorder, and cerebral palsy Brachial neuritis Pregnancy Breastfeeding Immunosuppression, including people with HIV (Tdap poses no known safety concern for immunosuppressed people; the immunogenicity of Tdap in people with immunosuppression has not been studied and could be suboptimal) Intercurrent minor illness Antimicrobial use

Guide to Contraindications and Precautions to Immunizations, 2018, continued

Vaccine	Contraindications	Precautions[a]	Conditions in Which Vaccines Should Be Given if Indicated
Varicella[h]	Pregnancy	Current moderate or severe acute illness with or without fever	Pregnancy of mother of recipient
	Severe allergic reaction (eg, anaphylaxis) after a previous dose or to a vaccine component	Recent receipt of Immune Globulin (see Table 1.13, p 40)	Immunodeficiency in a household contact
	Known severe immunodeficiency (hematologic and solid tumors, receipt of chemotherapy, long-term immunosuppressive therapy,[i] receipt of biologic response modifiers,[j] congenital immunodeficiency, or patients with HIV infection who are severely immunocompromised[k])	Family history of immunodeficiency[n]	HIV-infected children without evidence of varicella immunity and with a CD4+ T-lymphocyte percentage of 15% or greater
		Personal or family history of seizure if provided as MMRV (consider giving as separate administrations [MMR+V])	Household contact with HIV
		Receipt of specific antivirals (ie, acyclovir, famciclovir, or valacyclovir) 24 hours before vaccination; avoid use of these antiviral drugs for 21 days after vaccination	

DTaP indicates diphtheria and tetanus toxoids and acellular pertussis; DT, pediatric diphtheria-tetanus toxoid; Td, adult tetanus-diphtheria toxoid; Tdap, tetanus toxoid, reduced diphtheria toxoid, and acellular pertussis; IPV, inactivated poliovirus; MMR, measles-mumps-rubella; MMRV, measles-mumps-rubella-varicella; Hib, *Haemophilus influenzae* type b; HPV, human papillomavirus; DTP, diphtheria and tetanus toxoids and pertussis; GBS, Guillain-Barré syndrome; HIV, human immunodeficiency virus; PPD, purified protein derivative (tuberculin); PCV7 and PCV13, pneumococcal conjugate vaccine; PPSV23, pneumococcal polysaccharide vaccine.

[a] The events or conditions listed as precautions, although not contraindications, should be reviewed carefully. The benefits and risks of administering a specific vaccine to a person under the circumstances should be considered. If the risks are believed to outweigh the benefits, the immunization should be withheld; if the benefits are believed to outweigh the risks (eg, during an outbreak or foreign travel), the immunization should be administered. Whether and when to administer DTaP to children with proven or suspected underlying neurologic disorders should be decided on an individual basis.

[b] If a person reports a severe (anaphylactic) allergy to latex, vaccines supplied in vials or syringes that contain natural rubber should not be administered unless the benefits of immunization outweigh the risks of an allergic reaction to the vaccine. For latex allergies other than anaphylactic allergies (eg, a history of contact allergy to latex gloves), vaccines supplied in vials or syringes that contain dry natural rubber or latex can be administered.

cInfants weighing less than 2 kg at birth and born to hepatitis B surface antigen (HBsAg)-negative mothers should receive the first dose of HepB vaccine series starting at 1 month of chronologic age or at hospital discharge if before 1 month of chronologic age. All infants weighing less than 2 kg born to HBsAg-positive mothers should receive immunoprophylaxis (Hepatitis B Immune Globulin and vaccine) beginning as soon as possible after birth, and always within 12 hours after birth, followed by appropriate postimmunization testing and receipt of 3 doses of hepatitis B vaccine. All infants weighing less than 2 kg at birth and born to mothers with unknown HBsAg status should receive hepatitis B vaccine within 12 hours of birth; if status remains unknown by 12 hours of life or if maternal HBsAg is positive, Hepatitis B Immune Globulin should be given.

dAcetaminophen given before administering DTaP and thereafter every 4 hours for 24 hours may be considered for children with a personal or family (ie, siblings or parents) history of seizures.

eThe decision to give additional doses of DTaP should be made on the basis of consideration of the benefit of further immunization versus the risk of recurrence of GBS. For example, completion of the primary series in children is justified.

fEgg allergy is not considered a contraindication or precaution.

gRefer to Influenza chapter (p 476).

hThe administration of multiple live-virus vaccines within 28 days (4 weeks) of one another if not given on the same day may result in suboptimal immune response. Data substantiate this risk for MMR and possibly varicella vaccine, which should, therefore, be given on the same day or more than 4 weeks apart.

iImmunosuppressive steroid dose is considered to be 2 or more weeks of daily receipt of 20 mg prednisone or the equivalent. Vaccination should be deferred for at least 1 month after discontinuation of such therapy.

jRefer to Biologic Response Modifiers Used to Decrease Inflammation (p 85).

kEvidence of severe immunosuppression in HIV-infected children is CD4+ T-lymphocyte percentage less than 15% in children of any age, and CD4+ T-lymphocyte percentage less than 200 lymphocytes/mm³ in children 6 years and older. Severely immunocompromised HIV-infected infants, children, adolescents, and young adults should not receive measles virus-containing vaccine, because vaccine-related pneumonia has been reported. The quadrivalent measles-mumps-rubella-varicella (MMRV) vaccine should not be administered to any HIV-infected infant, regardless of degree of immunosuppression, because of lack of safety data in this population.

lA theoretical basis exists for concern that measles vaccine might exacerbate tuberculosis. Consequently, before administering MMR to people with untreated active tuberculosis, initiating antituberculosis therapy is advisable.

mMeasles immunization may suppress tuberculin reactivity temporarily. MMR vaccine may be given after, or on the same day as, tuberculin skin testing. If MMR has been given recently, postpone the tuberculin skin test until 4 to 6 weeks after administration of MMR. The effect of MMR on IGRA test results is unknown.

nVaricella vaccine should not be administered to a person who has a family history of congenital or hereditary immunodeficiency (such as parents or siblings) until the potential vaccinee's immune competence has been substantiated clinically or verified by a laboratory.

····························

APPENDIX VI

Prevention of Infectious Disease From Contaminated Food Products[1]

Foodborne diseases are associated with significant morbidity and mortality in people of all ages. The Centers for Disease Control and Prevention (CDC) estimates that there are 48 million cases of foodborne illness in the United States each year, resulting in approximately 128 000 hospitalizations and 3000 deaths.[2,3] Young children, the elderly, and immunocompromised people are especially susceptible to illnesses and complications caused by many of the organisms associated with foodborne illness. Norovirus is the most common cause of outbreaks of foodborne illness, as well as number of foodborne infections, in the United States.[3] The system for surveillance and reporting for norovirus infections is known as CaliciNet. Information about CaliciNet can be found at **www.cdc.gov/norovirus/reporting/calicinet/index.html.**

The Foodborne Diseases Active Surveillance Network (FoodNet) of the CDC's Emerging Infections Program conducts active, population-based surveillance in 10 states for all laboratory-confirmed infections with select enteric pathogens transmitted commonly through food. The FoodNet program conducts surveillance for illnesses attributable to *Campylobacter* species, *Listeria monocytogenes*, *Salmonella* species, Shiga toxin-producing *Escherichia coli* (STEC) O157:H7, *Shigella* species, *Vibrio* species, and *Yersinia enterocolitica* (since 1996); *Cryptosporidium* species and *Cyclospora* species (since 1997); and STEC non-O157 (since 2000). FoodNet also conducts surveillance for hemolytic-uremic syndrome (HUS), a complication of STEC infection. Additional information about FoodNet can be found at **www.cdc.gov/foodnet/index.html.**

Outbreak surveillance provides insights into the causes of foodborne illness, types of implicated foods, and settings where transmission occurs. The CDC collects data on foodborne disease outbreaks submitted from all states and territories (**www.cdc.gov/foodsafety/fdoss/index.html**). Public health, regulatory, and agricultural professionals can use this information when creating targeted control strategies and to support efforts to promote safe food preparation practices among food industry employees and the public. Data on foodborne disease outbreaks are available online through the Foodborne Outbreak Online Database (**wwwn.cdc.gov/foodborneoutbreaks**).

Four general rules should be followed to maintain safety of foods:
1. **Clean:** Wash hands and surfaces thoroughly and often.
2. **Separate:** Do not cross-contaminate.
3. **Chill:** Refrigerate foods promptly.

---

[1]Centers for Disease Control and Prevention. Diagnosis and management of foodborne illnesses: a primer for physicians. *MMWR Recomm Rep.* 2004;53(RR-4):1–33

[2]Centers for Disease Control and Prevention. Surveillance for foodborne disease outbreaks—United States, 2008. *MMWR Morb Mortal Wkly Rep.* 2011;60(35):1197-1202

[3]Centers for Disease Control and Prevention. Surveillance for foodborne disease outbreaks—United States, 1998–2008. *MMWR Morb Mortal Wkly Rep.* 2013;62(SS-2):1–34

4. **Cook:** Cook food to the proper temperature.

The following preventive measures can be implemented to decrease the risk of infection from specific foods.

Unpasteurized Milk and Milk Products

The American Academy of Pediatrics (AAP) endorses the use of pasteurized milk and recommends that parents be fully informed of the important risks associated with consumption of unpasteurized milk.[1] Interstate sale of unpasteurized (raw) milk and products made from unpasteurized milk (with the exception of certain cheeses) is banned by the US Food and Drug Administration (FDA). The most vulnerable populations, such as children, pregnant women, elderly people, and immunocompromised people, should not consume unpasteurized milk or products made from unpasteurized milk, including cheese, butter, yogurt, pudding, or ice cream, from any species, including cows, sheep, and goats. Serious infections attributable to *Salmonella* species, *Campylobacter* species, *Mycobacterium bovis*, *L monocytogenes*, *Brucella* species, *E coli* O157:H7, and *Y enterocolitica* have been linked to consumption of unpasteurized milk. Although some states allow the sale of raw milk that meets specific standards (certified milk), certified raw milk has also been linked to outbreaks. In particular, a number of outbreaks of campylobacter infection among children have been associated with school field trips to farms that include consumption of raw milk. School officials should take precautions to prevent raw milk from being served to children during educational trips. Cheeses made from unpasteurized milk also have been associated with illnesses attributable to *Brucella* species, *L monocytogenes*, *Salmonella* species, *Campylobacter* species, *Shigella* species, *M bovis*, and STEC.

Eggs

At-risk populations, including children, should not eat raw or undercooked eggs, unpasteurized powdered eggs, or foods that may contain raw or undercooked eggs. Ingestion of raw or improperly cooked eggs can result in severe illness attributable to *Salmonella* species. Examples of foods that may contain raw or undercooked eggs include some homemade frostings and mayonnaise, homemade ice cream, tiramisu, eggs prepared "sunny-side up," Caesar salad dressing, Hollandaise sauce, cookie dough, and cake batter.

Raw and Undercooked Meat

Children should not eat raw or undercooked meat or meat products. Various raw or undercooked meat products have been associated with harmful bacteria, including *Salmonella* species and *Campylobacter* species. Specific meat products have been linked with certain bacterial infections (pathogen-commodity pair): ground beef with STEC and *Salmonella* species; hot dogs with *L monocytogenes*; pork with *Trichinella* species; and wild game with *Brucella* species, *Francisella* species, STEC, and *Trichinella* species. Ground meats should be cooked to an internal temperature of 160°F; roasts and steaks should be cooked to an in-

---

[1]American Academy of Pediatrics, Committee on Infectious Diseases and Committee on Nutrition. Consumption of raw or unpasteurized milk and milk products by pregnant women and children. *Pediatrics*. 2014;
133(1):175-179

ternal temperature of 145°F; poultry should be cooked to an internal temperature of 165°F. Use of a food thermometer is the only sure way of knowing that meat has reached a high enough temperature to destroy bacteria. Color is not a reliable indicator that ground beef patties have been cooked to a temperature high enough to kill harmful bacteria. Knives, cutting boards, plates, and other utensils used for raw meats should not be used for preparation of fresh fruits or vegetables until they have been cleaned properly (see Web sites at end of this Appendix for details).

Unpasteurized Juices

Children should drink only fruit juice that has been pasteurized or that has been freshly squeezed from washed fruit. Consumption of packaged fruit juices that have not undergone pasteurization or a comparable treatment has been associated with foodborne illness attributable to *E coli* O157:H7 and *Salmonella* species. To identify a packaged juice that has not undergone pasteurization or a comparable treatment, consumers should look for a warning statement that the product has not been pasteurized.

Seed Sprouts

The FDA and the CDC have reaffirmed health advisories that people who are at high risk of severe foodborne disease, including children, people with compromised immune systems, and the elderly, should avoid eating raw seed sprouts (including alfalfa sprouts).[1] Raw seed sprouts have been associated with outbreaks of illness attributable to *Salmonella* species, STEC, and *L monocytogenes*.

Fresh Fruits and Vegetables and Raw Nuts

Many fresh fruits and vegetables have been associated with disease attributable to *Cryptosporidium* species, *Cyclospora* species, norovirus, hepatitis A virus, *Giardia* species, STEC, *Salmonella* species, *L monocytogenes*, and *Shigella* species. Raw shelled nuts, commercially processed vegetable snacks, spinach, lettuce, tomatoes, cucumbers, melons, basil, and cilantro have been associated with outbreaks of salmonellosis. Nuts that have been roasted or otherwise treated can minimize the risk of foodborne illness. Washing can decrease bacterial contamination of fresh fruits and vegetables. Knives, cutting boards, utensils, and plates used for raw meats should not be used for preparation of fresh fruits or vegetables until the utensils have been cleaned properly (see Web sites at end of this Appendix for details).

Raw Shellfish and Fish

Children should not eat raw shellfish. Raw shellfish, including mussels, clams, oysters, scallops, and other mollusks, can carry many pathogens, including norovirus, *Vibrio* species, and hepatitis A virus as well as foodborne toxins (see Appendix VII, p 1086). *Vibrio* species contaminating raw shellfish may cause severe disease in people with liver disease or other conditions associated with decreased immune function. Some experts caution

---

[1]For additional information, contact the FDA Food Information Line at 1-888-723-3366, the US Department of Agriculture (USDA) information line at 1-202-720-2791, the USDA Food and Poultry Hotline at 1-888-674-6854 (USDA Food) or visit the following Web sites: **www.foodsafety.gov** and **www.usda.gov**.

against children ingesting raw fish, which has been associated with transmission of parasites (eg, *Anisakis simplex*, *Diphyllobothrium latum*).

Honey

Children younger than 1 year should not be given honey. Honey has been shown to contain spores of *Clostridium botulinum*. No cases associated with light and dark corn syrup have been documented.

Powdered Infant Formula

For many reasons, infants should be fed human milk rather than infant formula whenever possible. Powdered infant formula is not commercially sterile and has been associated with severe illnesses attributable to *Cronobacter* species and *Salmonella* species. If infant formula must be used, caregivers can reduce the risk of infection by choosing sterile, liquid formula products rather than powdered products. This may be particularly important for those at greatest risk of severe infection, such as neonates and infants with immunocompromising conditions. Otherwise, water used for mixing infant formula must be from a safe water source, as defined by the state or local health department. If there are concerns or uncertainty about the safety of tap water, bottled water or cold tap water which has been brought to a rolling boil for 1 minute, then cooled to room temperature for no more than 30 minutes, may be used.

Prepared formula must be discarded within 1 hour after serving to an infant. Prepared formula that has not been given to an infant may be stored in the refrigerator for 24 hours.

Food Irradiation[1]

Irradiation of food can be an effective tool to control foodborne pathogens. Irradiation involves exposing food briefly to ionizing radiation (eg, gamma rays, x-rays, or high-voltage electrons). More than 40 countries worldwide, including the United States, have approved the use of irradiation for various types of foods. Every governmental and professional organization that has reviewed the efficacy and safety of food irradiation has endorsed its use. Meat, spices, shell eggs, seeds for sprouting, and some produce items may be irradiated for sale in the United States. The risk of foodborne illness in children could be decreased significantly with the routine consumption of irradiated meat, poultry, and produce.

In addition to the Web sites and phone numbers previously cited in this section, detailed information on food safety issues and practices, including steps which consumers can take to protect themselves, is available on the following Web sites:

- **www.foodsafety.gov**
- **www.fightbac.org**
- **www.cdc.gov/foodsafety**

---

[1]**www.fsis.usda.gov/wps/portal/fsis/topics/food-safety-education/get-answers/food-safety-fact-sheets/production-and-inspection/irradiation-resources/irradiation-resources**

·····································
APPENDIX VII

Clinical Syndromes Associated With Foodborne Diseases[1,2]

Foodborne disease results from consumption of contaminated foods or beverages and causes morbidity and mortality in children and adults. The epidemiology of foodborne disease is complex and dynamic because of numerous possible pathogens, the variety of disease manifestations, the increasing prevalence of immunocompromised children and adults, dietary habits changes, and trends toward centralized food production and widespread distribution. The cultural diversity of foods and food practices likely is another issue impacting the epidemiology of foodborne disease.

Consideration of a foodborne etiology is important in any patient with a gastrointestinal tract illness, as well as those with certain acute neurologic findings. A detailed history is invaluable, with important questions including time of onset of symptoms, history of recent travel or antimicrobial use, and presence of blood or mucus in stool. To aid in diagnosis, foodborne disease syndromes have been categorized by incubation period, predominant symptoms, causative agent, and foods commonly associated with specific etiologic agents (food vehicles) (see Table). Diagnosis can be confirmed by laboratory testing of stool, vomitus, or blood, depending on the causative agent. Sporadic (ie, non-outbreak associated) cases account for the majority of foodborne illnesses. In localized outbreaks that affect individuals who shared a common meal, the incubation period can be estimated. In more widely dispersed outbreaks and in sporadic cases, the incubation period typically is unknown.

An outbreak should be considered when 2 or more people who have ingested the same food develop an acute illness characterized by nausea, vomiting, diarrhea, or neurologic signs or symptoms. If an outbreak is suspected, public health officials should be notified immediately to initiate an epidemiologic investigation, including diagnostic and management interventions, to curtail the outbreak.

---

[1]Centers for Disease Control and Prevention. Surveillance for foodborne-disease outbreaks—United States, 2008. *MMWR Morb Mortal Wkly Rep*. 2011;60(35):1197-1202. Additional information can be found at **www.cdc.gov/foodsafety** and **www.fsis.usda.gov/wps/portal/fsis/home**

[2]Centers for Disease Control and Prevention. Surveillance for foodborne disease outbreaks—United States, 1998–2008. *MMWR Morb Mortal Wkly Rep*. 2013;62(SS-2):1-34

Table. Clinical Syndromes Associated With Foodborne Diseases

Clinical Syndrome	Incubation Period	Causative Agents	Commonly Associated Vehicles[a]
Nausea and vomiting	2–4 h	*Staphylococcus aureus* (preformed enterotoxins, A through V but excluding F)	Food contaminated by infected food handler that is not cooked or is improperly cooked and stored, including ham, poultry, beef, cream-filled pastries, potato and egg salads, mushrooms, unpasteurized cheese
	<1–6 h	Preformed *Bacillus cereus* (emetic toxin cereulide)	Contaminated food that is improperly stored after cooking, including rice
	<1 h	Heavy metals (copper, tin, cadmium, iron, zinc)	Acidic beverages, metallic container
	1 h	Vomitoxin (deoxynivalenol)	Foods made from grains such as wheat, corn, barley
	1–3 days	Rotavirus	Food contaminated by infected food handler
	3–4 days	Astrovirus	Bivalve mollusks grown in polluted waters, fresh produce (greens, berries) irrigated with contaminated water, food contaminated by infected food handler that is not cooked or is improperly cooked and stored (ready-to-eat salads/sandwiches)
	Varies	*Listeria monocytogenes*	Soft cheeses, raw milk, hot dogs, cole slaw, ready-to eat delicatessen meats, produce (eg, sprouts, cantaloupe)
Flushing, dizziness, burning of mouth and throat, palpitations, headache, gastrointestinal tract symptoms, urticaria	<1 h	Histamine (scombroid)	Fish (bluefish, bonita, mackerel, mahi-mahi, marlin, tuna, skipjack, and many other fish types)

Table. Clinical Syndromes Associated With Foodborne Diseases, continued

Clinical Syndrome	Incubation Period	Causative Agents	Commonly Associated Vehicles[a]
Diverse array of neurologic, gastrointestinal tract, and cardiovascular symptoms. Facial and extremity paresthesias and hot/cold temperature sensation reversal are characteristic	2–4 h	Ciguatera toxin	Large reef-dwelling carnivorous fish (eg, amberjack, barracuda, grouper, snapper)
Gastrointestinal tract and neurologic symptoms including paresthesia	Up to 18 h[b]	Neurotoxic shellfish toxin (brevetoxin)	Shellfish (eg, mussels, oysters, clams)
As above, and short-term memory loss	1 day[c]	Domoic acid (amnesiac shellfish toxin)	Mussels, clams
Neurologic, including confusion, salivation, hallucinations; gastrointestinal tract manifestations	0–2 h	Mycotoxins (shorter-acting)	Mushrooms
Neuromuscular weakness, symmetric descending paralysis, respiratory weakness, neurologic symptoms may be preceded by gastrointestinal tract manifestations	12–48 h	*Clostridium botulinum* (preformed toxin)	Home-canned vegetables, fruits and fish, salted fish, meats, bottled garlic, potatoes baked in aluminum foil, cheese sauce; honey-associated infantile botulism has a longer incubation period[d]
Neurologic, constipation	3–30 days	*Clostridium botulinum*	Honey
	10–45 min	Tetrodotoxin (ascending paralysis)	Puffer fish
Neurologic, gastrointestinal tract	0.5–3 h	Paralytic shellfish toxins (saxitoxins, etc)	Shellfish (clams, mussels, oysters, scallops, other mollusks)

Table. Clinical Syndromes Associated With Foodborne Diseases, continued

Clinical Syndrome	Incubation Period	Causative Agents	Commonly Associated Vehicles[a]
Abdominal cramps and watery diarrhea, vomiting	8–24 h	Bacillus cereus (diarrheal enterotoxin)	Meats, stews, gravies, vanilla sauce
	6–24 h	Clostridium perfringens	Meat, poultry, gravy, dried or precooked foods
	12–48 h	Norovirus	Feces-contaminated shellfish, salads, ice, cookies, water, sandwiches, fruit, leafy vegetables, ready-to-eat foods handled by infected food worker
	1–3 days	Rotavirus	Feces-contaminated salads, fruits, ready-to-eat foods handled by infected food worker
Abdominal cramps, watery diarrhea	1–4 days	Enterotoxigenic Escherichia coli	Feces-contaminated seafood, herbs, fruits, vegetables, water, often acquired abroad—"travelers' diarrhea"
	4–30 h	Vibrio parahaemolyticus	Shellfish, especially oysters
	1–5 days	Vibrio cholerae O1 and O139	Shellfish (including crabs and shrimp), fish, water
	1–5 days	V cholerae non-O1	Shellfish, especially oysters
	1–14 days	Cyclospora species	Raspberries, vegetables, water
	2–28 days	Cryptosporidium species	Vegetables, fruits, milk, water, in particular recreational water exposures
	1–4 wk	Giardia intestinalis	Water, ready-to-eat foods handled by infected food worker
Diarrhea, fever, abdominal cramps, blood and mucus in stools, bacteremia	6–48 h	Salmonella species (nontyphoidal)	Poultry; pork; beef; eggs; dairy products, including ice cream; raw vegetables (eg, alfalfa sprouts); fruit, including unpasteurized juices; peanut butter
	2–4 days	Shigella species	Feces-contaminated lettuce-based salads, potato and egg salads, salsas, dips, and oysters, ready-to-eat foods handled by infected food worker
	7–14 days	Salmonella typhi	Food contaminated by infected food handler (acutely ill or chronic carrier)
	2–4 wk	Amebiasis (Entameba histolytica)	Feces-contaminated food or water

Table. Clinical Syndromes Associated With Foodborne Diseases, continued

Clinical Syndrome	Incubation Period	Causative Agents	Commonly Associated Vehicles[a]
Bloody diarrhea, abdominal cramps, hemolytic-uremic syndrome (HUS)	1–10 days	Shiga toxin-producing *E coli*	Undercooked beef (hamburger); raw milk; roast beef; salami; salad dressings; lettuce and other leafy greens; game meats, unpasteurized juices, including apple cider; sprouts; water
Febrile diarrhea or, especially in older children, abdominal pain resembling that of appendicitis	4–6 days	*Yersinia enterocolitica*	Pork chitterlings, tofu, milk
Hepatorenal failure, watery diarrhea	6–48 h	Mushroom toxins (late onset)	Mushrooms (especially *Amanita* species)
Other extraintestinal manifestations	Varied, up to months (usually >30 days)	*Brucella* species	Goat cheese, queso fresco, raw milk, meats
Fever, chills, headache, pharyngitis, arthralgia	1–4 days	Group A *Streptococcus*	Egg and potato salad
Fever, malaise, anorexia, jaundice	15–50 days	Hepatitis A virus	Shellfish, raw produce (eg, strawberries, lettuce, green onions)
Meningoencephalitis, sepsis, fetal loss	2–6 wk	*Listeria monocytogenes*	Soft cheeses, raw milk, hot dogs, coleslaw, ready-to eat delicatessen meats, produce (eg, sprouts, cantaloupe)
Muscle soreness and pain	Varied, up to 4 wk	*Trichinella spiralis*	Wild game, pork, meat
Fever, lymphadenopathy, neurologic (reactivation)	5–23 days	*Toxoplasma gondii*	Undercooked meat (especially pork, lamb, and game meat), fruits, vegetables, raw shellfish
Sepsis, meningitis	Unknown	*Cronobacter (Enterobacter) sakazakii*	Powdered infant formula
	Unknown	*Salmonella* species	Powdered infant formula

Table. Clinical Syndromes Associated With Foodborne Diseases, continued

Clinical Syndrome	Incubation Period	Causative Agents	Commonly Associated Vehicles[a]
Seizures, behavioral disturbances, and other neurologic signs and symptoms	Months	*Taenia solium* (neurocysticercosis)	Food contaminated with feces from a human carrier of adult pork tapeworm
Epigastric discomfort, abdominal pain, cholangitis, obstructive jaundice, pancreatitis	Varied (several days to months)	*Clonorchis sinensis* (liver fluke) *Opisthorchis* species (liver fluke)	Fish Fish
Guillain-Barré syndrome (ascending paralysis)	2–10 days	*Campylobacter* species *Shigella* Enteroinvasive *E coli* *Yersinia enterocolitica* *Vibrio parahaemolyticus*	Poultry, raw milk, water Feces-contaminated food or water Vegetables, hamburger, raw milk Pork chitterlings, tofu, raw milk Fish, shellfish
Postdiarrheal HUS (acute renal failure, hemolytic anemia, thrombocytopenia)	7 days–2 wk after onset of diarrhea	Shiga toxin-producing *E coli* (especially serotype O157:H7)	Beef (hamburger); raw milk; roast beef; salami; salad dressings; lettuce and other leafy greens; unpasteurized juices, including apple cider; alfalfa and radish sprouts; water
	1–5 days after onset of diarrhea	*Shigella dysenteriae* type 1	Water, milk, other contaminated food, rare in the United States
Reactive arthritis	Varies Varies	*Campylobacter* species *Salmonella* species	Poultry, raw milk, water Poultry, pork, beef, eggs, dairy products, including ice cream; vegetables (alfalfa sprouts and fresh produce); fruit, including unpasteurized juices; peanut butter
	Varies Varies	*Shigella* species *Yersinia enterocolitica*	Feces-contaminated food or water Pork chitterlings, tofu, raw milk

[a]List of vehicles in several categories is not exhaustive, because any number of foods can be contaminated; current online literature may be helpful to sort through commonly associated vehicles.

[b]See **https://emergency.cdc.gov/agent/brevetoxin/pdf/brevetoxincasedef.pdf.**

[c]See **www.cdc.gov/mmwr/preview/mmwrhtml/rr5304a1.htm** and **www.cdc.gov/habs/illness-symptoms-marine.html.**

[d]Honey has been implicated in infant botulism but follows ingestion of spores with production of toxin in the intestine; longer incubation period.

APPENDIX VIII

Diseases Transmitted by Animals (Zoonoses)

Morbidity resulting from selected zoonotic diseases in the United States is reported annually by the Centers for Disease Control and Prevention (see "Summary of Notifiable Diseases" at **www.cdc.gov/mmwr/mmwr_nd/**). Information also can be obtained via the Web site of the National Center for Emerging and Zoonotic Infectious Diseases (**www.cdc.gov/ncezid/about-ncezid.html**) or through the main Centers for Disease Control and Prevention Web site (**www.cdc.gov**).

Table. Diseases Transmitted by Animals

Disease and/or Organism	Animal Sources/Reservoirs	Vector or Modes of Transmission
Bacterial Diseases		
Aeromonas species	Aquatic animals, especially shellfish, medical leeches	Wound infection, ingestion of contaminated food or water
Anthrax (*Bacillus anthracis*)	Herbivores (cattle, goats, sheep)	Direct contact with infected animals or their carcasses, or contact with products from infected animals (eg, meat, hides or hair) contaminated with *B anthracis* spores
Bartonellosis (*Bartonella* species)	Cats, dogs, body lice	Bites of arthropods suspected, but evidence is lacking in many species
Brucellosis (*Brucella* species)	Cattle, goats, sheep, pigs, dogs, elk, bison, deer, camels, rodents, marine mammals	Direct or indirect contact with aborted fetuses or tissues or fluids of infected animals; inoculation through mucous membranes, cuts or abrasions of the skin; inhalation of contaminated aerosols; ingestion of undercooked meat or unpasteurized dairy products.
Campylobacteriosis (*Campylobacter jejuni*)	Poultry, dogs (especially puppies), kittens, ferrets, pet rodents, cattle, sheep, birds	Ingestion of contaminated food, water, direct contact (particularly with animals with diarrhea), person-to-person (fecal-oral)
Capnocytophaga canimorsus	Dogs, rarely cats	Bites, scratches, and prolonged contact with dogs
Cat-scratch disease (*Bartonella henselae*)	Cats, infrequently other animals (less than 10%)	Scratches, bites; fleas play a role in cat-to-cat transmission (evidence for transmission from cat fleas to humans is lacking)
Erysipelothrix rhusiopathiae	Pigs, sheep, cattle, birds, fish, shellfish	Direct contact with animal or contaminated animal product, or water
Hemolytic-uremic syndrome (eg, Shiga toxin-producing *Escherichia coli*) (STEC)	Cattle, sheep, goats, deer	Ingestion of undercooked contaminated ground beef, unpasteurized milk, or other contaminated foods or water; contact with infected animals or their environments (eg, farms and ranches); contact with animals in public settings including petting zoos and agricultural fairs (fecal-oral)

Table. Diseases Transmitted by Animals, continued

Disease and/or Organism	Animal Sources/Reservoirs	Vector or Modes of Transmission
Leptospirosis (*Leptospira* species)	Dogs, rodents, livestock, other wild animals	Contact with or ingestion of water, food, or soil contaminated with urine or fluids from infected animals, or direct contact with infected animals
Lyme disease (*Borrelia burgdorferi*)	Mice, squirrels, shrews, and other small mammals and birds	Black-legged or deer tick bites (*Ixodes scapularis* or *Ixodes pacificus*)
Mycobacterium marinum	Fish (and cleaning aquaria)	Skin injury or contamination of existing wound
Mycobacterium bovis and *Mycobacterium tuberculosis*	Cattle, elephants, giraffes, rhinoceroses, bison, deer, elk, feral pigs, badgers, nonhuman primates	*M bovis* usually is transmitted from cattle through ingestion of contaminated food and unpasteurized milk, although airborne transmission from cattle or other species is possible; *M tuberculosis* is uncommon in most nonhuman species except for elephants and primates, and it is transmitted by the airborne route
Pasteurella multocida	Cats, dogs, other animals	Bites, scratches, licks
Plague (*Yersinia pestis*)	Rodents, cats, dogs, ground squirrels, prairie dogs	Bite of rodent fleas (especially Oriental rat fleas, *Xenopsylla cheopis*), direct contact with infected animal tissues, airborne from other human or animal (eg, cat) with pneumonic plague
Q fever (*Coxiella burnetii*)	Sheep, goats, cows, cats, dogs, wild rodents, birds	Contact with excreta (birth products, urine, feces, milk) of infected animals, inhalation of pathogen-contaminated dust, ingestion of unpasteurized milk, and fomite transmission (possible role of ticks not well defined)
Rat-bite fever (*Streptobacillus moniliformis*, *Spirillum minus*)	Rodents (especially rats, occasionally squirrels), gerbils	Bites, secretions, and contaminated food, milk, and water
Relapsing fever (tickborne) (*Borrelia* species)	Wild rodents	Soft tick bites (*Ornithodoros* species)

Table. Diseases Transmitted by Animals, continued

Disease and/or Organism	Animal Sources/Reservoirs	Vector or Modes of Transmission
Salmonellosis (*Salmonella* species)	Cattle, poultry, turtles, frogs, lizards, snakes, salamanders, geckos, iguanas, dogs, cats, hedgehogs, hamsters, guinea pigs, mice, rats and other rodents, ferrets, other wild and domestic animals	Ingestion of contaminated food (eg meat, poultry, dairy, eggs, produce, processed foods), unpasteurized milk and other raw dairy products, or contaminated water; contact with infected animals or their environments; animal products including dry dog and cat food and pet treats; contact with fecally contaminated surfaces
Streptococcus iniae	Fish grown by aquaculture	Skin injury during handling of fish
Tetanus (*Clostridium tetani*)	Any animal indirectly via soil containing animal feces	Wound infection, skin injury or soft tissue injury with inoculation of bacteria (as from soil or a contaminated object)
Tularemia (*Francisella tularensis*)	Sheep, cats, wild rabbits, hares, voles, muskrats, moles, hamsters	Wood tick bites (*Dermacentor andersoni*), dog tick bites (*D variabilis*), Lone-star tick bites (*Amblyomma americanum*), deerfly bites; direct contact with infected animal, ingestion of contaminated water, mechanical transmission from claws or teeth (cats), aerosolization of tissues or excreta
Vibrio species	Shellfish	Ingestion of contaminated food or water; skin injury or contamination of existing wound
Yersiniosis (*Yersinia enterocolitica*, *Yersinia pseudotuberculosis*)	Pigs, deer, elk, horses, goats, sheep, cattle, rodents, birds, rabbits	Ingestion of contaminated food (particularly pork products), water, or milk; rarely direct contact
Fungal Diseases		
Cryptococcosis (*Cryptococcus neoformans*)	Excreta of birds, particularly pigeons	Inhalation of aerosols from accumulations of bird feces
Histoplasmosis (*Histoplasma capsulatum*)	Excreta of bats, birds, particularly starlings	Inhalation of aerosols from accumulations of bat or bird feces
Ringworm/tinea corporis (*Microsporum* and *Trichophyton* species)	Cats, dogs, fowl, pigs, moles, horses, rodents, cattle, monkeys, goats	Direct contact

Table. Diseases Transmitted by Animals, continued

Disease and/or Organism	Animal Sources/Reservoirs	Vector or Modes of Transmission
Parasitic Diseases		
Angiostrongylus cantonensis	Rodents	Ingestion of larvae in raw or undercooked snails or slugs, or in contaminated raw vegetables
Anisakiasis (*Anisakis* species)	Saltwater and anadromous fish (migrating up rivers from the sea to spawn, eg, salmon)	Ingestion of larvae in raw or undercooked fish (eg, sushi)
Babesiosis (several *Babesia* species)	Mice and various other rodents and small mammals; wildlife	Tick bite (in the United States, *Babesia microti* is transmitted mainly by *Ixodes* scapularis; in Europe, *Babesia divergens* is mainly transmitted by *Ixodes* tick bites)
Balantidiasis (*Balantidium coli*)	Pigs	Ingestion of contaminated food or water
Baylisascariasis (*Baylisascaris procyonis*)	Raccoons	Ingestion of eggs shed in raccoon feces
Cryptosporidiosis (*Cryptosporidium* species)	Domestic animals (including cattle, sheep, goats, horses, pigs, dogs, cats), particularly young animals	Ingestion of contaminated water (especially groundwater) or foods
Cutaneous larva migrans (primarily *Ancylostoma* species)	Dogs, cats	Penetration of skin by larvae, which develop in soil contaminated with animal feces
Dog tapeworm (*Dipylidium caninum*)	Dogs, cats	Ingestion of fleas infected with larvae
Dwarf tapeworm (*Hymenolepis nana*) and rat tapeworm (*Hymenolepis diminuta*)	Rodents (humans are more important reservoirs than rodents for *H nana*; for *H diminuta*, rodents are primary and human infection is infrequent)	Ingestion of eggs from feces (contaminated food, water), animal-to-person (fecal-oral)
Echinococcosis, hydatid disease (*Echinococcus* species)	Dogs, foxes, possibly other carnivores, coyotes, wolves	Ingestion of eggs shed in animal feces
Fish tapeworm (*Diphyllobothrium latum*)	Saltwater and freshwater fish	Ingestion of larvae in raw or undercooked fish (eg, sushi)

Table. Diseases Transmitted by Animals, continued

Disease and/or Organism	Animal Sources/Reservoirs	Vector or Modes of Transmission
Giardiasis (*Giardia intestinalis*)	Wild and domestic animals, including dogs, cats, cattle, pigs, beavers, muskrats, rats, pet rodents, rabbits, nonhuman primates	Ingestion of contaminated water or foods, and animal-to-person (fecal-oral)
Scabies (*Sarcoptes scabeii* subspecies *canis*)	Dogs (with clinical mange)	Direct contact
Taeniasis/beef tapeworm (*Taenia saginata*)	Cattle (intermediate host)	Ingestion of larvae in raw or undercooked beef; cysticercosis in cattle is caused by ingestion of embryonated eggs excreted by humans with *Taenia* infection
Taeniasis and cysticercosis/pork tapeworm (*Taenia solium*)	Pigs (intermediate host)	Ingestion of larvae in raw or undercooked meat; cysticercosis in pigs is caused by ingestion of embryonated eggs excreted by humans with *Taenia* infection, or by autoingestion
Toxoplasmosis (*Toxoplasma gondii*)	Cats, livestock	Ingestion of infective oocysts from cat feces, consumption of cysts in raw or undercooked meat
Trichinellosis (*Trichinella spiralis* and other *Trichinella* species)	Pigs, bears, seals, horses, walruses	Ingestion of larvae in raw or undercooked meat
Ocular or visceral toxocariasis/larva migrans (*Toxocara canis* and *Toxocara cati*)	Dogs, cats	Ingestion of eggs, usually from soil contaminated by animal feces
Chlamydial and Rickettsial Diseases		
Human ehrlichiosis (*Ehrlichia chaffeensis* and *Ehrlichia ewingii*)	Deer, dogs, gray foxes; goats (*E ewingii*)	Tick bites (lone-star ticks, *Amblyomma americanum*)
Human anaplasmosis (*Anaplasma phagocytophilum*)	Deer, dogs, elk, wild rodents, horses, ruminants	Black-legged tick (*Ixodes scapularis*) and western black-legged tick (*I pacificus*) bites
Psittacosis (*Chlamydia psittaci*)	Pet birds (especially psittacine birds such as parakeets, parrots, macaws, and cockatoos) and poultry	Inhalation of aerosols from feces of infected birds

Table. Diseases Transmitted by Animals, continued

Disease and/or Organism	Animal Sources/Reservoirs	Vector or Modes of Transmission
Rickettsialpox (*Rickettsia akari*)	House mice	Mite bites (house mouse mite, *Liponyssoides sanguineus*)
Rocky Mountain spotted fever (*Rickettsia rickettsii*)	Dogs, wild rodents, rabbits	Tick bites (American dog tick, *Demacentor variabilis*; Rocky Mountain wood tick, *D andersoni*; and brown dog tick, *Rhipicephalus sanguineus*)
Rickettsia parkeri infection (Maculatum disease, American boutonneuse fever)	Unknown; perhaps cattle, dogs, small wild rodents	Gulf coast ticks, *Amblyomma maculatum*
Typhus, fleaborne endemic typhus, Murine typhus (*Rickettsia typhi*)	Rats, opossums, cats, dogs	Infected flea feces scratched into abrasions; oriental rat fleas (*Xenopsylla cheopis*) and cat fleas (*Ctenocephalides felis*) are vectors.
Typhus, louseborne epidemic typhus (*Rickettsia prowazekii*)	Flying squirrels	Person-to-person via body louse, contact with flying squirrels, their nests, or ectoparasites (role and species of ectoparasites undefined)
Viral Diseases		
B virus (formerly herpes B, monkey B virus, herpesvirus simiae, or herpesvirus B)	Macaque monkeys	Bite or exposure to secretions or tissues
Colorado tick fever	Rodents (squirrels, chipmunks)	Tick bites (Rocky Mountain wood tick, *Demacentor andersoni*)
Crimean Congo hemorrhagic fever	Small rodents, hares, farm animals	Animal slaughter, tick bites, person-to-person via contact (droplet, contact) with infectious blood or body fluids
Eastern equine encephalitis	Birds	Mosquito bites (*Coquillettidia* species, *Aedes* species, *Culex* species, *Ochlerotatus* species)
Ebola hemorrhagic fever	Bats; nonhuman primates may become infected	Contact with bats, contact with sick/dead nonhuman primates
Hantaviruses	Wild and peridomestic rodents	Inhalation of aerosols of infected secreta and excreta

Table. Diseases Transmitted by Animals, continued

Disease and/or Organism	Animal Sources/Reservoirs	Vector or Modes of Transmission
Hendra	Flying foxes; horses become infected	Contact with body fluids of infected horses, close contact with fruit bats
Novel influenza (H5N1, H7N9, H9N2, H3N2 variant)	Chickens, birds, pigs	Contact with infected animals or aerosols (markets, slaughter house)
Jamestown Canyon virus	Large mammals	Mosquito bites (*Culex* species, *Aedes* species, *Coquillettidia* species, and *Culiseta* species)
Japanese encephalitis	Pigs, birds	Mosquito bites (*Culex tritaeniorhynchus*)
Kyasanur forest disease/Alkhurma hemorrhagic fever	Primates, small mammals, possibly farm animals, camels	Primarily tick bites (*Haemaphysalis spinigera*), animal slaughter
La Crosse	Rodents (squirrels, chipmunks)	Mosquito bites (*Ochlerotatus triseriatus*)
Lassa fever	Multimammate rat (*Mastomys natalensis*)	Inhalation of aerosols or direct contact with infected secreta or excreta, consumption of food contaminated by rodents
Lymphocytic choriomeningitis (LCMV)	Rodents, particularly house mice and pet hamsters (includes feeder rodents used as reptile food), guinea pigs	Direct contact, inhalation of aerosols, ingestion of food contaminated with rodent excreta
Marburg hemorrhagic fever	Bats, infected nonhuman primates	Contact with fruit bats or their excreta (e.g. entering caves or mines inhabited by bats); contact with infectious blood or tissue of infected monkeys
Middle East respiratory syndrome (MERS-CoV coronavirus)	Uncertain, virus found in camels in several countries	Possible direct contact or droplet
Monkeypox	Prairie dogs, African rodents	Direct contact, bite, scratch
Nipah	Bats; pigs can become infected	Close contact with bats, consumption of bat contaminated fruit/sap; direct contact with infected pigs
Omsk hemorrhagic fever	Muskrats, other wild rodents	Handling infected muskrats (eg, hunting, trapping, skinning), and tick bites

Table. Diseases Transmitted by Animals, continued

Disease and/or Organism	Animal Sources/Reservoirs	Vector or Modes of Transmission
Orf (pox virus of sheep)	Sheep, goats	Contact with infected saliva, infected fomites
Powassan	Rodents (groundhogs, squirrels, mice)	Tick bites *(Ixodes cookei, Ixodes marxi, Ixodes scapularis)*
Rabies (Lyssavirus)	In the United States, primarily wildlife (bats, raccoons, skunks, foxes, coyotes, mongooses) or, less frequently, domestic animals (dogs, cats, cattle, horses, sheep, goats, ferrets)	Bites; rarely contact of open wounds, abrasions (including scratches), or mucous membranes with saliva or other infectious materials (eg, neural tissue)
Rift Valley fever	Cattle, sheep, goats	Animal slaughter, mosquito bites
Severe acute respiratory virus (SARS-CoV, coronavirus)	Bats, civet cats, potentially other animal species	Possible direct contact or droplet
South American arenaviruses (Junin, Machupo, Guanarito, Sabia, Chapare)	Rodents	Inhalation of aerosols of infected secretions or excreta, consumption of food or water contaminated with infected secretions or excreta, direct contact of abraded or broken skin with rodent excrement
St Louis encephalitis	Birds	Mosquito bites *(Culex species)*
Tickborne encephalitis	Rodents; goats and sheep become infected	Tick bites *(Ixodes ricinus, Ixodes persulcatus)*; infected milk products
Venezuelan equine encephalitis	Horses	Mosquito bites *(Psorophora species, Ochlerotatus species)*
West Nile	Birds	Mosquito bites *(Culex species)*
Western equine encephalitis	Birds	Mosquito bites *(Culex tarsalis)*
Yellow fever	Nonhuman primates (jungle and sylvatic cycles)	Mosquito bites *(Haemagogus species, Sabethes species, Aedes species)*

Index

Page numbers followed by "t" indicate a table. Page numbers followed by "f" indicate a figure.

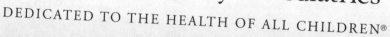

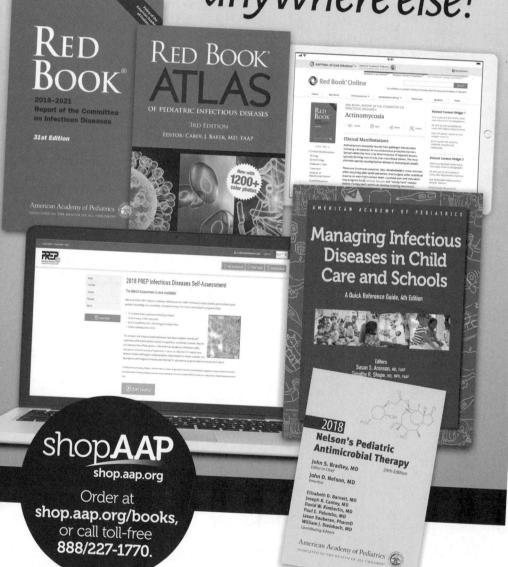